SBHMC BOOK
54009000229811

KU-406-572

Nuclear Medicine in Clinical Diagnosis and Treatment

Commissioning Editor: Geoffrey Nuttall
Project Editor: Lowri Daniels
Copy Editors: Andrew Gardiner, Helen McDonald, Robin Watson, Kathryn Whyman
Design Direction: Sarah Cape
Project Manager: Mark Sanderson
Sales Promotion Executive: Caroline Boyd

Nuclear Medicine in Clinical Diagnosis and Treatment

VOLUME 2

Edited by

I. P. C. Murray AM MD FRCP(Ed) FRACP FACR
Director of Nuclear Medicine, Prince of Wales Hospital; Associate Professor of Medicine, University of New South Wales, Sydney, New South Wales, Australia

P. J. Ell MD MSc PhD FRCR FRCP
Professor of Nuclear Medicine, University College London, London, UK

FOREWORD BY
H. William Strauss MD
Professor and Director of Nuclear Medicine, Division of Nuclear Medicine, Stanford University Medical Center, Stanford, California, USA

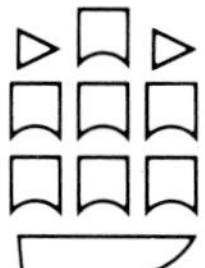

CHURCHILL LIVINGSTONE
EDINBURGH LONDON MADRID MELBOURNE NEW YORK AND TOKYO 1994

CHURCHILL LIVINGSTONE
Medical Division of Longman Group Limited

Distributed in the United States of America by Churchill Livingstone Inc., 650 Avenue of the Americas, New York, N.Y. 10011, and by associated companies, branches and representatives throughout the world.

First published 1994

ISBN 0 443 04710 3

British Library Cataloguing in Publication Data
A catalogue record for this book is available from the British Library.

Library of Congress Cataloging in Publication Data
A catalog record for this book is available from the Library of Congress.

The publisher's policy is to use **paper manufactured from sustainable forests**

Printed in Hong Kong

Contents

Contents

Contributors

Hussein Abdel-Dayem MD
Professor of Radiology, New York Medical College, Valhalla, New York; Chief, Nuclear Medicine, St. Vincent's Hospital & Medical Center of New York, New York, USA

Duncan Ackery MA MSc FRCR
Formerly Consultant and Honorary Clinical Professor, Department of Nuclear Medicine, Southampton University Hospitals, Southampton, UK

L. Barry Arkles FRACP
Chairman, Division of Radiation Sciences and Director, Department of Nuclear Medicine, Heidelberg Repatriation Hospital, Melbourne; Senior Associate, Department of Medicine, University of Melbourne, Melbourne, Victoria, Australia

Dale L. Bailey MAppSc
Senior Physicist, Department of Nuclear Medicine, Royal Prince Alfred Hospital, Sydney, New South Wales, Australia

Edward J. Baker MA MD MRCP
Senior Lecturer, United Medical and Dental Schools; Honorary Consultant Paediatric Cardiologist, Guy's and St. Thomas' Hospital, London, UK

Richmond J. Baker BSc(Hons) PhD
Radiochemist, Department of Nuclear Medicine, Prince of Wales Hospital, Randwick, New South Wales, Australia

J. J. Bax MD
Research Fellow, Department of Cardiology, Free University Hospital, Amsterdam, The Netherlands

George A. Beller MD
Ruth C. Heede Professor of Cardiology and Head, Cardiovascular Division, University of Virginia Health Sciences Center, Charlottesville, Virginia, USA

Simona Ben-Haim MD DSc
Senior Physician, Department of Medicine, Rambam Medical Centre, Haifa, Israel

Hans-J. Biersack MD
Professor and Chairman, Department of Nuclear Medicine, University of Bonn, Bonn, Germany

Gerald G. Blackwell MD
Assistant Professor of Medicine, Division of Cardiovascular Disease, University of Alabama at Birmingham, Birmingham, Alabama, USA

M. Donald Blaufox MD PhD
Professor and Chairman, Department of Nuclear Medicine and Professor of Medicine, Albert Einstein College of Medicine and Montefiore Medical Center, Bronx, New York, USA

Robert Bonow MD
Goldberg Professor of Medicine and Chief, Division of Cardiology, Northwestern University Medical School, Chicago, Illinois, USA

P. Bourgeois MD
Service of Nuclear Medicine, University Hospital Saint-Pierre, Université Libre de Bruxelles, Brussels, Belgium

R. E. Boyd BSc MACPSEM, AMCT
Senior Principal Research Scientist, Australian Nuclear Science & Technology Organisation, Lucas Heights, Sydney, New South Wales, Australia

Simon H. Braat MD
Associate Professor, Department of Cardiology, Academic Hospital Maastricht, University of Limburg, Maastricht, The Netherlands

Lawrence M. Brass MD
Associate Professor and Chief, Neurology Service, Yale University School of Medicine, West Haven, Connecticut, USA

Keith E. Britton MD MSc FRCR FRCP
Professor of Nuclear Medicine, St Bartholomew's Hospital and Medical College, London, UK

Stephen C. W. Brown MA MD FRCS
Senior Registrar in Urology, Manchester Central Hospitals and Community Care NHS Trust, Manchester, UK

Bernd R. Bubeck MD BSc
Professor, Department of Nuclear Medicine, University of Heidelberg, Heidelberg, Germany

R. E. Butler MB BS MRCPsych
Registrar in Psychiatry, UCL Medical School, London, UK

Maria Lucia Calcagni MD
Specialist in Nuclear Medicine, Institute of Nuclear Medicine, Catholic University of the Sacred Heart, Rome, Italy

Paolo G. Camici MD FESC FACC
Head of PET Cardiology, MRC Cyclotron Unit, Royal Postgraduate Medical School, Hammersmith Hospital, London, UK

Jean-François Chatal MD
Professor and Head of Department of Nuclear Medicine, University of Nantes, Nantes, France

Barry E. Chatterton MBBS FRACP DDU
Director of Nuclear Medicine, Royal Adelaide Hospital, Adelaide, South Australia, Australia

Susan E. M. Clarke MSc FRCP
Consultant Physician in Nuclear Medicine, Guy's and St Thomas' Hospital Trust and Lewisham Hospital, London; Senior Lecturer in Radiological Sciences, UMDS, London, UK

Tony Coakley MSc FRCP FRCR
Consultant in Nuclear Medicine, Kent & Canterbury Hospital, Canterbury, UK

John Cormack BSc(Hons) MSc
Chief Hospital Scientist, Department of Radiology, Flinders Medical Centre, Bedford Park, South Australia, Australia

Durval C. Costa MD MSc PhD
Senior Lecturer and Consultant Physician, Institute of Nuclear Medicine, UCL Medical School, London, UK

David B. Coupland MD FRCPC
Clinical Instructor, Division of Nuclear Medicine, Department of Radiology, University of British Columbia and Vancouver General Hospital, Vancouver, British Columbia, Canada

Magnus Dahlbom PhD
Assistant Professor, Division of Nuclear Medicine, Department of Molecular and Medical Pharmacology, UCLA School of Medicine, Los Angeles, California, USA

M. H. W. de Bois MD
Staff Rheumatologist, Department of Rheumatology, University Hospital, Leiden, The Netherlands

Jan de Kraker MD PhD
Consultant in Paediatric Oncology, Academic Medical Centre, Amsterdam, The Netherlands

Giuseppe de Rossi MD
Associate Professor of Nuclear Medicine, Faculty of Medicine, Catholic University; Assistant Director, Institute of Nuclear Medicine, A. Gemelli Hospital, Rome, Italy

Michael D. Devous Sr PhD
Associate Professor of Radiology; Associate Director, Nuclear Medicine Center; Director, Brain Imaging Core Laboratory, MHCRC, The University of Texas Southwestern Medical Center, Dallas, Texas, USA

Stefan Eberl BE MSc
Senior Hospital Scientist, Department of Nuclear Medicine, Royal Prince Alfred Hospital, Sydney, New South Wales, Australia

P. J. Ell MD MSc PhD FRCR FRCP
Professor of Nuclear Medicine, University College, London, UK

Keigo Endo MD
Professor of Nuclear Medicine, Gunma University School of Medicine, Gunma, Japan

Eugene J. Fine MD
Associate Professor of Nuclear Medicine, Albert Einstein College of Medicine, Bronx, New York, USA

Manfred Fischer MD
Professor and Head of Department of Nuclear Medicine, Staedt Kliniken, Kassel, Germany

Juan A. Flores MD
Associate Professor, Department of Nuclear Medicine, University of Vienna, Vienna, Austria

Maggie Flower BA MSc PhD
Lecturer in Medical Physics, Joint Department of Physics, Institute of Cancer Research and Royal Marsden Hospital, Sutton, Surrey, UK

John E. Freitas MD
Clinical Associate Professor of Internal Medicine, University of Michigan Medical School, Ann Arbor; Director, Nuclear Medicine Services, St Joseph Mercy Hospital, Ann Arbor, Michigan, USA

Roger Fulton MAppSc
Senior Hospital Scientist, Department of Nuclear Medicine, Royal Prince Alfred Hospital, Sydney, New South Wales, Australia

Stanley J. Goldsmith MD FACP FACC FACNP
Clinical Director, Nuclear Medicine Service, Memorial Sloan-Kettering Cancer Center, New York; Professor of Radiology, Cornell University Medical College, New York, USA

Isky Gordon FRCR
Consultant Radiologist, Hospitals for Sick Children, London; Honorary Senior Lecturer, Institute of Child Health, London, UK

Maria Granowska MD MSc
Senior Lecturer and Honorary Consultant in Nuclear Medicine, St Bartholomew's Hospital and Medical College, St Mark's Hospital, London, UK

Milton D. Gross MD
Professor, Division of Nuclear Medicine, Department of Internal Medicine, University of Michigan Medical Center, Ann Arbor; Director/Chief, Nuclear Medicine Service, Department of Veterans' Affairs Medical Center, Ann Arbor, Michigan, USA

Frank Grünwald MD
Privat-Dozent, Department of Nuclear Medicine, University of Bonn, Bonn, Germany

Wolf-Dieter Heiss MD
Professor and Chairman, Department of Neurology, University of Cologne and Max Planck Institute für Neurologische Forschung, Cologne, Germany

Sydney Heyman BSc MBChB MMed(Paed)
Professor of Radiology, University of Pennsylvania School of Medicine; Director, Division of Nuclear Medicine, Children's Hospital of Philadelphia, Philadelphia, Pennsylvania, USA

Rodney J. Hicks MBBS(Hons) FRACP
Director of Nuclear Cardiology, Heidelberg Repatriation Hospital, Melbourne, Australia

Andrew J. W. Hilson MB BChir MSc FRCP
Consultant in Nuclear Medicine, Royal Free Hospital and School of Medicine, London, UK

Cornelis A. Hoefnagel MD PhD
Consultant in Nuclear Medicine, Department of Nuclear Medicine, The Netherlands Cancer Institute, Amsterdam, The Netherlands

Brian F. Hutton MSc FACPSEM
Principal Hospital Scientist, Department of Nuclear Medicine, Royal Prince Alfred Hospital, Sydney, New South Wales, Australia

Kazuo Itoh MD PhD
Associate Professor, Department of Nuclear Medicine, Hokkaido University School of Medicine, Sapporo, Japan

Peter Jarritt BSc PhD MIPSM
Senior Lecturer, UCL Medical School, London, UK

Jack E. Juni MD
Director, Positron Diagnostic Center, Nuclear Medicine Department, William Beaumont Hospital, Royal Oak, Michigan, USA

Cornelius L. E. Katona MD(Cantab) MRCPsych
Professor of Psychiatry of the Elderly, University College London Medical School, Middlesex Hospital, London, UK

Robert Kerwin MA PhD MRCPsych
Senior Lecturer in Neuroscience and Honorary Consultant Psychiatrist, Institute of Psychiatry, London, UK

Chun Ki Kim MD
Associate Professor of Radiology, Division of Nuclear Medicine, Department of Radiology, Mount Sinai Medical Center, Mount Sinai School of Medicine, New York, USA

Edward Klemm MD
Department of Nuclear Medicine, University of Bonn, Bonn, Germany

F. F. (Russ) Knapp Jr PhD
Group Leader, Nuclear Medicine, Health Sciences Research Division, Oak Ridge National Laboratory, Oak Ridge, Tennessee, USA

Elissa Lipcon Kramer MD
Associate Professor of Clinical Radiology, New York University School of Medicine; Associate Director of Nuclear Medicine, New York University Medical Center, New York, USA

E. P. Krenning MD PhD
Professor of Nuclear Medicine, Erasmus University, Rotterdam; Head of Department of Nuclear Medicine, University Hospital, Rotterdam, The Netherlands

D. J. Kwekkeboom MD PhD
Clinical Research Associate, Department of Nuclear Medicine, University Hospital Rotterdam, Rotterdam, The Netherlands

Steven W. J. Lamberts MD PhD
Professor of Medicine, Department of Medicine III, Erasmus University, Rotterdam, The Netherlands

Steven M. Larson MD
Chief, Nuclear Medicine Service, Memorial Sloan-Kettering Cancer Center, New York; Professor of Radiology, Cornell University Medical College, New York, USA

Brian C. Lentle MD FRCPC
Professor and Head, Department of Radiology, University of British Columbia and Vancouver General Hospital, Vancouver, British Columbia, Canada

Jeffrey A. Leppo MD
Professor of Medicine and Nuclear Medicine and Director of Nuclear Cardiology, University of Massachusetts Medical Center, Worcester, Massachusetts, USA

Valerie J. Lewington BM MSc MRCP
Consultant in Nuclear Medicine, Southampton University Hospitals NHS Trust, Southampton, UK

Frederic T. Lovegrove MBBS FRACP MBA
Consultant Physician in Nuclear Medicine, St John of God Hospital and Sir Charles Gairdner Hospital, Nedlands, Western Australia, Australia

Val J. Lowe MD
Assistant Professor, Department of Medicine, Division of Nuclear Medicine, Saint Louis University Medical Center; Medical Director, Saint Louis University/Saint Louis VA Medical Center PET Imaging Facility, Saint Louis, Missouri, USA

Homer A. Macapinlac MD
Assistant Attending Radiologist, Nuclear Medicine Service, Department of Radiology, Memorial Sloan-Kettering Cancer Center; Assistant Member, Sloan-Kettering Institute; Assistant Professor of Radiology, Cornell University Medical College, New York, USA

Alexander J. B. McEwan MB FRCPC
Professor and Chair, Department of Radiology and Diagnostic Imaging, University of Alberta, Edmonton; Director, Nuclear Medicine, Cross Cancer Institute, Edmonton, Alberta, Canada

Andrew F. McLaughlin MBBS FRACP
Formerly Director of Clinical Nuclear Medicine, Royal Prince Alfred Hospital, Camperdown, Sydney; Physician, Nuclear Medicine Diagnostic Centre, Burwood, Sydney, New South Wales, Australia

Richard McLean MBBS FRACP
Consultant Physician in Nuclear Medicine, Sydney, New South Wales, Australia

Jamshid Maddahi MD
Professor of Molecular and Medical Pharmacology, UCLA School of Medicine, Los Angeles, California, USA

Marc André Mahé MD
Médécin Spécialiste des Centres de Recherche et de Lutte Contre le Cancer, Department of Radiation Therapy, Centre René Gauducheau, Nantes, France

John J. Mahmarian MD
Associate Professor of Medicine, Baylor College of Medicine, Texas, USA

Michael D. Mann PhD MMed(Paed) MMed(Nuc Med)
Associate Professor, Department of Paediatrics and Child Health, University of Cape Town; Head, Department of Nuclear Medicine, Red Cross Children's Hospital, Groote Schuur Hospital and University of Cape Town, Rondebosch, South Africa

Alan H. Maurer MD
Director, Nuclear Medicine, Professor, Diagnostic Imaging, Temple University School of Medicine, Philadelphia, Pennsylvania, USA

Bernard Mazière PhD
Professor, Head of Department of Research in Imaging, Physiology and Pharmacology, CEA-Orsay, France

Mariannick Mazière PhD
Directeur de Recherche Scientifique, Centre National de la Recherche Scientifique, Service Hospitalier Frédérick Joliot, Orsay, France

Steven R. Meikle BAppSc
Physicist, Department of Nuclear Medicine, Royal Prince Alfred Hospital, Sydney, New South Wales, Australia

Malcolm V. Merrick FRCP(Edin) FRCR
Consultant in Nuclear Medicine, Western General Hospital, Royal Infirmary and Royal Hospital for Sick Children, Edinburgh, UK

D. Douglas Miller MD
Associate Professor of Medicine, St. Louis University Medical Center, St. Louis, Missouri, USA

Chihoko Miyazaki MD
Chief of Diagnostic Radiology, Sapporo-City General Hospital; Attending Radiologist, Department of Nuclear Medicine, Hokkaido University School of Medicine, Sapporo, Japan

J. L. Moretti MD PhD
Professor, Université Paris 13, CHU Bobigny, France

P. J. Mountford BSc MSc PhD FInstP FIPSM
Consultant Medical Physicist, Department of Nuclear Medicine, Queen Elizabeth Hospital, Birmingham, UK

Roland Müller-Suur MD PhD
Associate Professor in Clinical Physiology and Consultant Nuclear Medicine Physician, Karolinska Institute, Departments of Clinical Physiology and Nuclear Medicine, Danderyd Hospital, Stockholm, Sweden

I. P. C. Murray AM MD FRCP(Ed) FRACP FACR
Director of Nuclear Medicine, Prince of Wales Hospital; Associate Professor of Medicine, University of New South Wales, Sydney, New South Wales, Australia

Sten Nilsson MD PhD
Associate Professor, Section of Nuclear Medicine, Depart-

ment of Oncology, University Hospital, Uppsala, Sweden

Michael J. O'Doherty MA MRCP MD
Consultant Physician, Department of Nuclear Medicine, Kent & Canterbury Hospital, Kent, UK

Hong-Yoe Oei MD PhD
Associate Professor of Nuclear Medicine, University Hospital Rotterdam-Dijkzigt, Rotterdam, The Netherlands

Christopher J. Palestro MD
Associate Professor of Nuclear Medicine and Radiology, Albert Einstein College of Medicine of the Yeshiva University, Bronx; Attending Physician and Chief, Division of Nuclear Medicine, Long Island Jewish Medical Center, New York, USA

J. Anthony Parker MD PhD
Radiologist, Beth Israel Hospital, Boston; Associate Professor of Radiology, Harvard Medical School, Boston, Massachusetts, USA

E. K. J. Pauwels DSc
Professor of Radiological Sciences (Nuclear Medicine), University Hospital, Leiden, The Netherlands

Dudley Pennell MA MD MRCP
Senior Lecturer and Honorary Consultant in Cardiac Imaging, Royal Brompton National Heart and Lung Hospital, London, UK

A. M. Peters MD MRCPath MRCP MSc(Nucl Med)
Reader in Nuclear Medicine, Department of Radiology, Hammersmith Hospital, London, UK

Matthias E. Pfisterer MD FESC FACC
Professor of Cardiology, Divisions of Cardiology and Nuclear Medicine, University Hospital, Basel, Switzerland

Lyn Sara Pilowsky BM BS MRCPsych
Wellcome Research Fellow and Honorary Lecturer, Institute of Psychiatry, London, UK

Ivo Podreka MD
Professor, University Department of Neurology, Vienna General Hospital, Vienna, Austria

Gerald M. Pohost MD
Professor of Medicine and Chief, Division of Cardiovascular Disease, University of Alabama at Birmingham, Birmingham, Alabama, USA

S. N. Reske MD
Professor of Nuclear Medicine, Head and Chief, Department of Radiology III, Nuclear Medicine, University of Ulm, Ulm, Germany

Jean-Claude Reubi MD
Professor and Head of the Division of Cell Biology and Experimental Cancer Research, Institute of Pathology, University of Berne, Berne, Switzerland

Pierre Rigo MD
Head, Nuclear Medicine Division, CHU, University of Liège, Liège, Belgium

Howard Ring BSc MBBS MRCPsych
Honorary Lecturer in Neuropsychiatry, Institute of Neurology, London, UK

Monica A. Rossleigh MBBS(Hons) FRACP
Senior Staff Specialist, The Prince of Wales Hospital, Sydney; Senior Lecturer in Medicine, The University of New South Wales, Sydney, New South Wales, Australia

Christopher C. Rowe MD FRACP
Director of Nuclear Medicine and Senior Consultant Neurologist, The Queen Elizabeth Hospital, Adelaide, South Australia, Australia

Charles D. Russell MD PhD
Professor of Radiology (Nuclear Medicine), University of Alabama School of Medicine, University of Alabama at Birmingham Medical Center; Veterans Affairs Medical Center, Birmingham, Alabama, USA

Seth Saverymuttu BSc MD MRCP
Consultant Gastroenterologist, Broomfield Hospital, Chelmsford, UK

Guy V. Sawle DM MRCP
Senior Lecturer in Neurology, Queens Medical Centre, Nottingham, UK

Heinrich R. Schelbert MD PhD
Professor and Vice Chair, Department of Molecular and Medical Pharmacology, UCLA School of Medicine; Chief, Cardiovascular Nuclear Medicine Section, The Laboratory of Nuclear Medicine, Los Angeles, California, USA

Andrew M. Scott MBBS FRACP DDU
Senior Lecturer in Medicine, University of Melbourne; Head, Tumour Targeting Program, Ludwig Institute Oncology Unit; Physician in Nuclear Medicine, Department of Nuclear Medicine, Austin Hospital, Heidelberg, Victoria, Australia

James E. Seabold MD
Associate Professor of Radiology, Division of Nuclear Medicine, University of Iowa Hospitals and Clinics, Iowa City, Iowa, USA

In Suk Seo MD
Director, Cardiac Imaging, The Brooklyn Hospital, Brooklyn, New York, USA

Brahm Shapiro MBChB PhD
Professor of Internal Medicine, Division of Nuclear Medicine, Department of Internal Medicine, University of Michigan Medical Center, Ann Arbor; Staff Physician, Nuclear Medicine Service, Department of Veterans Affairs Medical Center, Ann Arbor, Michigan, USA

David J. Silvester BSc PhD CChem FRSC
Head of Chemistry Section, MRC Cyclotron Unit, Hammersmith Hospital, London, UK

Helmut Sinzinger MD
Professor, Department of Nuclear Medicine, University of Vienna, Vienna, Austria

Richard C. Smart BSc MSc PhD
Principal Physicist, Department of Nuclear Medicine, St. George Hospital, Kogarah, Sydney, New South Wales, Australia

H. Dirk Sostman MD
Professor of Radiology, Duke University Medical Center, Durham, North Carolina, USA

Samuel Sostre MD PhD FACP
Associate Professor of Radiology, The Johns Hopkins Medical Institutions, Baltimore, Maryland, USA

Andrew E. Southee MBBS FRACP MRCP(UK)
Director of Nuclear Medicine, John Hunter Hospital and Hunter Area Health Service, Newcastle, New South Wales, Australia

Richard P. Spencer MD PhD
Professor and Chairman, Department of Nuclear Medicine, University of Connecticut Health Center, Farmington, Connecticut, USA

Terence J. Spinks PhD
Senior Scientist, PET Methodology, MRC Cyclotron Unit, Royal Postgraduate Medical School, Hammersmith Hospital, London, UK

Wilfrido M. Sy MD
Chairman, Department of Nuclear Medicine; Director Magnetic Imaging (MRI), The Brooklyn Hospital Center, Brooklyn, New York, USA

André Syrota MD PhD
Professor of Biophysics and Nuclear Medicine and Head of Service Frédérick Joliot, Commissariat à l'Energie Atomique, Orsay, France

Henrik S. Thomsen MD MSc
Lecturer in Radiology, Department of Diagnostic Radiology, University of Copenhagen, Herlev Hospital, Copenhagen, Denmark

Jocelyn E. Towson MA MSc
Radiation Safety Officer, Royal Prince Alfred Hospital, Sydney, New South Wales, Australia

Luigi Troncone MD
Associate Professor, Department of Nuclear Medicine, Policlinico 'A. Gemelli', Catholic University of the Sacred Heart, Rome, Italy

James E. Udelson MD
Assistant Professor of Medicine and Radiology, Tufts University School of Medicine; Director, Nuclear Cardiology Laboratory; Associate Director, Cardiac Catheterization Laboratory, New England Medical Center Hospitals, Boston, Massachusetts, USA

S. Richard Underwood MA MRCP
Senior Lecturer in Cardiac Imaging, National Heart & Lung Institute, London; Consultant in Charge, Department of Nuclear Medicine, Royal Brompton Hospital, London, UK

Renato A. Valdés Olmos MD
Consultant in Nuclear Medicine, The Netherlands Cancer Institute, Amsterdam, The Netherlands

Héric Valette MD
Maître de Conférence Universitaire; Praticien Hospitalier, Hôpital de Bicêtre, Bicêtre, France

Hans Van der Wall MBBS FRACP
Director of Nuclear Medicine, Concord Repatriation General Hospital; Deputy Director of Medical Imaging, Concord Repatriation General Hospital and Royal Prince Alfred Hospital, Sydney, New South Wales, Australia

Mario S. Verani MD
Professor of Medicine, Section of Cardiology, Baylor College of Medicine; Director, Nuclear Cardiology, The Methodist Hospital, Houston, Texas, USA

Alfons Michel Verbruggen PhD
Professor of Radiopharmaceutical Chemistry, Faculty of Pharmaceutical Sciences, Katholieke Universiteit Leuven, Leuven, Belgium

Nicolaas Paul L. G. Verhoeff MD PhD
Research Fellow, Department of Nuclear Medicine, Academic Medical Centre, Amsterdam; Lieutenant-Physician, Central Section for Individual Assistance, Utrecht, The Netherlands

F. C. Visser MD PhD
Cardiologist, Head of the Rehabilitation Department of Cardiology, Free University Hospital Amsterdam, Amsterdam, The Netherlands

Richard L Wahl MD
Professor of Internal Medicine and Radiology and Director, General Nuclear Imaging, University of Michigan, School of Medicine, Ann Arbor, Michigan, USA

Brenda Walker MSc
Senior Physicist, Department of Nuclear Medicine, Prince

of Wales Hospital, Sydney, New South Wales, Australia

S. Walton MD FRCP
Consultant Cardiologist, Aberdeen Royal Infirmary; Honorary Senior Lecturer in Medicine, University of Aberdeen, Aberdeen, UK

Daniel F. Worsley MD
Fellow, Division of Nuclear Medicine, Hospital of the University of Pennsylvania, Philadelphia, Pennsylvania, USA; Resident, Division of Nuclear Medicine, Vancouver General Hospital, Vancouver, British Columbia, Canada

Sinclair Wynchank MD DPhil FInstP
Head, Medical Biophysics Programme, Medical Research Council, Parow; Senior Lecturer, Department of Paediatrics and Child Health, University of Cape Town, Rondebosch, South Africa

Peter G. Yeates MPharm
Chief Radiopharmacist, Department of Nuclear Medicine, Royal Prince Alfred Hospital, Sydney, New South Wales, Australia

Liwa T. Younis MD PhD
Assistant Professor of Internal Medicine, Division of Cardiology, St. Louis University Health Sciences Center, St. Louis, Missouri, USA

Robert E. Zimmerman MSEE
Medical Physicist, Principal Associate in Radiology (Physics), Radiology Department, Harvard Medical School, Boston, Massachusetts, USA

Lionel S. Zuckier MD
Assistant Professor, Departments of Nuclear Medicine and Radiology, Albert Einstein College of Medicine, Bronx, New York, USA

Foreword

In the past we had a light which flickered, in the present we have a light which flames, and in the future there will be a light which shines over all the land and sea.

Sir Winston Churchill

The tracer principle was conceived of and tested by Von Hevesy. There is an apocryphal story about an early application of the tracer principle when Von Hevesy wanted to solve an important problem. As a student, he was living in a boarding house where he received his meals. He believed that his landlady was recycling the uneaten mashed potatoes to her boarders at a subsequent meal. One evening, so the story goes, Von Hevesy added a small amount of radioactive lead (radium-D) to his uneaten portion of mashed potatoes. When mashed potatoes were served again, he sequestered a small portion in his suitcase for measurement with an electroscope.[1] Voilà! He had the data. When he presented the evidence to his landlady, she was unimpressed and promptly threw him out of the boarding house. There are several morals to this tale: first, learning a scientific truth does not always lead to success; second, application of sophisticated technology does not always solve the fundamental problem; and third, when you have the evidence, you have to be careful about how and where you present it.

This humble and stormy beginning spawned the specialty of nuclear medicine. Investigators quickly realized the power of the tracer principle in elucidating many of the principles of physiology and biochemistry that are fundamental to modern medicine. In 1927, Herrman Blumgart measured the circulation time in man by injecting radon intravenously and measuring the time required to see tracks in a Wilson cloud chamber. While this was an early use of radionuclides in man, it did not signal the start of nuclear medicine. That event can probably be traced to a lecture delivered by Karl Compton, then president of MIT, in 1936.[2] In that lecture, Compton described the work of Von Hevesy using phosphorus-32 in biological systems. Drs John Means and Earle Chapman (who ran the well-known thyroid clinic at the Massachusetts General Hospital) were in the audience. They asked one of their colleagues, Robley Evans, if an isotope of iodine could be created for the purpose of studying thyroid function. Within a year, they had I-128 and began their famous studies on thyroid physiology. The subsequent development of I-131, with its longer half-life, made studies of the thyroid possible as a procedure to enable clinical decisions to be made. In the late 1940s, point counting of the thyroid gland with a highly collimated detector was employed to determine whether or not a palpable nodule was iodine-avid. Benedict Cassen was trying to simplify this measurement by mechanically moving a radiation detector over the thyroid gland[3] while creating an 'image' based on the level of activity found at each point over the gland. This 'scanner' was improved with the addition of a scintillation detector and a multi-hole focused collimator, so that in 1952 it was practicable to use this instrument for the evaluation of the thyroid on a routine basis. Nuclear medicine was born.

Over the next four decades, improvements in instrumentation, radiopharmaceuticals and the interest of commercial manufacturers contributed to the remarkable growth of the field. Nearly a century after the studies of Von Hevesy demonstrated the inseparable nature of isotopes, nuclear medicine remains the most sensitive approach to the measurement of in vivo physiology, biochemistry and metabolism. The continued expansion of the field indicates that effective patient care requires infor-

[1] Brucer M 1990 A chronology of nuclear medicine 1600–1989. Heritage Publications, St Louis, Missouri, p 141

[2] Brucer M 1990 A chronology of nuclear medicine 1600–1989. Heritage Publications, St Louis, Missouri, pp 223–224

[3] Brucer M 1990 A chronology of nuclear medicine 1600–1989. Heritage Publications, St Louis, Missouri, p 248

mation about these important parameters.

This text is an encyclopaedic compilation of the contemporary applications of nuclear medicine in the clinical and research environment. The contributors have been selected to permit each topic to be considered in depth and with expertise. There is, therefore, a remarkable international representation which reflects the mixture of well-known authorities and younger authors who have achieved particular renown in specialized aspects.

The text comprises 114 chapters organized into major sections dealing with acute care, renal disorders, gastrointestinal function, neurological and psychiatric studies, tumour diagnosis and therapy, examinations of bones and joints, nuclear cardiology and the basic sciences. To achieve a complete presentation of the clinical utility of radionuclide procedures in each area, the editors present each type of examination from an array of technical and clinical viewpoints. In this fashion, the reader gains specific information on the performance and interpretation of these tests and a panoramic view of their use. Study of acutely ill patients, for example, covers the unique attributes of the intensive care environment and the kind of information that nuclear medicine can provide about unstable patients. Performing the same procedure in a stable patient permits more detailed imaging and, when appropriate, interventional studies to define reserve function in the organ.

The authors and editors have laboured well to produce a book that is readable and easily understood. They have defined the technology and identified areas for its effective application. The text will stand as a landmark, defining the state of practice at a time when nuclear medicine is poised to enter the next century.

H.W.S

Preface

For those who had to endure the tedium of measuring basal metabolic rate or the enforced meticulous estimation of protein-bound iodine, the advent of radioiodine for the investigation of thyroid disease was revolutionary. The procedure offered a simple but accurate method of identifying changes in physiology with an even greater impact on clinical practice when it became feasible to obtain images of the distribution of altered function within the thyroid gland. This seminal use of a tracer radionuclide heralded a vista of entirely new diagnostic investigations. Succeeding years steadily unveiled the enormous potential of this clinical tool which even today is not fully fulfilled. Successive advances in instrumentation and radiopharmaceuticals have honed the diagnostic value and established nuclear medicine as a critical discipline in health care. From time to time, the advent of new imaging technologies have been accompanied by gloomy prognostications as to the future of the scintigraphic procedures, yet, on every occasion, subsequent experience has actually enhanced their status by establishing their complementary role to these new modalities. Indeed, as we look towards the next century, with ever-increasing sensitivity and speed of detecting equipment, the quintessential attribute of identifying altered physiology or biochemistry will undoubtedly burgeon, and an expanding range of the targeting radiopharmaceuticals developing from organ-specific to cell-specific and even disease-specific, is to be expected.

Nevertheless, even with this ever-increasing sophistication, it can never be forgotten that these procedures are merely clinical tools which must be applied appropriately to some particular clinical problem. Since there must be justification for the use of radiation in any individual, awareness of the likely advantages or limitations of any nuclear medicine investigation is critical in determining whether it should be undertaken. This text therefore aims to provide an understanding of the role of nuclear medicine in clinical practice. In emphasizing the clinical impact and demonstrating the input to the overall management of patients, it is divided into sections which, relating to the clinical presentation, highlight indications for various studies and guidelines to their interpretation. Over the years, a plethora of different uses have been advocated; many have gained a reliable diagnostic role while others have not found supportive protagonists. An attempt has been made, therefore, to ensure that the proportion of the text allocated to the various topics does bear a relationship to the relative contribution of each procedure to contemporary nuclear medicine. Even at the risk of repetition, attention is paid dominantly to those investigations which are of the greatest value in the most common clinical situations, although those which are less frequent but have a particular diagnostic value are also considered in detail.

This approach has also permitted consideration in the appropriate context of the therapeutic role of unsealed radionuclides. The growth of this aspect of the discipline has been, in recent years, rapid and exciting. However, there is the promise of even more effective applications of this form of treatment and this growing frontier is the subject of particular attention.

The referring physician and practitioner in nuclear medicine often has an uncertain understanding of the underlying scientific principles, many of which are unique to the field. Many may be daunted by the mathematical formulae, chemical equations and technological detail or confused by the jargon. The final section therefore has been conceived with a view to clarifying misconceptions, introducing concepts and, hopefully, encouraging better understanding and stimulating further reading. In maintaining a clinical orientation, particular attention has been paid to the practical application in relation to patients and staff of the principles of radiation safety.

The preparation of this book has occupied several years and would not have been possible without the assistance of many, varying from our Advisory Section Editors and our contributing colleagues, most of whom achieved the deadlines, to the staff of Churchill Livingstone, in particular Lowri Daniels, Senior Project Editor, who was ever ready to advise and also to chide the tardy authors. A full listing of acknowledgements would be 'Oscar-like' and, similarly, would be fraught with the embarrassment of omissions. However, we must express our particular thanks to Ms Jan Newman who, bearing the major burden of the immense intercontinental correspondence, typing and retyping innumerable chapters, and developing an eagle eye in the proofreading stage, continually displayed a dedication to the project and an unremitting and inspiring enthusiasm. Finally, we must certainly acknowledge our wives and families who experienced even more 'lost' weekends than they have had to endure for so many years.

Sydney and
London, 1994

I.P.C.M.
P.J.E.

SECTION 5

Nuclear medicine in tumour diagnosis and therapy

PART A

Diagnosis

55. Tumour-seeking radiopharmaceuticals: nature and mechanisms

Richard P. Spencer

Tumour imaging may be defined as non-invasive procedures for detecting and localizing 'abnormal' tissue (benign or malignant) in the intact living patient. While a number of modalities have been applied in an effort to achieve detection of tumours while they are small in size and localized, developments are still evolving. Radiopharmaceutical approaches for tumour imaging will be outlined with cross-reference to other techniques. Many are discussed in greater detail in the succeeding chapters.

It has become apparent that no one procedure is capable of detecting all tumours.[1] Maisey et al[2] have pointed out the possibility of 'synergistic imaging' or combining information when two or more imaging modalities are employed. For example, coupling data on perfusion and metabolism may be of value in following tumour response to therapy.

Approaches to tumour imaging have developed somewhat empirically. An initial classification of radiopharmaceuticals utilized for this purpose is therefore empirical as well (Table 55.1). As underlying principles become clarified, the classification can be revised.

Table 55.1 An empirical classification of the range of mechanisms by which radiopharmaceuticals have been employed in tumour detection

1. *Interference with a normal function*
   Example: 'negative defect' on radiocolloid scan of liver, due to intrahepatic tumour

2. *Altered perfusion/metabolism around a tumour*
   Example: positive bone scan surrounding a metastasis

3. *Non-specific binding or accumulation*
   Example: uptake of ^{99m}Tc diphosphonates by neuroblastomas and fibrohistiocytomas (perhaps related to iron or ferritin). Osteosarcomas, especially in areas away from bone, may reveal marked uptake of bone imaging agents

4. *Uptake without effective excretion*
   Examples: ^{131}I Rose Bengal or ^{99m}Tc-HIDA in hepatomas, ^{99m}Tc pertechnetate in Warthin's tumour

5. *Altered perfusion/metabolism within a tumour*
   a. Vasculature that differs from surrounding tissue, such as
      i) capillary haemangiomas
      ii) principally hepatic artery blood supply to intrahepatic tumours;
   b. markers of oxidative metabolism and hypoxia;
   c. PET metabolic intermediates;
   d. uptake of potassium and analogues (^{201}Tl, ^{99m}Tc isonitriles);
   e. active transport
      Example: radioiodide entry into differentiated thyroid tumours;
   f. MIBG;
   g. iodocholesterol;
   h. melanoma localization.

6. *Receptor or cell surface binding (± internalization)*
   a. ^{67}Ga and transferrin metabolism;
   b. labelled monoclonal antibodies against surface markers;
   c. radiolabelled hormones and receptor binding;
   d. labelled interleukins and white blood cells;
   e. liposomes;
   f. mitogens.

7. *Mixed cellular binding,* such as most antineoplastic agents
   Example: binding to DNA

INTERFERENCE WITH NORMAL FUNCTION

Radiopharmaceutical studies are often based on agents whose uptake is indicative of specific function. Decreased or absent function can thus be inferred to be indicative of interference with that function, such as caused by the presence of a tumour. For example, even 'minimal deviation hepatomas' have lost the ability to accumulate radiocolloids (that is reticuloendothelial cell activity is absent or non-functional). An example of a tumour replacing reticuloendothelial activity is presented in Figure 55.1. However, it is recognized that cysts and haematomas can produce similar 'negative defects'. It is here that diagnostic accuracy can be improved by coupling information. Thus, for example, imaging during the perfusion phase may be able to demonstrate whether there is blood flow to the lesion. Such flow would rule out a cyst or haematoma. A lesion within the liver that is 'negative' for radiocolloid uptake may be 'positive' for accumulation of red blood cells (capillary haemangioma, haemangiosarcoma or some hepatomas). An example is shown in Figure 55.2. It should be pointed out, however, that the manner of presentation of the patient may be quite different. Ultrasound, CT and MRI have been the principal tools for deter-

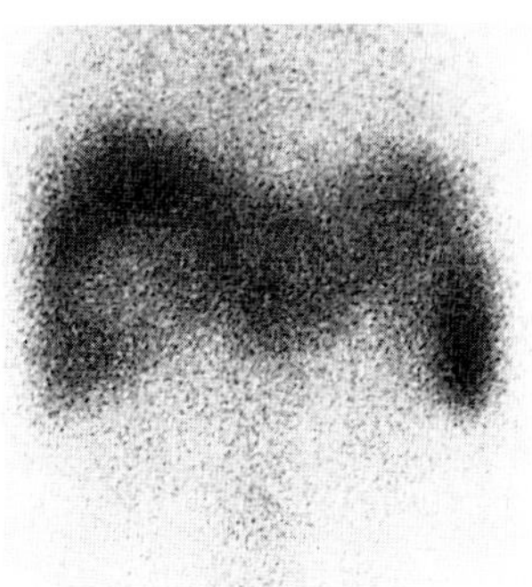

Fig. 55.1 This is an anterior abdominal gamma camera image, taken at 22 h after intravenous administration of autologous white blood cells labelled with In-111-oxine. A 'negative' defect in the right hepatic lobe can be noted, due to the presence of metastatic malignant melanoma in a 46-year-old woman.

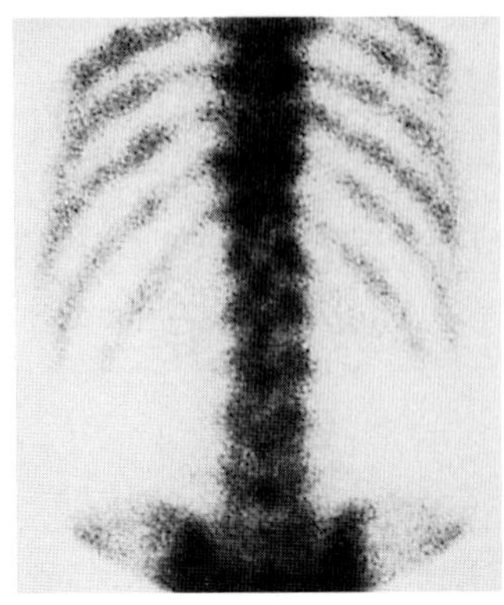

Fig. 55.3 A posterior thoracolumbar image was obtained at 2 h following the intravenous administration of ^{99m}Tc methylenediphosphonate in a 64-year-old man. The kidneys cannot be clearly delineated, while the vertebrae have intense uptake. Ribs demonstrate a quite uneven distribution in terms of both sites and degree of uptake. This represents a 'super scan', resulting from widely metastatic prostatic carcinoma. Bone avidity for the imaging agent reduced the quantity available for renal excretion.

mining the presence of a region that differs somehow ('tissue signature') from surrounding areas. It is then the responsibility of radiopharmaceutical studies to define further the nature of the region by identifying the functional status.

ALTERED PERFUSION/METABOLISM AROUND A TUMOUR

If a tumour cannot be detected directly, it can sometimes be localized by its effects on nearby cells. 'Early' tumours are marked by displacement of normal tissue, and the organ is still 'isovolumetric' prior to the tumour causing bulk changes. A variety of malignancies, metastatic to bone, do not have increased uptake of ^{99m}Tc diphosphonates within their substance. However, the osseous tissue surrounding the tumour can show marked uptake of the radiotracer, thus delineating the presence of abnormal cells (but not necessarily their intrinsic volume or metabolism). This is demonstrated in Figure 55.3.

The mechanisms of tumour–normal tissue interactions have yet to be defined in depth. Certainly tracers that localized angiogenesis factors or their vascular effects would be of value in defining tumours. The metabolic rate of a lesion may also be of some help in distinguishing these abnormal tissues. A well-known example occurs in the course of inflammation, when an infected region around the gall bladder results in hepatic tissue heating and compression, with the appearance of a 'rim sign' due to increased uptake of radiotracer at the site.[3]

NON-SPECIFIC BINDING OR ACCUMULATION

'Non-specific' means that the mechanism is uncertain and that the phenomenon can be found in a variety

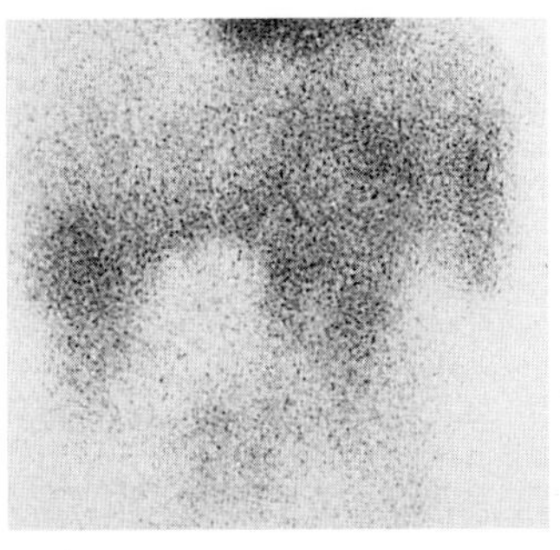

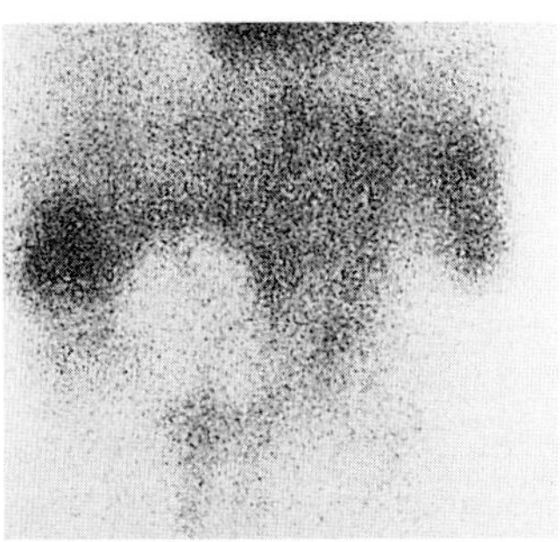

Fig. 55.2 These are anterior abdominal images in a 60-year-old woman, after intravenous administration of autologous red blood cells. These were labelled with ^{99m}Tc pertechnetate in vivo (following prior injection of stannous pyrophosphate). Left: View at 2 min. The cardiac blood pool is above. Right: View at 30 min. A large 'negative' defect is seen on both images. This was an intrahepatic cyst. The delayed image shows enhancement of an area in the lateral right hepatic lobe, as compared with the first view. This was an 'enhancing' intrahepatic capillary haemangioma.

of lesions. Perhaps the best documented of these occurrences is the uptake of ^{99m}Tc diphosphonates in a multitude of tumours (and other lesions as well). For example, bone imaging agents can be found to delineate many lesions, such as osteogenic sarcoma, in which the mechanism may be related to deposition on a bone-like surface. About one-third to one-half of neuroblastomas, and most fibrohistiocytomas will concentrate ^{99m}Tc diphosphonates.[4] Both of these tumours possess iron-containing compounds (ferritin, haemosiderin), which may be the basic cause of uptake of the bone imaging agents. Examples are shown in Figure 55.4. Many other cell types will also accumulate ^{99m}Tc diphosphonates. Particularly common is the detection of mucinous adenocarcinomas of the colon, metastatic to the liver.

UPTAKE WITHOUT EFFECTIVE EXCRETION

A recognized principle in positron emission tomography (PET) imaging is 'metabolic trapping'. For example, 2-deoxy-2-fluoroglucose is transported similarly to glucose and is then phosphorylated. However, the next enzyme in the metabolic pathway does not further process the substrate. Thus, it is trapped for a period of time and the F-18 analogue can be imaged. By analogy, there are several examples of tumour imaging based on uptake of a radiolabel but inefficient or absent further processing.

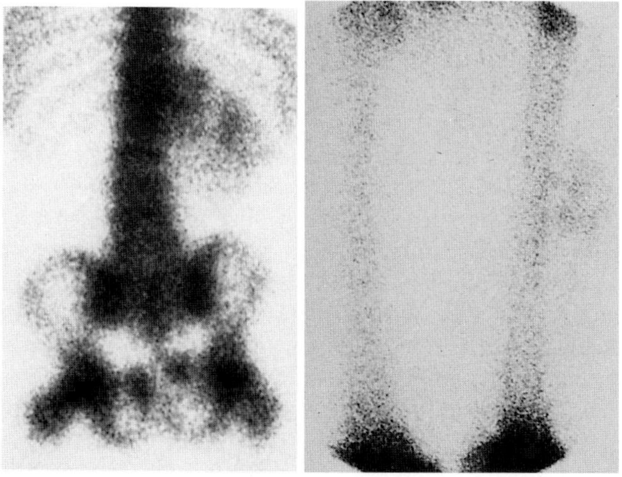

Fig. 55.4 ^{99m}Tc methylenediphosphonate uptake in malignancies. Left: Posterior thorax, lumbar region and pelvis in a 3.5-year-old girl. The left kidney was dysplastic and had no uptake of radiotracer. The right kidney can be seen, with activity also noted adjacent to the vertebral column. This was a neuroblastoma, with considerable concentration of the bone imaging agent. Right: Anterior view of the femurs in a 19-year-old male. Activity lateral to the left femur was within a fibrous histiocytoma. The tumour was not attached to the nearby bone.

Hepatobiliary agents that follow the pathway blood → hepatic parenchymal cells → bile are accumulated by some well-differentiated hepatomas. Both ^{131}I Rose Bengal[5] and ^{99m}Tc iminodiacetic acid derivatives share this property.[6] Hepatomas do not have a ductal system for excretion of those agents and it is uncertain if the biochemical excretory pathway is intact. Hepatoblastomas also possess the hepatobiliary uptake mechanism,[7] as apparently do some hepatocellular carcinomas.

A tumour of the salivary glands, oncocytoma, can accumulate ^{131}I sodium iodide. Again, without an efficient excretory system for the concentrated radiopharmaceutical, there is localized retention. Indeed, radioiodide uptake has been reported as a means of treating oncocytoma.[8] Also in this category may be ^{99m}Tc pertechnetate uptake by Warthin's tumour of the salivary glands. The accumulation is not coupled with an effective excretory pathway.

ALTERED PERFUSION/METABOLISM WITHIN A TUMOUR

This is a large and heterogeneous grouping and presently accounts for multiple radiopharmaceutical approaches to tumour imaging.

Vasculature

Radiolabelled antibodies or other markers for angiogenesis factors and endothelins are not yet available. However, use has been made of the properties of vessels which differ from those in their vicinity, as in the previous example of a capillary haemangioma, which slowly accumulated radiolabelled red cells (Figure 55.2). A second example involves tumours which have a principal arterial supply as contrasted with nearby venous inflow. Intrahepatic tumours are largely dependent on blood from the hepatic artery, as contrasted with the portal vein. Catheter placement into the artery supplying the tumour is followed by introduction of ^{99m}Tc microspheres (20 μm diameter). This should delineate the extent of the tumour, and also demonstrate whether there is shunting, in which case some of the labelled microspheres will pass to the lungs. The technique has had some clinical utilization[9] in preparation for arterial catheter introduction of chemotherapeutic agents into the tumour. Use of catheter delivery of radiating microspheres for internal irradiation of hepatocellular carcinoma has enjoyed only limited success thus far.[10] However, there may be a role here for pharmacological intervention. Adrenaline and noradrenaline are reported to vasoconstrict normal liver arterioles, while vessels in the tumour (without smooth musculature) do not respond.[11]

Markers of oxidative metabolism and hypoxia

For over 60 years it has been recognized that cells, in the presence of oxygen, are more sensitive to radiation. Perhaps this relates to the generation of oxygen radicals during radiation therapy, with increased cellular damage. At the opposite extreme, 'hypoxic radioresistance' has been noted in several animal tumours and in some human malignancies as well.[12] Hypoxic tumour cells are often those most distant from the blood supply, and thus radioimmunotherapy may be less effective since the labelled antibodies have to traverse a greater distance.[13] A major problem in vivo has been the lack of a non-invasive procedure for demonstrating tumour hypoxia. The proposal had been made that a method of searching for compounds more cytotoxic to hypoxic cells than aerobic ones is to examine for reductive metabolism.[14] There are at least two known classes of compounds which are stated to be cytotoxic to hypoxic cells.[15] The first class comprises quinone reductive–alkylating agents; mitomycin C is an example. A problem is that although activity is shown in vitro, there is less effect in vivo. The second class includes hypoxic cell sensitizers such as misonidazole. Studies have shown binding of tritiated misonidazole to hypoxic areas in both human and animal tumours. Whether enough of the compounds can be administered without toxic effects to increase radiosensitivity significantly has still to be determined clinically.

Markers of cellular hypoxia have a potential to delineate the underoxygenated portions of tumours, and hence to localize these regions during life. Figure 55.5 lists some radiolabelled compounds which have been reported, or hypothesized, to localize in hypoxic tumour sites in vivo or in vitro. The first is iodoazomycin arabinoside, labelled with ^{123}I.[16] The azomycin nucleosides are analogues of misonidazole. An initial study showed some concentration in human tumours (3/10) at 1 day post injection. The radiofluorine derivative of misonidazole has also been prepared.[12,17] The first study on patients showed slight tumour concentration of the radiolabel over plasma values, in two out of three cases.[12]

Glucarate is a dicarboxylic acid with four H–C–OH groupings, while gluconate is a monocarboxylic acid also with four H–C–OH groups and a terminal CH_2OH. Both of these compounds bind ^{99m}Tc. In addition, they have shown, in vitro, a two- to three-fold enhanced accumulation in hypoxic Chinese hamster ovary cells.[18] Addition of fructose to the medium reduced cellular uptake of the ^{99m}Tc derivative of both glucarate and gluconate; this suggested at least one shared step in uptake or concentration. Because of their ^{99m}Tc label, both of the compounds will be of interest; whether they are effective in delineating hypoxic areas in vivo has still to be determined.

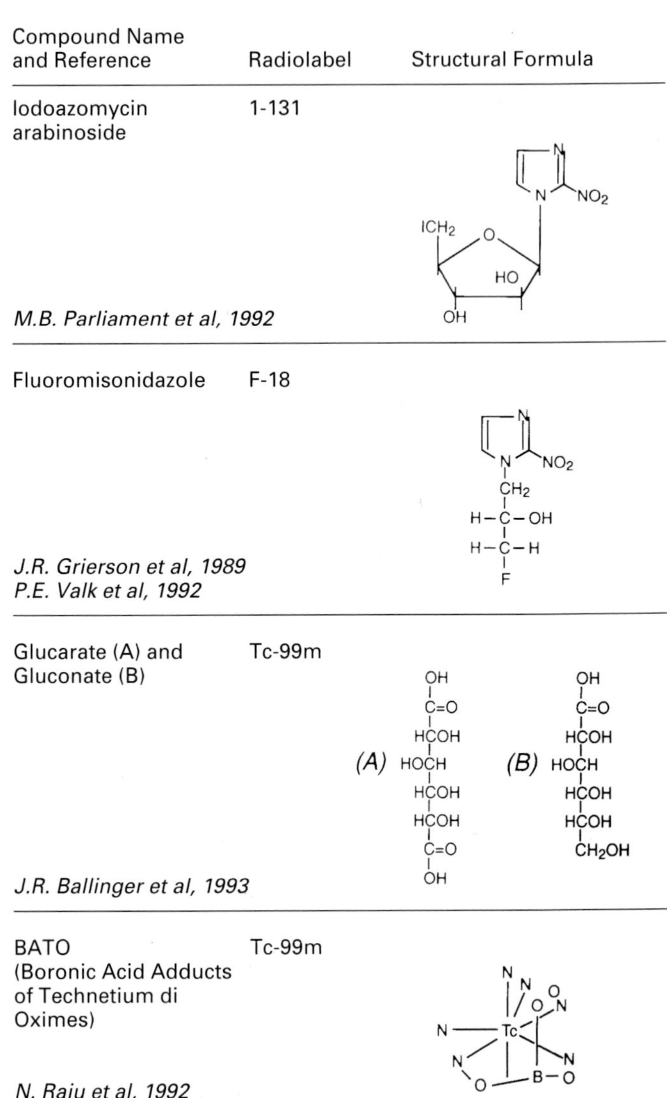

Fig. 55.5 Some compounds proposed for imaging of hypoxic areas.

A series of lipophilic boronic acid derivatives of nitromidazole has been prepared,[19] and shown to bind ^{99m}Tc. Whether, in practice, they do localize in hypoxic sites still has to be demonstrated in vivo. Another approach may be feasible. Acetate, labelled with positron-emitting ^{11}C, has been utilized as an indicator of oxidative metabolism. For example, the right ventricle has been studied by use of this tracer.[20] If applied to a tumour, or an area suspected of containing a tumour, variations in the oxidative metabolism gradient might be employed to point out sites with a low oxidative metabolism and possible anaerobic metabolism.

PET metabolic indicators

The glucose analogue, 2-fluoro-2-deoxy-D-glucose (^{18}F) had been employed in a number of studies which sought to monitor the effects of treatment on tumour metabolism.

Minn and Paul[21] summarized 15 studies up to 1991, which evaluated 176 patients. Unfortunately, a variety of tumours were involved, as well as a number of therapies, including chemotherapy, radiotherapy, transarterial embolization and hyperthermia. It is still uncertain if PET can meaningfully evaluate tumour metabolism before and after therapy. Efforts are being made, however, to sort out a number of variables, and to devise standardized protocols. Both kinetic and steady-state methods have been utilized in exploring fluorodeoxyglucose uptake in tumours.[22] There has been recognition that elevated blood glucose concentrations degrade PET images of fluorodeoxyglucose uptake in tumours.[23] Therefore, fasting has been suggested before these studies, and Fischman and Alpert[24] have discussed possible corrections to the crude data. It is also possible that account must be made of the plasma insulin level.[22]

While some tumours reveal significant uptake of radiolabelled fluorodeoxyglucose, others appear hypometabolic.[25] Not all tumours exhibit a decrease in uptake of the radiotracer after therapy. Indeed, in some an increase can be noted.[26] Haberkorn et al[27] reported that radiolabelled fluorodeoxyglucose studies showed that tumours were more sensitive to therapy than were the involved lymph nodes. The disassociation between PET metabolic results and other radiopharmaceutical imaging is perhaps best demonstrated by the report of Sasaki et al.[28] In two cases, ^{99m}Tc HMDP bone scintigraphy was negative. However, radiolabelled fluorodeoxyglucose imaging was positive in the bone tumours. This re-emphasized that bone imaging examines the metabolic response in the tissues around a lesion, while PET (fluorodeoxyglucose) can examine a lesion itself. With a known tumour type, for example gliomas, there is some evidence that glucose use, measured by fluorodeoxyglucose, corresponds with the grade of malignancy.[29]

PET technology also allows access to other classes of biologically relevant compounds. Ogawa et al[30] utilized ^{11}C methionine to study 50 patients with gliomas. The radiolabelled amino acid was taken up by 31/32 (97%) high-grade gliomas and 11/18 (61%) low-grade gliomas. Individually, it was difficult to assess the grade of malignancy from the extent of uptake of ^{11}C methionine. The PET study was stated to define the extent of the glioma more clearly than CT. Hence, a role in defining tumour extent, rather than grade of the glioma, may evolve. Of interest, the uptake of ^{11}C methionine in tumours but only slight accumulation in areas of radiation necrosis has suggested a role for this radioactive tracer in distinguishing recurrent tumour from radiation-related necrosis.

The presumed heavy intracellular traffic in DNA and RNA precursors, within tumours, may yield a meaningful approach to employing PET methodology. For example, a tritiated thymidine labelling index as well as flow cytometry has been used in predicting survival in non-Hodgkin's lymphoma.[31] ^{11}C thymidine can be synthesized, and the tracer has been employed in evaluating human head and neck tumours by means of PET.[32] Standards have been produced for ^{11}C carbon monoxide.[33] Upon inhalation, this positron-emitting radiotracer binds to haemoglobin and might be employed for delineating tumour blood pools before and after therapy. Positron-emitting ^{124}I ($t_{1/2}$ = 4.4 days, 26% yield of beta plus) has been utilized in quantitative studies on antibody distribution.[34]

Uptake of potassium and analogues

Following intravenous administration of radioactive potassium, there is wide distribution of tissue uptake. Availability to tissues is not in exact proportion to arterial blood flow, since at least two organs have a dual blood supply (liver – hepatic artery and portal vein; lungs – bronchial arteries and pulmonary artery). In addition, the kinetics of entry is different in tissues such as the brain and the testes. However, the cellular penetration of radiopotassium is recognized, and multiple studies have appeared on its use in the detection of intracranial tumours. The two available potassium radioisotopes are far from ideal for imaging (Table 55.2).

The finding that radiothallium (^{201}Tl monovalent) is 'potassium-like' in terms of cardiac uptake led to investigations of its potential in tumour detection. For example, Tonami & Hisada[35] were among the early investigators who noted that ^{201}Tl chloride had advantages in detecting lung and thyroid malignancies. Elgazzar et al[36] have provided a review of many pertinent aspects of the use of radiothallium for tumour localization. As a cationic radionuclide, with a single positive charge, ^{201}Tl is accumulated like potassium intracellularly via the ATP-dependent sodium–potassium pump; however, additional mechanisms of entry have not been excluded. Radiothallium is cleared from the myocardium more slowly than potassium, probably because of more avid binding to the ATPase enzyme. The basis for the use of radiothallium in tumour detection can be found in the following observations.

1. ^{201}Tl Cl is not accumulated in necrotic regions, perhaps because of lack of a functional ATPase. There is some uptake at inflammatory sites.
2. Normal tissue and malignancies do show some uptake of radiothallium.

Table 55.2 Characteristics of potassium radioisotopes

Radionuclide	Production	$t_{1/2}$ (h)	Beta minus	Gamma (mEv)
^{42}K	^{41}K (n, gamma)	12.4	Yes	1.52 (18%)
^{43}K	^{40}Ar (alpha, p)	22.4	Yes	0.36 (85%) 0.63 (81%)

3. In some instances, the malignant counterpart of a normal tissue accumulates more radiothallium. At the subcellular level, a portion of radiothallium within tumours can be noted to localize in mitochondrial and microsomal fractions. Sandrock et al[37] have provided histological evidence that the ability of dual radionuclide (^{201}Tl/^{99m}Tc) studies to detect parathyroid adenomas is partly dependent upon oxyphil cells rich in mitochondria and presumably in radiothallium avidity.

Radiothallium currently has three roles in tumour detection.

Localization of parathyroid adenomas

The rationale is that potassium-like radionuclides such as ^{201}Tl will enter tumours within the neck. When ^{99m}Tc pertechnetate is subsequently administered, it accumulates in functional thyroid tissue. Hence, by electronic subtraction 'non-thyroid' tissues in the area can be identified.[38] Many variants of the procedure have been described. Some groups prefer to utilise pertechnetate first, to localize the thyroid. Other workers, however, employ ^{201}Tl, since its emission has a lower energy and it is utilized in smaller amounts than pertechnetate. A variant of this (thyroid localization with radioiodide and use of a thallium 'analogue') is given in Figure 55.6. Sandrock et al[37] have provided a summary of much of the literature. In our experience, the procedure has worked well for detection of parathyroid adenomas. Limits to the success of the methodology have been the small size (or avidity) of some adenomas and the presence of thyroid lesions which either distort the image or which themselves accumulate radiothallium.

Intracranial lesions

Radiothallium concentrates in many intracranial malignancies. Further, radiothallium imaging has been reported to be superior to both CT and other single photon gamma-emitters in detecting recurrent brain tumours.[39] The technology is readily available and hence likely to be utilized in many centres, rather than PET methodologies, which are more limited in worldwide availability.

The wider use of radiothallium imaging of the brain may be in determining whether there is still viable tumour remaining after therapy, either surgery or, more particularly, external radiation. Yoshii et al[40] noted literature reports on the difficulty in distinguishing viable from non-viable tumour after therapy, because of necrosis and oedema. They discussed the utilization of radiothallium tomography; the assumption is that viable tumour cells will accumulate radiothallium. The method failed in the case of tumours under 1.5 cm in diameter and in the instance of a thin-rimmed tumour.

A further approach has been to use a dual radionuclide technique for determining whether viable intracranial tumour remains after radiation therapy. Dillehay[41] has summarized a portion of the pertinent literature. In brief, tomography with a perfusion agent such as ^{99m}Tc-HMPAO is utilized to determine if a region within the brain is perfused. Radiothallium is employed to estimate whether there is viable tissue within the space. Schwartz et al[42] describe the procedure in depth, as well as the experience of their group. An example of cranial cross-sectional imaging, with the use of radiothallium, is shown in Figure 55.7.

^{99m}Tc isonitriles have shown a similarity to ^{201}Tl chloride in terms of uptake into viable myocardial tissue. Previously, it was pointed out that radiothallium appeared to be concentrated in mitochondrial and microsomal fraction. Crane et al[43] have stated that over 90% of ^{99m}Tc isonitrile that entered the guinea pig myocardium is associated with the mitochondria. Since ischaemia resulted in loss of mitochondrial viability, they concluded

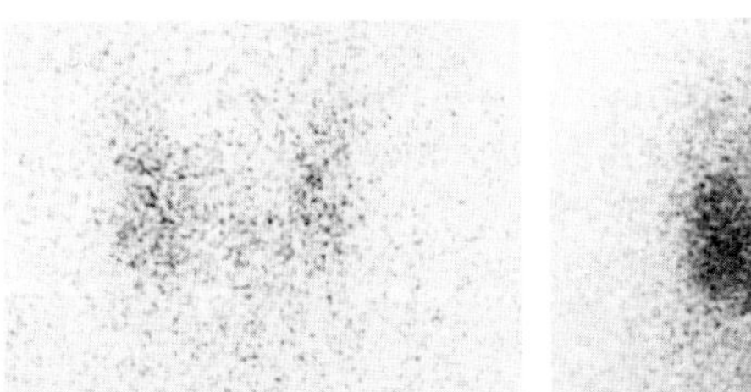

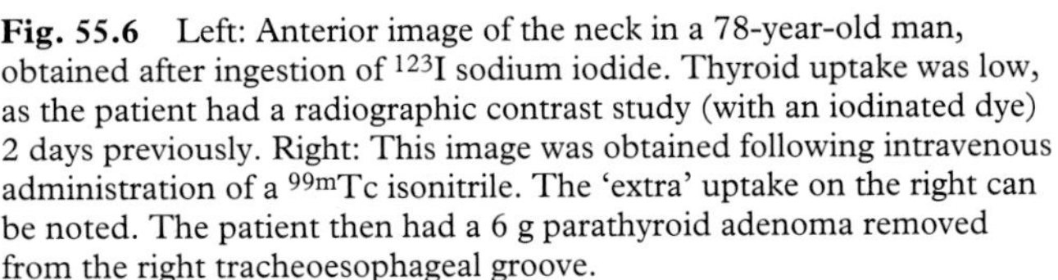

Fig. 55.6 Left: Anterior image of the neck in a 78-year-old man, obtained after ingestion of ^{123}I sodium iodide. Thyroid uptake was low, as the patient had a radiographic contrast study (with an iodinated dye) 2 days previously. Right: This image was obtained following intravenous administration of a ^{99m}Tc isonitrile. The 'extra' uptake on the right can be noted. The patient then had a 6 g parathyroid adenoma removed from the right tracheoesophageal groove.

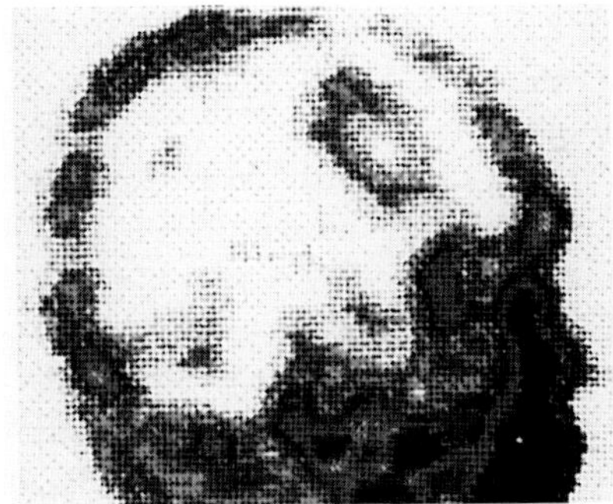

Fig. 55.7 A sagittal cross-section image (^{201}Tl thallous chloride) of the cranial region in a 37-year-old man. The patient had prior localized irradiation for a tumour in the frontal region. A small rim of radiothallium activity was seen around a 'cold' centre. Uptake was less than that in the skull away from the irradiated area. A perfusion study (^{99m}Tc HMPAO) revealed nearly absent perfusion of the site. Radiothallium uptake probably represented gliosis; there has been no evidence of tumour recurrence.

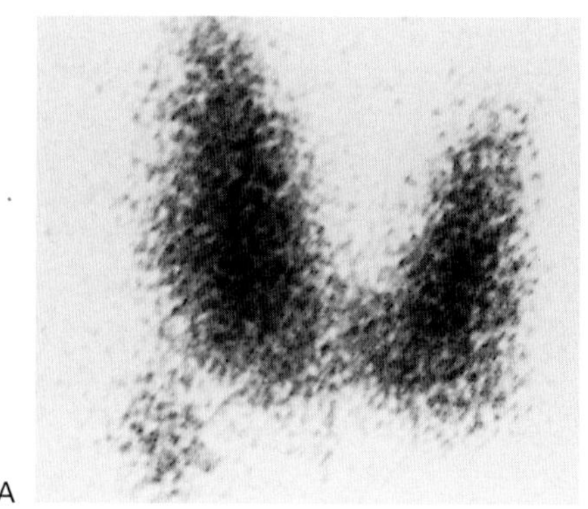

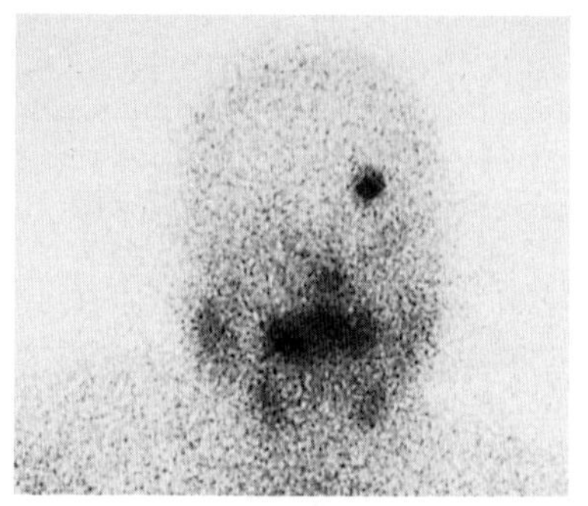

Fig. 55.8 Two presentations of thyroid carcinoma. (A) Neck image (^{123}I sodium iodide) in a 58-year-old woman. In addition to the well-formed thyroid lobes, an area of activity can be seen low in the right side of the patient's neck. This was uptake in a lymph node which had been largely replaced by papillary carcinoma of the thyroid. (B) Anterior view of the head and neck in a 56-year-old woman. This was obtained at 48 h after ingestion of 5 millicuries of ^{131}I sodium iodide. The patient had a prior thyroidectomy for follicular carcinoma. Intense localized uptake can be noted in a skull metastasis.

that ^{99m}Tc isonitriles should not accumulate in areas of infarction. Reports are beginning to accumulate on the uptake of ^{99m}Tc isonitriles within intracranial metastatic malignancies.[44] In addition, the ^{99m}Tc isonitriles are being explored for detection of other tumours, and for use in lieu of radiothallium in the search for parathyroid adenomas (Figure 55.6).

Determination of presence or viability of other tumours

Radiothallium has been employed for the detection of other types of tumours. A listing of some of these has been given by Mut et al.[44] Charkes et al[45] have described use of SPECT radiothallium imaging in detecting metastases from thyroid carcinoma. An additional use may be in following lymphomas. It can be expected that the ^{99m}Tc isonitriles may also have a role in these instances.

Active transport

When active transport can be employed to localize a tumour, advantage should be taken of the great specificity of the transport event and its ability to move molecules against a concentration gradient. The best example of this is radioiodide transport into well-differentiated thyroid malignancies. Not all thyroid malignancies demonstrate this property. It has been noted that most tumours of the thyroid will not show radioiodide uptake as long as a major portion of the normal gland is present. There are exceptions, shown for example in Figure 55.8A. A usual protocol when a thyroid mass is palpated is to perform needle biopsy.[46] A biopsy positive for a well-differentiated thyroid carcinoma is followed by total thyroidectomy. Shortly after this (and prior to starting administration of thyroid hormone), the patient is administered 185 MBq (5mCi) of ^{131}I sodium iodide orally. Whole-body imaging is carried out at 48 h (Figure 55.8B). In addition to a significant portion of papillary and follicular thyroid carcinomas, occasionally a medullary thyroid carcinoma may be found to concentrate radioiodide.[47] As previously discussed, radiothallium imaging can have a role in the detection of metastases from thyroid carcinoma.[45]

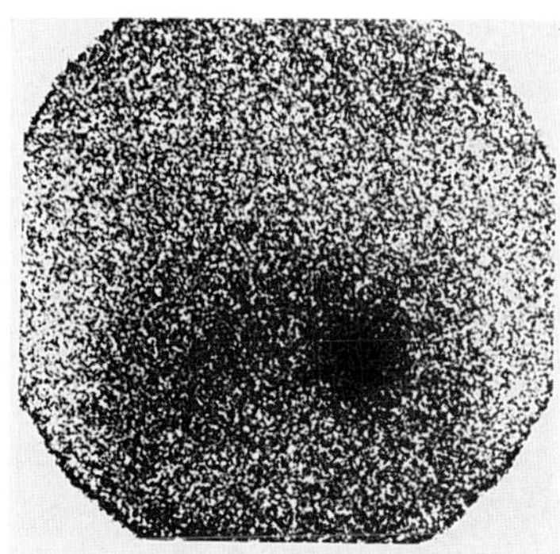

Fig. 55.9 An anterior thoracic abdominal ^{131}I MIBG image, obtained at only 18 h after intravenous administration (hence the high body background). A 47-year-old woman had a 7 cm left adrenal mass. This turned out to be a functional phaeochromocytoma. Uptake was so intense that it could be readily detected anteriorly.

MIBG

Metaiodobenzylguanidine is a noradrenaline analogue, initially synthesized at the University of Michigan. In the adrenal medulla, there is apparently an active uptake system residing in or near the cell membrane. Transfer of the compound into storage granules, often referred to as synaptosomes, then occurs. Neural crest tumours have these storage granules in abundance and MIBG, commonly labelled with ^{131}I, has been employed in localization of neural crest and related malignancies. Hoefnagel[48] has reviewed over 2400 cases of neural crest tumours reported in the literature, and noted the following sensitivities for MIBG; neuroblastoma 91%, phaeochromocytoma 88%, carcinoid 69%, medullary thyroid carcinoma 34%, other neural crest tumours 40%. Hence, while imaging with MIBG can be regarded as quite sensitive for localizing neuroblastomas and phaeochromocytomas, the procedure is less effective for the other neural crest tumours. Disadvantages of MIBG imaging include the need to administer iodide to block thyroid uptake of any liberated radioiodide and the frequent interference by medications.[49] The most intensely positive well-localized MIBG study we have encountered is shown in Figure 55.9. This, an anterior image obtained at only 17 h after intravenous administration of ^{131}I-MIBG, revealed intense uptake in a well-defined phaeochromocytoma. The radiolabelled compound also localizes in most metastatic phaeochromocytomas. An example is shown in Figure 55.10.

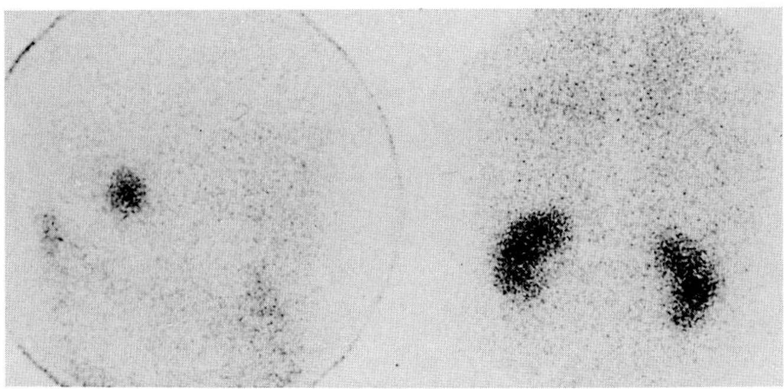

Fig. 55.11 Left posterior abdominal image at 72 h after intravenous administration of ^{131}I iodocholesterol. Faint activity can be seen in the liver and large bowel. A well-defined site to the left of the patient's midline can be noted. Right: renal study with ^{99m}Tc DTPA. This was obtained in order to localize the site of iodocholesterol uptake.

Iodocholesterol

The adrenal cortex is lipid rich, with a high content of cholesterol and its derivatives. Indeed, cholesterol is the starting point for synthesis of multiple adrenal hormones. The Michigan group studied the structural requirements for entry into the cholesterol-to-hormone metabolic pathway and produced compounds with the I-H_2C grouping at the 19 carbon ring position (19-iodocholesterol) and at the 6 position of the ring (6-beta-iodomethyl-19-norcholesterol).[50] This latter substance had considerably greater adrenal affinity. Proper use of the 6-beta compound is dependent upon knowledge of the biochemical output of the tumour being sought. The diagnosis is principally a biochemical one, with iodocholesterol being utilized to define the location and possible multiplicity of the tumour. For example, in Cushing's syndrome due to adrenal overproduction of glucocorticoids, the pituitary is suppressed and only the autonomous area(s) is defined (Figure 55.11). In other cases, external hormone must be administered to suppress the pituitary, such as when looking for aldosterone-secreting adrenal tumours.[51,52] In many cases, CT is used as the initial screen for adrenal masses[53] with scintigraphy being reserved for determining the functional status of the mass.

Melanoma localization

Several radiolabelled analogues of tyrosine, the melanin precursor, as well as inhibitors of tyrosinase have been examined. However, none exhibits satisfactory behaviour in patients with malignant melanoma. Michelot et al[54] described an iodobenzamide analogue which appeared more promising in initial studies. The mechanism

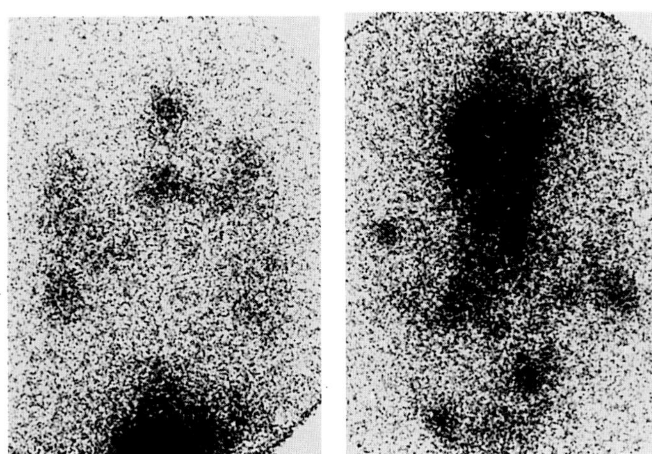

Fig. 55.10 Images, obtained at 48 h, in a 63-year-old woman with widely metastatic phaeochromocytoma. To the left is the anterior view of the neck and thorax. To the right is the abdomen and upper pelvis. There is such intense deposition in the metastatic sites that activity in the liver cannot be clearly defined.

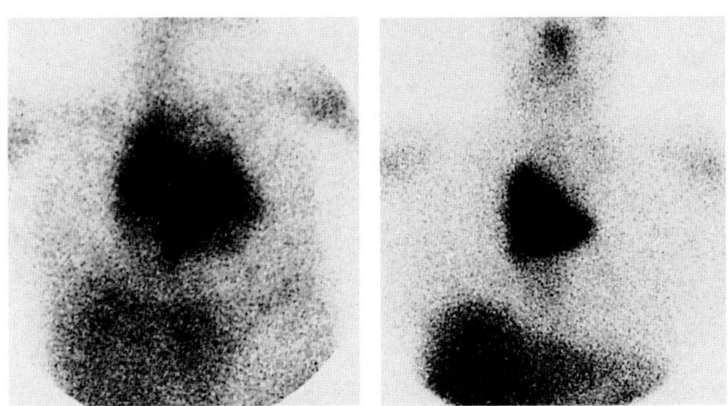

Fig. 55.12 Left: Anterior thoraco-abdominal view at 1 day after administration of radiogallium to a 12-year-old female with Hodgkin's disease. The massive intrathoracic activity provides a clear image. The lesion had greater uptake than the liver. Right: The corresponding image in a 17-year-old female with non-Hodgkin's lymphoma, taken 6 days after administration of the radiotracer. In this case, the lesion/background activity had improved markedly with time.

of uptake/binding is as yet not clarified. However, because of the ominous nature of malignant melanoma, in-depth studies are indicated. More recently, John et al[55] described an improved synthesis of the labelled compound.

RECEPTOR OR CELL-SURFACE BINDING (WITH OR WITHOUT INTERNALIZATION)

Multiple cellular events, from inward passage of selected nutrients to signalling by hormone molecules, depend upon interactions with the surface of a cell. The surface, with multiple transmembrane domains contributing to its topography, is a complex and key part of cellular activities. Some molecules bind to a surface receptor and, through the transmembrane portion of the receptor, activate an internal process. In other cases, the signalling molecule is actually internalized. These events, and their multiple variations, have provided a number of approaches to tumour imaging.

^{67}Ga and transferrin metabolism

The finding by Edwards and Hayes[56] that lymphomas and other tumours concentrate ^{67}Ga citrate initiated multiple studies as to the mechanisms of this uptake. It was soon noted that radiogallium concentration is not specific for tumours. Many inflammatory sites also accumulate the radiotracer. A second key observation was that when ^{67}Ga citrate was incubated with blood it had two major binding sites: leucocytes and the plasma protein transferrin. Thus, a complex distribution is involved, with cellular and soluble delivery components. Two patients were described with absent circulating polymorphonuclear leucocytes, in whom ^{67}Ga localized at inflammatory sites.[57] Thus, other pathways are sufficient to distribute the radiogallium. The binding of radiogallium to transferrin, and subsequent attachment to tumour cells, is probably related to iron metabolism. Iron–transferrin attaches to transferrin receptors. Recent studies have shed light on the process whereby part of the cell membrane (with transferrin and the receptors) is internalized and iron is then released into intracellular vesicles.[58] Many cells contain the protein lactoferrin, which has an even greater binding affinity for radiogallium than does transferrin.[59] Hence, the suggestion has been made that the concentration of lactoferrin may account for radiogallium binding in breast secretion, as well as in the liver and spleen, polymorphonuclear leucocytes and nasopharyngeal secretions.[60] The liver is the usual 'reference organ' for radiogallium uptake. Hepatic content of ^{67}Ga citrate can be reduced in several situations, such as following transfusion, possibly because of the loading, and after chemotherapy, likely from the result of sloughing of surface acceptor sites.[61] Quantities of administered stable gallium salts would possibly produce the same effect. Gallium nitrate has been utilized parenterally because of its antineoplastic effects.[62]

Several problems with radiogallium imaging of tumours include the binding to blood components, resulting in high background activity. Several days may have to pass before lesions become clearly defined (Figure 55.12). Liver and bowel uptake of radiogallium makes the radiotracer less useful in evaluating malignancies in the abdomen.

While some tumours such as lymphomas and hepatomas have high radiogallium uptake, others have less avid or minimal concentration of the radiotracer. This may be related to the content of transferrin receptors and internal depots. Transferrin has also been employed as a transport vehicle for other molecules. For example, transferrin that has been conjugated to adriamycin shows binding to transferrin receptors and cell killing in vitro.[63] A 'universal brain drug transport vector' has been described, in which an antibody to the transferrin receptor is employed.[64]

Labelled monoclonal antibodies against surface markers

A period of nearly 17 years elapsed between initial description of monoclonal antibodies[65] and release of the first of these materials for use in imaging in the USA. Thus, despite much promise, radiolabelled monoclonal antibodies are still awaiting a firm imaging role in the practice of oncology.

Several reasons may be cited for the slow development of scintigraphy utilizing monoclonal antibodies:

1. Tissues other than the tumour under study may contain receptors for the antibody. This raises the 'background' and makes tumour detection more difficult. When the antibody reacts with a blood-borne component (formed blood elements or soluble protein), detection efficiency is rapidly degraded.
2. Binding of antigen–antibody on the cell surface can be accompanied by sloughing of the complex (antigenic modulation). Hence, the marker is carried away from the target.
3. Injection of the antibody, seen by the body as a foreign protein, can be followed by production of antibodies against the molecule. Many available monoclonals are of murine origin. Human anti-mouse antibodies (HAMA) can be elicited.[66] Reaction by HAMA to a later injection of the antibody can produce effects varying from mild to quite severe.
4. There are concerns about transmitting slow-growing viruses when utilizing biological products.
5. Radiolabelling the antibody may distort the molecule, making it less reactive with the antigen.

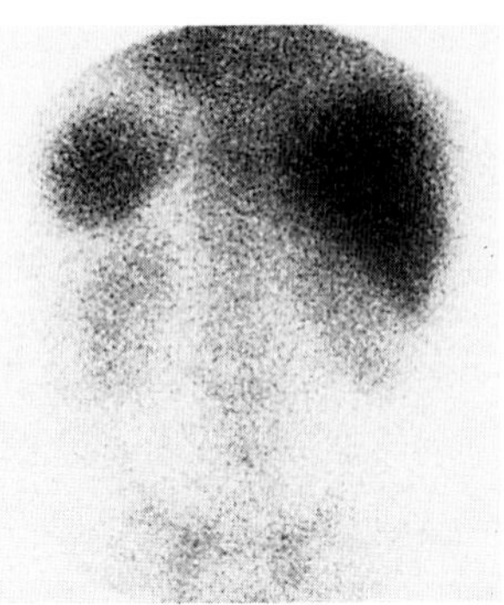

Fig. 55.13 Posterior abdominal image in a 66-year-old woman who had prior resection for carcinoma of the colon. The blood CEA level was rising, so this image was taken (at 48 h) in an effort to localize metastatic deposits. At the top of the image, the cardiac blood pool can be visualized. The radiopharmaceutical was ^{111}In CYT-103.

Approaches are being taken in an effort to avoid some of the problems enumerated. Chimeric antibodies have been described.[67] Molthoff et al[67] discussed MOv18, an antibody associated with ovarian cancer. The murine-derived binding site (variable region) of the antibody was coupled with a human constant region. The chimeric antibody, hopefully of lower antigenicity, was stated to be as effective as the original monoclonal.

Human–human monoclonal antibodies are difficult to produce, but some progress has been made. Ostberg[68] has looked at this from the broad perspective of tissue transplantation, and noted problems associated with making authentic human monoclonal antibodies. Erb et al[69] have described C-OU1, a human–human hybridoma antibody which is reactive with an antigen in colon tumours. The hybridoma was produced by fusing lymphocytes (from a lymph node of a patient with colon adenocarcinoma) with a human lymphoblastoid cell. Of interest, human–human hybridomas can apparently be derived from human tonsil lymphoid cells.[70]

Other approaches have been suggested. One involves bivalent or 'Janus' antibodies.[71] A single arm at the variable end of the antibody is designed to react with a tumour antigen, while the other arm is reactive with a radiolabelled antibody which is injected some time later. A system for synthetic generation of antibodies has been described ('antibodies without immunization').[72] Because of the great avidity of avidin for biotin, various schemes have been devised in which one component bound to an antibody is injected, followed subsequently by the second component carrying a radiolabel.[73,74]

The first monoclonal antibody for radiolabelling that has been released by the US Food and Drug Administration is termed CYT-103, which is a modified B72-3 antibody (OncoScint, Cytogen Corporation).[75,76] The oligosaccharides of the monoclonal are oxidized and the aldehydes produced are reacted with a linker containing a terminal DTPA. The reaction vial is added to ^{111}In. Normal distribution of the labelled monoclonal is shown in Figure 55.13. Uses of this radiolabelled antibody will be in the investigation of patients with carcinoma of the ovary or colon (for example, prior resection of tumour and new evidence of recurrence at one or more sites, as signalled by an increasing blood CEA level). CT has been reported to detect a larger proportion of metastases in the liver; the labelled antibody may be used in examining for tumour spread to the pelvis and to extrahepatic abdominal locales.[76] Petersen et al[77] provided data on the use of ^{111}In-CYT-103 in colon cancer, and gave values from which the accuracy of 87% could be calculated. Antibodies to the murine monoclonal antibody can be detected in some patients.[78]

The antibody B72-3 has also been labelled with ^{131}I.[79] Reilly et al[79] noted literature reports on B72-3 recognizing a tumour-associated glycoprotein antigen expressed in 85% of colon cancers, 95% of ovarian cancers and 70% of breast cancers. The target antigen (TAG-72) is shed by colon tumours and can be found in the bloodstream in 60% of colon cancer patients. The monoclonal B73-2 has also been labelled with radioyttrium (^{90}Y) in an effort to treat ovarian carcinomas.[80] This modification apparently speeds up the rate of plasma clearance, as compared with the ^{111}In-labelled antibody.[81]

Feggi et al[82] have described their experience with use of ^{99m}Tc-labelled anti-melanoma F(ab$'$)$_2$ fragments in 135 patients with malignant melanoma. The procedure was well tolerated. While the scintigraphy only had a 61.5% sensitivity in detecting lymph node involvement, it did better at other sites. From the viewpoint of the historical development of the area of immunoscintigraphy, attention must be paid to anti-CEA polyclonal and monoclonal antibodies. A recent generation antibody, carrying ^{99m}Tc as a radiolabel, is under investigation in several centres (Figure 55.14). Various groups are studying antibodies to B-cell lymphomas[83] and a variety of other malignancies. Of particular interest, the proto-oncogene c-*erb*-B2 has an extracellular product, transmembrane glycoprotein which

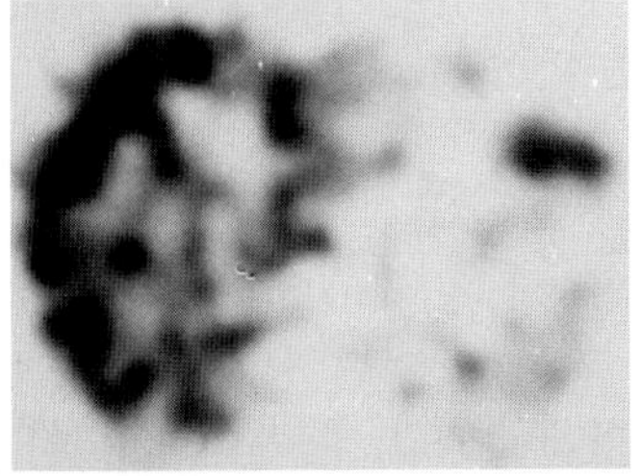

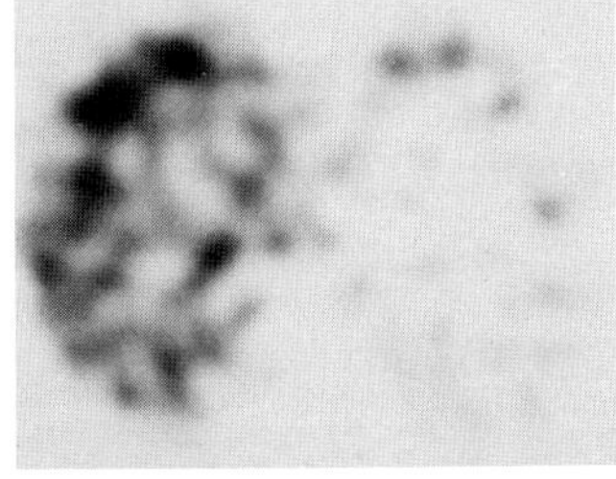

Fig. 55.14 Transverse cross sectional images of the liver, 1 cm thick (and separated by 1 cm). The patient was a 44-year-old woman who had prior surgery for adenocarcinoma of the rectosigmoid; the CEA level was now rising. The monoclonal antibody utilized was a Tc-99m-Fab anti-CEA. The uneven pattern of distribution, and its variation between nearby sections is apparent. (Courtesy of Dr. Gary M. Levine and the Garden State Medical Center at the Center for Molecular Medicine and Immunology, Newark, New Jersey).

can be recognized, allowing monoclonals to be constructed. At least two groups are investigating radiolabelled monoclonals which recognize this product.[84,85]

Radiolabelled hormones and receptor binding

Each cell carries a complement of surface receptors which are crucial to events involved in the interaction of the cell and its immediate environment. The transferrin receptor has been discussed above. For the purpose of tumour imaging, receptors which bind circulating hormones may offer some advantages.

A frequent cause of failure to respond to a hormone is a defect in the cellular binding site. Familial resistance to insulin has been described[86] and is usually related to a receptor mutation which interferes with hormone binding. In the Laron type of dwarfism, growth hormone is produced in adequate amounts, but a receptor defect is present in cells. Such cells would show reduced to absent binding of radiolabelled hormone and a 'negative defect' on imaging the malignancy. It is uncertain if such a situation can be exploited in specific tumours.

The opposite situation, namely overexpression of receptors for a hormone at a tissue site, or presence in the region usually devoid of such receptors, could be employed for tumour imaging. For example, the intact thyrotropin receptor has been reported to be overexpressed in a human thyroid cancer cell line.[87]

Somatostatin is a peptide with a variety of actions.[88] Somatostatin inhibits secretion of the pituitary hormones growth hormone and thyroid-stimulating hormone, as well as the gastrointestinal hormones insulin, glucagon, vasoactive intestinal peptide and secretin. There is also an effect of somatostatin on neurotransmission centrally. Somatostatin has been shown to inhibit various animal tumours. Receptors for somatostatin are present in some human tumours, in both primary sites and metastases. Reubi et al[88] have provided a table that lists the fraction of tumours of a particular type which express somatostatin receptors. Neuroendocrine tumours (pituitary adenomas, carcinoids, phaeochromocytoma, medullary thyroid carcinoma, etc.) have a high frequency of somatostatin receptors. Both lymphomas and certain central nervous system tumours (astrocytomas, neuroblastomas, meningiomas) also have a high rate of expression of somatostatin receptors. However, only about one-half of breast and ovarian tumours show these receptors, while prostate and pancreatic tumours do not reveal somatostatin binding. A radioindium-labelled somatostatin analogue has been employed in imaging tumours of malignant lymphoma lineage[89] as well as neuroendocrine tumours.[90]

Since tumours of the breast, ovary and other parts of the female reproductive system may demonstrate oestrogen and progesterone receptors, much effort has been devoted to synthesizing radiolabelled analogues of the compounds. For example, F-18-labelled oestrogens[91] and a progesterone analogue[92] have been described for potential use as receptor-binding agents. Such compounds also have implications in the delivery of therapeutic radiation to receptor-rich regions of tumours.[93] Tamoxifen, referred to as an anti-oestrogen (although it has some oestrogen-like characteristics) has been described as the most widely used hormonal therapy for carcinoma of the breast.[94] Halogenated analogues of tamoxifen have been synthesized,[95] but it is uncertain as to what role they might play in scintigraphy. Other halogenated anti-oestrogens have also been described,[96] and the area may evolve into one of clinical usefulness.

Labelled interleukins and white blood cells

With some degree of efficiency, white blood cells, either in their entirety or separated morphological types, can be radiolabelled. Among the most commonly employed radiopharmaceuticals are ^{111}In oxine (8-hydroxyquinoline) and ^{99m}Tc-HMPAO. However, simply labelling the cells does not impart any special preference for migration to tumour tissue. A number of strategies have been employed in an effort to direct labelled white blood cells to tumours in vivo.

1. Lymphocytes which have infiltrated tumours ('tumour-infiltrating lymphocytes' or TILs) may have been sensitized to one or more of the tumour's antigens.[97] Radiolabelled TILs have thus been studied as potential markers for the extent of such tumours. A problem has been obtaining TILs from tumour sections and then undertaking a cloning process. The TILs have also been tried in tumour therapy.[98]
2. Another approach to immunodetection of tumours is to harvest lymphocytes from peripheral blood and then co-culture them with sections of autologous

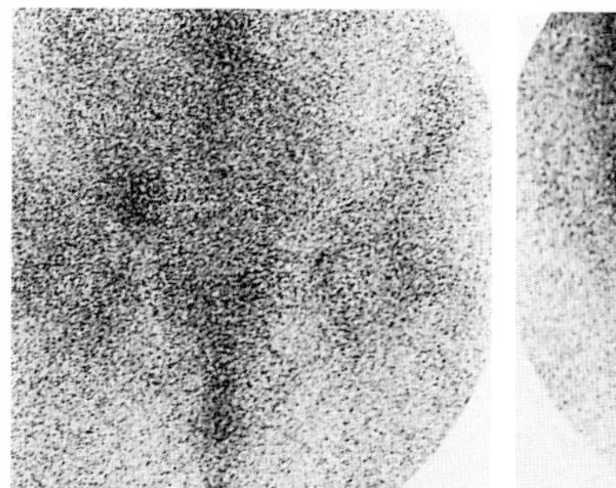
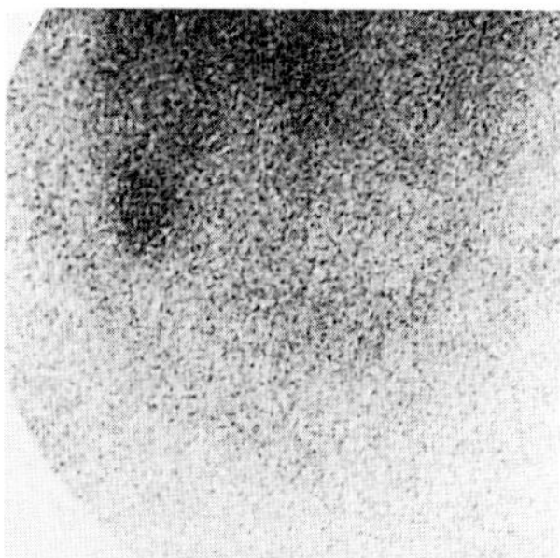

Fig. 55.15 Left: Posterior pelvic view at 48 h after intravenous administration of ^{67}Ga citrate in a 48-year-old woman with metastatic malignant melanoma. A focal deposit can be noted. Right: Many weeks later, the patient's white blood cells were grown in coculture with a sample of her tumour, and the white cells then cloned with interleukin 2. The cells were radiolabelled with ^{111}In oxine and injected intravenously. The same area shows focal uptake at 48 h.

tumour. The lymphocytes are then proliferated in the presence of interleukin 2. After radiolabelling, the 'activated' lymphocytes are reinjected (Figure 55.15). This procedure has had only modest success.[99] Whether injected intravenously as a lymphocyte mitogen, used in culture, or both, the role of interleukin 2 in detection or therapy of tumours is still under debate.[100]

3. White blood cells have receptors which, when activated, trigger a burst of metabolic activity. For example, neutrophils possess binding sites for certain *N*-formyl-peptides, such as *N*-formyl-Met-Leu-Phe. Binding produces chemotaxis as well as phagocytosis and release of lysosomal enzymes. Efforts have been made, by several groups, to produce radiolabelled analogues of the *N*-formyl-peptides. For example, phenylalanine in the molecule has been replaced by tyrosine, which can be iodinated. ^{75}Se selenomethionine analogues of the *N*-formyl-peptides can be constructed and have some affinity for white blood cell binding sites.[101] The problem, however, is that activated leucocytes do not appear to be attracted to tumours, and a further approach is required.
4. Immunostimulatory peptides can be isolated from human milk. Among these are Gly-Leu-Phe and Val-Glu-Pro-Ile-Pro-Tyr.[102] Interestingly, different cell types were involved in uptake. The Gly-Leu-Phe bound to polymorphonuclear leucocytes, while the second peptide bound to monocytes only. Since these originate in milk, studies are needed as to whether they show an affinity for milk fat globules or other components of secretion.
5. There have been two interesting developments that await further evaluation. Signore et al[103] have reported on the labelling of interleukin 2 with ^{123}I. In mice with pancreatic lymphocytic infiltration, the injected radiolabelled interleukin 2 showed a high concentration in the pancreas. Whether this would label tumour-infiltrating lymphocytes in vivo is unknown.

Interleukin 2-activated cells (lymphokine-activated killer cells or LAK) can be shown to be cytotoxic to many tumours in vitro. However, in vivo they are far less effective. Part of this might be related to lack of 'recruitment' of the injected activated cells to the tumour site. To improve recruitment, Takahashi et al[104] linked LAK cells with antibodies to a surface antigen of the tumour. Treated LAK cells, upon injection, had greater uptake in the tumours and also inhibited tumour growth. This approach might have both diagnostic and therapeutic implications.

Liposomes

Arshady[105] has described the term 'microsphere' as meaning those particles which are both spherical and of a small size. These are usually rigid and non-compressible, as contrasted with entities which have a membrane and are somewhat compressible, such as artificial cells and liposomes. Artificial cells have not been widely pursued as vehicles for tumour imaging agents. However, Gaze et al[106] have described use of multicellular spheroids of a human neuroblastoma cell line to study ^{131}I-MIBG uptake.

Liposomes are lipid vesicles which can carry aqueous solutions within their interiors. Thus, they behave as sacs for containing water-soluble materials, such as radiopharmaceuticals, within their lipid-rich external coating. Liposomes can be constructed in various diameters and can have a single coat (unilamellar) or be composed of many concentric layers (multilamellar) with aqueous medium between each layer. When administered intravenously, liposomes are usually accumulated by the reticuloendothelial system, reducing the amount available for accumulation in tumours. There are several approaches that have been tried in order to avoid or minimize reticuloendothelial uptake.

1. Oku et al[107] described 'RES-avoiding liposomes'. These were modified by palmityl-glucuronide, which apparently greatly delayed clearance from the bloodstream.
2. It has been pointed out that a major problem in tumour detection is the lag time between introduction of the radiopharmaceutical and actual imaging. The time is needed to clear the radioactive material from the bloodstream. ^{67}Ga citrate, for example, binds to both white blood cells and to the protein transferrin. Because of this background activity imaging may not be feasible for 48 hs or longer. Ogihara-Umeda et al[108] described a technique which may shorten this time period. They prepared liposomes and incorporated biotin into the coating. The liposomes contained ^{67}Ga desferrioxamine. This was given intravenously to mice bearing a sarcoma. 4 h later, avidin was given intravenously to form an avidin–biotin complex. The blood level of radioactivity fell to 5% of that in control animals. Hence, a high tumour/blood level of activity was achieved, although the reticuloendothelial system also had a high content of radioactivity.
3. Variations in the lipid coating of the liposomes might produce more rapid blood clearance. Kubo et al[109] described liposomes containing an ionophore (and EDTA plus ^{111}In internally) which had an initially rapid rate of clearance from the intravascular pool.

Multiple formulations of liposome membranes have been proposed, and these may have profound effects on delivery of the contained materials to tumours. Incorporating antibodies or antibody fragments in the lipid wall or the presence of a specific charge might aid in localization. Liposomes have been used for formulating drugs for external use, and such factors as leakage from the liposomes and aggregation/fusion have been discussed.[110] Liposomes also carry the potential for therapy, both in terms of drug delivery[111] and in bringing radiotracers to a specific tumour.

Mitogens

There are two distinct approaches for the use of mitogens in an effort to enhance tumour uptake of radiopharmaceuticals.

1. Most tumours are more active metabolically when stimulated by a mitogen. Use of this had been made, some years ago, in an effort to treat carcinoma of the prostate metastatic to bone. Testosterone was administered for tumour stimulation, followed by therapeutic amounts of ^{32}P sodium phosphate. The difficulty is that tumour spread may be stimulated, and growth of any tumour deposits can be associated with pain. However, this model when adapted to tumour stimulation and then imaging may prove to have some utility.
2. While there has been relatively little work on the area of radiolabelled mitogens for tumour imaging, Bitner et al[112] noted that pokeweed mitogen is a

Table 55.3 Some antineoplastic agents which have been, or could be, radiolabelled with gamma-ray-emitting nuclides

Compound	Possible or actual radiolabel	Comments
Bleomycin	^{57}Co	This compound has a long history as a potential tumour imaging agent.[113] However, the long half-life of ^{57}Co is a problem. Quantitation of ^{57}Co bleomycin entry into breast cancer has been reported.[114] Entry of the compound is likely different from that of ^{57}Co.[115] Iron–bleomycin has also been reported[116]
Iododoxorubicin	^{123}I ^{131}I	Anthracyclines have been utilized in the treatment of human malignancies. Iododoxorubicin is apparently less cardiotoxic than the hydroxy compound. Resistance can develop[117–119]
cis-Diamine-dichloroplatinum	^{193m}Pt ^{195m}Pt	This effective antineoplastic compound showed little accumulation in tumours on initial trials[120, 121]
5-Fluorouracil (5-FU)	^{18}F	This also has a long history. Uptake is greater in 5-FU-responsive tumours.[122] Metabolites can be followed
Iododeoxyuridine	^{125}I ^{131}I (Br)	Incorporated into DNA.[123] Dehalogenation may be a problem. Has been delivered to hepatic tumours by catheter[124]
Iodoaminopterin	^{131}I	This was the first active site directed gamma-ray-labelled enzyme inhibitor (against folate reductase). The label could be displaced from the enzyme by an even more avidly bound compound such as methotrexate[125]
Ruthenium	(Ru)	Ruthenium analogues of Pt compounds with antineoplastic effect are known,[126] and others can be synthesized. Postulated event is binding to tumour DNA. A ruthenium–transferrin complex can be formed
Adriamycin-Fe^{3+}	^{52}Fe ^{59}Fe	Only utilized in vitro thus far[127]
Growth factors, such as epidermal growth factor	^{123}I ^{131}I	Such compounds have been synthesized. Another possibility involves peptide-like molecules,[128] which potentially could carry a variety of radiolabels
Labels for protein	^{11}C (Pt)	Protein kinase C is involved in signal transduction. Both ^{11}C phorbol esters[129] and a Pt-labelled complex with ethanolamine have been described[130] as binding
Indium–manganese metalloporphyrin	^{111}In	Phorphyrins have an affinity for many types of malignant tumours. A porphyrin derivative has been labelled with In-111[131]
Boronated compounds activation	(B, neutron)	Phenylboronic acids have shown uptake in human tumours,[132] but the mechanism is not clear. Boron has been incorporated into antibodies[133] and other compounds, for uses in neutron capture therapy
DMSA	^{99m}Tc (V)	The compound localizes in a number of tumours, perhaps related to a resemblance to the phosphate ion[134]
Bromine analogues of ifosfamide	(Br)	Brominated analogues have been synthesized.[135] Biological testing with radiobromine has to be performed
Amino acids	^{75}Se ^{18}F	Selenomethionine was the first to be studied, but there are problems with the long half-life of ^{75}Se and lack of specificity.[136] Multiple fluorinated amino acids have been described[137,138]

biomodulator involved in cellular differentiation and cellular interactions. One effect is to alter rates of tissue clearance. Pokeweed mitogen was labelled with ^{99m}Tc and administered to tumour-bearing mice. Tumours could be visualized between 2 and 4 h post administration. Parallel studies showed that rates of clearance of other radiopharmaceuticals were also affected. This suggests the need for studies to maximize the effect, and to determine if other mitogens might have clinical utilization.

MIXED CELLULAR BINDING

A number of radiopharmaceuticals have demonstrated some effect in imaging selected tumours. Multiple mechanisms are probably involved. Table 55.3 shows a compilation of antineoplastic agents which have been, or could be, labelled with a gamma-ray-emitting radionuclide. Many of the compounds achieve a high concentration within tumours. For example, small amounts may block DNA uncoiling, damage the cell wall, or otherwise make the cell non-viable, without maintaining sufficient amounts to yield a high tumour–background ratio.

SUMMARY

Radiopharmaceuticals for tumour detection have evolved empirically. There are now a sufficient number of these agents available so that the underlying principles are coming to the forefront. Hence, there will be a better defined use of the available compounds as well as a more rigorous approach to the search for additional radiotracers. Efforts along this line will be spurred by the fact that radiopharmaceuticals which have a high tumour–background uptake ratio will be potential candidates for delivery of therapeutic radiation.

REFERENCES

1. Mauer A M 1992 Biologic markers for cancer: the search for the Holy Grail continues. J Lab Clin Med 120: 828–830
2. Maisey M N, Hawkes D J, Lukawiecki-Vydelingum A M 1992 Synergistic imaging. Eur J Nucl Med 19: 1002–1005
3. Busnell K D, Perlma S B, Wilson M A, Poleyn R E 1986 The rim sign: association with acute cholecystitis. J Nucl Med 27: 353–356
4. Spencer R P, Evans D D, Forouhar F, Fetters D V, Yeh S D J 1988 Tc-99m-diphosphonate uptake in malignant fibrous histiocytoma: a possible iron-related effect. Clin Nucl Med 13: 734–735
5. Shoop J D 1969 Functional hepatoma demonstrated with Rose Bengal scanning. AJR 107: 51–53
6. Lee V W, Shapiro J H 1983 Specific diagnosis of hepatoma using ^{99m}Tc-HIDA and other radionuclides. Eur J Nucl Med 8: 191–195
7. DeKraker J, Hoefnagel C A, Voûte P A 1989 I^{131} Rose Bengal therapy in inoperable hepatoblastoma. Med Pediat Oncol 17: 278
8. Kosuda S, Ishikawa M, Tamura K, Mukai M, Kubo A, Hashimoto S 1988 Iodine-131 therapy for parotid oncocytoma. J Nucl Med 29: 1126–1129
9. Kaplan W D 1984 Radionuclide delivery by hepatic artery catheter: diagnostic and therapeutic uses. In: Spencer R P (ed) Interventional nuclear medicine. Grune & Stratton, New York, pp 3–13
10. Shepherd F A, Rotstein L E, Houle S, Yip T C K, Paul K, Sniderman K W 1992 A phase I dose escalation trial of yttrium-90 microspheres in the treatment of primary hepatocellular carcinoma. Cancer 70: 2250–2254
11. Ackerman N B, Hechmer P A 1980 The blood supply of experimental liver metastases. V. Increased tumor perfusion with epinephrine. Am J Surg 140: 625–631
12. Valk P E, Mathis C A, Prados M D, Gilbert J C, Budinger T F 1992 Hypoxia in human gliomas: demonstration by PET with fluorine-18-fluoromisonidazole. J Nucl Med 33: 2133–2137
13. Langimuir V K, Mendonca H L 1992 The combined use of ^{131}I-labelled antibody and the hypoxic cytoxic SR-4233 in vitro and in vivo. Radiat Res 132: 351–358
14. Lin A J, Cosby L A, Shansky C W, Sartorelli A C 1972 Bioreductive alkylating agents. I Benzoquinone derivatives. J Med Chem 15: 1247–1252
15. Zeman E M, Brown J M, Lemmon M J, Hirst W K, Lee W W 1986 SR-4233: a new bioreductive agent with high selective toxicity for hypoxic mammalian cells. Int J Radiat Oncol Biol Phys 12: 1239–1242
16. Parliament M B, Chapman J D, Urtasun R C, McEwan A J, Golberg L, Mercer J R, Mannan R H, Wiebe L I 1992 Non-invasive assessment of human tumour hypoxia with ^{123}I-iodoazomycin arabinoside: preliminary report of a clinical study. Br J Cancer 65: 90–95
17. Grierson J R, Link J M, Mathis C A, Rasey J S, Krohn K A 1989 A radiosynthesis of fluorine-18 fluoromisonidazole. J Nucl Med 30: 343–350
18. Ballinger J R, Cowan D S M, Boxen I, Zhang Z M, Rauth A M 1993 Effect of hypoxia on the accumulation of technetium-99m-glucarate and technetium-99m-gluconate by Chinese hamster ovary cells in vitro. J Nucl Med 34: 242–245
19. Raju N, Ramalingam K, Nowotonik D P 1992 Syntheses of some nitroimidazole substituted boronic acids: precursors to technetium-99m complexes with potential for imaging hypoxic tissue. Tetrahedron 48: 10233–10238
20. Hicks R J, Kalff V, Savas V, Starling M R, Schwaiger M 1991 Assessment of right ventricular oxidative metabolism by positron emission tomography with C-11 acetate in aortic valve disease. Am J Cardiol 67: 753–757
21. Minn J, Paul R 1992 Cancer treatment monitoring with fluorine-18-2 fluoro-2-deoxy-D-glucose and positron emission tomography: frustration or future. Eur J Nucl Med 19: 921–924
22. Minn H, Leskinen-Kallio S, Lindholm P, Bergman J, Ruotsalainen U, Teras M, Haaparanta M 1993 (F-18) fluorodeoxyglucose uptake in tumors – kinetic versus steady-state methods with reference to plasma insulin. J Comput Asst Tomogr 17: 115–123
23. Lindholm P, Minn H, Leskinen-Kallio S, Bergman J, Ruotsalainen U, Joensuu, H 1993 Influence of the blood glucose concentration on FDG uptake in cancer – a PET study. J Nucl Med 34: 1–6
24. Fischman A J, Alpert M 1993 FDG-PET in oncology: there's more to it than looking at pictures. J Nucl Med 34: 6–11
25. Borbely K, Fulham M J, Brooks R A, DiChiro C 1992 PET-fluorodeoxyglucose of cranial and spinal neuromas. J Nucl Med 22: 1931–1934
26. Haberkorn J, Reinhardt M, Strauss L G et al 1992 Metabolic design of combination therapy: use of enhanced fluorodeoxyglucose uptake caused by chemotherapy. J Nucl Med 33: 1981–1987
27. Haberkorn U, Strauss L G, Dimitrakopoulou A et al 1993 Fluorodeoxyglucose imaging of advanced head and neck cancer after chemotherapy. J Nucl Med 34: 12–17

28. Sasaki M, Ichiya Y, Kuwabara Y et al 1993 Fluorine-18-fluorodeoxyglucose positron emission tomography in technetium-99m-hydroxymethylenediphosphate negative bone tumors. J Nucl Med 34: 288–290
29. DiChiro G, DeLaPaz R L, Brooks R A et al 1982 Glucose utilization of cerebral gliomas measured by ^{18}F-fluorodeoxyglucose and positron emission tomography. Neurology 32: 1323–1329
30. Ogawa T, Shishido F, Kanno I et al 1993 Cerebral glioma: evaluation with methionine PET. Radiology 186: 45–53
31. Costa A, Silvestrini R, Giardini R, Messinagabrielli G, Boracchi P, Veneroni S 1992 Contribution of H-3-thymidine labelling index and flow cytometric S-phase in predicting survival of patients with non-Hodgkin's lymphoma. Br J Cancer 66: 680–684
32. Venijkeren M E, Deschryver A, Goethals P, Poupeye E, Schelstraete K, Lamahieu I, Depotter C R 1992 Measurement of short-term C-11-thymidine activity in human head and neck tumours using positron emission tomography (PET). Acta Oncol 31: 539–543
33. Dunn B B, Channing M A, Kiesewetter D O 1992 USP standards for C-11 labelled carbon monoxide. Pharmacopeial Forum 18: 4414–4415
34. Bakir M A, Eccles S A, Babich J W, Aftab N, Styles J M, Dean C J, Ott R J 1992 C-erb2 protein overexpression in breast cancer as a target for PET using iodine-124-labeled monoclonal antibodies. J Nucl Med 33: 2154–2160
35. Tonami N, Hisada K 1977 Clinical experience of tumour imaging with ^{201}Tl-chloride. Clin Nucl Med 2: 75–81
36. Elgazzar A H, Fernandez-Ulloa M, Silberstein E B 1993 ^{201}Tl as a tumour-localizing agent: current status and future considerations. Nucl Med Comm 14: 96–103
37. Sandrock D, Merino M J, Norton J A, Neumann R D 1993 Ultrastructural histology correlates with results of thallium-201/technetium-99m parathyroid subtraction scintigraphy. J Nucl Med 34: 24–29
38. Ferlin G, Borsato N, Perelli R, Camerani M, Conte N, Manenten P, LoGiudice C 1981 Technetium–thallium subtraction scan: a new method in the preoperative localization of parathyroid enlargement. Eur J Nucl Med 6: A12
39. Kaplan W D, Takvorian T, Morris J H, Rumbaugh C L, Connolly B T, Atkins H L 1987 Thallium-201 brain tumor imaging: a comparative study with pathologic correlation. J Nucl Med 28: 47–52
40. Yoshii Y, Satou M, Yamamoto T et al 1993 The role of thallium-201 single photon emission tomography in the investigation and characterization of brain tumours in man and their response to treatment. Eur J Nucl Med 20: 39–45
41. Dillehay G L 1993 201-Tl imaging of brain tumours. Appl Radiol 22: 55–60
42. Schwartz R B, Carvalho P A, Alexander III E, Loeffler J S, Folkerth R, Holman B L 1992 Radiation necrosis vs high grade recurrent glioma: differentiation by using dual-isotope SPECT with ^{201}Tl and ^{99m}Tc-HMPAO. AJR 158: 399–404
43. Crane P, Laliberte R, Heminway S, Thoolen M, Orlandi C 1993 Effect of mitochondrial viability and metabolism on technetium-99m-sestamibi myocardial retention. Eur J Nucl Med 20: 20–25
44. Mut F, Bianco A, Nunez M, dePalma G, Touya E 1993 Tc-99m-isonitrile uptake in a brain metastatic lesion, comparison with Tc-99m DTPA using planar and SPECT imaging. Clin Nucl Med 18: 143–146
45. Charkes N D, Vitti R A, Brooks K 1990 Thallium-201 SPECT increases detectability of thyroid cancer metastases. J Nucl Med 31: 147–153
46. Mazzaferri E L 1993 Management of a solitary thyroid nodule. N Engl J Med 328: 553–559
47. Nusynowitz M L, Pollard E, Bennedetto A R, Lecklitner M L, Ware R W 1982 Treatment of medullary carcinoma of the thyroid. J Nucl Med 23: 143–146
48. Hoefnagel C A 1991 Radionuclide therapy revisited. Eur J Nucl Med 18: 408–431
49. Khafagi F A, Shapiro B, Fig L M, Mallette S, Sisson J C 1989 Labetalol reduces iodine-131 MIBG uptake by pheochromocytoma and normal tissues. J Nucl Med 30: 481–489
50. Beierwaltes W H, Wieland D M, Swanson D 1981 Adrenocortical compounds. In: Spencer R P (ed) Radiopharmaceuticals: structure–activity relationships. Grune & Stratton, New York, pp 395–412
51. Gross M D, Shapiro B, Freitas J E 1985 Limited significance of asymmetric adrenal visualization on dexamethasone-suppression scintigraphy. J Nucl Med 26: 43–48
52. Gross M D, Frietas J E, Swanson, D P, Woodburn M C, Schteingart D E, Beierwaltes W H 1981 Dexamethasone suppression adrenal scintigraphy in hyperandrogenism: concise communication. J Nucl Med 22: 12–17
53. Guerin C K, Wahner H W, Gorman C A, Carpenter P C, Sheedy II P F 1983 Computed tomographic scanning versus radioisotope imaging in adrenocortical diagnosis. Am J Med 75: 653–657
54. Michelot J M, Moreau M C, Labarre P G et al 1991 Synthesis and evaluation of new iodine-125 radiopharmaceuticals as potential tracers for malignant melanoma. J Nucl Med 32: 1573–1580
55. John C S, Saga T, Kinuya S et al 1993 An improved synthesis of [^{125}I]N-(diethylaminoethyl)-4-iodobenzamide: a potential ligand for imaging malignant melanoma. Nucl Med Biol 20: 75–79
56. Edwards C L, Hayes R L 1969 Tumor scanning with ^{67}Ga citrate. J Nucl Med 10: 103–105
57. Dhawan V M, Sziklas J J, Spencer R P 1978 Localization of Ga-67 in inflammations in the absence of circulating polymorphonuclear leukocytes. J Nucl Med 19: 292–294
58. Cammack R 1993 A new use for an old enzyme. Current Biol 3: 41–43
59. Hoffer P B, Huberty J P, Khayam-Bishi H 1977 The relative binding affinity of gallium-67 for lactoferrin and transferrin. J Nucl Med 18: 619
60. Hoffer P B, Huberty J, Khayam-Bashi H 1977 The association of Ga-67 and lactoferrin. Nucl Med 18: 713–717
61. Roswig D M, Spencer R P 1984 Decreased hepatic concentration of radiogallium-67 Ga. Semin Nucl Med 14: 57–58
62. Whelan H T, Schmidt M H, Anderson G S et al 1992 Antineoplastic effects of gallium nitrate on human medulloblastoma in vivo. Pediatr Neurol 8: 323–327
63. Berczi A, Barabas K, Sizensky J A, Faulk W P 1993 Adriamycin conjugates of human transferrin bind transferrin receptors and kill K 562 and HL60 cells. Arch Biochem Biophys 300: 356–372
64. Yoshikawa T, Pardridge W M 1992 Biotin delivery to brain with covalent conjugate of avidin and a monoclonal antibody to the transferrin receptor. J Pharm Exp Ther 263: 897–903
65. Kohler G, Milstein C 1975 Continous cultures of fused cells secreting antibody of predefined specificity. Nature 256: 495–497
66. Massuger L F A G, Thomas C M G, Segers M F G, Corstens F H M, Verheijen R H M, Kenemans P, Poels L G 1992 Specific and nonspecific immunoassays to detect HAMA after administration of indium-111-labeled OV-TL3 F(ab')$_2$ monoclonal antibody to patients with ovarian cancer. J Nucl Med 33: 1958–1963
67. Molthoff C F, Buist M R, Kenemans P, Pindoe H M, Boven E 1992 Experimental and clinical analysis of the characteristics of a chimeric monoclonal antibody, MOv18, reactive with an ovarian cancer-associated antigen. J Nucl Med 33: 2000–2008
68. Ostberg L 1992 Human monoclonal antibodies in transplantation. Transplant Proc 24 (suppl 2): 26–30
69. Erb K, Borup-Christensen P, Ditzel H, Chemnitz J, Haas H, Jensenius J C 1992 Characterization of a human–human hybridoma antibody, C-OU1, directed against a colon tumor-associated antigen. Hybridoma 11: 121–134
70. Massicotte H, Harley J B, Bell D A 1992 Characterization of human–human hybridoma monoclonal anti-R_0(SSA) autoantibodies derived from normal tonsil lymphoid cells. J Autoimmun 5: 771–785
71. Goodwin D A, Meares C F, McTigue M et al 1992 Pretargeted immunoscintigraphy: effect of hapten valency on murine tumor uptake. J Nucl Med 33: 2006–2013
72. Lerner R A, Kang A S, Bain J D, Burton D R, Barbas III C F 1992 Antibodies without immunization. Science 258: 1313–1314
73. Koch P, Macke H R 1992 ^{99m}Tc labeled biotin conjugate in a

tumor 'pretargeting' approach with monoclonal antibodies. Angew Chem Int-Ed Engl 31: 1507–1509

74. Hnatowich D J, Fritz B, Virzi F, Mardirossian G, Rusckowski M 1993 Improved tumor localization with (strept) avidin and labeled biotin as a substitute for antibody. Nucl Med Biol 20: 189–195
75. Abdel-Nabi H, Doerr R J, Chan H W, Blau D, Schmelter R F, Maguire R T 1990 In-111-labeled monoclonal antibody immunoscintigraphy in colorectal carcinoma: safety, sensitivity, and preliminary clinical results. Radiology 175: 163–171
76. Collier B D, Abdel-Nabi H, Doerr R J et al 1992 Immunoscintigraphy performed with In-111-labelled CYT-103 in the management of colorectal cancer: comparison with CT. Radiology 185: 179–186
77. Peterson Jr B M, Bass B L, Bates H R, Chandeysson P L, Harmon J W 1993 Use of the radiolabelled murine monoclonal antibody, ^{111}In-CYT-103 in the management of colon cancer. Am J Surg 165: 137–143
78. Doerr R J, Abdel-Nabi H, Krag D, Mitchell E 1991 Radiolabeled antibody imaging in the management of colorectal cancer. Ann Surg 214: 118–124
79. Reilly R M, Kirsch J, Gallinger S et al 1993 Compartmental analysis of the pharmacokinetics of radioiodinated monoclonal antibody B72-3 in colon cancer patients. Nucl Med Biol 20: 57–64
80. Rosenblum M G, Kavanagh J J, Burke T W, Wharton J T, Cunningham J E, Shanken L J, Silva E G, Thompson L, Cheung L, Lamki L, Murray J L 1991 Clinical pharmacology, metabolism, and tissue distribution of ^{90}Y-labeled monoclonal antibody B72-3 after intraperitoneal administration. J Natl Cancer Inst 83: 1629–1636
81. Zimmer A M, Kuzel T M, Spies W G et al 1992 Comparative pharmacokinetics of In-111 and Y-90 B72-3 in patients following single dose intravenous administration. Antibody, Immunoconjugates Radiopharm 5: 285–294
82. Feggi L, Indelli M, Pansini G C, Santini A, Prandini N, Virgili A R 1993 Immunoscintigraphy in malignant melanoma: a five year clinical experience. Nucl Med Comm 14: 145–148
83. Kaminski M S, Fig L M, Zasadny K R et al 1992 Imaging, dosimetry and radioimmunotherapy with Iodine 131-labeled anti-CD37 antibody in B-cell lymphoma. J Clin Oncol 10: 1696–1711
84. Saga T, Endo K, Akiyama T et al 1991 Scintigraphic detection of overexpressed c-erbB-2 protooncogene products by a class-switched murine anti-c-erbB 2 protein monoclonal antibody. Cancer Res 51: 990–994
85. Bakir M A, Eccles S A, Babich J W, Aftab N, Styles J M, Dean C J, Ott R M 1992 c-erbB 2 protein overexpression in breast cancer as a target for PET using iodine-124-labeled monoclonal antibodies. J Nucl Med 33: 2154–2160
86. Tanak K, Sugawara A, Sakamoto M et al 1992 Generalized resistance of thyroid hormone (GRTH) in a family – case studies. Endocrinol Jpn 39: 533–538
87. Namba H, Yamashita S, Usa T, Kimura H, Yokoyama N, Izumi M, Nagataki S 1993 Overexpression of the intact thyrotropin receptor in a human thyroid carcinoma cell line. Endocrinology 132: 839–845
88. Reubi J C, Laissue J, Krenning E, Lamberts S W J 1992 Somatostatin receptors in human cancer: incidence, characteristics, functional correlates and clinical implications. J Steroid Biochem Mol Biol 43: 27–35
89. Vanhagen P M, Krenning E P, Reubi J C et al 1993 Somatostatin analogue scintigraphy of malignant lymphomas. Br J Haematol 83: 75–79
90. Westlin J E, Janson E T, Ahlstrom H, Nilsson S, Ohrvall V, Oberg K 1992 Scintigraphy using a indium-111-labeled somatostatin analogue for localization of neuroendocrine tumors. Antibody Immunoconjugates Radiopharm 5: 367–384
91. French A N, Napolitano E, Vanbrocklin H F, Hanson R N, Welch M J, Katzenellenbogen J A 1993 Synthesis, radiolabeling and tissue distribution of 11 β-fluoroalkoxy-substituted estrogens: target tissue uptake selectivity and defluorination of a homologous series of fluorine-18-labelled estrogens. Nucl Med Biol 20: 31–47
92. Verhagen A, Elsinga P H, deGroot T J, Paans A M J, deGoij C C J, Sluyser M, Vaalburg W 1991 A fluorine-18 labeled progestin as an imaging agent for progestin receptor positive tumors with positron emission tomography. Cancer Res 51: 1930–1932
93. DeSombre E R, Shafii B, Hanson R N, Kuivanen P C, Hughes A 1992 Estrogen receptor directed radiotoxicity with Auger electrons: specificity and mean lethal dose. Cancer Res 52: 5752–5758
94. Sunderland M C, Osborne C K 1991 Tamoxifen in premenopausal patients with metastatic breast cancer: a review. J Clin Oncol 9: 1283–1297
95. Yang D J, Tewson T, Tansey W et al 1992 Halogenated analogues of tamoxifen: synthesis, receptor assay and inhibition of MCF7 cells. J Pharm Sci 81: 622–625
96. Levesque C, Merand Y, Dufour J M, Labrie C, Labrie F 1991 Synthesis and biological activity of new halo-steroidal antiestrogens. J Med Chem 34: 1624–1630
97. Hom S S, Rosenberg S A, Topaliani S L 1993 Specific immune recognition of autologous tumor by lymphocytes infiltrating colon carcinoma: analysis by cytokine secretion. Cancer Immunol Immunother 36: 1–8
98. Favrot M C, Phillip T, Merrouche Y et al 1992 Treatment of patients with advanced cancer using tumor infiltrating lymphocytes transduced with the gene of resistance to neomycin. Hum Gene Ther 3: 533–542
99. Mukherji B, Spitznagle L A, Spencer R P, Arnbjanarson O, Ergin M T 1986 Tumor imaging by In-111 labelled lymphocytes after sensitization to autologous tumor and expansion with interleukin-2. J Nucl Med 27: 970–971
100. Maas R A, Dullens H F J, Denotter M 1993 Interleukin-2 in cancer treatment – disappointing or (still) promising – a review. Cancer Immunol Immunother 36: 141–148
101. Sripada P K, Spencer R P, Vitkauskas G, Becker E L 1979 Studies on the binding of a chemotactic factor N-formyl-selenomethionine-methionine to rabbit neutrophils. J Nucl Med 20: 681
102. Jazir M, Migliore-Samouk D, Casabianca-Pignede M R, Keddad K, Morgat J L, Jolles P 1992 Specific binding sites on human phagocytic blood cells for gly-leu-phe and val-glu-pro-ile-pro-tyr, immunostimulating peptides from human milk proteins. Biochim Biophys Acta 1160: 251–261
103. Signore A, Chianelli M, Toscano A et al 1992 A radiopharmaceutical for imaging areas of lymphocytic infiltration: ^{123}I-interleukin-1. Labelling procedure and animal studies. Nucl Med Comm 13: 713–722
104. Takahashi H, Nakada T, Puisieux I 1993 Inhibition of human colon cancer growth by antibody-directed human LAK cells in SCID mice. Science 259: 1460–1463
105. Arshady R 1993 Review: microspheres for biomedical applications: preparation of reactive and labelled microspheres. Biomaterials 14: 5–15
106. Gaze M N, Mairs R J, Boyack S M, Wheldon T E, Barrett A 1992 ^{131}I-meta-iodobenzylguanidine therapy in neuroblastoma spheroids of different sizes. Br J Cancer 66: 1048–1052
107. Oku N, Takeda A, Toyota T, Namba Y, Sakakibara T, Ito F, Okada S 1992 Preparation of RES-avoiding liposomes. J Pharmacobio Dyn 15: S-69
108. Ogihara-Umeda I, Sasaki T, Nishigori H 1993 Active removal of radioactivity in the blood circulation using biotin-bearing liposomes and avidin for rapid tumour imaging. Eur J Nucl Med 20: 170–172
109. Kubo A, Nakamura K, Sammiya T et al 1993 Indium-111-labelled liposomes: dosimetry and tumour detection in patients with cancer. Eur J Nucl Med 20: 107–113
110. Talsma H, Crommelin D J A 1993 Liposomes as drug delivery systems. Part 3. Stabilization. Biopharmacy 6: 40–46
111. Zeisig R, Fichtner I, Arndt D, Jungmann S 1991 Antitumor effects of alkylphosphocholines in different murine tumor models: use of liposomal preparations. Anti-Cancer Drugs 2: 411–417
112. Bitner D M, Mann P L, D'Souza P et al 1993 Enhanced tumor imaging with pokeweed mitogen. Nucl Med Biol 20: 203–210
113. Hall J N, Woolfenden J M, Chen J D, Patton D D 1977 Cobalt-

bleomycin A2: a better radiolabelled tumor localizing agent. J Nucl Med 18: 617–618
114. Pace L, D'Aiuto G, Acampora C et al 1993 Tumour uptake of 57-cobalt-bleomycin in patients with breast cancer. Eur J Cancer 29A: 195–198
115. Kasten V, Hartwig A, Beyersmann D 1992 Mechanisms of cobalt (II) uptake into V79 Chinese hamster cells. Arch Toxicol 66: 592–597
116. Huttenhofer A, Hudson S, Noller H R, Mascharak P K 1992 Cleavage of tRNA by Fe(II)-bleomycin. J Biol Chem 267: 24471–24475
117. Farina A, Quaglia M G, Bossu E, Melchiorre P 1991 Analysis of iododoxorubicin and its major impurity. J Pharm. Biomed. Analysis 9: 1165–1168
118. Mross K, Mayer U, Zeller W, Becker K, Hossfeld D K 1992 Pharmacodynamic and pharmacokinetic aspects of iodo-doxorubicin. Oncol Res 4: 227–231
119. Friche E, Danks M K, Beck W T 1992 Characterization of tumor cell resistance to 4′-deoxy-4′-iododoxorubicin developed in Ehrlich ascites cells in vivo. Cancer Res 52: 5701–5706
120. Lange R C, Spencer R P, Harder H C 1973 The antitumor agent cis-$Pt(NH_3)_2Cl_2$: distribution studies and dose calculations for 193mPt and 195mPt. J Nucl Med 14: 191–195
121. Lippert B 1992 From cisplatin to artificial nucleases – the role of metal ion-nucleic acid interactions in biology. Biometals 5: 195–208
122. Wolf W, Shani J, Young D, Vine E 1977 Radiopharmacokinetics of antitumor agents: Fluorine-18 5-fluorouracil. J Nucl Med 18: 617
123. Scherberg N, Dzekhtser S 1992 Preparation of I-125-2′-deoxyuridine triphosphate and incorporation of the labeled nucleotide into DNA by the polymerase chain reaction. Bioorganicheskaya Khimiya 18: 1104–1107
124. Taniguchi H, Daidoh T, Shioaki Y, Takahasi T 1993 Blood supply and drug delivery to primary and secondary human liver cancers studied with in vivo bromodeoxyuridine labeling. Cancer 71: 50–55
125. Johns D G, Spencer R P, Chang P K, Bertino J R 1968 ^{131}I-iodoaminopterin: a gamma-labeled active-site directed enzyme inhibitor. J Nucl Med 9: 530–536
126. Sava G, Pacor S, Bregant F, Ceschia V 1991 Metal complexes of ruthenium: a potential class of selective anticancer drugs. Anticancer Res 11: 1103–1108
127. Miura T, Muraoka S, Ogiso T 1993 Inhibitory effect of urate on oxidative damage induced by adriamycin-Fe^{3+} in the presence of H_2O_2. Res Commun Chem Pathol Pharmacol 79: 75–85
128. Kleinert H D, Baker W R, Stein H H 1993 Orally available peptide like molecules: a case history. Biopharmacy 6: 36–41
129. Ohmori Y, Imahori Y, Ueda S, Fujii R, Ido T, Wakita K, Nakahashi H 1993 Protein kinase C imaging using carbon-11-labeled phorbol esters: 12-deoxyphorbol 13-isobutyrate-2-[1-^{11}C] butyrate as the potential ligand for positron emission tomography. J Nucl Med 34: 431–439
130. Mikhaevich I S, Vlasenkova N K, Gerasimova G K 1992 Antiproliferative effect of complexes of platinum (II) with plasmanyl-(N-acyl)-ethanolamine, an inhibitor of protein kinase C. Anti-Cancer Drugs 3: 513–517
131. Nakajima S, Yamauchi H, Sakata I et al 1993 ^{111}In-labelled Mn-metalloporphyrin for tumor imaging. Nucl Med Biol 20: 231–237
132. Kinsey B M, Kassis A I 1993 Synthesis and biological activity of $^{125}I/^{127}I$-phenylboronic acid derivatives. Nucl Med Biol 20: 13–22
133. Ranadive G N, Rosenzweig H S, Epperly M W, Bloomer W D 1993 A technique to prepare boronated B72.3 monoclonal antibody for boron neutron capture therapy. Nucl Med Biol 20: 1–6
134. Chauhan U P S, Babbar A, Kashyap R, Prakash R 1992 Evaluation of a DMSA kit for instant preparation of ^{99m}Tc-(V)-DMSA for tumour and metastasis scintigraphy. Nucl Med Biol 19: 825–830
135. Glazmankusnierczyk H, Matuszyk J, Radzikowski C 1992 Antitumor activity evaluation of bromine-substituted analogues of ifosfamide. 1. Stereodifferentiation of biological effects and selection of the most potent compounds. Immunopharmacol Immunotoxicol 14: 883–912
136. Douglas J G, Zambartas C N, Sumerling M D, Finlayson N D C 1981 ^{75}Se-selenomethionine in the diagnosis of hepatocellular carcinoma. Eur J Nucl Med 6: 91–92
137. Nakamichi H, Murakami M, Miura S, Kondoh Y, Mizusawa S, Ono Y 1993 L-[2.F-18]fluorophenylalanine and L-[U-C-14]phenylalanine – a comparative study of their transport to rat brain. Nucl Med Biol (Part B) 20: 95–100
138. Xu Y, Abeles R H 1993 Inhibition of tryptophan synthase by (1-fluorovinyl) glycine. Biochemistry 32: 806–811

56. The nodule in the neck: the role of thyroid scanning

R. McLean K. Endo

INTRODUCTION

The introduction of studies with ^{131}I provided a major advance in studying iodine metabolism and thus in the assessment of thyroid dysfunction. However, the simple quantitation of function did not assist in diagnosing the nature of palpable thyroidal abnormalities. This was initially achieved by time-consuming mapping of the distribution of radioiodine in the neck using Geiger counters. This crude introduction of radionuclide organ imaging was the impetus to the introduction of the rectilinear scanner. Thyroid imaging was further simplified by the gamma-camera (Fig. 56.1) and, indeed, early instruments were dedicated to this purpose.[1]

Because of the variety of pathology which can lurk within the thyroid, radionuclide imaging retains a valuable role despite the availability of ultrasound and fine needle aspiration. All provide complementary information which will assist in heightening or lowering the suspicion of malignancy which arises on discovery of a thyroid nodule.

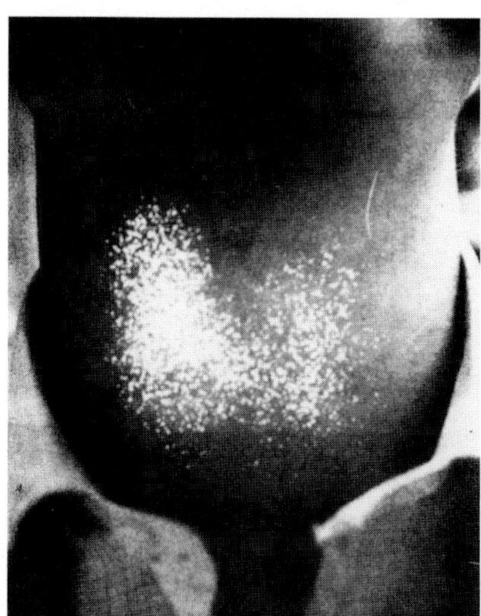

Fig. 56.1 A thyroid scintigram performed in the early 1960s using ^{131}I and small gamma-camera. For reference, the scan is superimposed on a picture of the patient's neck.

Considerations of radiation burden have resulted in ^{131}I being largely replaced by ^{123}I or ^{99m}Tc. However, although sensitive in demonstrating function, scans with these radionuclides are of low specificity and a variety of other radionuclides have been utilized as supplementary investigations. The effort is worthwhile not only because of the need to identify cancer but also because of the desirability of avoiding unnecessary operations for benign lesions.

INVESTIGATIONAL APPROACHES – AN OVERVIEW

A variety of procedures may be employed, either singly or sequentially, in the assessment of a patient in whom a nodule in the thyroid is observed (Fig. 56.2). Frequently, the individual may be unaware of the presence of the abnormality until comment is passed. Occasionally, there may be symptoms which assist in ascertaining the nature of the nodule, such as rapid onset as occurs in intrathyroidal haemorrhage, or the acute pain, fever and malaise typical of focal thyroiditis. Concern regarding possible malignancy will be raised by symptoms such as hoarseness, palpatory findings of fixation and hardness of the nodule, local lymphadenopathy or a history of previous irradiation to the head and neck. Age and sex must also be considered, malignancy being more frequently found in the solitary nodule in a male. Associated symptoms such as diarrhoea may cause suspicion of medullary thyroid carcinoma and indicate particular investigations as are discussed in Chapter 57.

Following palpation of the neck it may be considered that the nodule is solitary, with such confidence that it may be believed that the only subsequent procedure required is a fine needle aspiration. Occasionally, apparently solitary nodules may be shown to be part of a multinodular goitre. This may be apparent on palpation but is readily demonstrated by scintigraphy with ^{99m}Tc. Such a finding does reduce concern since the incidence of malignancy is lower in a multinodular goitre. Nevertheless, if the scan does show the palpated nodule to be very

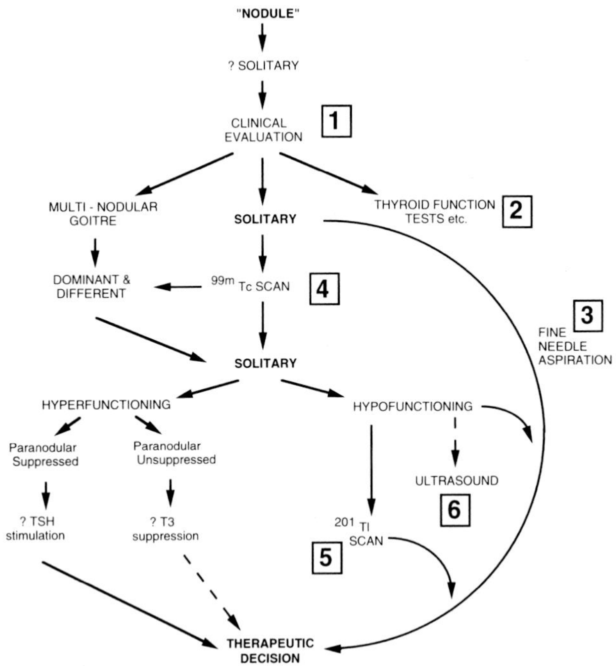

Fig. 56.2 Diagnostic algorithm for the investigation of the nodule in the neck. The boxed numbers refer to numbered sections in the text.

dominant and different in appearance from the rest of the goitre, it must undergo the same further investigations as if the ^{99m}Tc scan had shown it to be solitary.

The major benefit of a ^{99m}Tc scan will be to identify whether the nodule is hyperfunctioning or hypofunctioning. If the former, appropriate supplementary investigations will be required to ascertain whether abnormal secretion of thyroid hormones is occurring and affecting the metabolic status of the patient. While this is likely to eventuate in a proportion of such nodules, the increase in function may not have progressed to a stage to produce hyperthyroidism in a particular individual. This is particularly probable if there is only partial suppression of paranodular tissue. The prognosis can possibly be assessed by undertaking a further ^{99m}Tc scan following suppression with triodothyronine to establish that the nodule is autonomous. When there is total suppression of paranodular tissue, consideration can be given to further scintigraphy following stimulation with TSH to evaluate the nature of the paranodular tissue. If this does identify marked multinodular changes, an operation might well be considered preferable to ^{131}I therapy.

The demonstration that a solitary nodule is hypofunctioning is associated with a risk that it is malignant. Accordingly, many believe that this finding is an immediate indication for fine needle aspiration. Although this procedure is of extreme value, it cannot be totally relied upon and difficulties can be encountered. Supplementary investigations do therefore retain a role. Ultrasound can, for example, discriminate between solid and cystic lesions but does lack further specificity. ^{201}Tl scanning has been applied for many years since preferential accumulation in a nodule is associated with increased cellularity, thus heightening suspicion of malignancy. It does therefore retain popularity.

AGENTS

The major radionuclides which may be employed in thyroid scanning are shown in Table 56.1, along with their main applications.[2] The most commonly used are the isotopes of iodine and ^{99m}Tc. The dosimetry associated with these is important in determining their popularity (Table 56.2).[3]

Radioiodine and ^{99m}Tc imaging

^{131}I was, for many years, the only radionuclide suitable for thyroid scanning, but it does result in a relatively high radiation dose to the patient. When ^{99m}Tc became widely available it rapidly gained fairly universal use because of

Table 56.1 Radiopharmaceuticals and their uses

Radiopharmaceutical	Use
^{99m}Tc pertechnetate	Routine thyroid scanning
^{123}I	Thyroid scanning when an isotope of iodine is required
^{131}I	Investigation of thyroid cancer or if ^{123}I is unavailable
^{201}Tl chloride	Detection of differentiated carcinoma, investigation of thyroid nodules, demonstration of suppressed thyroid tissue
^{67}Ga citrate	Detection of lymphoma, anaplastic carcinoma, thyroiditis, abscess
^{99m}Tc(V) DMSA	
^{131}I-MIBG	Detection of medullary carcinoma

Adapted from Fogelman et al[2].

Table 56.2 Radionuclide physical characteristics and thyroid dosimetry

Radionuclide	^{123}I	^{131}I	^{99m}Tc
Mode of decay	Electron capture	Beta minus	Isomeric transition
Physical half-life	13.2 h	8.06 d	6.03 h
Decay constant	0.0533 h^{-1}	0.0860 d^{-1}	0.1149 h^{-1}
Photon energy MeV (mean no. per disintegration)	0.028 (0.867) 0.159 (0.836) 0.529 (0.011)	0.030 (0.046) 0.080 (0.026) 0.284 (0.058) 0.364 (0.820) 0.637 (0.065) 0.723 (0.017)	0.0186 (0.077) 0.1405 (0.879)
Thyroidal absorbed dose* (Gy/MBq administered)	2.0	216.2	0.06

*15% RAIU (radioactive iodine uptake), 19.6 g gland in a euthyroid adult. Adapted from Freitas et al[3].

the markedly lesser radiation burden and the high quality of the images that could be obtained much sooner after its administration. Unlike iodine, it is not organified after trapping. There are occasions, albeit rare, when a nodule appears functioning on a ^{99m}Tc image but, lacking organification ability, is non-functioning on an iodine scan (Fig. 56.3). Approximately 3–8% of thyroid nodules will exhibit this discordance.[4,5] Such a problem is overcome by using ^{123}I which does provide excellent images and, having a higher target:non-target ratio than achievable with ^{99m}Tc, is particularly useful when the gland function is low or in evaluating a retrosternal goitre. It also permits the use of physiological interventional studies such as perchlorate discharge test. However, it has disadvantages of high cost and uncertain and limited availability. In addition, the necessity for imaging at least 4 h after administration is inconvenient compared to the early imaging with ^{99m}Tc. A study comparing ^{99m}Tc and ^{123}I in 316 patients was reported by Kusic et al.[6] Iodine scans were preferred but the differences were small. Discrepancies between the images were found in 5–8% of cases. In the 12 carcinomas present, there was no discrepancy between the scans. Therefore, ^{99m}Tc deserves its place as the most universally used tracer for thyroid scanning.

There is one clinical context in which radioiodine may be preferred over ^{99m}Tc. If a retrosternal goitre is suspected, this may be better visualized with ^{131}I. Park et al[7] in 54 consecutive cases of suspected upper mediastinal masses, found retrosternal goitres in 42. Thirty nine (93%) were demonstrated by thyroid scanning using radioiodine. In addition, the authors showed that the attenuation of ^{131}I photons by the sternum was less than half of that for ^{99m}Tc photons. Therefore, if an initial scan with ^{99m}Tc is negative or equivocal, a repeat study with ^{131}I is justified.

Excess non-radioactive iodine will competitively inhibit uptake of all these tracers by the thyroid. Apart from excess dietary iodine, for example in the form of kelp tablets, and therapeutic medications containing iodine such as amiodarone, the commonest clinical situation is that following a radiological procedure involving iodine. Examples include an oral cholecystogram and a CT scan with iodinated intravenous contrast media. Although a recent study by Laurie et al[8] found lower levels of free iodide than might have been expected, clinical experience suggests that it is desirable to permit an interval of 4 weeks following such contrast media before undertaking thyroid scanning. A similar period should be allowed following cessation of treatment with thyroid hormones unless the study is being undertaken to assess whether a therapeutic response to suppression has been achieved.

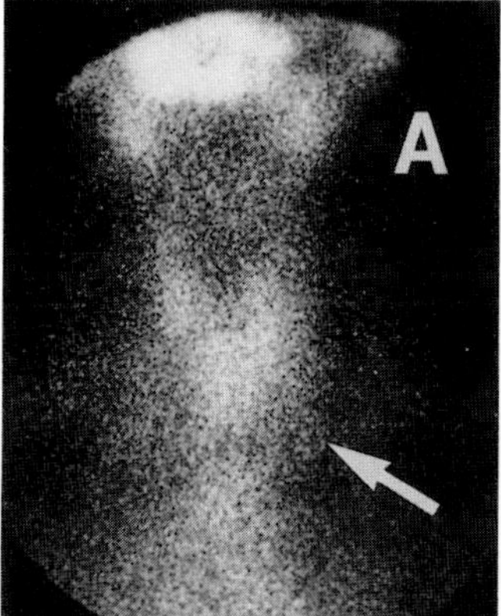

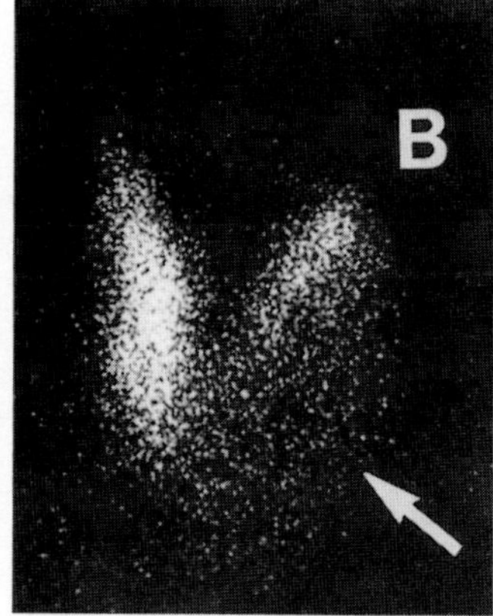

Fig. 56.3 Thyroid follicular adenoma showing discordant images. ^{99m}Tc image (A) demonstrates uptake in the region of the nodule (arrowed) but no uptake is seen on the ^{123}I image (B).

^{201}Tl imaging

Although ^{201}Tl has gained increasing acceptance for the investigation of a wide range of malignancies in recent years (Chapter 63), it has been employed in the investigation of thyroid nodules for a long time with varying popularity (Fig. 56.4). The early studies of Hisada et al[9] and Tonami et al[10] engendered enthusiasm although subsequently differing reliability was experienced.[11] The use of early and delayed ^{201}Tl imaging was suggested by Ochi et al[12] since they found that persistence of uptake favoured malignancy and yielded a sensitivity of 94% and a specificity of 90%. Although this approach was not confirmed by Henze et al[13] nor Bleichrodt et al,[14] it has recently been advocated once more by El-Desouki.[15] Nineteen out of 20 malignant nodules had increased uptake in early and late images whereas no increase was demonstrated in 35 out of 38 benign lesions. Improved discrimination was also achieved by Höschl et al[16] by grading the intensity of the ^{201}Tl uptake in nodules shown to be non-functioning with ^{99m}Tc (Fig. 56.5). They showed the predictive value of a negative test to be 90%. Emphasizing the nature of ^{201}Tl as a potassium analogue and its uptake, therefore, being an indicator of cellular metabolism, they pointed out that, while preferential uptake merely indicated a hypercellular nodule, marked accumulation significantly heightened suspicion of malignancy. ^{201}Tl scanning retains this role and is therefore of value in assisting the reaching of a therapeutic decision.

A further role for ^{201}Tl is in the detection of thyroid tissue suppressed by an autonomous nodule.[17] It is important to determine the presence of normal but suppressed thyroid tissue so that radioiodine treatment can be given with the confidence that suppressed tissue will subsequently function normally and hypothyroidism will not occur. ^{201}Tl scanning can also be used in focal subacute thyroiditis to confirm the presence of non-involved but suppressed thyroid tissue (Fig. 56.6).

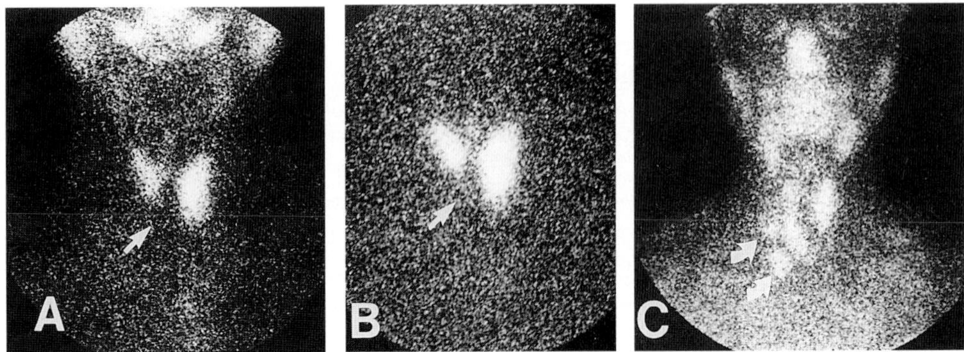

Fig. 56.4 Papillary thyroid cancer. The palpable nodule at the lower pole of the right lobe (arrowed) shows no uptake on ^{99m}Tc (A) or ^{123}I (B) scans but increased uptake of ^{201}Tl (C) is present in the nodule and in metastatic lymph nodes (arrowed).

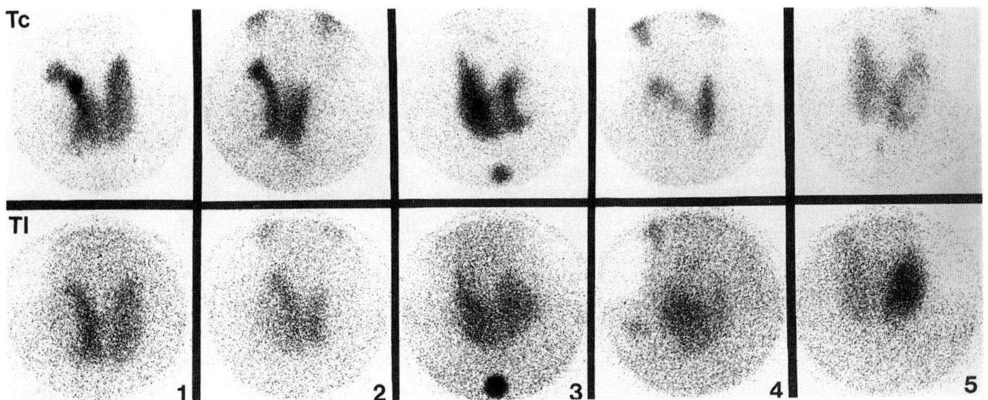

Fig. 56.5 A series of ^{99m}Tc and ^{201}Tl scans in patients with thyroid nodules. All nodules are hypofunctioning on ^{99m}Tc scans (upper row) but demonstrate a range of ^{201}Tl uptake (1 = no uptake, 2 = reduced uptake, 3 = similar uptake to paranodular tissue, 4 = mildly increased uptake, 5 = markedly increased uptake in comparison with paranodular tissue). See text for value of grading.

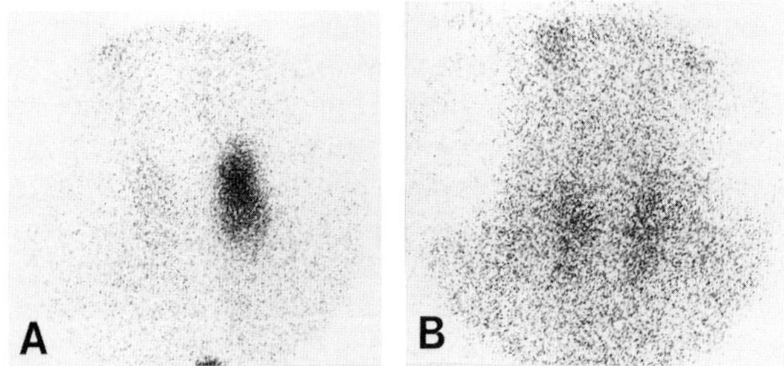

Fig. 56.6 Subacute thyroiditis. ^{99m}Tc (A) scan shows marked hypofunction in right thyroid lobe. Normal uptake is shown on ^{201}Tl scan (B).

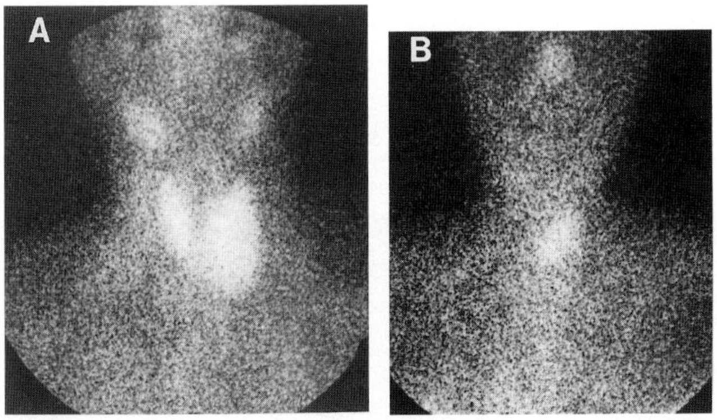

Fig. 56.7 Non-Hodgkin's lymphoma of the thyroid in a patient with chronic thyroiditis developing as a solitary nodule in the left lobe. ^{201}Tl image (A) demonstrates uptake in the nodule as well as in the normal right thyroid lobe. ^{67}Ga image (B) demonstrates uptake only in the nodule.

^{67}Ga imaging

^{67}Ga imaging in the evaluation of thyroid malignancy has recently been reviewed by Higashi et al.[18] They have shown that the tracer is valuable in suspected anaplastic carcinoma and malignant lymphoma of the thyroid, in the detection of metastases and in the evaluation of therapy. Further roles include the assessment of suspected metastases to the thyroid from other malignancies and the differentiation of malignant lymphoma from chronic

Table 56.3 Differential diagnosis of thyroid nodule

- Common
  - Colloid (adenomatoid) nodule
  - Cyst
    - simple
    - mixed
    - haemorrhagic
  - Adenoma
    - macrofollicular
    - microfollicular
    - embryonal
    - Hürtle cell
  - Carcinoma
    - papillary
    - follicular
    - mixed
  - Nodule as part of unrecognized multinodular goitre
- Uncommon
  - Post-surgical hypertrophy
  - Thyroiditis
    - subacute
    - Hashimoto's
  - Carcinoma
    - medullary
    - anaplastic
    - metastatic
    - lymphoma
  - Graves' disease
    - asymmetric thyroid
    - superimposed cold nodule
    - Marine-Lenhart syndrome
  - Extra thyroidal cause
    - lymph node
    - tortuous carotid artery
  - Abscess
  - Developmental abnormality
    - unilateral agenesis
    - cystic hygroma

Table 56.4 Clinical evaluation of solitary thyroid nodules – important historical and physical examination features

1. Age <20 or >60	5. Compression symptoms (dysphagia, etc.)
2. Male sex	6. Rapid growth
3. Family history of thyroid carcinoma	7. Single nodule
4. Exposure to ionizing radiation	8. Lymphadenopathy

Adapted from Mazzaferri et al[19].

Table 56.5 Relation between clinical findings and malignant thyroid tumours in 169 patients with nodular thyroid disease

Suspected likelihood of cancer	% of patients	% with malignant tumour	Clinical findings
Low	44	11	No suspicious symptoms or signs
Moderate	38	14	Age <20 or >60 years History of head or neck irradiation Male sex Dubious nodule fixation Nodule >4 cm in diameter and partially cystic
High	18	71	Rapid tumour growth Very firm nodule Fixation to adjacent structures Vocal-cord paralysis Enlarged regional lymph nodes

Adapted from Mazzaferri et al[20].

thyroiditis (Fig. 56.7A and B). They noted that, in general, ^{67}Ga uptake is more avid in malignant lymphoma than in anaplastic carcinoma. Although approximately 50% of patients with chronic thyroiditis will show some gallium uptake, a negative gallium scan will rule out lymphoma.

The use of ^{99m}Tc(V)DMSA and ^{131}I-MIBG in medullary thyroid cancer is described in Chapter 57.

ROLE AND INTERPRETATION

In the patient presenting with a thyroid nodule the differential diagnosis must be considered (Table 56.3) and appropriate investigations undertaken. A suggested diagnostic algorithm is given in Fig. 56.1. The various steps in the algorithm are described below:

1. Clinical examination

There are a number of clinical features which increase the likelihood that a nodule is a carcinoma (Table 56.4).[19] The relationship between these clinical features and final pathology in 169 patients is shown in Table 56.5.[20] Although 71% of those with a high clinical suspicion had cancer, 11% of those with low clinical suspicion (44% of total population) also had malignant tumours. This indicates that clinical judgement, although being valuable, is inadequate by itself.

The frequency of clinically apparent thyroid nodules increases throughout life, reaching approximately 5–6% at the age of 60 years. Nodules are about four times more common in women than men but are 10 times more frequent when the gland is examined at autopsy, during surgery or by ultrasonography.[20] Therefore, many clinically solitary nodules are in fact part of a multinodular process.

Just as there are many 'silent' thyroid nodules, there are many 'silent' carcinomas. The prevalence of occult thyroid cancer detected at autopsy varies from country to country. Estimates range from approximately 4% in the US to 21.5% in Japan. Other countries have intermediate prevalences.[19]

Of surgically removed nodules, 42–77% are colloid nodules, 15–40% are adenomas and 8–17% are carcinomas.[19]

2. In vitro testing of thyroid function

In general this is most easily performed at the time of the clinical examination. Estimation of serum TSH will usually be sufficient to confirm euthyroidism. If hyperthyroidism is suspected on clinical grounds, serum thyroxine estimation is often adequate. Occasionally the first evidence of metabolic dysfunction will be alteration of triiodothyronine levels. If triiodothyronine suppression studies are to be undertaken, awareness of the hormone levels is essential since, because of the autonomy of the nodule, the administration of this hormone may precipitate a hyperthyroid state. Approximately one-third of apparently solitary nodules have been shown by scintigraphy to be part of a multinodular goitre[21,22] and, if suppressive thyroxine therapy is contemplated on a long-term basis, baseline thyroid function tests are useful. Ancillary investigations such as an ESR may be indicated in circumstances such as suspected subacute thyroiditis.

3. Fine needle aspiration (FNA)

There is a wide body of opinion which considers that a FNA should be the initial investigation in all nodules and that it is sufficient to reach a diagnosis. This view exists not only because the technique is safe, quick and inexpensive but also is based on the high sensitivity reported in many series, well reviewed by Mazzaferri et al.[19] FNA may yield four results – inadequate, benign, indeterminate/suspicious, malignant. The frequency of inadequate results varies from series to series but decreases with experience and the number of samples taken, ranging from 5%[23] to 20%.[4] Of the remainder, 60–75% are benign, 5–20% are malignant and about 20% are indeterminate.

The reported accuracy of FNA depends on how the suspicious lesions are handled. If the suspicious lesions are included with the malignant lesions, the sensitivity increases to over 95% but the specificity decreases to about 70%. If the suspicious lesions are not included, the sensitivity is reduced to below 90% but specificity increases to over 90%. Some studies using FNA have shown a marked reduction in the surgical rate for nodules yet an increased incidence of malignancy.[25,26]

False-positive and false-negative rates average 10%.[19] False-positive results occur with highly cellular tumours and hyperfunctioning nodules, as well as in Hashimoto's thyroiditis.[23,27,28] False-negative results may be due to sample errors, particularly in large (> 4 cm) or small (< 1 cm) nodules or haemorrhagic lesions. This problem would not arise if these nodules were shown to be hyperfunctioning by scanning prior to deciding on FNA since the incidence of malignancy in these cases is low.[23] Although it has been advocated that nodules with indeterminate cytology should be scanned subsequently, Gordon et al[29] have shown FNA can alter the scan pattern, in particular by reducing the uptake in 'warm' nodules. Nevertheless, a cost–benefit analysis[23] which considered several diagnostic strategies including radionuclide scan, FNA and ultasound, concluded that the most cost effective procedure was FNA followed by a radionuclide scan.

4. ^{99m}Tc thyroid scan

In some patients there may be a very strong clinical suspicion of malignancy such as that arising from a history of previous radiation treatment to the head and neck. An increasing incidence of development of nodules, in up to 37% of patients who have had such treatment, occurs over the subsequent 15–25 years with carcinoma being identifiable in approximately 10%.[30] Findings on examination such as lymphadenopathy and vocal cord palsy will engender concern.

FNA may be easily justified as the initial investigation but in most subjects a thyroid scan is warranted. This will immediately identify whether the nodule is solitary or does arise in a multinodular gland (Fig. 56.8). The latter finding decreases the possibility of malignancy unless the nodule is dominant and non-functioning when it must be assessed as if it were solitary. The scan may reveal the patterns of Plummer's disease varying from a single hyperfunctioning nodule in a multinodular gland to multiple clearly defined toxic nodules throughout the gland.

Ross[4] has suggested a number of other reasons for performing a scan before FNA. Firstly, patients may be extremely apprehensive regarding FNA. As approximately 5% of solitary nodules are autonomous, these patients can avoid the trauma of the procedure if thyroid function tests and thyroid scan are first performed. Secondly, those patients with 'suspicious' FNA results and subsequent

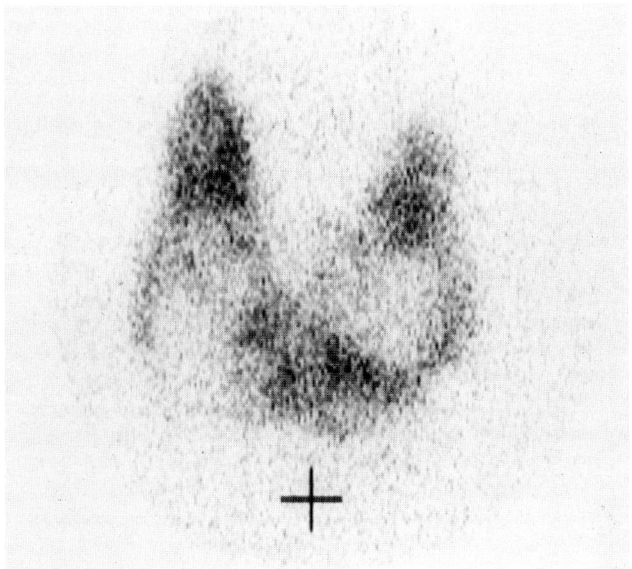

Fig. 56.8 Typical multinodular goitre with areas of increased and decreased uptake in both thyroid lobes.

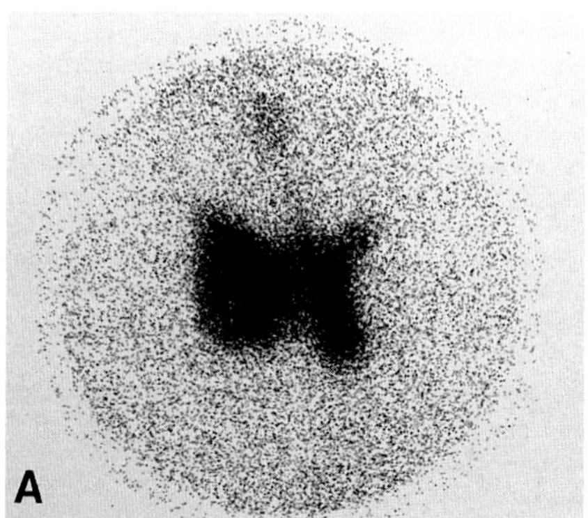

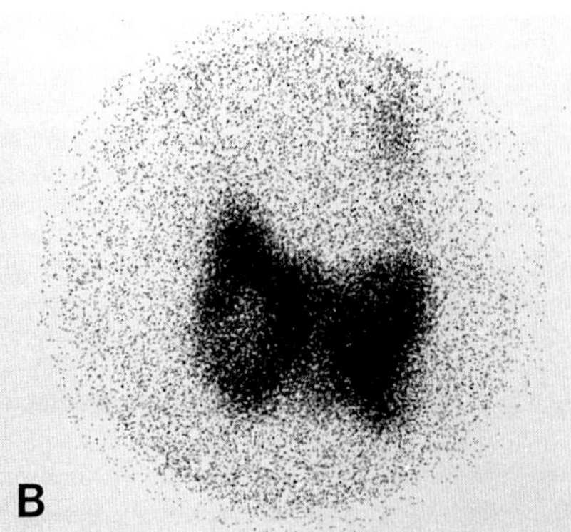

Fig. 56.9 Anterior and RAO pinhole images of the thyroid in a patient with nodules in both thyroid lobes. The non-functioning nodule in the right thyroid lobe is not well appreciated on the anterior image (A) but is clearly seen on the RAO image (B).

demonstration of autonomy on the thyroid scan may feel the (unnecessary) need to proceed to surgery. Thirdly, approximately 5% of patients with a 'thyroid nodule' may have an asymmetrically enlarged thyroid lobe and positive antimicrosomal antibodies, indicating Hashimoto's thyroiditis. A thyroid scan and thyroid function test prior to FNA will indicate that it is unnecessary. Further, if one is performed, cytological interpretation can be difficult due to the presence of oxyphil change. Finally, if the nodule is a non-dominant lesion in a multinodular goitre, FNA may not be necessary unless the nodule changes clinically.

A separate group of patients with thyroid nodules who deserve a thyroid scan before FNA is children. These patients may be very apprehensive and may be uncooperative, leading to a traumatic procedure. Hung et al[31] reported a series of 71 children with solitary thyroid nodules. All underwent thyroid scintigraphy and 16 (22.5%) demonstrated normal or excessive function; none was malignant on excision. Fifty five patients had hypofunctioning nodules and 14 (22.5%) were malignant.

Autonomous nodules

In a review of 22 series in which radioiodine scans were obtained and all patients underwent operation regardless of functional status of the nodule, 10.5% were warm and 5.5% were hot.[23] Malignancy was found in 9% of warm nodules and 4% of hot nodules. A warm or hot nodule therefore reduces the likelihood of, but does not exclude, malignancy. However, as discussed by Ross,[4] there are two situations in which an apparent functioning nodule is demonstrated and a thyroid cancer subsequently found on pathological examination. Firstly the cancer may be distant from the nodule, occult and of uncertain significance. Secondly the area of autonomy may be adjacent to the cancer. Scintigraphy is a two-dimensional scanning procedure and its limitations result from the superimposition of abnormal nodular and normally functioning thyroid tissue. Nodular tissue can distort thyroid architecture. If, for example, it causes a local area of increased anteroposterior dimension of normal thyroid tissue, this may appear warm or hot on a scan. These difficulties may be reduced by routinely obtaining oblique views using a pinhole collimator (Fig. 56.9). In one study, 16% of cancers histologically determined were found in a region in the thyroid distant from the palpated nodule and most were occult papillary cancers less than 1 cm.[4] Careful palpation at the time of the scan and the use of a radioactive marker to localize any nodule is mandatory.

As mentioned previously, there may be a difference between ^{99m}Tc pertechnetate and radioiodine scans

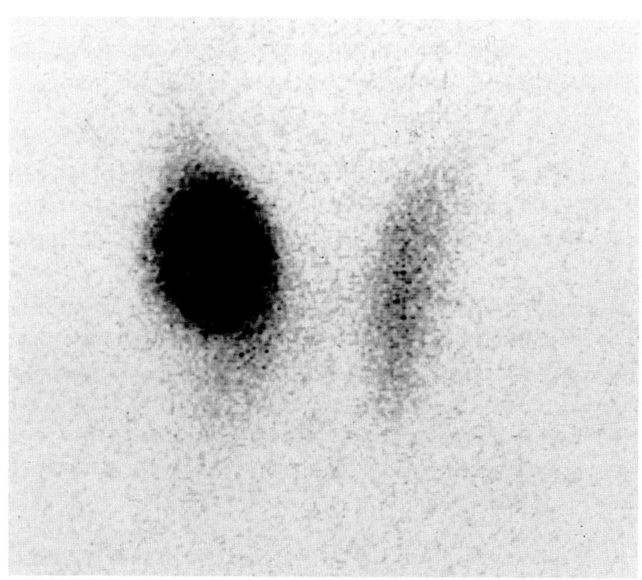

Fig. 56.10 Hyperfunctioning nodule in the right thyroid lobe. Slight uptake is present in the remainder of the right lobe and in the left lobe.

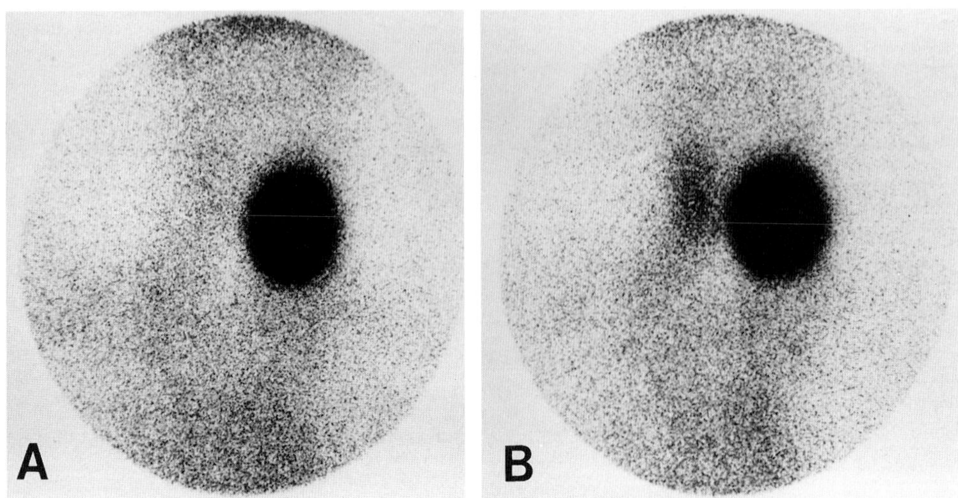

Fig. 56.11 Toxic nodule in the left thyroid lobe without evidence of functioning thyroid tissue in the right thyroid lobe (A). Following TSH stimulation, the right thyroid lobe is visualized (B).

with approximately 5% of nodules concentrating ^{99m}Tc but failing to organify radioiodine and therefore appearing warm or hot on ^{99m}Tc scans but cold on radioiodine scans. There are several reports of such occurrences in thyroid carcinoma.[32-34] Even more uncommon is the finding of a carcinoma concentrating both ^{99m}Tc and ^{131}I.[35]

If a hyperfunctioning thyroid nodule is present on a thyroid scan, it may be autonomous or non-autonomous. An autonomous nodule will not be suppressed by triiodothyronine administration and will remain hyperfunctioning on the scan. It should be noted, however, that most autonomous functioning nodules are not toxic. A large review by Hamburger[36] showed that less than 20% were toxic. Toxic nodules were more likely in patients over 60 years of age when in males and more than 3 cm in diameter. Approximately half of the toxic nodules produced predominantly triiodothyronine. Only about 10% became toxic within 1–6 years. The scan reflects the degree of hyperfunction and at an early stage there may be preferential uptake in the nodule but inadequate production of hormone to induce suppression of the remaining gland which is still demonstrable (Fig. 56.10). In these circumstances, if ^{131}I therapy is contemplated, triiodothyronine suppression is essential to protect the normal tissue. With development of total autonomy, only the hyperfunctioning nodule will be demonstrated. If it is felt desirable to evaluate the remaining gland, a further scan can be undertaken after TSH stimulation (Fig. 56.11A and B). Visualization of the paranodular tissue can also be achieved with a ^{201}Tl scan. This may also be of use in showing the absence of any contralateral lobe and thus identifying that unilateral uptake is due to thyroid hemiagenesis.

Thyroid nodules and biochemical hyperthyroidism

In a review of 872 patients with hyperthyroidism,[37] 84% were found to have Graves' disease, 12% had autonomous functioning nodules, 3% had Graves' disease in a multinodular gland and 1% had no clear diagnosis, probably hyperthyroidism due to thyroiditis or the Jod-Basedow phenomenon. It was noted that in 20 out of 63 patients with a single autonomous functioning nodule, the initial clinical assessment was incorrect. In a cohort of patients receiving treatment for hyperthyroidism, the same group also reported that 13 out of 63 patients with a single autonomous functioning nodule and 10 out of 41 patients with multiple functioning nodules received incorrect treatment prior to a thyroid scan.[38] This suggests that the thyroid scan helps to reduce inappropriate treatment.

Belfiore et al[39] reported on the occurrence of thyroid cancer in hyperthyroid patients. Twenty four cancers were identified in 359 hyperthyroid patients, in 9.8% of patients operated on for Graves' disease and in 3.9% of patients operated on for autonomous thyroid hyperfunction. In those with Graves' disease, most malignant nodules were clinically 'silent' but, in the group of 24 patients with Graves' disease and a coincidental palpable thyroid nodule, 11 were malignant. In general, these carcinomas were more aggressive with extra-thyroidal invasion, multiple foci, lymph node involvement and distant metastases. Only one of 227 patients who underwent surgery for an autonomous hyperfunctioning nodule had a clinically apparent carcinoma of greater than 1.5 cm in diameter. Livadas et al[40] reported 65 hyperthyroid patients with a cold nodule on thyroid scanning, 21.5% being found to be malignant at surgery.

There is certainly a role for FNA in these circumstances since some non-functioning nodules occurring in a toxic gland are TSH-dependent and will function after radioiodine treatment, the Marine-Lenhart syndrome.[41]

Other conditions presenting with palpable thyroid abnormality and hyperthyroidism

These include a unilateral multinodular toxic goitre,[42] subacute thyroiditis, silent thyroiditis and Hashimoto's thyroiditis.[43] In the latter disorder there can be a variety of scan abnormalities including a pattern identical to Graves' disease, a multinodular gland with high tracer uptake, an enlarged gland with normal tracer uptake, a multinodular gland with normal tracer uptake, a single non-functioning nodule, low tracer uptake, or a normal scan.

Hypofunctioning nodules

The essential objective of thyroid scanning is to identify whether a nodule is hypofunctioning not only because this is the most likely finding but because a solitary nodule is associated with a probability of malignancy. The incidence varies considerably in the literature but is such that it must be excluded in every nodule shown to be non-functioning. In the large series of 8177 patients reviewed by Ashcraft & Van Herle,[23] 88.3% of solitary nodules were non-functioning. Malignancy was present in 983 (16.8%) of these 5856 patients, a fairly typical incidence.

The likelihood of malignancy in a non-functioning nodule in a multinodular goitre has generally been thought to be low. However, several recent series have questioned this belief. McCall et al[44] found that the incidence of carcinoma in multinodular goitres was 13% (compared with 17% in patients with a solitary cold nodule) while Belfiore et al[45] found the incidence in multinodular goitres to be 4.1%, very similar to the incidence of 4.7% in patients with a solitary nodule. Most studies primarily refer to clinical multinodular goitres rather than multinodular goitres incidentally detected on radionuclide scanning or ultrasound examinations.

5. ^{201}Tl scanning

Evidence of diminished function in a ^{99m}Tc scan is an indication for FNA of a nodule. However, as discussed, difficulties may be encountered. ^{201}Tl scanning can often be useful in providing evidence of the degree of cellularity and therefore assist in decision making.

6. Ultrasound

It is generally agreed that the routine use of ultrasound in the evaluation of thyroid nodules is not cost effective.[46,47] It is clear that high resolution ultrasound can detect cysts of 2 mm diameter and solid lesions of 4 mm diameter, much smaller than nodules which can be detected by radionuclide scanning.[48] Brander et al,[49] comparing clinical and ultrasound examination of the thyroid in clinical practice, have shown that only one-third of clinically solitary nodules are solitary on ultrasound examination. Approximately one-third of clinically 'silent' nodules were greater than 2 cm in diameter.

While ultrasound patterns may be suggestive of certain pathologies they are not diagnostic. Hypoechoic lesions are more likely to be malignant while hyperechoic lesions and those with a complete halo are likely to be benign, but the specificity is inadequate for diagnostic purposes.

Similarly the detection of a cystic lesion on ultrasound does not confirm its benign nature. Some series have reported a malignancy rate of less than 3%, yet others have reported much higher rates. Ashcraft & Van Herle[23] reviewed about 1000 patients with thyroid nodules. 80% were solid or mixed solid/cystic while 20% were cystic. Overall, 17% of all lesions were malignant but 20% of lesions initially thought to be cystic were also malignant. Evans[50] found that in 110 cases of cancer, ultrasound showed a cystic lesion in 19%.

Although ultrasound detects many lesions not detected by scintigraphy, the reverse may also occur. Abdel-Nabi et al[51] reviewed 60 patients with non-functioning nodules on ^{123}I scan and found that ultrasound missed surgically proven nodules in 32% of cases.

The main roles for thyroid ultrasound are in precise determination of thyroid volume and thyroid nodule size together with assessment of response of these parameters to therapy.

REFERENCES

1. Murray P, Thomson J A 1963 The use of the gamma camera in the investigation of thyroid disorders. Am J Roentgenol 90: 345–351
2. Fogelman I, Maisey M N 1989 The thyroid scan in the management of thyroid disease. Freeman L M, Weissmann H S, eds. Nucl Med Ann, Raven Press, New York, pp 1–48
3. Freitas J E, Gross M D, Ripley S, Shapiro B 1985 Radionuclide diagnosis and therapy of thyroid cancer: current status report. Semin Nucl Med 15: 106–130
4. Ross D S 1991 Evaluation of the thyroid nodule. J Nucl Med 32: 2181–2192
5. Szonyi G, Bowers P, Allwright S et al 1982 A comparative study of ^{99m}Tc and ^{131}I in thyroid scanning. Eur J Nucl Med 7: 444–446
6. Kusic Z, Becker D V, Saenger E L et al 1990 Comparison of technetium-99m and iodine-123 imaging of thyroid nodules: correlation with pathologic findings. J Nucl Med 31: 393–399
7. Park H, Tarver R D, Siddiqui A R, Schauwecker D S, Wellman H N 1987 Efficacy of thyroid scintigraphy in the diagnosis of intrathoracic goiter. AJR 148: 527–529
8. Laurie A J, Lyon S G, Lasser E C 1992 Contrast material iodides: potential effects on radioactive iodine thyroid uptake. J Nucl Med 33: 237–238
9. Hisada K, Tonami N, Miyamae T et al 1978 Clinical evaluation of tumor imaging with Tl-201 chloride. Radiology 129: 497–500

10. Tonami N, Bunko H, Michigishi T, Kuwajima A, Hisada K 1978 Clinical application of Tl-201 scintigraphy in patients with cold thyroid nodules. Clin Nucl Med 3: 217–221
11. Harada T, Ito Y, Shimaoka K, Taniguchi T, Matsudo A, Senoo T 1980 Clinical evaluation of 201-chloride scan for thyroid nodule. Eur J Nucl Med 5: 125–129
12. Ochi H, Sawa H, Fukuda T et al 1982 Thallium-201-chloride thyroid scintigraphy to evaluate benign and/or malignant nodules. Cancer 50: 236–240
13. Henze E, Roth J, Boerer H, Adam W E 1986 Diagnostic value of early and delayed Tl–201 thyroid scintigraphy in the evaluation of cold nodules for malignancy. Eur J Nucl Med 211: 413–416
14. Bleichrodt R P, Vermey A, Piers D A et al 1987 Early and delayed thallium 201 imaging: diagnosis of patients with cold thyroid nodules. Cancer 60: 2621–2623
15. El-Desouki M 1991 Tl–201 thyroid imaging in differentiating benign from malignant thyroid nodules. Clin Nucl Med 16: 225–230
16. Höschl R, Murray I P C, McLean R G, Choy D, Indyk J S 1984 Radiothallium scintigraphy in solitary nonfunctioning thyroid nodules. World J Surg 8: 956–962
17. Corstens F, Huysmans D, Kloppenborg P 1988 Thallium–201 scintigraphy of the suppressed thyroid. An alternative for iodine-123 scanning after TSH stimulation. J Nucl Med 29: 1360–1363
18. Higashi T, Ito K, Nishikawa Y et al 1988 Gallium-67 imaging in the evaluation of thyroid malignancy. Clin Nucl Med 13: 792–799
19. Mazzaferri E L, de los Santos E T, Rofagha-Keyhani S 1988 Solitary thyroid nodule: diagnosis and management. Med Clin North Am 72: 1177–1211
20. Mazzaferri E L 1993 Management of solitary thyroid nodule. N Eng J Med 328: 553–559
21. Alderson P I, Sumner H W, Siegel B A 1976 The single palpable thyroid nodule. Cancer 37: 258–262
22. Maxon H R, Hertzberg V, Vasavada P, Yao Pu M, Volarich D 1985 The continuing impact of thyroid scintigraphy on the diagnosis of thyroid enlargement. Clin Nucl Med 10: 306–307
23. Ashcraft M W, Van Herle A J 1981 Management of thyroid nodules. II. Scanning tehniques, thyroid suppressive therapy, and fine-needle aspiration. Head Neck Surg 3: 297–322
24. Gharib H, Goellner J R, Zunsmeister A R, Grant C S, Heerden J A V 1984 Fine needle aspiration biopsy of the thyroid. (The problem of suspicious cytological finding). Ann Intern Med 10: 25–28
25. Al Sayer H M, Krukowski Z H, Williams V M et al 1985 Fine-needle aspiration cytology in isolated thyroid swellings: a prospective two year evaluation. Br Med J 290: 1490
26. Reeve T S, Delbridge L, Sloan D, Crummer P 1986 The impact of fine-needle aspiration biopsy on surgery for single thyroid nodules. Med J Aust 145: 308–311
27. Hall T L, Layfield L J, Philippe A, Rosenthal D L 1989 Sources of diagnostic error in fine needle aspiration of the thyroid. Cancer 63: 718–725
28. Walfish P G, Strawbridge H T G, Rosen I B 1985 Management implications from routine needle biopsy of hyperfunctioning thyroid nodules. Surgery 98: 1179–1187
29. Gordon D L, Wagner R, Dillehay G L et al 1993 The effect of fine-needle aspiration biopsy on the thyroid scan. Clin Nucl Med 18: 495–497
30. Schneider A B, Recant W, Pinsky S M, Yun U, Bekerman C, Shore-Freedman E 1986 Radiation-induced thyroid carcinoma: clinical course and results of therapy in 296 patients. Ann Intern Med 105: 405–412
31. Hung W, Anderson K D, Chandra R S et al 1992 Solitary thyroid nodules in 71 children and adolescents. J Pediatric Surg 27: 1407–1409
32. Turner J W, Spencer R P 1976 Thyroid carcinoma presenting as a pertechnetate 'hot' nodule, but without ^{131}I uptake: case report. J Nucl Med 17: 22–23
33. O'Connor M K, Cullen M J, Malone J F 1977 A kinetic study of (^{131}I) iodide and (^{99m}Tc) pertechnetate in thyroid carcinomas to explain a scan discrepancy: case report. J Nucl Med 18: 796–798
34. Ikekubo K, Hino M, Ito H et al 1989 Thyroid carcinoma in solitary hot thyroid lesions on Tc-99m sodium pertechnetate scans. Ann Nucl Med 3: 31–36
35. Tech K E, David L, Dworkin H 1991 Papillary thyroid carcinoma concentrating both Tc-99m sodium pertechnetate and I-131 iodide: case report and review of the literature. Clin Nucl Med 16: 497–500
36. Hamburger J I 1980 Evolution of toxicity in solitary nontoxic autonomously functioning thyroid nodules. J Clin Endocrinol Metab 50: 1089–1093
37. Fogelman I, Cooke S G, Maisey M N 1986 The role of thyroid scanning in hyperthyroidism. Eur J Nucl Med 11: 397–400
38. Cooke S G, Ratcliffe G E, Fogelman I, Maisey M N 1985 Prevalence of inappropriate drug treatment in patients with hyperthyroidism. Br Med J 291: 1491–1492
39. Belfiore A, Garofalo M R, Giuffrida D et al 1990 Increased aggressiveness of thyroid cancer in patients with Graves' disease. J Clin Endocrinol 70: 830
40. Livadas D, Psarras A, Koutras D A 1976 Malignant cold thyroid nodules in hyperthyroidism. Br J Surg 63: 726–728
41. Charkes N D 1972 Graves' disease with functioning nodules (Marine-Lenhart syndrome). J Nucl Med 13: 885–892
42. DeRubertis F R, Geyer S J 1986 Case report: unilateral multinodular toxic goiter: scintiscan mimicking solitary toxic nodule. Am J Med Sci 291: 183–186
43. Ramtoola S, Maisey M N, Clarke S E M, Fogelman I 1988 The thyroid scan in Hashimoto's thyroiditis: the great mimic. Nucl Med Commun 9: 639–645
44. McCall A, Jarosz H, Lawrence A M, Paloyan E 1986 The incidence of thyroid carcinoma in solitary cold nodules and in multinodular goiters. Surgery 100: 1128–1131
45. Belfiore A, La Rosa G L, La Porta G A et al 1992 Cancer risk in patients with cold thyroid nodules: relevance of iodine intake, sex, age and multinodularity. Am J Med 93: 363–369
46. Van Herle A J, Rich P, Ljung B E, Ashcraft M W, Solomon D H, Keeler E B 1982 The thyroid nodule. Ann Int Med 96: 221–232
47. Rojeski M T, Gharib H 1985 Nodular thyroid disease: evaluation and management. N Eng J Med 313: 428–436
48. Scheible W, Leopold G R, Woo V L, Gosink B B 1979 High-resolution realtime ultrasonography of thyroid nodules. Radiology 133: 413–417
49. Brander A, Viikinkoski P, Tuuhea J, Voutilainen L, Kivisaari L 1992 Clinical versus ultrasound examination of the thyroid gland in common clinical practice. J Clin Ultrasound 20: 37–42
50. Evans D M 1987 Diagnostic discriminants of thyroid cancer. Am J Surg 153: 569–570
51. Abdel-Nabi H, Falko J M, Olsen J O, Freimanis A K 1984 Solitary cold thyroid nodule: cost ineffectiveness of ultrasonography. South Med J 77: 1146–1148

57. Medullary thyroid cancer

S. E. M. Clarke

Medullary thyroid cancer (MTC) is rare, accounting for about 10% of all thyroid malignancies. The first report of 'a malignant thyroid with amyloid' appeared in the literature at the beginning of this century.[1] Initially the tumour was believed to be a variant of an anaplastic cancer of the thyroid, and it was only in 1955 that Hazard[2] first described the major histological features of the tumour, including the presence of amyloid.

In 1961, Sipple[3] described the high incidence of carcinoma of the thyroid in patients with phaeochromocytoma. Subsequently it was recognized that carcinoma of the thyroid occurring with phaeochromocytoma was always of the medullary type.[4] In 1963 Manning et al[5] reported on the association of phaeochromocytoma hyperparathyroidism and MTC, and the familial nature of the syndrome was soon established by several investigators.[6,7] A second familial syndrome was also recognized at this time, which included MTC, phaechromocytoma, gastrointestinal neuromatosis and Marfanoid habitus.[8] In 1968, Steiner et al[9] introduced the term multiple endocrine neoplasia type 2 (MEN-2) in order to distinguish this combination of tumours from Vermer's syndrome, which had been given the name MEN-1. MEN-2 has subsequently been divided into MEN-2a with MTC phaeochromocytoma and hyperparathyroidism and MEN-2b, which refers to the less common syndrome associated with neuromata (Table 57.1). It is now known that only 10% of all medullary thyroid carcinomas are familial, inherited as an autosomal dominant trait with high penetrance and variable expression. C-cell hyperplasia is now recognized as a premalignant condition in these patients. On the basis of Knudson's two-mutation event theory of carcinogenesis,[10] Jackson et al[11] postulated that C-cell hyperplasia was the result of the first inherited genetic mutational event and that a subsequent somatic mutation led to the transformation of hyperplastic to malignant cells. In recent years the MEN-2a gene has been mapped to the pericentromeric region of chromosome 10.

Table 57.1 Multiple endocrine neoplasia syndrome type 2

MEN-2a	MEN-2b
Medullary thyroid carcinoma Phaeochromocytoma Hyperparathyroidism	Medullary thyroid carcinoma Phaeochromocytoma Neuromata Marfanoid habitus

PATHOLOGY

MTC arises from the C cells or parafollicular cells of the thyroid. These cells make up less than 1% of the thyroid cells mass and are found in parafollicular, interfollicular or intrafollicular locations. They are predominantly situated in the parenchyma of the middle third of each thyroid lobe and are polygonal or spindle shaped with large nuclei. They are characterized by large mitochondria and electron-dense secretory granules 200–300 Å in diameter.[13,14] C cells are derived from neural crest tissue and have the characteristics of the amine precursor uptake and decarboxylation (APUD) series of cells.

C cells secrete the polypeptide hormone calcitonin, which is composed of 32 amino acids. As well as calcitonin, MTC may secrete a wide variety of peptide and non-peptide substances. Patients with MTC may secrete ACTH with resultant Cushing's syndrome in 1–2% of cases.[15] Calcitonin gene-related peptide (CGRP) levels are also elevated in patients with MTC.[16] Other peptides secreted include somatostatin[17] and substance P.[18] Carcinoembryonic antigen (CEA) levels are also frequently elevated in patients with MTC.[19]

Although only 10% of all MTCs are familial in origin, first-degree relatives of all newly diagnosed patients should be screened for elevated levels of calcitonin. As 30% of patients with MTC have normal basal calcitonin levels,[20] several provocative agents have been used to promote the secretion of calcitonin by MTC.[21–23] At the present time a rapid intravenous injection of pentagastrin (0.5 μg/kg over 5–10 s) is used, which produces greater stimulation of calcitonin within a shorter time compared with other provocative techniques.[24]

CLINICAL FEATURES

Clinically, most patients with MTC present with a slowly growing lump in the thyroid, which is generally painless.[25] Palpable cervical lymphadenopathy at the time of presentation is not uncommon,[26] and diarrhoea occurs in about a quarter of patients at the time of presentation.[27] The presence of diarrhoea correlates with advanced disease and is thought to be caused by a humoral agent secreted by the tumour. MTC is a slowly growing tumour that metastasizes initially to local cervical lymph nodes and then to mediastinal nodes. Distant metastases may be found in the liver, skeleton, lungs and, uncommonly, in the brain. Owing to the slow-growing nature of the tumour, patients may survive many years despite widespread metastatic disease.

In patients with the syndromes MEN-2a and -2b, symptoms of phaeochromocytoma may also be experienced. The phaeochromocytomas may precede the development of the MTC by a number of years or may develop subsequently. Patients with MEN-2b generally present in childhood or early adulthood and have a classical facies. These children may also present with intestinal problems secondary to intestinal neuromatosis.

MANAGEMENT

Since most patients with MTC present with a thyroid nodule, the initial management is concerned with establishing the diagnosis. A raised serum calcitonin level is diagnostic of MTC and a calcitonin estimation should be performed on any patient presenting with a neck nodule and a history of diarrhoea. The presence of bilateral non-functioning nodules in the thyroid should also raise the possibility of a familial form of MTC. Fine-needle aspiration is a rapid and effective method of diagnosing MTC. Frequently though the diagnosis is only established at the time of surgery.

Although surgery remains the only treatment option in the majority of patients, the extent of surgery remains a subject of debate. While some surgeons advocate an aggressive approach including thorough neck dissection, sternal splitting and node dissection to the aortic arch, others adopt a more conservative approach involving thyroidectomy and dissection of clinically involved nodes only.[28,29,30]

The use of ^{131}I to ablate any remnant thyroid is a further subject for discussion. Unlike patients with follicular thyroid cancer, ^{131}I has no long-term role in the follow-up and treatment of patients with MTC. It is usually uncertain at the time of initial surgery whether the patient has the sporadic form of the disease or the familial form, and there are therefore pragmatic reasons for completely destroying all thyroid tissue since recurrence may occur at the site of C-cell hyperplasia in patients with familial disease.

However aggressive the surgery, there remains a significant group of patients who will have a persistently elevated calcitonin level post-operatively. Radiotherapy and chemotherapy have not been shown to have any impact on the progression of disease[30] and further surgery remains the main therapeutic option. The accurate localization of missed or recurrent disease is fundamental if surgery is to achieve its aim of a disease-free interval.

IMAGING TECHNIQUES IN MTC

Computerized tomography (CT)

Assessment of the extent of MTC in the neck may be effectively undertaken using CT imaging with and without contrast. CT will identify both primary tumour within the thyroid gland and also diagnose involved lymph nodes provided they exceed 1 cm in size. CT will also identify tracheal and oesophageal invasion by tumour if present. Vascular invasion may also be demonstrated. Post-operatively, CT may also be used to investigate persistent or rising calcitonin levels. Distortion of normal anatomy, particularly if significant node dissection has been undertaken, may make image interpretation difficult and therefore reduces the sensitivity of the test. The lung fields and liver may also be imaged with CT if disease is suspected clinically at these sites. Whole-body information cannot readily be obtained with CT however.

^{99m}Tc pertechnetate

In a patient with a palpable nodule in the thyroid, the simple technique of imaging the thyroid using ^{99m}Tc

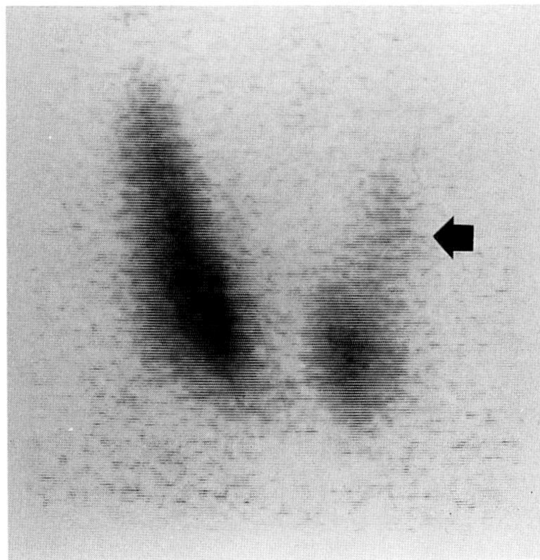

Fig. 57.1 ^{99m}Tc pertechnetate scan of the thyroid in a patient with a thyroid nodule. At surgery this was discovered to be a medullary thyroid carcinoma.

pertechnetate will identify whether the palpable nodule is functioning or non-functioning. Function within a thyroid nodule virtually excludes the possibility of malignancy.

If a non-functioning nodule is visualized, ultrasound will be required to define the cystic or solid nature of the lesion. Fine-needle aspiration may be undertaken in solid lesions to obtain a histological diagnosis (Fig. 57.1).

If bilateral non-functioning nodules are identified on the ^{99m}Tc pertechnetate thyroid scan, the possibility of MTC associated with MEN-2a or MEN-2b should be considered.[31]

^{99m}Tc(V) dimercaptosuccinic acid

^{99m}Tc(V) dimercaptosuccinid acic (DMSA) was initially developed in Japan as a general tumour-imaging agent.[32] It rapidly became apparent that its main clinical use is in patients with MTC. Sensitivities ranging from 50%[33] to 80%[34,35] have been reported in patients with primary and recurrent MTC. Images should be acquired 2–3 h after injection and uptake may be observed in both soft-tissue and bone metastases (Fig. 57.2). Recent studies indicate that SPECT imaging of the neck and mediastinum improves the sensitivity of tumour detection further (Fig. 57.3).

The method of manufacture of ^{99m}Tc(V)-DMSA appears critical to successful imaging. It has been demonstrated by Blower et al[36] that ^{99m}Tc(V)-DMSA exists in three isomeric forms, and the biodistribution of the individual isomers differs from the whole radiopharmaceutical.[37] It has also been demonstrated by Blower et al[37] that the isomeric mix of ^{99m}Tc(V)-DMSA varies when it is prepared using different commercially available DMSA kits. The Amersham DMSA kit would appear to yield the most successful tumour-imaging results. It is suspected that the poor sensitivity results reported by some workers may be due to the isomeric composition of their manufactured product. A further explanation for some of the poor results reported may be the patient selection. There is a well-recognized subset of patients in whom the calcitonin level is elevated but stable and in whom no focal disease can be demonstrated for several years. Imaging with ^{99m}Tc(V)-DMSA in this subset will yield a significantly lower sensitivity for tumour detection.

The normal biodistribution of ^{99m}Tc(V)-DMSA is seen at 2 h to be in the nasal mucosa and faintly in the skeleton.

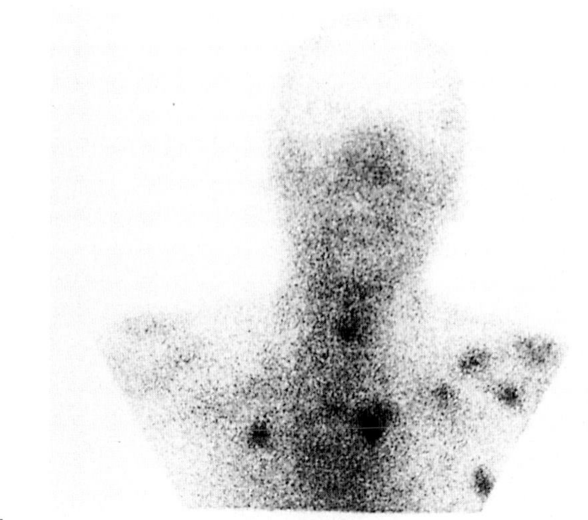

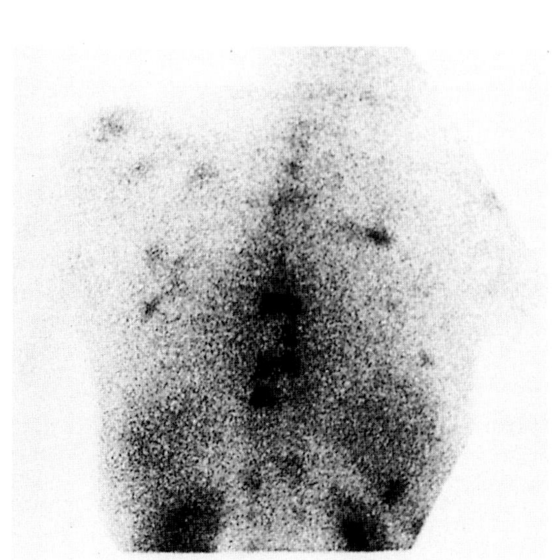

Fig. 57.2 ^{99m}Tc(V)-DMSA whole-body scan in a patient with known medullary thyroid carcinoma. The scan (**A**) shows local soft-tissue recurrence in the neck, anterior mediastinum and skeleton. The posterior scan (**B**) shows uptake in multiple bone metastases.

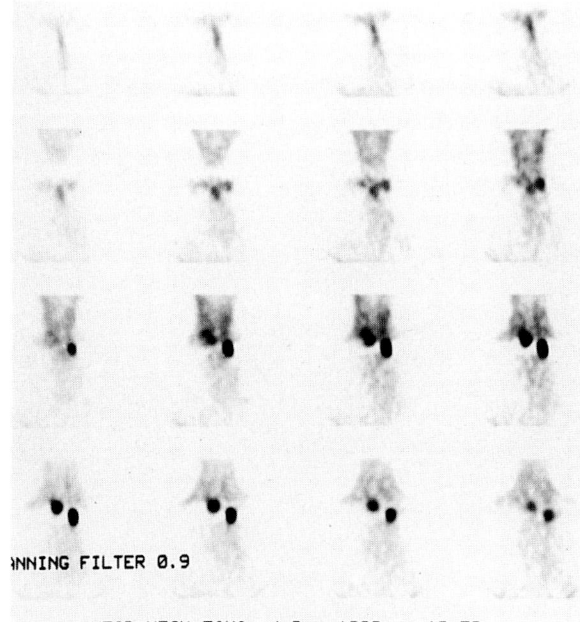

Fig. 57.3 ^{99m}Tc(V)-DMSA coronal SPECT scan of the neck demonstrating local neck recurrence in a patient with MTC.

Breast uptake may be noted in women. Blood pool activity persists at 2 h and the blood pool of the heart, liver and spleen may be identified on whole-body imaging. There is no non-specific tracer uptake observed in the liver, making ^{99m}Tc(V)-DMSA one of the few tumour-imaging agents that is able to reliably detect liver metastases. Pituitary uptake may be seen in some patients.

Uptake in sites of MTC ranges from intense to faint with uptake ratios of greater than 30:1 observed in some patients with neck recurrence (Fig. 57.4). Uptake in soft-tissue sites appears more intense than is observed in sites of bone metastases. Image quality is generally good, although the lack of non-specific uptake may make localization of an identified lesion difficult. Recent studies using the principle of image registration have permitted the merger of image data from the ^{99m}Tc(V)-DMSA image with the data from an anatomically precise MRI image. This merged image gives clinically useful information to the surgeon prior to surgery. Image registration also raises the sensitivity of both imaging modalities by increasing the confidence with which small lesions may be diagnosed[38] (Fig. 57.5). The role of ^{99m}Tc(V)-DMSA in the clinical management of patients with MTC is now established with its prime role being in the follow-up of patients after surgery.[39]

In primary MTC, the main role that ^{99m}Tc(V)-DMSA can play is to confirm a clinical suspicion of MTC while the calcitonin results are awaited. Papillary and follicular tumours of the thyroid do not take up ^{99m}Tc(V)-DMSA, and positive uptake in a cold nodule on a ^{99m}Tc pertechnetate scan is strongly suggestive of MTC. ^{99m}Tc(V)-DMSA whole-body imaging is also useful when planning surgery to stage the disease. It is probably the most effective imaging agent for demonstrating soft-tissue and bone metastases. SPECT imaging will increase the sensitivity of lesion detection and will also define the extent of the primary tumour more accurately.[39]

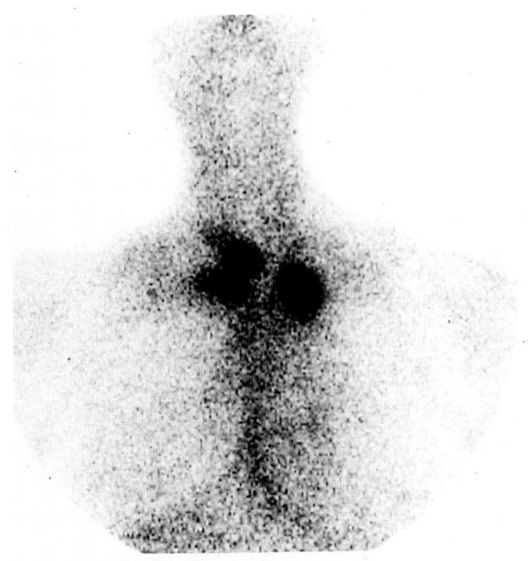

Fig. 57.4 ^{99m}Tc(V)-DMSA planar scan of the neck in a patient with local recurrence of MTC showing high tracer uptake.

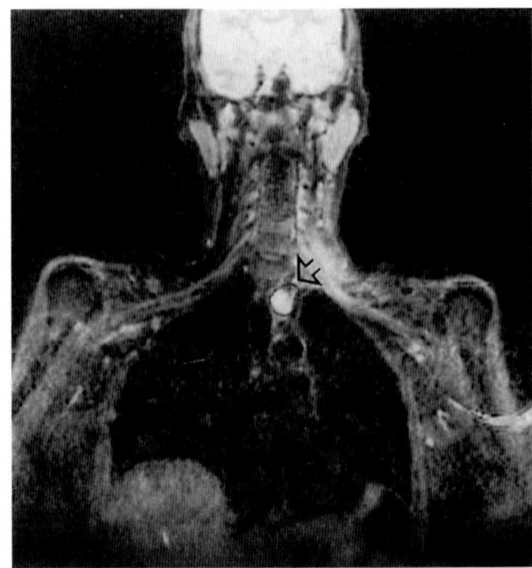

Fig. 57.5 MRI STIR (T1 weighted fat suppression) coronal scan of neck and chest with lesion identified on ^{99m}Tc(V)-DMSA registered and identified as a region of interest on the MRI scan confirming a mediastinal metastasis.

Immediately following surgery, ^{99m}Tc(V)-DMSA imaging may be useful in determining whether residual tumour is present (Fig. 57.6). It is essential that the patient is imaged prior to surgery when there is large bulk disease to assess whether the primary tumour takes up the agent. In longer term follow-up, ^{99m}Tc(V)-DMSA imaging can be used to determine the site of recurrence in patients in whom the post-operative calcitonin level starts to rise. Again SPECT imaging will increase the sensitivity of lesion detection, particularly in patients with small-volume recurrent mediastinal deposits.

Recent work has been published confirming the successful labelling of DMSA with rhenium-186.[40] The physical characteristics of ^{186}Re are shown in Table 57.2. Preliminary clinical experience with this new radiopharmaceutical confirms that its biodistribution resembles that of ^{99m}Tc(V)-DMSA, although renal retention is greater (Fig. 57.7). Therapy trials with this new agent are now in progress.[41]

Thallium-201

Thallium-201 has been recognized as a tumour-imaging agent since 1976 when Cox et al[42] first demonstrated ^{201}Tl uptake in a bronchial carcinoma included inadvertently in the field of view during a myocardial stress study. Since then, ^{201}Tl uptake has been described in breast carcinomas, lymphomas, osteosarcomas, Ewing's sarcomas and oesophageal cancers.[43–46](See Chapter 63.)

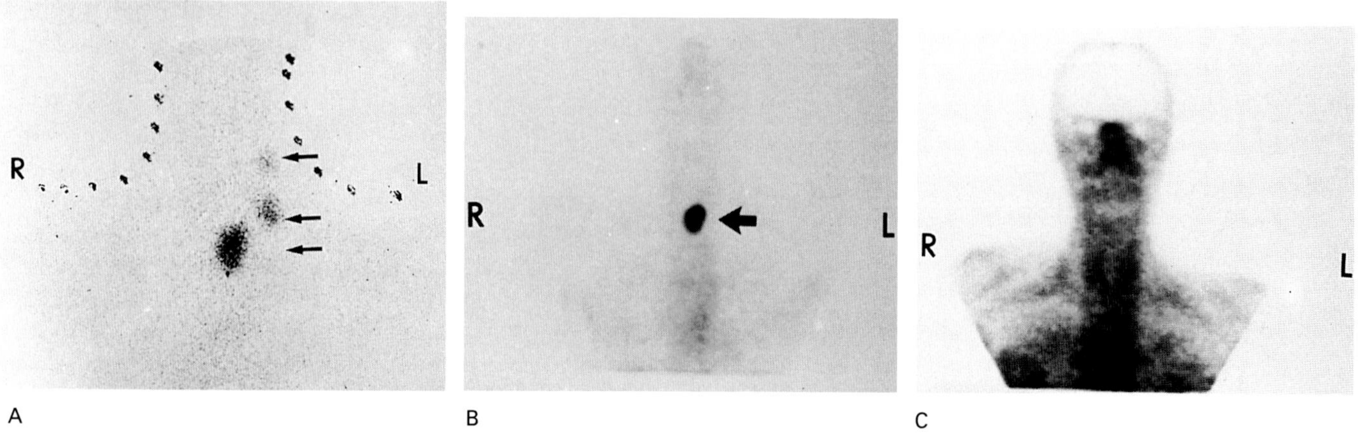

Fig. 57.6 ^{99m}Tc(V)-DMSA scan of a patient with rising calcitonin levels following surgery to a primary MTC. The scan (A) shows three sites of uptake in the left side of the neck (arrows). Following further surgery, a repeat scan (B) shows a persistent focus of activity in the suprasternal notch region. Further surgery located this area of recurrence and a final scan (C) confirms successful removal of tumour.

Table 57.2 Physical characteristics of rhenium-186

Half-life	3.72 days
Gamma-energy	137 keV
Beta E_{max}	1.07 MeV

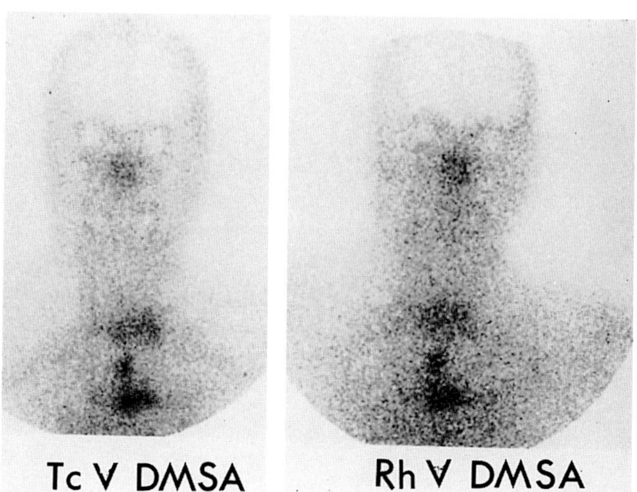

Fig. 57.7 ^{99m}Tc(V)-DMSA image on the left in a patient with locally recurrent MTC. The image on the right was acquired using ^{186}Re(V)-DMSA and shows an identical distribution.

In 1978, Tonami et al[47] described the use of ^{201}Tl in investigating patients with cold thyroid nodules. However, Harada et al[48] demonstrated that ^{201}Tl could not distinguish between benign and malignant nodules.[48] In 1980, Parthasarathy et al[49] first described the accumulation of ^{201}Tl in an MTC primary lesion, and subsequently uptake has been reported in both primary and recurrent lesions[50–52] with sensitivities of up to 91% reported and specificities of 100%. The poor imaging characteristics of ^{201}Tl are not a problem in visualizing neck recurrence, but limit the value of this agent in detecting distant metastases (Fig. 57.8). The non-specific uptake of this tracer in the liver and lungs and its uptake in the myocardium reduce its sensitivity in detecting liver and lung metastases.

^{201}Tl provides a cheap, rapid method of evaluating patients with suspected recurrent MTC and has the advantage over ^{99m}Tc(V)-DMSA in that no radiopharmaceutical preparation is necessary and images may be obtained using 74 MBq of ^{201}Tl within an hour of injection.

A summary of the advantages and disadvantages of the various radiopharmaceuticals used to image patients with MTC is given in Table 57.3.

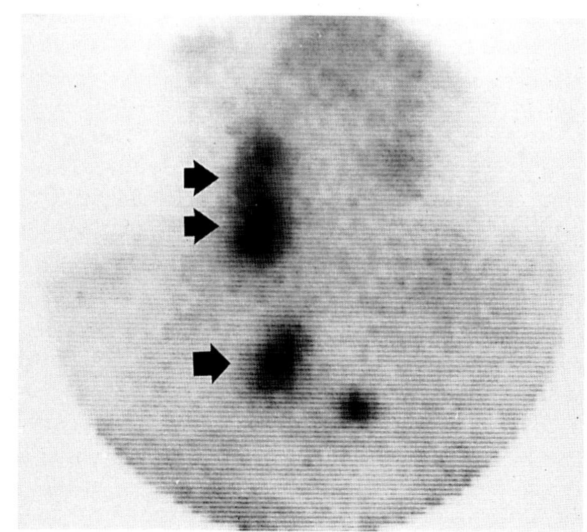

Fig. 57.8 ^{201}Tl scan of the neck in a patient with recurrent MTC. The scan identifies three foci of tumour, subsequently confirmed at surgery.

Table 57.3 Comparison of radiopharmaceuticals available for imaging MTC

Radiopharmaceutical	Advantages	Disadvantages
^{99m}Tc pertechnetate	Cheap Available	Non-specific
^{99m}Tc(V)-DMSA	Cheap Available Sensitive Specific Good images	Complex preparation
^{201}Tl	Cheap Sensitive	Non-specific Poor imaging characteristics
^{123}I/^{131}I-MIBG	Specific in neck with good thyroid block	Poor sensitivity Expensive
^{123}I/^{131}I/^{111}In antibodies	Moderate sensitivity	Expensive Limited availability
^{123}I/^{111}In octreotide	Sensitive Moderate specificity	Expensive

Iodine-123/131 metaiodobenzylguanidine (MIBG)

Following successful imaging of the adrenal medulla by Wieland et al[53] in 1980, many groups have studied the uptake of the guanethidine analogue metaiodobenzylguanadine in neuroectodermally derived tumours including MTC. (See Chapter 65.)

Nakajo et al[54] in 1983 studied a number of patients with neuroectodermal tumours, including one patient with MTC. They reported no uptake in MTC. The first positive case of ^{131}I-MIBG uptake in a patient with MEN-2a was reported by Endo et al[55] in 1984. Uptake in both the primary medullary carcinoma and the coexistent phaeochromocytoma was observed. In the same year Connell et al[56] also described ^{131}I-MIBG uptake in a patient with familial MTC and a primary tumour. The first report of uptake in metastatic MTC was made by Sone et al[57] in 1985, who studied a non-familial case of MTC with bone and liver metastases. Uptake was seen in all sites of known disease.

Following the publication of these case reports a number of series of cases have been reported. Poston et al[58] in 1985 studied six patients, three with sporadic MTC, two with MEN-2a and one with MEN-2b. Although all patients studied were post-operative with calcitonin evidence of recurrence, only one patient had a positive study. Hoefnagel et al[59] in 1985, Hilditch et al[60] in 1986, Clarke et al[61], Moll et al[62] in 1987, and Verga et al[63], Troncone et al[64] and Sandrock et al[65] in 1989 have all published the results of series of MTC patients studied with MIBG. The later series have been performed with ^{123}I-MIBG with its increased resolution, but none of the studies has utilized SPECT. In most studies a sensitivity of 30% is reported, and this is confirmed when the cumulative experience is reviewed.

Several studies have been undertaken to compare the sensitivities of different radiopharmaceuticals in MTC. Clarke et al[66] in 1988 compared the uptake of ^{99m}Tc(V)-DMSA, ^{131}I-MIBG and ^{99m}Tc-MDP in patients with MTC and showed that ^{99m}Tc(V)-DMSA was the most sensitive agent for detecting sites of MTC. Verga et al[63] in 1989 compared ^{99m}Tc(V)-DMSA and ^{123}I- or ^{131}I-MIBG and again confirmed that ^{99m}Tc(V)-DMSA was the more sensitive agent.

The technical aspects of ^{123}I- or ^{131}I-MIBG imaging in MTC need to be considered. In patients with primary disease or suspected neck recurrence who have not undergone total thyroidectomy, it is essential to block the thyroid prior to administration of MIBG. Unless adequate blockade with potassium iodate is achieved, interpretation of uptake in the neck will be extremely difficult. Whole-body images at 4 and 24 h should be acquired, and SPECT imaging of the neck and liver at 24 h will increase lesion detection in patients imaged with ^{123}I-MIBG

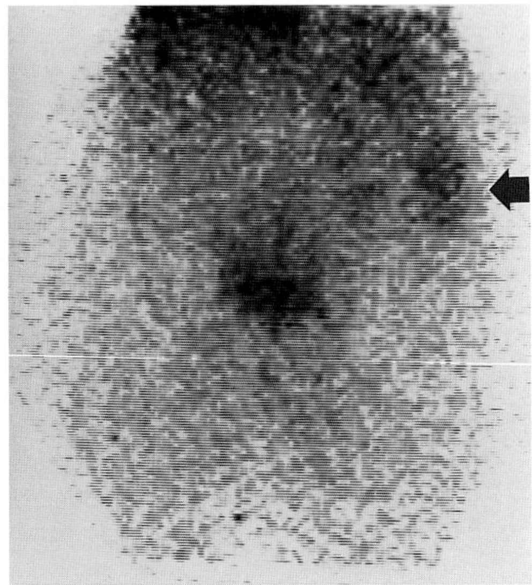
A

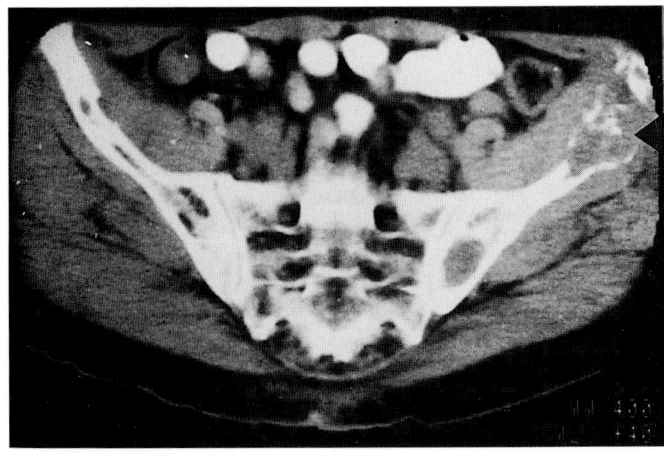
B

Fig. 57.9 ^{131}I-MIBG scan (A) in a patient with MTC and iliac crest pain. The scan shows ^{131}I-MIBG uptake in the iliac crest and CT (B) confirms a lytic lesion at this site.

(Fig. 57.9). There is no role for ^{131}I-MIBG in diagnostic imaging.

Although ^{131}I- and ^{123}I-MIBG have been shown to have an unacceptably low sensitivity for diagnostic imaging, the therapeutic potential of ^{131}I-MIBG in those patients in whom good uptake is demonstrated should be recognized. A number of patients with MTC have now been treated with ^{131}I-MIBG[67] and a palliative response has been achieved in about 50% of patients treated. Partial response has been observed in a further 25% of patients with response times lasting up to 18 months. (See Chapter 74.)

Monoclonal antibodies

Several monoclonal antibodies have been used to image patients with MTC. These include ^{123}I, ^{131}I and ^{111}In CEA,[64,65,68,69] both whole antibody and fragments, and ^{111}In anti-calcitonin antibody.[70] Results from imaging with monoclonal antibodies have been varied, ranging from 0% with anti-calcitonin antibody[70] to 78% with ^{131}I anti-CEA antibody.

The results of imaging with monoclonal antibodies in patients with MTC have been compared with imaging with other radiopharmaceuticals by a number of groups. Cabezas et al[69] compared imaging with ^{131}I anti-CEA antibody and ^{131}I-MIBG and showed significantly higher lesion detection with the antibody. They also compared the relative sensitivity of CT imaging compared with the two radionuclide techniques and showed that CT imaging was also inferior to ^{131}I anti-CEA imaging.[69] Sandrock et al[65] compared the results of imaging with ^{131}I-MIBG, ^{201}Tl and ^{111}In anti-CEA antibody. They also concluded that imaging with the antibody yielded the best results. Troncone et al[64] evaluated ^{99m}Tc(V)-DMSA, ^{131}I-MIBG and ^{131}I anti-CEA antibody. They showed that the sensitivity of imaging with ^{99m}Tc(V)-DMSA and ^{131}I anti-CEA antibody was similar and was far superior to imaging with MIBG.

^{123}I/^{111}In octreotide

A recent advance in tumour imaging has been the development of somatostatin receptor imaging using a radiolabelled octopeptide labelled with either ^{123}I- or ^{111}In-DTPA. (See Chapter 66.) Somatostatin is a neuropeptide which was discovered in 1978[71] and has been found to have an inhibitory effect on growth hormone receptors. In animals this peptide appears to inhibit the growth of various malignant tumours.[72] A number of neuroectodermally derived tumours express somatostatin receptors, including MTC (Yamada 1977).

The normal biodistribution of ^{111}In-DTPA octreotide (Pentetreotide) is in the liver, spleen and kidneys with faint accumulation in the pancreas and thyroid. This biodistribution makes the ^{111}In-labelled agent preferable to the ^{123}I-labelled agent as there is no non-specific bowel accumulation due to hepatobiliary excretion.

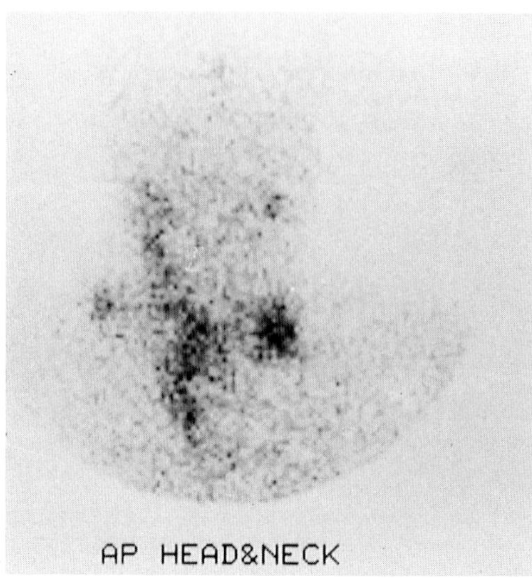

Fig. 57.10 ^{111}In octreotide scan of the neck in patient with recurrent MTC showing uptake of tracer in tumour sites.

250–300 MBq of ^{111}In-DTPA octreotide is administered intravenously and imaging is performed at 4 and 24 h after injection (Fig. 57.10). SPECT imaging will enhance lesion detection in the neck and liver. Sensitivities of 65% have been reported in detecting MTC lesions, although the sensitivity is lower in the liver as a result of non-specific uptake.[73]

Since some therapeutic response in MTC has been reported using a somatostatin analogue,[74] the ability to demonstrate which MTC patients may respond to this new therapeutic agent should prove of great benefit given the high cost of treatment.

CONCLUSIONS

The main therapeutic tool in patients with MTC remains that of surgery. If surgery is to have maximum efficacy, accurate demonstration of all tumour sites must be achieved. Although non-nuclear medicine techniques have a significant role to play in the preoperative assessment of patients, the non-specificity of these techniques may cause problems in image interpretation.

Radionuclide techniques provide an adjunctive method of imaging patients, and a surprising number of radiopharmaceuticals are now being used in this rare tumour. The combined information provided by an anatomically precise study together with a physiologically based study give optimum sensitivity and specificity for lesion detection. This accurate identification of disease facilitates surgery and improves the prognosis of patients.

Radionuclide therapy is still the subject of research programmes, but some encouraging results have been achieved in patients with inoperable disease. The possibility of using nuclear medicine therapies earlier in the history of the disease is now being explored.

REFERENCES

1. Burk W 1901 Uber Einen Amyloid-Tumor mit metastasen. PhD dissertation. Pietzcker, Tubingen
2. Hazard J B 1955 Neoplasms of the thyroid. Arch Pathol 59: 502–511
3. Sipple J H 1961 The association of phaeochromocytoma with carcinoma of the thyroid gland. Am J Med 31: 163–166
4. Cushman P 1960 Familial endocrine tumours – Report of two unrelated kindreds affected with phaeochromocytoma and also with multiple thyroid carcinoma. Am J Med 32: 352–360
5. Manning P, Molnar G, Marden Black B, Priestlly J T, Wooler L B 1963 Phaeochromocytoma, hyperparathyroidism and thyroid carcinoma occurring coincidentally. N Engl J Med 268: 68–71
6. Nourok D S 1964 Familial phaeochromocytoma and thyroid carcinoma. Ann Intern Med 60: 1028–1033
7. Sarosa G, Doe R P 1968 Familial occurrence of parathyroid adenomas, phaeochromocytoma and medullary carcinoma of the thyroid with amyloid? Am Intern Med 68: 1305–1309
8. Gortin R J 1968 Multiple mucosal neuromas, phaeochromocytomas and medullary carcinomas of the thyroid – a syndrome. Cancer 22: 293–296
9. Steiner A L, Goodman A D, Powers S R 1968 Study of a kindred with phaeochromocytoma, medullary carcinoma, hyperparathyroidism and Cushings disease, multiple endocrine neoplasia, Type 2. Medicine 47: 371–409
10. Knudson A G, Stron L C, Anderson D F 1973 Prog Med Genet 9: 133–141
11. Jackson C E, Block M A, Greenwald K A, Tashjian A H 1979 Two mutational-event theory in medullary thyroid carcinoma. Am J Hum Genet 31: 704–711
12. Ponder B A J et al 1989 Molecular genetics of MEN 2a. H Ford Hosp Med J 37: 205
13. Bordi C, Anversa P, Vitali-Mazzal 1972 Ultrastructural study of a calcitonin secreting tumour. Virchows Arch (Pathol Anat) 357: 145–161
14. Braumstein H, Stephens C L, Gibson R L 1968 Secretory granules in medullary carcinoma of the thyroid. Arch Pathol Lab Med 85: 306–308
15. Donahaver G F, Schumacher O P, Hazard J S 1968 Medullary carcinoma of the thyroid – a cause of Cushing's syndrome. Report of two cases. J Clin Endocrinol 28: 1199
16. Fischer J A, Rink H, Born W 1989 Diagnostic relevance of calcitonin gene production in MTC patients. H Ford Hosp Med J 37: 204
17. O'Brien D S, DeLellis R A, Wolfe H J, Tashjian A H, Reichlin S 1987 Somatostatin immunoreactivity in human c-cell hyperplasia and medullary thyroid carcinoma. J Lab Clin Med 109: 320–326
18. Skrabanek P, Cannon D, Dempsey J, Kirrane J, Neligan M, Powell D 1979 Substance P in medullary carcinoma of the thyroid. Experentia 35: 1295–1297
19. Ishikawa N, Hamada S 1976 Association of MCT with CEA. Br J Cancer 34: 111–113
20. Jackson C E, Tashjian A H, Block M A 1973 Detection of medullary thyroid carcinoma by calcitonin assay in families. Ann Intern Med 78: 845–849
21. Nelvin K E W, Miller H H, Tashjian A H 1971 Early diagnosis of medullary carcinoma of the thyroid glands by means of calcitonin assay. N Engl J Med 285: 1115–1118
22. Wells S A, Baylin S B, Linehan W H, Farrell R E, Cox E B, Cooper C W 1978 Provocative agents and the diagnosis of carcinoma of the thyroid gland. Ann Surg 188: 139–142
23. Dymling J F, Ljunberg O, Hillyard C J, Greenberg P B, Evans I M A, Macintyre I 1976 Whisky – a new provocative test for calcitonin secretion. Acta Endocrinol 83: 500–504
24. Hennessey J H, Wells S A, Ontjes D A, Cooper C W 1974 A comparison of pentagastrin injection and calcium infusion as provocative agents for the detection of medullary thyroid carcinoma. J Clin Endocrinol Metastasis 39: 487–494
25. Saad M F, Ordonez N G, Rashidir K, Guido J J, Stratton-Hill C, Hickey R, Samaan N 1984 A study of the clinical features and prognostic factors in 161 patients. Medicine 63: 319–327
26. Chang G C, Beahrs O H, Sizemore G W, Woolner L H 1975 Medullary carcinoma of the thyroid gland. Cancer 35: 695–695
27. Bernier J J, Ramband J C, Cotton D, Prost A 1969 Diarrhoea associated with MCT. Gut 10: 980
28. Brunt L M, Wells S A 1987 Advances in the diagnosis and treatment of medullary thyroid cancer. Surg Clin N Am 67: 263–279
29. Tissel L E, Hausson G, Jansson S, Salander H 1986 Reoperation in the treatment of asymptomatic metastasizing medullary thyroid carcinoma. Surgery 99: 60–66
30. Samaan N A, Yang K-P, Schultz P, Hickey R C 1989 Diagnosis, management, and pathogenetic studies in medullary thyroid carcinoma syndrome. H Ford Hosp Med J 37: 134–137
31. Anderson R J, Sizemore G W, Wahner H W 1978 Thyroid scintigraphy in familial medullary carcinoma of the thyroid gland. Clin Nucl Med 3: 148
32. Ohta H, Yamamoto K, Endo K 1984 A new imaging agent for medullary thyroid cancer. J Nucl Med 323–325
33. Verga V, Muratori F, Sacco G, Banfi F, Libroia A 1989 Role of ^{131}Iodine MIBG and ^{99m}Tc (V)DMSA in the diagnostic value of MTC. H Ford Hosp Med J 37: 175–177
34. Clarke S E M, Fogelman I, Lazarus C R, Edwards S, Maisey M N 1987 A comparison of ^{131}Iodine-MIBG and ^{99m}Tc-pentavalent-DMSA for imaging patients with medullary carcinoma of the thyroid. In: Schmidt H A E, Emrich D (eds) Nuklearmedizin – nuclear medicine in research and practice. Schattauer, Stuttgart, pp 375–378
35. Guerra U P, Pizzocara C, Terzi A 1989 New tracers for imaging MTC. Nucl Med Comm 10: 285–295
36. Blower P, Singh J, Clarke S E M, Bisnnaden M, Went M 1990 Pentavalent ^{186}Rhenium DMSA: a possible tumour therapy agent. J Nucl Med 31: 768–770
37. Blower P J, Singh J, Clarke S E M 1991 The chemical identity of pentavalent technetium 99m-dimercaptosuccinic acid. J Nucl Med 32: 845–849
38. Chaudhuri A R, Lewis M K, Bingham J B, Clarke S E M 1993 Registration of MR and SPECT images in medullary thyroid carcinoma. Nucl Med Comm 14: 256
39. Clarke S E M, Lazarus C R, Maisey M N 1989 Experience in imaging medullary thyroid carcinoma using ^{99m}Tc (V) dimercaptosuccinic acid (DMSA). H Ford Hosp Med J 37: 167–168
40. Singh J, Powell A K, Clarke S E M, Blower P J 1991 Crystal structure and isomerism of a tumour targetting radiopharmaceutical: [ReO(dmsa)2] – (H2dmsa=meso-2,3-dimercapto succinic acid) J Chem Soc Chem Comm 16: 1115
41. Allen S, Blake G M, McKenney D B et al 1990 ^{186}Re-V-DMSA: dosimetry of a new radiopharmaceutical for therapy of medullary carcinoma of the thyroid. Nucl Med Commun 11: 220–221
42. Cox P H, Belfer A J, Van der Pompe W B 1976 Thallium 201 uptake in tumours, a possible complication in heart scintigraphy. Br J Radiol 49: 767–768
43. Hisada K, Tonami N, Miyamae T et al 1978 Clinical evaluation of tumour imaging with 201-Tl chloride. Radiology 129: 497–500
44. Salvatore M, Carratu L, Porta E 1976 Thallium-201 as a positive indicator for lung neoplasms: preliminary experiments. Radiology 121: 487–488
45. Marks D S, Caroll K L 1978 ^{201}Tl-chloride uptake by non-Hodgkin's lymphoma: radiographic exhibit. H Ford Hosp Med J 26: 56–57
46. Terui S, Oyamada H, Nishikawa K, Beppu Y, Fukuma H 1984 Tl-201 chloride scintigraphy for bone tumours and soft part sarcomas (abstract). J Nucl Med 25: P114
47. Tonami N, Bunko H, Mishigishi T, Kuwajima A, Hisada K 1978 Clinical application of ^{201}Tl scintigraphy in patients with cold thyroid nodules. Clin Nucl Med 3: 217–221
48. Harada T, Ito Y, Shimaoka K, Taniguchi T, Matsudo A, Senoo T 1980 Clinical evaluation of ^{201}Tl-chloride scan for thyroid nodule. Eur J Nucl Med 5: 125–130
49. Parthasarathy K L, Shimaoka K, Bakshi S P, Razack M S 1980 Radiotracer uptake in medullary carcinoma of the thyroid. Clin Nucl Med 5: 45–48

50. Senga O, Miyakawa M, Shirota H, Makiuchi M, Yano K, Miyazawa M, Takizawa M 1982 Comparison of ^{201}Tl-chloride and ^{67}Ga-citrate scintigraphy in the diagnosis of thyroid tumour: concise communication. J Nucl Med 23: 225–228
51. Arnstein N B, Juni J E, Sisson J C, Lloyd R V, Thompson N W 1986 Recurrent medullary carcinoma of the thyroid demonstrated by Thallium-201 scintigraphy. J Nucl Med 27: 1564–1568
52. Hoefnagel C A, Delprat C C, Marcuse H R 1984 T1-201 total body scintigraphy in postoperative follow up of thyroid carcinoma. In: Schmidt H A E, Vauramo D E (eds) Nuklearmedizin – nuclear medicine in research and practice. Schattauer, Stuttgart, pp 584–587
53. Wieland D M, Win J L, Brown L E 1980 Radiolabelled adrenergic neuroblocking agents: adrenomedullary imaging with Iodine-131 meta iodobenzyl guanidine. J Nucl Med 21: 349–353
54. Nakajo M, Shapiro B, Copp J 1983 The normal and abnormal distribution of the adrenomedullary imaging agent *M*-[I-131] re Meta [I131] iodobenzylguanidine in man: evaluation by scintigraphy. J Nucl Med 24: 672
55. Endo K, Shiomi K, Kasagi K, Konishi J, Torizuka K, Nakao K, Tanimura H 1984 Imaging of medullary thyroid carcinoma with ^{131}Iodine-MIBG. Lancet 2: 233–235
56. Connell J M C, Hilditch T E, Elliott A, Semple P F 1984 ^{131}I-MIBG and medullary carcinoma of the thyroid. Lancet 2: 1273–1274
57. Sone T, Fukunaga M, Otsuka N et al 1985 Metastatic medullary thyroid cancer: localization with ^{131}Iodine metaiodobenzylguanidine. J Nucl Med 26: 604–608
58. Poston G J, Thomas A M, Macdonald D W et al 1986 Imaging of the medullary carcinoma of the thyroid with ^{131}Iodine metaiodobenzylguanidine. Nucl Med Commun 7: 215–221
59. Hoefnagel C A, deKraker J, Marcuse H R, Voûte P A 1985 Detection and treatment of neural crest tumours using ^{131}I MIBG. Eur J Nucl Med 11: A73
60. Hilditch T E, Connell J M C, Elliot A T, Murray T, Reed N S 1986 Poor results with ^{99m}Tc-V-DMS and ^{131}Iodine MIBG in the imaging of medullary thyroid carcinoma. J Nucl Med 27: 1150–1153
61. Clarke S E M, Lazarus C R, Edwards S 1987 Scintigraphy and treatment of MTC with 131 Iodine MIBG. J Nucl Med 28: 1820–1825
62. Moll L, McEwan A J, Shapiro B, Sisson J, Gross M D, Lloyd R, Beals E, Beierwaltes W H, Thompson N W 1987 Iodine^{131} MIBG scintigraphy of neuroendocrine tumours other than phaeochromocytoma and neuroblastoma. J Nucl Med 28: 979–988
63. Verga V, Muratori F, Sacco G, Banfi F, Libroia A 1989 Role of ^{131}I MIBG and ^{99m}Tc(V) DMSA in the diagnosis of MTC. H Ford Hosp Med J 37: 175–177
64. Troncone L, Rufini V, De Rosa G, Testa A 1989 Diagnostic and therapeutic potential of new radiopharmaceutical agents in medullary thyroid carcinoma. H Ford Hosp Med J 37: 178–184
65. Sandrock D, Blossey H C, Bessler M J, Steinroder M, Muntz D 1989 Contribution of different scintigraphic techniques to the management of MTC. H Ford Hosp Med J 37: 173–174
66. Clarke S E M, Lazarus C R, Wraight P, Sampson C, Maisey M N 1988 Pentavalent ^{99m}Tc DMSA, ^{131}I MIBG, and ^{99m}Tc MDP – an evaluation of three imaging techniques in patients with medullary carcinoma of the thyroid. J Nucl Med 29: 33–38
67. Clarke S E M 1991 131 I Meta iodobenzylguanidine therapy in MTC: Guy's Hospital experience. J Nucl Med Biol 35: 323–327
68. Reiners C, Eilles C, Spiegel W, Becker W, Boerner W 1986 Immunoscintigraphy in MTC using 123I or 111In labelled monoclonal anti CEA antibody fragment. J Nucl Med 25: 227–231
69. Cabezas R C, Berna L, Estorch M, Carrio I, Garcia-Ameijeiras A 1989 Localisation of metastases from medullary thyroid carcinoma using different methods. H Ford Hosp Med J 37: 169–172
70. Guilloteau D, Baulieu J-L, Besnard J C 1985 Medullary thyroid carcinoma imaging in an animal model: use of radiolabelled anti-calcitonin F(ab')2 and metaiodobenzyl guanidine. Eur J Nucl Med 11: 198–200
71. Guillemin R 1978 Peptides in the brain: the new endocrinology of the neuron. Science 202: 390–402
72. Lamberts S W J, Koper J W, Reubi J C 1987 Potential role of the somatostatin analogues in the treatment of cancer. Eur J Clin Invest 17: 281–287
73. Krenning E P, Lamberts S W J, Reubi J C et al 1991 Somatostatin receptor imaging in medullary thyroid carcinoma. Thyroid 1 (Suppl 1): 564
74. Libroia A, Verga U, Di Sacco G, Piolini M, Muratori F 1989 Use of somatostatin analog SMS 201- 995 in MTC, H Ford Hosp Med J 37: 151–153

58. Parathyroid imaging

M. J. O'Doherty   A. J. Coakley

Parathormone (PTH) is essential for the control of calcium metabolism and is secreted by the parathyroid glands. Oversecretion may result in symptomatic hypercalcaemia. With the increasing frequency of biochemical screening of patients, asymptomatic hypercalcaemia is being found and hyperparathyroidism is more commonly diagnosed.

ANATOMY OF THE PARATHYROID GLANDS

There are normally two pairs of parathyroid glands, the upper and lower pairs, which are located to the dorsal side of the thyroid gland. Approximately 6% of normal individuals have one or more of the glands sited in ectopic positions, and occasionally there may be more than four glands. Ectopic glands can be found in a wide range of sites but most commonly are in the neck, thymus, carotid sheath and mediastinum. Glands at any of these sites may become autonomous.

CAUSES OF HYPERPARATHYROIDISM

Hyperparathyroidism may be due to either primary or secondary causes. Some 80% of cases of primary hyperparathyroidism are due to solitary parathyroid adenomas. 10–15% of cases are due to hyperplasia of more than one gland, commonly all four. Parathyroid carcinoma accounts for 3–4% of cases of primary disease. Secondary hyperparathyroidism is due to a need for compensatory hyperproduction of PTH in diseases which can affect calcium metabolism leading to hypocalcaemia. The most common cause is chronic renal failure, but osteomalacia, malabsorption syndromes and renal tubular disorders can also predispose to the condition. In some cases of secondary hyperparathyroidism, glands may develop autonomous function resulting in tertiary hyperparathyroidism.

TREATMENT FOR HYPERPARATHYROIDISM

Surgical removal of parathyroid tissue is the only effective means of treatment of symptomatic hyperparathyroidism. There remains debate over which asymptomatic patients should undergo parathyroidectomy, although most physicians would advise this for the younger age group and more severe biochemical disease. In an experienced parathyroid surgeon's hands 90–95% of parathyroid adenomas will be localized during an initial neck exploration.[1,2] There is no doubt, however that failure of parathyroidectomy is more common with surgeons who only occasionally perform the operation. Moreover, after failed parathyroidectomy in relatively inexperienced hands, the missed adenoma is subsequently often found in the neck or accessible from a neck incision, and frequently is in a normal site.[3] The well-known possibility of parathyroid adenomas being situated close to the aortic arch or elsewhere in the lower mediastinum is in fact extremely rare. Reoperation is technically more difficult than the first operation with a higher associated morbidity. These factors point to the importance of the surgeon being able to localize and remove the abnormal glands at the first operation.

LOCALIZATION OF THE PARATHYROID GLAND

It is against this background that a variety of imaging techniques have been developed to help localize the abnormal gland(s) prior to surgery. The accuracy of these techniques assumes even greater importance in patients who have already undergone exploratory neck surgery. Techniques used include high-resolution ultrasound, computerized tomography (CT), magnetic resonance imaging (MRI), selective venous sampling and a variety of nuclear medicine techniques. Unfortunately, all the available imaging methods have some limitations. The use of high-resolution ultrasonography has reported sensitivities between 43 and 75%.[4] It is not capable of distinguishing thyroid from parathyroid adenomas and is particularly difficult when previous neck surgery has been performed and in thymic and upper mediastinal lesions. CT has a reported sensitivity of 76%[5] but probably has its major use in examining the mediastinum. Venous sampling is a relatively invasive technique requiring a high degree of operator dependency. MRI has a reported sensitivity of 50–93%[6] but still needs further evaluation. These techniques therefore have similar ranges of sensitivity of detection, and this is partly determined by the size of the lesion. However, it is noticeable that with all the techniques there is a wide variation in accuracy of localization between different centres reporting results.

Over the last three decades a number of methods have been used to localize parathyroid glands with radionuclides. Initially radiocyanocobalamin (^{57}Co vitamin B_{12})[7] and ^{75}Se selenomethionine on its own[8] or in combination with thyroid subtraction techniques[9,10] were used with varying success.

A major advance occurred when the technique of thallium-201–technetium-99m subtraction scanning was described.[11] The method relies on the fact that thallium is taken up by thyroid and parathyroid tissue whereas ^{99m}Tc pertechnetate is only taken up by the thyroid. The thallium may be given either before or after the injection of ^{99m}Tc pertechnetate for imaging purposes, and the images are acquired on to a computer using either a converging or a pinhole collimator. It is important to keep a patient still during the procedure and to check for patient movement when processing the images.

This method became the accepted radionuclide technique, but as with other imaging techniques there was wide variation in the sensitivity and specificity between centres. Many reported sensitivities of detection of lesions of 85–95% for adenomas. However, other centres have not been able to reproduce these results and others have reported unacceptably low sensitivity.[12] One consistent finding is that the sensitivity of detection is much lower for hyperplastic glands than for primary adenomas. Gland size appears to be an important factor,[4,13] with glands over 500 mg usually being detected, with a much lower sensitivity for those less than 300 mg. However even large glands are sometimes not identified.[14] The explanation for the differences in reported sensitivities[12,15–18] remain unclear. Different patient referral patterns may be one explanation.[19] The differences in imaging protocols[20–22] has also been postulated, although this seems less likely as good results have been obtained with a variety of scanning methods. Scan interpretation also plays a part, especially with upper pole adenomas frequently prolapsing caudally (to a middle or lower pole position) (Fig. 58.1) and therefore may be misreported as arising from the lower pole.[23]

False-positive images have been described and the most common cause of these is with solid thyroid nodules whether solitary or in multinodular glands (Fig. 58.2).

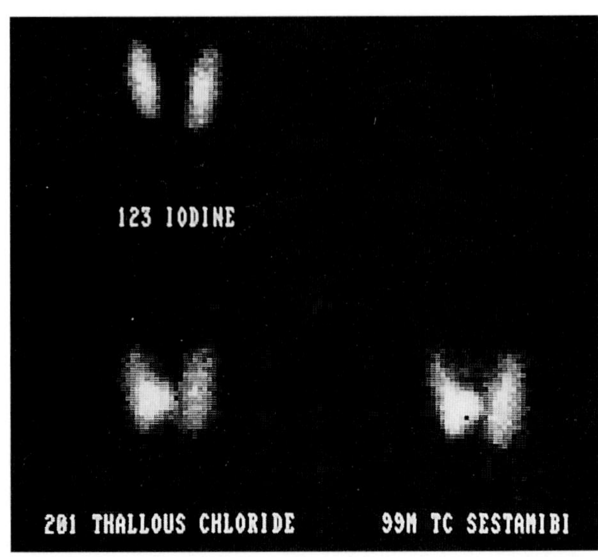

Fig. 58.1 ^{201}Tl and ^{99m}Tc sestamibi images show increased uptake in the medial side of the right lobe of the thyroid at the mid-pole. This was a prolapsed right upper pole parathyroid adenoma.

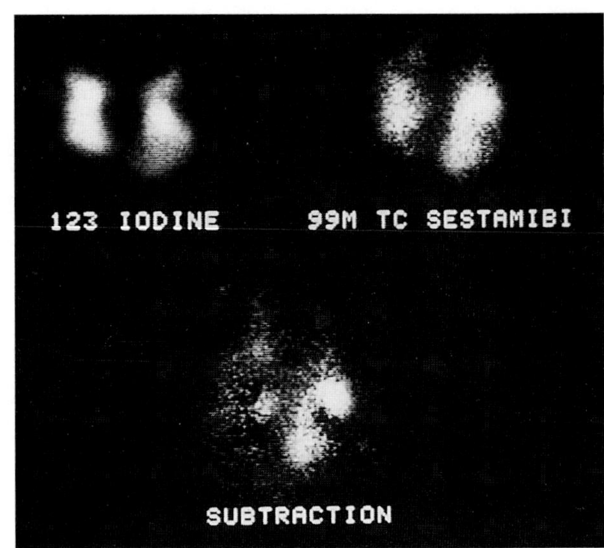

Fig. 58.2 Images in a multinodular thyroid. The subtraction scan showed at least four areas of selective ^{99m}Tc sestamibi accumulation. At surgery the parathyroid adenoma was the lower area on the left, the others being thyroid nodules.

Interpretation of images is also difficult in patients who are taking thyroxine when the thyroid may not be visualized. Other false positives have been described with sarcoidosis,[24] thyroid carcinoma[25] and lymphoma.[26]

Recently ^{99m}Tc sestamibi has been described as an alternative to thallium-201 for parathyroid localization. ^{99m}Tc sestamibi is a cationic complex which has been developed for studying myocardial perfusion and as a possible substitute for thallium. ^{99m}Tc sestamibi appears useful for parathyroid localization either as a combined subtraction procedure with ^{123}I[27,28] (Figs 58.3 and 58.4), with ^{99m}Tc pertechnetate[29] or indeed as a sole agent.[30] The compound has different biokinetic handling in thyroid and parathyroid tissue[28,30] enabling the possibility of single agent use if delayed imaging is performed. The difference in uptake may be explained by the number of mitochondria in the cells since adenomas have a large number,[31] and Chiu et al[32] have suggested that ^{99m}Tc sestamibi is sequestered in the cytoplasm and mitochondria. Initial reports show that the agent is at least as sensitive as thallium-201 and can at least on some occasions localize lesions that the latter has missed.[28]

This evidence, together with the more favourable radiation dosimetry (Table 58.1) and better physical characteristics, mean that ^{99m}Tc sestamibi may well replace thallium for the localization of parathyroid glands. In patients who have had previous surgery with failure of localization of the parathyroid gland our practice is to use a larger dose of sestamibi (300–350 MBq) and to scan the patients with both a pinhole and a parallel-hole collimator to include the mediastinum. Mediastinal adenomas may thus be located and other ectopic glands found (Fig. 58.5). These encourage the correct surgical exploration, especially if the scan is convincingly positive and initial exploration may not show the gland (Fig. 58.6).

Given the inherent problems with the various imaging modalities other techniques are being explored. Parathyroid-specific antibodies have been labelled and shown to have uptake in the parathyroid gland in animal studies.[33,34] Human studies have not yet been performed. Although the use of ^{131}I toluidine blue has been reported as a successful parathyroid localizing agent[35] a similiar compound, ^{123}I methylene blue, has proven unsuccessful.[36] The development of new cationic complexes and other compounds which may have differential metabolism in the thyroid and parathyroid glands may help further improve localizing techniques.

Table 58.1 Dosimetry associated with parathyroid imaging

Radiopharmaceutical	Activity (MBq)	EDE (mSv)
^{99m}Tc (pertechnetate)	75	1.0
^{123}I	20	3.0
^{99m}Tc sestamibi	200	
(Males)		2.4
(Females)		3.0
$^{201}T1$	75	25

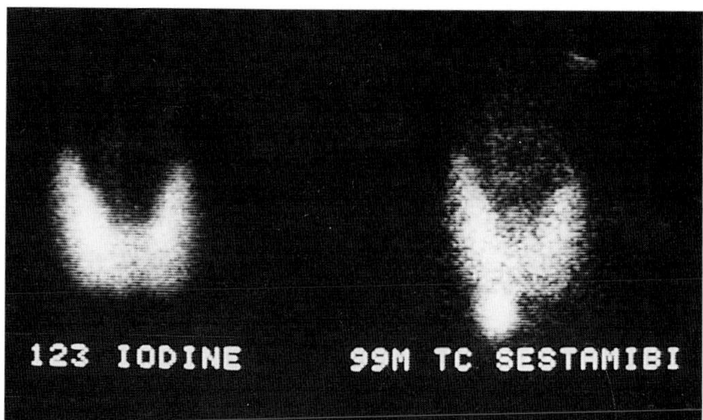

Fig. 58.3 Selective ^{99m}Tc sestamibi accumulation is seen just below the lower pole of the right lobe of the thyroid. Computer subtraction was not necessary to localize this adenoma.

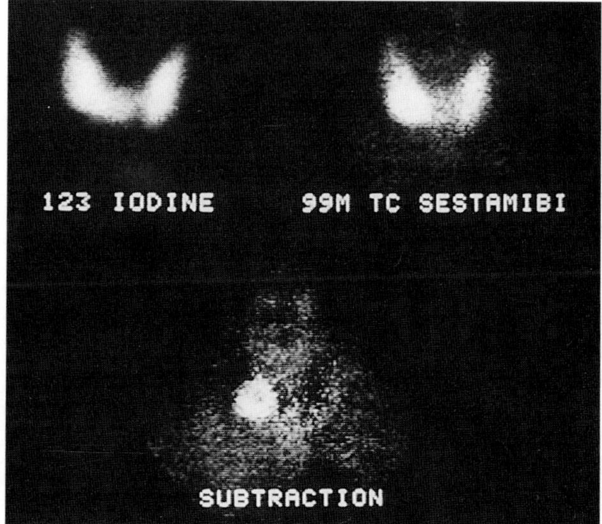

Fig. 58.4 An intrathyroid parathyroid adenoma in the lower pole of the right lobe of the thyroid is enhanced by the subtraction procedure.

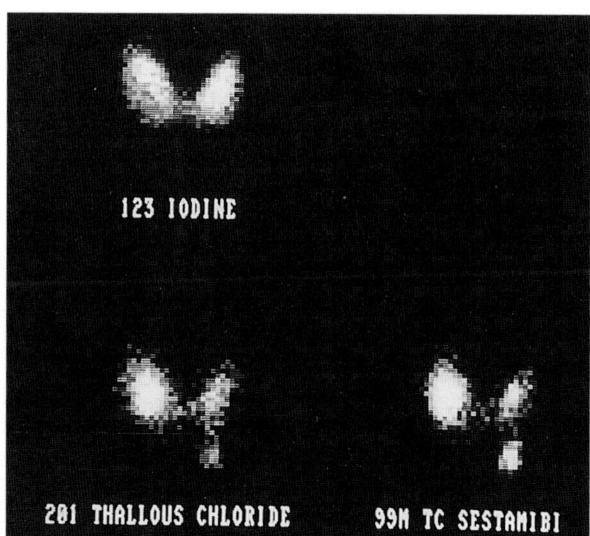

Fig. 58.5 Scans in patients with four-gland hyperplasia. The left lower gland was sited ectopically in the thymus.

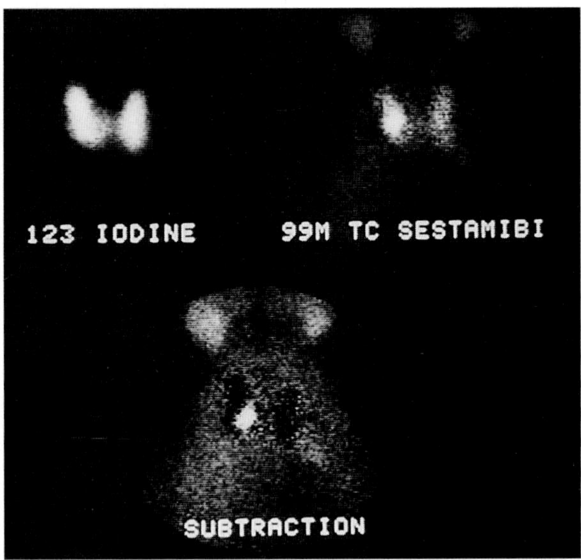

Fig. 58.6 A clear area of increased uptake is shown close to the lower pole of the thyroid. This proved difficult to find at surgery, but was eventually localized deep to the thyroid attached to paratracheal tissue.

CONCLUSION

In defining the role of parathyroid imaging two factors are of crucial importance. The first is the attitude of the surgeon as to the desirability of preoperative localization. The second is the local expertise in performing the imaging procedures. The Consensus Development Conference Panel[37] believe that imaging of the parathyroid glands prior to an initial neck exploration is not necessary, although they conceded that some surgeons found preoperative imaging useful in planning the sequence of the operation. None of the existing techniques exceeds the 95% 'sensitivity' of detecting adenomas at the first operation with experienced surgeons. Certainly the lower sensitivity of detection rate when hyperplasia is expected means that it is inappropriate to attempt localization. If the patient has had a failed surgical procedure then there is general agreement that every attempt should be made to accurately localize the gland before further surgery. Unless local expertise is lacking, radionuclide imaging utilizing ^{99m}Tc sestamibi (or thallium-201) would seem to be the first approach and, if there remains a doubt or further evidence is needed, a CT scan of the neck and mediastinum or MRI should be considered.

REFERENCES

1. Fine E J 1987 Parathyroid imaging: its current status and future role. Semin Nucl Med 17: 350–359
2. Krubsack A J, Wilson S D, Lawson T L et al 1989 Prospective comparison of radionuclide, computed tomographic, sonographic and magnetic resonance localisation of parathyroid tumours. Surgery 106: 639–646
3. Edis A J, Sheedy P F, Beahrs O H, van Heerden J A 1978 Results of re-operation for hyperparathyroidism, with evaluation of pre-operative localisation studies. Surgery 84: 384–393
4. Goris M L, Basso L V, Keeling C 1991 Parathyroid imaging. J Nucl Med 32: 887–889
5. Stark D D, Gooding G A W, Moss A A, Clark O H, Ovenfors C O 1983 Parathyroid imaging: comparison of high-resolution CT and high-resolution sonography. AJR 141: 633–638
6. Miller D L, Doppman J L, Krudy A G et al 1987 Localisation of parathyroid adenomas in patients who have undergone surgery. Part 1. Non-invasive imaging methods. Radiology 162: 133–137
7. Sisson J C, Beierwaltes W H 1962 Radiocyanocobalamine ($Co^{57}B_{12}$) concentration in the parathyroid glands. J Nucl Med 3: 160–162
8. Potchen E J, Wilson R E, Dealy J B 1965 External parathyroid scanning with Se-75 selenomethionine. Ann Surg 162: 492
9. Ell P J, Todd-Pokropek A, Britton K E 1975 Localisation of parathyroid adenomas by computer-assisted parathyroid scanning. Br J Surg 62: 553–555
10. Robinson R J 1982 Parathyroid scintigraphy re-visited. Clin Radiol 33: 37–41
11. Ferlin G, Borsato N, Camerani M et al 1983 New perspectives in localising enlarged parathyroids by technetium–thallium subtraction scan. J Nucl Med 24: 438–441
12. Sandrock D, Merino M J, Norton J A, Neumann R D 1990 Parathyroid imaging by Tc/T1 scintigraphy. Eur J Nucl Med 16: 607–613
13. Gimlett T M D, Brownless S M, Taylor W H, Shields R, Simkin E P 1986 Limits to parathyroid imaging with thallium-201 confirmed by tissue uptake and phantom studies. J Nucl Med 27: 1262–1265
14. Coakley A J 1991 Parathyroid imaging – how and when. Eur J Nucl Med 18: 151–152
15. Corcoran M O, Seifacian M A, George S L, Milroy S E 1983 Localisation of parathyroid adenomas by thallium-201 and technetium-99m subtraction scanning. Br Med J 286: 1751–1752
16. Miller D L, Doppman J L, Shawker T H et al 1987 Localisation of parathyroid adenomas in patients who have undergone surgery. 1. Noninvasive imaging methods. Radiology 136: 133–137
17. MacFarlane S D, Hanelin L G, Taft D A, Ryan Jr J A, 1984 Fredlund P N. Localisation of abnormal parathyroid glands using thallium-201. Am J Surg 148: 7–12
18. Okerlund M D, Sheldon K, Corpuz S et al 1984 A new method with high sensitivity and specifity for localisation of abnormal parathyroid glands. Ann Surg 200: 381–388
19. Sandrock D, Dunham R G, Neumann R D 1990 Simultaneous dual energy acquisition for ^{201}T1/^{99m}Tc parathyroid subtraction scintigraphy: physical and physiological considerations. Nucl Med Commun 11: 503–510
20. Fogelman I, McKillop J H, Bessent R G et al 1984 Successful localisation of parathyroid adenomata by thallium-201 and technetium-99m subtraction scintigraphy: description of an improved technique. Eur J Nucl Med 9: 545–547
21. Percival R C, Blake G M, Urwin G H et al 1985 Assessment of thallium-pertechnetate subtraction scintigraphy in hyperparathyroidism. Br J Radiol 58: 131–135
22. Percival R C, Blake G M, Urwin G H et al 1985 Thallium–technetium subtraction scintigraphy as an aid to parathyroid surgery. Br J Urol 57: 133–136
23. Tindale W B, Everett K, Harding L K 1987 Upper pole parathyroid adenomas: a problem for nuclear medicine (abstract). Nucl Med Commun 8: 251
24. Young A E, Gaunt J I, Croft D N et al 1983 Location of parathyroid adenomas by thallium-201 and technetium-99m subtraction scanning. Br Med J 286: 1384–1386
25. Intenzo C, Park C H 1985 Co-existent parathyroid adenoma and thyroid carcinoma. Clin Nucl Med 10: 560–561

26. Punt J A, De Hooge P, Hoekstra J B L 1985 False positive subtraction scintigram of the parathyroid glands due to metastatic tumour. J Nucl Med 26: 155–156
27. Coakley A J, Kettle A G, Wells C P, O'Doherty M J, Collins R E C 1989 ^{99m}Tc-sestamibi – new agent for parathyroid imaging. Nucl Med Commun 10: 791–794
28. O'Doherty M J, Kettle A G, Wells P C, Collins R E C, Coakley A J 1992 Parathyroid imaging with technetium-99m-sestamibi: preoperative localisation and tissue uptake studies. J Nucl Med 33: 313–318
29. Carroll M J, Solanki K K, Britton K E, Besser G M 1991 Change detection and movement correction for parathyroid imaging with Tc-99m MIBI (abstract). J Nucl Med 32: 1011
30. Taillefer R, Boucher Y, Potviuc C, Lambert R 1992 Detection and localisation of parathyroid adenomas in patients with hyperparathyroidism using a single radionuclide imaging procedure with ^{99m}Tc sestamibi (double phase study). J Nucl Med 33: 1801–1807
31. Sandrock D, Merino M J, Norton J A, Neumann R D 1993 Ultrastructural histology correlates of thallium-201/technetium-99m parathyroid subtraction scintigraphy. J Nucl Med 34: 24–29
32. Chiu M L, Kronange J F, Piwnica-Worms D 1990 Effect of mitochondrial and plasma-membrane potentials on accumulation of hexakis (2-methoxyisobutylisonitrile) technetium in cultured mouse fibroblasts. J Nucl Med 31: 1646–1653
33. Cance W G, Otsuka F L, Dilley W F et al 1988 A potential new radiopharmaceutical for parathyroid imaging: radiolabeled parathyroid-specific monoclonal antibody. I. Evaluation of ^{125}I-labelled antibody in a nude mouse model system. Int J Radiat Appl Instrum 15: 299–303
34. Otsuka F L, Cance W G, Dilley W G et al 1988 A potential new radiopharmaceutical for parathyroid imaging: radiolabeled parathyroid-specific monoclonal antibody. II. Comparison of ^{125}I and ^{111}In-labeled antibodies. Int J Radiat Appl Instrum 15: 305–311
35. Zwas S T, Czerniak A, Boruchowsky S, Itamar A, Wolfstein I 1987 Preoperative parathyroid localisation by superimposed iodine-131 toluidine blue and technetium-99m pertechnetate imaging. J Nucl Med 28: 298–307
36. Blower P J, Kettle A G, O'Doherty M J, Collins R E C, Coakley A J 1992 ^{123}I-methylene blue: an unsatisfactory parathyroid imaging agent. Nucl Med Commun 13: 522–527
37. Consensus Development Conference Panel 1991 Diagnosis and management of asymptomatic primary hyperparathyroidism: consensus development conference statement. Ann Intern Med 114: 593–597

59. Scintigraphic diagnosis of tumours of the liver

Brian C. Lentle   David B. Coupland

In the past, liver imaging with radiocolloids was used extensively to detect metastatic disease. With the emergence of ultrasonography, computed tomography and magnetic resonance imaging as alternative methods by which to image liver morphology, radionuclide imaging has come to be used more appropriately to identify function and tissue-specific characteristics related to liver lesions. Often the presence but not the nature of these has been suspected from the use of other diagnostic methods.

PROCEDURAL ASPECTS

Because the diagnosis of liver tumours depended previously in large part on anatomical display, the major role in diagnosis has been provided by the use of radiocolloids such as ^{99m}Tc sulphide colloid or ^{113m}In hydroxide colloid. As the role of radionuclide imaging has come to focus instead upon tissue specificity and the functional implications of tumours, so other radiopharmaceuticals have come into use. Chief among these are ^{99m}Tc iminodiacetic acid analogues and ^{99m}Tc-labelled red blood cells. These radiotracers respectively are extracted by hepatic polygonal cells or label the blood pool, whereas radiocolloids are taken up by the reticuloendothelial (Kupffer) cells in the liver.

While high count density planar images may suffice for diagnosis, there is ample evidence that single photon emission computed tomography (SPECT) increases the sensitivity of liver imaging, for example in the detection of small haemangiomas.[1] Sensitivity can also be improved by interrupting imaging while the patient breathes or by having the patient erect during count acquisition, which reduced artefact due to respiratory motion. Without such unusual strategies the typical reported sensitivity and specificity of liver imaging in detecting masses such as 'cold' lesions is 0.79 and 0.85 respectively, compared with figures of 0.86 and 0.88 in the same patients using SPECT.[2] Low-energy high-resolution collimators are preferred for liver imaging with ^{99m}Tc-labelled agents. The use of a costal margin marker may sometimes be of assistance in relating the findings on clinical examination to those evident scintigraphically.

Positron emission tomography (PET) has been used with ^{13}N ammonia, among other PET methods, to examine the metabolic characteristics of tumours. It has, for example, been suggested that this method might contribute to the distinction between metastases and hepatomas.[3]

SCINTIGRAPHIC FINDINGS

The patterns of radionuclide findings observed in the different types of liver tumours are summarized in Table 59.1. While magnetic resonance imaging of the liver may prove to be relatively specific in this context, the expense involved leaves a rational and justifiable role for scintigraphic diagnosis.[4]

Metastases

Liver metastases can be identified as focal lesions with no uptake of radiotracer either ^{99m}Tc radiocolloids or ^{99m}Tc iminodiacetic acid analogues (Fig. 59.1A and B), although this finding is not specific, occurring also as a result of liver cysts and other diseases. Such lesions must be about 2.0 cm in diameter to be consistently detectable,[5] although sensitivities are greater, as is depth detection, if SPECT is used (Fig. 59.2A and B).[2] Such metastases are well known to be more common in patients with cancers of the bowel, breast and lung as well as melanomas. Although not a specific finding, it has been noted that metastases from breast cancer and melanoma are apt to appear as widespread multifocal disease as distinct from larger more solitary focal lesions.[6]

Positive uptake of various radiotracers is found in liver metastases for both non-specific and specific reasons. In the former context, tracers such as ^{99m}Tc chelates with longer residence times in the blood, for example ^{99m}Tc

Table 59.1 Scintigraphic patterns in hepatic lesions

	Hepatoma	Metastasis	Haemangioma	Adenoma	Focal nodular hyperplasia	Regenerative nodule	Fatty degeneration
Flow (irrespective of type of tracer)	++ (arterial) +++	0 (usually) ↓ +	0	0	0 ↓ ++	0	0
Blood pool (immediate)	++	0 ↓ ±	0 (in very small lesions and in children may be +)	0	±	0	0
Delayed blood Pool(^{99m}Tc RBC)	++	0	+++ (1 h plus)	0	0	0	0
Extraction of ^{99m}Tc sulphur colloid	0	0	0 (+ 'reportable')	0	0 ca 50% + ca 30% ++ ca 20%	+ (usually)	± (irregular pattern of distribution)
Extraction of ^{99m}Tc-IDA	± (with stasis: also reported in lung metastases, etc)	0	0	0 (usually) +	+ or 0	+	± (irregular pattern of distribution)
^{67}Ga citrate ^{75}Se selenomethionine ^{111}In chloride	+++ (not necessarily uniformly)	0, + or ++	0	+	+	0 or +	0 (^{127}Xe, ^{133}Xe ++)

0 → +++: increasing degree to which the radiotracer is found in the respective lesions

phosphates, may leak detectably into those metastases with an expanded interstitial space.[7] Occasionally other mechanisms may also operate, such as the localization of this bone-seeking radiopharmaceutical in calcified metastases, such as those from mucus-producing adenocarcinomas.[8] More specific mechanisms operate in the uptake of tracers such as metaiodobenzylguanidine (labelled with either ^{123}I or ^{131}I), octreotide (labelled with ^{123}I or ^{111}In) or monoclonal antibodies (variously labelled).

In considering specific methods for the detection of liver metastases using the tracers noted above, it has to be remembered that such tracers often localize in normal liver. Thus, for a lesion of given size, the conspicuousness of a lesion in the liver will be less than that for a similar lesion elsewhere. Thus, almost prospective studies of labelled monoclonal antibodies, for example, have found lower sensitivities in detecting liver lesions compared with those elsewhere. However, one recent report is an exception to this.[9]

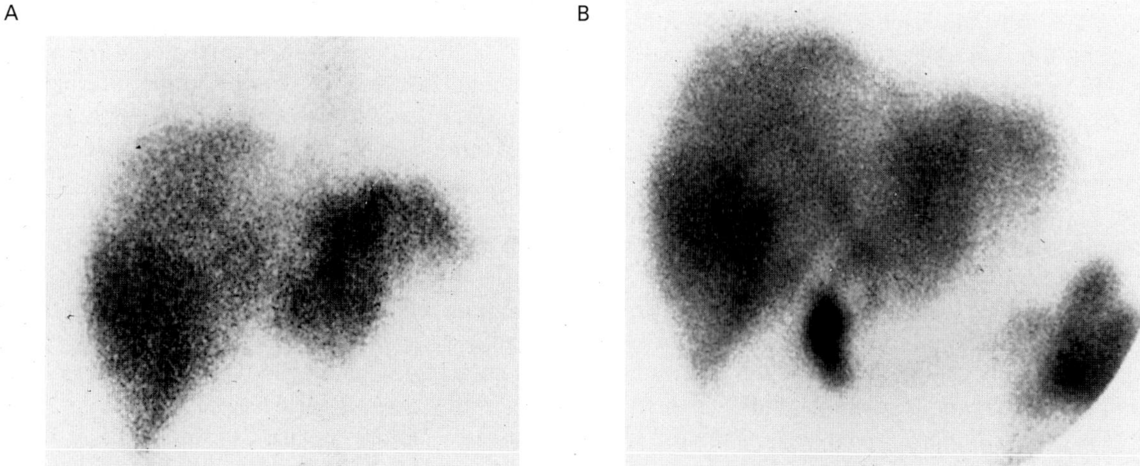

Fig. 59.1 Anterior images of the liver of a patient with metastatic breast carcinoma. Focal defects in uptake of both ^{99m}Tc sulphide colloid (A) and ^{99m}Tc-IDA (B) are evident in scans undertaken a few days apart.

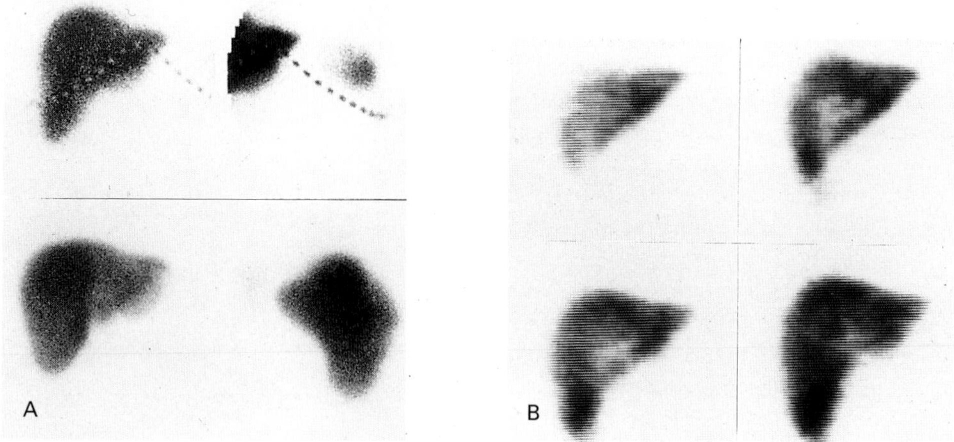

Fig. 59.2 Planar (A) and tomographic (B) images of the liver in the same patient. Only the tomographic images reveal the metastatic disease (^{99m}Tc sulphide colloid).

Hepatoma and hepatic adenoma

Hepatomas often declare themselves on dynamic imaging of the liver because of their marked vascularity. Reflecting this and the fact that tumours of the liver typically have a blood supply derived from the hepatic artery, there is a phase shift on dynamic images with the tumour blood flow preceding the blood supply to the rest of the (normal) liver, which is in large part derived from the portal circulation (Fig. 59.3).

Historically, ^{67}Ga citrate and ^{75}Se selenomethionine were used to examine the liver in patients in whom hepatoma (hepatocellular carcinoma) was suspected. Perhaps more importantly in the context of what radio-

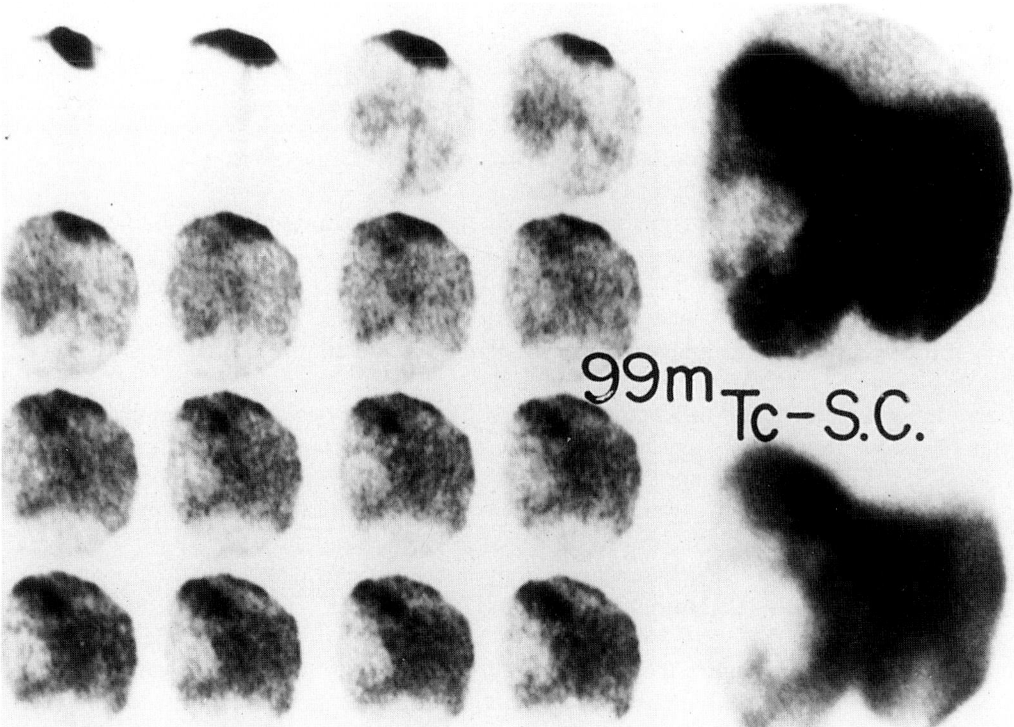

Fig. 59.3 Dynamic and static scintigraphy in a patient with multifocal hepatoma. The arterial blood supply to the tumour is seen on early images and the defect in uptake of ^{99m}Tc sulphide colloid on the later ones.

nuclide imaging might achieve in cancer diagnosis, it is of interest to note that uptake of agents extracted by hepatocytes, such as ^{99m}Tc iminodiacetic acid (IDA) analogues, may be used to measure the relative degree of differentiation of the tumour cells.[10,11] A role for ^{67}Ga citrate scintigraphy in the follow-up of patients having had a resection of hepatocellular carcinoma is suggested by evidence that this method may aid in the early detection of recurrent disease.[12]

The diagnosis of hepatoma complicating hepatic cirrhosis can be difficult when using any imaging technique, but this is a context in which the tissue specificity of radionuclide imaging may be particularly of value.

Adenomas do not contain Kupffer cells, and in this may differ from focal nodular hyperplasia.[13,14] They appear as defects on radiocolloid images of the liver. Hepatic adenomas are related to oral contraceptive use, a relationship which is much less well established in respect of focal nodular hyperplasia.

Focal nodular hyperplasia

These lesions have somewhat variable appearances on radionuclide imaging.[13,14] However, the majority reveal focal hypofixation of radiocolloids. In some patients there is uptake, and this is greater than in normal liver in about 10%. There may or may not be uptake of ^{99m}Tc-IDA analogues, and this specific appearance may sometimes make other diagnostic measures unnecessary (Fig. 59.4A and B).[15]

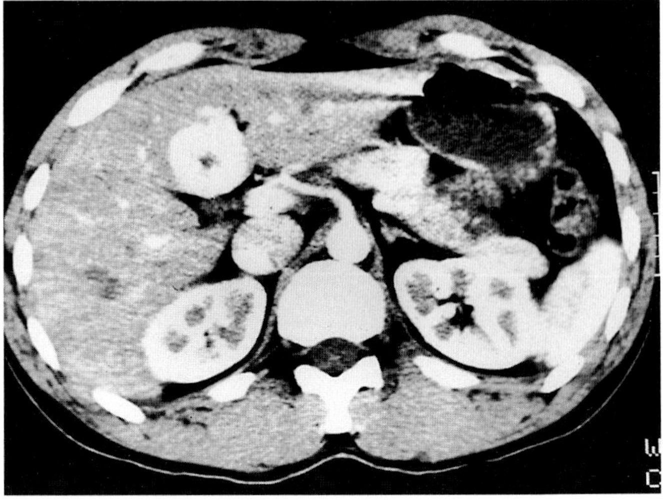

A

3 4 7 8

B

Fig. 59.4 CT (A) and ^{99m}Tc sulphide colloid SPECT (B) in a patient with focal nodular hyperplasia of the liver. The lesion shows non-specific contrast enhancement in the former and intense hyperfixation of colloid in the latter.

Haemangioma

Haemangiomas of the liver are not uncommon, occurring in between 0.5% and 5% of the population. As such, they are frequently suspected when the liver is being examined by ultrasonography or computed tomography in the search for metastatic lesions.[16]

The characterization of lesions as haemangiomas is, therefore, one of the commoner indications at present for examining mass lesions of the liver by radionuclide methods. These lesions are deficient in Kupffer cells and have low rates of blood flow but a large blood volume. These facts result in the characteristic appearance of such a lesion in delayed images 2–3 h after injection of ^{99m}Tc-labelled red blood cells (Fig. 59.5A and B). A sensitivity of 89% can be achieved with planar imaging,[17] but the detection of small lesions and those at depth is enhanced by tomography.[2]

The radionuclide findings are highly specific although some isolated false-positive examinations have been reported.[18] The findings are in fact more specific than those obtained using computed tomography (CT).[19] This is due to the lack of blood volume contrast marker for use with CT, the existing contrast agents being too rapidly eliminated through the kidneys to permit consistent opacification of lesions by equilibration of the contrast in the vascular space. However, the smallest lesions detectable using SPECT are at least 1 cm in diameter.[1] There is as yet no indication that magnetic resonance imaging will prove diagnostically superior to ^{99m}Tc SPECT.[20]

Larger lesions, rather arbitrarily designated as giant haemangiomas, may require images at delays greater than 1 h to permit equilibration of the labelled red blood cells throughout the locally expanded red cell space.[21]

RADIONUCLIDE THERAPY

Reference has been made above to the arterialization of liver tumours (whether primary or secondary) as distinct from the predominantly portal venous blood supply of normal liver. This physiological fact has been exploited by injecting not only radiotracers with particulate emissions (e.g. ^{90}Y), but also embolic materials and chemotherapeutic drugs directly into the hepatic artery after its

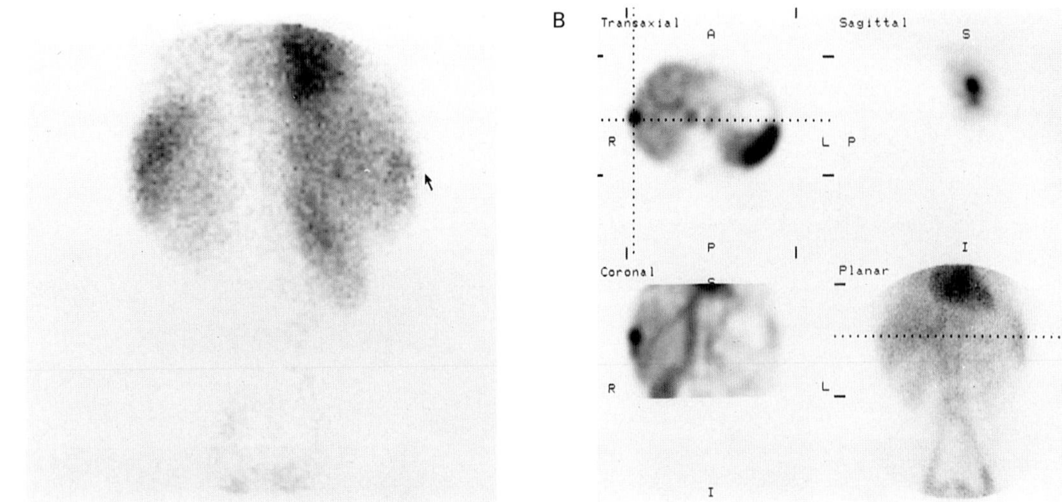

Fig. 59.5 ^{99m}Tc red blood cell scintigraphy in a patient with a hepatic haemangioma. The lesion is barely seen in the posterior planar image (A) at 2 h but is very evident in all planes with SPECT (B).

catheterization. There is a proportionately greater effect upon the tumour than upon normal liver.

It has been necessary to develop an agent for local radiotherapy that is not appreciably leached out to irradiate other than the target tissue. ^{90}Y-labelled microspheres and ^{131}I ethiodol have been used as such agents.[22,23] A preliminary injection of ^{99m}Tc albumin macroaggregates is used to rule out anomalous distribution of blood from the hepatic artery, e.g. into the duodenum through the duodenogastric vessel, which might result in unacceptable radiation doses to that or other structures. This agent may also be used to map the distribution of any treatment and exclude the presence of vascular shunting. Certainly radiation duodenitis and even perforation have been observed as a complication of intra-arterial radiotherapy of the liver. With these precautions, which have not been insuperable, substantial degrees of palliation may be achieved in patients with inoperable liver metastases.[22] This therapeutic approach is considered in more detail in Chapter 000.

REFERENCES

1. Brunetti J C, Van Heertum R L, Yudd A P, Cooperman A M 1988 The value of SPECT imaging in the diagnosis of hepatic hemangioma. Clin Nucl Med 13: 800–804
2. Brendel A J, Leccia F, Drouillard J et al 1984 Single photon emission computed tomography (SPECT), planar scintigraphy, and transmission computed tomography: a comparison of accuracy in diagnosing focal hepatic lesions. Radiology 153: 527–532
3. Shibata T, Yamamoto K, Hayashi N et al 1988 Dynamic positron emission tomography with ^{13}N-ammonia in liver tumors. Eur J Nucl Med 14: 607–611
4. Reinig J W 1991 Differentiation of hepatic lesions with MR imaging: the last word? Radiology 179: 601–602
5. Ruiter D J, Byck W, Pauwels E K J et al 1977 Correlation of scintigraphy with short interval autopsy in malignant focal liver disease. Cancer 39: 172–175
6. Drum D E, Beard J M 1976 Scintigraphic criteria for hepatic metastases from cancer of the colon and breast. J Nucl Med 17: 677–680
7. Worsley D F, Lentle B C 1993 Uptake of technetium-99m MDP in primary amyloidosis with a review of the mechanisms of soft tissue localization of gene-seeking radiopharmaceuticals. J Nucl Med 34: 1612–1615
8. Guilberteau M J, Potsaid M S, McKusick K A 1976 Accumulation of Tc-99m-diphosphonate in four patients with hepatic neoplasm: case report. J Nucl Med 17: 1060–1061
9. Divgi C R, McDermott K, Johnson D K et al 1991 Detection of hepatic metastases from colorectal carcinoma using indium-111 (^{111}In) labeled monoclonal antibody (mAb): MSKCC experience with mAb ^{111}In-C110. Int J Radiat Appl Inst 18: 705–710
10. Calvet X, Pons F, Bruix J et al 1988 Technetium-99m DISIDA hepatobiliary agent in diagnosis of hepatocellular carcinoma: relationship between detectability and tumor differentiation. J Nucl Med 29: 1916–1920
11. Hasegawa Y, Nakano S, Hiyama T et al 1991 Relationship of uptake of technetium-99m(Sn)-N-pyridoxyl-5-methyltryptophan by hepatocellular carcinoma to prognosis. J Nucl Med 32: 228–235
12. Serafini A N, Jeffers L J 1988 Early recognition of recurrent hepatocellular carcinoma utilizing gallium-67 citrate scintigraphy. J Nucl Med 29: 712–716
13. Casarella W J, Knowles D M, Wolff M, Johnson P M 1978 Focal nodular hyperplasia and liver cell adenoma; radiologic and pathologic differentiation. AJR 131: 393–402
14. Salvo A F, Schiller A, Athanasoulis C et al 1977 Hepatoadenoma and focal nodular hyperplasia; pitfalls in radiocolloid imaging. Radiology 125: 451–455
15. Biersack H J, Thelen M 1980 Focal nodular hyperplasia of the liver as established by Tc-99m sulfur colloid and HIDA scintigraphy. Radiology 137: 187–190
16. Nelson R C, Chezmar J L 1990 Diagnostic approach to hepatic hemangiomas. Radiology 176: 11–13
17. Engel M A, Marks D S, Sandler M A, Shetty P 1983 Differentiation of focal intrahepatic lesions with ^{99m}Tc-red blood cell imaging. Radiology 146: 777–782
18. Ginsberg F, Slavin Jr J D 1986 Hepatic angiosarcoma: mimicking of angioma on three-phase technetium-99m red blood cell scintigraphy. J Nucl Med 27: 1861–1863
19. Brodsky R I, Friedman A C, Maurer A H et al 1987 Hepatic cavernous hemangioma: diagnosis with Tc-99m-

labeled red cells and single-photon emission CT AJR 1987 148: 125–129

20. Brown R K J, Gomes A 1987 Hepatic hemangiomas: evaluation by magnetic resonance imaging and technetium-99m red blood cell scintigraphy. J Nucl Med 28: 1683–1687
21. Lisbona R, Derbekyan V 1989 Scintigraphic and ultrasound features of giant hemangioma of the liver. J Nucl Med 30: 181–186
22. Nakajo M, Kobayashi H 1988 Biodistribution and in vivo kinetics of iodine-131 lipiodol infused via the hepatic artery of patients with hepatic cancer. J Nucl Med 29: 1066–1077
23. Blanchard R J W, Morrow I M, Sutherland J B 1989 Treatment of liver tumors with yttrium-90 microspheres alone. J Can Assoc Radiol 40: 206–210

60. Lymphoscintigraphy in adult malignancy

P. Bourgeois

The diagnosis of lymph node metastases is important in adult malignancies, both for the choice of therapy and for the prediction of prognosis. Generally, lymph nodes draining a tumour are removed at the same time as the primary e.g. the axillary nodes in breast cancer. However, due to the complications related to these lymphadenectomies (such as limb oedema) and the low a priori probability of lymph node invasion in several subgroups of patients, the trend in the case of several carcinomas is moving towards surgical therapies which are either more limited, or more selectively defined. On the other hand, some groups of nodes either cannot be easily investigated (the intra-thoracic and intra-abdominal) or are not usually removed at the time of surgery e.g. the internal mammary or retroparasternal nodes in breast cancer. As a result, various techniques have been developed for demonstrating those nodes which may harbour the cancer or the metastatic deposits and for diagnosing their pathological status. X-ray lymphangiography is the oldest and best-known technique in this field, but it is being used less and less. Computed tomography, ultrasonography and nuclear magnetic resonance imaging are now routinely used to demonstrate enlarged invaded nodes. Some nuclear medicine techniques (gallium scanning, immunoscintigraphy, etc.) also allow involved lymph nodes to be demonstrated specifically in the general management of several cancers. In this chapter, the applications, results and contributions of the 'classical' lymphoscintigraphies (i.e. those not using labelled antibodies) in adult malignancies will be reviewed.

The radionuclide counterpart of X-ray lymphangiography, the lymphoscintigraphic technique, represents a simple and less traumatic way of investigating the lymphatic system and evaluating lymph node status. Indeed, labelled molecules not injected intravenously in a given territory are, if of adequate size, simply removed by the lymphatic termini and drained through the lymphatic vessels towards the lymph nodes, at which point, if colloidal they are trapped, phagocytosed by the reticuloendothelial cells. From a purely anatomical point of view, the lymphatic drainage pathway(s) of a tumour can thus be easily demonstrated after peri- or intra-tumoural injection of the tracer. With regard to the lymph node stätus, the fact of their being invaded or tumourous may be suggested either when they are visible where they are expected to be present (Fig. 60.1), or when they exhibit modifications (see Fig. 60.2) of their scintigraphic aspect. Their 'normal' variation in anatomical distribution the inflammatory or fibrotic nodes represent the main causes of false positive diagnosis. Lymphoscintigraphies thus provide anatomical and diagnostic information that can be used in the management of various cancers.

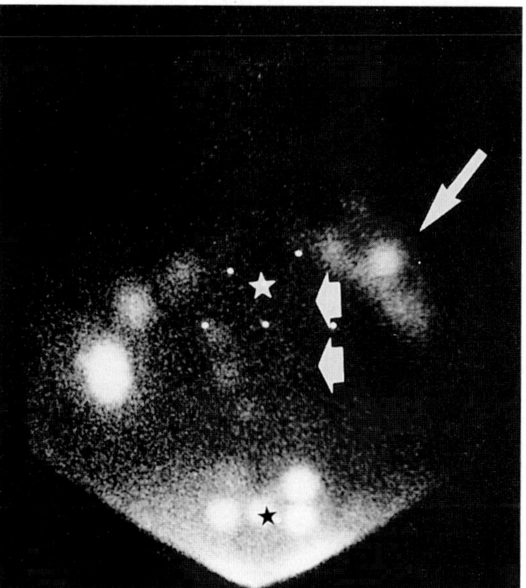

Fig. 60.1 Combined internal mammary and axillary lymphoscintigram obtained postoperatively (radical mastectomy with 'complete' axillary nodes dissection) in a patient who presented with one left mammary carcinoma (clinical Stage 2, T2N1bMO). The picture is centred on the thorax and includes both axillae. White star: sternal notch. Black star: xyphoid. No internal mammary nodes can be demonstrated left where they are expected to be visualized (thick, short arrows), which suggests the invasion of the parasternal chain. No axillary node was visualized after the intercostal injection but well after the interdigital one (oblique arrow).

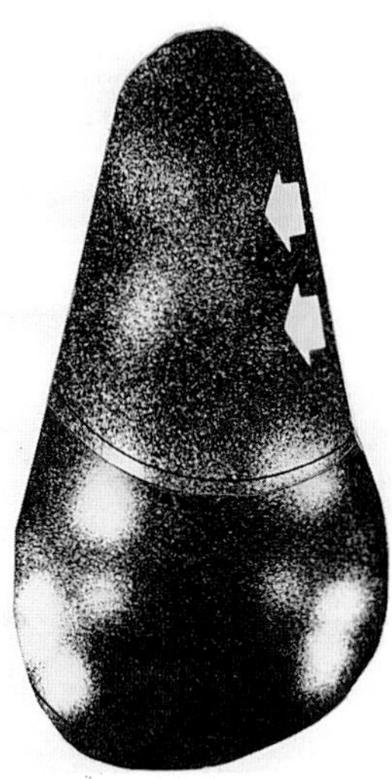

Fig. 60.2 Lower limb bipedal radionuclide lymphangiogram obtained in a patient with Hodgkin's lymphoma. Left iliac and lumboaortic nodes (thick arrows) are hypoactive when compared to the right ones. X-ray bipedal lymphangiography confirmed that they were tumorous.

LYMPHOSCINTIGRAPHIES IN BREAST CANCER (see Fig. 60.3)

In the breast, lymph – and in the case of mammary carcinoma – metastatic cells drain from all parts of the organ towards the axillary (Ax) and internal mammary (IM) nodes.[1] Whilst the former are usually removed at the same time as the mammary tumour, the latter are not. However, according to the largest series,[2–4] they are invaded in between 16.8 and 32.5% of the patients and the importance of their status for the prognosis[2,3,5,6] as well as of their adequate irradiation–treatment[7–10] has been well demonstrated.

Internal mammary lymphoscintigraphy (IMLSc)

Introduced by Schenck et al[11] and Rossi et al[12] in 1966, and further developed by Ege since 1972,[13–16] IMLSc can be considered amongst the non-traumatic investigations of these nodes,[17] as being the one which has best demonstrated its diagnostic value, its prognostic implications and its importance in X-ray treatment planning. The following published findings illustrate these features:

- The study by Matsuo[19] compares the results of preoperative IMLSc to the anatomopathologically (AP)-established status of the resected IM nodes and documents extremely well the reliability of IMLSc in predicting their neoplastic involvement: 90% true positive, 100% true negative.
- The conclusions of all large series[14–16, 19–22] using

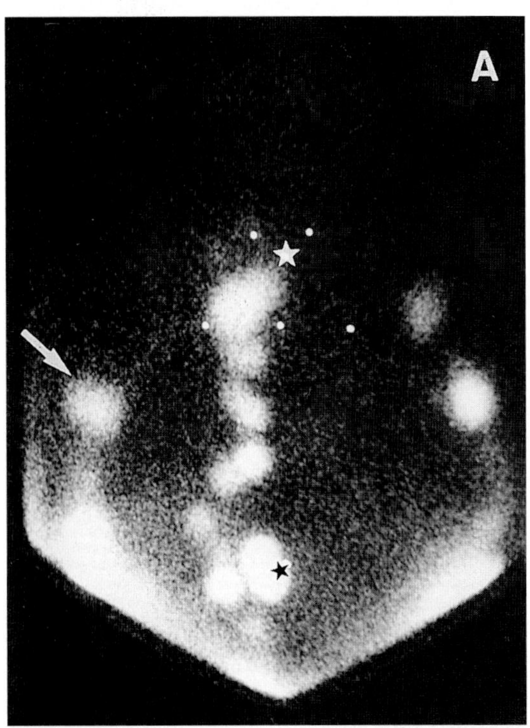

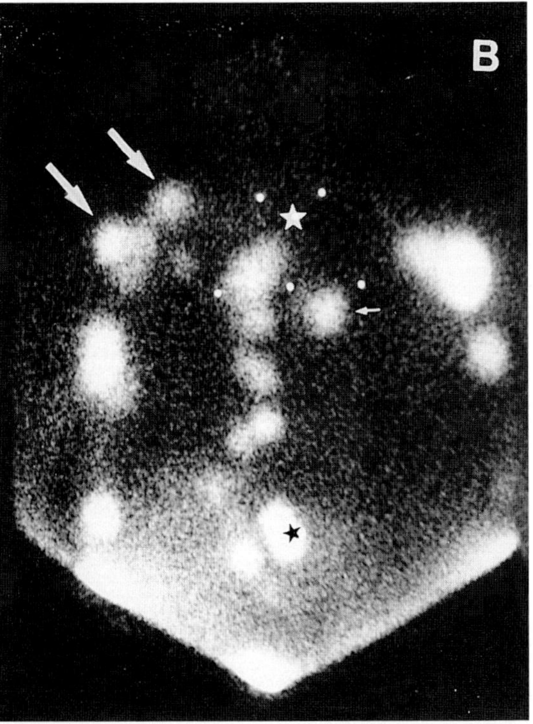

Fig. 60.3 Combined two-stage internal mammary and axillary lymphoscintographies (for the technique, see ref. 37), performed postoperatively (radical mastectomy with 'complete' axillary nodes dissection) in a patient who presented one right mammary carcinoma (clinical Stage 2, T1N1bMO). The pictures are centred on the thorax and include both axillae. White stars: sternal notch. Black stars: xyphoid. A All the right retrosternal (paramedian) internal mammary nodes are visualized from the xyphoid level to the sternal notch level. Whereas axillary lymph nodes draining the chest wall are well visualized on the left, none was theoretically to be expected from the right intercostal injection. However, at least one node (oblique arrow) can be observed. B The left internal mammary chain is now visualized (constituted by a single node (small arrow) in the second intercostal space). Additional axillary nodes are demonstrated right by the interdigital injection (oblique arrows).

IMLSc to diagnose IM node invasion (pathological findings in around 30% of the cases; percentage increasing with the stage of the tumour, its size and the extent of the disease in the axilla) which concern the previous conclusions based on surgical removal of these nodes.

- The prognostic value of a pathological IMLSc – performed pre- or post-operatively is also well established. In one population of 520 patients with no Ax node involvement, Ege and Elhakim[23] have reported 3-year relapse rates (local or distant) significantly higher in cases with pathological IMLSc (15% and 25%) than in cases with normal IMLSc (6% and 8%). Large series[14,21,24] have demonstrated that the percentage of treatment failure increases with the (AP-established) Ax node, and the (LSc-evaluated) IM status: IM-Ax- < IM+Ax- = IM-Ax+ < IM+Ax+ (see Fig. 60.4). Five-year survival rates have also been demonstrated[25] to be significantly worse in cases of pathological IMLSc than in cases of normal IMLSc, even when other prognostic factors such as clinical staging (Stage 1: 87.2% vs 98.6%, Stage 2: 70.3% vs 87.2%), clinical size (T1: 82.3% vs 96.1%, T2: 68.2% vs 86.9%) or oestrogen receptivity (48.7% vs 73.2% for ER−) are also taken into account. In a multivariate analysis of the prognostic factors for the free disease interval and the generalization performed on our population of 1154 patients with a median follow-up of 48 months, IMLSc results featured after the clinical size of the tumour and just after or with the same value as the AP Ax nodes status.[25] Consequently, it has been proposed[26] that the classical (T)N (M) staging be modified to take into account the information provided by IMLSc and not considered in several therapeutic trials, which might explain some unexpected results.
- With regard to the problems of IM node irradiation–treatments, it has been demonstrated[20,22] using IMLSc that these nodes were included within the 'classical' en-face limits of the so-called 'direct' internal mammary irradiation field in only 47% of cases. The nodes – usually retroclavicular (see Fig. 60.3) were outside the field in 34% and borderline in 19%. With regard to according to Baclesse[28] or McWhirter[29] only 78% came within the field (outside 15% – usually related to crossed drainage phenomena from one chain to the heterolateral one, or to single heterolateral IM chain – and borderline in 7%). In the case of tangential fields,[29] Recht et al[30] have also shown that the percentage of patients with at least one node missed–underdosed also varied with the medial entrance point of the field (17% if 3 cm across the midline, 34% if 2 cm, 52% if 1 cm and 80% if 0 cm) even if the nodes were within the 'en-face' limits of the field drawn on the patient. Consequently, IMLSc is currently used in order to modify and to adapt irradiation fields according to the particular anatomy of each patient.[31–33]

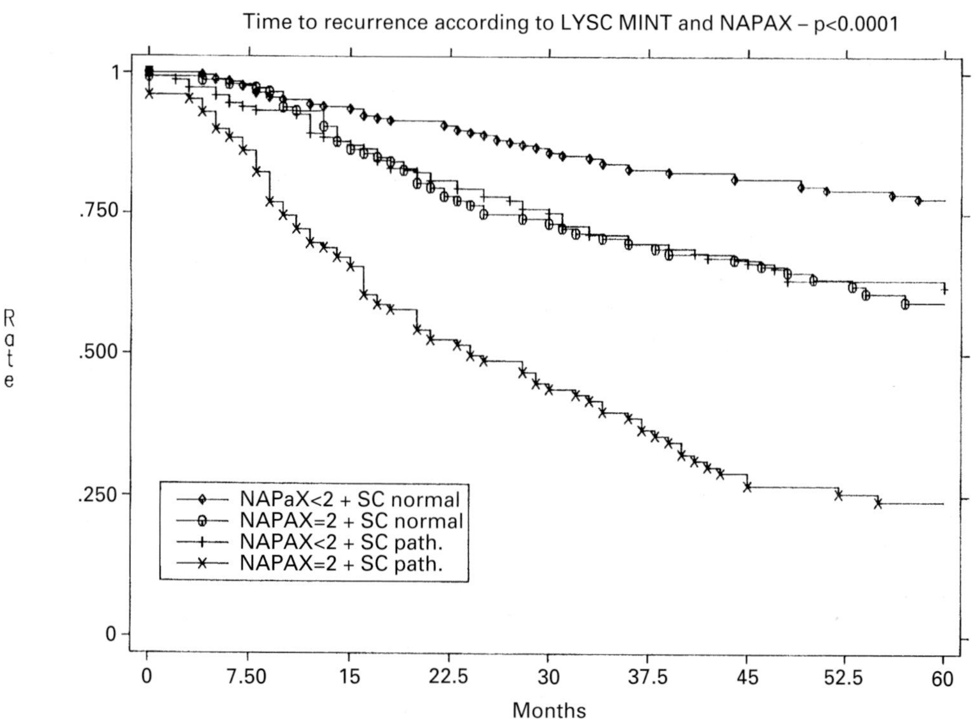

Fig. 60.4 Recurrence rate curves or free-disease interval curves according to the anatomopathologically established axillary nodes status ('NAPAX < 2' = less than 4 nodes positive, 'NAPAX = 2' = more than 3 nodes positive) and according to the result of the internal mammary scintigram (SC normal or pathological).

(Pre- and post-operative) axillary lymphoscintigraphies (AxLSc)

With regard to the Ax nodes, several techniques (depending on the site of injection: arm, intratumoural, periareolar, combined or not combined with interdigital) have been proposed for preoperative evaluation. Black et al,[34] in a study of 25 patients, reported a sensitivity of 90% and a specificity of 93%. Hill et al[35] found AxLSc accurate in 94% of the normal axillae but in only 67% of the abnormal cases. These values are the same as those of Matsuo[19] (accuracy of AxLSc = 69% if metastases were found in the axilla and = 100% if not). More interestingly (because with clear prognostic implications), Gabelle et al[36] have demonstrated in 270 patients that they found more than 3 nodes invaded in the Ax piece of dissection in 80% of the patients where preoperatively the intratumoural injection of 99mTc rhenium colloid had led to the visualization of less than 2 foci of radioactivity in the axilla (against only 15.1% of the patients with 2 or more). These results might explain the prognostic weight observed by McLean and Ege[37] for pathological AxLSc in patients with small tumours, where no axillary dissection was performed.

Used post-operatively (where it also represents a simple method of 'quality control' for surgery (see Figs 60.1 and 60.3), the two stage LSc investigations of the axilla[38–41] have proven useful in establishing the presence of residual Ax nodes draining the chest wall (in 12.5% of patients), as well as the interruption of the lymphatic drainage of the upper limb (in 40.6% of cases), these percentages varying according to the experience of the surgeon. It has indeed been demonstrated[38] that the risk of nodal relapse was higher in the former group (18% as against 5%), and that upper limb oedema occurred more frequently in the latter (24.5% as against 16%).

LYMPHOSCINTIGRAPHIES IN MELANOMAS

In these cases, lymphoscintigraphy is of limited value for the diagnosis of nodal invasion. The technique, however, has found a critical place in the management of melanomas of the head, neck and trunk because lymphatic drainage in watershed areas such as near the mid-line or near the Sappey's line can be unpredictable and may occur towards more than one adjacent group. Melanomas located on shoulders, proximal arms and lower extremities can also cause many dilemmas. For example, a tumour located on the shoulder can drain to the ipsilateral, supraclavicular or infraclavicular Ax nodes, or to some combination of the three. In such cases, LSc following peritumoural injection of the labelled tracer, permits the determination of the lymph node groups at greatest risk of harbouring metastatic deposits. In a review paper covering five series,[42] 40% of the patients exhibited lymphatic drainage towards more than one group and nodal metastases were consequently found in 26 of the 58 patients of the series in which results of the lymphadenectomies were reported. This type of preoperative LSc evaluation of lymph node groups at risk may also lead to the extension of nodal resection to more groups than expected or, on the other hand, to the limitation of dissection. In this light, Eberbach et al[43] documented lymphatic flow in 75% of the cases (18 out of 24) to more than a single adjacent predictable nodal group. As a consequence, surgical treatment was extended in 9 out of 19 cases and limited in 1. The discovery of metastatic disease in one patient was clearly attributable to LSc. More recently, Blesin et al[44] reported their experience of 124 stage II patients on whom they performed 'continuity dissection' including all scintigraphically-detected lymph vessels and lymph nodes. The survival rates of these patients (without relapse) were 93% respectively at 2 and 3 years, percentages which are higher than those found in the literature. Such a result needs confirmation, but it underlines the clinical value of scintigraphy-guided surgical treatment.

However, even if it does not lead to a more extensive nodal resection, LSc represents in all these patients a way to define the nodal group(s) at risk of relapse and requiring to be monitored during subsequent evaluations. For example, Rees et al,[44] in a large series, as well as Berqvist et al[45] in a more limited one, found no lymph node metastases during follow-up in areas other than those indicated by LSc. It has to be stressed at this point that the lymphatic drainage may vary depending on the times at which it is studied: before or just after excisional biopsy, after large resection of the tumour or after nodal resection. In the last case, collateralization pathways towards lymph node groups (other than those expected) may be observed (and have been demonstrated using LSc), which explain nodal relapses in unexpected sites.[46,47]

LYMPHOSCINTIGRAPHIES IN SUBDIAPHRAGMATIC CANCERS

From a methodological point of view, two techniques related to the sites of injection must be identified: first, the 'classical' bipedal (BP) LSc[48,49] obtained after subcutaneous injection(s) of the tracer in the feet, leading to the visualization of the femoroinguinal, external iliac, common iliac and lumboaortic nodes (see Fig. 60.2), and, secondly, the 'ilio-pelvic' (IP) LSc obtained after intraprostatic,[50–52] perianal (or ischiorectal) or paracervical injections,[53–59] which facilitates investigation of the internal iliac, common iliac, sacral, pararectal and lumboaortic nodes. These two techniques, which have been combined by several authors, are discussed in detail in Chapter 33.

In non-lymphomatous diseases,[48,53–59] the reported

sensitivities and specifities are highly variable (from 62% to 100% and from 46% to 83% respectively), depending on the technique(s) used and the site(s) of injections as well as the kind and stage of tumours studied. However, it has to be noted that Feigen et al[58] found IP LSc more sensitive but less specific than X-ray lymphangiography or computed tomography.

In lymphomatous diseases, BPLSc has been compared to its radiological counterpart and to lymph node biopsies.[49,55] The reported percentage agreement or predictive value were respectively 80%–84% and 88%–91% for positive scans and 64% and 57% for negative ones. In his biopsy-proven series, Glassburn et al[49] also reported a 91% sensitivity for BPLSc (39 out of 43) and noted only 1 false positive scan in 9 negative X-ray lymphangiograms.

LYMPHOSCINTOGRAPHY AND SURGERY OR LYMPHOSCINTIGRAPHY-ASSISTED SURGERY?

Lymphoscintigraphies have also been used to demonstrate, preoperatively, the nodes to be resected. In cases of carcinomas of the cervix uteri, Gitsch et al,[60] performing lymphadenectomies under the gamma-camera control of the lymph nodes to be removed (and visualized after injection of labelled colloids in the second and third interdigital space of the feet) showed that they increased their rate of lymphadenectomy with an increased survival rate at 3 years as a consequence. Such 'intra-operative lymph node imaging' has also been used successfully in the surgical treatment of breast cancer and of testicular cancer.[62]

MISCELLANEOUS

Contributions from lymphoscintigraphic investigations have also been reported in cases of head and neck carcinomas,[64,65] lung[65–67] and pleural[65] carcinomas and of testicular carcinomas.[68]

CONCLUSIONS

Lymphoscintigraphies in adult malignancies represent a simple and relatively nontraumatic way of demonstrating which lymph nodes are at risk of harbouring tumours or metastatic deposits. They can be used either by the surgeon or by the radiotherapist to evaluate their treatments or to modify them. They allow the diagnosis of lymph node involvement and have demonstrated their prognostic value in several cancers. They can also be used to define the nodes at risk of nodal relapse.

REFERENCES

1. Hultborn R A, Larsson L G, Ragnhult I 1955 The lymph drainage from the breast to the axillary and parasternal lymph nodes studied with the aid of colloidal 198Au. Acta Radiol 43: 52–64
2. Haagensen C D 1969 Metastasis of carcinoma of the breast to the periphery of lymph nodes filter. Ann Surg 169: 174–190
3. Urban J A, Marjani M A 1971 Significance of internal mammary lymph node metastases in breast cancer. AJR III: 130–136
4. Morrow M, Foster R S 1981 Staging of breast cancer: a new rationale for internal mammary node biopsy. Arch Surg 116: 748–751
5. Livingston S F, Arlen M 1974 The extended extrapleural radical mastectomy: its role in the treatment of carcinoma of the breast. Ann Surg 179: 260–265
6. Veronesi U, Cascinelli N, Greco M et al 1985 Prognosis of breast cancer patients after mastectomy and dissection of internal mammary nodes. Ann Surg 202: 702–707
7. Fletcher G H, Montague E D 1978 Does adequate irradiation of the internal mammary chain and supraclavicular nodes improve survival rates? Int J Radiation Oncol Biol Phys 4: 481–492
8. Strender L E, Wallgren A, Arndt J, Arner O, Bergström J, Blomstedtt B, Granberg P O, Nilsson B, Räf L, Silfverswärd C 1981 Adjuvant radiotherapy in operable breast cancer. Correlation between dose in internal mammary nodes and prognosis. Int J Radiat Oncol Biol Phys 7: 1319–1325
9. Lê M G, Arriagada R, De Vathaire F, Dewar J, Fontaine F, Lacour J, Contesso G, Tubiana M 1990 Can internal mammary chain treatment decrease the risk of death in patients with medial breast cancers and positive axillary lymph nodes? Cancer 66: 2313–2318
10. Arrigada R, Lê M G, Mouriesse H et al 1988 Long term effect of internal mammary chain treatment. Results of a multivariate analysis of 1195 patients with operable breast cancer and positive axillary nodes. Radiother Oncol 11: 213–222
11. Schenck P, Zum Winkel K, Becker J 1966 Die szintigraphie des parasternalen lymphsystems. Nucl Med 5: 388–396
12. Rossi R, Ferry O, Trevellini G 1966 Etude de la chaine lymphatique mammaire interne par 198Au colloidal. J Chir 95: 79–96
13. Ege G N 1976 Internal mammary lymphoscintigraphy. Radiology 118: 101–107
14. Ege G N 1978 Internal mammary lymphoscintigraphy: a rationale adjunct to the staging management of breast carcinoma. Clin Radiol 29: 453–456
15. Ege G E, Clarek R M 1980 Internal mammary lymphoscintigraphy in the conservative surgical management of breast carcinoma. Clin Radiol 31: 559–563
16. Ege G N 1983 Lymphoscintigraphy: techniques and applications in the management of breast carcinoma. Semin Nucl Med XIII: 26–33
17. Turoglu H T, Janjan N A, Thorsen M K et al 1992 Imaging of regional spread of breast cancer by internal mammary lymphoscintigraphy, CT and MRI. Clin Nucl Med 17: 482–484
18. Bourgeois P, Fruhling J, Henry J 1983 Postoperative axillary lymphoscintigraphy in the management of breast cancer. Int J Radiat Oncol Biol Phys 9: 29–32
19. Matsuo S 1974 Studies of the metastasis of breast cancer to lymph nodes – II Diagnosis of metastasis to internal mammary nodes using radiocolloid. Acta Medica Okayama 28: 361–371
20. Bourgeois P, Fruhling J 1980 Internal mammary lymphoscintigraphy in the diagnosis and treatment of breast cancer. J Belge Radiol 63: 669–677
21. Bourgeois P, Fruhling J 1983 Internal mammary lymphoscintigraphy: current status in the treatment of breast cancer. CRC Crit Rev Oncol Hematol 1: 21–47
22. Ege G N 1980 Radiocolloid lymphoscintigraphy in neoplastic disease. Cancer Res 40: 3065–3071
23. Ege G N, Elhakim T 1984 The relevance of internal mammary lymphoscintigraphy in the management of breast carcinoma. J Clin Oncol 7: 774–781
24. Casara D, Rubello D, Saladini G, Masarotto G, Calzavara F 1993 Significance of internal mammary lymphoscintigraphy in clinical staging and prognosis of breast cancer. Eur J Lymphol Rel Prob 3: 103–109
25. Bourgeois P, Fruhling J Internal mammary lymphoscintigraphy in the prognosis of breast cancer: a multivariate analysis (in press)

26. Ege G N, Clark R M 1985 Internal mammary lymphoscintigraphy in the conservative management of breast carcinoma: an update and recommendations for a new TNM staging. Clin Radiol 36: 469–472
27. Bourgeois P, Fruhling J, Piron A, Renaud A, Henry J 1980 The role of internal mammary lymphoscintigraphy in the management of breast cancer. J Nucl Med 21: 496–497
28. Baclesse F 1949 Roentgen therapy as the sole method of treatment of cancer of the breast. AJR 62: 311–319
29. McWhirter R 1948 The value of simple mastectomy and radiotherapy in the treatment of cancer of the breast. Br J Radiol 21: 599–617
30. Recht A, Siddon R L, Kaplan W D, Andersen J W, Harris J H 1988 Three-dimensional internal mammary lymphoscintigraphy: implications for radiation therapy treatment planning for breast cancer. Int J Radiat Oncol Biol Phys 14: 477–481
31. Rose C M, Kaplan W D, Marck A, Bloomer W D, Hellman S 1979 Parasternal lymphoscintigraphy: implications for the treatment planning of internal mammary nodes in breast cancer. Int J Radiat Oncol Biol Phys 5: 1849–1853
32. Hoefnagel C A, Bartelink H, Heidendal-Jeune M, Marcuse H R 1982 Internal mammary lymphoscintigraphy for radiation therapy planning breast carcinoma. J Eur Radiother 3: 35–42
33. Hunt M A, Shank B S, McCormick B, Yahalom J, Graham M, Jutcher G J 1989 The use of lymphoscintigraphy in treatment planning of primary breast cancer. Int J Radiat Oncol Biol Phys 17: 597–606
34. Black R B, Merrick M V, Taylor T V 1980 Prediction of axillary metastases in breast cancer by lymphoscintigraphy. Lancet 2: 15–17
35. Hill N S, Ege G N, Greyson N D et al 1983 Predicting by lymphoscintigraphy of nodal metastases in breast cancer. Can J Surg 26: 507–509
36. Gabelle P, Comet M, Bouchet Y 1984 Lymphocintigraphie mammaire préopératoire dans le cancer du sein (abstract). 1st Congress of the European Lymphology Group, Brussels, 1984
37. McLean R G, Ege G N 1986 Prognostic value of axillary lymphoscintigraphy in breast carcinoma patients. J Nucl Med 27: 1116–1124
38. Fruhling J, Bourgeois P, Mattheiem W 1982 Postoperative axillary lymphoscintigraphy: a qualitative approach of modified radical mastectomy (abstract). 1st Congress of the European Society of Surgical Oncology, Athens, 1982
39. Mattheiem W, Bourgeois P, Delcorde A, Stegen M, Fruhling J 1989 Axillary dissection in breast cancer revisited. Eur J Surg Oncol 15: 490–495
40. Fruhling J, Bourgeois P 1983 Axillary lymphoscintigraphy: current status in the treatment of breast cancer. CRC Crit Rev Oncol Hematol 1: 1–20
41. Bennet L R, Lago G 1983 Cutaneous lymphoscintigraphy in malignant melanoma. Semin Nucl Med 13: 61–69
42. Blesin H J, Buchali K, Winter H, Schürer M 1990 Lymph drainage scintigraphy in malignant melanoma: evaluation of clinical efficiency. Eur J Lymphol Rel Prob 1: 41–43
43. Eberbach M A, Wahl R L, Argenta L C, Froelich J, Niederhuber J E 1987 Utility of lymphoscintigraphy in directing surgical therapy for melanomas of the head, neck and upper thorax. Surgery 102: 433–442
44. Rees W V, Robinson D S, Holmes E C, Morton D L 1980 Altered lymphatic drainage following lymphadenectomy. Cancer 45: 3045–3049
45. Berqvist L, Strand S E, Hafström L, Jönsson P E 1984 Lymphoscintigraphy in patients with malignant melanoma: a quantitative and qualitative evaluation of its usefelness. Eur J Nucl Med 9: 129–135
46. Hoefnagel C A, Jonk A, Kroon B B R 1989 Contralateral lymph node metastasis in patients with melanoma of the lower extremity: a lymphoscintigraphic explanation (abstract). J Nucl Med 30: 912
47. Gest J, Debouche F 1963 Die indirekte lymphographie met radioaktieven isotopen. J Radiol 44: 86–90
48. Glassburn J R, Prasha-Svinichia S, Nuss R C, Croll M N, Brady L W 1972 Correlation of 198Au abdominal lymph scan with lymphangiograms and lymph node biopsies. Radiology 105: 93–97
49. Collette J M, Darras T, Bourgeois P, Lardinois J, Peetroons P, Dondelinger R F, Kurdziel J C 1988 Imagerie actuelle du système lymphatique. Encycl Méd Chir (Paris, France) Radiodiagnostic III, 32290 A10, 2-1988, 22 pp
50. Stone A R, Merrickx M V, Chisholm G D 1979 Prostatic lymphoscintigraphy. Br J Urol 51: 556–560
51. Zuckier L S, Finkelstein M, Stone F, Freed S Z, Bard R, Blaufox M D, Freeman L M 1986 Tc99m antimony sulfide colloid lymphoscintigraphy of the prostate by direct transrectal injection (abstract). J Nucl Med 27: 1034
52. Horenblas S, Nuyten M J, Hoefnagel C A, Moonen L M, Delemarre J F 1992 Detection of lymph node invasion in prostatic carcinoma with iliopelvic lymphoscintigraphy. Br J Urol 69: 180–182
53. Ege G N, Cummings B J 1980 Interstitial iliopelvic lymphoscintigraphy: technique, anatomy and clinical applications. Int J Radiat Oncol Biol Phys 6: 1483–1490
54. Ege G N 1982 Augmented ilio-pelvic lymphoscintigraphy: application in the management of genito-urinary malignancy. J Urol 127: 265–269
55. Croll M N, Brady L W, Dadparvar S 1983 Implications of lymphoscintigraphy in oncologic practice: principles and differencies vis-a-vis other imaging modalities. Semin Nucl Med 13: 4–8
56. Bloomer W D 1983 Lymphoscintigraphy in gynecologic malignancies. Semin Nucl Med 13: 54–60
57. Kaplan D W 1983 Iliopelvic lymphoscintigraphy. Semin Nucl Med 13: 42–53
58. Feigen M, Crocker E F, Read J, Crandon A J 1987 The value of lymphoscintigraphy, lymphangiography and computer tomography scanning in the preoperative assessment of lymph nodes involved by pelvic malignant conditions. Surg Gynecol Obstet 105: 107–112
59. Demirkiran F, Cepni I, Önsel C et al 1993 Preoperative assessment of lymph nodes metastases in gynecologic malignancies by pelvic lymphoscintigraphy. Eur J Lymphol Rel Prob 3 (in press)
60. Gitsch E, Philipp K, Pateisky N 1984 Intraopeartive lymph scintigraphy during radical surgery for cervical cancer. J Nucl Med 25: 486–489
61. Gitsch E, Philipp K, Kubista E 1983 Die intraoperative lymphszintigraphie bei der radikaloperation des Mamma-karzinomas. Geburtshilfe Frauenheilkd 43: 112–115
62. Kuber W, Leodolster S 1980 Radioisotopenlymphonodektomie bei malignen hodentumoren. Urologe A 19: 25–31
63. Munz D L, Jung H 1985 Peritumoral interstitial double-nuclide double-compound lymphoscintigraphy (PIDDL) in squamous cell carcinoma of the oral cavity. J Nucl Med 26: 65
64. Jackson B S, Rosenthall L, Attia E 1981 Laryngeal lymphoscintigraphy. Laryngoscope 91: 2085–2088
65. Bourgeois P 1981 Internal mammary lymphoscintigraphy in lung and pleural carcinomas (abstract). VIIIth Congress of the International Society of Lymphology, 1981
66. Andrieu M, Boneu A, Carles P, Lenot H, Combes P F, Bollinelli R. La lymphoscintigraphie médiastinale indirecte: note préliminaire. Nouv Presse Méd 10: 2989–2990
67. Bethune D C, Mulder D S, Chiu R C 1978 Endobronchial lymphoscintigraphy (EBLS): new diagnostic modality. J Thorac Cardiovasc Surg 76: 446–452
68. Spaventi S, Agbaba M, Bosnar M, Paic G, Keros P 1979 Selective scintigraphic lymphography of the testis. Nukl Med 2: 148–153

61. Marrow scintigraphy

S. N. Reske

ANATOMY OF NORMAL BONE MARROW

The tissue mass of normal bone marrow in the adult is 1600–3600 g (mean 2700 g).[1] One-half of this is haematopoietic marrow, the other half being mostly fat or yellow marrow.[1] Blood is supplied to the bone from nutrient arteries and from a periosteal capillary network which feeds blood into venous sinuses. These are drained into a large central venous vessel.[2] In the endothelial cells lining the myeloid sinuses there are randomly distributed small fenestrations which are spanned by diaphragms.[2] These are sites at which particulate material or macromolecules may penetrate the endothelial lining more easily. There is no distinct basal lamina beneath the sinuses. With positron emission tomography marrow blood flow was measured at 10.0 ml/min 1 ± 3.0 (SD) cm^3 in controls and was shown to be markedly elevated in polycythaemia vera, myelofibrosis and chronic granulocytic leukaemia.[3]

RADIOPHARMACEUTICALS

Based on the target cell system, bone marrow scintigraphy may be divided into three categories: imaging of (a) erythropoietic precursor cells, (b) the reticulohistiocytic system (RHS);[4] and (c) granulopoietic bone marrow.[5]

Iron-52 is used for erythropoietic marrow imaging and ^{99m}Tc-labelled colloids for RHS imaging. The exact target cells of indium-111 have not been identified[4] and its use as a marrow imaging agent will not be discussed. Recently ^{99m}Tc-labelled monoclonal antibodies (^{99m}Tc-MAb) directed against non-specific cross-reacting antigen 95 (NCA-95), a differentiation antigen of granulopoiesis,[6] have been developed and clinically applied for imaging granulopoietic marrow in man.[5]

Using ^{99m}TcMAb bone marrow scans of improved quality without significant superposition of liver or spleen radioactivity have been obtained.[5,7] ^{99m}Tc-MAb uptake in haematopoietic marrow was 2–4 times higher than that of ^{99m}Tc microcolloid.[8] Healthy controls consistently showed scans of excellent image quality with homogeneous tracer uptake in haematopoietic bone marrow (Fig. 61.1).

EXAMINATION TECHNIQUE AND SCAN EVALUATION

400–740 MBq of ^{99m}Tc microcolloid or ^{99m}Tc-MAb is injected intravenously.[9,10] Whole-body or overlapping gamma-camera spot views are obtained, beginning 20–

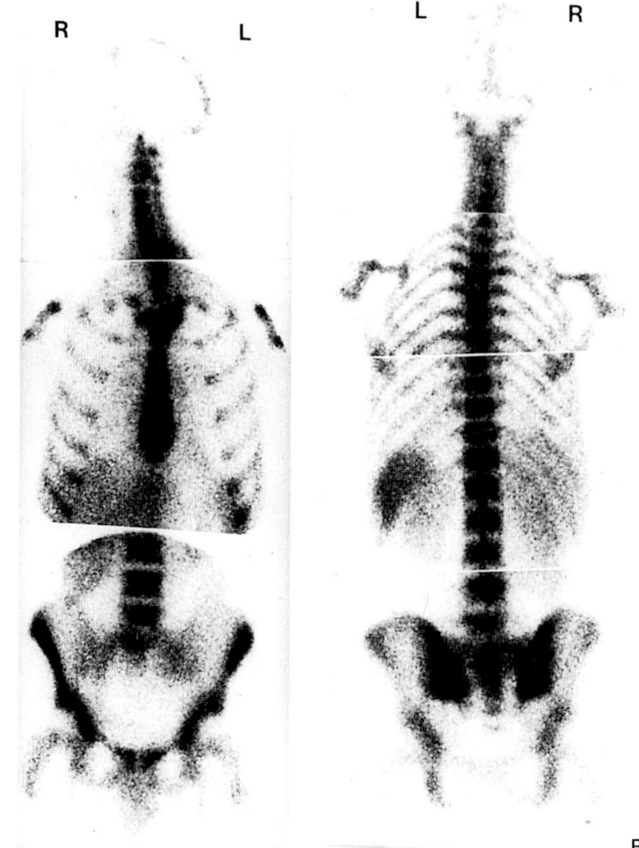

Fig. 61.1 Normal bone marrow immunoscan with ^{99m}Tc-MAb: anterior (A) and posterior (B) views.

Table 61.1 Radiation exposure of ^{99m}Tc-labelled microcolloids and anti-granulocytic anti-myelocytic antibodies (mGy/MBq)

	Microcolloid	Antibody
Red marrow	0.015	0.029
Liver	0.07	0.022
Spleen	0.07	0.029
Effective dose	0.014	0.005
Equivalent (mSv/MBq)		

30 min after injection for microcolloid scans or 3–4 h post injection for immunoscans of bone marrow. The scans are evaluated for homogeneity and intensity of radioactivity uptake in normally haematopoietic marrow-containing structures, the presence and extent of peripheral marrow expansion, central marrow depletion and focal marrow defects.

CLINICAL APPLICATIONS

Bone marrow scintigraphy has been mostly used for evaluating the presence and extent of bone marrow involvement in circulatory, inflammatory and haematological diseases and in malignant infiltration originating from multiple myeloma, Hodgkin's disease, non-Hodgkin's lymphoma and various carcinomas (Table 61.2).

Circulatory marrow disorders

Bone marrow scanning with radiocolloids has been used in conjunction with bone scanning and/or gallium-67 scanning to differentiate infarct from osteomyelitis.[11]

Table 61.2 Clinical applications of bone marrow scanning

Circulatory disorders
Marrow infarct
Avascular necrosis of the hip
Inflammation
Spondylitis
Spondylodiscitis
Osteomyelitis
AIDS
Blood and lymphoid organs
Polycythaemia vera
Myelofibrosis, osteomyelosclerosis
Aplastic anaemia and myelodysplastic syndromes
Haemolytic anaemias
Leukaemias
Multiple myeloma
Hodgkin's disease and non-Hodgkin's lymphomas
Metastases
Breast
Prostate
Lung
Kidney and bladder
Others
Miscellaneous
Post-irradiation fibrosis
Psoriasis
Progressive systemic sclerosis

Marrow infarcts are characterized by concordant defects on marrow and bone or gallium-67 scans. Osteomyelitis can be identified by combined sequential marrow and bone scanning within 6 days after the onset of acute clinical symptoms:[12] in active osteomyelitis, the marrow scan may be normal or show decreased radiocolloid uptake, whereas bone scans reveal increased tracer uptake in the same skeletal region.[12,13] Similarly, gallium-67 uptake is incongruently increased in osteomyelitis at the symptomatic site.[11] Follow-up bone marrow studies in asymptomatic patients with old marrow infarcts may show normalization of marrow defects after several months, indicating repopulation of active bone marrow.[14]

Bone marrow scanning has traditionally been used for detecting *avascular necrosis of the hip*.[4] Asymmetric radiocolloid uptake in the femoral heads, however, was observed in about 45% of adult patients,[15,16] posing a significant diagnostic dilemma.

INFLAMMATION

^{99m}Tc microcolloids and Tc-MAb have been used for localization and assessment of activity of skeletal inflammatory diseases. The mechanisms involved are microcolloid extravasation and, conceivably, phagocytosis by tissue macrophages or in vivo labelling of granulocytes infiltrating the inflammatory sites.[17,18]

For the differential diagnosis of marrow defects, it is worthwhile noting that subacute and chronic spondylitis as well as spondylodiscitis usually cause clearly defined radiocolloid or Tc-MAb marrow uptake defects in the corresponding vertebral bodies or the vertebrae adjacent to the inflamed intervertebral disc.[19]

HAEMATOLOGICAL DISORDERS

In the early stages of *polycythaemia vera* bone marrow scans generally may be normal. This has been found with iron-52 and PET,[20] radiocolloids[4] and ^{99m}Tc-MAb. Peripheral expansion may be noted in patients with active disease (Fig. 61.2). ^{99m}Tc-MAb uptake in the spleen is moderately increased. This is probably related to myeloid metaplasia of the red pulp (neoplastic extramedullary haematopoiesis)[1]. Progression to myelofibrosis and myeloid metaplasia is associated with peripheral expansion.[4,21]

Myelofibrosis shows trilineage hyperplasia, reactive marrow fibrosis (myelofibrosis) and prominent myeloid metaplasia, which includes the spleen, liver and lymph nodes.[1] It involves particularly the central flat and proximal long bones. Osteosclerosis, i.e. thickening of bony trabeculae, may be present.[1] Normal radiocolloid marrow scans are observed in the early stages, but usually show massive spleen and moderate liver enlargement and

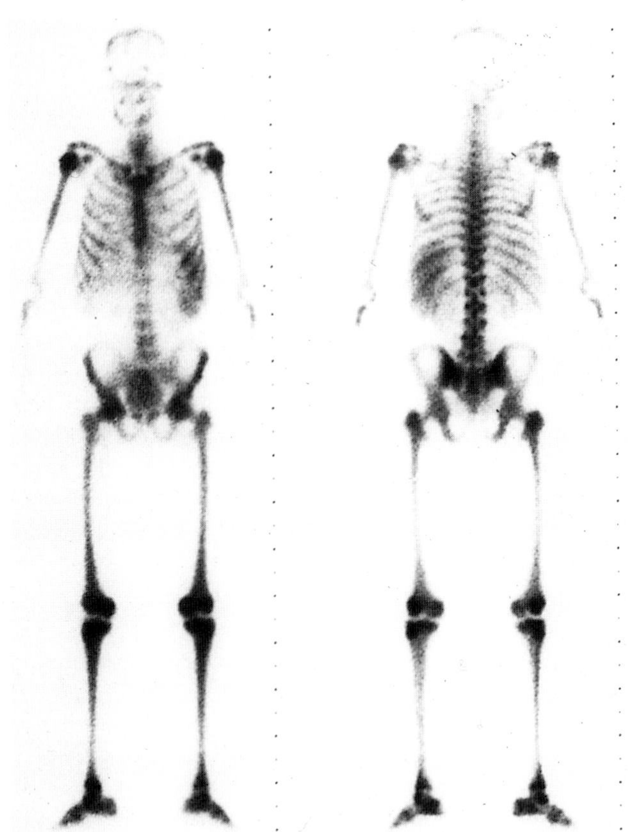

Fig. 61.2 Marked peripheral bone marrow expansion in polycythaemia vera.

peripheral expansion. Deficient radiocolloid marrow uptake is found in advanced osteomyelosclerosis.

Using ^{99m}Tc-MAb marrow and bone scans, a nearly pathognomonic scan pattern was observed in our laboratory in osteomyelosclerosis: the bone scan showed a pattern similar to a superscan with diffusely increased tracer uptake probably related to osteosclerosis and virtually lacking visualization of the kidneys. The antibody marrow scan demonstrated decreased or, in advanced stages, even deficient central activity, marked peripheral expansion and massively increased uptake in the spleen, probably related to extramedullary haematopoiesis.[22]

In *aplastic anaemia*, hypocellularity of the bone marrow is reflected by a highly reduced or virtually deficient marrow uptake of any marrow scanning agent.[4]

Myelodysplastic syndromes are characterized by ineffective haematopoiesis or increased intramedullary destruction of mature haematopoietic cells.[1] We have observed in this entity generalized diffusely distributed small, focal defects on ^{99m}Tc-MAb bone marrow scans without indication of extramedullary haematopoiesis or peripheral expansion.

As pointed out by Datz & Taylor,[4] marrow scans are usually normal in acute *haemolytic disorders*, whereas peripheral expansion is found in chronic haemolytic states.

In *multiple myeloma*, most authors have found peripheral expansion on radiocolloid marrow scans.[23] Focal defects in the axial skeleton have been observed in 40–50% of patients. Using ^{99m}Tc-MAb as marrow scanning agent, the author's group observed bone marrow expansion in 6 of 10 patients and focal defects also in 60%. Marrow scanning revealed in these patients a significantly more extended skeletal involvement as compared with bone scanning (19.7% *vs.* 4.7%, *P*<0.001).

In *leukaemia*, especially in acute disease, highly variable scan patterns have been observed.[4,21] Most authors found peripheral expansion. Occasionally, generalized reduced or deficient radiocolloid marrow uptake and focal defects have been noted in acute and chronic myeloid or lymphatic leukaemia.

Bone marrow involvement is found in *Hodgkin's disease* in about 10% of patients.[1] Focal, multifocal or diffuse infiltration of bone marrow may be observed.

In *Non-Hodgkin's lymphoma (NHL)* bone marrow involvement depends on the cell type, being 50–70% in the small cleaved type and 5–10% in the large cell type in the bone marrow. The initial involvement is usually focal, but multifocal or diffuse patterns with marrow replacement may be seen.[1] Bone marrow expansion has been observed on microcolloid scans in 33–81% of patients, with Hodgkin's disease as well as NHL.[23] Focal lesions were found in 19–90%. Occasional central marrow depletion or even deficient marrow radiocolloid uptake has been reported during the fulminant course of high-grade NHL. Linden et al[24] found a sensitivity of 50% with the marrow scan in Hodgkin's disease, 75% in high-grade NHL and 30% in low-grade NHL using iliac crest biopsy as gold standard. However, a significant sampling error in the blind biopsy must be considered. Thus, the ultimate

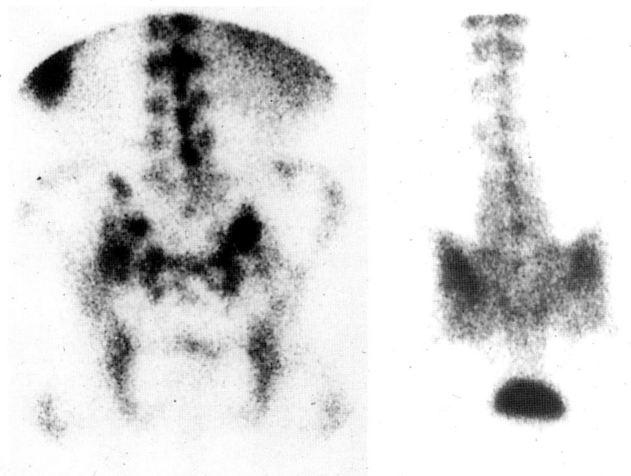

Fig. 61.3 Bone marrow infiltration due to NHL. The lower lumbar spine and pelvis are shown in posterior views. The marrow immunoscan (A) shows multiple marrow defects, verified by bone marrow biopsy, whereas the bone scan (B) is essentially normal.

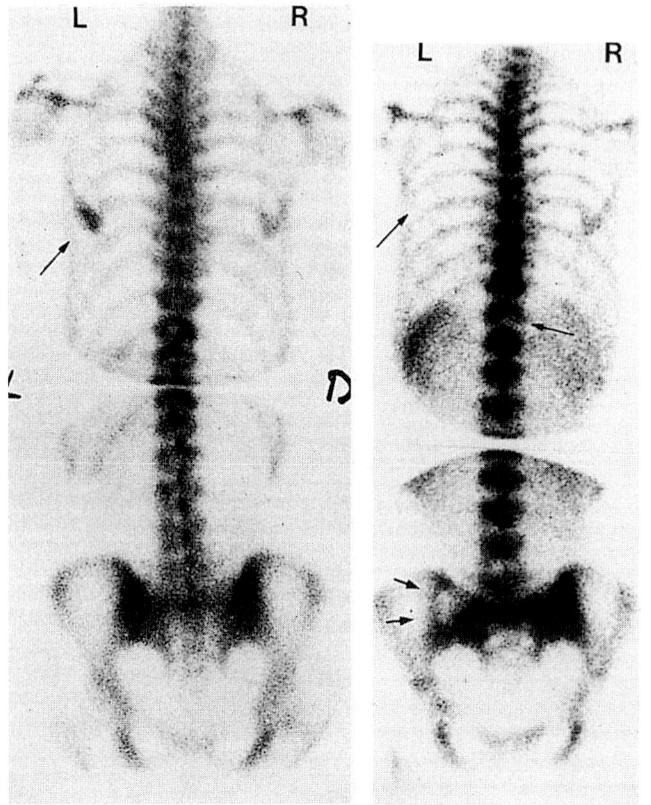

Fig. 61.4 Bone marrow metastases due to breast carcinoma. Bone (A) and marrow immunoscan (B) of the axial skeleton in posterior view are shown. A large lytic lesion in the left pelvis is demonstrated on the marrow scan (double arrow and a minor lesion in T11 (arrow) with normal findings on the bone scan. Concordant lesion in left scapula.

value of bone marrow scanning in malignant lymphoma may be higher than currently appreciated. In support of this view, when comparing ^{99m}Tc-MAb marrow scanning with iliac or sternal marrow biopsy or aspiration cytology, positive concordance in 14 of 36 patients with malignant lymphoma was observed, and negative concordance in 17.[23] ^{99m}Tc-MAb scans showed more widespread involvement of the skeletal system than bone scanning in these patients (39% *vs.* 10.6% of the skeleton) (Fig. 61.3).

METASTATIC TUMOURS

The bone marrow is a frequent site of metastatic tumours. About 90% of metastases develop in the distribution of the haematopoietic bone marrow. Metastases below the elbows and knees are distinctly uncommon.

Focal marrow defects are the major criterion for detecting skeletal metastases.[23] Marrow expansion was observed in 75.6% of patients with and in 50% of patients without skeletal metastases.[25] The sensitivity of marrow scanning for detecting skeletal metastases in breast cancer was 80.5%;[25] the negative predictive value in this study was 91%. False-negative findings were reported in locations devoid of haematopoietic marrow after irradiation and due to superposition of radiocolloid uptake in the liver and spleen.[25]

In patients with carcinoma of the breast, prostate, lung, kidney or bladder significantly more lesions compared with skeletal scintigraphy were observed[23] (Fig. 61.4). Duncker et al[26] concluded that marrow scanning with ^{99m}Tc-MAb is a sensitive method for the early detection of bone invasion in these patients.

Occasionally, general marrow carcinosis is observed on marrow scans of patients with virtually normal bone scans.[23]

MISCELLANEOUS

Clearly defined tracer uptake defects with sharp borders in haematopoietic bone marrow are found at the radiation ports after irradiation. Peripheral marrow expansion and central depletion have been reported in psoriasis and progressive systemic sclerosis respectively. Failure of radiocolloid marrow uptake is occasionally observed in association with concomitant chemotherapy.[21]

REFERENCES

1. Bonner H 1988 The blood and the lymphoid organs. In: Rubin E, Farber J L (eds) Pathology. Lippincott, Philadelphia, p 1014
2. De Bruyn P P H 1981 Structural substrates to bone marrow function. Semin Hematol 18: 179
3. Martiat P H, Ferrant A, Cogneau M et al 1987 Assessment of bone marrow blood flow using positron emission tomography: no relationship with marrow cellularity. Br J Haematol 66: 307
4. Datz F L, Taylor Jr A 1985 The clinical use of radionuclide bone marrow imaging. Semin Nucl Med XV: 239
5. Reske S N, Karstens J H, Glöckner W, Schwarz A, Steinsträsser A, Ammon J, Büll U 1989 Radioimmunoimaging of bone marrow. Results in patients with breast cancer and skeletal metastases and patients with malignant lymphomas. Lancet 2: 299
6. Wahren B, Gahrton G, Hammerstroem S 1980 Non-specific cross-reacting antigen in normal and myeloid cells and serum of leukemic patients. Cancer Res 40: 2039
7. Reske S N, Sohn M, Karstens J H, Bares R, Buell U 1990 Immunoscintigraphy of bone marrow with Tc-99m labelled NCA-95/CEA antibodies (TcNCAA). Comparison with bone scanning, plain radiographs and HAMA-response (abstract). J Nucl Med 31: 751
8. Munz D L, Sandrock D, Rilinger N 1990 Comparison of immunoscintigraphy and colloid scintigraphy of bone marrow (letter). Lancet 1: 258
9. Hotze A, Loew A, Mahlstedt J, Wolf F 1984 Kombinierte Knochenmark- und Skelettszintigraphie bei ossaeren und myelogenen Erkrankungen. Fortschr Roentgenstr 140: 717
10. Hotze A, Mahlstedt F, Wolf F 1984 Bone marrow imaging. Technique, findings, interpretation. GIT Ernst Giebeler, Darmstadt
11. Kahn C E, Ryan J W, Hatfield M K, Martin W B 1988 Combined bone marrow and gallium imaging. Differentiation of osteomyelitis and infarction in sickle cell hemoglobinopathy. Clin Nucl Med 13: 443
12. Kim H C, Alavi A, Russel M O, Schwartz E 1989 Differentiation of bone and bone marrow infarcts from osteomyelitis in sickle cell disorders. Clin Nucl Med 14: 249

13. Southee A E, Lee K J, Rossleigh M A, Morris J G 1988 Extensive pelvic infarction diagnosed by radionuclide skeletal and bone marrow imaging. Clin Nucl Med 13: 613
14. Alavi A, Heyman S, Kim H C 1987 Scintigraphic examination of bone and marrow infarcts in sickle cell disorders. Semin Roentgenol 12: 213
15. Munz D L, Hör G 1983 Symmetric visualization of femoral heads in reticuloendothelial bone marrow scanning in adults: correlation with peripheral expansion of the bone marrow organ. Eur J Nucl Med 8: 109
16. Spencer R P, Lee Y S, Sziklas J J, Rosenberg R J, Krimeddini M K 1983 Failure of uptake of radiocolloids by the femoral heads: diagnostic problem (concise communication). J Nucl Med 24: 116
17. De Schrijver M, Streule K, Senekovitch R, Fridrich R 1987 Scintigraphy of inflammation with nanometer-sized coloidal tracers. Nucl Med Commun 8: 895
18. Joseph K, Höffken H, Bosslet K, Schorlemmer H U 1988 In vivo labelling of granulocytes with Tc-99m anti-NCA monoclonal antibodies for imaging inflammation. Eur J Nucl Med 14: 367
19. Reske S N, Zillkens K M, Glöckner M W, Buell U 1989 Localisation of subacute and chronic inflammatory lesions by means of Tc-99m labelled murine monoclonal anti-NCA-antibodies (abstract). J Nucl Med 30: 797
20. Ferrant A, Rodhain J, Leners N, Cogneau M, Verwilghen R L, Michaux J L, Sokal G 1985 Quantitative assessment of erythropoiesis in bone marrow expansion areas using Fe-52. Br J Hematol 62: 247
21. Munz D L 1984 Knochenmarkszintigraphie: Grundlagen und klinische Ergebnisse. Der Nuklearmediziner 4: 251
22. Reske S N, Grimmel S, Buell U 1991 Typical bone and bone marrow scan pattern in osteomyelofibrosis. (abstract 747). J Nucl Med 32: 1085
23. Reske S N 1991 Recent advances in bone marrow scanning. Europ J Nucl Med 18: 203–221
24. Linden A, Zankovitch R, Theissen P, Diehl V, Schicha H 1989 Malignant lymphoma: bone marrow imaging versus biopsy. Radiology 173: 335
25. Bourgeois P, Gassavelis C, Malarme M, Feremans W, Frühling J 1989 Bone marrow scintigraphy in breast cancer. Nucl Med Commun 10: 389–400
26. Duncker C M, Carrio I, Berna L, Estorch M, Alonso C, Ojeda B, Blanco R, Germa J R, Ortega V 1990 Radioimmune imaging of bone marrow in patients with suspected bone metastases from primary breast cancer. J Nucl Med 31: 1450

62. Gallium scintigraphy in tumour diagnosis and management

Andrew F. McLaughlin   Andrew E. Southee

Nuclear medicine has an unparalleled capacity to monitor and measure responses to intervention and therapy non-invasively. No other modality has this capability. Gallium (^{67}Ga) scintigraphy has the unique ability to localize in viable cells of a variety of tumours. Hence, it offers the medical oncologist a valuable tool to stage, restage, detect relapse, and predict response to therapy and outcome. These are key issues to be addressed in the management of all cancer patients.

Anatomical imaging modalities, computerized tomography (CT), magnetic resonance imaging (MRI) and others are incapable of reliably distinguishing inactive disease or scar from active, viable tumour in residual masses (or normal sized lymph nodes), post-therapy. They are, therefore, of limited value to the oncologist faced with the management dilemma of the residual mass, post-therapy. Does the patient require further therapy? Should it be alternate or salvage? Current nuclear medicine techniques, in particular ^{67}Ga, are the only methods that partly go toward solving this problem, at least in the malignant lymphomas.[1]

The use and role of ^{67}Ga in the management of the malignant lymphomas, at least up to the 1980s, has been controversial. Even now, it is still not widely used in staging, restaging, detecting relapse and predicting outcome and response to therapy despite strong evidence to the contrary in lymphoma.[2–10] The evidence for a valuable clinical role in other malignancies is less well defined and often confusing. For example, it has recently been shown to have an important role in determining the response to therapy of metastatic and recurrent soft tissue sarcomas,[11] but has a less reliable role in bone sarcomas.[12]

It cannot be emphasized enough that the accuracy and usefulness of ^{67}Ga studies is contingent on optimal technique. This necessitates a satisfactory technical performance of the study, which includes using an adequate dose, performing appropriate non-standard views such as lateral views or single photon emission computerized tomography (SPECT). An accurate assessment of the clinical significance of scan abnormalities can then only be made in full knowledge of all relevant clinical, radiological and pathological data.

MECHANISM OF GALLIUM UPTAKE

The mechanism of ^{67}Ga uptake by tumours continues to be incompletely understood and debatable. There is both experimental evidence and inferential patient data that ^{67}Ga uptake reflects metabolic activity/tumour viability. It has been shown that ^{67}Ga uptake correlates with metabolic activity and with histological viability in an animal tumour model. Hammersley & Zivanovic[13] have shown by in vitro study of regenerating liver that increased ^{67}Ga uptake is associated with G2 or the protein synthesis phase of the cell cycle. They and others have presented evidence from animal studies that increased ^{67}Ga uptake is related to the proliferation of ribosomal protein synthesizing structures, both in vivo and in vitro.

After intravenous (IV) injection of carrier-free ^{67}Ga, over 90% of the tracer in the circulation is in plasma and is almost all protein-bound, predominantly to transferrin. Increase in citrate or carrier ^{67}Ga decreases both plasma protein binding and tumour uptake. While ^{67}Ga competes with iron for binding to transferrin, it has less affinity for the molecule. Iron saturation has marked effects on ^{67}Ga kinetics, including binding, plasma clearance, tissue retention and whole body retention. In normal tissues, such as liver, ^{67}Ga is localized mainly in lysosomes. In animal tumours, ^{67}Ga binds to lysosome-like bodies, which are different from the sites of binding in normal tissue. Some disagreement exists that lysosomes are the site of accumulation, but this has been attributed to faulty experimental technique.

Gallium has also been shown to bind to macromolecules within the intracellular organelles in tumours. Major controversy exists as to the exact means by which ^{67}Ga penetrates tumour cells. An adequate blood supply is one requirement for tumour uptake, particularly as tumour perfusion is often relatively greater than surrounding normal tissue. The increase in capillary permeability due to neovascularization in tumours is also likely to be involved.

Hoffer[14] speculated that ^{67}Ga uptake in tumours may be receptor-mediated. Based on in vitro evidence of enhancement of ^{67}Ga uptake in tumour cells by low concentrations of transferrin, Larson et al[15] postulated the transferrin receptor hypothesis for ^{67}Ga uptake by tumours. They proposed that ^{67}Ga binds to transferrin in the immediate extracellular space or plasma. The ^{67}Ga-transferrin complex binds to a cell surface transferrin receptor and is taken into the cell, probably by absorptive endocytosis. It is transported to the lysosome, where ^{67}Ga is released and binds to acceptor molecules which are probably intracellular proteins. While transferrin receptors have been widely demonstrated on proliferating tumour cells, results of in vivo studies of the effect of transferrin on tumour uptake are conflicting. Adding to the uncertainty about the role of transferrin is the observation that tumour cells do take up ^{67}Ga even in the absence of transferrin.

Some tumours are infiltrated by inflammatory cells, which also accumulate ^{67}Ga. This may contribute further to ^{67}Ga localization in malignant tissues.

INSTRUMENTATION

Gallium scintigraphy is a technically demanding imaging procedure for two main reasons. Firstly, the target to background ratio is sometimes low, depending on the particular tumour under investigation. Secondly, ^{67}Ga has a range of gamma emissions (93 keV, 40%; 184 keV, 24%; 296 keV, 22%; 388 keV, 7%) which have different counting efficiencies and scattering properties. The higher energy emissions are more likely to penetrate the collimator septa, resulting in image degradation, yet it was recognized at an early stage that there was a need to include more than the most abundant photo peak to increase counting statistics. Use of medium energy collimators only partially limits the amount of septal penetration. This, along with triple pulse height analysis has, in general, been adopted as the imaging method of choice.

The performance characteristics of current generation gamma-cameras in ^{67}Ga imaging are poorly documented. In particular, the effect of scattered photons on resolution and contrast for the three principle emissions is not well understood. It has been shown that there may be a slight loss of contrast with inclusion of the 296 keV window with a very limited gain in useful counts.[16] The fact that apparent scatter in the 296 keV window was higher than in the lower energy windows contradicts common belief. Scatter was very much reduced in the 93 keV window; however, there were still significant wings on the point spread function in the 296 keV window, presumably due to septal penetration through the medium energy collimator. These results raise some concern as to whether the inclusion of the third window provides any real benefit. The authors have ceased using the 296 keV photo peak.

There are two ways in which ^{67}Ga image quality may be significantly improved: contrast enhancement using tomographic techniques and scatter reduction. SPECT ^{67}Ga studies have met with mixed success largely due to the poor statistics. However, SPECT does result in improved contrast with more certain lesion recognition and localization. Surprisingly, scatter correction has not been widely applied to ^{67}Ga studies. However, the recent introduction of energy-weighted acquisition[17] on some cameras offers very encouraging results. Preliminary work has indicated an improvement in lesion contrast of up to 30%.[18] Use of the technique or alternative methods of

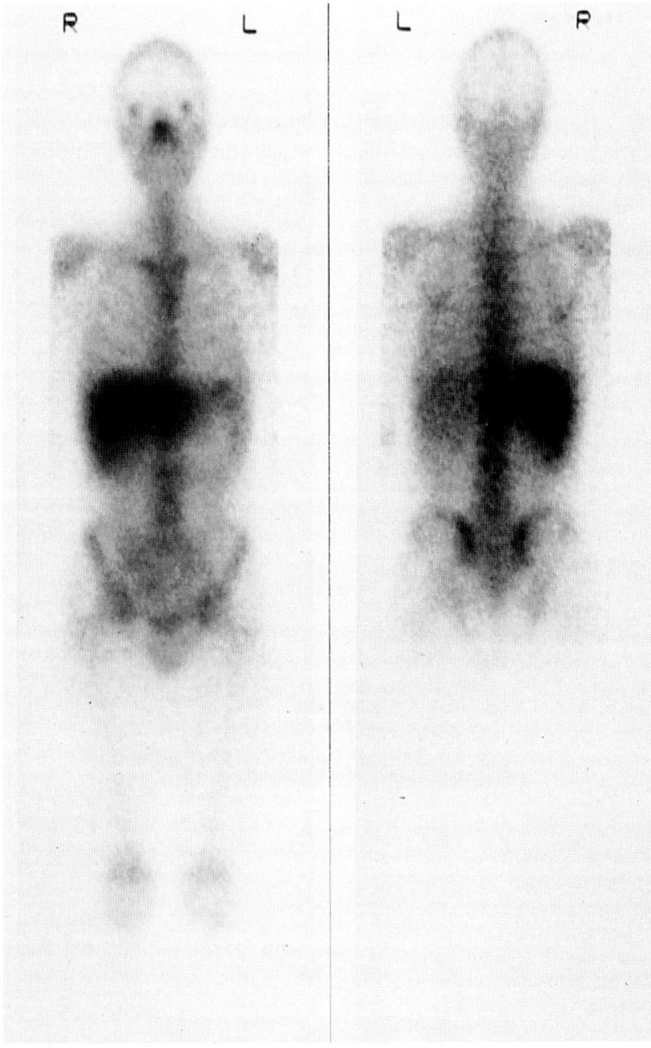

Fig. 62.1 Distribution of ^{67}Ga. The normal biodistribution of ^{67}Ga is shown in (A) anterior (left) and posterior (right) whole body sweeps. The most intense accumulation is demonstrated in the liver and spleen with uptake present in the lacrimal and salivary glands as well as in bone.

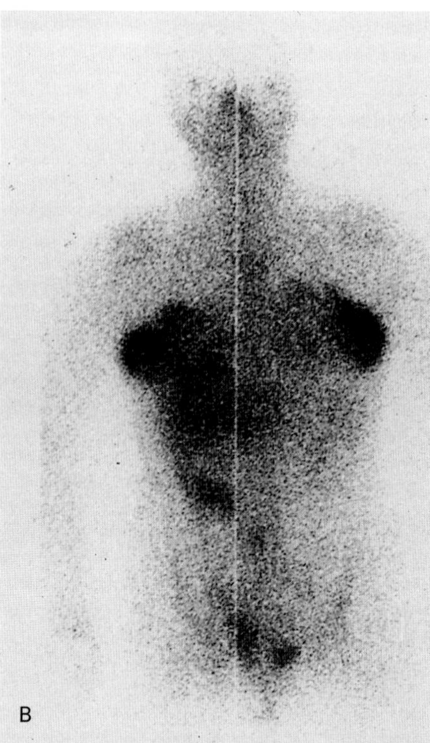

Fig. 62.1 (B) demonstrates intense breast accumulation of activity in addition to the normal biodistribution. This was due to elevated prolactin levels from a secretory pituitary tumour.

scatter correction may also improve the quality of ^{67}Ga SPECT.

NORMAL DISTRIBUTION, PITFALLS AND EFFECTS OF THERAPY

Normal biodistribution

The principal sites of localization of ^{67}Ga are in liver, spleen, bone marrow and bone. Colonic accumulation is also prominent but is transient. Lesser accumulation may be seen in the lacrimal and salivary glands, nasal mucosa, external genitalia and in breast tissue (Fig. 62.1). Rarely, gastric accumulation may also be demonstrated, and is of questionable significance. While uptake in these latter organs is faint under normal conditions, it may be considerably enhanced by a number of situations. Infants demonstrate significant activity in the base of the skull and epiphyses, as do children.

Pitfalls

Radiation therapy and chemotherapy may lead to sialoadenitis, resulting in enhanced uptake in the salivary glands. Chemotherapy may lead to thymic rebound in children, resulting in increased mediastinal uptake which, however, has a characteristic pattern (Fig. 62.2). Rarely, faint hilar uptake may be seen in normal patients and is of dubious significance. Uncomplicated surgical wounds also exhibit uptake for about 2 weeks after surgery. Intense renal accumulation can be due to a number of mechanisms. A list of factors that can alter the pattern of uptake under various conditions is provided in Table 62.1.

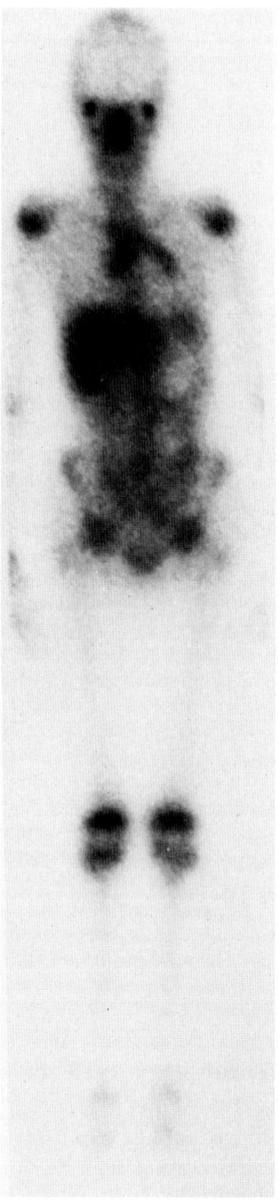

Fig. 62.2 Thymic hyperplasia. Planar image in a child treated for Burkitt's lymphoma reveals increased accumulation in a bilobed structure in the mediastinum, subsequently confirmed to be due to thymic hyperplasia following chemotherapy. The distribution of ^{67}Ga is otherwise physiological, with uptake also being present in the epiphyseal growth plates. Persistent colonic activity is visualized.

Although tumour uptake of ^{67}Ga is maximal within 24 h, scanning is delayed to 48 h or later to improve lesion contrast by the progressive clearance of activity from blood and other tissues. Between 9% and 15% of ^{67}Ga is colonically excreted, making interpretation of delayed scans difficult. Some workers have advocated bowel

Table 62.1 Conditions leading to altered distribution of ^{67}Ga

Alteration	Cause
Breast tissue uptake	Lactation Pregnancy Hormones (e.g. oral contraceptive)
Salivary gland uptake	Radiotherapy Chemotherapy Sjögren's syndrome
Salivary and lacrimal gland uptake	Sarcoidosis ('Panda' sign)
Pulmonary hilar uptake	Idiopathic Bronchitis Chemotherapy Sarcoidosis ('Lambda' sign)
Increased bone uptake	Recent chemotherapy AIDS Iron overload
Renal uptake	Interstitial nephritis (e.g. chemotherapy) Blood transfusion (iron overload) Hepatic failure Chronic anaemia Pyelonephritis Glomerulonephritis
Reduced soft tissue & hepatic uptake	Chemotherapy Blood transfusion (iron overload) AIDS
Prominent colonic activity	Cathartics Constipation
Wound uptake	Recent surgery
Absent tumour uptake	Recent chemo/radiotherapy MRI contrast administration Non-^{67}Ga avid tumour
Diffuse lung uptake	Chemotherapy Opportunistic infection Interstitial alveolitis Contrast lymphangiography

preparation in order to improve the detection of abdominal disease. However, Zeman & Ryerson,[19] in a retrospective study, showed no benefit from any form of artificial bowel clearance, although this is often undertaken. If evaluation of possible intra-abdominal disease is critical, further images at 72–96 h or even 7–14 days may be worthwhile. A high roughage diet can be of value.

Effects of therapy

Recent prior chemotherapy and radiotherapy are known to reduce tumour uptake of ^{67}Ga. Noujaim et al[20] showed decreased uptake experimentally up to 1 week after cisplatin. Animal and patient data suggest this is related to increased binding of iron to transferrin, displacing ^{67}Ga. Bone marrow iron uptake is also reduced after irradiation. Various chemotherapeutic agents, including methotrexate, fluorouracil, actinomycin D, hydroxyurea, galactoflavin and nitrogen mustard have been shown to have similar effects, possibly by different mechanisms. Scandium and gadolinium contrast agents have also been reported to alter ^{67}Ga distribution. A strategy to overcome the risk of false-negative studies due to therapy is to delay injection and imaging until immediately before the next cycle of therapy is due (usually 3–4 weeks after the last cycle). Under extreme conditions, injection of ^{67}Ga may be given 24 h before therapy, followed by imaging after therapy.

Deliberate alterations in iron kinetics also alters ^{67}Ga uptake. Parenteral iron injection prior to ^{67}Ga administration may improve imaging by reducing tissue uptake more than tumour uptake. These observations have made no clinical impact.

SCANNING TECHNIQUE

Ideally, all patients should have SPECT examination of the thorax and abdomen at 48–72 h post-injection. Careful imaging of the superficial lymph node groups is also important. Attention to positioning can prove rewarding, e.g. the axillae are best imaged with the shoulders abducted fully and the elbows flexed to allow the detector to get close access. Most departments, however, do not have the luxury of time or instrumentation available to study all patients in this ideal fashion. A more practical compromise is to perform whole-body planar views with a 500 mm field of view gamma-camera and SPECT only in special, difficult circumstances, e.g. distinguishing superficial from deep structures such as in the abdomen. An appropriate lateral view of the thorax is better than an oblique view to define 'soft' hilar or mediastinal disease seen on a planar anterior or posterior view (Fig. 62.3). Similarly, a planar view of the chest with the liver out of the field of view and acquisition of over 1 million counts may obviate the need for more time-consuming SPECT studies.

Patients should have abdominal scans at up to 10–14 days post-injection to allow the clearance of activity from the colon in order to clearly visualize abdominal disease, although by this time the residual activity is unlikely to be adequate to permit SPECT studies of a quality to identify clearly aspects such as para-aortic lymphadenopathy.

LYMPHOMA

It would be an oversight not to mention the contribution of Edwards & Hayes to the clinical usefulness of ^{67}Ga in lymphoma.[21] Theirs was a landmark paper. Not only did they observe clear ^{67}Ga localization in the diseased lymph nodes of several patients with Hodgkin's disease (HD) and non-Hodgkin's lymphoma (NHL), but also that chemotherapy affects the uptake in some way and may be a marker or predictor of response to therapy.

Subsequently, a variety of tumours were studied, as well as lymphoma.[22–31] Gallium was hailed as a 'magic bullet' for detecting cancer. However, it was subsequently shown experimentally to be a non-specific tumour-seeker that also localized at sites of inflammation.[32,33] It, therefore, was more an 'all purpose' disease finder.[25] Interest in the use of ^{67}Ga was revived in the early 1980s when excellent results in both HD and NHL were reported.[2,4–10] With the salient exception of Turner's work,[25,34,35] most of the early studies utilized outmoded equipment and poor scintigraphic techniques. The modification of instruments to acquire the three gamma emissions of ^{67}Ga made an enormous difference.[34,35] The introduction of large field gamma-cameras, with triple pulse height analysis and higher doses of ^{67}Ga, increasing photon yield, all led to better images.[4,36] In particular, change in dosage from 3–5 mCi (111–185 MBq) to 10 mCi (370 MBq) together with newer imaging techniques has improved the sensitivity of the technique in the detection of abdominal disease as well as in non-Hodgkin's lymphoma.[3] SPECT has been shown to offer additional benefit in certain situations, particularly in assessing the mediastinum.[5]

The detectability of lesions in lymphoma depends on a number of factors inherent to the disease process itself. Cell type is important, with almost all Burkitt's lymphoma, virtually all HD and large cell lymphomas being detected by ^{67}Ga. The sensitivity of the technique is somewhat poorer in the detection of the small cell lymphomas.

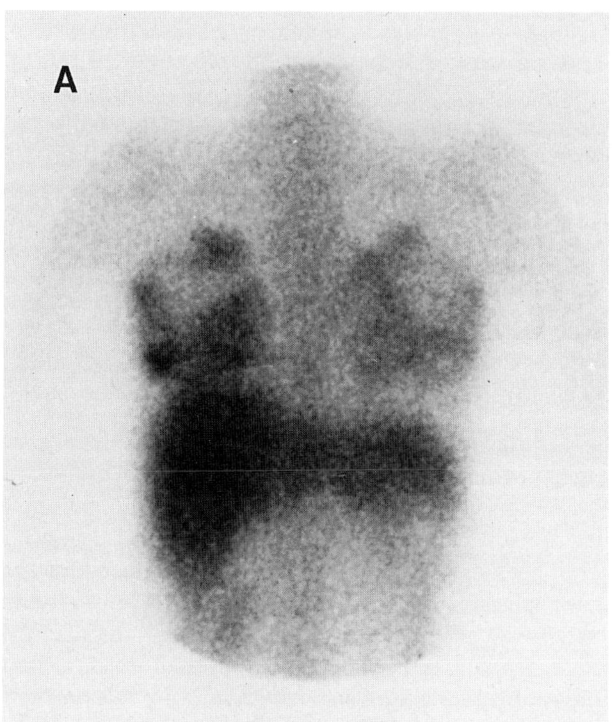

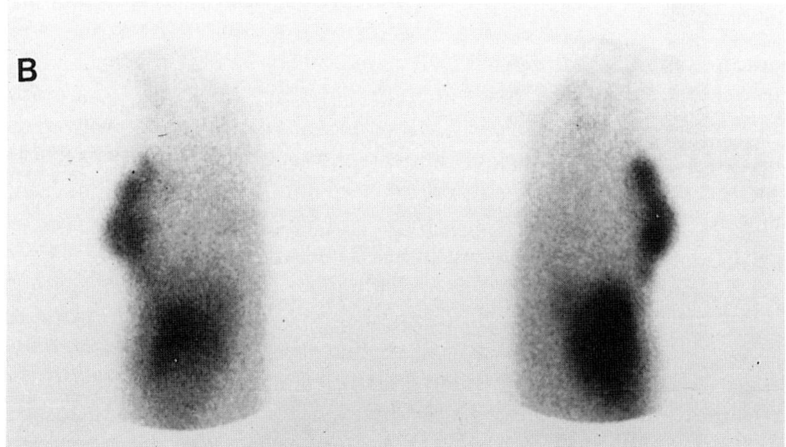

Fig. 62.3 The value of lateral views: The anterior image of the chest and abdomen (**A**) shows normal uptake in the liver with markedly increased intake in the chest bilaterally. The patient had been previously treated for mediastinal Hodgkin's disease and was lactating at the time of this ^{67}Ga study. The lateral views of the chest (**B**) clearly show there is no ^{67}Ga avid disease in the mediastinum and that the abnormal activity is confined to the breast. Lactating breasts have a high affinity for ^{67}Ga. Appropriate radiation safety advice therefore needs to be given to the mother.

Staging

The outcome in HD, and to a lesser extent in NHL (cell type being more important), is dependent on stage or extent of the disease. It is therefore essential that the extent of disease in an individual patient is carefully documented so that the correct treatment options are chosen (radiation, chemotherapy or a combination of both). It is important to determine, from diagnosis, whether a patient's disease is ^{67}Ga avid, which allows the patient to act as their own control for follow-up studies.[37] The ^{67}Ga scan is ideally suited for use as a staging procedure. It is non-invasive, examines the whole body, has no morbidity and can be performed as an outpatient, prior to costly hospital admission. It was, for these reasons, advocated in staging strategy as long ago as 1970 by Edwards & Hayes.[22] However, for optimal use it requires meticulous attention to dosage and technique and frequent return visits for up to 10 or more days post-injection.[16] The use of high ^{67}Ga dose and tomographic imaging can provide high sensitivity and specificity in both HD and NHL. In three well-conducted series[3,4,16] of over 170 patients, the overall sensitivity for HD was 93% and for NHL 89%, while the specificity was 100% in both instances.

Lymphangiography (LAG) was a long established staging procedure for the assessment of abdominal nodal disease until the work of first McCaffrey et al[38] and then Rudders et al.[39] They found that ^{67}Ga and LAG had similar accuracy (87% and 88% respectively) but LAG's had a false-positive rate of 9% whereas ^{67}Ga had no false positives. The LAG also suffers from 'blind spots' – pelvic and some retroperitoneal nodes. Gallium has the added advantage of being non-invasive, while LAG has significant morbidity. Current data indicates that there is no longer justification for LAG, although it is still practised in some centres.

Laparotomy was a traditional part of staging HD for many years. It too is a procedure where the evidence for discontinuance is strong. It has significant morbidity and mortality.[37] In 1984, Gomez et al[40] studied 104 patients with early-stage HD in a prospective, randomized trial of laparotomy and no laparotomy (76 *vs.* 28 patients). It was shown that there was no benefit from laparotomy in terms of remission, survival numbers or abdominal relapses. Blackwell et al[37] also confirmed this. They studied 16 early-stage HD patients prospectively with ^{67}Ga scintigraphy and abdominal CT scanning. All patients were subjected to laparotomy with a follow-up of 12–36 months. All had normal ^{67}Ga, CT and laparotomy findings. Three patients in the series relapsed outside the abdomen. They concluded that reliance on non-invasive investigations carries no adverse risk to outcome from inaccurate staging nor affects the choice of therapy, and that the laparotomy only increases the morbidity and mortality.

It is also vital to use ^{67}Ga scintigraphy as part of the staging procedure because of its proven impact on management as a result of altering staging. It significantly changes radiation therapy planning. Jochelson et al[41] looked at the role of ^{67}Ga in the planning of mantle irradiation in 26 patients. They compared it with CT scanning and plain X-ray. Three of the 26 patients had the iradiation fields altered as a result of the ^{67}Ga findings over and above the abnormalities demonstrated on the CT scan. The CT scan gave no additional information. It demonstrated the clinical utility of ^{67}Ga as an initial staging tool, prior to radiation planning.

Gallium scintigraphy provides a whole-body image, which is a major advantage over all other staging procedures. It is the one test that clearly identifies those patients with stage IV disease[16] and should therefore be regarded as an essential staging procedure in HD and NHL.

Restaging

It is vital for the oncologist to know if a patient is in complete remission at the end of treatment. However, establishing this in practice can be difficult. The subsequent clinical course is often the only reliable method available, with all its inherent disadvantages and uncertainties. The conundrum for the clinician is whether to cease, continue therapy, or institute alternate or salvage therapies for resistant or residual disease.

The advantages of routine ^{67}Ga scanning in this setting are therefore manifold. Henkin et al[26] made this point in 1974. They were the first to report the use of ^{67}Ga as a restaging procedure and made the important observation that different diagnostic problems exist before and after therapy, and that it may be difficult to determine either relapse or residual progressive disease. They invoked the need for a simple screening test to replace the complex and often invasive diagnostic strategy for staging and restaging. They confirmed that the ^{67}Ga scan is often the first and only objective evidence of residual, progressive or relapsed disease.[31] It has been further validated by many investigators.[42–46] Two series of over 50 patients[16] found ^{67}Ga to be the most specific predictor of residual disease at approximately 95%. The presence of persistent ^{67}Ga positivity after five cycles of chemotherapy in diffuse large cell NHL was also shown to be a grave prognostic sign in 11 patients, with eight deaths in this group. It suggests the necessity of alternate therapy if the scan remains positive after 3–5 cycles of therapy.

The residual mass dilemma

The residual mass, following therapy, falls into a new category of unconfirmed/uncertain complete remission – CR[u]. This has recently been introduced to accommodate the problem of residual, anatomical masses at restaging which lead to uncertainty over the need for alternate or salvage therapy. Both CT and MRI have a limited capacity to differentiate residual, active disease from fibrosis or scar, independent of a residual mass. Gallium scintigraphy goes a long way toward solving this problem.[1] Figures 62.4–62.7 give examples of this dilemma. Figures 62.4 and 62.5 show pre- and post-treatment CXR and ^{67}Ga scans with a persisting mediastinal mass after therapy but negative ^{67}Ga. Figures 62.6 and 62.7 show pre- and post-treatment CXR and ^{67}Ga with no persisting mediastinal mass after therapy but a positive ^{67}Ga scan. Figure 62.8 clearly shows active, viable tumour with areas of necrosis which appear relatively uniform on MRI. It emphasizes the importance of not only correlative imaging (Fig. 62.9) but also that ^{67}Ga SPECT is even more sensitive than planar studies (Fig. 62.10).[5]

The use of ^{67}Ga to distinguish tumour recurrence from post-radiation fibrosis was suggested by Paterson & McCready in 1975.[23] Anderson et al[4] found ^{67}Ga to be superior to all other modalities in predicting active from inactive disease in residual masses post-therapy. Southee et al[6] and Wylie et al[7] examined 39 patients with

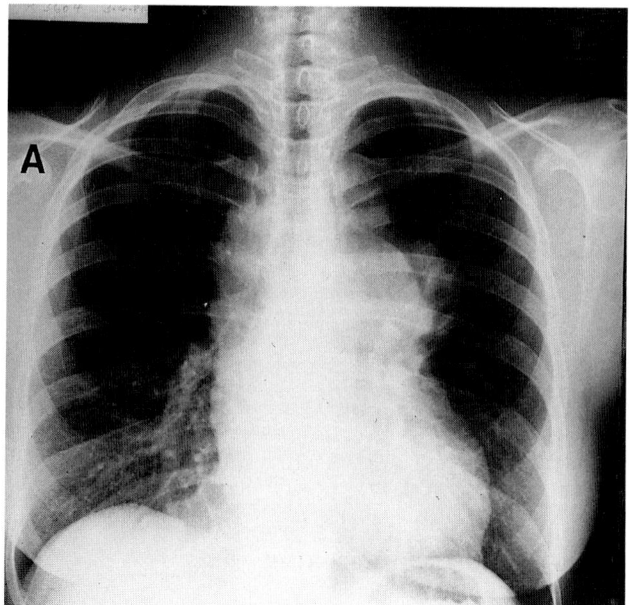

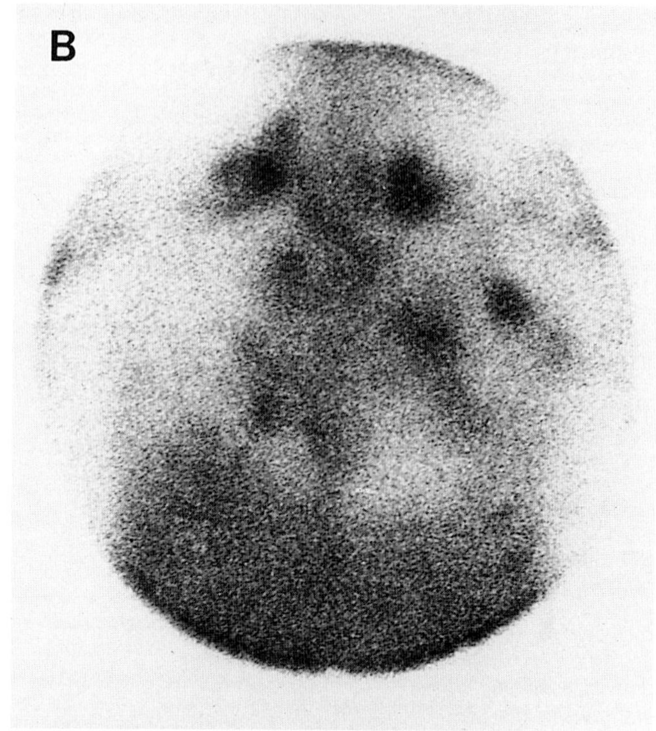

Fig. 62.4 Staging. Staging chest X-ray (A) of a young woman with a large mediastinal mass and palpable lymph nodes in the neck, supraclavicular fossae and axillae. Staging ^{67}Ga scan (B) of the anterior thorax of the same patient shows avid ^{67}Ga uptake in the mediastinal mass, both hilar regions and the sites of palpable lymph node enlargement in the neck and axillae.

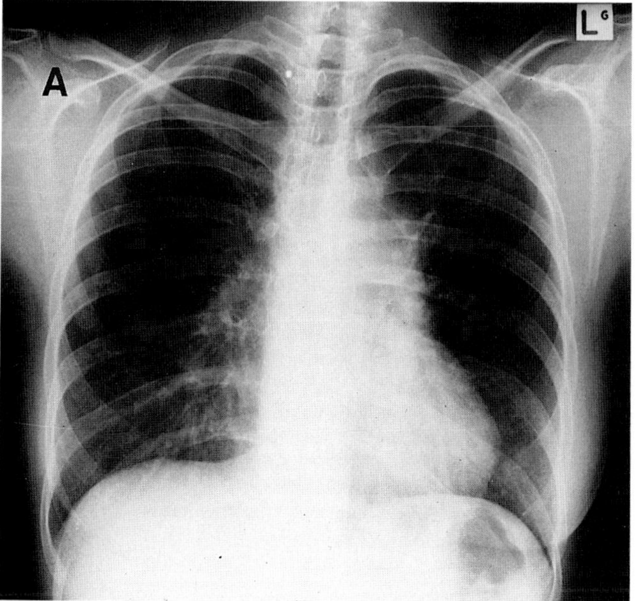

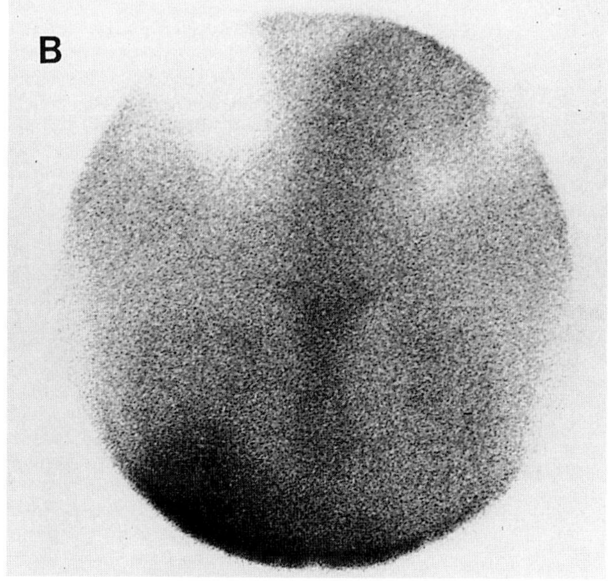

Fig. 62.5 Residual mass dilemma. Restaging chest X-ray (A) of the same patient as in Figure 62.4 showing a residual mediastinal mass following apparently successful therapy. Normal restaging ^{67}Ga scan (B) of the anterior thorax indicating no active viable tumour in the residual mass.

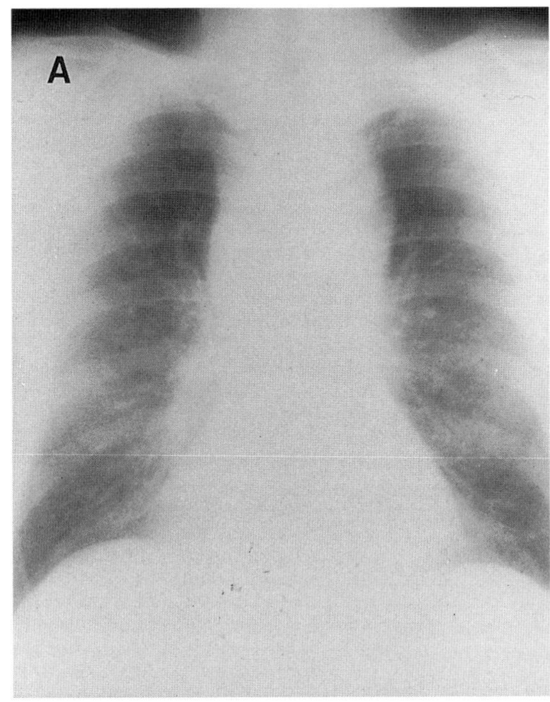

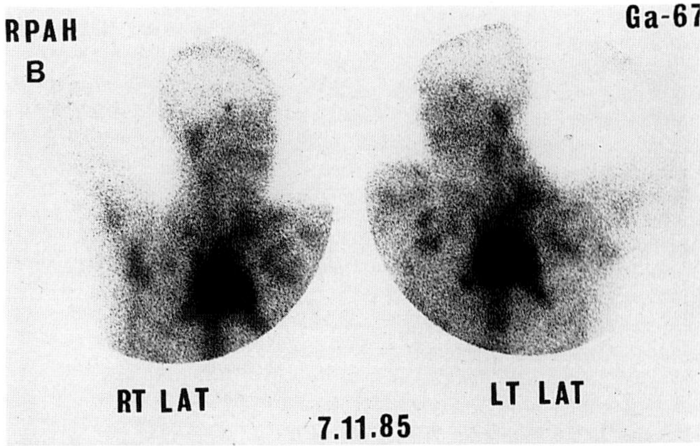

Fig. 62.6 Staging. Staging CXR (A) of a young man with a large superior mediastinal mass and palpable nodes in the neck, supra and infraclavicular fossae and axillae. Staging ^{67}Ga scan (B) of the axillae and anterior thorax. This shows very avid ^{67}Ga uptake in the mediastinal mass, both hilar regions and the sites of lymph node enlargement. Note also the abducted upper arms giving the best views of the axillae.

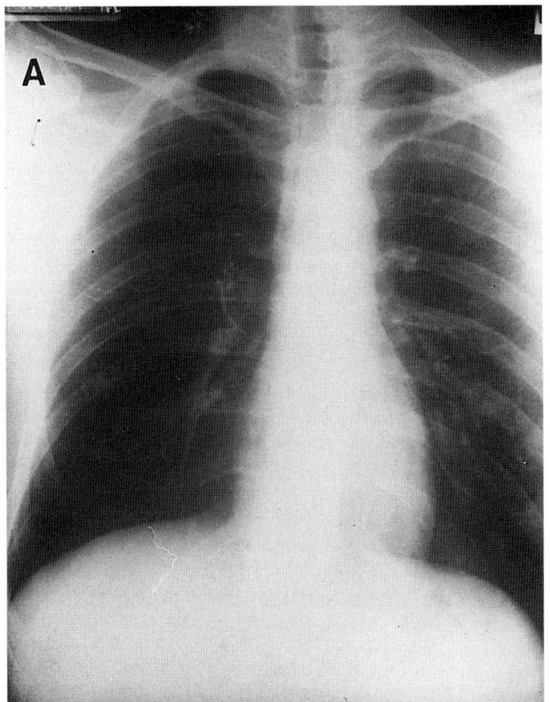

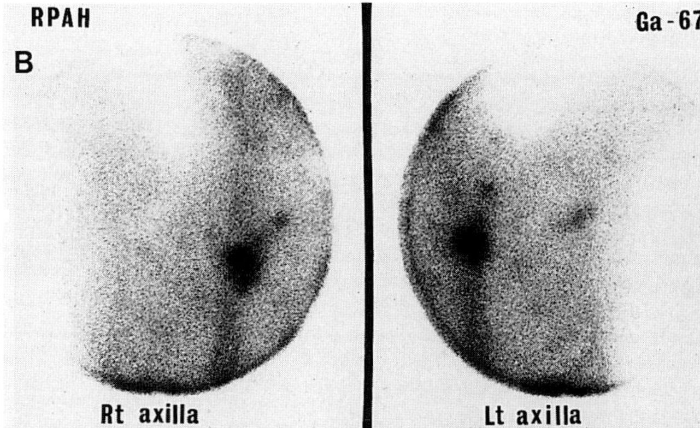

Fig. 62.7 Prognostic value at restaging. Restaging chest X-ray (A) of the same patient as Figure 62.6 showing no residual mediastinal mass following apparently successful therapy. Restaging ^{67}Ga Scan (B) of the axillae and anterior thorax showing persisting avid ^{67}Ga uptake (in the absence of anatomical masses) in the superior mediastinum, left infraclavicular region and left axillae. The patient subsequently relapsed and went on to autologous bone marrow transplantation.

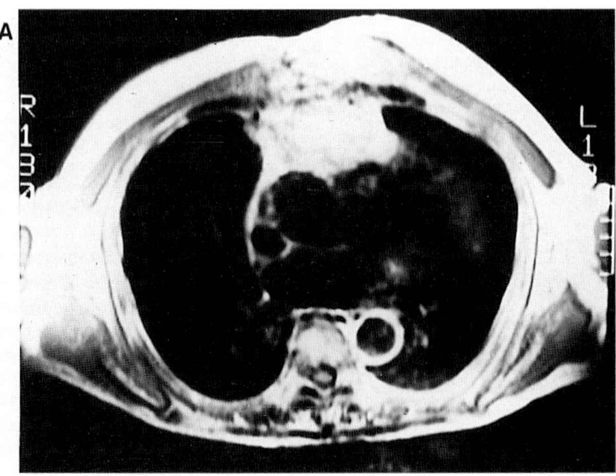

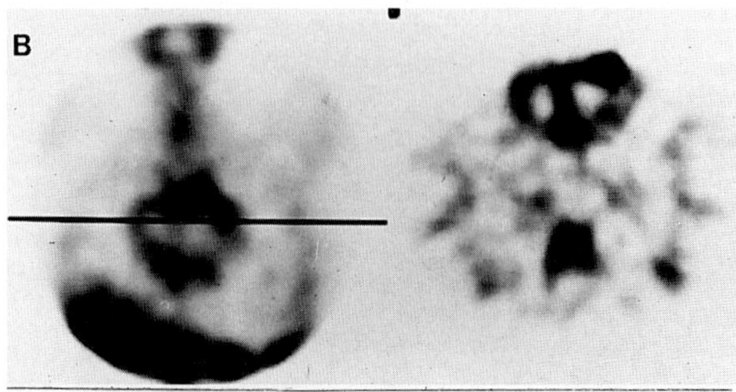

Fig. 62.8 Detection of tumour viability. SPECT ^{67}Ga scan of the thorax – coronal reference image on the left and transaxial slice on the right through a heterogeneous mass on MRI (A). The ^{67}Ga slice (B) clearly shows areas of ^{67}Ga avid, active tumour growth with central photopenia shown to be necrotic tumour at autopsy.

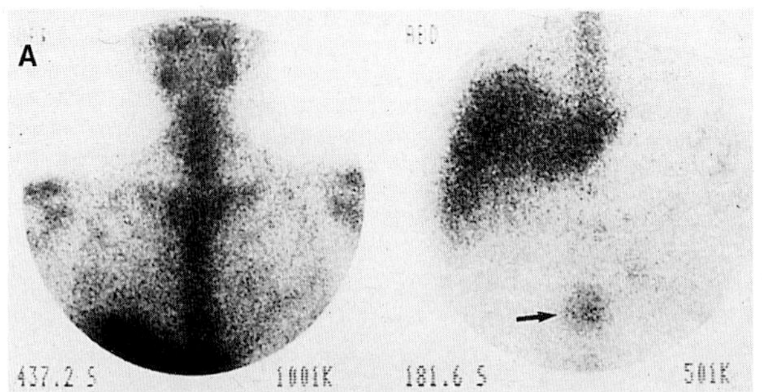

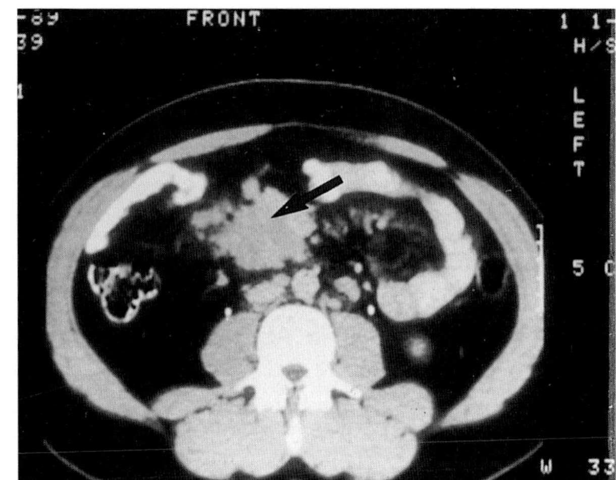

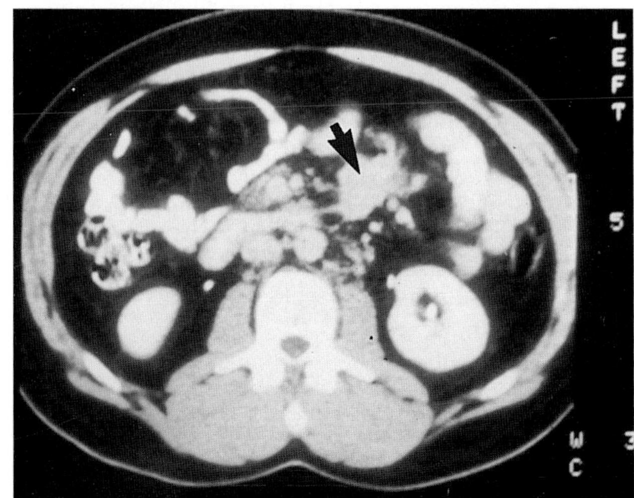

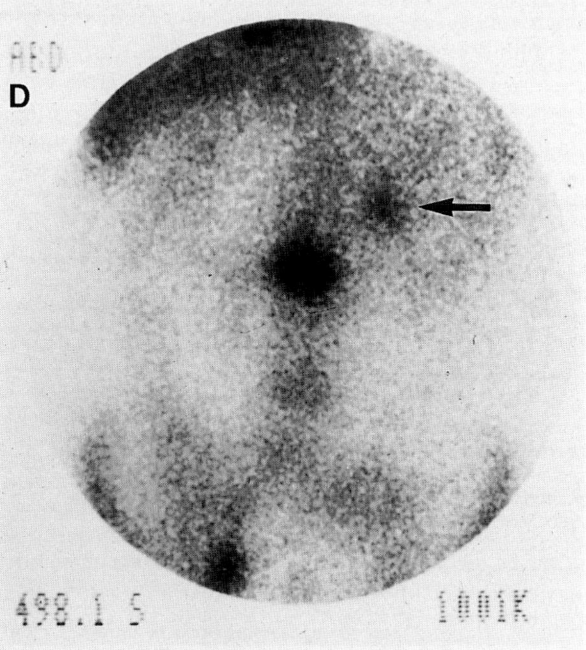

Fig. 62.9 The value of correlative imaging. The initial anterior abdominal image shown in (A) demonstrates moderately increased ^{67}Ga avidity in the mid abdomen. This corresponds to the abnormality seen in the CT scan (B). However, a higher CT slice shown in (C) reveals a second area of disease in the upper left abdomen. A further image taken for 1 million counts (D) quite clearly demonstrates a second area of increased uptake in the left upper abdomen. This example clearly shows the dangers in reporting nuclear medicine studies blindly without other radiographic or clinical information. SPECT or alteration of the threshold on digital image would probably have given the same information.

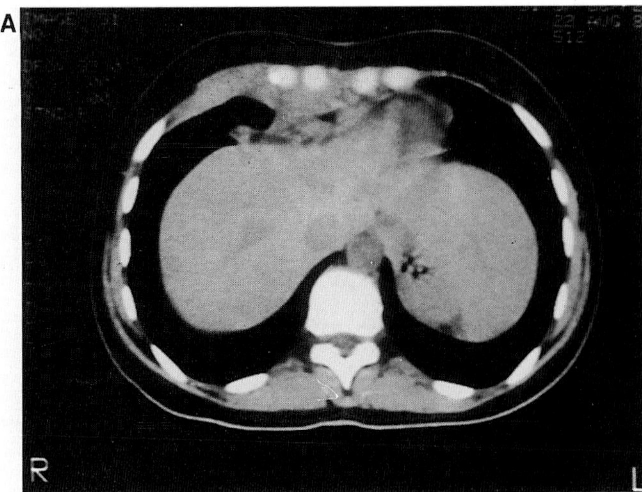

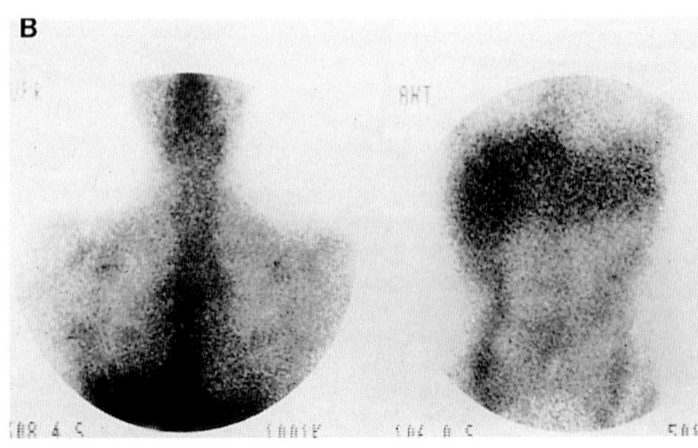

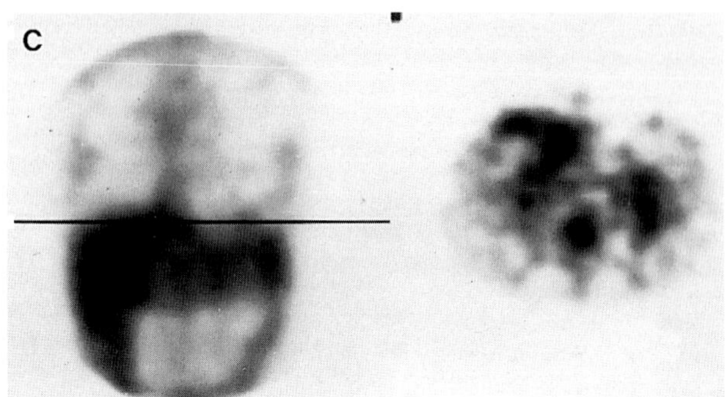

Fig. 62.10 The value of SPECT. This patient with known recurrence of sarcoma was considered clinically to have residual active disease in a mass anterior to the liver shown on the CT scan (A). The planar anterior abdominal view (B) showed equivocal increased uptake related to the superomedial aspect of the liver. SPECT transverse reconstructions (C) show the large area of residual ^{67}Ga avid disease anterior to the liver.

mediastinal HD, 17 of whom had a residual mass after the completion of apparently successful therapy. They found that disease activity correlated with positive ^{67}Ga uptake and was independent of the presence or absence of a residual mediastinal mass. Israel et al[8] studied 25 patients pre- and post-treatment. They found ^{67}Ga was the most specific test for residual disease at 95%, while CT at 57% and plain chest X-ray at 55% had low specificities due to their inability to distinguish tumour from fibrosis. These results were validated by Kostakoglu et al.[46] Gallium SPECT was used in a retrospective study of 30 patients at restaging of HD after therapy, correlating CT and SPECT findings with biopsy results. SPECT had an overall accuracy of 93% and correctly identified active disease in 96% of proven residual disease, confirming the high sensitivity of ^{67}Ga SPECT. Israel et al[47] also reported two cases of residual masses that were completely resected post-therapy, both of which were ^{67}Ga negative and contained no residual tumour.

Predicting response to therapy and outcome

Edwards & Hayes[21,22] observed that the alteration of ^{67}Ga uptake, by radio- and chemotherapy, may be a marker or predictor of response to treatment. This has been confirmed by many investigators.[7,9,44,48] It is a signal to the oncologist to consider alternate or salvage therapy. This role of ^{67}Ga was emphasized by Kaplan.[49]

Henkin et al[26] correctly predicted that residual ^{67}Ga uptake, post-therapy, may be of prognostic significance. It is the only diagnostic modality that has been shown to predict outcome accurately.[7–9,48,50] Detection of unsuspected stage IV disease at initial staging is also a grave prognostic sign, as is failure to convert to a negative ^{67}Ga, mid-cycle, in diffuse large cell NHL.[9] This has also been shown to be the case in HD.[48] Two studies of 25 patients[6,7] found that ^{67}Ga scanning correctly predicted residual disease in 89% of patients.

Appropriate summary statistics for the sensitivity of ^{67}Ga scanning in the various clinical settings of lymphoma are presented in Table 62.2.

SOFT-TISSUE SARCOMA

Soft-tissue sarcomas are ^{67}Ga avid tumours[11,31,51–59] with sensitivities reported to reach 96%.[11,58,59] Although the

Table 62.2 Summary of statistics for ^{67}Ga in lymphoma

Clinical setting	Sensitivity	Specificity
Overall		
Hodgkin's disease	93%	100%
Non-Hodgkin's lymphoma	89%	100%
Chest disease		
Planar	66%	66%
SPECT	96%	100%
Abdominal disease		
Planar	69%	87%
SPECT	85%	100%

accuracy in recent papers appears to be similar to that in intermediate grade lymphomas, ^{67}Ga studies in soft-tissue sarcoma are underutilized. This is mainly because of poor results from early studies,[51] which used inferior imaging techniques.

Like lymphomas,[60] uptake is in general related to tumour grade with high grade tumours demonstrating more avidity than low grade tumours.[11] This probably explains why some early series showed selective cell types (liposarcomas, synovialsarcomas, and rhabdomyosarcomas) as being ^{67}Ga negative.[52,54] Most cell types have been reported to give ^{67}Ga negative results on occasions. Microscopic tumour, following excision biopsy, will also usually be ^{67}Ga negative. Kaposi's sarcoma, which biologically behaves very differently from other sarcomas, is always ^{67}Ga negative[61] and this feature can be used to advantage in differentiating Kaposi's sarcoma in the lung from infection.

A recent series of 56 patients was reported using optimal planar technique in metastatic or recurrent disease.[11] Many had received chemotherapy and radiotherapy. There was no difference in the ability to detect metastatic (Fig. 62.11) or recurrent sites which were both detected with a high degree of reliability, 93% of patient studies being ^{67}Ga positive. Liver metastases were detected poorly (56% sensitivity) but all other sites were reliably detected (91% pre- and 92% post-therapy). Small (1–2 mm) lesions in the chest, seen only on CT, were not detected but otherwise the actual size of lesions had no relationship to detectability. In another series of 55 patients,[59] large and small sarcomas were detected with a sensitivity of 96%. However, this high sensitivity was at the expense of a lower than usually reported specificity (87%).

Gallium has an important adjunctive role at staging for the detection of clinically or radiographically occult disease in 9%[11] to 13%[59] of patients. It also has a role in restaging and in the detection of local recurrence of primary lesions following treatment.[55] As in lymphoma, it is able to identify foci of active tumour within residual post-treatment masses.[11]

MELANOMA

The clinical utility of ^{67}Ga in melanoma staging and restaging is controversial. There is no doubt that melanoma avidly concentrates ^{67}Ga.

In a series of 67 patients, the sensitivity was 89% and the specificity 99%.[62] Another series of 41 (sensitivity 80%, specificity 75%) suggested the use of ^{67}Ga to identify patients with regional lymph node metastases.[63]

A recent series of 222 patients showed only a 0.5% incidence of unsuspected disease in a group of patients with no apparent clinical disease screened with ^{67}Ga. The positive predictive value was only 20%.[64] In a subgroup where there was high clinical or radiographic suspicion of disease there was a high false-negative rate which caused a negative predictive value of only 32%. Although the authors claimed considerable ^{67}Ga expertise, they admitted some sites of abnormality were positive on ^{67}Ga in retrospect. Four adrenal metastases were ^{67}Ga negative.

It has been previously emphasized that particular care is needed to optimize ^{67}Ga scintigraphy, as it is in lymphoma studies. Recent biopsy as well as injection sites of BCG (adjuvant immunotherapy) should be identified so that they are not mistaken for active tumour.[31]

The major role for ^{67}Ga in melanoma is probably in evaluating residual scarring/tumour post-treatment.[31,63–65] However, there is currently insufficient data to confirm this.

LUNG CANCER

All histological types of bronchogenic carcinoma are associated with a relatively high affinity for gallium.[66] Sensitivity is reported between 85 and 97%. Gallium has been used as a screening investigation for distal metastases with 80% accuracy when combined with a chest X-ray alone. Identification of unexpected distal metastases may avoid needless thoracotomy.[66] In addition, the documentation of extensive disease may have important prognostic value.

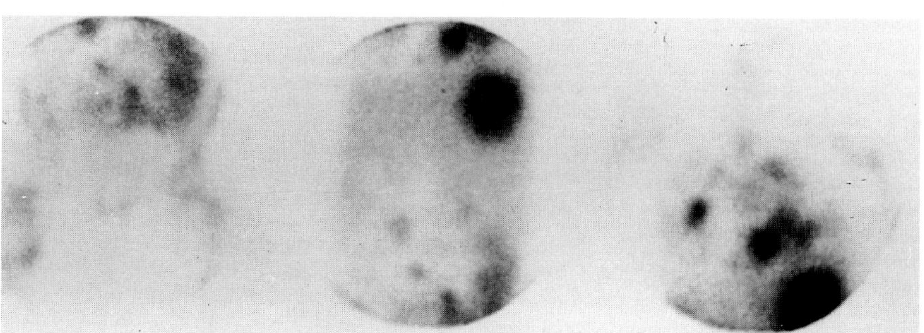

Fig. 62.11 Widespread metastatic sarcoma. There are multiple areas of increased ^{67}Ga uptake of varying size and avidity. Most of the sites were undetected clinically or radiographically.

Gallium has been utilized to assess mediastinal spread of the primary tumour and the accuracy in this situation has been quite variable. Some groups reported a high sensitivity[67–69] while others noted a low sensitivity,[70] but high specificity. It seems that, if the mediastinum is assessed separately from the hilum, the sensitivity for detection of metastatic disease is low but the specificity high. When hilum and mediastinum are considered together sensitivity is high but specificity is low.[72] The logical conclusion is that, using the published data, ^{67}Ga cannot be recommended to evaluate mediastinal spread routinely in lung cancer patients.[65] There is no data yet available using the optimal technique of a multi-headed SPECT device.

Some early studies showed ^{67}Ga to be superior, overall, to CT.[71,73] According to one group CT added little in the staging of bronchogenic carcinoma but ^{67}Ga was useful if it was positive in the mediastinum.[71] A more recent study compared standard staging of CT of the chest and upper abdomen, chest X-ray and history and examination with whole-body ^{67}Ga scans.[74] Gallium identified unexpected metastases in 5% of cases. However, the authors state that, in an additional 3% of cases, metastases were identified which 'probably would not have been overlooked' by clinical examination or other tests. They also admit additional metastatic sites were identified in hindsight. This brings into question whether an optimal technique was used. The authors did not conclude whether the additional relatively low yield of ^{67}Ga scanning justified its use. However, ^{67}Ga was clearly shown to have a secondary role to CT at staging and this now seems to be the view held at most cancer centres. In a recent series of 38 patients using SPECT, 201-thallium chloride (^{201}Tl) was found to be superior to ^{67}Ga both for evaluation of the primary lesion and for lymph node metastases.[75]

Whilst the routine use of ^{67}Ga to stage lung cancer anatomically probably cannot be justified, there is evidence to suggest that it offers important prognostic information which CT cannot provide. Increasing ^{67}Ga avidity correlates with the incidence of metastases and a shorter patient survival.[76] As with other ^{67}Ga avid tumours, ^{67}Ga has a unique role in assessing post-treatment masses.[66,74,77]

OTHER TUMOURS

Myeloma

The sensitivity of ^{67}Ga for myeloma sites is well documented to be poor (25–40%). This compares to 50–60% sensitivity for the bone scan and 80% for radiographs.[78,79] However, ^{67}Ga does appear to offer important prognostic information in that, in one series all five patients who had avid ^{67}Ga uptake, which was significantly more intense than the uptake ratio on bone scintigraphy, died within 3 months.[79]

Mesothelioma

^{67}Ga scanning can be used to help differentiate benign mesothelioma from malignant disease both in the chest and in the abdomen.[55,57] However, ^{67}Ga uptake is variable and, unlike most other ^{67}Ga avid tumours, may not be related to cell type.[11] Although there is no conclusive data to recommend routine use of ^{67}Ga, there is evidence of its utility as an adjunct to CT in identifying the sites which are most suitable for biopsy, if there is a suspicion of recurrence after decortication surgery, radio- or chemotherapy.[11]

Testicular tumours

Testicular tumours appear to be ^{67}Ga avid according to cell type with embryonal cell carcinoma being most ^{67}Ga avid and teratoma positive in only 25% of cases in the early reports.[80,81] An accuracy of 92% has been reported in detecting nodal metastases.[80,82] Following the success of ^{67}Ga in the assessment of post-treatment tumour viability in lymphoma, several centres are looking prospectively at the problem of recurrence of testicular cancer which is a common diagnostic dilemma.

Breast carcinoma

In the breast, only 25% of primary tumours will be ^{67}Ga avid and ^{201}Tl appears to be a more useful tumour marker with a 96% sensitivity for palpable breast abnormalities.[83]

Brain tumours

Although 80% of brain tumours will be ^{67}Ga avid, CT is the investigation of choice at staging. As far as tumour recurrence after treatment is concerned it has been shown that there is a complementary role for ^{201}Tl. This is because CT or MRI cannot reliably differentiate necrosis, fibrosis and active tumour. In that series of 29 patients ^{67}Ga was found to be inferior to ^{201}Tl in identifying viable tumour. The authors postulated that this was probably because of an effect of steroid therapy on ^{67}Ga uptake.[84]

Head and neck carcinoma

Detection of head and neck tumours is poor.[85] However, as in multiple myeloma recurrent lesions which demonstrate ^{67}Ga avidity are an ominous sign for poor short-term survival.[86]

Colorectal carcinoma

Gallium uptake in colorectal carcinoma has been found to be poor, with sensitivity of up to 65%.[86] There are technical problems due to ^{67}Ga excretion in the colon. Abnormal accumulation is difficult to distinguish from normal physiological excretion, particularly in constipated patients. Delayed images, up to 2 weeks after initial injection, may be necessary.

Hepatoma

Hepatomas are ^{67}Ga avid, and this property has been used to distinguish these tumours, which are frequently multifocal in a cirrhotic liver, from regenerative cirrhotic nodules which are ^{67}Ga negative.[65] However, ^{67}Ga is taken up by normal liver which may make interpretation difficult. Gallium uptake in an area of reduced uptake on the colloid scan is a positive study.[88] Unfortunately the test lacks specificity as metastatic liver disease, abscess and benign adenomas may also be ^{67}Ga avid and hence biopsy is often unavoidable.

Bone sarcoma

Gallium has a high degree of accuracy in detection of bone sarcomas, approaching 100% sensitivity.[12,56,89] In one series of 37 patients with osteogenic sarcoma, all patients had ^{67}Ga positive studies.[89] Predominantly lytic lesions were found in patients with minimal uptake and blastic lesions were associated with avid uptake as were hypervascular tumours. The authors did not identify the total number of metastatic sites evaluated but stated that only two of four pulmonary metastases were detected (bone scans were negative in all four). In general, those tumours with high ^{67}Ga affinity responded more favourably to treatment. In another series all 38 patients with a variety of bone sarcomas were ^{67}Ga positive, including 18 with osteogenic sarcoma.[12] On repeat studies 6 weeks following chemotherapy, ^{201}Tl was found to be a better predictor of tumour necrosis than ^{67}Ga. This was no doubt due to the bone seeking properties of ^{67}Ga with avid uptake by healing bone, ^{201}Tl not having this property.

REFERENCES

1. Canellos G P 1988 Residual mass in lymphoma may not be residual disease (Editorial). J Clin Oncol 6: 931–933
2. McLaughlin A F, Chu J, Howman-Giles R 1981 Whole body gallium scanning in malignant lymphoma – its role in 1980. Aust NZ J Med 11: 436
3. Kaplan W D, Anderson K C, Leonard R C F 1983 High dose gallium imaging in the evaluation of lymphoma. J Nucl Med 24: 50
4. Anderson K C, Leonard R C F, Canellos G P, Skarin A T, Kaplan W D 1983 High dose gallium imaging in lymphoma. Am J Med 75: 327–331
5. Tumeh S S, Rosenthal D S, Kaplan W D, English R J, Holman B L 1987 Lymphoma: evaluation with Ga-67 SPECT. Radiology 164: 111–114
6. Southee A E, Wylie B R, McLaughlin A F, Joshua D E, Kronenberg H, Morris J G 1988 Gallium scintigraphy in the management of mediastinal Hodgkin's disease. Aust NZ J Med 18: 508
7. Wylie B R, Southee A E, Joshua D E et al 1989 Gallium scanning in the management of mediastinal Hodgkin's disease. Eur J Haematol 42: 344–347
8. Israel O, Front D, Menachem L et al 1988 Gallium-67 imaging in monitoring lymphoma response to treatment. Cancer 61: 2439–2443
9. Kaplan W D, Jochelson M S, Herman T S et al 1990 Gallium-67 imaging: a predictor of residual tumor viability and clinical outcome in patients with diffuse large-cell lymphoma. J Clin Oncol 8: 1966–1970
10. Israel O, Front D, Epelbaum R et al 1990 Residual mass and negative gallium scintigraphy in treated lymphoma. J Nucl Med 31: 365–368
11. Southee A E, Kaplan W D, Jochelson M S et al 1992 Gallium imaging in metastatic and recurrent soft-tissue sarcoma. J Nucl Med 33: 1594–1599
12. Ramanna L, Waxman A, Binney G, Waxman S, Mirra J, Rosen G 1990 Thallium-201 scintigraphy in bone sarcoma: comparison with gallium-67 and technetium-MDP in the evaluation of chemotherapeutic response. J Nucl Med 31: 567–572
13. Hammersley P A G, Zivanovic M A 1976 Gallium-67 uptake in the regenerating rat liver. J Nucl Med 17: 226
14. Hoffer P B 1978 Mechanisms of localization. In: Hoffer P B, Bekerman C, Henkin R E, eds Gallium-67 imaging. John Wiley, New York. pp 4–8
15. Larson S M, Rasey J S, Allen D R et al 1980 Common pathway for tumour cell uptake of gallium-67 and iron-59 via a transferrin receptor. J Natl Cancer Inst 64: 41–53
16. McLaughlin A F, Magee M A, Greenough R et al 1990 Current role of gallium scanning in the management of lymphoma. Eur J Nucl Med 16: 755–771
17. DeVito R P, Stoub E W, Siegel M E 1986 Weighted acquisition using finite spatial filters for real-time scatter removal. J Nucl Med 27: 960
18. Siegel M E, Lee K H, DeVito R P, Chen O, Chen D C P 1986 Weighted acquisition: a method for improving bone and gallium images. J Nucl Med 27: 988
19. Zeman R K, Ryerson T W 1977 The value of bowel preparations in Ga-67 citrate scanning: concise communication. J Nucl Med 18: 886–889
20. Noujaim A A, Turner C J, Van Niewwenhuyze B M, Terner U, Lentle B C 1981 An investigation of the mechanism of cis-diamine dichloroplatinum (cis-pt) interference with radiogallium uptake in tumors. Aust NZ J Med 11: 437
21. Edwards C L, Hayes R L 1969 Tumor scanning with 67-Ga citrate. J Nucl Med 10: 103–105
22. Edwards C L, Hayes R L 1970 Scanning malignant neoplasms with gallium-67. J Am Med Assoc 212: 1182–1190
23. Paterson A H G, McCready V R 1975 The current status of gallium 67 scanning. Br J Radiol 48: 944
24. Pinsky S M, Henkin R E 1976 Gallium-67 tumour scanning. Semin Nucl Med 4: 397–409
25. Turner D A, Fordham E W, Ali A, Slayton R E 1978 Gallium-67 imaging in the management of Hodgkin's disease and other malignant lymphomas. Semin Nucl Med 8: 205–218
26. Henkin R E, Polcyn R E, Quinn J L III 1974 Scanning treated Hodgkin's disease with 67-Ga citrate. Radiology 110: 151–154
27. Silbertstein E B 1976 Cancer diagnosis, the role of tumour-imaging radiopharmaceuticals. Am J Med 60: 226–236
28. Kaplan W D, Adelstein S J 1976 The radionuclide identification of tumors. Cancer 37: 487–495

29. Halpern S, Hagan P 1980 Gallium-67 citrate imaging in neoplastic and inflammatory disease. In: Freemen L M, Weissman H S, eds. Nuclear Medicine Annual 1980. Raven Press, New York. p. 219
30. Hoffer P B 1980 Status of gallium-67 in tumour detection. J Nucl Med 21: 394–398
31. Bekerman C, Hoffer P B, Bitran J D 1985 The role of gallium-67 in the clinical evaluation of cancer. Semin Nucl Med 15: 72–103
32. Ito Y, Okuyama S, Sato K, Takahashi K, Sato T, Kanno I 1971 67-Ga tumor scanning and its mechanism studied in rabbits. Radiology 100: 357–362
33. Lavender J P, Lowe J, Barker J R, Burn J I, Chaudhri M A 1971 Gallium-67 scanning in neoplastic and inflammatory lesions. Br J Radiol 44: 361–366
34. Turner D A, Pinsky S M, Gottschalk A, Hoffer P B, Ultmann J E, Harper P V 1972 The use of 67-Ga scanning in the staging of Hodgkin's disease. Radiology 103: 97–101
35. Turner D A, Gottschalk A, Hoffer P B, Harper P V, Morgan E, Ultmann J E 1973 Gallium-67 scanning in the staging of Hodgkin's disease. IAEA, Vienna. pp 615–629
36. Turner D A, Fordham E H, Slayton R E 1978 Malignant lymphoma. In: Hoffer P B, Bekerman C, Henkin R E, eds. Gallium-67 imaging. Wiley, New York. pp 95–112
37. Blackwell E A, Joshua D E, McLaughlin A F, Green D, Kronenberg H, May J 1986 Early supra-diaphragmatic Hodgkin's disease. High dose gallium scanning obviates the need for staging laparotomy. Cancer 58: 883–885
38. McCaffrey J A, Rudders R A, Kahn P C, Harvey H A, De Lellis R A 1976 Clinical usefulness of 67-gallium scanning in the malignant lymphomas. Am J Med 60: 523–530
39. Rudders R, McCaffrey J A, Kahn P 1977 The relative roles of gallium-67 citrate scanning and lymphangiography in the current management of malignant lymphoma. Cancer 40: 1439–1443
40. Gomez G A, Reese P A, Nava H et al 1984 Staging laparotomy and splenectomy in early Hodgkin's disease, no therapeutic benefit. Am J Med 77: 205–210
41. Jochelson M S, Herman T S, Stomper P C, Mauch P M, Kaplan W D 1988 Planning mantle radiation therapy in patients with Hodgkin's disease: role of gallium-67 scintigraphy. Am J Roentg 151: 1229–1231
42. Caride V J, Gottschalk A 1977 Recent advances in cancer diagnosis in nuclear medicine techniques. Cancer 40: 495–499
43. Herman T, Jones S 1976 Systematic restaging in patients with Hodgkin's disease: a southwest oncology group study. Cancer 42: 1976–1982
44. Front D, Isreal O 1989 Nuclear medicine in monitoring response to cancer treatment (Editorial). J Nucl Med 30: 1731–1736
45. Front D, Israel O, Epelbaum R et al 1990 Ga-67 SPECT before and after treatment of lymphoma. Radiology 175: 515–519
46. Kostakoglu L, Heh S D J, Portlock C et al 1992 Validation of gallium-67-citrate single photon emission computed tomography in biopsy-confirmed residual Hodgkin's disease in the mediastinum. J Nucl Med 33: 345–350
47. Israel O, Front D, Epelbaum R et al 1990 Residual mass and negative gallium scintigraphy in treated lymphoma. J Nucl Med 31: 365–368
48. Southee A E, McLaughlin A F, Joshua D E et al 1989 Gallium scanning as a predictor of outcome in mediastinal Hodgkin's disease. Eur J Nucl Med 15: 547
49. Kaplan W D 1990 Residual mass and negative gallium scintigraphy in treated lymphoma: when is the gallium scan really negative? (Editorial). J Nucl Med 31: 369–371
50. Huys J, Schelstraete K, Simons M 1982 Gallium-67 imaging in Hodgkin's disease. Clin Nucl Med 7: 174–179
51. Lepanto P B, Rosenstock J, Littman P, Alavi A, Donaldson M, Kuhl D E 1976 Gallium-67 scans in children with solid tumours. AJR 126: 179–186
52. Bitran J D, Bekerman C, Golomb H M, Simon M A 1978 Scintigraphic evaluation of sarcomata in children and adults by Ga-67 citrate. Cancer 42: 1760–1765
53. Kirchner P T, Simon M A 1984 The clinical value of bone and gallium scintigraphy for soft tissue sarcomas of the extremities. J Bone Joint Surg 66: 319–327
54. Finn H A, Simon M A, Martin W B, Darakjian H 1987 Scintigraphy with gallium-67 citrate in staging of soft tissue sarcomas of the extremity. J Bone Joint Surg 69: 886–891
55. Wentz von K-U, Irngartinger A, Georgi P, Van Kaick A, Kleckow M, Vollhaber H H 1986 Malignant pleural mesothelioma – accuracy of Ga-67 scintigraphy vs. computed tomography. ROFO 145: 61–66
56. Howman-Giles R, Stevens M, Bergin M 1982 Role of gallium-67 in management of paediatric solid tumours. Aust Ped J 18: 120–125
57. Armas E R, Goldsmith S J 1985 Gallium scanning in peritoneal mesothelioma. AJR 144: 563–565
58. Kaufman J H, Cedermark B J, Parthasarathy K L, Didolkar M S, Bakshi S P 1977 The value of Ga-67 scintigraphy in soft tissue sarcoma and chondrosarcoma. Radiology 123: 131–134
59. Schwartz H S, Jones C K 1992 The efficacy of gallium scintigraphy in detecting malignant soft tissue neoplasms. Ann Surg 215: 78–82
60. Chen D C, Hung G L, Levine A, Siegel M E 1986 Correlation of gallium uptake and degree of malignancy in non-Hodgkin's lymphoma. J Nucl Med 27: 1031 (Abstract)
61. Krishnamurthy G T, Singhi V, Taylor R D, Ranganath K, Blabd W H 1976 Radionuclide scanning in the evaluation of Kaposi sarcoma. Arch Intern Med 136: 400–403
62. Kirkwood J M, Myers, Vlock D R et al 1982 Tomographic gallium-67 citrate scanning: useful new surveillance for metastatic melanoma. Ann Intern Med 97: 694–699
63. Rossleigh M A, McCarthy W H, Milton G W et al 1984 The role of gallium-67 studies in the management of malignant melanoma. Med J Aust 140: 401–404
64. Kagan R, Witt T, Bines S, Mesleh G, Economou S 1988 Gallium-67 scanning for malignant melanoma. Cancer 61: 272–274
65. Neumann R D, Hoffer P B 1988 Gallium for detection of malignant disease. In: Gottschalk A, Hoffer P B, Potchan, Berger, eds. Diagnostic nuclear medicine, 2nd ed. Williams and Wilkins pp 1076–1089
66. Bekerman C, Caride V J, Hoffer P B, Boles C A 1990 Non-invasive staging of lung cancer. Indications and limitations of gallium-67 citrate imaging. Radiol Clin North Am 28: 497–510
67. Alazraki N P, Ramsdell J W, Taylor A, Friedman P J, Peters R M, Tisi G M, 1978 Reliability of gallium scan, chest radiography compared to mediastinoscopy for evaluating mediastinal spread of lung cancer. Am Rev Respir Dis 117: 415–420
68. Lesk D M, Wood T E, Carrol S E, Reese L 1978 The application of Ga-67 scanning in determining the operability of bronchogenic carcinoma. Radiology 129: 707–709
69. Fosberg R G, Hopkins G B, Kan M K 1979 Evaluation of the mediastinum by gallium-67 scintigraphy in lung cancer. J Thorac Cardiovasc Surg 77: 76–82
70. DeMeester T R, Golomb H M, Kirchner P et al 1979 The role of gallium-67 scanning in the clinical staging and preoperative evaluation of patients with carcinoma of the lung. Ann Thorac Surg 18: 451–464
71. Richardson J V, Zenk B A, Rossi N P 1980 Preoperative non-invasive mediastinal staging in bronchogenic carcinoma. Surgery 88: 382
72. Waxman A D, Julien P J, Brachman M B et al 1984 Gallium scintigraphy in bronchogenic carcinoma: the effect of tumor location on sensitivity and specificity. Chest 86: 178
73. Hirleman M T, Yiu-Chiu V S, Chiu L C 1980 The resectability of primary lung carcinoma: a diagnostic staging review. J Comput Tomogr 4: 146
74. MacMahon H 1989 Efficacy of computed tomography of the thorax and upper abdomen and whole-body gallium scintigraphy for staging of lung cancer. Cancer 64: 1404–1408
75. Matsuno S, Tanabe M, Kawasaki Y et al 1992 Effectiveness of planar image and single photon emission tomography of thallium-201 compared with gallium-67 in patients with primary lung cancer. Eur J Nucl Med 19: 86–95
76. Higashi T, Wakao H, Nakamura A 1982 Quantitative gallium-67 scanning for predictive value in primary lung carcinoma. Clin Nucl Med 7: 553
77. Hatfield M K, MacMahon H, Ryan J W et al 1986 Post operative recurrence of lung cancer: detection by whole-body gallium scintigraphy. Am J Radiol 147: 911–916

78. Hubner K F, Andrews G A, Hayes et al 1977 The use of rare-earth radionuclides and other bone seekers in the evaluation of bone lesions in patients with multiple myeloma or solitary plasmacytoma. Radiology 125: 171–176
79. Waxman A, Siemsen J, Levin A M 1981 Radiographic and radionuclide imaging in multiple myeloma: the role of gallium scintigraphy. Concise communication. J Nucl Med 22: 232–236
80. Patterson A H, Peckham M J, McCready V R 1976 Value of gallium scanning in seminoma of the testis. Br Med J 1: 1118–1121
81. Sauerbrunn B, Andrews G, Hubner K 1978 Ga-67 citrate imaging in tumours of the genitourinary tract: report of co-operative study. J Nucl Med 19: 470–475
82. Pinsky S M, Bailey T B, Blom J, Grove R B, Borski A, Johnson M C 1973 Ga-67 citrate in the staging of testicular malignancies. J Nucl Med 14: 439
83. Waxman A D, Ramanna L, Memsic L D et al 1993 Thallium scintigraphy in the evaluation of mass abnormalities of the breast. J Nucl Med 34: 18–23
84. Kaplan W D, Takvorian T, Morris J H, Rumbaugh C L, Connolly B T, Atkins H L 1987 Thallium-201 brain tumour imaging: a comparative study with pathologic correlation. J Nucl Med 28: 47–52
85. Teates C D, Preston D F, Boyd C M 1980 Gallium-67 imaging in head and neck tumours. Report of co-operative study . J Nucl Med 21: 622
86. Silberstein E B, Kornblut A D, Shumrick D A 1974 Ga-67 as a diagnostic agent for detection of head and neck tumours and lymphomas. Radiology 110: 605
87. Sumi Y, Ozaki Y, Amemiya K, Shirakata F, Tamamoto F, Katayama H 1992 Reappraisal of clinical usefulness of Ga-67 citrate scintigraphy for primary colorectal carcinoma: with evaluation of scintigram obtained from resected specimens. Ann Nucl Med 6: 137–145
88. Lomas F R, Dibos P E, Wagner H N 1972 Increased specificity of liver scanning with the use of gallium-67 citrate. N Engl J Med 286: 1323
89. Yeh S D J, Rosen G, Capattos B, Benua R S 1984 Semiquantitative gallium scintigraphy in patients with osteogenic sarcoma. Clin Nucl Med 9: 175–183

63. Thallium-201 chloride: a tumour imaging agent

Hussein Abdel-Dayem Steven M. Larson Homer Macapinlac Andrew Scott

Thallium-201 (^{201}Tl) is a monovalent cationic radioisotope with biological properties similar to those of potassium.[1–3] As early as 1975 Lebowitz et al[2] suggested that because of the similarity of thallium to alkali metals such as caesium, which has been shown to concentrate in tumours, the use of radiothallium should be evaluated for the purpose of tumour imaging. The primary role of ^{201}Tl in nuclear medicine is its use for myocardial perfusion and, recently, for myocardial viability. Non-cardiac imaging applications include parathyroid and tumour imaging. The role in parathyroid imaging is declining because of better success with ^{99m}Tc sestamibi.[4,5] The role in imaging viable tumours is increasing because of the problems encountered by magnetic resonance imaging (MRI) and X-ray CT, especially after surgical, radiation or chemotherapy treatment, in differentiating post-therapy changes from residual viable tumour tissue, local recurrence or necrosis.[6]

MECHANISM OF INTRACELLULAR THALLIUM UPTAKE

There are different theories for the intracellular accumulation of thallium. Mullins and More[7] suggested that it is driven by the transmembrane electropotential gradient. Other theories suggest that the action on the cell membrane of the ATPase system, that extrudes sodium from the cell and allows potassium ion to enter, is an important mechanism.[8–10] However, the uptakes of ^{201}Tl and potassium in the cell are not identical. Thallium appears to bind to two sites on the enzyme system compared with the one site for potassium.[8] This may explain the more prolonged clearance of thallium from the myocardium compared with potassium.[11] The cellular uptake of thallium is inhibited by ouabain, digitalis and frusemide, which block the sodium–potassium pump.[9,12] In the Ehrlich ascites tumour cell model developed by Sessler et al[9] it was found that frusemide inhibits a co-transport system involving potassium and sodium, as well as chloride ion, and that there is an additive effect of frusemide and ouabain on the inhibition of thallium uptake. Accordingly, Sessler et al[9] postulated that there are at least two transport systems involved in the uptake of thallium by tumour cells. In his results the co-transport system for thallium showed a significant increase from 6-day- to 12-day-old Ehrlich cells. In contrast, the ATPase system became less important as the cells became older. The dominant mode of cellular transmission using this model was found in the frusemide-sensitive group, indicating that co-transport plays a dominant role in cellular transport of thallium. After inhibition of the ATPase system, as well as the co-transport system, a minimal rest flow for ionic transport was noted. This flow was attributed to a calcium-dependent ion channel.

The biodistribution of ^{201}Tl in tumour-bearing animals was investigated by Ando et al,[13] who found that thallium was mainly accumulated by viable tumour tissue, less in connective tissue which contained inflammatory cells and was barely detectable in necrotic tissue. Absence of thallium uptake in areas of necrosis may be due to the non-functioning ATPase cell membrane pump activity and no active transport into necrotic tumour cells. This group also found that, regardless of the time after administration, ^{201}Tl mainly existed in the free form in the fluid of the tumour. They also found that a small fraction of thallium was localized in the nuclear, mitochondrial and microsomal fractions of these tissues and that it was bound to protein in these fractions.

Venuta et al[14] studied thallium uptake in rat thyroid tissue and found that transformed cells took up thallium faster and concentrated it more than normal cells. They also found that, when normal epidural cells grew at different rates, the faster growing cells took up thallium quicker than the slow-growing ones. Ando et al[15,16] also found that the distribution and accumulation mechanisms of thallium and ^{67}Ga in tumour cells are different. They found that ^{67}Ga accumulates avidly in inflammatory tissue, less in tumours and scarcely at all in necrotic tissue. Accordingly, they concluded that ^{201}Tl is better than ^{67}Ga for the visualization of viable tumours.

In a review of thallium applications in clinical oncology, Waxman[17] summarized the possible factors influencing ^{201}Tl uptake by tumour cells: blood flow, viability, tumour type, sodium–potassium, ATPase system, co-transport system, calcium ion channel system, vascular immaturity due to 'leakage' and increased cell membrane permeability. Sehweil et al[12] and Caluser et al[18] had shown in clinical studies that, although blood flow is important for the delivery of thallium to the tumour cells, it is not the only factor responsible for thallium uptake in tumour cells. Sehweil et al[12] also demonstrated that, as in cultured myocardial cells, the addition of digoxin blocks thallium uptake in cultured breast carcinoma cells.

OPTIMUM TIME FOR IMAGING

The optimum time for tumour imaging following the i.v. injection of thallium has been studied by Sehweil et al.[19] In this study dynamic imaging over the tumour and myocardium showed that both had the same time–activity curves for the initial uptake. The highest tumour–background ratio was achieved between 11 and 20 min. Imaging can be performed between 20 and 60 min following the i.v. injection. During this time there were minimal changes in tumour-to-background ratio. They also demonstrated that the majority of tumours show variable thallium washout around 25% over a 2 h period, yet some tumours had more thallium uptake over the same time period. This phenomenon of thallium washout from tumours is complicated and needs more investigation.

Because the blood pool activity decreases with time and the tumour background contrast gets better, Chen et al[20] recommended delayed thallium imaging at 3 h in lymphoma because delayed images have better resolution than earlier ones at 20 min. With planar and SPECT scintigraphy, Ganz et al[21] imaged 33 patients with soft-tissue or osseous masses 5 min and 1–4 h following i.v. injection of thallium. Uptake was quantitated on all images against the contralateral side. In all patients with proven malignancy there was an increase in the ratio from early to late images except for the patients who had a biopsy 1 day prior to scan or who had a superimposed linear fracture. All benign conditions had decreasing ratios over time except for a non-united fracture, which had an increasing linear pattern of uptake. Similar observations have been found in AIDS patients, in whom thallium is used to differentiate pulmonary Kaposi's sarcoma from other opportunistic infections or malignant lymphoma. When comparing early and delayed lesions with background ratios, the ratio increases with time and lesions are better visualized in Kaposi's sarcoma and malignant lymphoma. In other opportunistic infections the ratio decreases with time and the lesions become less well visualized. More work is needed in order to decide whether early or late images alone are enough for accurate interpretation or if there is need for both.

LIMITATIONS OF THALLIUM IMAGING

The limitations of ^{201}Tl chloride in tumour imaging are related to its physical, biological or economic properties. The poor physical characteristics and long half-life (73 h) limit the injected adult dose to between 3 and 5 mCi. The low photon energy (80 kEv) is reflected by the poor resolution, especially for planar images. The normal uptake of thallium in the lacrimal glands, salivary glands, thyroid, myocardium, liver, spleen, kidneys, splanchnic areas and muscles limits the use of thallium for tumour localization in these locations and surrounding areas. Thallium uptake in tumours is usually lower than in these normal organs. The resolution depends upon the tumour-to-background ratio. Thallium-avid tumours cannot be identified in the proximity of high-thallium uptake in the normal organs. In the author's experience thallium tumour imaging in the abdominal or pelvic region has no value. It has limited use in the mediastinum. SPECT imaging is essential in imaging intracranial and intrathoracic lesions.[22] Recent developments of multi-head gamma-camera systems have improved the resolution of thallium SPECT imaging and made it easier and faster.

COMPARISON WITH GALLIUM-67 CITRATE

Since cellular uptake of ^{201}Tl is ATPase dependent, it has several advantages over ^{67}Ga citrate for tumour imaging. These include the shorter waiting time for ^{201}Tl imaging of about 20 min versus 48–96 h for gallium. Also, thallium is more specific for differentiating tumours from acute inflammatory lesions and the intracellular thallium uptake is not affected by steroid administration, chemotherapy or radiation therapy.[23,34] There is minimal thallium uptake in comparison with increased gallium uptake in healing surgical wounds. The lower energy of thallium permits three-phase bone scans to follow thallium studies on the same day using ^{99m}Tc radiopharmaceuticals for patients with bone and soft-tissue tumours. Conversely, problems with ^{67}Ga are related to the fact that its intracellular uptake is related to transferrin binding and transferrin receptors over the cell membrane. It is influenced by several factors affecting this binding affinity, such as blood transfusions, chemotherapy, steroid therapy and/or radiation therapy. Gallium uptake is non-specific for tumour tissue. Inflammatory and autoimmune diseases also show positive gallium uptake.

Different reports exist as to the relationship between ^{201}Tl and ^{67}Ga uptake and histological type of tumours. Tagawa et al[25] reported two cases of adenocarcinoma of the lung in which thallium gave better delineation of metastatic lesions than ^{67}Ga. They also reported that thallium–gallium ratios are high for adenocarcinoma (2 ± 1.55) but low for epidermoid (0.47 ± 0.30) and small-cell carcinoma (0.37 ± 0.05), indicating that adenocarcinoma and oat cell carcinoma take up more ^{201}Tl than ^{67}Ga.[26] Rageb et al[27] found that ^{67}Ga uptake is higher than ^{201}Tl uptake in all types of non-small-cell lung cancer and that there is no relationship between ^{201}Tl and ^{67}Ga uptake intensity and the histological type of the tumour except for higher ^{67}Ga uptake in undifferentiated carcinomas. Kaplan et al[28] compared ^{201}Tl and ^{67}Ga uptake in non-Hodgkin's lymphoma. They found that ^{201}Tl uptake is higher than ^{67}Ga uptake in low-grade lymphoma, while ^{67}Ga uptake is higher in high-grade lymphoma. The ^{67}Ga uptake in inflammatory cells was higher than the specific uptake of thallium by tumour cells and there was no uptake of ^{201}Tl in inflammatory cells.

In the author's experience there are variations between thallium and gallium uptake in various tumours. For example, a tumour might be highly positive for thallium and negative for gallium. The case in Figure 63.1 is that of soft-tissue sarcoma of the right lower leg that demonstrates high thallium uptake and low gallium uptake [positive ^{18}F image fluorodeoxyglucose (FDG)] before chemotherapy. After chemotherapy, repeat thallium images show no response to the treatment and there was an increase in gallium uptake.

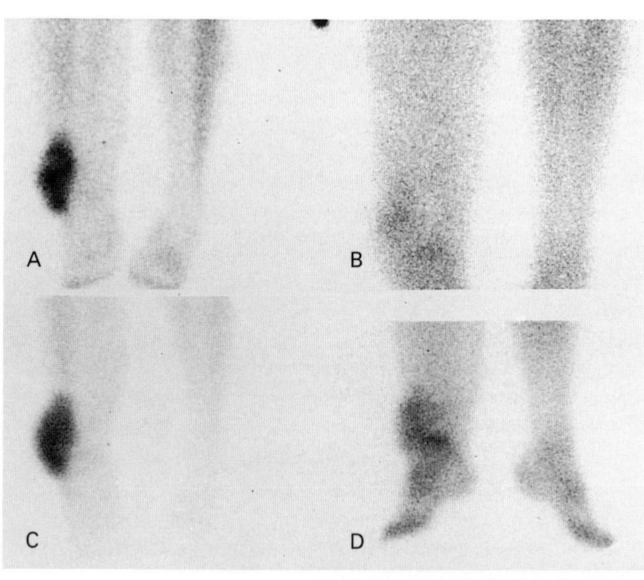

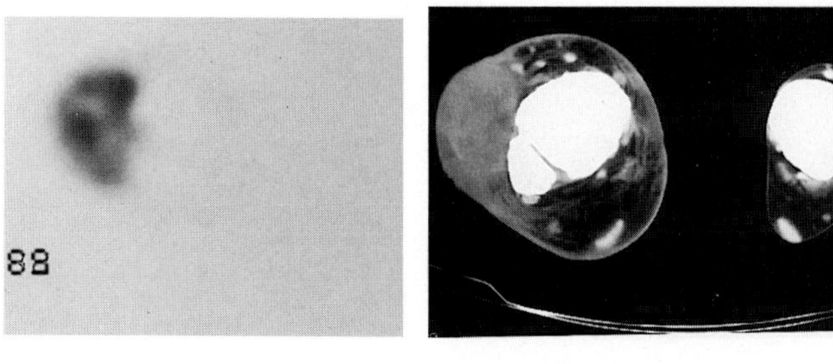

Fig. 63.1 A 28-year-old male with embryonal rhabdomyosarcoma of the soft tissues of the right ankle. (A) ^{201}Tl anterior planar image showing intense accumulation in the right ankle soft tissues. (B) ^{67}Ga scan showing slight uptake in the right ankle tumour. (C) ^{201}Tl images showing no significant change after a full course of chemotherapy. (D) ^{67}Ga scan showing interval appearance of uptake in the right ankle tumour after chemotherapy. (E) ^{18}FDG PET before chemotherapy showing hypermetabolism in the right ankle soft-tissue tumour and the corresponding CT scan (F).

Ramanna et al[29] compared ^{201}Tl, ^{67}Ga and ^{99m}Tc-MDP bone scanning agent for evaluating the response of bone and soft-tissue sarcomas to preoperative chemotherapy. They found that thallium was the most reliable of the three and was more accurate than X-ray CT or MRI.

OBJECTIVES FOR USE OF THALLIUM-201 FOR TUMOUR IMAGING

^{201}Tl chloride for tumour imaging has been tried at various locations. Its use is justified whenever there are clinical problems that cannot be accurately solved by other imaging modalities. These are mainly the following: differentiating benign from malignant lesions, determining the grade of malignancy of the tumour, predicting the response to preoperative treatment, detecting and differentiating local recurrence from radiation necrosis or fibrosis. X-ray CT and MRI have limitations in addressing these clinical problems.[6] Positron emission tomography (PET) using ^{18}F-FDG or ^{11}C-L-methionine, ^{11}C-D-glucose or ^{68}Ga-EDTA is more helpful than X-ray or CT in these situations.[30–38] However, there are limitations for its widespread use. Comparison between ^{201}Tl and ^{18}F-FDG in brain tumour imaging was done by Macapinlac et al[39] and Hoh et al.[40] There was good correlation between ^{201}Tl chloride and ^{18}F-FDG. Both are highly reliable in supratentorial tumours and have limitations in infratentorial lesions. Accordingly, ^{201}Tl chloride can substitute for PET for those who cannot afford the latter. However, it has the limitations of poor resolution, lack of quantitation and restrictions for imaging intra-abdominal and pelvic tumours. Figures 63.2 and 63.3 demonstrate comparisons between MRI, ^{18}F-FDG and ^{201}Tl scans in a successfully treated brain tumour (Fig. 63.2) and in a recurrent brain tumour (Fig. 63.3).

For the above objectives, ^{201}Tl chloride has been used in tumour imaging in order to:

1. Differentiate benign from malignant diseases and localize sites for biopsy. The most common organs reported in literature have been thyroid,[41–51] bones and soft tissue,[21,52–54] lung,[24,25,55,56] brain[57,58] and breast.[56,59–61,64]
2. To determine the grade of malignancy of the tumour. The most common sites for this have been reported for the brain[57,58,62–65] and soft tissue.[53]
3. To evaluate the response of preoperative chemotherapy or radiotherapy, and to determine the

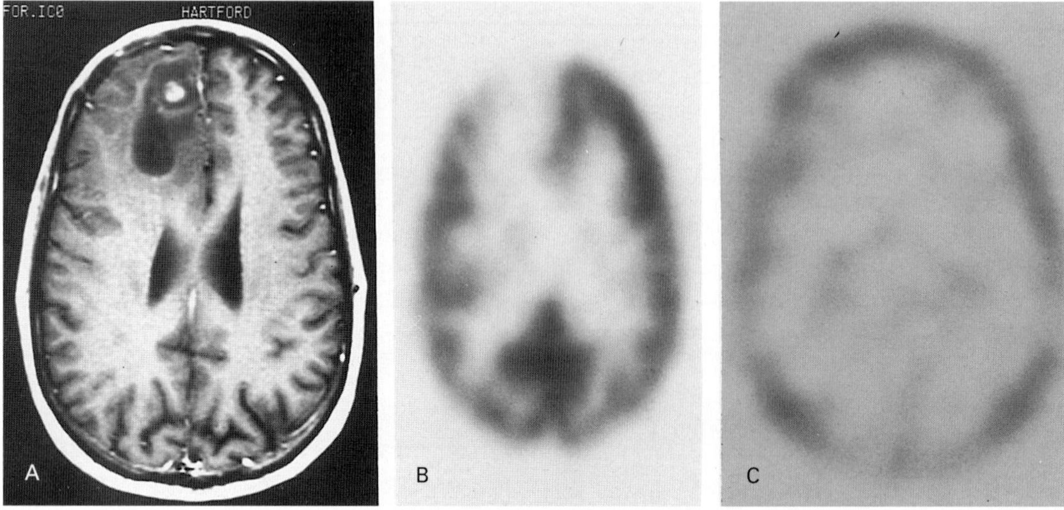

Fig. 63.2 A 29-year-old male with a mixed anaplastic oligodendroglioma resected 1 year previously and with treatment by procarbazine, CCNU and vincristine 6 months later. He was referred for evaluation of residual disease. (A) ^{201}Tl-weighted Gd-DTPA-enhanced MRI showing enhancement in the right frontal lobe. (B) ^{18}F-FDG PET showing hypometabolism of the left frontal lobe. (C) ^{201}Tl SPECT showing no significant uptake in the brain. The patient did well on conservative management.

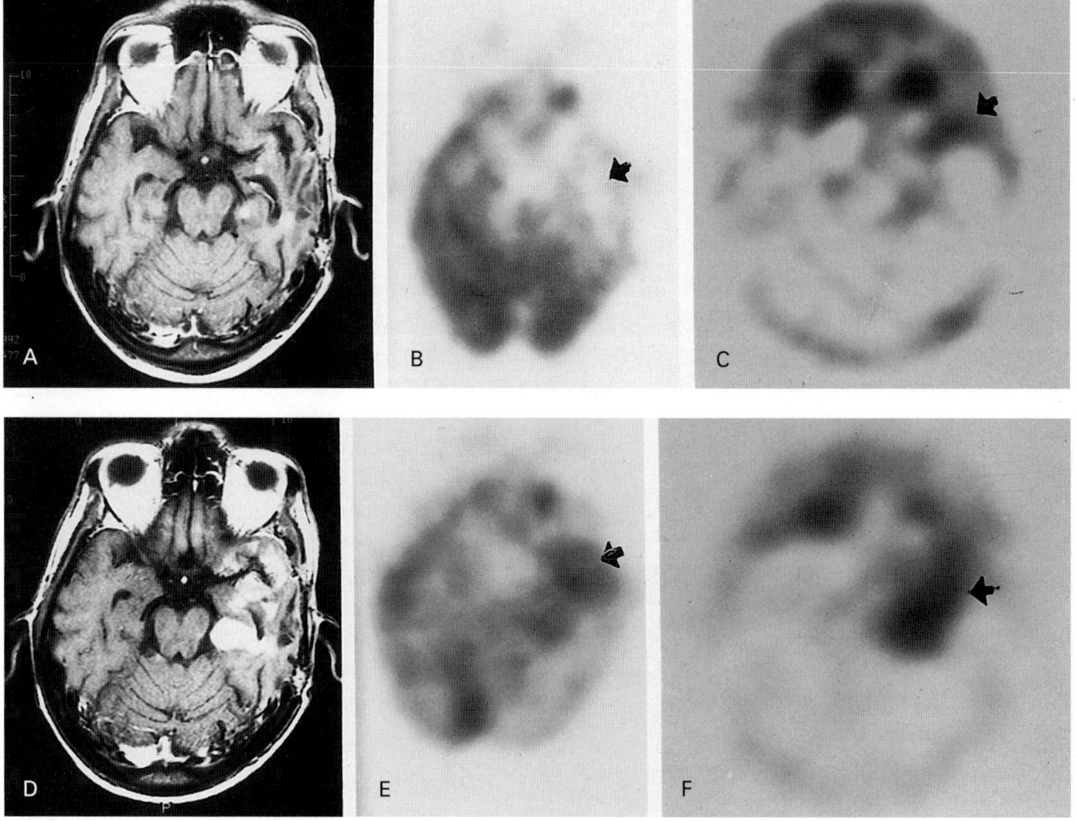

Fig. 63.3 A 52-year-old male with left temporal glioblastoma multiform post resection and recurrent tumour (1 year ago), with recurrent tumour resected 6 months ago, being studied for baseline evaluation following four courses of BCNU therapy. (A) ^{201}Tl-weighted Gd-DTPA-enhanced MRI showing multiple areas of enhancement not specific for residual tumour. (B) ^{18}F-FDG PET showing hypometabolism of the left temporal lobe. (C) ^{201}Tl SPECT at the same level (note activity in the scalp and eye muscles) showing abnormal activity in the medial aspect of the left temporal lobe. Ratio: 4:1. The same patient was evaluated months later, re-evaluated for increasing confusion and overall clinical deterioration. (D) ^{201}Tl-weighted Gd-DTPA enhanced MRI showing new enhancement in the left temporal lobe. (E) ^{18}F-FDG PET showing hypermetabolism in the left temporal lobe extending towards the midline. (F) ^{201}Tl SPECT showing more extensive increased uptake in the left temporal lobe. Ratio: 10:1.

presence of residual tumour and/or local occurrence. The most common sites are the brain,[62–64] bones and soft tissue[30,65] and lung.[27,67]

4. To differentiate post-therapy tissue necrosis or fibrosis from local recurrence. Most common locations are the brain,[62,63,68–70] bones and soft tissue[53,70] and head and neck cancer.[71]

QUANTITATION OF THALLIUM UPTAKE

Comparison of thallium uptake between tumour and adjacent normal or background tissue or contralateral normal tissue has been recommended by various authors in order to differentiate benign from malignant lesions. The values of these ratios vary according to the identification of the region of interest, the location, size of the lesion and whether or not there is central necrosis. Some recommend drawing the region of interest over the highest pixel counts of thallium uptake, while others recommend drawing a region of interest over the inner or outer border of the tumour and averaging the pixel counts.[21,52,58,62,64,65] Ratios above 1.6–2.4 are reported to indicate malignant lesions and lower ratios to indicate either benign lesions or early recurrence. It is reported that the higher the ratio, the higher the grade of malignancy in brain, bone or soft-tissue sarcomas. In the author's judgement, although the ratios are only suggestive of the nature of these lesions, it should not be considered as an absolute indicator. It should always be interpreted with many reservations. There is an overlap between the benign and malignant lesions.[21,52] The normal uptake in the surrounding tissues increases the background counts and decreases the tumour ratio. Ratios are more important if the lesions have not been previously treated. For a thallium-avid lesion that has been previously treated and became thallium negative on follow-up studies, any low level of ^{201}Tl uptake is an indicator of tumour recurrence no matter how low this ratio is. With time this ratio increases as the tumour grows in size. Lower thallium uptake is also observed in the early follow-up studies after surgical excisions and/or aggressive chemotherapy. This is due to granulation tissue and associated new vascularity. A lower ratio for thallium uptake due to granulation tissue should disappear with repeated follow-up thallium studies. In order to increase the specificity of thallium studies in this complex situation, especially in brain and soft-tissue tumours, early and delayed thallium imaging at 30 min and 2–3 h is recommended. Thallium activity due to new vascularity and granulation tissue decreases in the delayed images. The use of combined ^{201}Tl and ^{99m}Tc-HMPAO for brain tumours has been recommended.[68,69,72] ^{99m}Tc-HMPAO uptake ratios over the lesion and the cerebellum were calculated compared with thallium ratios in normal tissue or calvarium ratios. Lesion-to-cerebellum HMPAO ratios higher than 0.5 indicated tumour recurrence, while lower ratios indicated tumour necrosis.

Van der Wall et al[54] reported that, for identification of malignancy in bone lesions, thallium scanning was found to have a sensitivity of 88%, specificity of 94%, positive predictive value of 88% and a negative predictive value of 94%. Thallium uptake with lower tumour–background ratios has been reported in certain benign lesions, such as tuberculosis,[52] sarcoidosis,[56,73] villonodular synovitis[74] and cerebral candidiasis.[75] Thallium uptake should be considered as a reflection of tissue metabolism and ATPase activity irrespective of whether the lesion is benign or malignant. A correlation between thallium uptake and the histological appearance of the lesion, i.e. vascularity, nature of intercellular matrix and density of viable cells, helps in most cases to explain the intensity of thallium uptake in the lesion. For example, in acute abscesses there is no thallium uptake in the centre of the lesion where the tissues are necrotic. Minimal thallium uptake is noted at the periphery of abscesses where there is an ongoing healing process.[76] The same observation has been noted in rapidly growing brain tumour with necrotic centres in AIDS patients.

In order to increase the specificity for differentiating benign from malignant lesions, Caluser et al[77] studied 37 patients in 47 studies with treated and untreated bone and soft-tissue sarcomas. The tumour–background ratios obtained from thallium studies were compared with the same ratios obtained from the blood pool image of the three-phase bone scans done immediately following the thallium studies.[77] They found that when the thallium ratio was higher than the blood pool ratio the lesions were all malignant, with a specificity of 100% (20 lesions). However, the reverse was not true. If the blood pool ratio was higher than the thallium ratio, it was not specific for a benign lesion.

USE OF THALLIUM FOR STAGING MALIGNANT DISEASE

There are controversial reports in the literature about the use of thallium for staging of malignant disease of the chest. Sehweil et al[78] found that planar thallium has low sensitivity for staging of lung cancer, breast cancer and mediastinal lymphoma. However, Matsuno et al[67] found that thallium SPECT imaging was superior to ^{67}Ga for evaluation of the primary lesion and lymph nodes when both were compared in 38 patients scanned before surgery. The results were correlated with pathological findings after thoracotomy. On the other hand, it was found[27] that planar gallium is more sensitive than thallium for determining the local extent of the disease in 70 patients with non-small-cell lung cancer. However, both were less sensitive than X-ray CT. Tonami et al[79,80] reported that the accuracy of ^{201}Tl SPECT for mediastinal involvement is 88%.

I agree with the early findings reported by Sehweil et al.[78] Even with better resolution multidetector systems, detection of mediastinal nodal disease is less sensitive than X-ray CT or MRI. However, for the evaluation of therapy or for follow-up, radionuclide procedures might be more specific than X-ray CT or MRI.

ROLE OF THALLIUM IN AIDS PATIENTS

Thallium imaging has a significant role in differentiating malignant from inflammatory lesions or Kaposi's sarcoma in AIDS patients. Lee et al[81,82] reported that pulmonary Kaposi's sarcoma lesions are thallium positive, gallium negative. Figure 63.4 shows an example of pulmonary Kaposi's sarcoma. Other neoplastic lesions such as lymphoma are thallium and gallium positive. Acute opportunistic infection lesions are gallium positive, thallium negative. This approach of sequential thallium and gallium scans in AIDS patients was evaluated and it was found that the accuracy of thallium- and gallium-negative lesions for the diagnosis of Kaposi's sarcoma is 88%. Chronic inflammatory or TB lesions are thallium and gallium positive. *Pneumocystis carinii* pneumonia shows diffuse increased thallium uptake if imaged 30 min after the injection. This uptake decreases in imaging 2 h later.

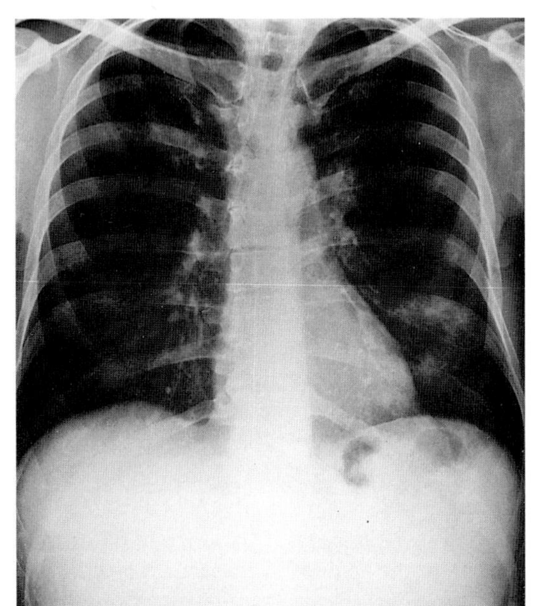

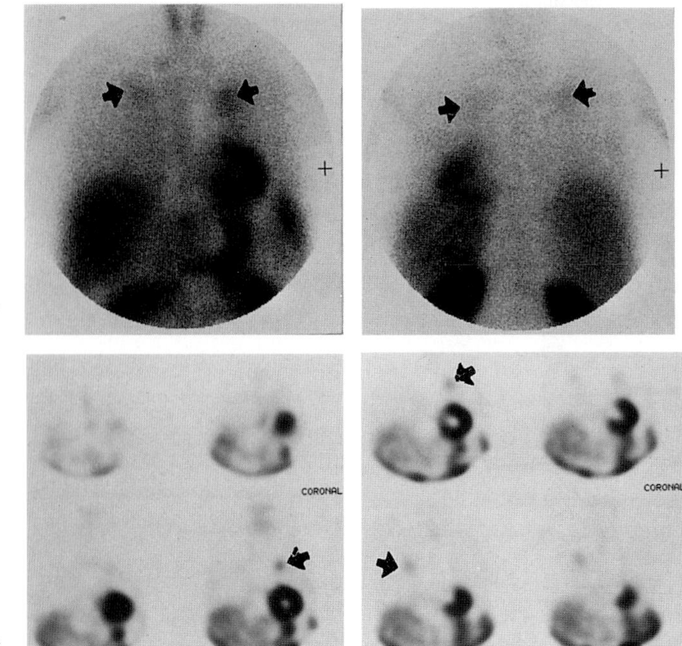

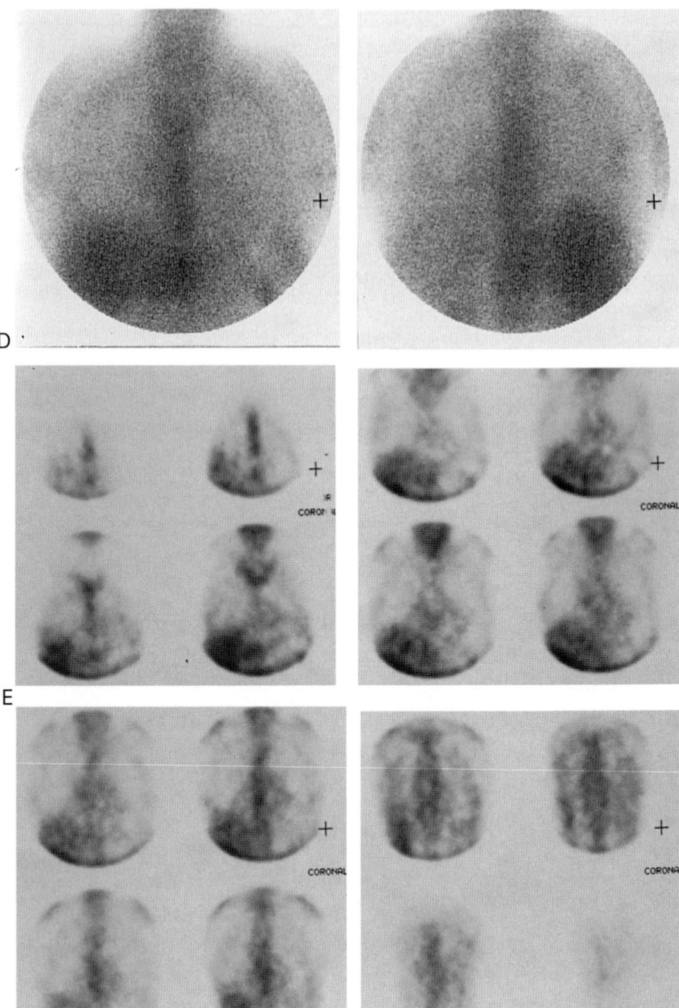

Fig. 63.4 A 51-year-old male patient suffering from AIDS had cutaneous Kaposi's sarcoma lesions. Chest (**A**) is normal. ^{201}Tl scan, planar (**B**) and SPECT (**C**) show lesions in both left upper and right upper lungs. ^{67}Ga scans [planar (**D**) and SPECT (**E**)] are negative. Findings are suggestive of Kaposi's sarcoma.

COMPARISON BETWEEN THALLIUM-201 AND TECHNETIUM-99m SESTAMIBI

^{99m}Tc methoxy-methylpropyl isonitrile (sestamibi,

Cardiolite) has been in use for myocardial perfusion imaging. Whether it will substitute for thallium in non-cardiac applications is still under investigation. Promising results in parathyroidal localization have been reported by Taillefer and others.[4,5] The mechanism of cellular uptake is different from thallium. The cellular membrane transport of sestamibi is affected by the electric potential across the cell membrane, the blood flow and probably the metabolic activity of the cell itself.[83] Sestamibi becomes attached to an intracellular protein, fixed inside the cell and does not wash out from the cells as does ^{201}Tl. Intracellular sestamibi uptake is not affected by drugs that work on the ATPase system. Hassan et al[84] studied the kinetics of initial uptake of ^{99m}Tc sestamibi in benign and malignant lesions and found it to be similar to thallium. It peaked at the same time with the myocardial uptake. Macapinlac et al[85] compared thallium and sestamibi in brain tumour. Thallium was more useful. Sestamibi has normal uptake in the pituitary gland and choroid plexus which is not blocked by i.v. atropine, oral potassium perchlorate or i.v. diamox. Low-grade malignant lesions close to the choroid plexus were not visualized with sestamibi while they were seen with thallium. There are reports of sestamibi uptake in benign and malignant lesions in thyroid, lung and brain lesions.[86–90] Further work is needed for comparison between ^{201}Tl and sestamibi.

In summary, the indications for ^{201}Tl chloride in tumour imaging are: (1) differentiating benign from malignant lesions, (2) providing a guide to the grade of malignancy of the lesions, (3) evaluation of chemotherapy and (4) differentiating tissue necrosis or fibrosis from tumour recurrence. The areas in which thallium is currently considered clinically useful are, in order of importance: (1) brain, (2) peripheral bone and soft-tissue sarcomas, (3) Kaposi's sarcoma and AIDS-related chest problems (Ch. 80). Many consider it to have a role in the differentiation of the thyroid module (Ch. 56), the detection of medullary thyroid carcinoma (Ch. 57) and the postoperative follow-up of differentiated thyroid carcinoma (Ch. 72). There are limited indications for thallium in the following locations: (1) breasts, (2) mediastinal lymphoma, (3) lung carcinoma, (4) head and neck cancer. No indications for thallium in tumour imaging exist in the following locations: (1) abdominal and pelvic regions, (2) spinal cord, vertebral column, either in bones or soft tissues.

In these days of cost containment it is important that the test is used only if it will help solve a clinical problem and will add valuable information that will help in patient management.

REFERENCES

1. Gehring P J, Hammand P B 1967 The interrelationship between thallium and potassium in animals. J Pharmacol Exp Ther 155: 187–201
2. Lebowitz E, Greene M W, Fairchild et al 1975 Thallium-201 for medical use. I. Nucl Med 16: 151–155
3. Bradley-Moore P R, Lebowitz E, Greene M W, Atkins H L, Ansari A N. Thallium-201 for medical use. II. Biologic behavior. J Nucl Med 16: 156–160
4. Taillefer R, Boucher Y, Potvin C, Lambert R 1992 Detection and localization of parathyroid adenomas in patients with hyperparathyroidism using a single radionuclide imaging procedure with technetium-99m-SestaMIBI (double-phase study). J Nucl Med 33: 1801–1807
5. Coakley A J, Kettle A G, Wells C P, O'Doherty M J, Collins R E C 1989 Tc-99m SestaMIBI, a new agent for parathyroid imaging. Nucl Med Commun 10: 791–794
6. Wallner K E, Galieich J H, Malkin M G, Arbit E, Korl G, Rosenblum M K 1989 Inability of computed tomography appearance of recurrent malignant astrocytoma to predict survival following reoperation. J Clin Oncol 7: 1492–1496
7. Mullins L J, More R D 1960 The movement of thallium ions in muscle. J Gen Physiol 43: 759–773
8. Britten J S, Blamk M 1968 Thallium activation of the (Na^+–K^+) activated ATPase of rabbit kidney. Biochim Biophys Acta 159: 160–166
9. Sessler M J, Geck P, Maul F D et al 1986 New aspects of cellular Tl-201 uptake: T+NA+-2CL- cotransport is the central mechanism of ion uptake. Nucl Med 25: 24–27
10. Muranake A 1981 Accumulation of radioisotopes with tumor affinity. II. Comparison of the tumor accumulation of Ga-67 citrate and thallium-201 chloride in vitro. Acta Med Okayama 35: 85–101
11. Strauss H W, Pitt B 1977 Thallium-201 as a myocardial imaging agent. Semin Nucl Med 7: 49–58
12. Sehweil A M, McKillop J H, Milroy R et al 1989 Mechanism of Tl-201 uptake in tumors. Eur J Nucl Med 15: 376–379
13. Ando A, Ando I, Katayama M et al 1987 Biodistribution of Tl-201 in tumor bearing animals and inflammatory lesions induced animals. Eur J Nucl Med 12: 567–572
14. Venuta S, Ferraiuolo R, Morrone G et al 1979 The uptake of Tl-201 in normal and transformed thyroid cell lines. J Nucl Med Allied Sci 23: 163–166
15. Ando A, Ando I, Sanada S et al 1984 Study of the distribution of tumor affinity metal compounds and alkaline metal compounds in the tumor tissues by macroautoradiography. Int J Nucl Med Biol 11: 195–201
16. Ando A, Ando I, Sanada S et al 1985 Tumor and liver uptake models of Ga-67 citrate. Eur J Nucl Med 10: 262–268
17. Waxman A D 1991 Thallium-201 in nuclear oncology. In: Freeman L M (ed) Nuclear Medicine Annual. Raven Press, New York, pp 193–209
18. Caluser C, Macapinlac H, Healy T et al 1992 The relationship between thallium uptake, blood flow and blood pool activity in bone and soft tissue tumors. Clin Nucl Med 17: 565–571
19. Sehweil A, McKillop J H, Ziada G, Al-Sayed M, Abdel-Dayem H, Omar Y T 1988 The optimum time for tumor imaging with thallium-201. Eur J Nucl Med 13: 527–529
20. Chen D C P, Ma G Q, Ansari A et al 1992 Optimal imaging time for thallium as a tumor agent in patients with lymphoma (abstract 844). J Nucl Med 33 & 44
21. Ganz W I, Nguyen T Q, Benedetto M P et al 1993 Use of early, late and SPECT thallium imaging in evaluating activity of soft tissue and bone tumors (abstract). J Nucl Med 34: 33p
22. Holman B L, Tumeh S S 1990 Single-photon emission computed tomography (SPECT): applications and potential. JAMA 263: 561–564
23. Kaplan W D, Takuovian T, Morris J H et al 1987 Thallium-201 brain tumor imaging: a comparative study with pathologic correlation. J Nucl Med 28: 47–52
24. Editorial 1990 Systemic evaluation of primary brain tumors. J Nucl Med 31: 969–971
25. Tagawa T, Yui N, Koakutsu M et al 1989 Two cases of adenocarcinoma of the lung in which thallium-201 gave a better

delineation of metatastic lesions than gallium-67. Clin Nucl Med 14: 197–201
26. Tagawa T, Suzuki A, Kato K et al 1985 Relation between Tl-201 to gallium-67 uptake ratio and histological type in primary lung cancer. Eur J Cancer Clin Oncol 28: 925–930
27. Rageb A, El-Gazzar A H, Abdel-Dayem H M et al 1993. A comparative study between planar Ga-67, Tl-201, chest X-ray and X-ray CT scans in inoperable non-small cell carcinoma of the lung. Eur J Nucl Med 20: 838 (Abstract)
28. Kaplan W D, Southee M L, Annese M S et al 1990 Evaluating low and intermediate grade non-Hodgkin's lymphoma (NHL) with gallium-67 (Ga) and thallium-201 (tl) imaging (abstract). J Nucl Med 31: 793
29. Ramanna L, Waxman A D, Binney G, Waxman S, Mirra J, Rosen G 1990 Tl-201 scintigraphy in bone sarcoma: comparison with Ga-67 and Tc-99m MDP in the evaluation of chemotherapeutic response. J Nucl Med 31: 567–572
30. Alavi J B, Alavi A, Chawluk J et al 1988 Positron emission tomography in patients with glioma. A predictor of prognosis. Cancer 62: 1074–1078
31. Patronas N J, DiChiro G, Kufta C et al 1985 Prediction of survival in glioma patients by means of positron emission tomography. J Neurosurg 62: 816–822
32. Glantz M J, Hoffman J M, Coleman R E et al 1991 Identification of early recurrence of primary central nervous system tumors by [18F] fluorodeoxyglucose positron emission tomography. Ann Neurol 29: 347–355
33. Valk P E, Budinger T F, Levin V A, Silver P, Gutin P H, Doyle W K 1988 PET of malignant cerebral tumors after interstitial brachytherapy. Demonstration of metabolic activity and correlation with clinical outcome. J Neurosurg 69: 830–838
34. Doyle W K, Budinger T F, Valk P E, Levin V A, Gutin P H 1987 Differentiation of cerebral radiation necrosis from tumor recurrence by F-18-FDG and Rb-82 positron emission computed tomography. J Comput Assist Tomogr 11: 653–670
35. Kim E E, Chung S K, Haynie T P et al 1992 Differentiation of residual or recurrent tumors from post-treatment changes with F-18 FDG PET. Radiographics 12: 269–279
36. Lilja A, Lundqvist H, Olsson Y, Spannare B, Guilberg P, Langstrom B 1989 Positron emission tomography and computed tomography in differential diagnosis between recurrent or residual glioma and treatment-induced brain lesions. Acta Radiol 30: 121–128
37. Ericson K, Lilja A, Bergstrom M et al 1985 Positron emission tomography with ([11C]methyl)-L-methionine, [11C]D-glucose and [68Ga]EDTA in supratentorial tumors. J Comput Assist Tomogr 9: 683–689
38. Dichiro G, De La Paz R L, Brooks R A et al 1982 Glucose utilization of cerebral glioma patients by means of positron emission tomography. Neurology 32: 1323–1329
39. Macapinlac H, Finlay J, Yeh S D J et al 1992 Comparison of Tl-201 SPECT and F-18 FDG PET imaging with MRI (Gd-DTPA) in the evaluation of recurrent supratentorial and infratentorial brain tumors. J Nucl Med 33: 867
40. Hoh C K, Khannas, Harris G C et al 1992 Evaluation of brain tumor recurrence with Tl-201 SPECT studies: correlation with FDG PET and histological results. J Nucl Med 33: 867
41. Harada T, Ito Y, Shimaoka K et al 1980 Clinical evaluation of thallium-201 chloride scan for thyroid nodule. Eur J Nucl Med 5: 125–130
42. Nemec J, Zamrazil V, Pohunkova D et al 1984 The rational use of Tl-201 scintigraphy in the evaluation of differentiated thyroid cancer. Eur J Nucl Med 9: 261–264
43. Ochi H, Sawa H, Fukuda T 1982 Thallium-201 chloride thyroid scintigraphy to evaluate benign and/or malignant nodules. Cancer 50: 236–240
44. El-Desouki M 1991 Tl-201 thyroid imaging in differentiating benign from malignant thyroid nodules. Clin Nucl Med 16: 425–430
45. Henze E, Roth J, Boerer H et al 1986 Diagnostic value of early and delayed Tl-201 thyroid scintigraphy in the evaluation of cold nodules for malignancy. Eur J Nucl Med 211: 413–416
46. Bleichrodt R P, Vezmey A, Piers D A et al 1987 Early and delayed thallium-201 imaging: Diagnosis of patients with cold thyroid nodules. Cancer 60: 2621–2623
47. Tonami N, Bunko H, Michigishi T et al 1978 Clinical evaluation of tumor imaging with Tl-201 chloride. Radiology 129: 497–500
48. Eguchi S, Matsumura T, Nomura Y et al 1979 Thyroid scanning with Tl-201 chloride. Otologia (Fukuoka) 24: 353–359
49. Palermo F, Bruniera F, Caldatr L et al 1979 Scintigraphic evaluation of the cold thyroid areas. Eur J Nucl Med 4: 43–48
50. Tennvall J, Palmer J, Bjorklund A et al 1984 Kinetics of Tl–201 uptake in adenomas and well-differentiated carcinomas of the thyroid. A double isotope investigation with Tc-99m and Tl-201. Acta Radio Oncol 23: 55–95
51. Hardoff R, Baron E, Sheinfeld M 1991 Early and late lesion to non-lesion ratio of thallium-201 chloride uptake in the evaluation of cold thyroid nodules. J Nucl Med 32: 1873–1876
52. Elgazzar A H, Malki A, Abdel-Dayem H M 1989 Role of thallium-201 in the diagnosis of solitary bone lesions. Nucl Med Commun 10: 477–485
53. Ramanna L, Waxman A D, Weiss A, Rosen G 1992 Thallium-201 (Tl-201) scan patterns in bone and soft tissue sarcoma (abstract 843). J Nucl Med 33: 843
54. Van der Wall H, Murray I P C, Huckstep R L, Philips R L 1993 The role of thallium scintigraphy in excluding malignancy in bone. Clin Nucl Med 18: 551–557
55. Tonami N, Yokoyama K, Taki J et al 1990 Tissue characterization of suspected malignant pulmonary lesions with Tl-201 SPECT. J Nucl Med 31: 766
56. Sehweil A 1988 Thallium kinetics in malignant tumors. PhD Thesis, Glasgow University
57. Kaplan W D, Takvorian T, Morris J H et al 1987 Thallium-201 brain tumor imaging: a comparative study with pathologic correlation. J Nucl Med 28: 47–52
58. Black K L, Hawkins R A, Kim K T et al 1989 Use of thallium-201 SPECT to quantitate malignancy grade of gliomas. J Neurosurg 71: 432–436
59. Waxman A, Ramanna L, Memsic A et al 1990 Thallium scintigraphy in the determination of malignant from benign mass abnormalities of the breast. J Nucl Med 31: 767
60. Sluyser M, Hoefnagel C 1988 Breast carcinomas detected by thallium-201 scintigraphy. Cancer Letters 40: 161–168
61. Waxman A D, Ramanna L, Memsic L D et al 1993 Thallium scintigraphy in the evaluation of mass abnormalities of the breast. J Nucl Med 34: 18–23
62. Kim K T, Black K L, Marciano D et al 1990 Thallium-201 SPECT imaging of brain tumors. Methods and results. J Nucl Med 31: 965–969
63. Sizofski W J, Krishna L, Chevres S J et al 1991 SPECT thallium index and brain tumors. J Nucl Med 32: 1138
64. Sjöholm B A, Elonquist D, Rehncrona S, Rosen I, Salford L 1992 Thallium-201 and SPECT distinguishes high-grade from low-grade gliomas (abstract). J Nucl Med 33: 868
65. Kosuda S, Aoki S, Suzuki K, Nakamura O, Shidara N 1992 Re-evaluation of quantitative thallium-201 brain SPECT for brain tumors (abstract). J Nucl Med 33: 844
66. Nishizawa K, Okunieff P, Elmaleh D et al 1991 Blood flow of human soft tissue sarcomas measured by Tl-201 scanning: prediction of tumor response to radiation. Int J Radiat Oncol 20: 593–597
67. Matsuno S, Tanabe M, Kawasaki Y et al 1992 Effectiveness of planar image and single photon emission tomography of thallium-201 compared with gallium-67 in patients with primary lung cancer. Eur J Nucl Med 19: 86
68. Carvalho P A, Schwartz R B, Alexander III E et al 1992 Detection of recurrent gliomas with quantitative Tl-201/Tc-99m HMPAO SPECT. J Neurosurg 77: 565–570
69. O'Tuama L A, Janicek M J, Barnes P D et al 1991 Tl-201/Tc-99m HMPAO SPECT imaging of treated childhood brain tumors. Pediatr Neurol 7: 249–257
70. Podoloff D, Haynie T, Kim E et al 1991 Thallium-201 SPECT tumor imaging in differentiation of recurrent metastatic disease from post therapy complication. J Nucl Med 32: 962
71. Elgazzar A H, Sehweil A, Rageb A, Abdel-Dayem H M, Mahmoud A, Omar Y T 1988 Experience with thallium-201 imaging in head and neck cancer. Clin Nucl Med 13: 286–290

72. Schwartz R B, Carvalho P A, Alexander III E, Loeffler J S, Folkerth R, Holman B L 1991 Radiation necrosis vs high-grade recurrent glioma: Differentiation by using dual-isotope SPECT with Tl-201 and Tc-99m HMPAO. AJR 12: 1187–1192
73. Waxman A D, Goldsmith M S, Grief M et al 1987 Differentiation of tumor versus sarcaridosis using thallium-201 in patients with hilar adenopathy (abstract P). J Nucl Med 28: 561
74. Caluser C, Healey T, Macapinilac H et al 1992 Tl-201 uptake in recurrent pigmented villonodular synovitis. Correlation with three-phase bone imaging. Clin Nucl Med 17: 751–753
75. Tonami N, Matasuda H, Ooba H et al 1990 Thallium-201 accumulation in cerebral candidiasis: Unexpected finding on SPECT. Clin Nucl Med 15: 397–400
76. Krisha L, Slizofski W J, Katsetos C D et al 1992 Abnormal intracerebral thallium localization in bacterial abscess. J Nucl Med 33: 2017–2019
77. Caluser C, Abdel-Dayem H M, Macapinlac H A et al 1992 The value of thallium and three phase bone scans in the evaluation of soft tissue and bone sarcomas. Radiology 185: 315
78. Sehweil A M, McKillop J H, Milroy et al 1990 Tl-201 scintigraphy in the staging of lung cancer, breast cancer and lymphoma. Nucl Med Commun 11: 263–269
79. Tonami N, Shuke N, Yokoyama K et al 1989 Thallium-201 single photon emission computed tomography in the evaluation of suspected lung cancer. J Nucl Med 30: 907–1004
80. Tonami N, Yokoyama K, Taki J et al 1991 Pre-operative assessment for mediastinal involvement of lung cancer using Tl-201 SPECT. J Nucl Med 32: 961
81. Lee V W, Rosen M P, Baum A et al 1988 AIDS-related Kaposi's sarcoma. Findings on thallium-201 scintigraphy. Am J Radiol 151: 1233–1235
82. Lee V W, Fuller J D, O'Brien M J et al 1991 Pulmonary Kaposi's sarcoma in patients with AIDS: Scintigraphy diagnosis with sequential thallium and gallium scanning. Radiology 180: 409–412
83. Piwinca-Worms D, Kronauge I F, Holman B C, Lister-James J, Davison A, Jones A G 1988 Hexakis (carbomethoxy isopropyl isonitrile) technetium 1, a new myocardial perfusion agent; binding characteristics in cultured chick heart cells. J Nucl Med 29: 55–61
84. Hassan I M, Sehweil A, Constantinides C et al 1989 Uptake and kinetics of Tc-99m-Hexakis 2-methoxy isobutyl isonitrile in benign and malignant lesions in the lungs. Clin Nucl Med 14: 333–340
85. Macapinlac H, Scott A, Caluser C et al 1992 Comparison of Tl-201 and Tc-99m 2-methoxyisobutyl isonitrile (MIBI) with MRI in the evaluation of recurrent brain tumors (abstract). J Nucl Med 33: 867
86. Muller S T, Reiner C, Paas M et al 1989 Tc-99m-MIBI and Tl-201 uptake in bronchial carcinoma. J Nucl Med 30: 845
87. Muller S T, Guth-Taugelides B, Creutzig H. Imaging of malignant tumors with Tc-99m-MIBI SPECT. J Nucl Med 28: 562
88. O'Tuama L A, Packard A B, Treves S T 1990 SPECT imaging of paediatric brain tumor with hexakis (methoxyisobutyl isonitrile) technetium (I). J Nucl Med 31: 2040–2041
89. Caner B, Kitapci M, Anas T, Erbengi G, Ugur O, Bekdik C 1991 Increased accumulation of hexakis (2-methoxyisobutyl isonitrile) Technetium (I) in osteosarcoma and its metastatic lymph nodes. J Nucl Med 32: 1977–1978
90. Aktolun C, Bayhan H, Celasun B, Kir M K 1991 Unexpected uptake of lymph node hyperplasia of the mediastinum (Castleman's disease). Eur J Nucl Med 18: 856–859

64. Adrenocortical scintigraphy

Brahm Shapiro Milton D. Gross

Adrenal scintigraphy antedates both adrenal CT and MRI. Despite the relatively low spatial resolution of scintigraphy, it continues to provide unique in vivo functional imaging data on the adrenal cortex which the high spatial resolution of the anatomical modalities cannot replace.[1–3]

IMAGING THE ADRENAL GLANDS: COMPARISON OF MODALITIES

The adrenal glands are inaccessible to clinical examination and thus require medical imaging for their depiction.[1–3] All major radiological techniques have been applied and their relative advantages, disadvantages, risks and costs are compared in Table 64.1. Currently, CT, MRI and scintigraphy are most widely employed while there is a limited role for ultrasound and venous sampling.[1–3] In the adrenocortical hypersecretory syndromes imaging should not be performed until a firm diagnosis has been made on the basis of the history and physical examination and confirmed by the appropriate biochemical investigations.[2] Anatomical imaging (usually CT), which includes the adrenals, is often performed to locate or stage known or suspected malignancy or to investigate abdominal pain. Adrenal masses discovered in these circumstances may be further characterized by scintigraphy.[4]

FUNCTIONAL ADRENAL SCINTIGRAPHY: UNDERLYING PRINCIPLES

Radiolabelled cholesterol analogues when administered intravenously are incorporated into low-density lipoprotein (LDL) and enter the tissues by LDL receptor-mediated transport. Cholesterol is the substrate for adrenal steroid hormone synthesis and is normally derived from LDL (although de novo synthesis from acetate may also occur).[3,5] The radiolabelled cholesterol analogues undergo esterification and storage in the intracellular lipid droplet pool but are not further metabolized.[3,5] There are thus no radiolabelled steroid hormone analogues synthesized. Cholesterol analogues taken up by liver LDL receptors are excreted unchanged and also undergo metabolism to bile acid analogues, which are both excreted in the bile and subject to enterohepatic circulation.[3,5,6] Adrenocortical radiopharmaceutical uptake is modulated by the factors which act on the hypothalamic–pituitary–adrenal (CRF–ACTH–cortisol) axis and the renin–angiotensin–aldosterone axis.[3,5]

An alternative elegant approach to adrenocortical scintigraphy has been to radiolabel compounds which bind to and inhibit specific adrenal hormone biosynthetic enzymes (e.g, metyrapone and its analogues). These tracers have shown promise in animal studies.

RADIOPHARMACEUTICALS

The first adrenocortical-avid radiopharmaceutical introduced into practice was ^{131}I 19-iodocholesterol (see Fig. 64.1). A second-generation radiopharmaceutical, ^{131}I 6-beta-iodomethyl-norcholesterol (NP59) was identified as a contaminant of 19-iodocholesterol preparations and has at least a fivefold greater affinity for adrenocortical uptake.[3,5] The closely related radiopharmaceutical, ^{75}Se 6-beta-selenomethyl-norcholesterol, has very similar properties to NP59 and the ^{75}Se label may provide the marginal advantages of longer shelf-life and the ability to image as late as 14 days post injection, when non-adrenal background is negligible.[7,8]

The dosimetry of adrenocortical radiopharmaceuticals is relatively high (see Table 64.2).

Adrenocortical imaging procedures

Adrenocortical imaging is performed in two ways: (1) baseline or non-suppression imaging[3,5] and (2) in the face of dexamethasone suppression, which decreases pituitary ACTH and thus tracer uptake by the glucocorticoid-synthesizing component of the adrenal cortex.[3,5,9] This enhances the detection of mineralocorticoid and androgen-secreting adrenal adenomas and their differentiation from bilateral hyperplasia. The most widely employed dexamethasone suppression regimen is 1 mg q.i.d. for 7 days before tracer injection continued throughout the imaging

Table 64.1 A comparison of adrenal gland imaging techniques

Technique	Underlying principle	Advantages	Disadvantages	Comments	Relative cost
Abdominal radiography	X-ray attenuation, depicts anatomy	Widely available. Cheap	Very insensitive	Obsolete	+
Retroperitoneal gas insufflation	X-ray attenuation with gas contrast, depicts anatomy	High contrast. Excellent depiction	Invasive. Risk of gas embolus Risk of infection	Obsolete	++
Intravenous urography with nephrotomography	X-ray attenuation with iodinated contrast, depicts anatomy	Widely available	Insensitive. Risks of contrast	Obsolete	++
Ultrasound	Reflection of ultrasound, depicts anatomy	Widely available	Limited resolution. Interference by fat and bowel gas	Limited utility	++
Angiography	X-ray attenuation with iodinated contrast, depicts vascular anatomy	Detailed depiction of vascular anatomy	Invasive (arterial puncture). Technically demanding. May cause adrenal haemorrhage or infarction. Risks of contrast	Generally obsolete	++++
Venography with venous sampling	Hormone assay. X-ray attenuation with iodinated contrast, depicts venous anatomy	Characterization of hormonal secretory state (gold standard). Depiction of venous anatomy	Invasive (venous catheterization). Technically demanding. Requires multiple hormonal measurements. May cause adrenal haemorrhage or infarction. Risks of contrast	Still occasionally valuable when non-invasive studies are equivocal	+++++
Adrenal CT	X-ray attenuation, depicts anatomy (iodinated contrast may be used)	Highest resolution. Widely available	May fail in post-operative or very thin patients	Very widely employed	++++
Adrenal MRI	Radiofrequency signal elicited by protons in magnetic field following radiofrequency stimulus	High resolution. No ionizing radiation. Some degree of tissue characterization	Limited specificity of tissue characterization. Resolution less than CT	Limited advantages over CT	+++++
Adrenal scintigraphy	External detection of radio-pharmaceutical uptake, depicts adrenal cholesterol uptake and storage	Non-invasive. Functional in vivo depiction of physiology. Potentially quantifiable	Only moderate resolution. Delay from tracer injection to imaging. Limited availability in USA	Underutilized. Often complementary to CT or MRI	+++

Table 64.2 Radiation dosimetry of adrenocortical radiopharmaceuticals (rad/mCi)

Organ	19-Iodocholesterol	NP59	^{75}Se selenomethyl-norcholesterol
Whole body	0.94	1.2	8.5
Adrenal cortex*	49.0	26.0	20–100
Ovary	20.7	8.0	9.5
Testis	4.8	2.3	–
Liver	7.1	2.4	13.5

*Baseline unsuppressed state (adrenal radiation dose reduced by at least 50% by dexamethasone suppression) (data from Gross et al[3] and Shapiro et al[5])

period.[9] With ^{131}I-labelled tracers thyroidal uptake of free ^{131}I is blocked by iodides. Typical doses of NP59 and 19-iodocholesterol are 1 mCi, which may be scaled to body weight or surface area (1 mCi per 1.73 m^2 or 1 mCi per 70 kg body weight).[2,3,5] The dose of ^{75}Se selenomethyl-nor-cholesterol is 200–250 μCi.[7,8] Posterior and lateral images are obtained in analogue and digitized computer-stored format in the posterior and lateral projections (the anterior is also occasionally useful) for 50 000–100 000 counts. With unsuppressed NP59 studies imaging is performed at 5 and/or 7 days, and 7 and/or 14 days with selenomethyl-

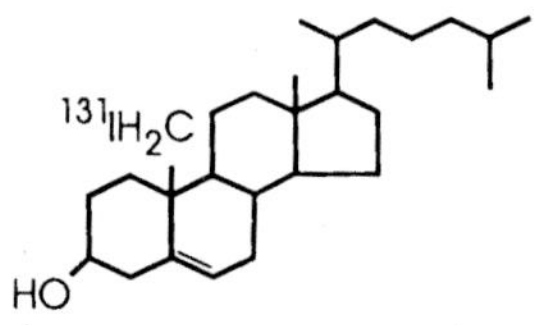

^{131}I-19-Iodocholesterol
(^{131}I-19-Iodocholest-5(6)-en-3β-ol)

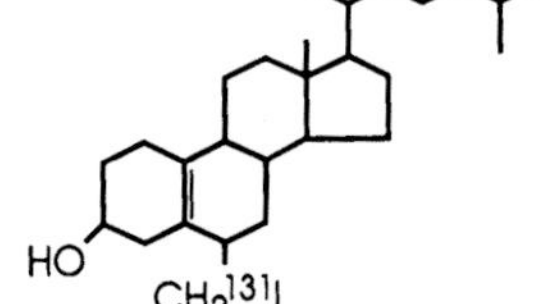

^{131}I-NP-59
(6β-^{131}I-Iodomethyl-19-Nor cholest-5(10)-en-3β-ol)

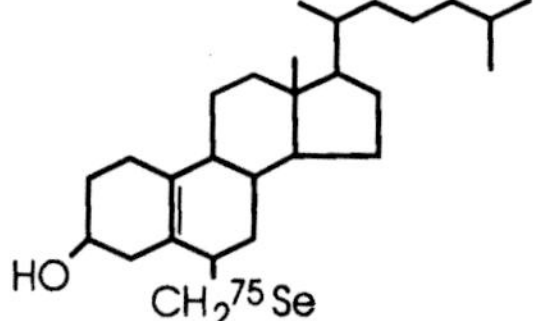

Scintadren®
(6β-^{75}Se-Seleno Methyl-19-Nor cholest-5(10)-en-3β-ol)

Fig. 64.1 Chemical structures of the three adrenal cortex-avid radiopharmaceuticals in general use.

norcholesterol.[3,5,7,8] Dexamethasone suppression scintigraphy imaging is performed on days 3–5 and, possibly, day 7. The computer-acquired data can also be used with depth correction and phantom calibration to provide background-subtracted quantitative adrenal uptake measurements.[3,5]

NORMAL TRACER DISTRIBUTION

Features of normal adrenocortical radiopharmaceutical biodistribution include prominent liver uptake and excretion into the bile.[3,5,6] Occasionally visualization of the gall bladder may be confused with right adrenal uptake but comparison with anterior and lateral views should eliminate ambiguity. The gall bladder will also empty in response to a fatty meal or cholecystokinin.[9] Radioactivity in the gut may overlap the adrenal region and interfere with diagnosis, and thus laxatives are routinely prescribed.[10] Normal adrenal glands are depicted as symmetrical foci of uptake; the right often appears slightly more prominent than the left (because of high liver background) and is somewhat more cephalad and deeper than the left adrenal (see Fig. 64.2A).[3,5,11] The normal degree of right-to-left asymmetry is 0.9–1.2. Baseline adrenal uptake is greater than that on dexamethasone suppression (0.15 ± 0.04% vs. 0.04 ± 0.01% of the administered dose).[3,5] Earliest visualization is at 2–3 days in the unsuppressed state and 5 days or later in the face of dexamethasone suppression.[3,5,9]

PATHOLOGICAL TRACER DISTRIBUTIONS

In most instances the qualitative imaging pattern, when interpreted in the light of the clinical and biochemical profile, is diagnostic. Objective quantification of uptake has been used to distinguish subtle degrees of asymmetry and mild bilateral hyperplasia from normal.[3,5]

Hypersecretory syndromes

It is a central tenet of endocrine radiology that imaging should not be performed unless hormonal hypersecretion is first suspected on clinical grounds and the diagnosis confirmed by appropriate hormonal measurements.[1–3,5] Because adrenocortical scintigraphy traces LDL receptor-mediated cholesterol uptake by adrenocortical tissue, a fundamental early step in all steroid hormone biosynthesis, this technique provides a graphic, in vivo depiction of the sites of abnormal hormonal secretion in most instances of Cushing's syndrome, hyperaldosteronism and adrenal hyperandrogenism (Table 64.3).[3,5,9]

Cushing's syndrome

Adrenocortical scintigraphy has been used in all forms of Cushing's syndrome.[2,3,5,11] In ACTH-dependent syndromes, Cushing's disease and ectopic ACTH syndrome,

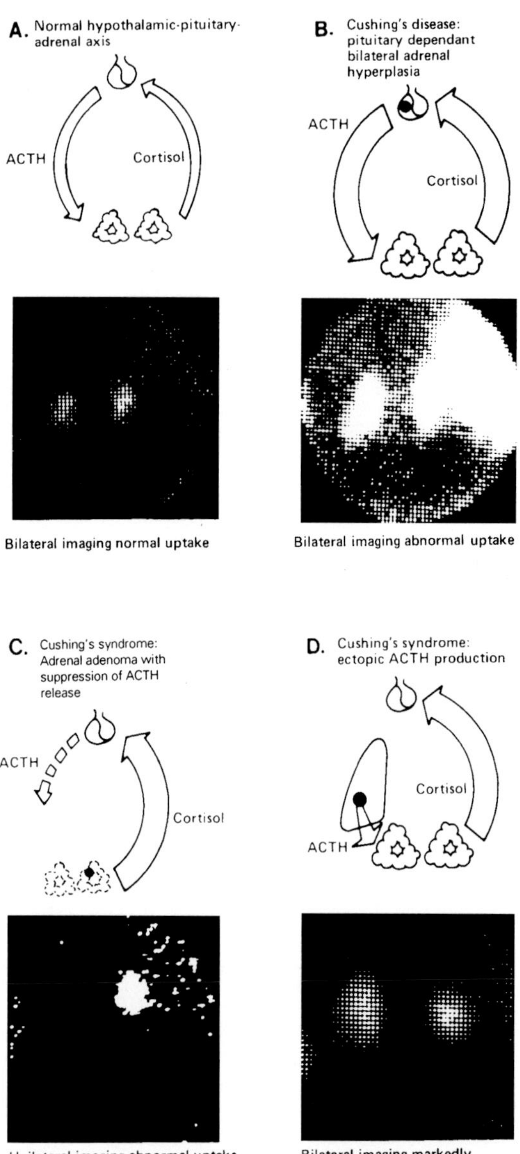

Fig. 64.2 Imaging patterns in Cushing's syndrome. Depiction of the NP59 imaging patterns and diagrams of the underlying physiology in (A) normal subjects, (B) pituitary-dependent Cushing's disease, (C) adrenal adenoma and (D) ectopic ACTH syndrome. (Reproduced with permission from Gross et al[11]).

there is symmetrical humoral stimulation of both adrenals which is reflected as bilateral symmetrical increased tracer uptake. This is generally greatest in ectopic ACTH syndromes where the stimulus is greatest (see Fig. 64.2B and D). While this is a graphic demonstration of the adrenal pathophysiology, the fundamental problem is to locate the source of the ACTH. Adrenocortical scintigraphy has greatest practical value in ACTH-independent Cushing's syndrome (Table 64.3).[3,5,11,12] In adrenal adenoma there is intense tracer uptake by the tumour and none by the normal adrenal cortex owing to prolonged suppression of ACTH with resultant atrophy and hypofunction (see Fig. 64.2C).[3,5,11,12] Almost all adreno-

Table 64.3 Imaging patterns in Cushing's syndrome (performed without dexamethasone suppression) and aldosteronism (performed with dexamethasone suppression)

Scintigraphic pattern	Type of disease
Cushing's syndrome	
1. Bilateral symmetrical imaging	ACTH dependent; hypothalamic; pituitary Cushing's disease; ectopic ACTH syndrome
2. Bilateral asymmetrical imaging	ACTH-independent nodular hyperplasia*
3. Unilateral imaging	Adrenal adenoma†; adrenal remnants‡; ectopic adenocortical tissue‡
4. Bilateral non-visualization	Adrenal carcinoma†§; severe hypercholesterolaemia¶
Aldosteronism	
1. Symmetrical early imaging (before day 5)	Bilateral autonomous hyperplasia; secondary aldosteronism‖
2. Unilateral early imaging (before day 5)	Unilateral adenoma (Conn's tumour)
3. Symmetrical late imaging (on or after day 5); non-diagnostic pattern	Normal adrenals; dexamethasone-suppressible aldosteronism**

*Almost always asymmetrical.
†Cortisol-secreting lesions suppress tracer uptake by contralateral gland.
‡Usually only one focus present, occasionally more than one focus may be present.
§Very rarely tumours will take up enough tracer to image.
¶A potential cause of interference with effectiveness of study.
‖Should be excluded by measurement of renin and aldosterone levels and should not require imaging.
**Dexamethasone suppression interferes with diagnosis in this setting.

cortical carcinomas have insufficient tracer uptake for in vivo imaging. As with adenoma, the normal adrenal cortex also fails to visualize (see Fig. 64.3).[3,5,11,12] Scintigraphy is thus useful in the preoperative characterization of larger adrenal masses which might be either carcinoma or adenoma. Modern CT is highly accurate (~100%) in lateralizing adenomas and carcinomas but frequently fails to correctly disclose the bilateral nature of ACTH-independent hyperplasia in up to 40% of cases.[2,3,5,12] Not infrequently the largest nodule is misclassified by CT as a unilateral adenoma. In contrast, scintigraphy clearly depicts the process as a bilateral, often asymmetrical, imaging pattern in all cases (see Fig. 64.4).[3,5,11,12] These three imaging patterns are observed in between 95 and 100% of patients with ACTH-independent Cushing's syndrome.[2-4,8,11-20] Finally, adrenocortical scintigraphy may be used to locate adrenal remnants causing recurrent Cushing's syndrome following bilateral adrenalectomy (see Fig. 64.5).[3,5,11]

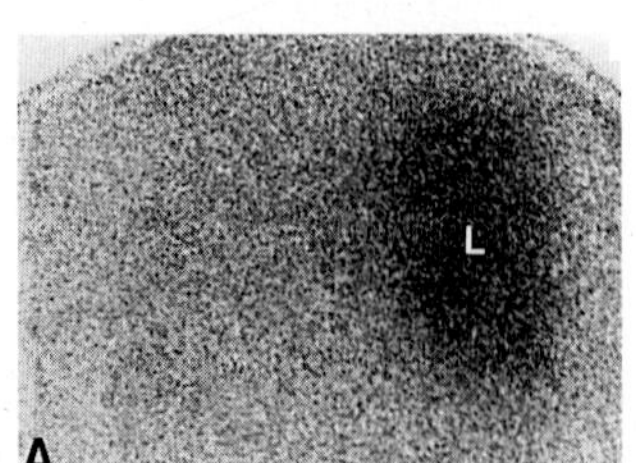

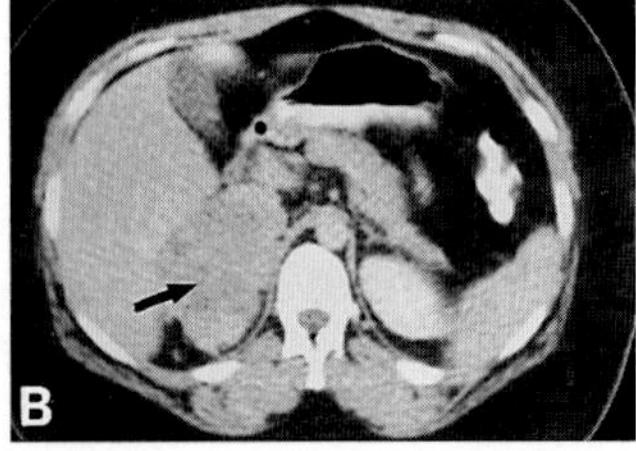

Fig. 64.3 Adrenocortical carcinoma causing Cushing's syndrome. (A) NP59 scintigraphy demonstrates no uptake by the carcinoma; the contralateral normal adrenal cortex is not visualized because of suppression of ACTH. Normal liver uptake=L. (B) Large hypersecretory adrenocortical carcinoma (arrow). (Reproduced with permission from Fig et al.[12])

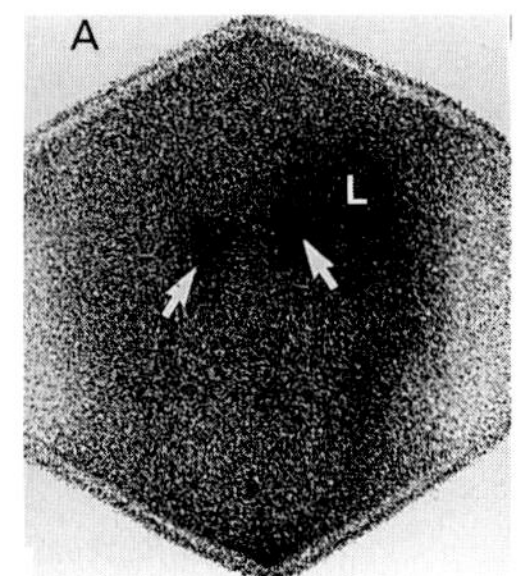

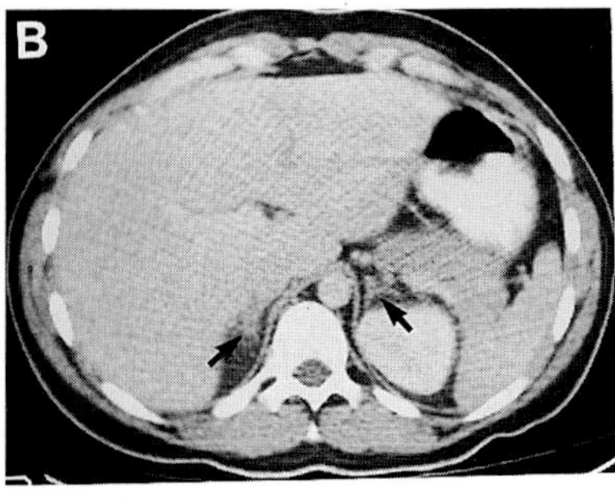

Fig. 64.4 ACTH-independent bilateral macronodular adrenal hyperplasia. (A) NP59 scintigraphy clearly depicts the bilateral nature of the autonomous adrenal hyperfunction (white arrows) despite only minimal enlargement of the right adrenal and a morphologically normal left adrenal on CT (B, black arrows). (Reproduced with permission from Fig et al.[12])

Aldosteronism

In primary aldosteronism, baseline adrenocortical scintigraphy may be used to distinguish an asymmetrical imaging pattern in adenoma (Conn's tumour) from symmetrical

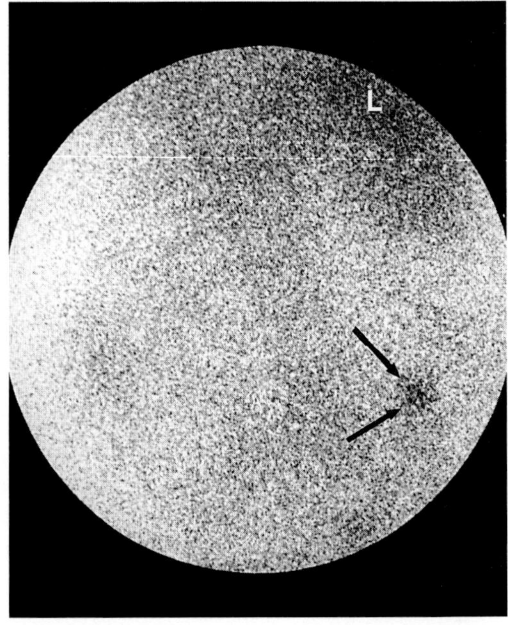

Fig. 64.5 Post-adrenalectomy adrenal remnants. A small focus of abnormal NP59 uptake to the right of the midline in the lower abdomen (arrow) due to an adrenal remnant in the retroperitoneum in a patient with recurrent Cushing's syndrome several years after a bilateral adrenalectomy. Normal liver uptake=L.

increased tracer uptake in bilateral hyperplasia. Because the deviations from normal may be subtle, quantification has been advocated as an adjunct.[3,5,7,8] Suboptimal sensitivity of baseline imaging results from the high background tracer uptake by the zona fasciculata. The administration of dexamethasone to suppress ACTH and reduce this component of tracer uptake enhances sensitivity. The hallmark of pathology is early visualization before the fifth post-injection day. In contrast, normal adrenal glands are not visualized before the fifth day (Table 64.3 and Fig. 64.6).[3,5,9,37]

It is essential that primary aldosteronism be diagnosed before scintigraphy because secondary hyperaldosteronism produces a bilateral imaging pattern indistinguishable from primary autonomous bilateral hyperplasia.[3,5,9] It is also essential that all drugs which may disturb the renin–angiotensin–aldosterone axis be withdrawn to prevent distortion of the imaging pattern.[3,5,9]

CT has been shown to be effective in disclosing most Conn's tumours, but the diagnosis of bilateral hyperplasia is usually inferred from the absence of an adenoma. In contrast, the functional depiction by scintigraphy provides a specific diagnostic pattern in bilateral hyperplasia (Table 64.3).[3,5] Furthermore, some smaller adenomas which are not clearly visualized by CT can be depicted by scintigraphy and thus the technique retains considerable utility in primary aldosteronism, having an overall accuracy of 80–95%.[2,3,5,8,11,15,17,20,22–26]

Hyperandrogenism

Adrenal hyperandrogenism presents imaging patterns similar to those in primary aldosteronism, asymmetrical baseline imaging in the presence of adenoma and symmetrical increased uptake in bilateral hyperplasia. Dexamethasone suppression scintigraphy demonstrates patterns analogous to those in primary aldosteronism.[2,3,5,9] Where cortisol synthesis is impaired (e.g. 21-hydroxylase deficiency), baseline imaging may depict the ACTH-mediated bilateral adrenocortical hyperfunction, but this may normalize in the face of dexamethasone suppression.

NP59 scintigraphy has also depicted ovarian lesions causing hyperandrogenism. Experience is limited but anterior pelvic as well as adrenal imaging is probably warranted in such cases.[27]

PRIMARY ALDOSTERONISM — SCAN PATTERN

1. ADRENAL ADENOMA

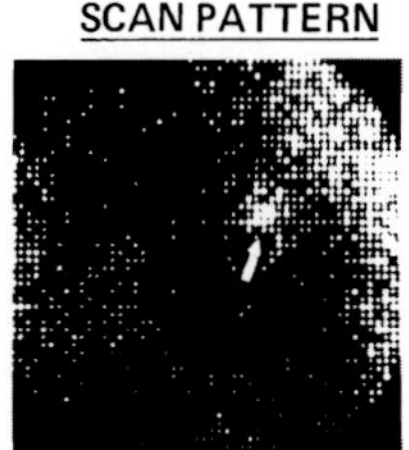

EARLY UNILATERAL ACTIVITY (DAY 3)

2. BILATERAL ADRENAL HYPERPLASIA

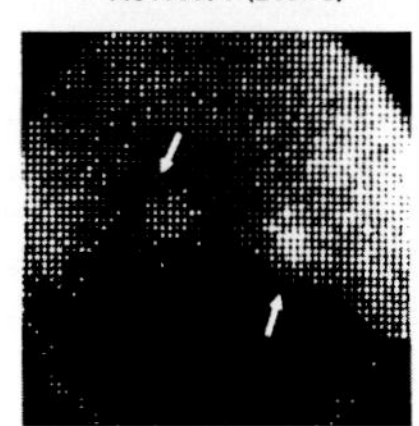

EARLY BILATERAL ACTIVITY (DAY 3)

Fig. 64.6 The characteristic imaging patterns of dexamethasone suppression NP59 scintigraphy in primary aldosteronism. Top (1): Unilateral early imaging of an adrenal adenoma. Bottom (2): Bilateral early imaging of bilateral hyperplasia. (Reproduced with permission from Gross et al[11])

Quantitative relationships

Quantitative NP59 uptake is significantly correlated with urinary free cortisol in Cushing's syndrome, urinary aldosterone in primary aldosteronism and 17-ketosteroid excretion in adrenal hyperandrogenism. This confirms the close functional relationship between adrenal radiopharmaceutical uptake and the synthesis of adrenal steroid hormones.[28–30] Adrenal uptake is reduced in hypercholesterolaemia and in extreme cases the glands may not be visualized. The mechanisms for this are unclear but may include tracer dilution and down-regulation of LDL receptors.[31]

Non-hypersecretory syndromes

For many years adrenocortical scintigraphy was employed primarily for hypersecretory endocrine syndromes, but the technique also has a role in depicting the function of adrenocortical tissue in euadrenal or Addisonian patients.[1–4]

'Incidentalomas'

The widespread utilization of abdominal CT has led to the recognition that between 2 and 9% of patients without clinical evidence of adrenal disease have adrenal mass lesions ('incidentalomas').[2–4] The commonest circumstances in which this occurs are CT scans performed for abdominal pain or the diagnosis or staging of known or suspected non-adrenal malignancies.[4,32] Most metastases to the adrenals occur with widespread tumour dissemination, but in a minority isolated adrenal metastases may radically alter tumour staging and therapy. In most cases, the morphology of the mass does not disclose the nature of the lesion. Screening biochemistry should be performed to exclude subclinical hypersecretory adrenal syndromes, which, if present, are treated on their own merits.[3–5] If adrenal function is normal, there is considerable controversy as to the further management of such cases. Approaches include: surgical resection of masses >5 cm; serial follow-up CT with resection of lesions showing growth; tissue characterization by MRI; and CT-guided needle biopsy.[2–4,32,33] As the vast majority of lesions are benign, non-hypersecretory adenomas, resection on the basis of size alone (even for lesions >5 cm) will result in many unnecessary operations. Tissue characterization by MRI is currently unreliable and needle biopsy is invasive, potentially dangerous and may not provide clear cytological differentiation between adenoma and adrenocortical carcinoma.[2,3,5]

Adrenocortical scintigraphy has been used to characterize the nature of incidentalomas in a fashion analogous to thyroid scintigraphy for thyroid nodules.[32–35] There are three imaging patterns:

1. 'Concordant' imaging, in which the lesion shows increased tracer uptake and is due to a benign non-hypersecretory adrenal adenoma. The contralateral gland may show variable degrees of suppression and some cases may eventually evolve to autonomous cortisol hypersecretion. [The analogy with euthyroid warm or hot thyroid nodules is striking (Fig. 64.7).]
2. A 'discordant' pattern in which there is absent, decreased or distorted tracer uptake on the side of the adrenal mass, many of which are due to destructive and malignant processes (Fig. 64.8).
3. A normal, non-lateralizing symmetrical pattern. If the mass lesion is >2 cm, serious consideration should be given to the lesion being a pseudoadrenal mass which arises from another organ (e.g. stomach, pancreas, kidney). Owing to the limited resolution of scintigraphy, some masses <2 cm may yield a non-lateralizing pattern in the presence of benign adenomas and malignant lesions.[3]

Thus for lesions >2 cm, adrenal scintigraphy provides a highly effective, non-invasive means to characterize incidentalomas (see Table 64.4).[32,33,35] Specificity decreases for lesions <2 cm, but high-resolution imaging using a pinhole collimator may be helpful (M Nakajo, personal communication, 1993).

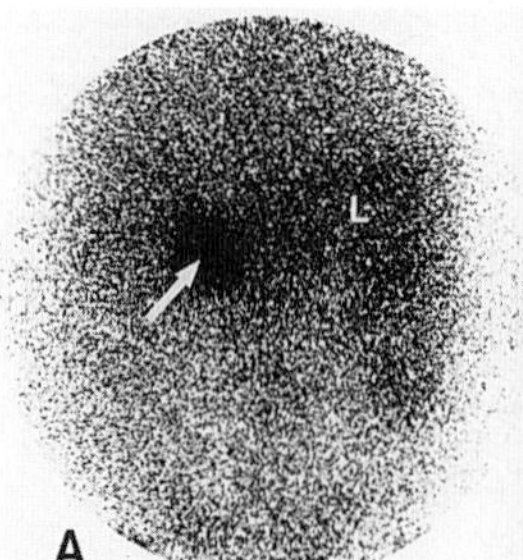

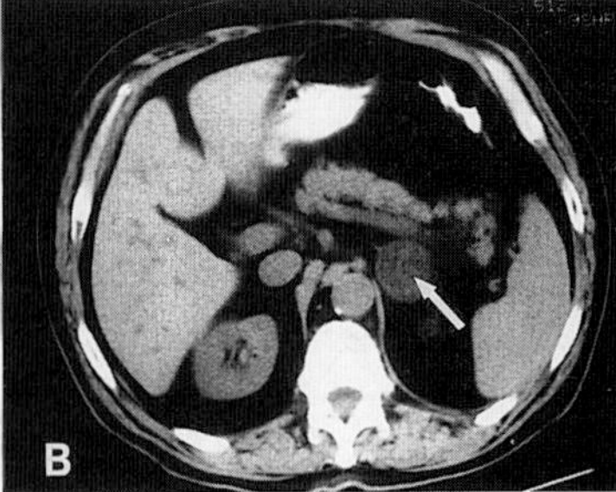

Fig. 64.7 Incidentally discovered adrenal mass lesion: concordant scintigraphic pattern. A CT performed for abdominal pain revealed a 3 cm left adrenal mass (B, arrow). All biochemical studies of adrenal cortical and medullary function were normal. Posterior abdominal NP59 scan performed 5 days after injection shows increased tracer uptake by the lesion (A, arrow), which proved to be a benign adrenocortical adenoma.

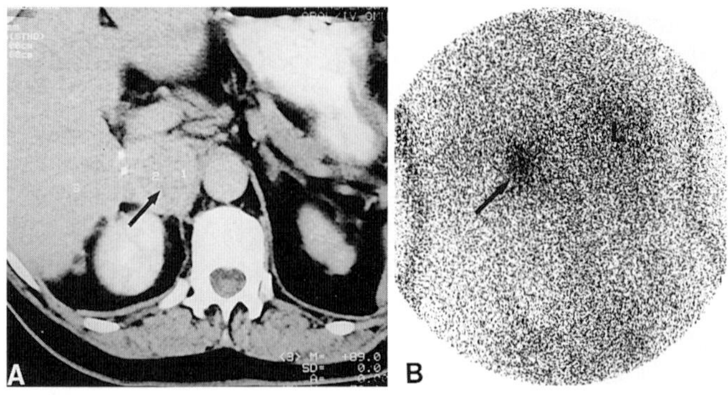

Fig. 64.8 Incidentally discovered adrenal mass lesion: discordant scintigraphic pattern. A CT scan in a man with Crohn's disease and abdominal pain was performed and revealed a 4 cm right adrenal mass (A, arrow). Indices of adrenocortical and medullary function were normal. A posterior abdominal NP59 scan (B) revealed no tracer uptake by the right adrenal. There is normal left adrenal uptake (arrow) and faint liver uptake (L); the body is outlined by a surface marker. Surgery revealed an adrenocortical carcinoma.

Table 64.4 Results of scintigraphy for incidentally discovered adrenal masses (Data from Gross et al[35])

Scintigraphic pattern	Diagnosis
Concordant NP59 uptake = 156	Benign non-hypersecretory adenoma = 156/156
Discordant NP59 uptake = 44	Metastatic lung cancer = 17 Metastatic colon cancer = 2 Lymphoma = 3 Adrenocortical cancer = 7 Fibrous histiocytoma = 2 APUDoma = 3 Ganglioneuroma = 1 Myelolipoma = 2 Adrenal cyst = 7
Symmetrical non-lateralizing uptake = 6 (mass > 2 cm)	Gastric varix = 1 Renal cysts = 2 Gastric leiomyoma = 1 Para-adrenal lymph node metastases = 2
Symmetrical non-lateralizing uptake = 17 (mass < 2 cm)	Benign non-hypersecretory adenoma = 14 Metastatic cancer = 3

Adrenal insufficiency

In the case of bilateral adrenal destruction due to autoimmune, infective or neoplastic processes, adrenal radiopharmaceutical uptake is absent or markedly decreased despite markedly elevated ACTH levels.[3,5,9] Exogenous ACTH does not stimulate adrenocortical tracer uptake when the gland has been destroyed but will do so if there is functional suppression (as in the case of the contralateral adrenal in Cushing's syndrome due to a unilateral adenoma).[3,5,9,36]

ACKNOWLEDGEMENT

This chapter is based in part on a presentation at an International Symposium 'Thomas Addison and his diseases: 200 years on' in London, May 1993.

REFERENCES

1. Dunnick N R 1990 Adrenal imaging: current status. AJR 154: 927–936
2. Francis I R, Korobkin M, Quint L, Gross M D, Shapiro B 1992 Integrated imaging of adrenal disease. Radiology 182: 1–13
3. Gross M D, Falke T H M, Shapiro B, Sandler M D 1992 Adrenal glands. In: Sandler M D, Patton J A, Gross M D, Shapiro B, Falke T H M (eds) Endocrine imaging. Appleton & Lange, Connecticut, pp 271–349
4. Gross M D, Shapiro B, Bouffard J A et al 1988 Distinguishing benign from malignant euadrenal masses. Ann Intern Med 109: 613–618
5. Shapiro B, Fig L M, Gross M D, Khafagi F 1989 Radiochemical diagnosis of adrenal disease. Crit Rev Clin Lab Sci 27: 265–298
6. Lynn M D, Gross M D, Shapiro B 1986 Enterohepatic circulation and distribution of I-131-6-iodomethyl-19-norcholesterol (NP-59). Nucl Med Comm 7: 625–630
7. Hawkins L A, Britton K E, Shapiro B 1980 Selenium 75 selenomethyl cholesterol: A new agent for quantitative functional scintigraphy of the adrenals: physical aspects. Br J Radiol 53 (633): 833–889
8. Shapiro B, Britton K E, Hawkins L A, Edwards C E 1981 Clinical experience with 75 Se-selenomethylcholesterol adrenal imaging. Clin Endocrinol 15: 19–27
9. Gross M D, Valk T W, Swanson D P et al 1981 The role of pharmacologic manipulation in adrenal cortical scintigraphy. Semin Nucl Med 9: 128–148
10. Shapiro B, Nakajo M, Gross M D, Freitas J E, Copp J E, Beierwaltes W H 1983 Value of bowel preparation in adrenocortical scintigraphy with NP-59. J Nucl Med 24: 732–734
11. Gross M D, Shapiro B, Beierwaltes W H 1983 Functional characterization of the adrenal gland by quantitative scintigraphy. In: Winshell S, Lawrence J (eds) Recent Adv Nucl Med 6: 83–115
12. Fig L M, Gross M D, Shapiro B et al 1988 Adrenal localization in ACTH-independent Cushing's syndrome. Ann Intern Med 109: 547–553
13. Moses D C, Schteingart D E, Sturman M R et al 1974 Efficacy of radiocholesterol imaging of the adrenal glands in Cushing's syndrome. Surg Gynecol Obstet 139: 201–204
14. Barliev G B 1979 Adrenal scintigraphy with 131-I-19 iodocholesterol in the diagnosis of Cushing's syndrome associated with adrenal tumor. Eur J Nucl Med 4: 449–451
15. Leger F A, Requeda E, Reach G et al 1981 Scintigraphie cortico-surrenalienne. Nouv Press Med 10: 395–399
16. Baba H 1982 CT of the normal adrenal glands and image diagnosis of the adrenal diseases. Nippon Acta Radiol 42: 938–960
17. Guerin C K, Wahner H W, Gorman C A et al 1983 Computed tomographic scanning vs. radioisotope imaging in adrenocortical diagnosis. Am J Med 75: 653–657
18. Lindberg S, Ernest I, Fjalling M et al 1985 Adrenal scintigraphy in Cushing's syndrome caused by bilateral hyperplasia, adenoma, or carcinoma. Nucl Med Commun 6: 31–36
19. Sarkar S, Simmons B, Kazam E 1987 Iodocholesterol scintigraphy and computed tomography (CT) in Cushing's syndrome and primary aldosteronism (abstract). J Nucl Med 28: 640A
20. Reschini E, Catania A 1991 Clinical experience with the adrenal scanning agents iodine 131-19-iodocholesterol and selenium 75-6-selenomethyl cholesterol. Eur J Nucl Med 18: 817–823
21. Gross M D, Thompson N W, Beierwaltes W H 1982 Scintigraphic approach to the localization of adrenal lesions causing hypertension. Urol Radiol 3: 241–244
22. Conn J W, Cohen E L, Herwig K R 1976 TA dexamethasone-modified adrenal scintiscans in hyporeninemic aldosteronism (tumor v. hyperplasia): a comparison with adrenal venography and adrenal venous aldosterone. J Lab Clin Med 88: 841–855
23. Freitas J E, Grekin R J, Thrall J H et al 1979 Adrenal imaging with iodomethyl-norcholesterol (I-131) in primary aldosteronism. J Nucl Med 20: 7–12
24. Gross M D, Shapiro B, Grekin R J et al 1984 The scintigraphic localization of the adrenal lesion in primary aldosteronism. Am J Med 77: 839–844
25. Pendergrass P W, Scofield R H, Leonard J L 1991 Utility of iodocholesterol scanning in primary aldosteronism (abstract). Clin Nucl Med 16: 219
26. Ishimura J, Fukuchi M 1992 High diagnostic accuracy of qualitative adrenal SPECT imaging without dexamethasone suppression in primary aldosteronism (abstract). J Nucl Med 33: 384
27. Mountz E M, Gross M D, Shapiro B et al 1988 Scintigraphic localization of ovarian dysfunction 131-I-6-beta-iodomethyl-norcholesterol (NP-59). J Nucl Med 29: 1644–1650
28. Gross M D, Valk T, Freitas J E et al 1981 The relationship of adrenal iodomethylnorcholesterol uptake to indices of adrenal cortical function in Cushing's syndrome. J Clin Endocrinol Metab 52: 1062–1066
29. Gross M D, Shapiro B, Grekin R J, Meyers L J, Swanson D P, Beierwaltes W H 1983 The relationship of adrenal gland iodomethyl-norcholesterol uptake to zona glomerulosa function in primary aldosteronism. J Clin Endocrinol Metab 57: 477–481
30. Gross M D, Shapiro B, Freitas J E et al 1984 The relationship of 131-I-6-iodomethyl-19-norcholesterol (NP-59) adrenal cortical uptake to indices of androgen secretion in women with hyperandrogenism. Clin Nucl Med 9(5): 264–270
31. Lynn M D, Gross M D, Shapiro B, Bassett D 1986 The influence of hypercholesterolemia on the adrenal uptake and metabolic handling of I-131-6-iodomethyl-19-norcholesterol (NP-59). Nucl Med Commun 7: 631–637
32. Francis I R, Smid A, Gross M D, Shapiro B, Naylor B, Glazer G M 1988 Adrenal masses in oncologic patients: functional and morphologic evaluation. Radiology 166: 353–356
33. Gross M D, Wilton G P, Shapiro B et al 1987 Functional and scintigraphic evaluation of the silent adrenal mass. J Nucl Med 28: 1404–1407
34. Gross M D, Shapiro B, Freitas J 1990 Scintigraphic endocrine mimicry. Clin Nucl Med 15: 457–464
35. Gross M D, Shapiro B, Francis I R et al 1993 International Symposium: Thomas Addison and his diseases: 200 years on. Guys Hospital, London, United Kingdom, May 25–27, 1993. J Endocrinol (in press)
36. Nakajo M, Sakata H, Shirona K, Shimabukuro K, Onohara S, Shinohara S 1983 Application of ACTH stimulation to adrenal imaging with radiocholesterol. Clin Nucl Med 8: 112–120

65. Radiolabelled metaiodobenzylguanidine in the diagnosis of neural crest tumours

Luigi Troncone

Radioiodinated metaiodobenzylguanidine (MIBG), first developed in 1980 for imaging the adrenal medulla and its diseases,[1–4] was subsequently shown to depict neuroblastomas[5] and a wide range of tumours originating from the neural crest of the amine precursor uptake and decarboxylation series (APUDomas).[6–11] At the present time, its field of application is still expanding. 'In vivo' studies are being developed to assess the functional status of the adrenergic autonomic innervation of several organs, especially the salivary glands, heart, lung and spleen,[12–17] in relation to uptake and storage in adrenergic storage vesicles within the nerve endings of these tissues.[1–18] Nevertheless, the principal application of MIBG imaging is still the diagnostic investigation of neural crest tumours, and ample coverage is given in literature. Because of its good, selective uptake and retention by these tumours,[19] careful consideration is also being given to the therapeutic potential of radiolabelled MIBG; several malignancies of this group have been given therapeutic doses of ^{131}I-MIBG, with encouraging results[20] (see also Ch 74).

RADIOIODINATED METAIODOBENZYLGUANIDINE

Chemical and biological characteristics

Radiolabelled MIBG represents a combination of the benzyl group of bretylium and the guanidine group of guanethidine.[21] It shares structural features with the hormone adrenergic neurotransmitter norepinephrine (NE) and to some extent shares its biological behaviour in that it is taken up, at the low concentration used in scintigraphy, predominantly by the active, sodium- and energy-dependent (type 1) amine uptake mechanism in the cell membrane of sympathomedullary tissues. Once within the cytoplasm, it is then transported into the intracellular catecholamine storage vesicles.[3,18,22] However, extravesicular storage seems also to contribute to MIBG retention in some neuroblastomas.[23] It is this uptake process that enables MIBG to enter into the NE pathways, and the prolonged storage within the vesicles is the major component permitting the high 'specific uptake' and imaging.[18] Radiolabelled MIBG differs from NE in that it does not bind well to post-synaptic receptors and is metabolized to only a minor extent. The majority of the tracer is excreted unaltered via the kidneys (85% of the radioactivity is excreted within 4 days; 55% within the first 24 h); 1–4% of it has been found to be excreted in the faeces, while some tracer can be detected in the saliva, sweat and exhaled breath.[3,18]

Interfering drugs

Drugs which interfere with the type 1 uptake mechanism (i.e. labetalol, tricyclic antidepressants, cocaine, etc.) or vesicular storage (i.e. reserpine, sympathomimetics, etc.) also interfere with MIBG uptake and retention. Although nifedipine has been reported to prolong retention in malignant phaeochromocytomas,[24] many drugs are known to or are expected to reduce MIBG uptake[25] (Table 65.1). Care must be taken to ensure that such agents are withdrawn prior to imaging.

Labelled radiopharmaceuticals

^{131}I-MIBG and ^{123}I-MIBG are both available today for diagnostic purposes (Table 65.2). Theoretical considerations (half-life 13.2 h, fewer particulate emissions which lead to favourable dosimetry, etc) and clinical experience indicate that the ^{123}I-labelled agent is a superior radiopharmaceutical, better suited to gamma-cameras.[18] It allows better quality images, better photon detection and greater sensitivity. The higher photon flow allows SPECT to be carried out, which may be an advantage.[26–28] Nevertheless, because of its lower cost, easier availability, longer (2 weeks) shelf-life and the possibility of obtaining delayed scans ^{131}I-MIBG is still used for most routine applications.[18,28]

^{125}I-MIBG is also available, but it is reserved for in vitro experiments and biodistribution studies in animals

Table 65.1 Drugs known or expected to reduce MIBG uptake (From Khafagi et al[25])

	Drug	Mechanism
(a) *Known*		
	Antihypertensive/cardiovascular	
	Labetalol	Uptake-1 inhibition Depletion of storage vesicle contents
	Reserpine	Depletion of storage vesicle contents Inhibition of vesicle active transport
	Calcium channel blockers	Uncertain (Also enhance retention of previously stored NE and MIBG by blocking Ca^{2+}- mediated release from vesicles.)
	Diltiazem Nifedipine Verapamil	
	Tricyclic antidepressants	Uptake-1 inhibition
	Amitriptyline and derivatives Imipramine and derivatives Doxepin Amoxapine Loxapine (antipsychotic agent)	
	Sympathomimetics	Depletion of storage vesicle contents
	Phenylephrine Phenylpropanolamine Pseudoephedrine, ephedrine	These drugs occur in numerous non-prescription decongestants and 'diet aids' – their use should be ruled out
	Cocaine	Uptake-1 inhibition
(b) *Expected*		
	Antihypertensive/cardiovascular	
	Adrenergic neurone blockers	Depletion of storage vesicle contents Competiton for transport into vesicles
	Bethanidine, debrisoquine Bretylium Guanethidine	
	Atypical antidepressants	Uptake-1 inhibition
	Maprotiline Trazolone	
	Antipsychotics ('major tranquillizers')	Uptake-1 inhibition
	Phenothiazines Chlorpromazine*, triflupromazine*, promethazine* Fluphenazine, acetophenazine, perphenazine* Prochlorperazine*, thiethyl-perazine, trifluoperazine Thioridazine, mesoridazine	
	Thioxanthines Chlorprothixene Thiothixene	
	Butyrophenones Droperidol Haloperidol Pimozide	
	Sympathomimetics	Depletion of storage vesicle contents
	Amphetamine and related compounds Amphetamine and derivatives Diethylpropion Fenfluramine Mazindol Methylphenidate Phenmetrazine and derivatives Phentermine and derivatives	
	Beta-sympathomimetics† Albuterol (salbutamol) Isoetharine Isoproterenol Metaproterenol Terbutaline	
	Dobutamine Dopamine Metaraminol	

*Frequently used as antiemetic/antipruritic agents.
†Systemic use. Effect unlikely with aerosol administration in conventional doses.

Table 65.2 Technical and dosimetric data on the diagnostic use of radiolabelled MIBG

Agent	Injected activity (MBq)	Patient preparation	Imaging time	Dosimetry (cGy/3.7 MBq)*						
				WB	AM	H	L	S	O	Thy
^{131}I-MIBG	18.5–37	Lugol's solution	24, 48 (72) h Delayed scan (6–8 days)	0.1	100	0.7	0.4	1.6	1.0	35
^{123}I-MIBG†	75–300	Lugol's solution	6, 24 (48) h SPECT (24 h)	0.02	0.80	0.03	0.05	0.14	0.06	2.20

*From Swanson et al[30].
†Pure ^{123}I-MIBG
WB, whole body; AM, adrenal medulla; H, heart; L, liver; S, spleen; O, ovary; Thy, thyroid

because of its physical properties. Some authors also consider it a potential agent for therapy in special conditions.[29]

Radiation dosimetry

When using ^{131}I-MIBG the adrenal medulla exposure is not negligible but is similar to that of the other diagnostic modalities.[18,30] The dosimetry of ^{123}I-MIBG is far more favourable, especially that of the 'pure' agent, i.e. not containing ^{124}I as a contaminant of ^{123}I synthesis: it allows the administration of 37 MBq of ^{123}I-MIBG with a radiation dose no higher than that of 1.8 MBq of ^{131}I-MIBG.[18,26,30] The radiation dosimetry of ^{131}I-MIBG and ^{123}I-MIBG is shown in Table 65.2.

THE SCINTIGRAPHIC TECHNIQUE

Technique

Essentially the following procedure is followed[18,31] for both ^{131}I-MIBG and ^{123}I-labelled MIBG. 18.5–37 MBq1.7 m^2 body surface area of ^{131}I-MIBG (specific activity >74 MBq/mg) or 74–300 MBq of ^{123}I-MIBG (specific activity 100–300 MBq/mg) are injected intravenously after thyroid blockade with Lugol's solution (1–2 mg/kg per day of potassium iodide beginning 2 days before tracer injection and continued for 7 days). Imaging is performed using an LFOV gamma-camera equipped with a high-energy (^{131}I-MIBG) or low-energy (^{123}I-MIBG) parallel-hole collimator interfaced with a minicomputer. Planar whole-body images are obtained at 24, 48 and occasionally 72–120 h (delayed scan) post injection when ^{131}I-MIBG is used, and at 4, 24 and occasionally 36 h when ^{123}I-MIBG is administered (Table 65.2).[18,31]

SPECT is carried out at 4–24 h after ^{123}I-labelled agent administration, using a rotating gamma-camera equipped with a parallel-hole, low- or medium-energy collimator with 64 projections obtained over 360° at 30–40 s per projection. The anatomical orientation of radioiodinated MIBG scans is derived from radioactive surface markers or the simultaneous imaging of various other systems (skeleton, kidneys, etc.).[18,26]

Quantitative measurements of ^{123}I-MIBG to calculate the adrenal medullary uptake have been performed to study adrenomedullary pathophysiology,[32] and concentration measurements have been taken for dosimetric purposes in candidates for ^{131}I-MIBG therapy.[18,33]

The normal scintigraphic pattern

In normal subjects the heart and lungs are currently visualized at early imaging; salivary glands, liver, spleen and bladder are visualized throughout the entire examination.[34] Colonic activity is also observed in later images in 20% of patients.[35] Normal adrenomedullary glands,

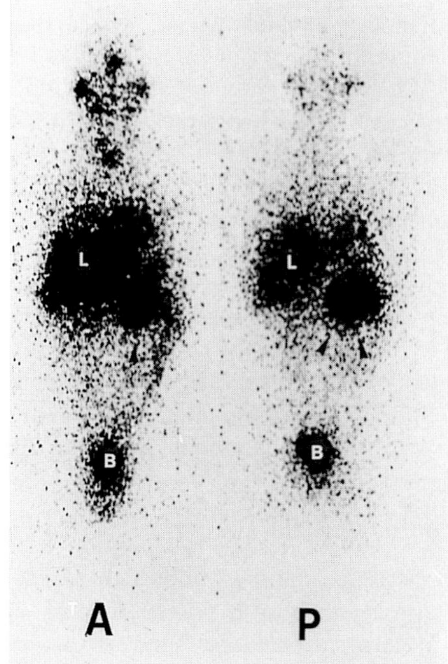

Fig. 65.1 ^{131}I-MIBG whole-body imaging (A, anterior view; P, posterior view) showing a left adrenal phaeochromocytoma, which intensely takes up the tracer. Arrows mark the tumour (L, liver; B, urinary bladder).

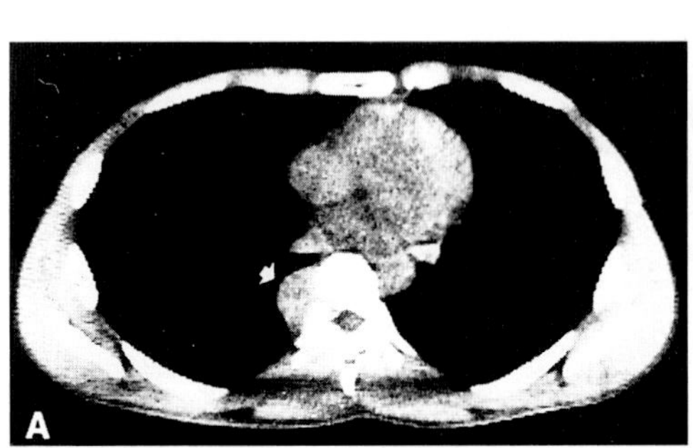

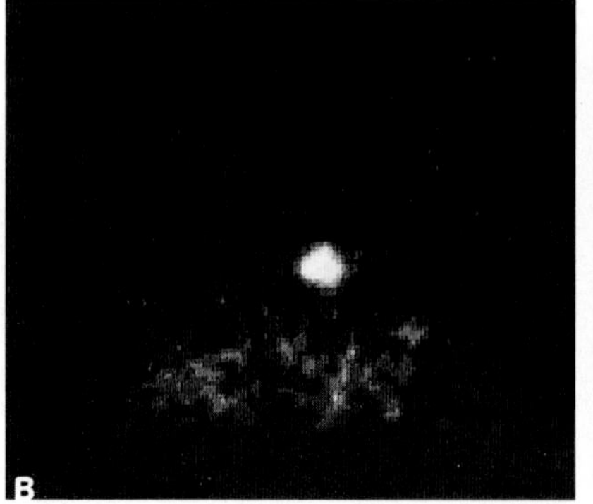

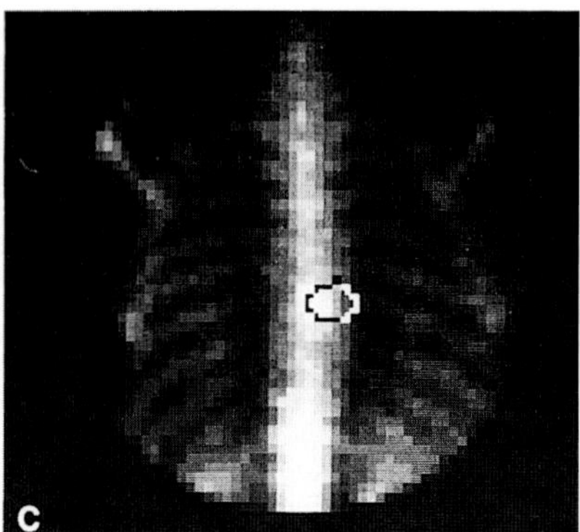

Fig. 65.2 Extra-adrenal malignant phaeochromocytoma. (A) CT scan showing a right paraspinal mass (arrow) infiltrating the VIII dorsal vertebra. (B) ^{131}I-MIBG scan (posterior view of the chest) showing an area of abnormal uptake. (C) The region of interest selected over the focus of abnormal MIBG uptake is superimposed on the bone scan and it appears localized in the right side of spine (VIII dorsal vertebra). (From Troncone et al[43] with permission.)

seldom seen with ^{131}I-MIBG (2% of patients at 24 h and 16% at 48 h post injection),[34] are frequently recognized when ^{123}I-MIBG is used. The latter agent can image the kidneys and lacrimal glands as well.[18] No bone activity is ever evident, not even in children. The vertebral column of a child is represented by a vertical photopenic strip and the joints are seen as photon-deficient areas surrounded by background muscle activity.[18,26–28,34,36]

DIAGNOSTIC APPLICATIONS OF RADIOLABELLED MIBG

Adrenal medullary hyperplasia

The first diagnostic application of ^{131}I-MIBG[37] was in multiple endocrine neoplasia (MEN 2A and MEN 2B syndromes), in which adrenomedullary hyperplasia is expected to occur. MIBG imaging was also found to be useful in hypertensive patients in whom hyperplasia could potentially represent a micronodular phase in the natural history of phaeochromocytoma.[38,39] Hyperplasia is imaged as an increased adrenomedullary bilateral uptake occurring throughout the 2- to 3-day examination period, while no, or only a transient, visualization occurs in normal subjects.[37] MIBG scintigraphy can play a useful role in the diagnostic work-up as CT and MRI are not able to detect adrenal medullary hyperplasia until it is very advanced, i.e. when the cortex to medulla ratio is reversed to 1 : 10.[40]

Phaeochromocytoma

Phaeochromocytoma, the most important adrenomedullary disease, is also referred to as chromaffinoma and, when occurring in extra-adrenal sites such as the sympathetic paraganglia, as paraganglioma. Its prevalence is estimated to be 0.1–0.4% of hypertensive patients, but this could be twice as high.[41] Approximately 60% of phaeochromocytoma-bearing patients present sustained hypertension (even though this is associated with distinct paroxysms in half of them); the other 40% show increased blood pressure only during an attack.[41] A proteiform symptomatology correlated with the excess catecholamines secreted and their pharmacological effects on the adrenergic receptors is usually associated. Nevertheless, a considerable number of phaeochromocytomas are asymptomatic and may be found only at autopsy.[42] Most phaeochromocytomas are larger than 2 cm in diameter and reside in the

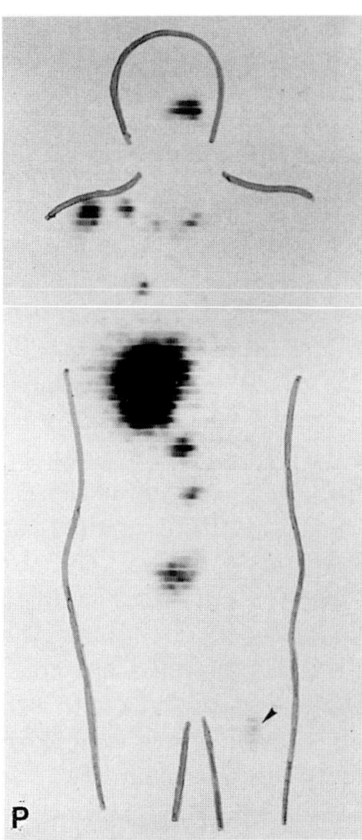

Fig. 65.3 ^{131}I-MIBG whole-body scan (posterior view) showing the large primary tumour (malignant phaeochromocytoma) and multiple areas of abnormal uptake corresponding to multilocular metastatic dissemination (secondaries in the cerebral posterior fossa and in the skeleton).

Table 65.3 ^{131}I scintigraphy in phaeochromocytomas: data analysis of the major reported series

Reference	Year	No. of studies	TP	FP	TN	FN	Sens.	Spec.	–PDA	+PDA	Prev.
18	1982–89	600	152	3	424	21	88	99	95	98	29
49	1984	46	21	1	21	3	88	95	88	95	52
50*	1984	99	42	2	51	4	91	96	95	93	46
51	1984	129	36	–	91	2	95	100	98	100	29
52	1984	97	30	–	60	7	82	100	90	100	38
53	1985	42	15	1	22	4	79	96	85	94	45
54	1985	94	41	2	47	4	91	96	92	95	48
55	1985	16	15	–	–	1	94	–	–	100	–
43†	1986–90	74	34	1	36	3	92	95	92	97	50
56	1989	19	17	–	1	1	94	–	–	100	94
57	1989	45	9	4	30	2	82	88	94	69	24
58	1993	36	24	–	7	5	83	100	58	100	80
Total		1297	436	12	790	57	88	98	93	97	

*Equivocal negative added to TN and equivocal positive added to TP.
†Including a few cases imaged with ^{123}I-MIBG
TP, true positives; FP, false positives; TN, true negatives; FN, false negatives; Sens., sensitivity; Spec., specificity; –PDA, negative predictive diagnostic accuracy; +PDA, positive predictive diagnostic accuracy; Prev, prevalence.

adrenal gland; a substantial fraction (10%) are multiple, extra-adrenal (mostly abdominal, 1% thoracic, 1% within the bladder and less than 1% in the neck) or malignant.[40–42] Phaeochromocytoma may be an inherited disease (familial syndromes) transmitted as an autosomal dominant trait, either alone or in combination with other abnormalities such as multiple endocrine neoplasia (MEN).[41,42]

Worldwide experience has proved the ability of ^{131}I-MIBG scintigraphy to locate phaeochromocytomas of all types, including sporadic intra-adrenal (Fig. 65.1)[3,4,43] and extra-adrenal lesions (Fig. 65.2),[3,4,43] malignant metastatic disease (Fig. 65.3)[3,18,31,39,43] as well as various familial syndromes associated with phaeochromocytomas, including MEN 2A and 2B,[3,37] von Hippel–Lindau syndrome,[3] von Recklinghausen's neurofibromatosis[3,44] and simple familial phaeochromocytomas.[3,45] Even non-functional paragangliomas may be visualized, as reported by several authors.[9,48,49] Radiolabelled MIBG uptake by the heart (and to a lesser extent by the salivary glands) was found to be decreased in the presence of hypercatecholaminaemia, as occurs in phaeochromocytoma-bearing patients.[48] Thus, the intensity of cardiac MIBG uptake may be a helpful adjunct in the diagnosis of phaeochromocytoma.

The overall diagnostic sensitivity of ^{131}I-MIBG imaging when evaluating the combined data reported in major series[43,49–58] is approximately 88% (Table 65.3). In malignant phaeochromocytomas the sensitivity is higher: 92.4%.[39] The prevalence of the metastatic disease was found to be 46%,[40] compared with the 10% rate usually reported.[40,41] In only 21% of these patients was the disease detected at the time of the primary operation; in the remainder, diagnosis was after a prolonged follow-up with the help of the MIBG imaging. This suggests that all patients submitted to surgery for the removal of a 'benign' phaeochromocytoma[40] should receive an annual MIBG scan.

Sensitivity improves still further with ^{123}I-MIBG (and with SPECT performed in certain circumstances).[59,60] In fact, ^{123}I-MIBG can visualize a number (~8%) of low MIBG-concentrating phaeochromocytomas which cannot be visualized with ^{131}I-MIBG (uptake capacity is reported to vary from 0.1% to 8%).[26,28,53,59–61]

Radiolabelled MIBG imaging is highly specific: it gives very few (1–5%) false-positive results (i.e. as a result of retention of radioactivity in the urinary tract, adrenal hyperplasia or the presence of other neuroendocrine tumours) and has a high tissue specificity, which permits the nature of the mass to be elucidated.[40,43]

When compared with high-resolution imaging modalities, the effectiveness of radiolabelled MIBG appears to be superior to traditional radiographs and ultrasound,[38] and equivalent to CT and MRI.[54,56,58,62–66] CT and MRI sensitivity is higher than that of ^{131}I-MIBG, but similar to that of ^{123}I-MIBG.[61,65] Scintigraphy has the advantage of tissue specificity and can easily screen the whole body. However, MRI with paramagnetic contrast media shows interesting discriminatory possibilities between phaeochromocytomas and other adrenal masses, such as non-hyperfunctioning adenomas and cysts, but not malignant lesions.[38] The complementary role played by CT, MRI and radiolabelled MIBG in the localization of phaeochromocytomas has been emphasized: the first two techniques provide mainly anatomical information and the last primarily functional information. Therefore when ^{123}I-MIBG is used as a first-choice imaging technique, as has been proposed,[62,64,65] a detailed anatomical focus of MIBG uptake is derived from MIBG-directed imaging procedures (CT, MRI and occasionally angio–raphy).[39,62–65]

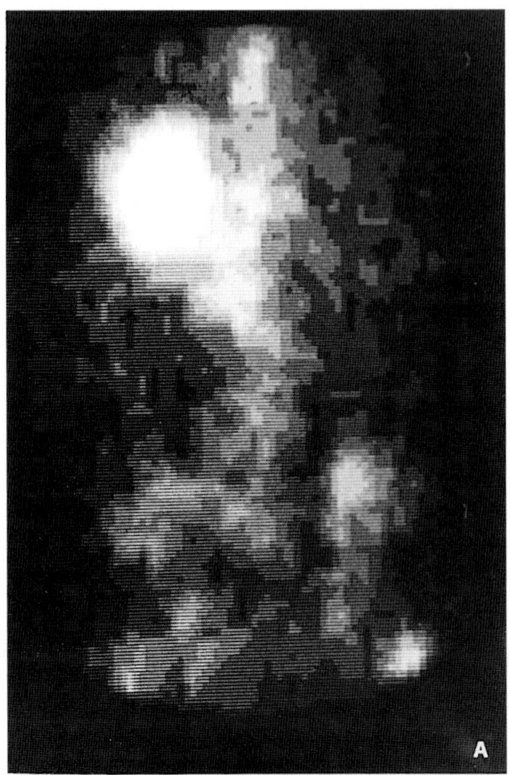

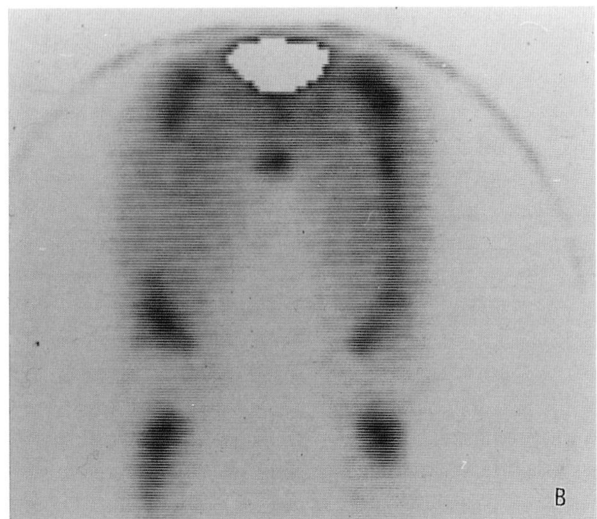

Fig. 65.4 A stage IV neuroblastoma. (A) ^{131}I-MIBG imaging in a 7-year-old child (posterior view of abdomen) visualizing a left adrenal primary neuroblastoma. The spine as well as the pelvis show an intense uptake consistent with the massive bone marrow infiltration. (B) ^{123}I-MIBG scintigraphy in a 2-year-old child (anterior view of lower extremities) showing high intensity bony uptake foci with an asymmetrical distribution of the tracer; they are indicative of bone metastases as well as bone marrow involvement.

On the whole, radiolabelled MIBG provides a safe, efficacious, non-invasive technique, potentially the best initial procedure for patients suspected of having phaeochromocytoma. It is especially indicated for (1) extra-adrenal phaeochromocytomas; (2) malignant phaeochromocytomas, both at presentation to assess the extent

Table 65.4 Results of radiolabelled MIBG scintigraphy for suspected neuroblastoma

Reference	Year	Case (studies)	TP	FP	TN	FN	Sens.	Spec.	–PDA	+PDA	Prev.
67	1987	37 (121)	33	–	1	3	92	100	–	100	97
68	1989	102 (410)	83	–	15	4	95	100	79	100	85
69	1988	69 (115)	36	–	22	11	77	94	67	110	67
70	1989	63 (96)	45	2	9	7	87	82	56	83	83
71	1986	26 (26)	17	–	9	–	100	100	100	100	65
72	1986–90	58 (160)	111	–	40	5	93	100	82	100	72
73	1988	35 (63)*	40	–	15	8	83	100	65	100	76
74–85	1985–90	200	159	–	22	19	89	100	54	100	89
Total		590 (1191)	524	2	133	57	**90**	**99**	70	100	49

*Five cases of ganglioneuroma not included
TP, true positives; FP, false positives; TN, true negatives; FN, false negatives; Sens., sensitivity; Spec., specificity; –PDA, negative predictive diagnostic accuracy; +PDA, positive predictive diagnostic accuracy; Prev., prevalence.

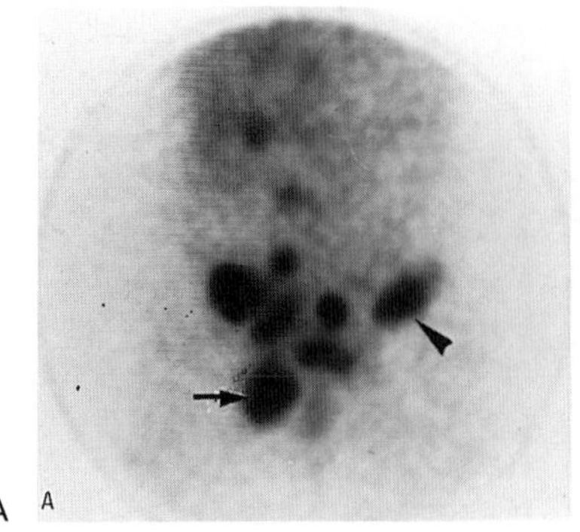

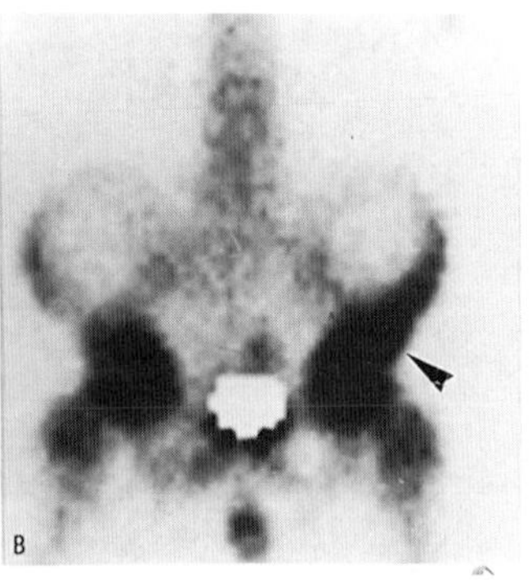

A B

Fig. 65.5 Stage IV neuroblastoma in a 9-year-old boy. ^{123}I-MIBG imaging (anterior view of abdomen and pelvis) showing a voluminous post-surgical residual tumour in the right side of the pelvis (arrow) as well as extensive abdominal and pelvic lymph node involvement and a large bone deposit in the lower left ilium (A). The bone deposit is confirmed by a ^{99m}Tc MDP bone scan (arrowheads) (B).

of the disease and at post-operative follow-up, for the early detection of a residual/recurrent disease; (3) after surgery when anatomical alterations or the presence of metallic clips allow only suboptimal results from anatomical imaging modalities; and (4) as a prelude to ^{131}I-MIBG therapy, to evaluate the concentration and retention of the agent in the lesions.[18,43,63]

Neuroblastoma

Radiolabelled MIBG imaging is now a well-established examination in the diagnosis and follow-up of neuroblastoma (NB), the most common (1–1.4/10 000 population) extracranial, highly malignant, solid childhood tumour (see Ch. 67). Whole-body scintigraphy (limbs and skull have to be included as frequent metastatic sites) depicts primary and residual/recurrent NBs, as well as lesions in bone, soft tissue and even in bone marrow when extensively infiltrated (Fig. 65.4). The overall accuracy in detecting the disease is ~90% (Table 65.4) according to the cumulative findings reported in the literature.[67–86] MIBG imaging is positive not only in NB-bearing patients with high levels of urinary catecholamines and metabolites, but also in those patients (~80%) with normal levels.[68,72] The highest sensitivity is shown in the detection of bone deposits (91–97%), where it reveals more lesions (10–40% more) than bone scintigraphy with ^{99m}Tc-MDP.[69,70,72] A few lesions, however, are detected by the latter technique only.[70,74] MIBG scintigraphy is less effective in disclosing soft-tissue metastases (Fig. 65.5) (sensitivity 60–70%).[69–72]

False-negative results can depend on several factors, including tumour heterogeneity, inadequate tumour uptake,[87] lesions (e.g. in lymph nodes) smaller than the resolving power of the method, sites of physiological MIBG uptake (e.g. masking liver metastases) and the presence of voluminous NB masses which surround or hide the lesions. Low, or no, MIBG uptake was found in the NB lesions of stage IVS children and in adults, in whom the disease may be encountered rarely.[72] Uptake by the lesions may also be poor during or immediately after chemotherapy or external radiation therapy.[67,72]

^{123}I-MIBG associated with SPECT guarantees a more favourable dosimetry and an improvement in sensitivity.[61,67,88] Soft-tissue metastases (liver, lymph nodes) and small lesions (1–2 cm) in which the ^{131}I-MIBG scan may fail are those that gain particular advantage.[61,70,88]

The efficacy of MIBG scintigraphy is similar or even superior to the combination of current imaging procedures, which are rather imperfect.[40,61,72,81] Nevertheless, because a sufficient number of lesions may be false negative, MIBG imaging complements rather than replaces such standard procedures including bone scan, CT and MRI.[70,72] Good correlation was found between MIBG imaging and immunoscintigraphy, which however is still being investigated. Nevertheless, it seems that when the former fails, the latter could be diagnostic.[89]

MIBG imaging is highly specific, with practically no false-positive results. It permits the diagnosis of the nature of the neoplastic lesions imaged, thus allowing the differential diagnosis of Wilms' tumour, Ewing's sarcoma, rhabdomyosarcoma, lymphoblastic leukaemia and other round-cell tumours that do not take up this tracer.[63,67–70,73]

On the whole, MIBG imaging is today considered to be the most effective indicator of NB. It plays an important role (first-choice modality) in: (1) NB staging at presentation (sometimes characterizing undiagnosed tumours as being NB) and restaging after treatment; (2) the search for post-surgical residual tumours; (3) monitoring the effect of treatment; and (4) the early diagnosis of recurrence at follow-ups; it is essential as a prelude to ^{131}I-MIBG therapy.[63,69–73]

IMAGING OF OTHER NEUROENDOCRINE TUMOURS

Other tumours may arise from the APUD cells, which are embryologically of neural crest origin and then differentiate throughout the body structure. Most of them are metabolically active in association with the presence of vesicles. The successful use of MIBG imaging in phaeochromocytomas and NBs has led to its application in a variety of APUDomas, assuming that these tumours may also be detected by radiolabelled MIBG scintigraphy. Worldwide experience with MIBG imaging in these tumours is still limited. In general it may be said that their sensitivity is far less than that of phaeochromocytomas and NBs.

Medullary thyroid carcinoma

Medullary thyroid carcinoma (MTC) is distinctly different from other thyroid malignancies; it derives from C cells, which originate embryologically from the neural crest. The reported prevalence is 3–12% of thyroid cancers. MTC may occur in either sporadic or familial (genetic) forms. The latter (~20% of cases) tend to present in association with MEN 2A and 2B.[90] MTC does not metabolize iodine (radioiodine uptake must be regarded as an exception) to produce the thyroid hormones, nor does it produce thyroglobulin. Determination of calcitonin, either with or without stimulation by pentagastrin or calcium infusion [and carcinoembryonic antigen (CEA)], is essential from a diagnostic standpoint, as is the demonstration of calcitonin within the cells by means of immunohistochemical techniques.[90,91] However, a number of radiopharmaceuticals which selectively concentrate in MTC have recently been developed. These include

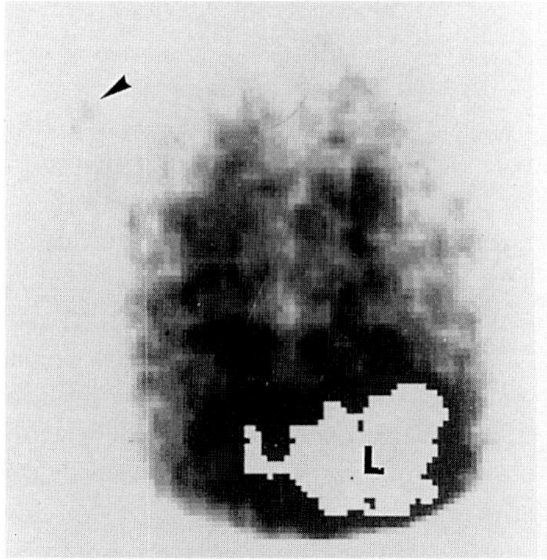

Fig. 65.6 Post-operative study of a medullary thyroid carcinoma in MEN 2B (posterior view of the chest). ^{131}I-MIBG scintigraphy showing a widespread intense uptake in the lungs consistent with bilateral pulmonary metastases and a faint area of abnormal uptake in the left shoulder, corresponding to bone metastasis (arrowhead).

Table 65.5 Diagnostic sensitivity of ^{123}I-MIBG, ^{131}I-MIBG, ^{99m}Tc(V)-DMSA and ^{201}Tl scintigraphy in medullary thyroid carcinoma

Reference	Year	^{123}I/^{131}I-MIBG	^{99m}Tc(V)-DMSA	^{201}Tl
95	1988	33.3%	80.0%	–
96	1988	27.2%	–	92.0%
97	1989	41.6%	84.0%	–
91, 98	1989–90	45.0%	77.0%	86.0%

radioiodinated MIBG and represent new diagnostic potential in the field.[91]

After the first encouraging reports concerning one or more MTC patients,[7,8,91] rather disappointing results followed.[91–97] Specificity is usually high (>95%), but sensitivity is only approximately 34%.[91] These inconsistent representations of MTC lesions cannot yet be convincingly explained. They may be due to the histological heterogeneity of MTC and/or the possible anaplastic transformation of the metastases.[91] However, MIBG uptake has been found to be high enough to warrant attempts at therapy.[91,96] MIBG imaging has been reported to give a more positive outcome in patients with familial disease with elevated calcitonin levels,[94] and to reveal otherwise undetected residual/recurrent lesions (Fig. 65.6)[91] and unsuspected liver metastases.[96] It is also helpful in identifying and locating phaeochromocytomas in MEN syndromes, as previously mentioned.[91,94] ^{123}I-MIBG with SPECT may improve efficacy, particularly in detecting small residual/recurrent lesions.[91]

Nowadays, however, other radiopharmaceuticals, such ^{201}Tl chloride and ^{99m}Tc(V) DMSA (Table 65.5) (although specific) and radiolabelled anti-CEA monoclonal antibodies (still under investigation), seem to be significantly better (70–80% sensitivity) than radiolabelled MIBG in the diagnostic scintigraphy of MTC.[91,95–98] On the basis of the overall data, MIBG imaging appears to have only a complementary role in the diagnosis of MTC. Its indications are, firstly, to elucidate the nature of the lesions revealed by other radiopharmaceuticals; to complement the outcome of other diagnostic modalities by disclosing residual/recurrent tumours; to detect phaeochromocytomas or adrenomedullary hyperplasia in familial MTC; and as a prelude to ^{131}I-MIBG therapy.

Carcinoid tumours

Carcinoids account for 55% of the small group (2%) of neuroendocrine tumours of the gut and pancreas: the annual incidence is 1.5–2% per 100 000 population.[99] Only in 10–40% of patients do symptoms occur (carcinoid syndrome, diarrhoea, flushing, dyspnoea and bronchospasm). Metastases are present at the time of initial detection in about 30% of patients, the regional lymph nodes being most frequently involved. Liver metastases have been recorded in 20–60% of patients, their preva-

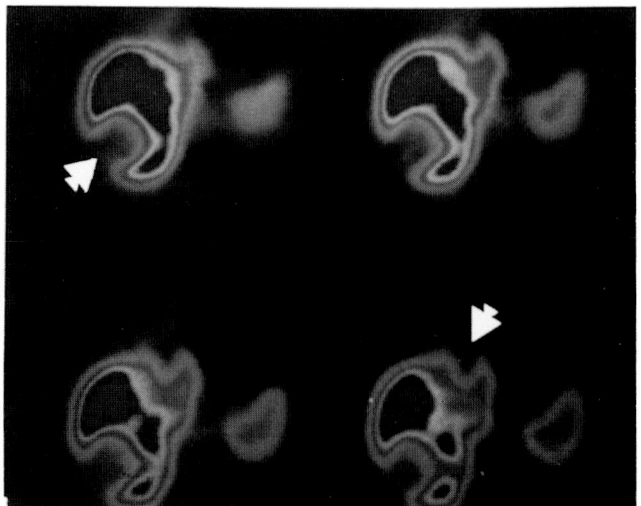

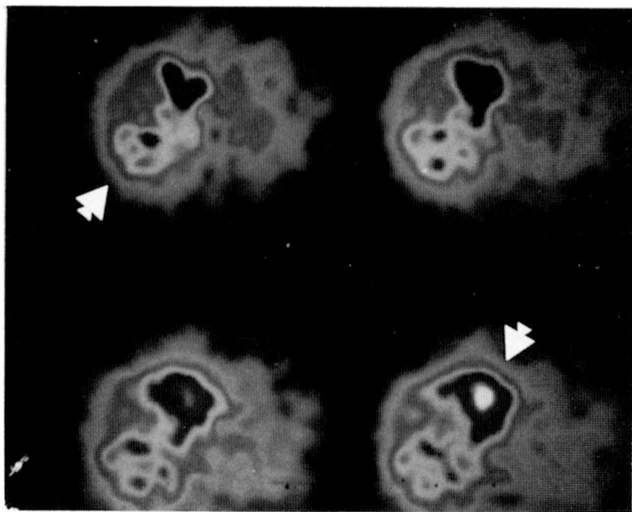

Fig. 65.7 Liver metastases from gastric carcinoid (relapsed after gastrectomy) in a 51-year-old man. The cold defects of uptake demonstrated on ^{99m}Tc colloid liver SPECT (transaxial sections) in both lobes (A) and on ^{123}I-MIBG SPECT appear to take up the tracer intensively, though inhomogeneously (B). (Also shown in colour on Plate 17.)

lence being related to the size of the primary tumour. The diagnosis is based on clinical features and supported by the presence of high levels of the principle metabolite, 5-hydroxyindolacetic acid (5-HIAA) in urine.[99,100]

A review of the series reported in literature shows that approximately 50–60% of carcinoids are able to concentrate radiolabelled MIBG.[43,94,100–105] It is not yet known which factors determine this ability. MIBG uptake apparently correlates with the urinary excretion of 5-HIAA, although this is denied by some.[100]

The most frequently occurring *midgut* carcinoids (appendix and distal ileum) probably concentrate the radiolabelled MIBG more readily than those in the *hindgut* (rectum) and *foregut* (oesophagus, stomach, duodenum, pancreas, biliary tract, larynx, bronchus and thymus).[100] Primary and residual tumours are sometimes visualized,[40,100] but the most striking imaging is that of carcinoid metastases in the peritoneum and liver (provided that ^{131}I-MIBG delayed scans are performed, because of the different pharmacokinetics between normal and tumoral liver tissue). Lymph node involvement, bone deposits and ovary metastases have been reported as imaging well. Because the uptake varies from 0.2% to 5% of the injected activity[100] additional tumoral lesions can be seen with therapeutic doses of ^{131}I-MIBG,[100] as well as with the higher activities of ^{123}I-MIBG[61]. SPECT may also help in improving efficacy in the detection of small primary/residual/recurrent tumours and lymph node involvement (Fig. 65.7). Furthermore, it can demonstrate the possible simultaneous presence of MIBG-positive and -negative metastases.[61]

MIBG imaging cannot generally be relied upon either to detect a carcinoid, or to rule out the disease. When a strongly suspect carcinoid has been diagnosed, however, the test can be worthwhile: (1) to disclose any residual/recurrent tumour, in the event that it is not shown by other techniques; (2) to better define the staging; and (3) as a prelude to ^{131}I-MIBG therapy.

Other neural crest tumours

Worldwide experience in the detection of tumours other than phaeochromocytomas, NBs, MTCs and carcinoids is very limited. Nevertheless, a wide range of single or sporadic case reports has been investigated. Only a few of these tumours showed some MIBG uptake, thus allowing imaging, and demonstrated a wide disparity in MIBG uptake between the different tumour sites. ^{131}I-MIBG scintigraphy visualized more than half the benign or malignant chemodectomas[10,106] and ganglioneuromas investigated[43,73,81,82,107,108] as well as a few cases of schwannoma,[10,107,110] Merkel cell tumour,[10] retinoblastoma,[107,109] islet cell tumours[107,110] and APUDomas of unknown origin.[111] Only 1 out of about 30 cases of oat cell carcinoma was imaged.[107,112–114] Liver metastases from only 1 out of 17 melanomas showed ^{131}I-MIBG uptake.[107,115] Most of the peripheral and cranial nerve tumours in a case of neurofibromatosis (generally considered to be MIBG negative), were recently visualized with MIBG imaging.[116]

There was hardly any radioiodinated MIBG uptake in most of the tumours investigated that were not of neural crest origin.[43,107] MIBG concentration was observed only in the metastatic lesions of a chorioncarcinoma[18] and in a parathyroid adenoma.[117]

CONCLUSIONS

MIBG imaging plays a prominent role in diagnosing

phaeochromocytomas (including non-functional paragangliomas) and NBs. It may be regarded as a first-choice imaging technique as it presents a wide range of clinical advantages in both the diagnosis and follow-up of these tumours. MIBG scintigraphy still plays a more limited role in the detection of MTCs and carcinoids. It can usefully complement other diagnostic modalities. This imaging technique also has a potential diagnostic application in a few other tumoral diseases (chemodectomas, ganglioneuromas, schwannomas, neurofibromatosis), but these still need further investigation.

The number of MIBG-negative studies especially in neural crest tumours other than phaeochromocytomas and NBs is challenging. Several factors are advocated as a justification. Nevertheless, rather than erroneous results perhaps they should be considered an expression of the fact that each individual histotype falls into a different subgroup with varying structural and ultrastructural characteristics, some of which can be differentiated and imaged by the tracer. If so, MIBG imaging may help stimulate further search to broaden knowledge of the most intimate structure of APUDomas.

REFERENCES

1. Wieland D M, Wu J L, Brown L E, Mangner T J, Swanson D P, Beierwaltes W H 1980 Radiolabeled adrenergic neuron blocking agents: adrenomedullary imaging with 131-I-iodobenzylguanidine. J Nucl Med 21: 349–353
2. Beierwaltes W H 1987 Clinical applications of 131-I-labeled meta-iodobenzylguanidine. J L Quinn III Memorial Essay. In: Hoffer R B (ed) Yearbook of nuclear medicine. Yearbook Medical Publishers, Chicago, pp 17–34
3. McEwan A J, Shapiro B, Sisson J C et al 1985 Radioiodobenzyl guanidine for the scintigraphic location and therapy of adrenergic tumors. Semin Nucl Med 5: 132–153
4. Sisson J C, Frager M S, Walk T W et al 1981 Scintigraphic localization of pheochromocytoma. N Engl J Med 305: 12–17
5. Kimmig B, Brandeis W E, Eisenhut A, Bubeck B, Hermann H S, zumWinkel K 1984 Scintigraphy of neuroblastoma with 131-I-meta-iodobenzylguanidine. J Nucl Med 25: 773–775
6. Fischer M, Kamanabroo D, Sonderkamp H, Proske T 1984 Scintigraphic imaging of carcinoid tumors with 131-I-MIBG. Lancet 2: 165
7. Endo K, Shiomi K, Kasagi K et al 1984 Imaging of medullary carcinoma of the thyroid with 131-I-MIBG. Lancet 2: 233
8. Connell J M C, Hilditch T E, Elliott A, Semple P F 1984 131-I-MIBG and medullary carcinoma of the thyroid. Lancet 2: 1273–1274
9. Smit A J, vanEssen L H, Hollema H et al 1984 131-I-MIBG uptake in a non-secreting paraganglioma. J Nucl Med 25: 984–986
10. Von Moll L, McEwan A J, Shapiro B et al 1987 Iodine I-131-MIBG scintigraphy of neuroendocrine tumors other than pheochromocytoma and neuroblastoma. J Nucl Med 28: 979–988
11. Hoefnagel C A, Voûte P A, De Kraker J, Marcuse H R 1987 Radionuclide diagnosis of neural crest tumors using 131-I-metaiodobenzylguanidine. J Nucl Med 28: 308–314
12. Sisson J C, Shapiro B, Meyers L et al 1987 Metaiodobenzylguanidine to map scintigraphically the adrenergic nervous system in man. J Nucl Med 28: 1625–1636
13. Sisson J C, Wieland D M, Jaques Jr S et al 1987 Radiolabeled meta-iodobenzylgaunidine and the adrenergic neurons of salivary glands. Am J Physiol Imaging 2: 1–9
14. Kline R C, Swanson D P, Wieland D M, Thrall J H, Gross M D, Pitt B, Beierwaltes W H 1981 Myocardial imaging in man with 123-I-metaiodobenzylguanidine. J Nucl Med 22: 129–132
15. Henderson E B, Kahn J K, Corbett R et al 1988 Abnormal 123-I-metaiodobenzylguanidine myocardial wash out and distribution may reflect myocardial adrenergic derangement in patients with congestive cardiomyopathy. Circulation 78: 1192–1194
16. Slosman D O, Donath A, Alderson P O 1989 131-I-metaiodobenzylguanidine and 125-I-iodoamphetamine. Parameters of lung endothelial cell function and pulmonary vascular area. Eur J Nucl Med 15: 207–210
17. Giordano A, Calcagni M L, Troncone L et al 1993 Inhaled 123-I-Metaiodobenzylguanidine for the evaluation of pulmonary adrenergic system function. Eur J Nucl Med 20: 826
18. Shapiro B, Gross M D 1991 Radioiodinated MIBG for the diagnostic scintigraphy and internal radiotherapy of neuroendocrine tumors. In: Troncone L (ed) I tumori della cresta neurale. Arcadia, Modena, Italy, pp 65–94
19. Sisson J C, Shapiro B, Beierwaltes W H et al 1984 Radiopharmaceutical treatment of malignant pheochromocytoma. J Nucl Med 25: 197–206
20. Troncone L, Galli G (eds) 1991 The role of 131-I-MIBG in the treatment of neural crest tumor. Proceedings of an International Workshop. Rome, September 6–7. J Nucl Biol Med 35: 177–363
21. Short J H, Darby T D 1967 Sympathetic nervous system blocking agents. III. Derivates of benzylguanidine. J Med Chem 10: 833–840
22. Jaques Jr S, Tobes M C, Sisson J C, Backer J A, Wieland D M 1984 Comparison of the sodium dependency of uptake of meta-iodobenzylguanidine and norepinephrine into cultured bovine adrenomedullary cells. Mol Pharmacol 26: 539–546
23. Smets L, Loesberg L, Janssen M, Metwally E, Huiskamp R 1989 Active uptake and extravesicular storage of metaiodobenzylguanidine in human SK-N-SH cells. Cancer Res 49: 2941–2944
24. Blake G M, Lewington V J, Fleming J S, Zivanovic M A, Ackery D M 1988 Modification by nifedipine of ^{131}I-Meta-iodobenzylguanidine kinetics in malignant phaeochromocytoma. Eur J Nucl Med 14: 345–348
25. Khafagi F A, Shapiro B, Fig L M, Mallette S, Sisson J C 1989 Labetalol reduces iodine-131-MIBG uptake by pheochromocytoma and normal tissues. J Nucl Med 30: 481–489
26. Lynn M D, Shapiro B, Sisson J C et al 1984 Portrayal of pheochromocytoma and normal human adrenal medulla by ^{123}I metaiodobenzylguanidine (^{123}I-MIBG): concise communication. J Nucl Med 25: 436–440
27. Shulkin B L, Shapiro B, Tobes M C et al 1986 Iodine-123-4-amino-3-iodobenzylguanidine, a new sympatho-adrenal imaging agent: comparison with iodine-131-metaiodobenzylguanidine. J Nucl Med 27: 1138–1142
28. Shapiro B, Gross M D 1987 Radiochemistry, biochemistry and kinetics of ^{131}I-MIBG and ^{123}I-MIBG. Med Pediatr Oncol 15: 170–177
29. Sisson J C, Shapiro B, Hutchinson R J et al 1991 Treatment of neuroblastoma with ^{125}I-metaiodobenzylguanidine. J Nucl Biol Med 35: 255–259
30. Swanson D P, Carey J E, Brown L E et al 1981 Human absorbed dose calculations for Iodine-131 and Iodine-123 labeled metaiodobenzylguanidine (mIBG): a potential myocardial and adrenal medulla imaging agent. In: Proceedings of the 3rd International Radiopharmaceutical Dosimetry Symposium. Health and Human Services Publication FDA 81-81-66, Rockville, Maryland, pp 213–224
31. Troncone L, Maini C L, De Rosa G et al 1984 Scintigraphic localization of a disseminated malignant pheochromocytoma with the use of ^{131}I-meta-iodobenzylguanidine. Eur J Nucl Med 9: 429–432
32. Bomanji J, Flatman W D, Hornee T et al 1987 Quantitation of Iodine-123 MIBG uptake by normal adrenal medulla in hypertensive patients. J Nucl Med 28: 319–324
33. Shulkin B L, Sisson J C, Koral K E et al 1988 Conjugate view

gammacamera method for estimating tumor uptake of iodine-131 meta-iodobenzylguanidine. J Nucl Med 29: 542–548

34. Nakajo M, Shapiro B, Copp J et al 1983 The normal and abnormal distribution of the adrenomedullary imaging agent in ^{131}I-iodobenzylguanidine (^{131}I-MIBG) in man: evaluation by scintigraphy. J Nucl Med 24: 672–682
35. Geatti O, Shapiro B, Hutchinson R J, Sisson J C 1988 Gastrointestinal ^{131}I-MIBG activity. Ann J Physiol Imaging 3: 188–201
36. Shulkin B L, Shen S W, Sisson J C, Shapiro B 1987 Iodine ^{131}I-MIBG scintigraphy of the extremities in metastatic pheochromocytoma and neuroblastoma. J Nucl Med 28: 315
37. Valk T W, Frager M S, Gross M D et al 1981 Spectrum of pheochromocytoma in multiple endocrine neoplasia. Ann Intern Med 94: 762–767
38. De Maria M, Barbiera F, Bonadonna F, Marozzi P, Tese', L 1992 Diseases of the adrenal medulla. In: Troncone L, Danza F M (eds) Diagnostic imaging of adrenal diseases. Rays 17: 62–86
39. Shapiro B, Copp J E, Sisson J C, Eyre P L, Wallis J, Beierwaltes W H 1985 131-Iodine-metaiodobenzylguanidine for the locating of suspected pheochromocytoma: experience in 400 cases. J Nucl Med 26: 576–585
40. Beierwaltes W H 1991 Endocrine imaging: parathyroid, adrenal cortex and medulla, and other endocrine tumors. Part II. J Nucl Med 32: 1627–1639
41. Landsberg L, Young J B 1987 Pheochromocytoma. In: Braunvald E, Isselbacher K J, Petersdorf R G, Wilson J D, Martin J B, Fanci AS (eds) Harrison's principles of internal medicine, 11th edn. McGraw-Hill, New York, pp 1775–1778
42. Minno A M, Bennett W A, Kvale W F 1954 Pheochromocytoma. A study of 15 cases diagnosed at autopsy. N Engl J Med 251: 959–965
43. Troncone L, Rufini V, Montemaggi P, Danza F M, Lasorella A, Mastrangelo R 1990 The diagnostic and therapeutic utility of radioiodinated metaiodobenzylguanidine (MIBG): 5 years of experience. Eur J Nucl Med 16: 325–335
44. Kalff V, Shapiro B, Lloyd R V et al 1982 The spectrum of pheochromocytoma in hypertensive patients with neuro-fibromatosis. Arch Int Med 142: 2092–2098
45. Glowniak J Y, Shapiro B, Sisson J C et al 1985 Familial extra-adrenal pheochromocytoma: a new syndrome. Arch Int Med 145: 257–261
46. Khafagi F, Egerton-Vernon J, Vandoorn T, Foster W, McPhee I B, Allison R W G 1987 Localization and treatment of familial malignant non functional paraganglioma with 131-Iodine-MIBG: report of two cases. J Nucl Med 28: 528–531
47. Baulieu J L, Guilloteau D, Fetissof F et al 1984 Paragangliomas sympathiques: utilization de la meta-iodobenzylguanidine pour leur exploration scintigraphique. Press Med 13: 1679–1682
48. Nakajo M, Shapiro B, Glowniak J Y, Sisson J C, Beierwaltes W H 1983 Inverse relationship between cardiac accumulation of meta 131-I-Iodobenzylguanidine (1-131-MIBG) and circulating catecholamines in suspected pheochromocytomas. J Nucl Med 24: 1127–1134
49. Ackery D M, Tippet P A, Condon B R, Sutton H E, Wyeth P 1984 New approach to the localization of pheochromocytoma: imaging with iodine-131-meta-iodobenzylguanidine. Br Med J 288: 1587–1591
50. Baulieu J L, Guilloteau D, Viel C et al 1984 Scintigraphie à la meta-iodobenzylguanidine: bilan d'une première année d'experience. Biophys Med Nucl 8: 27–33
51. Fischer M, Wetter M, Winterberg B et al 1984 Scintigraphic localization of pheochromocytomas. Clin Endocrinol 20: 1–7
52. Mahlstedt J, Hotze A, Pichl J, Wolf F et al 1984 Ergebnisse szintigraphischer Untersuchungen mit 131-I-meta-Benzylguanidin (MIBG) bei Raumforderungen neuroektodermaier Herkunft. Nucl Med 23: 257–264
53. Swansen S J, Brown M L, Sheps S G et al 1985 Use of 131-I-MIBG scintigraphy in the evaluation of suspected pheo-chromocytoma. Mayo Clin Proc 60: 299–304
54. Chatal J F, Charbonnel B 1985 Comparison of Iodobenzyl-guanidine imaging with computed tomography in locating pheochromocytoma. J Clin Endocrinol Metab 61: 769–772
55. Jakubowski W, Feltynowsky T, Januszewicz W, Graban W, Leowska L, Pacho R 1985 131-I-metaiodobenzylguanidine in localization and treatment of pheochromocytoma. Nucl Med Commun 6: 586
56. Welchik M G, Alavi A, Kressel H Y, Engelman K 1989 Localization of pheochromocytoma: MIBG, CT and MRI correlation. J Nucl Med 30: 328–336
57. Warren M J, Shepstone B J, Soper N 1989 Iodine-131-metaiodobenzylguanidine (131-I-MIBG) for the location of suspected pheochromocytoma. Nucl Med Commun 10: 467–475
58. Maurea S, Cuocolo A, Reynolds J C et al 1993 Iodine-131-metaiodobenzylguanidine scintigraphy in preoperative and post-operative evaluation of paragangliomas: comparison with CT and MRI. J Nucl Med 34: 173–179
59. Shulkin B, Shapiro B, Francis I, Dorr R, Shen S W, Sisson J C 1986 Primary extraadrenal pheochromocytoma: a case of positive 123-I-MIBG scintigraphy with negative 131-I-MIBG scintigraphy. Clin Nucl Med 11: 851–854
60. Horne F, Hawkins L A, Britton K E, Granowska M, Bouloux P 1984 Imaging of pheochromocytoma and adrenal medulla with 123-I-Metaiodobenzylguanidine. Nucl Med Commun 5: 763–768
61. Troncone L, Rufini V, Daidone M S, Giordano A, Saletnich I, Pantusa M 1993 Diagnostica dei tumori neuroendocrini con MIBG radioiodata: ruolo della 123-I-MIBG associata alla SPECT. Acta Med Rom 31: 371–377
62. Francis I R, Glazer G M, Shapiro B, Sisson J C, Gross M D 1983 Complementary roles of CT scanning and 131-I-MIBG scintigraphy in the diagnosis of pheochromocytoma. AJR 141: 719–725
63. Shapiro B, Gross M D, Sandler M P 1987 Adrenal scintigraphy revisited: a current status report on radiotracer, clinical utility and correlative imaging. In: Freeman L M, Weissmann H S (eds) Nuclear Medicine Annual 1987. Raven Press, New York, pp 193–232
64. Quint L E, Glazer G M, Francis I R, Shapiro B, Chenevert T L 1987 Pheochromocytoma and paraganglioma: comparison of MR imaging with CT and I-131-MIBG scintigraphy. Radiology 165: 89–93
65. Rufini V, Troncone L, Valentini A L, Danza F M 1988 Comparison of radiolabeled MIBG scintigraphy with computed tomography in the localization of pheochromocytomas. Radiol Med 76: 466–470
66. Lynn M D, Braunstein E M, Wahl R L, Shapiro B, Gross M D, Rabbani R 1986 Bone metastases in pheochromocytoma: comparative studies of efficacy in imaging. Radiology 160: 701–706
67. Feine U, Müller-Schauenburg W, Treuner J, Klin-gebiel T H 1987 Metaiodobenzylguanidine (MIBG) labeled with 123-I/131-I in neuroblastoma. Med Pediatr Oncol 15: 181–187
68. Hoefnagel C A 1989 Neuroblastoma: addendum. In: The clinical use of 131-I-metaiodobenzylguanidine (MIBG) for the diagnosis and treatment of neural crest tumors. Academisch proefschrift. Koninklijke drukkerij Callenbach, Nijkerk, The Netherlands, pp 98–114
69. Lumbroso J D, Guermazi F, Hartmann O et al 1988 Metaiodobenzylguanidine (MIBG) scans in neuroblastoma: sensitivity and specificity. A review of 115 scans. In: Evans A E, D'Angio G J, Knudson A G, Seeger R C (eds) Advances in neuroblastoma research, Vol 2. Alan R. Liss, New York, pp 689–705
70. Shapiro B, Khafagi F, Gross M D, Sisson J C 1989 MIBG in the management of neuroendocrine tumors. In: A Sagripanti, A Carpi, B Grassi (eds) Advances in management of malignancies. Monduzzi Editore, Bologna, pp 203–208
71. Harris R E, Gelfand M J 1986 Sensitivity and utility of the 131-I-MIBG scan in childhood neuroblastoma. Proc Am Soc Clin Oncol 5: 825
72. Troncone L, Rufini V, Danza F M et al 1990 Radioiodinated Metaiodobenzylguanidine (*I-MIBG) scintigraphy in neuroblastoma a review of 160 studies. J Nucl Med Allied Sci 34: 279–288
73. Claudiani F, Garaventa A, Scopinaro G et al 1988 Diagnostic and therapeutic use of 131-I-Metaiodobenzylguanidine in children with neuroblastoma. J Nucl Med Allied Sci 32: 1–6

74. Bouvier J F, Ducrettet T, Philip T, Brunat-Mentigny M, Chauvot P, Lahneche B E 1987 MIBG neuroblastoma diagnosis: value and limits. Proceedings of the MIBG and Catecholamines Workshop, Tours, March 16–17, 1987. Book of Abstracts. Laboratoire de Biophysique Medicale, UER de Médecine, Tours, p 42
75. Ythier H, Marchandise X, Deveaux M et al 1987 Results of scintigraphy with m-123-I-iodobenzylguanidine in neuroblastoma in children. Int J Rad Appl Instrum 14(2): 107–112
76. Lastoria S, Barile V, Salvatore M 1987 131-I-MIBG scintigraphy for diagnosis of neuroblastoma. Nucl Med 26: 40–42
77. Munkner T 1985 131-I-iodobenzylguanidine scintigraphy of neuroblastomas. Semin Nucl Med 15: 154–160
78. Yeh S D J, Helson L, Benua R S 1986 Metaiodobenzylguanidine (MIBG) imaging in neuroblastoma. J Nucl Med 27: 947–948
79. Heyman S, Evans A E 1986 I-131-metaiodobenzylguanidine (I-131-MIBG) in the diagnosis of neuroblastoma. J Nucl Med 27: 931–932
80. Hakvoort-Cammel F G A J, Ausema L, Krenning E P, Van Zanen G E 1987 123-I-Metaiodobenzylguanidine for diagnosis and follow-up of neuroblastoma. Proceedings of the International Conference on Pediatric Oncology, New Developments and Opinions. Nijmegen, June 1–3, 1987. Book of Abstracts. University Hospitalsint Radboud, Nijmegen, The Netherlands, p 77
81. Miceli A, Nespoli L, Burgio G R, Aprile C, Carena M, Saponaro M 1986 The role of meta-iodo-131-I-benzylguanidine (MIBG) in the diagnosis and follow-up of neuroblastoma. Pediatr Haemat Oncol 3: 37–47
82. Hibi S, Todo S, Imashuku S, Miyazaky T 1987 131-I-metaiodobenzylguanidine scintigraphy in patients with neuroblastoma. Pediatr Radiol 17: 308–313
83. Hadley G P, Rabe E 1986 Scanning with iodine-131-MIBG in children with solid tumors: an initial appraisal. J Nucl Med 27: 620–626
84. Edeling C J, Buchler Frederiksen P, Kamper J, Jeppesen P 1986 Diagnosis and treatment of neuroblastoma using 131-I iodobenzylguanidine. Nucl Med 25: 172–175
85. Gerrard M, Eden O B, Merrick H V 1986 Imaging and treatment of disseminated neuroblastoma with 131-I-meta-iodobenzylguanidine. Br J Radiol 60: 393–395
86. Gordon I, Peters A M, Gutman A, Morony S, Dicks-Mireaux C, Pritchard Y 1990 Skeletal assessment in neuroblastoma. The pitfalls of Iodine-123-MIBG scans. J Nucl Med 31: 129–134
87. Moyes J S E, Babich J W, Carter R, Meller S T, Agrawal M, McElwain T J 1989 Quantitative study of radiolabeled metaiodobenzylguanidine uptake in children with neuroblastoma: correlation with tumor histopathology. J Nucl Med 30: 474–480
88. Corbett R P, Fullbrook A, Meller S T 1990 123-I-metaiodobenzylguanidine (MIBG) SPECT in the assessment of neuroblastoma (abstract). Nucl Med Commun 11: 224–225
89. Yeh S D J, Larson S M, Burch L et al 1991 Radioimmunodetection of neuroblastoma with Iodine 131-3F8: Correlation with biopsy, iodine-131-metaiodobenzylguanidine and standard diagnostic modalities. J Nucl Med 32: 769–776
90. Melvin K E V 1986 Medullary carcinoma of the thyroid. In: Ingbar S H, Braverman L E (eds) Werner's the thyroid. Lippincott, Philadelphia, pp 1349–1362
91. Troncone L, Rufini V 1992 Medullary thyroid cancer: new trends in diagnosis and therapy. In: Carpi A, Sagripanti A, Mittermayer C H (eds) Progress in clinical oncology. Sympomed, Munchen, pp 227–250
92. Poston G J, Thomas A M K, McDonald W R et al 1986 Imaging of metastatic medullary carcinoma of the thyroid with 131-I-metaiodobenzylguanidine. Nucl Med Commun 7: 215–221
93 Hilditch T E, Connell J M C, Elliott A T et al 1986 Poor results with technetium-99m(V)DMSA and iodine-131 MIBG in the imaging of medullary thyroid carcinoma. J Nucl Med 27: 1150–1153
94. Baulieu J L, Guilloteau D, Delisle M J et al 1987 Radioiodinated meta-iodobenzylguanidine uptake in medullary thyroid cancer. A French cooperative study. Cancer 60: 2189–2194
95. Clarke S E M, Lazarus C R, Wraight P et al 1988 Pentavalent 99m-Tc-DMSA, 131-I-MIBG, and 99mTc-MDP. An evaluation of three imaging techniques with medullary carcinoma of the thyroid. J Nucl Med 29: 33–38
96. Hoefnagel C A, Delprat C C, Zanin D, Van der Schoot J B 1988 New radionuclide tracers for the diagnosis and therapy of medullary thyroid carcinoma. Clin Nucl Med 13: 159–165
97. Guerra U P, Pizzocaro L, Terzi A et al 1989 New tracers for the imaging of the medullary thyroid carcinoma. Nucl Med Commun 5: 285–295
98. Troncone L, Rufini V, De Rosa G, Testa A 1989 Diagnostic and therapeutic potential of new radiopharmaceutical agents in medullary thyroid carcinoma. Henry Ford Hosp Med J 37: 178–184
99. Zarrilli L, Marzano L A, Porcelli A, D'Avanzo A, Misso C 1991 The surgical management of carcinoid tumors. J Nucl Biol Med 35: 341–342
100. Hoefnagel C A, Den Hartog Jager F C A, Taal B G, Abeling N G G M, Engelsman E E 1989 The role of 131-I-MIBG in the diagnosis and therapy of carcinoids; and Addendum. In: The clinical use of 131-I-metaiodobenzylguanidine for the diagnosis and treatment of neural crest tumours. Academisch proefschrift. Koninklijke drukkerij, Callenbach. Nijkerk, The Netherlands, pp 117–130
101. Sinzinger H, Renner F, Granegger S 1985 131-I-MIBG imaging of carcinoids and apudomas. Eur J Nucl Med 1985; 11: A 17
102. Feldman J M, Blinder R A, Lucas K J, Coleman R E 1986 Iodine-131 metaiodobenzylguanidine scintigraphy of carcinoid tumors. J Nucl Med 27: 1691–1696
103. McEwan A J, Catz Z, Field S et al 1987 I-131-metaiodobenzylguanidine (mIBG) in the diagnosis and treatment of carcinoid syndrome. J Nucl Med 28: 658
104. Jodrell D J, Irvine A T, McCready V R, Woodcraft E, Smith I E 1988 The use of 131-I-MIBG in the imaging of metastatic carcinoid tumors. Br J Cancer 58: 663–664
105. Castellani M R, Di Bartolomeo M, Maffioli L, Zilembo N, Gasparini M, Buraggi G L 1991 131-I-MIBG therapy in carcinoid tumors. J Nucl Biol Med 35: 349–351
106. Van Gils A P G, Van Der May A G L, Hoosma R P J M et al 1989 Jodium 123-MIBG scintigraphie bij chemodectomen: een opvallend resultaat. Nucl Geneeskd Bull 11: 61
107. Hoefnagel C A 1989 Use of 131-I-meta-iodobenzylguanidine in other neuroendocrine tumors. In: The clinical use of 131-I-metaiodobenzylguanidine (MIBG) for the diagnosis and treatment of neural crest tumors. Academisch proefschrift. Koninklijke drukkerrij Callenbach. Nijkerk, The Netherlands, pp 149–161
108. Caballero O, Ferris J, Verdeguer A, Esquembre C, Castel V 1986 Visualization of ganglioneuroma by means of scintigraphy with 131-I-MIBG. Eur J Nucl Med 12: 351–352
109. Bomanji J, Kingston J E, Hungerford J L, Britton K E 1989 123-I-meta-iodobenzylguanidine scintigraphy of ectopic intracranial retinoblastoma. Medical and Pediatric Oncology 17: 66–68
110. Geatti O, Shapiro B, Barillari B 1989 Scintigraphic depiction of an insulinoma by I-131-metaiodobenzylguanidine. Clin Nucl Med 14: 903–906
111. Somers G, Houte K V, Segers O, Bossuyt A 1988 Iodine-123-MIBG imaging in a generalized pancreatic polypeptide-gastrin-serotonin secreting tumor. Clin Nucl Med 13: 352–355
112. Nakajo M, Taguchi M, Shimabukuro K, Shinohara S 1986 Iodine-131-MIBG uptake in a small cells carcinoma of the lung. J Nucl Med 27: 1785–1786
113. Vincent M D, Babich J, Irvine A, McCready V R, Smith I E 1987 Failure of Iodine-131-MIBG imaging in a small cell lung carcinoma. J Nucl Med 28: 1230
114. Wadler S, Tai K, Chervu L R et al 1989 Iodine-131-MIBG scintigraphy in small cell lung cancer. Eur J Nucl Med 15: 108–110
115. Fischer M, Vetter W, Winterberg B, Frieman J, Vetter H 1983 131-I-metaiodobenzylguanidin szintigraphie zum Nachweis eines Phaeochromocytomas. Nucl Compact 14: 356–360
116. Rufini V, Daidone M S, Teofili L, Nicoletti G, Leone G, Troncone L 1991 An unusual association of neurofibromatosis (NF) and neuroblastoma (NB) investigated with 131-I-MIBG. Eur J Nucl Med 18: 684
117. Hayward R S, Bowering C K, Warshawski R S 1988 I-131-metaiodobenzylguanidine uptake in a parathyroid adenoma. Clin Nucl Med 13: 632–634

66. Somatostatin receptor scintigraphy with [^{111}In-DTPA-D-Phe^{1}]octreotide

Eric P. Krenning   Dik J. Kwekkeboom   Jean-Claude Reubi
Steven W. J. Lamberts

SOMATOSTATIN AND SOMATOSTATIN RECEPTORS

Somatostatin membrane receptors have been identified on many cells and tumours of neuroendocrine origin, such as the somatotroph cells of the anterior pituitary and pancreatic islet cell tumours (Fig. 66.1).[1,2] However, cells and tumours not known to be of classically neuroendocrine origin, for example activated lymphocytes, lymphomas and breast cancer, may also possess these receptors.[4–9] The somatostatin analogue octreotide, which is eight amino acids long, has been shown to bind to somatostatin

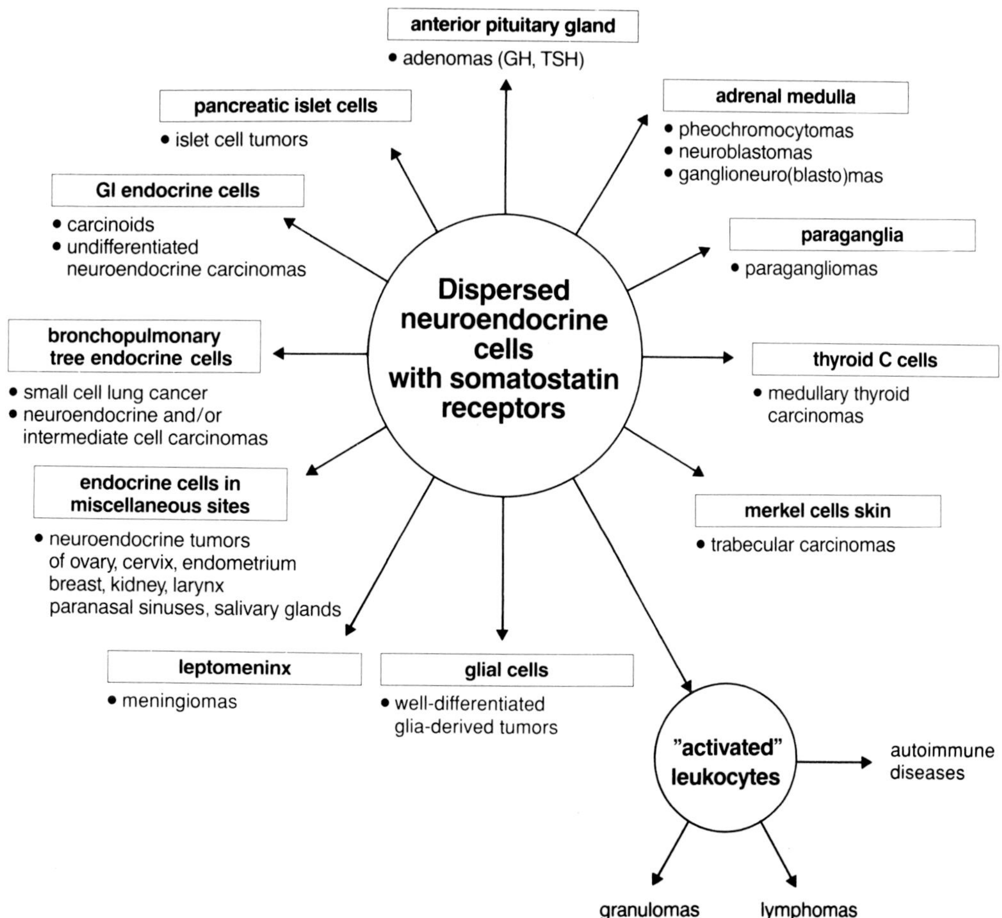

Fig. 66.1 Tumours and diseases in which neuroendocrine cells and/or activated leucocytes have an increased density of somatostatin receptors, which can be visualized with [^{111}In-DTPA-D-Phe^{1}]octreotide scintigraphy. (modified from Lamberts et al.[3])

receptors on both tumorous and non-tumorous tissues. Because of its relatively long effective half-life, [^{111}In-DTPA-D-Phe^{1}]octreotide is a radiolabelled somatostatin analogue which can be used to visualize somatostatin receptor-bearing tumours efficiently after 24 and 48 h, when interfering background radioactivity is minimized by renal clearance.[10]

APPLICATION OF ^{111}IN OCTREOTIDE SCINTIGRAPHY

^{111}In octreotide scintigraphy based on over 1000 patients indicates that this technique is without side-effects and very sensitive in the localization of even very small somatostatin receptor-positive lesions, for example neuroendocrine tumours and granulomatous diseases involving activated lymphocytes. An overview of our results in patients in whom the diagnosis was unequivocal is given in Table 66.1. The results of imaging in vivo correlated very well with the somatostatin receptor status on the tumours in vitro, as identified with [^{125}I-Tyr^{3}]octreotide autoradiography (Table 66.1). In this chapter more specific information is provided about patient groups that have been investigated in more detail (Fig. 66.2).

Table 16.1 Results of [^{111}In-DTPA-D-Phe^{1}]octreotide scintigraphy in various diseases as compared with in vitro somatostatin receptor autoradiography. In vivo and in vitro data are from different patient groups

	Results of			
	In vivo scintigraphy		In vitro receptor status	
GH-producing pituitary tumour	7/10	70%	45/46	98%
Non-functioning pituitary tumour	12/16	75%	12/22	55%
TSH-producing pituitary tumour	2/2	100%	2/2	100%
Gastrinoma	12/12	100%	6/6	100%
Insulinoma	14/23	61%	8/11	72%
Glucagonoma	3/3	100%	2/2	100%
Unclassified APUDoma	16/18	89%	4/4	100%
Paraganglioma	33/33	100%	11/12	92%
Medullary thyroid carcinoma	20/28	71%	10/26	38%
Neuroblastoma	8/9	89%	15/23	65%
Phaeochromocytoma	12/14	86%	38/52	73%
Carcinoid	69/72	96%	54/62	88%
Merkel cell tumour	4/5	80%	–	
Small-cell lung cancer	34/34	100%	4/7	57%
Non-small-cell lung cancer	36/36	100%	0/25	0%
Breast cancer	47/69	68%	33/72	46%
Breast cancer follow up*	8/28	29%	–	
Exocrine pancreatic carcinoma	0/24	0%	0/12	0%
Non-Hodgkin's lymphoma	59/74	80%	26/30	87%
Hodgkin's disease	23/24	96%	2/2	100%
Meningiomas	12/12	100%	54/55	98%
Grawitz tumours	2/4	50%	28/39	72%
Rheumatoid arthritis	15/15	100%	2/2	100%
Sarcoidosis	23/23	100%	3/3	100%
Tuberculosis	6/6	100%	2/2	100%
Graves' disease: thyroid	9	†	1/1	
Graves' ophthalmopathy	25	‡	–	

*Second [^{111}In-DTPA-D-Phe^{1}]octreotide scintigraphy, at least 2 years after first scintigraphy, only in patients with a positive initial scintigram.
† Increased accumulation of radioactivity in the thyroid gland in untreated hyperthyroidism.
‡Correlation with clinical activity score of orbital inflammation.

PITUITARY TUMOURS

Somatostatin receptors were demonstrated in vitro on virtually all growth hormone (GH)-producing pituitary adenomas. In vivo somatostatin receptor imaging was positive in most cases (Table 66.1). A close correlation between the presence of somatostatin receptors on GH-producing pituitary tumours in vitro and the preoperative in vivo sensitivity of tumorous GH secretion to octreotide has been reported.[11] Likewise, scan positivity or negativity during in vivo octreotide scintigraphy is linked to the sensitivity of GH release to suppression by octreotide.[12,13]

A group of patients with clinically non-functioning pituitary adenomas have been studied extensively.[14] Virtually all these tumours secrete gonadotrophins or their subunits, although this is seldom reflected in elevated serum concentrations. The adenomas from six of the seven patients were somatostatin receptor positive both in vivo and in vitro. However, long-term high-dose octreotide treatment in four of these patients resulted in some reduction of tumorous gonadotropin secretion in two patients, and improvement of visual field defects in three patients, but not in substantial reduction of tumour size in any of the patients.

Not only GH-producing or clinically non-functioning pituitary adenomas, but also TSH-secreting pituitary tumours can be visualized using octreotide scintigraphy (Table 66.1). In addition, other intra- or parasellar tumours, e.g. pituitary metastases from somatostatin receptor-positive neoplasms such as breast cancer, parasellar meningiomas or lymphomas, may be positive. The diagnostic value of octreotide scintigraphy in pituitary tumours does therefore appear to be limited.

ENDOCRINE PANCREATIC TUMOURS

Most peptide hormone-producing endocrine tumours stem from the islet cells of the pancreas, but they may also occur elsewhere in the gastrointestinal tract. These tumours are named after the hormone(s) they secrete, e.g. gastrinomas, insulinomas, glucagonomas. Octreotide has been shown to be of special benefit in the treatment of the clinical syndromes caused by hypersecretion of these hormones.[15,16] Surgery is the treatment of choice in most patients, but the localization of the primary as well as metastatic tumours may prove very difficult or even impossible with conventional imaging means.[17]

The majority of the endocrine pancreatic tumours can be visualized using [^{111}In-DTPA-D-Phe^{1}]octreotide scintigraphy (Table 66.1) (Fig. 66.3). Octreotide scintigraphy can therefore be of great value in localizing tumour

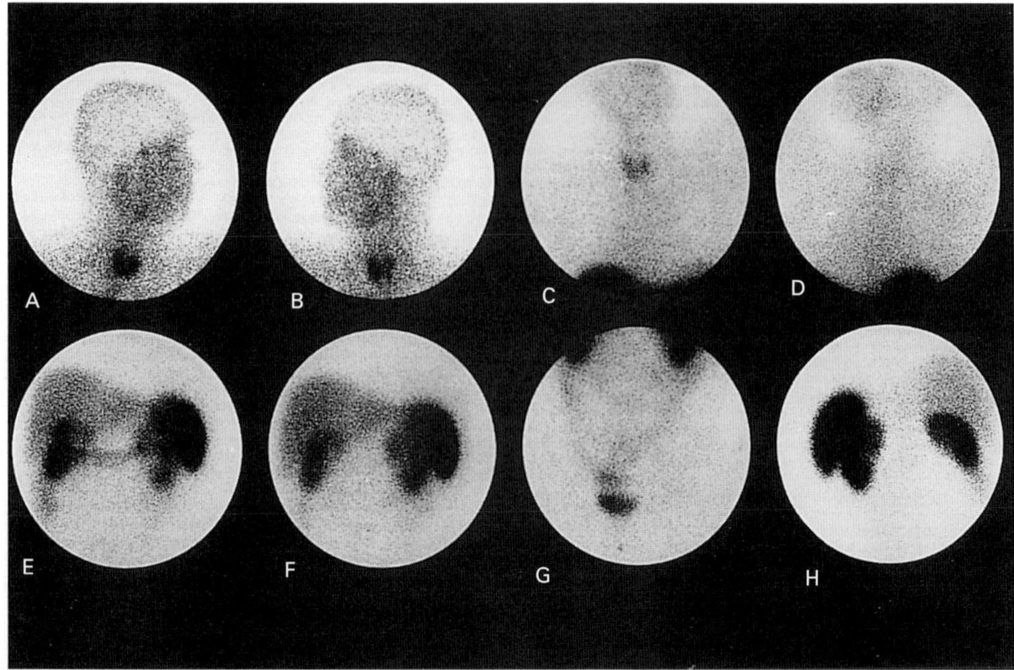

Fig. 66.2 Normal scintigraphic distribution of [^{111}In-DTPA-D-Phe^1]-octreotide in man 24 h after i.v. injection (except F). Usually the pituitary, thyroid gland, liver, spleen, kidneys, and urinary bladder are visualized. Views: right (A) and left (B) lateral part of the head, and anterior (C) and posterior (D) view of the thorax, anterior abdomen after 24 (E) and 48 h (F; note the disappearance of bowel activity due to the use of laxatives), (G) anterior view of the lower abdomen with activity in the kidneys, bowel and bladder, and (H) posterior view of the upper abdomen.

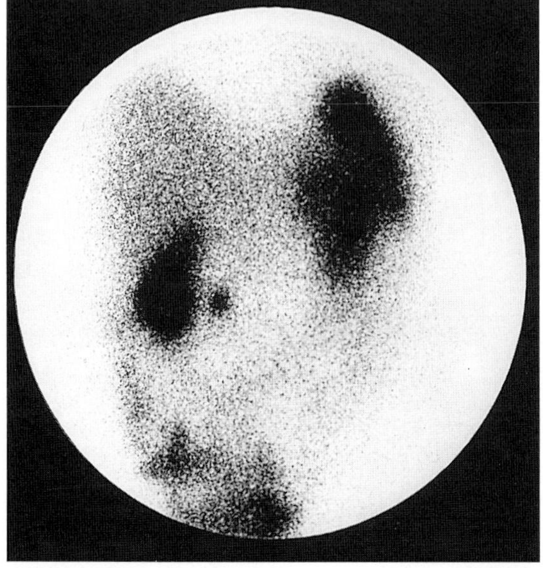

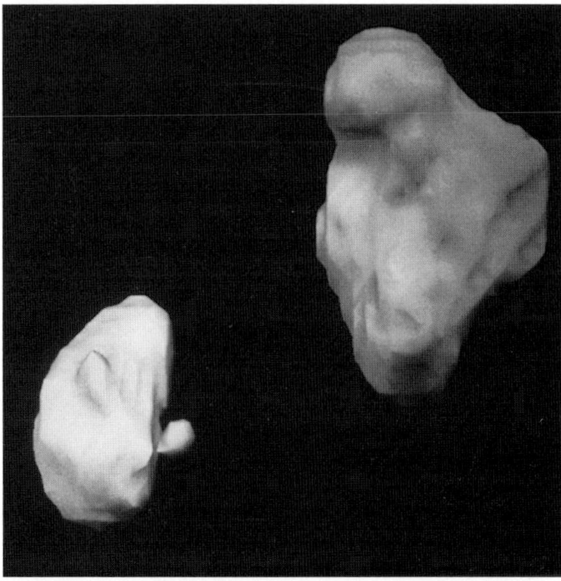

Fig. 66.3 (A) Anterior planar view of the abdomen of a patient with an insulinoma, 24 h after injection of [^{111}In-DTPA-D-Phe^1]octreotide. There is normal accumulation of radioactivity in the liver, spleen and kidneys. Also, activity in the bladder and some bowel contamination can be seen in the lower part of the image. Medial to the right kidney the insulinoma is visualized. (B) Three-dimensional reconstruction from a three-head camera (Picker Prism 3000) of the abdomen of the same patient. The spleen and left kidney are depicted in green, the insulinoma and right kidney in pink. (Part B also shown in colour in Plate 17.)

sites, particularly in those patients in whom surgery is indicated but in whom no tumour can be found with conventional imaging modalities.

Using ultrasound, CT, MRI and/or angiography, endocrine pancreatic tumours can be localized in about 50% of cases.[18,19] Recently, Rösch et al,[20] using endoscopic ultrasound, reported the detection of 32 of 39 (82%) endocrine pancreatic tumours which could not be localized with CT or transabdominal ultrasound. Although the described group contained very few extrapancreatic tumours, which are known to be more difficult to localize with other techniques, these results are impressive. A study comparing the value of endoscopic ultrasonography with octreotide scintigraphy in the same patients would be valuable. However, even if these two techniques were shown to have an equal sensitivity, octreotide scintigraphy would probably be preferred in most clinics, as endoscopic ultrasonography needs particular skill, and also might miss extrapancreatic metastases.

PARAGANGLIOMAS

Using [^{111}In-DTPA-D-Phe^1]octreotide scintigraphy, 50 of 53 (94%) known localizations in 25 well-documented patients with paragangliomas were visualized (Fig. 66.4).[21] In two patients, three localizations were missed during octreotide scintigraphy. Unexpected additional paraganglioma sites not detected or not investigated with conventional imaging techniques were found in 9 of 25 patients (36%) with known paragangliomas. In four of these, the reputed tumour localizations were subsequently also demonstrated with other imaging modalities.

High-resolution CT scanning in combination with MRI, with and without gadolinium-DTPA enhancement, is an effective imaging regimen for paragangliomas.[22] However, this type of imaging is usually limited to the site where a paraganglioma is clinically suspected. In our series, CT scanning or MRI of the site where a paraganglioma was primarily expected was in most cases combined with ultrasound of the neck, in order to detect multicentricity. With ^{111}In octreotide scintigraphy, however, unexpected additional paraganglioma sites not detected or not investigated with conventional imaging techniques were found in one-third of the patients with known paragangliomas. This finding is of special interest since multicentricity and distant metastases have each been reported to occur in only 10% of patients based on information from conventional imaging techniques.[23] The true frequency of multifocality may therefore have been previously underestimated. In this respect, one of the major advantages of octreotide scintigraphy is in identifying possible tumour sites in the whole body. It could thus be used as a screening test, to be followed by CT scanning, MRI or ultrasound of the sites at which abnormalities are found.

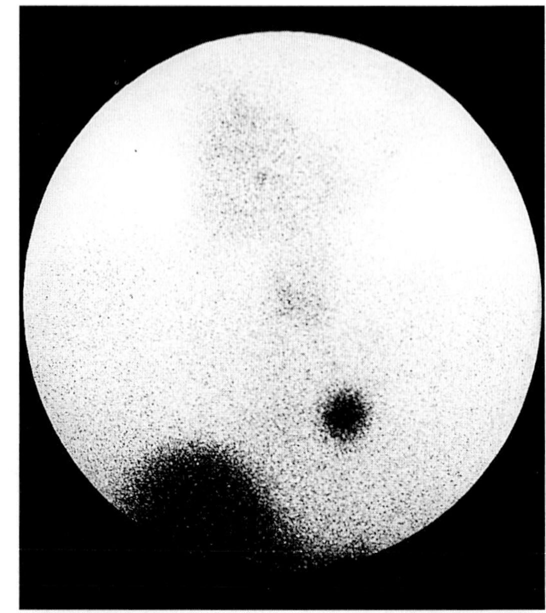

A

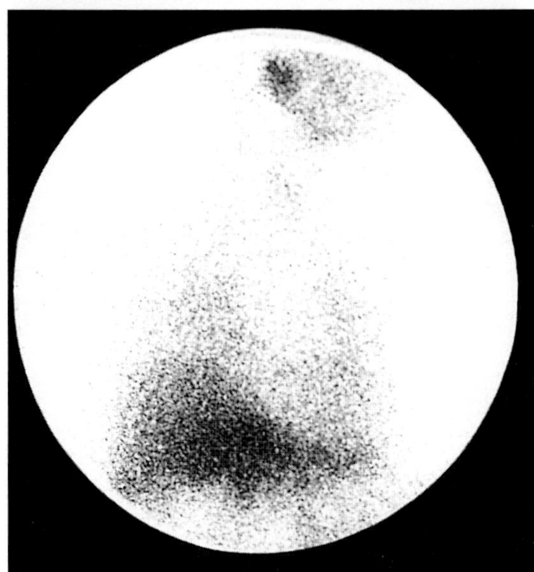

B

Fig. 66.4 (A) Anterior thoracic image of a patient with a dopamine-producing paraganglioma, 24 h after injection of [^{111}In-DTPA-D-Phe^1]octreotide. The tumour is clearly visualized. (B) Same view as in A, after ^{123}I-MIBG. No visualization of the tumour.

MEDULLARY THYROID CARCINOMA

In 11 of 17 (65%) well-documented patients with medullary thyroid carcinoma (MTC), tumour localization was demonstrated using ^{111}In octreotide scintigraphy.[24] Tumour localization in the liver in seven patients and in the thyroid in one patient was not detected during octreotide scintigraphy, most probably because of normal uptake of labelled octreotide in the surrounding tissue in these organs. It can thus be concluded that in the majority of patients with metastatic MTC tumour sites can be visualized using octreotide scintigraphy (Fig. 66.5), although this technique is insensitive in detecting liver metastases or intrathyroidal tumour when no subtraction techniques are applied.

Serum calcitonin (CT) and carcinoembryonic antigen (CEA) concentrations are used as tumour markers in

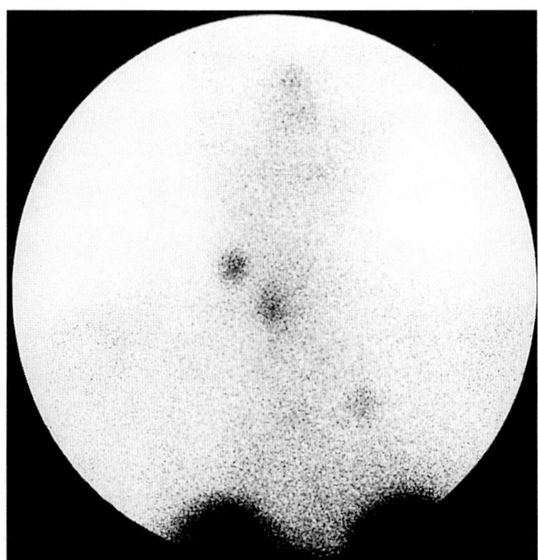

Fig. 66.5 Anterior thoracic image of a patient with medullary thyroid carcinoma, 24 h after injection. The upper edges of the liver and spleen are seen in the lower border of the image. Note the absence of thyroid accumulation due to thyroidectomy and abnormal accumulation of labelled octreotide in right supraclavicular area, in the mediastinum and in the left lung.

MTC. In the follow-up of patients with MTC, progressive disease and poor prognosis are correlated with a rise in serum CEA, while serum CT levels follow a non-parallel course.[25] In our series, neither serum CT nor CEA concentrations differed significantly between patients whose tumours were visualized during octreotide scintigraphy and those whose tumours were not. However, the ratio of CT to CEA was significantly higher in patients in whom octreotide scintigraphy was successfully applied. This may imply that somatostatin receptors can be detected in vivo on the more differentiated forms of MTC.

Long-term high-dose octreotide treatment in patients with MTC has been reported in two series. Mahler et al[26] reported a beneficial effect on symptoms and a lowering of CT and CEA levels by 45–80% in three patients with metastatic MTC who were treated with up to 2000 μg of octreotide daily. However, the suppression of serum tumour markers became less pronounced as therapy continued. Modigliani et al[27] observed a decrease in serum CT, but not CEA, concentrations in 4 of 14 patients with MTC who were treated with 500 μg of octreotide per day. Beneficial effects of octreotide treatment may be expected in patients with MTC who have tumours bearing somatostatin receptors. Apart from its merit in tumour localization, one of the major advantages of octreotide scintigraphy in MTC may be that the investigation can be used to select those patients who have somatostatin receptor-positive tumours, i.e. patients who could potentially benefit from octreotide treatment. Other tracers for MTC are described in Chapter 57.

CARCINOIDS

Scintigraphy with [^{123}I-Tyr^3]octreotide and [^{111}In-DTPA-D-Phe^1]octreotide was performed in 52 patients diagnosed as, suspected of, or at risk of having carcinoid tumours.[28] In 32 of 37 (86%) patients in whom histologically proven carcinoids were still present, known tumour sites were visualized (Fig. 66.6). Using [^{123}I-Tyr^3]octreotide, 24 of 40 (60%) known extrahepatic sites were visualized, whereas all of 12 (100%) extrahepatic lesions were visualized after injection of [^{111}In-DTPA-D-Phe^1]octreotide.

A

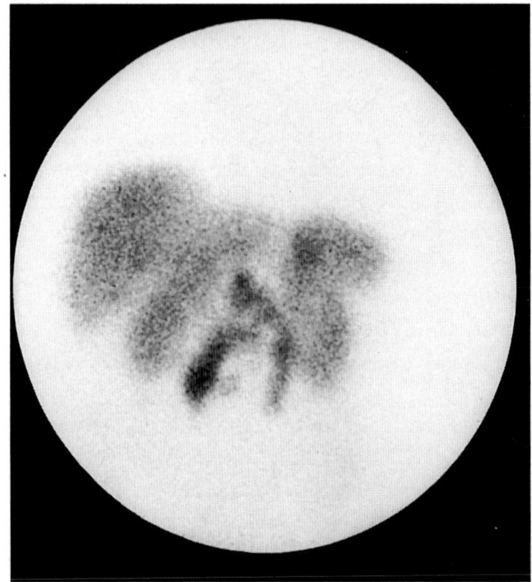

B

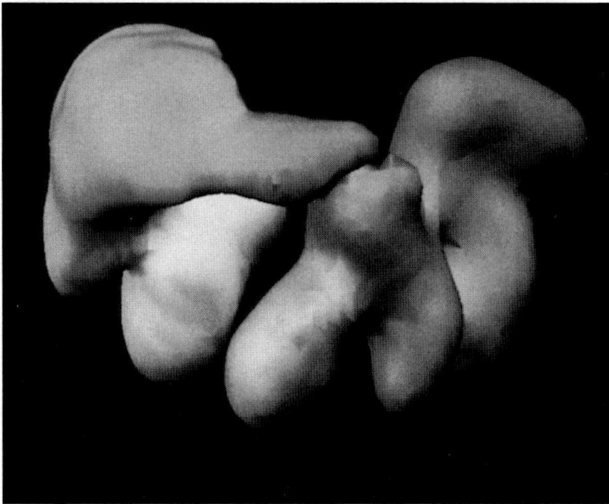

Fig. 66.6 (A) Anterior planar view of the abdomen in a patient with a carcinoid, 24 h after injection of [^{111}In-DTPA-D-Phe^1]octreotide. There is normal accumulation of radioactivity in the liver, spleen and kidneys. Abnormal uptake of labelled octreotide is seen in two strings between both kidneys, representing carcinoid-invaded retroperitoneal lymph nodes. (B) Three-dimensional reconstruction from a three-head camera (Picker Prism 3000) of the abdomen of the same patient. The liver, right kidney, spleen and left kidney are in orange, yellow, green and green–blue respectively. The tumour mass in purple to blue is also clearly visualized. (Part B also shown in colour on Plate 17.)

Known liver metastases were not distinctly visualized with octreotide scintigraphy in 12 of 24 patients. In all but two of these, a homogeneous distribution of radioactivity in the liver was observed. This is most probably because these liver metastases accumulated about as much radioactivity as does normal liver tissue. Subtraction techniques and/or SPECT studies might be useful in this respect, as an irregular distribution of radioactivity on the SPECT images was observed in several patients in whom planar images showed an even uptake of liver radioactivity.

Previously unsuspected extrahepatic localizations or sites not recognized with other imaging techniques were found in 20 of the 37 patients. In 3 of 11 patients who were thought to have been surgically cured, and in four of four patients who were suspected of having carcinoids, octreotide scintigraphy showed abnormal accumulation of radioactivity. Histological or radiological evidence that additional sites noticed on octreotide scintigrams did indeed represent tumour tissue has been obtained in 10 patients so far.

Unfortunately, our series included only two patients with a carcinoid of the appendix. Recurrence of these tumours after appendectomy has been reported to depend on the size of the tumour. In a long-term study of 150 patients with carcinoid tumours of the appendix, Moertel et al[29] found no metastases from tumours <2.0 cm in largest dimension, whereas metastases were observed from 3 of 14 lesions ≥ 2 cm and four of nine lesions ≥ 3 cm. The authors conclude that right hemicolectomy seems justified in young patients with tumours ≥ 2 cm who have a low risk of operative morbidity or mortality. Octreotide scintigraphy in these patients might provide useful additional information.

Visualization of extrahepatic carcinoid localizations did not depend on the site of the tumour or on the presence or absence of hormonal hypersecretion, as measured by urinary 5-HIAA and serum α-subunit concentrations.

Treatment with octreotide may cause a relief of symptoms and a decrease of urinary 5-HIAA levels in patients with the carcinoid syndrome.[30,31] In patients with the carcinoid syndrome, octreotide scintigraphy, because of its ability to demonstrate somatostatin receptor-positive tumours, could be used to select those patients who are likely to respond favourably to octreotide treatment.

MERKEL CELL TUMOURS

Trabecular carcinomas of the skin, or Merkel cell tumours, are aggressive neoplasms which tend to occur in the sun-exposed skin. These tumours metastasize and, despite therapy, disease-related death is high. Ultrastructurally and immunocytochemically, the majority of these tumours have neuroendocrine characteristics.

In four of five patients studied with octreotide scintigraphy in whom tumour had also been detected by CT and/or ultrasound, these sites were recognized on the scintigrams. In one patient, a tumour with a diameter less than 0.5 cm was missed with these techniques. In two of these five patients octreotide scintigraphy demonstrated more metastatic tumour localizations than previously recognized.[32]

Regional lymph node dissection and radiotherapy are generally not employed for Merkel cell tumours which have not disseminated. However, the metastatic potential of these carcinomas mandates that an early and accurate staging be made. From our data we conclude that octreotide scintigraphy has an equal or greater sensitivity for detecting Merkel cell tumours and their metastases than CT scanning and ultrasound. If octreotide scintigraphy were performed in patients with Merkel cell tumours, the sites of abnormal accumulation of radioactivity could thereafter be visualized using CT scanning or ultrasound, and biopsies be taken. Establishing the extent of the disease in this way may ensure an optimal choice of treatment for these tumours.

LUNG TUMOURS

[^{111}In-DTPA-D-Phe^1]octreotide scintigraphy revealed the primary tumour and its metastases (e.g. in the brain) in all of 34 patients with small-cell lung cancer (SCLC), whereas only the primary tumour could be visualized in all of 36 patients with non-SCLC. As somatostatin receptors are absent on most non-SCLC investigated thus far, their in vivo visualization is probably due to uptake of radioactivity by somatostatin receptor-positive tissue surrounding the tumour. This could be caused by infiltration of activated lymphocytes or a hyperplasia of neuroendocrine cells.

Because of the whole-body information it provides, octreotide scintigraphy may be useful as a staging technique in patients with proven SCLC. In particular, the early detection of brain metastases, present in several of our patients, may have therapeutic consequences, i.e. early brain irradiation. In cultured SCLC cells, treatment with somatostatin analogues results in a reduced growth, possibly as a consequence of a reduced secretion from these cells of autocrine growth factors.[33–35] If, in the future, treatment with somatostatin analogues is considered in patients with SCLC, octreotide scintigraphy could be used to select the patients with somatostatin receptor-positive tumours.

BREAST CANCER

As is clear from Table 66.1 the tumours can be visualized in about 70% of patients with breast cancer. Axillary lymph node metastases were identified in one-third of the patients with non-palpable axillary lymph node metastases. In 29% of patients with a somatostatin receptor-positive primary tumour who had undergone operations, a second octreotide scintigraphy detected recurrence of breast cancer 2–3 years after the primary operation. The majority of these patients were symptom-free.

MALIGNANT LYMPHOMAS

In the first 10 patients with Hodgkin's disease or non-Hodgkin's lymphoma, the lymphoma deposits were visualized with ^{111}In octreotide scintigraphy (Fig. 66.7).[36] In four patients, previously unrecognized additional tumour localizations were found. In four cases tissue biopsies were taken and confirmed by autoradiography to be somatostatin receptor positive. The role of ^{111}In octreotide scintigraphy in staging Hodgkin's disease and non-Hodgkin's lymphoma is presently being investigated in larger groups of patients.

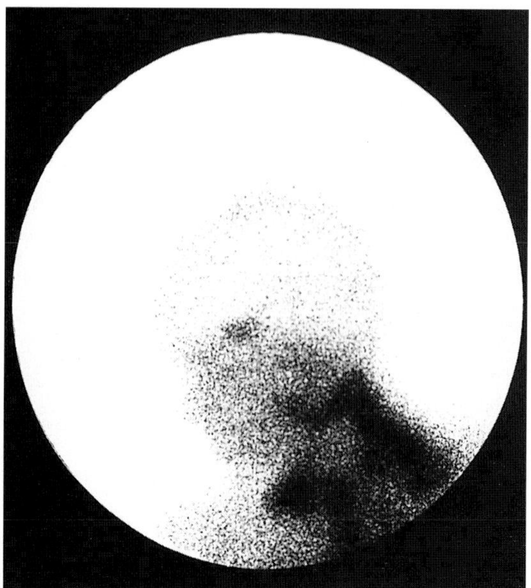

Fig. 66.7 Left lateral image of the head and neck of a patient with non-Hodgkin's lymphoma. Note the uptake in the pituitary. Also, there is substantial uptake of labelled octreotide in lymphoma deposits bilaterally in the neck.

GRANULOMATOUS DISEASES

In vivo somatostatin receptor imaging was positive in sarcoidosis and other granulomatous diseases, such as tuberculosis, Wegener's granulomatosis, DeQuervain's thyroiditis and aspergillosis. It is expected that octreotide scintigraphy may contribute to a more precise staging and a better evaluation of several of these granulomatous diseases. More importantly, it may be a sensitive indicator of the activity of sarcoidosis and of the efficacy of its therapy with corticosteroids.

GRAVES' DISEASE

The thyroid gland in untreated Graves' disease shows an increased accumulation of [^{111}In-DTPA-D-Phe^1]-octreotide. In most patients with Graves' disease who are treated with methimazole, the thyroidal uptake remains elevated. In patients who become hypothyroid after radioiodine treatment, there is no visible accumulation of radioactivity in the thyroid. In clinically active Graves' ophthalmopathy the orbits show accumulation of radioactivity 4 h and 24 h after injection of labelled octreotide. SPECT is needed for a proper interpretation of this orbital scintigraphy. The value of [^{111}In-DTPA-D-Phe^1]-octreotide scintigraphy in Graves' disease has yet to be established. Possibly this technique could select those patients with Graves' ophthalmopathy who might benefit from treatment with octreotide[37] and/or immunosuppressive agents.

SUMMARY

^{111}In octreotide scintigraphy is a simple and sensitive technique to demonstrate somatostatin receptor-positive localizations in the majority of patients with neuroendocrine tumours, and also in patients with lymphomas, granulomas or diseases in which activated lymphocytes play a role. Apart from its merit in tumour localization, in vivo somatostatin receptor imaging, as a result of its ability to demonstrate somatostatin receptor-positive tumours, can be used to select those patients with neuroendocrine tumours who are likely to respond favourably to octreotide treatment. This pertains to patients with endocrine pancreatic tumours, carcinoid syndrome and metastatic medullary thyroid carcinoma. Further, if treatment with octreotide were considered in patients with other somatostatin receptor tumours, such as SCLC and breast cancer, octreotide scintigraphy could also be used to identify patients with somatostatin receptor-positive tumours. In addition, octreotide scintigraphy may be used to monitor the efficacy of therapy. This may be of special interest in patients with autoimmune diseases.

Strong arguments in favour of [^{111}In-DTPA-D-Phe^1]-octreotide scintigraphy as a first localization technique, especially in neuroendocrine tumours, include both its harmless, non-invasive performance of whole-body scintigraphy and the ease of interpretation. Accordingly, it can be concluded that in many instances octreotide scintigraphy can replace invasive tumour localization methods such as angiography.

REFERENCES

1. Patel Y C, Amherdt M, Orci L 1982 Quantitative electron microscopic autoradiography of insulin, glucagon and somatostatin binding sites on islets. Science 217: 1155–1156
2. Reubi J C, Maurer R 1985 Autoradiographic mapping of somatostatin receptors in the rat CNS and pituitary. Neuroscience 15: 1183–1193
3. Lamberts S W J, Krenning E P, Reubi J-C 1991 The role of somatostatin and its analogs in the diagnosis and treatment of tumors. Endocrinol Rev 12: 450–482
4. Sreedharan S P, Kodama K T, Peterson K E, Goetzl E J 1989 Distinct subsets of somatostatin receptors on cultured human lymphocytes. J Biol Chem 264: 949–953
5. Reubi J C, Kvols L K, Waser B et al 1990 Detection of somatostatin receptors in surgical and percutaneous needle biopsy samples of carcinoids and islet cell carcinomas. Cancer Res 50: 5969–5977
6. Reubi J C, Lang W, Maurer R et al 1987 Distribution and biochemical characterization of somatostatin receptors in tumors of the human central nervous system. Cancer Res 47: 5758–5765
7. Reubi J C, Waser B, Foekens J A et al 1990 Somatostatin receptor incidence and distribution in breast cancer using receptor autoradiography: relationship to EGF-receptors. Int J Cancer 46: 416–420
8. Reubi J C, Waser B, Sheppard M, Macaulay V 1990 Somatostatin receptors are present in small-cell but not in non-small-cell primary lung carcinomas: relationship to EGF receptors. Int J Cancer 45: 269–274
9. Reubi J C, Waser B, vanHagen M et al 1992 In vitro and in vivo detection of somatostatin receptors in human malignant lymphomas. Int J Cancer 50: 895–900
10. Krenning E P, Bakker W H, Kooij P P M et al 1992 Somatostatin receptor scintigraphy with [^{111}In-DTPA-D-PHE^{1}]octreotide in man: metabolism, dosimetry and comparison with [^{123}I-Tyr-3]octreotide. J Nucl Med 33: 652–658
11. Reubi J C, Landolt A M 1989 The growth hormone responses to octreotide in acromegaly correlate with adenoma somatostatin receptor status. J Clin Endocrinol Metab 68: 844–850
12. Faglia G, Bazzoni N, Spada A et al 1991 In vivo detection of somatostatin receptors in patients with functionless pituitary adenomas by means of a radioiodinated analog of somatostatin ([^{123}I]SDZ 204-090). J Clin Endocrinol Metab 73: 850–856
13. Ur E, Mather S J, Bomanji J et al 1992 Pituitary imaging using a labelled somatostatin analogue in acromegaly. Clin Endocrinol 36: 147–150
14. de Bruin T W A, Kwekkeboom D J, Van't Verlaat J W et al 1992 Clinically nonfunctioning pituitary adenoma and octreotide response to long term high dose treatment, and studies in vitro. J Clin Endocrinol Metab 75: 1310–1371
15. Maton P M, O'Dorisio T M, Howe B A 1985 Effect of a long-acting somatostatin analogue (SMS 201-995) in patiens with pancreatic cholera. N Engl J Med 312: 17–21
16. Wood S M, Kraenzlin M E, Adrian T E, Bloom S R 1985 Treatment of patients with pancreatic endocrine tumours using a new long-acting somatostatin analogue SMS 201-995: symptomatic and peptide responses. Gut 26: 438–444
17. Moertel C G 1987 An odyssey in the land of small tumours. J Clin Oncol 5: 1503–1522
18. Lunderquist A 1989 Radiologic diagnosis of neuroendocrine tumors. Acta Oncol 28: 371–372
19. Doherty G M, Doppman J L, Shawker T H et al 1991 Results of a prospective strategy to diagnose, localize, and resect insulinomas. Surgery 110: 989–997
20. Rösch T, Lightdale C J, Botet J F et al 1991 Localization of pancreatic endocrine tumours by endoscopic ultrasonography. N Engl J Med 326: 1721–1726
21. Kwekkeboom D J, Van Urk H, Pauw K H et al 1993 Octreotide scintigraphy for the detection of paragangliomas. J Nucl Med 34: 873–878
22. Som P M, Sacher M, Stollman A L et al 1988 Common tumors of the parapharyngeal space: refined imaging diagnosis. Radiology 169: 81–85
23. Grufferman S, Gillman M W, Pasternak L R et al 1980 Familial carotid body tumors: case report and epidemiologic review. Cancer 46: 2116–2122
24. Kwekkeboom D J, Reubi J C, Lamberts S W J et al 1993 In vivo somatostatin receptor imaging in medullary thyroid carcinoma. J Clin Endocrinol Metab 76: 1413–1417
25. Saad M F, Fritsche Jr H A, Samaan N A 1984 Diagnostic and prognostic values of carcinoembryonic antigen in medullary carcinoma of the thyroid. J Clin Endocrinol Metab 58: 889–894
26. Mahler C, Verhelst J, De Longueville M, Harris A 1990 Long-term treatment of metastatic medullary thyroid carcinoma with the somatostatin analogue octreotide. Clin Endocrinol 33: 261–269
27. Modigliani E, Cohen R, Joannidis S et al 1992 Results of long-term continuous subcutaneous octreotide administration in 14 patients with medullary thyroid carcinoma. Clin Endocrinol 36: 183–186
28. Kwekkeboom D J, Krenning E P, Bakker W H et al 1993 Somatostatin analogue scintigraphy in carcinoid tumors. Eur J Nucl Med 20: 283–292
29. Moertel C G, Weiland L H, Nagorney D M, Dockerty M B 1987 Carcinoid tumor of the appendix: treatment and prognosis. N Eng J Med 317: 1699–1701
30. Kvols L K, Moertel C G, O'Connell M J et al 1986 Treatment of the malignant carcinoid syndrome. N Eng J Med 315: 663–666
31. Vinik A I, Tsai S T, Moattari A R et al 1986 Somatostatin analogue (SMS 201-995) in the management of gastroentero-pancreatic tumors and diarrhea syndromes. Am J Med 81 (suppl 6B): 23–40
32. Kwekkeboom D J, Hoff A M, Lamberts S W J et al 1992 Somatostatin analogue scintigraphy: a simple and sensitive method for the in vivo visualization of Merkel cell tumours and their metastases. Arch Dermatol 128: 818–821
33. Moody T W, Pert C B, Gazdar A F, Carney D N et al 1981 High levels of intracellular bombesin characterize human small-cell lung carcinoma. Science 214: 1246–1248
34. Cuttitta F, Carney D N, Mulshine J et al 1985 Bombesin-like peptides can function as autocrine growth factors in human small-cell lung cancer. Nature 316: 823–826
35. Macaulay V M, Everard M J, Teale J D et al 1990 Autocrine function for insulin-like growth factor I in human small cell lung cancer cell lines and fresh tumor cells. Cancer Res 50: 2511–2517
36. van Hagen P M, Krenning E P, Reubi J C et al 1993 Somatostatin analogue scintigraphy of malignant lymphomas. Br J Haematol 83: 75–79
37. Chang T C, Kao S C S, Huang K M 1992 Octreotide and Graves' ophthalmopathy and myxoedema. Br Med J 304: 158
38. Hoefnagel C A 1994 MIBG and somatostatin in oncology: role in the management of neural crest tumours. Eur J Nucl Med (in press)

67. Childhood neoplasia

C. A. Hoefnagel J. de Kraker

In recent years the contribution of nuclear medicine has been of increasing interest to paediatric oncology, in particular in imaging for diagnosis, staging and follow-up, in quantitative function analysis of organs at risk during oncological therapy, as well as in radionuclide therapy.

In tumour imaging the trend has been to use more or less specific tumour-seeking radiopharmaceuticals, which depict the tumour as a 'hotspot' on scintigraphy. A great number of these agents have become and are steadily becoming available, exploiting various metabolic and biological properties of individual tumours. Parallel to these developments radionuclide therapy becomes more widely used, whenever its success is envisaged on the basis of a good and selective uptake and long retention of the radiopharmaceutical in the tumour. Table 67.1 shows a list of currently available tumour-seeking radiopharmaceuticals which are applicable in paediatric oncology. Adequate tumour imaging in children requires special considerations regarding the performance of the procedure and the attitude of the attending staff.[1]

^{67}Ga citrate has been used for many years in the detection of lymphoma, more recently also for the staging, follow-up and early recognition of response to chemotherapy or radiotherapy[2] (Ch. 62).

^{201}Tl chloride scintigraphy, in conjunction with thyroglobulin assays in serum, has become a reliable alternative to the use of ^{131}I iodide in the follow-up of differentiated thyroid carcinoma, particularly as the procedure and radiation dose to the child compares favourably with that of ^{131}I.[3] ^{131}I maintains its role in radionuclide therapy of thyroid carcinoma and the selection of patients for this treatment. Both ^{67}Ga citrate and ^{201}Tl chloride, being non-specific tumour-seeking tracers, may also be used in other tumours.[4,5] (Ch. 63).

In differentiated osteosarcoma ^{99m}Tc diphosphonate may, as a result of the targeting of the tumour-produced osteoid, visualize not only the primary bone tumour and its skeletal metastases, but also the extra osseous metastases (Ch. 80).[6,7] For therapy of skeletal lesions beta-emitting bone-seeking agents, such as ^{89}Sr chloride, ^{186}Re-HEDP and ^{153}Sm-EDTMP, are available.

Table 67.1 Tumour-seeking radiopharmaceuticals and their indications in paediatric oncology

	Radiopharmaceutical	Indication
Imaging	^{67}Ga citrate	Lymphoma
	^{201}Tl chloride	Differentiated thyroid carcinoma
		Osteosarcoma,
		Brain tumours
	^{99m}Tc diphosphonate	Osteosarcoma
	^{99m}Tc pentavalent DMSA	Medullary thyroid carcinoma (MEN 2 syndromes)
	^{123}I/^{131}I-MIBG	Neuroblastoma, phaeochromocytoma, ganglioneuroma
	^{111}In pentetreotide	Neuroendocrine tumours, lymphoma
	^{99m}Tc-HIDA derivatives	Hepatoblastoma
	^{111}In anti-myosin Fab	Rhabdomyosarcoma
Therapy	^{131}I iodide	Differentiated thyroid carcinoma
	^{131}I-MIBG	Neuroblastoma
	^{125}I-MIBG	Neuroblastoma
	^{131}I-3F8 antibodies	Neuroblastoma
	^{131}I Rose Bengal	Hepatoblastoma
	^{131}I anti-ferritin	Hepatoblastoma
	^{89}Sr chloride	Osteosarcoma

When children are involved in the family screening of MEN 2 syndromes, a variety of tracers can be used to demonstrate medullary thyroid carcinoma: ^{201}Tl chloride, ^{99m}Tc pentavalent DMSA, ^{123}I-MIBG, ^{131}I-MIBG, ^{111}In pentetreotide and ^{131}I-labelled anti-CEA and anti-calcitonin antibodies (Ch. 57).

^{123}I/^{131}I metaiodobenzylguanidine (MIBG) has established its role in the diagnosis, staging and follow-up of neuroblastoma and other neural crest tumours,[8] and both ^{131}I-MIBG and ^{125}I-MIBG are used for the treatment of this condition (Ch. 74).

The somatostatin analogue ^{111}In pentatreotide may also be used for diagnostic scintigraphy of neuroendocrine tumours and lymphoma.[9]

Scintigraphy using hepatobiliary agents, such as ^{99m}Tc-

HIDA derivatives, may demonstrate uptake in hepatoblastoma, and by the same mechanism therapy, using ^{131}I Rose Bengal is feasible.[10]

Radiolabelled antibodies are also used in paediatric oncology: examples are radioimmunoscintigraphy using ^{111}In anti-myosin Fab fragments in rhabdomyosarcoma,[11] therapy of hepatic malignancies with ^{131}I anti-ferritin antibodies,[12] which might be used for hepatoblastoma, and the use of radiolabelled 3F8, UJ13A and BW575/9 antibodies in the diagnosis and therapy of neuroblastoma.[13]

This chapter will focus on the use of specific radionuclide tracers in diagnostic scintigraphy of neuroblastoma, hepatoblastoma and rhabdomyosarcoma.

NEUROBLASTOMA

The disease

Neuroblastoma is a malignant tumour of the sympathetic nervous system, occurring most frequently in early childhood. The incidence in US children has been reported to be around 5 per million population per year, with a slight preponderance of males and whites. In white and black children it is respectively the second and third most frequent solid tumour after CNS and Wilms' tumours.[14] 50% of neuroblastoma patients are younger than 2 years, 75% are younger than 4 and the disease is rare after the age of 14.

The tumour is of neural crest origin: the cells which form the sympathetic nervous system, called sympathogonia, migrate from the neural crest to the adrenal medulla, the paraganglion of Zuckerkandl and a large number of paraganglia retroperitoneally along the aorta down into the pelvis. The pluripotential sympathogonia differentiate into ganglion cells, neurofibrous and chromaffin cells, and tumours arising from these cells can be classified as neuroblastoma (sympathicoblastoma), ganglioneuroma, neurofibroma and phaeochromocytoma respectively. Because of this development neuroblastoma has the potential ability to mature into ganglioneuroma, ganglioma and phaeochromocytoma.[15]

On microscopy neuroblastomas may present as highly cellular tumours with undifferentiated sympathogonia and mitoses, or, as they become more differentiated, as groups of cells organized in rosettes and as ganglion cells with nerve fibres or immature chromaffin cells respectively. Electron microscopy reveals the characteristic ultrastructural features of neurotubules and neurosecretory granules in the cytoplasm. Chromaffin cells stain dark upon exposure to dichromate salts as a result of an oxidation process of the intracellular catecholamine stores.

The site of the primary tumour varies: 70% of all tumours originate in the retroperitoneal region, including around 30% in the adrenal gland and 10% in the abdominal sympathetic side chain, and 8% occur in the cervical, 17% in the thoracic and 5% in the pelvic sympathetic side chain. This is in contrast with the distribution of phaeochromocytoma, of which extra-adrenal occurrence is reported in only 10% of adults and 25% of children with this tumour.

Metastases may be found in two patterns: diffuse metastases in the liver (Pepper type), are seen in the youngest patients with stage IVs disease and may be accompanied by subcutaneous metastatic nodules, or metastases to the regional lymph nodes, bone, bone marrow and soft tissues (Hutchison type). Other organs, such as brain, heart and lungs, are rarely affected.

The symptomatology of this disease depends on the site and size of the primary tumour and its metastases and on the excessive production and excretion of catecholamines.

More than 90% of neuroblastomas produce the catecholamines dopamine, noradrenaline and noradrenaline in excess; these products and their metabolites can be monitored in serum and urine. The degree of malignancy and the prognosis are correlated with the pattern and rate of excretion. Other tumour markers for neuroblastoma are neuron-specific enolase (NSE), ferritin and gangliosides G_{D2}, which can all be determined in serum.[16]

Prognostic factors in the treatment of neuroblastoma are the stage of disease, the patient's age, the site of the primary tumour, the pattern and rate of catecholamine excretion, the serum ferritin level at diagnosis, the tumour histology and the amplification of the N-*myc* oncogene.[17]

Staging and therapy

Accurate staging of disease is essential for the prognosis and the choice of treatment. According to the 1985 UICC TNM description,[18] five stages of neuroblastoma can be distinguished. The staging criteria of Evans[19] are also frequently used. In an attempt to standardize the staging, the International Neuroblastoma Staging System (INSS) was formulated.

For staging and follow-up, a number of diagnostic procedures are used. Plain radiographs of the thorax and abdomen may show the primary tumour by the finding of calcifications. Intravenous pyelography may show displacement of the kidney and ureter. Ultrasonography is a most informative, non-invasive and inexpensive method of visualizing paediatric tumours and monitoring tumour size during treatment. Computerized tomography (CT) and magnetic resonance imaging (MRI) are more invasive techniques for young children, but provide better anatomical detail and information about the tumour's attachment to surrounding tissue. This is essential for the determination of resectability/operability. Myelography should be performed when intraspinal extension of the tumour is suspected. Bone scintigraphy, using ^{99m}Tc diphosphonates has always been the most sensitive technique to

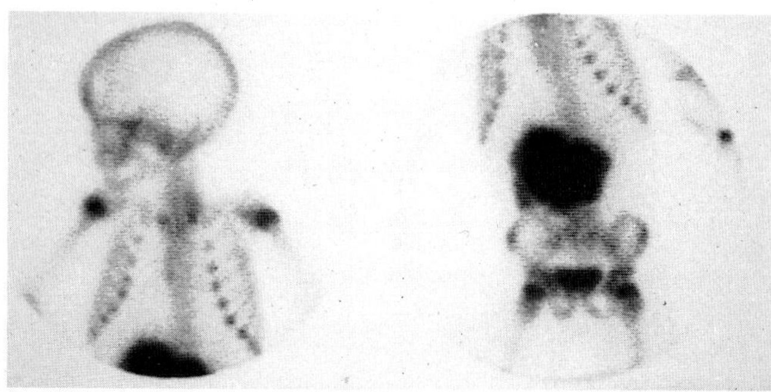

Fig. 67.1 Intense accumulation of ^{99m}Tc-MDP in the primary neuroblastoma on the bone scintigram.

detect skeletal metastases, although in children discrete lesions near the epiphyses may be more difficult to interpret, and its findings lack the specificity of ^{131}I-MIBG scintigraphy. Occasionally also the primary tumour may be visualized on the bone scintigram (Fig. 67.1). Bone marrow aspiration, together with ^{131}I-MIBG scintigraphy remains the most reliable proof of bone marrow infiltration, especially if multiple samples are taken by trephine and immunohistochemical staining techniques are applied.[20]

The choice of treatment and the prognosis of neuroblastoma depends on the stage of disease: localized disease without distant metastases (TNM stages I and II) is treated by complete surgical excision and has a good prognosis (2-year survival rates of 90%). Lymph node metastases and spread to other organs (TNM stages III–V) are correlated with a poor prognosis and is treated by combination chemotherapy preceding surgery for the primary tumour; this is followed by post-operative chemotherapy, sometimes including high-dose chemotherapy requiring allogenic or autologous bone marrow transplantation. Radiation therapy may be added to these regimens. New approaches to diagnosis and therapy of neuroblastoma include targeting of radionuclides via the immunological (monoclonal antibodies) and metabolic (MIBG) route.

^{131}I-MIBG scintigraphy

After the initial studies at the University of Michigan demonstrated a strong affinity of ^{131}I metaiodobenzylguanidine (^{131}I-MIBG) for the adrenal medulla and adrenergic nerve tissue, the successful scintigraphic localization of phaeochromocytoma with this agent was reported.[21] It was expected, therefore, that other tumours that are derived from the neural crest, and that may present the characteristic features of an active uptake-1 mechanism at the cell membrane and storage granules in the cytoplasm, responsible for the uptake and retention of ^{131}I-MIBG respectively, could also be detected in this way. After initial reports of ^{131}I-MIBG uptake in neuroblastoma[22,23] successful use of this tracer in a small series of patients was described.[24–26]

Table 67.2 Results of ^{131}I-MIBG diagnostic scintigraphy in neuroblastoma patients

	Positive scintigram	Negative scintigram	Total
Neuroblastoma +	129	5	134
Neuroblastoma –	0	16	16
Total	129 (96%)	21	150
Tumour localization			
Thoracic/abdominal tumour			
Primary tumour		54	
Tumour residue		19	
Local recurrence		12	
Metastases:			
Bone		75	
Bone marrow		44	
Lymph nodes		24	
Liver		8	
Lung/pleura		5	
Soft tissue		5	
Scrotum		1	

In general 18.5 MBq (0.5 mCi) of ^{131}I-MIBG is administered by slow intravenous injection and scintigraphy of the whole body is performed after 24, 48 and 72 h, using a gamma-camera with a high-energy collimator and set for the 364 keV photon energy peak. Delayed imaging may be done up to a week after administration.

As the number of patients imaged with ^{131}I-MIBG grew, the unique role of this technique in the management of neuroblastoma emerged. At The Netherlands Cancer Institute 745 scintigraphic studies using ^{131}I-MIBG have been done in 150 patients (143 children) with neuroblastoma between 1984 and 1993. Table 67.2 shows the results and the location of the primary tumours, recurrences and metastases which were correctly identified by ^{131}I-MIBG scintigraphy. 16 patients who were in a complete remission at the time of scintigraphy showed no pathological concentration of ^{131}I-MIBG, but merely the normal uptake in the salivary glands, myocardium, liver, gut and bladder (Fig. 67.2). The ^{131}I-MIBG scintigram was positive in 129 of 134 patients with manifest disease (96%), detecting multiple tumour sites regardless of the location (Fig. 67.2). Among these patients were 10 with a normal urinary excretion of catecholamine metabolites and nine patients with negative bone marrow aspirations, in whom ^{131}I-MIBG scintigraphy revealed bone marrow infiltration, which was subsequently confirmed (Fig. 67.3). Tumour concentration of ^{131}I-MIBG ranged from 0.05 to 27.8% of dose, and the calculated effective half-life was 2.6–8.0 days. There were false-negative results in four adults and one child with neuroblastoma, all of whom had normal catecholamine levels in urine, which raises the question of whether these neuroblastomas are truly tumours of the

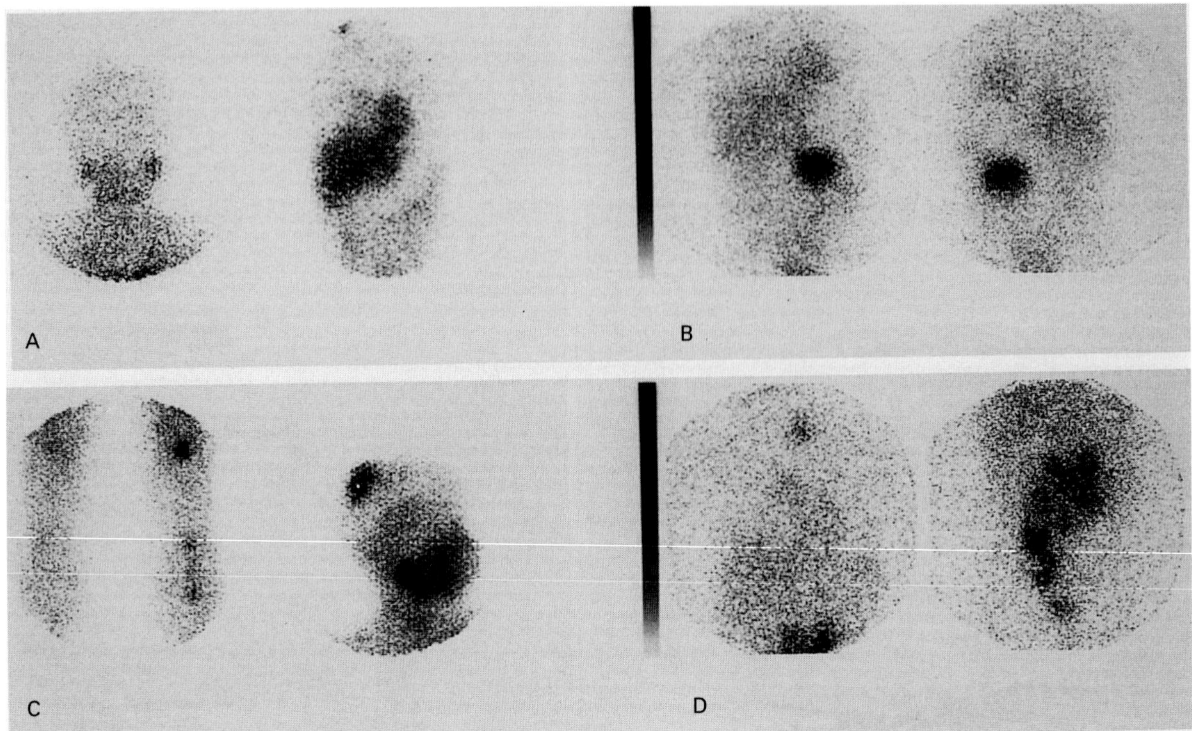

Fig. 67.2 Compilation of scintigraphic appearances of neuroblastoma. (a) Normal distribution of ^{131}I-MIBG showing uptake in the salivary glands, myocardium, liver and bowel. (b) ^{131}I-MIBG concentration in a primary tumour with decreased uptake in heart and liver. (c) Skeletal metastases in the skull, femora and left tibia. (d) Multiple metastases in abdominal lymph nodes.

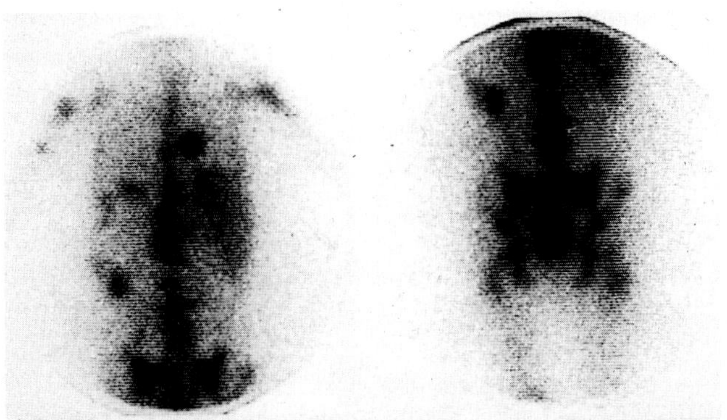

Fig. 67.3 Intense concentration of ^{131}I-MIBG throughout the bone marrow, indicating diffuse bone marrow invasion by neuroblastoma; although four consecutive bone marrow aspirates were negative for tumour, the involvement was confirmed when bone marrow was harvested for transplant.

sympathetic nervous tissue. It is not possible to differentiate between neuroblastomas of different nervous tissues on morphologic criteria. Consistent with the observation of rapid ^{131}I-MIBG clearance from the heart in phaeochromocytoma,[27] an inverse relationship between myocardial and tumour activities was found in neuroblastoma patients (Fig. 67.2).[8]

The cumulative findings of ^{131}I-MIBG scintigraphy in this institute and in major series reported in the world literature (Table 67.3), involving 776 patients,[28–41] indicate

Table 67.3 ^{131}I-MIBG scintigraphy in neuroblastoma: cumulative sensitivities, reported in the literature

Centre	Year	No. of patients	Sensitivity (%)	Specificity (%)	Reference
NKI, Amsterdam	1993	150	96.3	100	–
Scandinavia	1989	71	94.0	88	28
Villejuif	1987	69	76.6	100	29
Gemelli Rome	1990	43	92.0	100	30
MSK New York	1986	38	87.5	100	31
University of Michigan	1986	34	94.1	–	32
Other centres (26)	1989	370	90.6	99	33–41

Total: 776 patients, cumulative sensitivity 91.5%.

that 91.5% of neuroblastomas concentrate ^{131}I-MIBG, making ^{131}I-MIBG scintigraphy and urinalysis for catecholamine metabolites the most sensitive and highly specific indicators of neuroblastoma. This has the following clinical implications:

1. The uptake of ^{131}I-MIBG is so tissue specific that in a child presenting with a tumour of unknown origin ^{131}I-MIBG scintigraphy can non-invasively establish the diagnosis of neuroblastoma and rule out differential diagnoses such as Wilms' tumour, Ewing's sarcoma, rhabdomyosarcoma, osteosarcoma and malignant lymphoma (Fig. 67.4).

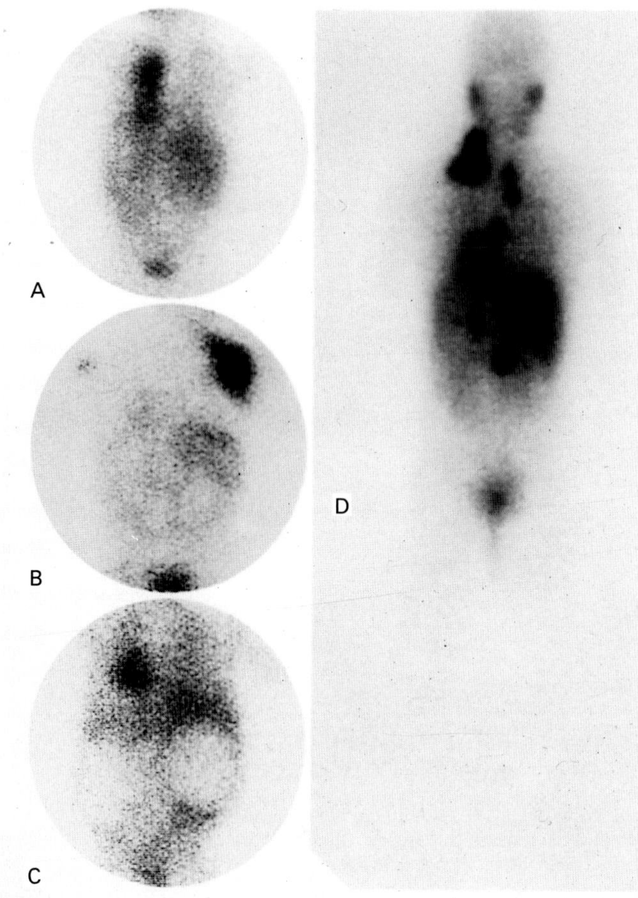

Fig. 67.4 Pathology in vivo: ^{131}I-MIBG scintigraphy non-invasively establishes the diagnosis of neuroblastoma in children presenting with (A) an unknown tumour in the chest, (B) a bone tumour of the right scapula thought to be Ewing's sarcoma and (C) a lymphoma in the neck. (D) In contrast, bilateral Wilms' tumours show no ^{131}I-MIBG uptake at all (c).

2. The enchanced detection of metastases anywhere in the body in a single procedure influences the staging of disease, frequently by upgrading the stage (Fig. 67.5).
3. The findings of post-operative or post-chemotherapy ^{131}I-MIBG scintigraphy should be included in the criteria of response (Figs 67.6 and 67.7).
4. The good concentration and the relatively long biological half-life of ^{131}I-MIBG at tumour sites in comparison with normal tissues enable therapy with this radiopharmaceutical; in analogy with the use of ^{131}I in thyroid cancer, ^{131}I-MIBG tracer studies can reveal which patients might benefit from this form of treatment.

Few comparative studies of MIBG scintigraphy and other nuclear medicine imaging techniques for neuroblastoma have been reported. Hibi et al[39] comparing ^{131}I-MIBG, ^{67}Ga citrate and ^{99m}Tc-HMDP in the detection of primary tumours and metastases before treatment, preoperatively after chemotherapy and post-operatively, found ^{131}I-MIBG scintigraphy to be the most sensitive and most specific procedure, although in one case a MIBG-negative bone metastasis was found to be positive on bone scintigraphy. In other studies[25,29,33,38–41] discrepant findings of MIBG and bone scintigrams have also been described, favouring either the former or of the latter technique. As a positive finding on an MIBG scintigram is a more specific one, certainly for bone lesions located near the epiphyses of long bones,[42] most authors favour the initial use of ^{131}I-MIBG scintigraphy, bearing in mind that complementary bone scintigraphy may be indicated (Fig. 67.8).

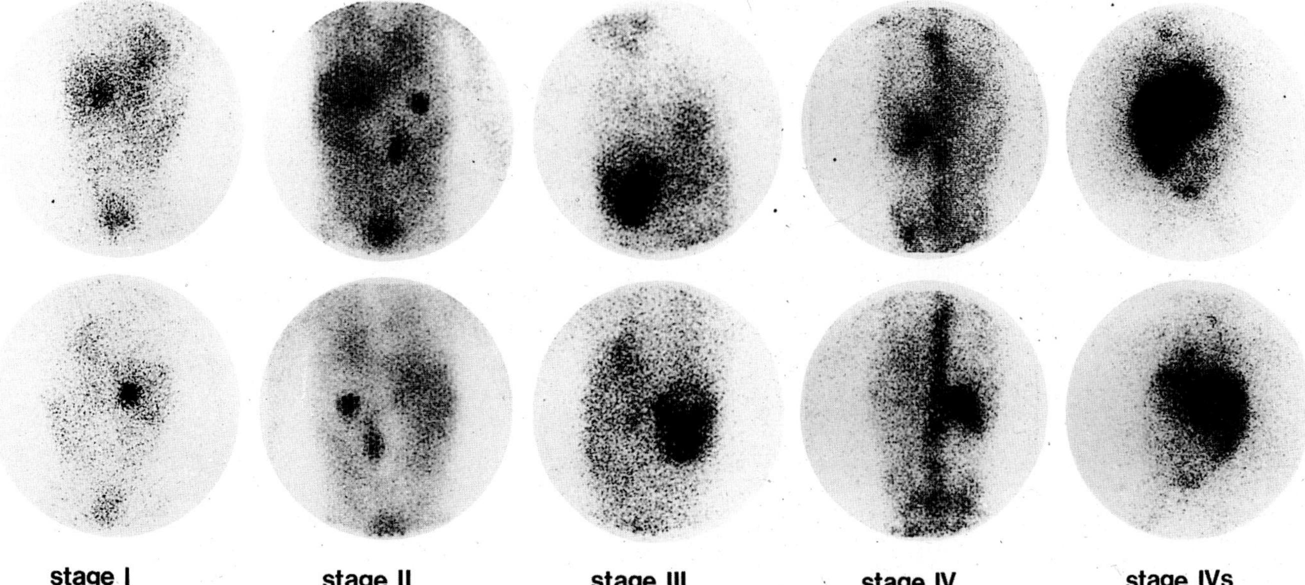

Fig. 67.5 Portrayal of the stages of neuroblastoma (according to Evans' criteria[19]) on ^{131}I-MIBG scintigrams: anterior view (top) and posterior view (below) images.

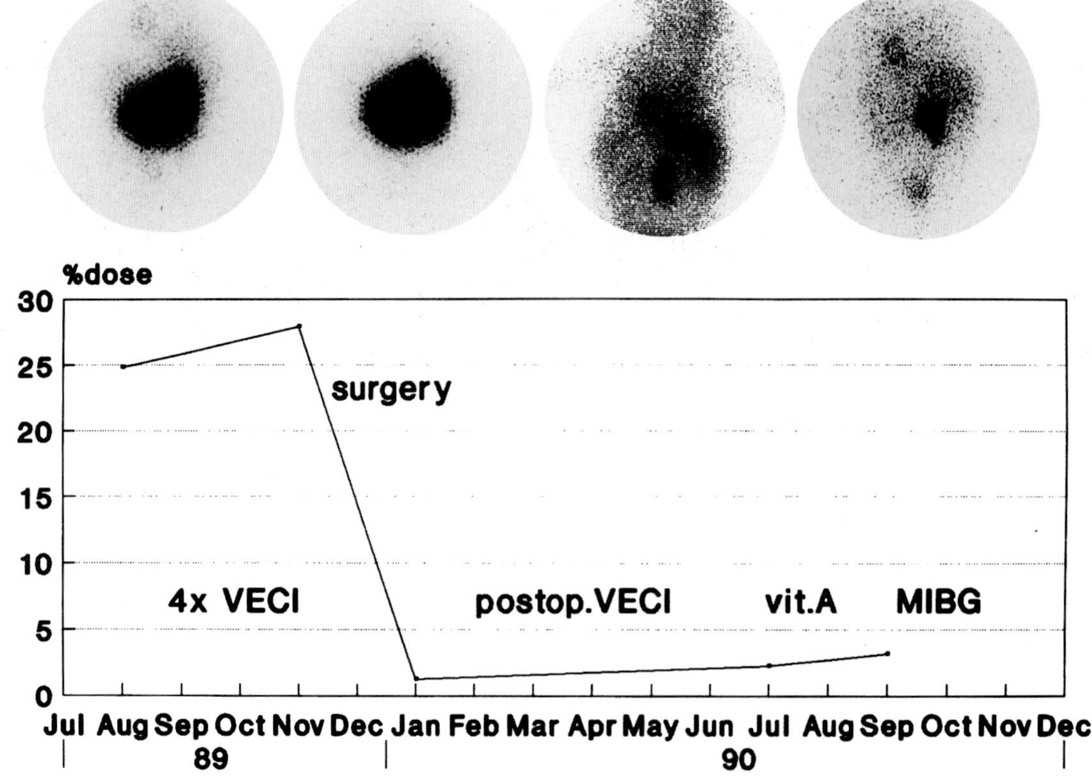

Fig. 67.6 Follow-up scintigraphy using ^{131}I-MIBG in a 1-year-old girl with a 12 × 12 × 10 cm neuroblastoma in the abdomen concentrating 24.8% of the administered dose. During preoperative chemotherapy the uptake increases; after surgery a tumour residue with 1.3% dose uptake persists, gradually increasing during post-operative chemotherapy.

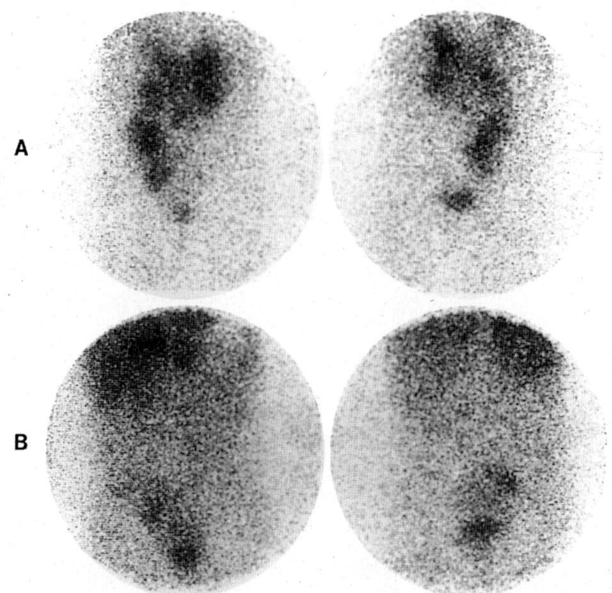

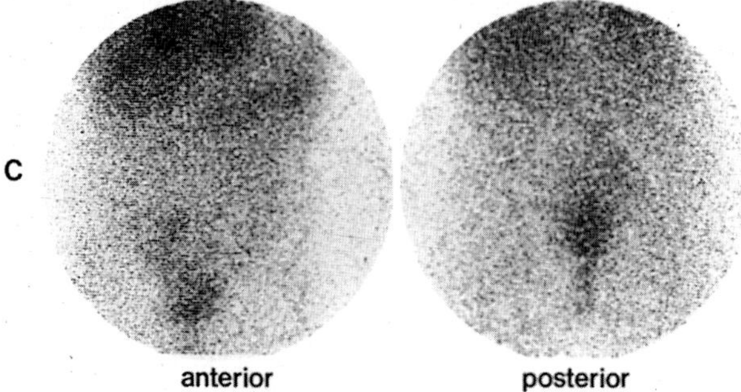

Fig. 67.7 ^{131}I-MIBG scintigraphic confirmation of response. This 10-year-old girl underwent treatment for multiple abdominal localizations of neuroblastoma (A). After chemotherapy and surgery all parameters were negative, indicating a complete remission; the ^{131}I-MIBG scintigram, however, revealed a tumour residue in the right lower abdomen (B). A further laparotomy was performed and a nodule of viable tumour, measuring 1 cm in diameter, was removed. The patient was then truly in complete remission and continues to be 7 years later (C).

^{123}I-MIBG scintigraphy

More recently ^{123}I-MIBG has also been used for diagnostic scintigraphy of phaeochromocytoma[43] and neuroblastoma. 111–185 MBq (3–5 mCi) is usually administered to children and scintigraphy can be performed as early as 4–24 h after injection. Owing to the relatively short physical half-life (13.2 h) and the lack of beta-particles, the radiation dose per MBq to the patient is lower than with ^{131}I. However, this benefit is given up by administering a higher dose. A clear advantage, however, is the greater photon flux with a photon energy peak of 159 keV, which better meets the characteristics of the most widely available equipment and enables images of superior quality as well

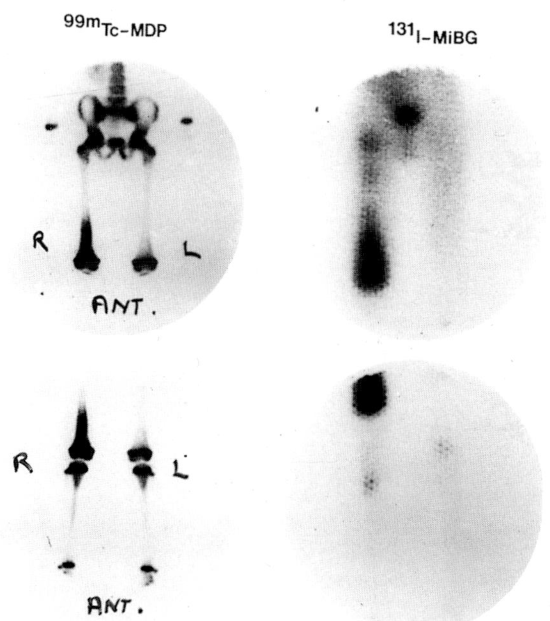

Fig. 67.8 Comparison of bone scintigraphy and ^{131}I-MIBG scintigraphy in a 4-year-old boy with skeletal metastases from neuroblastoma: the bone scintigram (left) shows a solitary lesion in the distal right femur; the ^{131}I-MIBG scintigram (right) provides a better assessment of the extension of the skeletal metastases in the right femur and shows additional lesions near the epiphyses, which are difficult to distinguish on the bone scintigram. (Reproduced with permission from Voûte et al.[15])

as single photon emission tomography. Nevertheless, using the appropriate dose of ^{131}I-MIBG and 364 keV photon energy peak, optimal images can be obtained.

When comparing ^{123}I- and ^{131}I-MIBG scintigrams it should be remembered that the optimal intervals between administration of these radiopharmaceuticals and scintigraphy differ, and that these images may therefore reflect a different distribution of the tracer. Delayed imaging for additional diagnostic information and dosimetry requires the use of ^{131}I-MIBG. A comparative study using both ^{123}I-MIBG and ^{131}I-MIBG in 37 neuroblastoma patients demonstrated that both tests were equally sensitive, but that, in general, the image quality was slightly better when ^{123}I-MIBG was used.[44] Although it never occurred that scintigraphy with one tracer was positive and negative with the other, the number of lesions detected was discrepant in 11 of 48 comparative studies: six times in favour of ^{123}I-MIBG and five times in favour of ^{131}I-MIBG. Figure 67.9 demonstrates the good image quality which can be obtained using ^{123}I-MIBG.

Precautions with MIBG scintigraphy

As the majority of neuroblastoma patients are young children, several precautions must be taken to ensure that scintigraphy is successful, safe and patient friendly. This means adequate explanation of the procedure to child and parents, dose adjustment and use of paediatric needles.

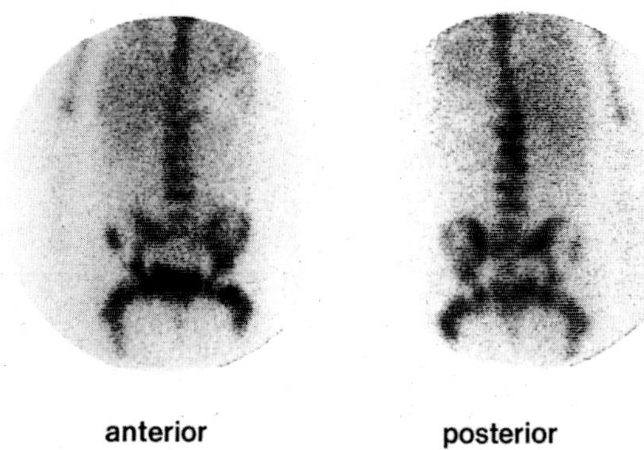

Fig. 67.9 Scintigrams using ^{123}I-MIBG showing diffuse bone marrow involvement of neuroblastoma with improved resolution.

Throughout the imaging period the child should be immobilized and kept amused, e.g. by video films or stories. If possible, the gamma-camera is positioned under rather than above the patient. It is important to complete the most essential images first. If these conditions are provided, sedation of the patient is hardly ever required. Potassium iodide (100 mg) must be administered orally for 5 or 2 days, starting on the day before the administration of ^{131}I-MIBG or ^{123}I-MIBG respectively, in order to block the thyroid for circulating free radioactive iodine.

A great number of drugs are known or may be expected to interfere with the uptake and/or retention of ^{131}I-MIBG[45] (Ch. 64). Although not frequently used in children with neuroblastoma, these drugs are to be avoided, or discontinued 2 weeks prior to scintigraphy.

Pitfalls in MIBG interpretation

As MIBG is normally concentrated in the myocardium and the liver, and as there may be scintigraphic evidence of bladder and bowel activity due to renal and biliary excretion of the tracer, the detection of recurrent or metastatic neuroblastoma in the vicinity of these structures may at times be difficult. Single photon emission tomography may assist in the detection and accurate localization of these tumours (Fig. 67.10).[46] Subtraction imaging may also be helpful in this respect (e.g. using ^{99m}Tc colloid to subtract liver and spleen, ^{99m}Tc-DMSA to subtract renal parenchyma and ^{99m}Tc-DTPA to subtract kidneys and bladder activity).

Other pitfalls in the interpretation of MIBG scintigrams may be increased activity in a hyperplastic residual adrenal gland after contralateral adrenalectomy, accumulation of activity in the renal pelvis in case of hydronephrosis, urine contamination on the skin or in clothes or nappies, residual activity in the reservoir of an implanted i.v. administration system or uptake in the thyroid when it has not been blocked adequately. Although a pathological lesion taking up ^{131}I-MIBG in a child is most likely to be

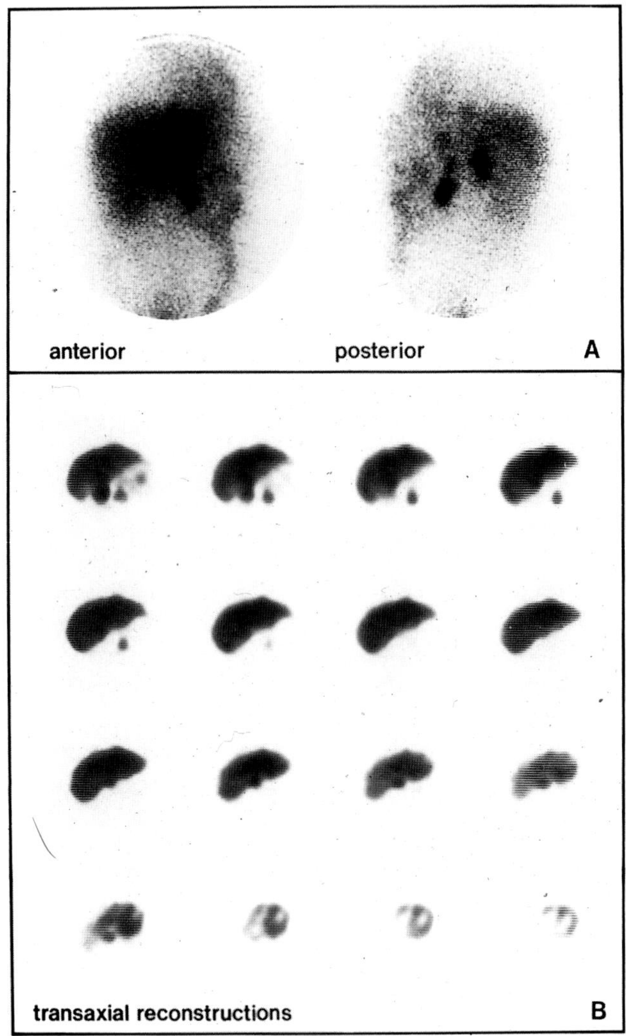

Fig. 67.10 Single photon emission tomography 72 h after a therapeutic dose of ^{131}I-MIBG. (A) Planar anterior and posterior view images showing multiple tumour localization behind and below the liver. (B) Transaxial reconstructions. (Reproduced with permission from Hoefnagel et al.[46])

neuroblastoma, other benign and malignant tumours, such as ganglioneuroma, phaeochromocytoma, paraganglioma, retinoblastoma and medullary thyroid carcinoma, must also be considered.

Octreotide

The somatostatin analogue octreotide, labelled with ^{123}I or ^{111}In, has been reported to be a successful imaging agent for the detection of neuroendocrine tumours and lymphoma by its binding to the somatostatin receptors[9] (Ch. 66) and has also been used in small numbers of neuroblastoma patients: scintigraphy was positive in eight of nine cases of neuroblastoma (E P Krenning, personal communication). Figure 67.11 shows an example of a neuroblastoma imaged with ^{111}In pentatreotide.

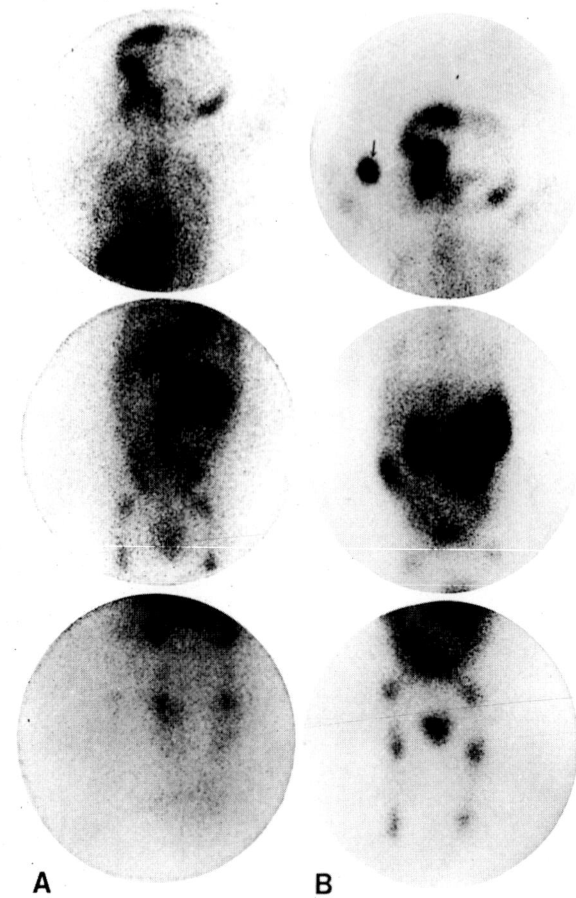

Fig. 67.11 Scintigraphy using ^{123}I-MIBG (A) and ^{111}In-pentetreotide (B) in a child with neuroblastoma in the left abdomen metastatic to the bone and bone marrow. Although the lesions in the extremities are shown better by the somatostatin analogue, the normal accumulation in the kidneys and liver obscures the primary tumour. (Courtesy of EP Krenning.)

Antibodies

Radioimmunoscintigraphy has also been used in children with neuroblastoma. Originally immunolocalization using the ^{131}I-labelled monoclonal antibody UJ13A was reported[47] and, after Cheung et al[48] had described the anti-GP_{D2} ganglioside monoclonal antibody 3F8, neuroblastoma was successfully imaged with ^{131}I-3F8 as well.[49] A comparative study of ^{131}I-labelled 3F8 antibodies and ^{131}I-MIBG in 41 patients with neuroblastoma demonstrated both studies to be abnormal in 27 patients, but ^{131}I-3F8 detected more lesions.[50] In addition, there were three abnormal radioimmunoscintigrams in patients with normal ^{131}I-MIBG, but the administered dosage of ^{131}I differed considerably in favour of the antibody. Both ^{131}I-UJ13A and ^{131}I-3F8 antibodies have been used in therapy trials of neuroblastoma patients.[131] Smolarz et al[51] used ^{99m}Tc-labelled BW575 monoclonal antibody fragments to image neuroblastoma, and Bihl & Matzku[52] reported comparative measurements of ^{125}I-BW575/9 and ^{131}I-MIBG in neuroblastoma xenografts.

HEPATOBLASTOMA

The disease

Hepatoblastoma is a rare tumour in infancy and childhood, accounting for less than 2% of all malignant tumours in this age group.[53] On microscopy the tumour contains mesenchymal elements and vascular lakes, which are characteristic, and immature or abortive forms of bile ducts are often found. The clinical course and prognosis largely depend on the resectability of the tumour. If unresectable, tumours may be made operable by pretreatment with chemotherapy and/or radiotherapy. However, drawbacks of external beam radiotherapy are the damage to normal liver tissue and impairment of growth of the surrounding structures in young children. Radiation may be delivered more specifically and at higher doses to the tumour by targeting radionuclides at the tumour cells, either via the immunological (anti-ferritin antibodies) or via the metabolic (hepatobiliary agents) route.

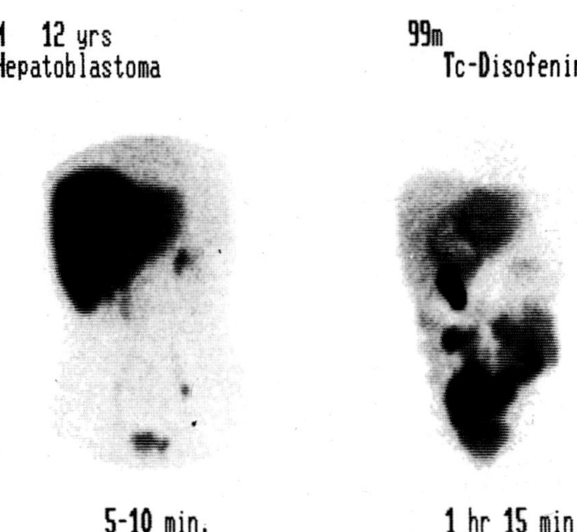

Fig. 67.12 Hepatobiliary scintigraphy using ^{99m}Tc disofenin in a 12-year-old boy with hepatoblastoma. At 5–10 min most of the radiopharmaceutical is located in the hepatocytes; an hour later hepatobiliary excretion into the bowel has taken place, but some of the activity is trapped in the tumour localizations. (Reproduced with permission from De Kraker et al.[10])

Hepatobiliary agents

After observations of hepatobiliary tracers being taken up by hepatoma and hepatocellular carcinoma in adults,[54–56] diagnostic scintigraphy using ^{99m}Tc-IDA, ^{99m}Tc-PIPIDA and ^{99m}Tc disofenin was applied in children with hepatoblastoma.[57–59] Ohshiro et al[60] describe tumour uptake of ^{99m}Tc *N*-pyridoxyl-5-methyltryptophan (PMT) in a boy with hepatoblastoma. The hypothesis for the targeting mechanism is that hepatobiliary agents are metabolically taken up in hepatocytes and hepatoblastoma cells and that, because of the abnormal and non-communicating bile ducts in the tumour, delayed excretion from the tumour in comparison with normal liver tissue will occur. De Kraker et al[10] demonstrated specific uptake and retention of ^{99m}Tc disofenin in two of six cases of hepatoblastoma (Fig. 67.12), and reported the therapeutic use of ^{131}I Rose Bengal in a 5-month-old boy with hepatoblastoma showing a tumour uptake of 21.6% of dose at 24 h and a long retention. This radiopharmaceutical, which was used in the past for the detection of biliary atresia in newborns, is not associated with the limiting side-effects of radiolabelled antibodies and may yield considerably higher tumour concentrations.

RHABDOMYOSARCOMA

Rhabdomyosarcoma (RMS) is a tumour arising from primitive mesenchymal tissue that mimics normal striated muscle.[61] Pathologically the tumour is thought to develop from primitive rhabdomyoblasts or pluripotential mesenchymal cells. It is the most common soft-tissue sarcoma in children, representing approximately 10% of all paediatric tumours. There are two peaks in the incidence, one at the age of 2–6 years and a second one at the age of 18 years.[62]

The primary tumour site may be located in the head and neck region, the pelvis, the orbit and the limbs. Metastases to regional lymph nodes are common. Haematogenous metastatic sites are the lungs, bone and bone marrow. 10% of the patients already have metastases at the time of presentation.

Reliable techniques to exclude metastases are essential for the planning of surgical management of this disease, and, in view of the improved survival rates, for the early detection of recurrence and metastases during follow-up. Bone scintigraphy is regarded useful for the detection of RMS skeletal metastases.[63] Weinblatt & Miller[64] reported a sensitivity of 76% and an 85% specificity in their series of 46 cases. Soft-tissue sarcomas may also be imaged with ^{67}Ga citrate[65] and ^{201}Tl chloride,[66] but these tumour-seeking radiopharmaceuticals are not specific for RMS. However, Cogswell et al[67] found that ^{67}Ga scans detected the primary RMS tumour in 25/29 (86%) children. They noted that bone scans were more sensitive than ^{67}Ga for the detection of skeletal metastases with sensitivities of 100% and 87% respectively. ^{67}Ga was, however, far superior in identifying soft-tissue metastases if the primary was gallium avid, the sensitivity being 84%.

The pathological diagnosis of RMS relies upon the immunohistochemical demonstration of myosin and myoglobin in the tumour tissue.[68] Anti-myosin monoclonal antibodies or fragments labelled with ^{111}In are successfully used for the detection of myocardial disease, such as infarction,[69] myocarditis,[70] heterologous cardiac transplant rejection[71] and anthracycline cardiotoxicity.[72] These antibodies may provide a specific tool for the scintigraphic detection of myosin-containing tumours, assuming that there is damage to the tumour cell membrane permitting the antibody to pass through and bind to intracellular myosin or for the myosin to be exposed. After Hoefnagel et al[73] had demonstrated the feasibility of ^{111}In anti-myosin imaging in children with rhabdomyosarcoma, there were several preliminary reports of the use of this technique in a variety of soft-tissue tumours.[74–77] However, most series included few cases of rhabdomyosarcoma and no children.

Between January 1987 and January 1992 a radioimmunoscintigraphic study was performed in 30 patients with histologically proven myosarcomas, among whom 21 were children with ages ranging from 3 to 14 years.[11] 27 patients had rhabdomyosarcoma (RMS), two leiomyosarcoma (LMS) and one alveolar soft-part sarcoma. Commercially available Fab fragments of the monoclonal antibody R11D10, directed against the heavy chain of cardiac myosin, were used, labelled with ^{111}In. Children received 0.25 mg of anti-myosin Fab fragments labelled with 37 MBq of ^{111}In by slow intravenous injection and whole-body scintigraphy was performed 24 and 48 h thereafter.

The imaging results are listed in Table 67.4, together with the observed tumour localizations. No adverse reactions were observed. In patients who were in a complete remission (seven RMS and one LMS) no pathological accumulations were found. Normal tracer accumulation was seen in the kidneys, liver and, to a lesser extent, in bone marrow and the heart. ^{111}In anti-myosin uptake into normal smooth and skeletal muscle was not apparent.

Table 67.4 Results of radioimmunoscintigraphy using ^{111}In anti-myosin Fab fragments in rhabdomyosarcoma patients[11]

	Positive scintigram	Negative scintigram	Total
Rhabdomyosarcoma +	22	4	26
Rhabdomyosarcoma –	3	7	10
Total (sensitivity 85%, specificity 70%)	25	11	36
Tumour localization			
Primary tumour		7/10	
Tumour residue			
Local recurrence		8/9	
Metastases:			
Bone		6/7	
Bone marrow		0/1	
Lymph nodes		7/8	
Lung		3/3	
Soft tissue		1/2	

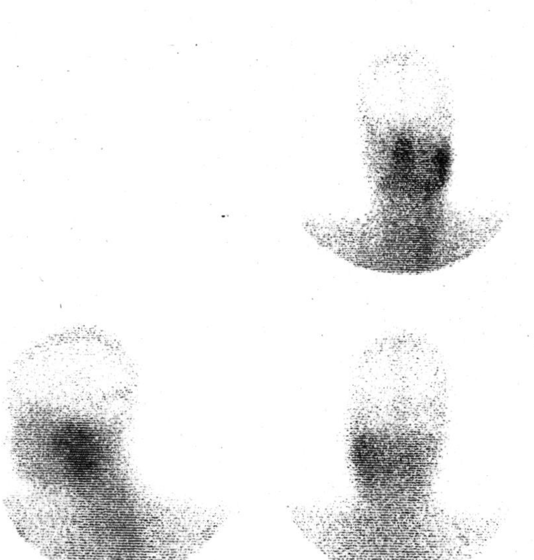

Fig. 67.13 Anterior, left lateral and posterior view ^{111}In antimyosin scintigrams of a 4-year-old girl, showing a local recurrence of rhabdomyosarcoma in the left cheek. (Reproduced with permission from Hoefnagel et al[11]).

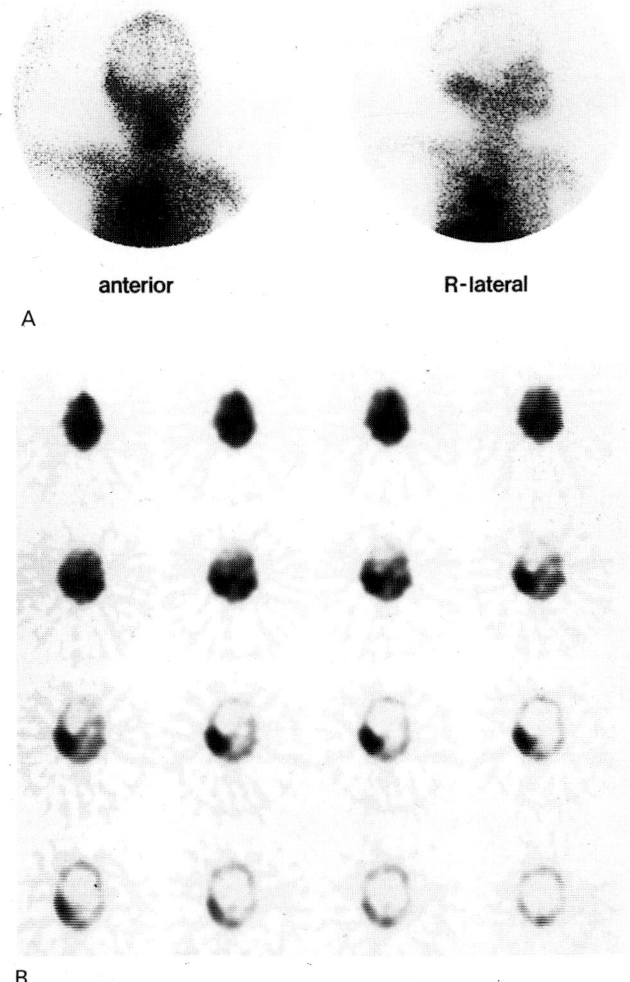

Fig. 67.14 (A) Radioimmunoscintigraphy using ^{111}In anti-myosin Fab fragments in a 4-year-old girl, showing grade 2 uptake in lung metastases of rhabdomyosarcoma and detecting a local recurrence in the right temporo-occipital area of the skull, which was clinically unsuspected. (B) Single photon emission tomography confirms this localization and the intracranial extension of the lesion. (Reproduced with permission from Hoefnagel et al.[11])

^{111}In anti-myosin scintigraphy correctly identified tumour localizations in 22 of 26 cases of RMS, as well as one of two leiomyosarcomas. Figure 67.13 shows uptake in primary RMS located in the left cheek. False-negative results occurred in five patients. In two of these cases this may be attributed to the fact that chemotherapy had been started only days before the scintigram; in two other cases a tumour residue measuring only a few millimetres in diameter was missed, one of which was of a different tumour type (alveolar soft-part sarcoma). The three false-positive findings were due to wound healing after surgery in two cases and sinusitis in another patient.

Single photon emission tomography was useful for discriminating between tumour and bladder/bowel activity in the pelvis, and to show the site and extension of intracranial lesions (Fig. 67.14). In five patients who were scanned both before and after chemotherapy the scintigram was correctly converted from positive to negative in three cases (complete remission) and indicated considerable improvement in two patients attaining a partial remission (Fig. 67.15).

Combining the results of three series[11,75,76] the overall sensitivity of RMS (31 patients) is 86% and for LMS (11 patients) 50%, i.e in the case of RMS a relatively high sensitivity for radioimmunoscintigraphy. Although the numbers of patients in complete remission of RMS are rather small, the specificity of ^{111}In anti-myosin scintigraphy was not as high as one would expect (70%). False-positive results due to wound healing and sinusitis, and the fact that also other soft-tissue sarcomas[76] and breast carcinoma (C A Hoefnagel, personal communication) may accumulate ^{111}In anti-myosin Fab, suggest that this technique is not entirely specific for rhabdomyosarcoma.

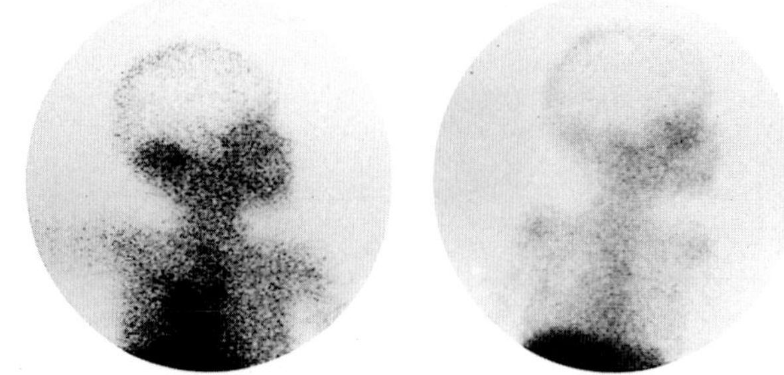

Fig. 67.15 Anti-myosin radioimmunoscintigraphy in follow-up of rhabdomyosarcoma: scintigrams before (left) and after two cycles of combination chemotherapy (right) demonstrates a marked decrease in pathological accumulation, indicating a favourable response. (Reproduced with permission from Hoefnagel et al.[11])

Considering the clinical role of ^{111}In anti-myosin imaging, it is concluded from this study that this technique is useful for the confirmation of RMS, the early detection of tumour recurrence and metastases, and for monitoring the response to chemotherapy. The non-invasiveness of the procedure makes it an easily applicable parameter in the follow-up. However, it cannot be used to exclude disease, and because of the suboptimal specificity positive findings need to be confirmed. Potential pitfalls of anti-myosin imaging are confusion with wound healing, infection, contamination, bladder or bowel activity and residual activity in PorthaCath reservoir or intravenous lines.

Extrapolating these results to potential radioimmunotherapy, the limited intensity of the tumour uptake does not appear to be a favourable dosimetric prerequisite.

REFERENCES

1. Piepsz A, Gordon I, Hahn K 1991 Paediatric nuclear medicine. Eur J Nucl Med 18: 41–66
2. McLaughlin A, Magee M A, Greenough R et al 1990 Current role of gallium scanning in the management of lymphoma. Eur J Nucl Med 16: 755–771
3. Hoefnagel C A, Delprat C C, Marcuse H R, de Vijlder J J M 1986 Role of Thallium-201 total-body scintigraphy in follow-up of thyroid carcinoma. J Nucl Med 27: 1854–1857
4. Kaplan W D, Takvorian T, Morris J H, Rumbaugh C L, Connolly B T, Atkins H L 1987 Thallium-201 tumor brain imaging: a comparative study with pathologic correlation. J Nucl Med 28: 47–52
5. Ramanna L, Waxman A, Binney G, Waxman S, Mirra J, Rosen G 1990 Thallium-201 scintigraphy in bone sarcoma: comparison with Gallium-67 and Technetium-MDP in the evaluation of chemotherapeutic response. J Nucl Med 31: 567–572
6. Hoefnagel C A, Bruning P F, Cohen P, van der Schoot J B, Marcuse H R 1981 Detection of lung metastases from osteosarcoma by scintigraphy using Tc-99m methylene diphosphonate. Diagn Imag 50: 277–284
7. McKillop J H, Erlinda E, Goris M L 1981 Indications and limitations of bone scintigraphy in osteogenic sarcoma: review of 55 patients. Cancer 48: 1133–1138
8. Hoefnagel C A, Voûte P A, de Kraker J, Marcuse H R. Radionuclide diagnosis and therapy of neural crest tumours using Iodine-131 metaiodobenzylguanidine. J Nucl Med 28: 308–314
9. Lamberts S W J, Bakker W H, Reubi J C, Krenning E P 1990 Somatostatin receptor imaging in the localization of endocrine tumours. N Engl J Med 323: 1246–1249
10. De Kraker J, Hoefnagel C A, Voûte P A 1991 ^{131}I-Rose Bengal therapy in hepatoblastoma patients. Eur J Cancer 27: 613–615
11. Hoefnagel C A, Kapucu Ö, de Kraker J, Voûte P A 1993 Radioimmunoscintigraphy using ^{111}In-antimyosin Fab fragments for the diagnosis and follow up of rhabdomyosarcoma. Eur J Cancer 29A: 2096–2100
12. Order S E, Stillwagon G B, Klein J L et al 1985 Iodine 131 antiferritin, a new treatment modality in hepatoma: a Radiation Therapy Oncology Group study. J Clin Oncol 3: 1573–1582
13. Miraldi F 1989 Monoclonal antibodies and neuroblastoma. Semin Nucl Med 19: 282–294
14. Young Jr J L, Miller R W 1975 Incidence of malignant tumors in U.S. children. J Pediatr 86: 254–258
15. Voûte P A, de Kraker J, Hoefnagel C A 1992 Tumours of the sympathetic nervous system. Neuroblastoma, ganglioneuroma and phaeochromocytoma. In: Voûte P A, Barrett A, Lemerle J (eds) Cancer in chidren: clinical management. Springer, Berlin, pp 226–243
16. Ninane J, Vermylen C, Cornu G 1988 Tumour markers for neuroblastoma. In Sluyser M, Voûte P A (eds) Molecular biology and genetics of childhood cancer: Approaches to neuroblastoma. Ellis Horwood, Chichester; pp 13–25

17. Evans A E, D'Angio G J, Propert K et al 1987 Prognostic factors in neuroblastoma. Cancer 59: 1853–1859
18. UICC 1985 TNM-atlas, illustrated guide to the TNM/pTNM classification of malignant tumours, 2nd edn. UICC, Geneva
19. Evans A E 1980 Staging and treatment of neuroblastoma. Cancer 45: 1799–1802
20. Schoemaker J H, Hoefnagel C A, van der Schoot C E, van Leeuwen E F 1992 Diagnosis of bone marrow involvement in neuroblastoma; the complementary role of 3 different methods. Med Pediatr Oncol 20: 427
21. Sisson J C, Frager M S, Valk T W et al 1981 Scintigraphic localization of pheochromocytoma. N Engl J Med 305: 12–17
22. Kimmig B, Brandeis W E, Eisenhut M, Bubeck B, Hermann H J, zum Winkel K 1984 Scintigraphy of a neuroblastoma with I-131-meta-iodobenzylguanidine. J Nucl Med 25: 773–775
23. Feine U, Treuner J, Niethammer D et al 1984 Erste Untersuchungen szintigraphischen Darstellung von Neuroblastomen mit ^{131}I-meta-Benzylguanidin. Nucl Compact 15: 23–26
24. Hoefnagel C A, Voûte P A, de Kraker J, Marcuse H R 1985 Total body scintigraphy with ^{131}I-meta-iodobenzylguanidine for detection of neuroblastoma. Diagn Imag Clin Med 54: 21–27
25. Geatti O, Shapiro B, Sisson J C et al 1985 Iodine-131-Metaiodobenzylguanidine scintigraphy for the location of neuroblastoma: preliminary experience in ten cases. J Nucl Med 26: 736–742
26. Munkner T 1985 ^{131}I-Meta-iodobenzylguanidine scintigraphy of neuroblastomas. Semin Nucl Med 15: 154–160
27. Nakajo M, Shapiro B, Glowniak J, Sisson J C, Beierwaltes W H 1983 Inverse relationship between cardiac accumulation of meta-^{131}I-iodobenzylguanidine and circulating catecholamines in suspected pheochromocytoma. J Nucl Med 24: 1127–1134
28. Schmiegelow K, Siimes M A, Agerloft L et al 1989 Radioiodobenzylguanidine scintigraphy of neuroblastoma: conflicting results when compared with standard investigations. Med Fed Onc 17: 126–130
29. Lumbroso J, Guermazi F, Hartmann O et al 1987 Interêt clinique de la scintigraphie des neuroblastomes par la mIBG marquée a l'iode 123. Proceedings of the MIBG and Catecholamines Workshop, Tours, 1987. J-L Baulieu, Tours
30. Troncone L, Rufini V, Montemaggi P, Danza F M, Lasorella A, Mastrangelo R 1990 The diagnosis and therapeutic utility of radioiodinated metaiodobenzylguanidine (MIBG). 5 year's experience. Eur J Nucl Med 16: 325–335
31. Yeh S D J, Helson L, Benua R S 1986 Metaiodobenzylguanidine (MIBG) imaging in neuroblastoma. J Nucl Med 27: 947
32. Beierwaltes W H 1987 Update on basic research and clinical experience with metaiodobenzylguanidine. Med Pediatr Oncol 15: 163–169
33. Heyman S, Evans A E, D'Angio G J 1988 I-131 Metaiodobenzylguanidine: Diagnostic use in enuroblastoma patients in relapse. Med Pediat Oncol 16: 337–340
34. Harris R E, Gelfand M J 1986 Sensitivity and utility of the I-131 MIBG scan in childhood neuroblastoma. Proc Am Soc Clin Onc 5: 825
35. Feine U, Müller-Schauenburg W, Treuner J, Klingebiel T H 1987 Meta-iodobenzyl-guanidine (MIBG) labeled with ^{123}I/^{131}I in neuroblastoma. Med Pediatr Oncol 15: 181–187
36. Miceli A, Nespoli L, Burgio G R, Aprile C, Carena M, Saponaro R 1986 The role of meta-iodo[^{131}I]benzylguanidine (MIBG) in the diagnosis and follow-up of neuroblastoma. Pediatr Hematol Oncol 3: 37–47
37. Hadley G P, Rabe E 1986 Scanning with Iodine-131 MIBG in children with solid tumors: an initial appraisal. J Nucl Med 27: 620–626
38. Bouvier J F, Ducrettet F, Philip T, Brunat-Mentigny M, Chauvot P, Lahneche B E 1987 MIBG neuroblastoma diagnosis: value and limits. Proceedings of the MIBG and Catecholamines Workshop, Tours, 1987. J-L Baulieu, Tours
39. Hibi S, Todo S, Imashuku S, Miyazaki T 1987 ^{131}I-meta-iodobenzyl-guanidine scintigraphy in patients with neuroblastoma. Pediatr Radiol 17: 308–313
40. Hoefnagel C A 1989 The clinical use of ^{131}I-meta-iodobenzylguanidine (MIBG) for the diagnosis and treatment of neural crest tumors. University of Amsterdam, p 99
41. Gordon I, Peters A M, Gutman A, Morony S, Dicks-Mireaux C, Pritchard J 1990 Skeletal assessment in neuroblastoma – the pitfalls of Iodine-123-MIBG scans. J Nucl Med 31: 129–134
42. Shulkin B L, Wei Chen S, Sisson J C, Shapiro B 1987 Iodine-131 MIBG scintigraphy of the extremities in metastatic pheochromocytoma and neuroblastoma. J Nucl Med 28: 315–318
43. Lynn M D, Shapiro B, Sisson J C et al 1984 Portrayal of pheochromocytoma and normal human adrenal medulla by m-[^{123}I]Iodobenzylguanidine (concise communication). J Nucl Med 25: 436–440
44. Sinon B, Hoefnagel C A, de Kraker J, van Steeg G, Valdés Olmos R A 1992 ^{123}I-MIBG or ^{131}I-MIBG for imaging of neuroblastoma? A comparative study. Eur J Nucl Med 19: 589
45. Khafagi F A, Shapiro B, Fig L M, Mallette S, Sisson J C 1989 Labetalol reduces iodine-131 MIBG uptake by pheochromocytoma and normal tissues. J Nucl Med 30: 481–489
46. Hoefnagel C A, Klumper A, Voûte P A 1987 Single photon emission tomography using meta-[^{131}I]iodobenzylguanidine in malignant pheochromocytoma and neuroblastoma: case reports. J Med Imag 1: 57–60
47. Goldman A, Vivian G, Gordon I et al 1984 Immunolocalization of neuroblastoma using radiolabelled monoclonal antibody UJ13A. J Pediatr 105: 252–256
48. Cheung N K V, Saarinen U M, Neely J E et al 1985 Monoclonal antibodies to a glycolipid antigen on human neuroblastoma cells. Cancer Res 45: 2642–2649
49. Miraldi F D, Nelson A D, Kraly C et al 1986 Diagnostic imaging of human neuroblastoma with radiolabeled antibody. Radiology 161: 413–418
50. Yeh S D J, Larson S M, Burch L et al 1991 Radioimmunodetection of neuroblastoma with Iodine-131-3F8: correlation with biopsy, iodine-131-metaiodobenzylguanidine and standard diagnostic modalities. J Nucl Med 32: 769–776
51. Smolarz K, Waters W, Sieverts H et al 1989 Immunoscintigraphy using Tc-99m-labeled monoclonal antibody BW575 compared with I-131-MIBG scintigraphy in neuroblastoma. Radiology 152: 173
52. Bihl H, Matzku S 1990 A comparison of MIBG and monoclonal antibody uptake in neuroblastoma xenografts. J Nucl Med 31: 741
53. Kasai M, Watanabe I 1992 Liver tumours. In: Voûte P A, Barrett A, Lemerle J (eds) Cancer in children: clinical management. Springer, Berlin, pp 256–268
54. Shoop J D 1969 Functional hepatoma demonstrated with rose bengal scanning. Am J Roentgenol 107: 51–53
55. Belfer A J, Grijm R, van der Schoot J B 1979 Hepatic adenoma: imaging with different radionuclides. Clin Nucl Med 4: 375–378
56. Lee V W, Shapiro J H 1983 Specific diagnosis of hepatoma using Tc-99m HIDA and other radionuclides. Eur J Nucl Med 8: 191–195
57. Miller J H, Greenspan B S 1985 Integrated imaging of hepatic tumours in childhood. I. Malignant lesions (primary and metastatic). Radiology 154: 83–90
58. Diament M J, Parvey L S, Tonkin I L D, Johnson K D, Bernstein R, Webber B 1982 Hepatoblastoma: Technetium sulfur colloid uptake simulating focal nodular hyperplasia. AJR 139: 168–171
59. De Kraker J, Hoefnagel C A, Voûte P A 1989 ^{131}I-Rose bengal therapy in inoperable hepatoblastoma. Med Pediatr Oncol 17: 278
60. Ohshiro K, Hanashiro Y, Shimabukuro K et al 1991 A hepatobiliary study with Tc-99m N-pyridoxyl-5-methyltryptophan (PMT) in a patient with hepatoblastoma. Clin Nucl Med 16: 10–12
61. Raney R B, Hays D M, Tefft M, Triche J T 1989 Rhabdomyosarcoma and undifferentiated sarcomas. In: Pizzo P A, Poplack D G (eds) Principles and practice of pediatric oncology. Lippincott, Philadelphia, pp 635–658
62. Flamant F, Voûte P A, Sommelet D 1992 Rhabdomyosarcoma. In: Voûte P A, Barrett A, Lemerle J (eds) Cancer in children: Clinical management. Springer, Berlin, pp 314–324
63. Oates E, Sarno C I 1987 Imaging of pelvic rhabdomyosarcoma by bone scintigraphy. Eur J Nucl Med 13: 297–299
64. Weinblatt M E, Miller J H 1981 Radionuclide scanning in children with rhabdomyosarcoma. Med Pediat Oncol 9, 293–301

65. Bekerman C 1978 Childhood malignancies. In: Hoffer P B, Bekerman C, Henkin R E (eds) Gallium-67 imaging. Wiley, New York, p 145
66. Ramanna L, Waxman A D, Waxman S et al 1988 Tl-201 scintigraphy in bone and soft tissue sarcoma: evaluation of tumor and mass and viability. J Nucl Med 29: 854
67. Cogswell A, Howman-Giles R, Bergin M 1994 Bone and gallium scintigraphy in children with rhabdomyosarcoma: a 10-year review. Med Pediatr Oncol 22: 15–21
68. Scupham R, Gilbert E F, Wilde J, Wiedrich T A 1986 Immunohistochemical studies of rhabdomyosarcoma. Arch Pathol Lab Med 110: 818–821
69. Khaw B A, Yasuda T, Gold H K et al 1987 Acute myocardial infarct imaging with ^{111}In-labeled monoclonal antimyosin Fab. J Nucl Med 28: 1671–1678
70. Yasuda T, Palacios I F, Dec G W et al 1987 In-111 monoclonal antimyosin imaging in the diagnosis of acute myocarditis. Circulation 76: 306–311
71. Carrio I, Bern L, Ballester M et al 1988 In-111 antimyosin scintigraphy to assess myocardial damage in patients with suspected myocarditis and cardiac rejection. J Nucl Med 29: 1893–1900
72. Estorch M, Carrio I, Bern L et al 1990 Indium-111 antimyosin scintigraphy after doxorubicin therapy in patients with advanced breast cancer. J Nucl Med 31: 1965–1969
73. Hoefnagel C A, Voûte P A, de Kraker J, Behrendt H 1987 Scintigraphic detection of rhabdomyosarcoma. Lancet i: 921
74. Hoefnagel C A, de Kraker J, Voûte P A, Behrendt H 1988 Tumor imaging of rhabdomyosarcoma using radiolabelled fragments of monoclonal anti-myosin antibody. J Nucl Med 29: 791
75. Cox P H, Verweij J, Pillay M, Stoter G, Schonfeld D 1988 Indium-111 antimyosin for the detection of leiomyosarcoma and rhabdomyosarcoma. Eur J Nucl Med 14: 50–52
76. Kairemo K J A, Wiklund T A, Liewendahl K et al 1990 Imaging of soft tissue sarcomas with In-111-labeled monoclonal antimyosin Fab fragments. J Nucl 31: 23–31
77. Reuland P, Koscelniak E, Ruck P, Treuner J, Feine U 1991 Application of an anti-myosin for scintigraphic differential diagnosis of infantile tumors. Int J Rad Appl Istrum [B] 18: 89–93

68. The diagnostic role of radiolabelled antibodies

K. E. Britton Maria Granowska

GENERAL PRINCIPLES

The cancer cell differs from normal cells of the same tissue in a number of subtle ways. These differences are exploitable by nuclear medicine both for imaging and therapy. This tissue characterization of cancer may be through surface receptors using binding agents such as the radiolabelled somatostatin analogues, or through surface components that are antigenic. These antigenic differences, both qualitative and quantitative, may be demonstrated by means of a large variety of monoclonal antibodies, each selected for a particular tumour-associated antigen. The techniques of using radiolabelled monoclonal antibodies for imaging in vivo is called radioimmunoscintigraphy (RIS) and for therapy radioimmunotherapy (RIT). The monoclonal antibody, its derived fragments and genetically engineered single chain or molecular recognition units have the property of specific and selective binding to an epitope, the binding part of an antigen. This ability distinguishes it from other radiopharmaceuticals. How to make best use of this important property in the management of patients with cancer is the subject of this section.

Clinical role

One might have thought that with the introduction of X-ray computerized tomography (CT), ultrasound, and nuclear magnetic resonance imaging (MRI) there was no need for another method of imaging cancer. Yet none of those techniques is able to demonstrate cancer cells in a specific way. For example, lymph node size may be used as an indicator of malignant involvement, yet this purely physical approach can neither show cancer cells in a normal sized node nor that an enlarged node does or does not contain cancer cells. RIS has the potential to do this.

The first clinical question that RIS is designed to answer is the demonstration of subclinical, subradiological disease. Unlike radiological techniques flat plaques of tumour are just as visible by RIS as spherical lesions. Bowel gas or lack of fat are not problems, but lack of clear anatomical landmarks may be.

Serum markers are used to detect cancer but for a serum marker to be elevated, there must be a certain size of tumour present able to release sufficient antigen to cause a rise in the serum level above a 'normal range'. To do this, distribution of the serum marker antigen in lymphatics and extracellular fluid must be extensive. Biological variation and other causes, such as cigarette smoking and release of the antigen due to inflammation, must be overcome. RIS is directed at imaging the tumour in situ and is able to be positive for cancer before serum markers are elevated, both in primary and in recurrent malignancy. If serum markers for cancer are elevated, RIS is able to demonstrate the site of cancer using a radiolabelled antibody either against the serum marker or one more specific for the cancer in question, even when radiology is negative.

When following up a patient with cancer, who may have had extensive surgery and/or radiotherapy, a mass for example in the pelvis may be evident clinically or radiologically. X-ray, CT, ultrasound and MRI may be unable to distinguish whether such a mass is due to post-surgical fibrosis, inflammatory reaction or truly viable tumour. The presence of viable tumour will be shown by RIS in this situation. Present methods of detecting the effectiveness of chemotherapy have included second look laparotomy or laparoscopy. RIS is able to demonstrate in a non-invasive way, the presence of viable tumour that has relapsed after chemotherapy.

Lastly RIS is able to show in a recurrent cancer, for which immunotherapy or RIT is considered, that the target antigen is present and accessible – for the demonstration of the presence of the antigen on a tissue section immunohistologically does not always predict that specific uptake of the chosen monoclonal antibody will take place in vivo.

The important roles of RIS in cancer outlined above should not be taken to imply that RIS should be used clinically in isolation from or in competition with other established diagnostic modalities. Rather RIS can take the diagnostic process forward non-invasively and help to overcome the lack of cancer specificity of radiological and other nuclear medicine techniques. For example, in screening well women the ultrasound positive pelvic mass can be shown to be benign or malignant by RIS. However, it must be stressed that the 'rules' of radioimmunoscintigraphy must be obeyed, conditions for optimal use of the selectivity and specificity of RIS must be met and the limitations of this approach, as any other, must be understood.

Tumour uptake: requirements and limitations

Tumour antigens

It remains almost true to say that there are no unique cancer antigens. The oncogene–proto-oncogene anti-oncogene theory of cancer implies that there are different DNA sequences in cancer cells as compared to normal cells. Therefore there are likely to be resultant oncoproteins that have cancer specificity. In practice, it appears that there are either excesses of oncogene or deletions of anti-oncogenes, most of which are very closely related to, but qualitatively and quantitatively different from, normal genetic material. Oncogene markers, such as k-ras for colorectal cancer, point the way towards the establishment of cancer specific antigens. In another future approach, anti-sense oligonucleotides against, for example, growth control related genes are being introduced into therapy and the development of radiolabelled anti-sense oligonucleotides for diagnosis and therapy is underway.

The antigens used for RIS may be classified (Table 68.1), together with examples of monoclonal antibodies that have been used clinically for RIS. This gives only a small selection of antibodies used in vivo in patients for each category. There are many more in use in vitro, in cell classification in immunohistochemistry, or experimentally in cell cultures or animals. The requirements for the ideal antigen are: that it is abundant with at least 5000 surface epitopes per cell accessible to antibody; that it is present in all malignant cells of the cancer under consideration; and that it is stable. Whereas the first requirement is usually met, the others are often not. Some whole tumours may not express the antigen, for example TAG72 against which B72.3 reacts, is not found in up to 20% of colorectal cancers. More often its antigen expression is heterogenous with some cells having high expression and others poor or no expression. This heterogeneity is not distributed evenly through the tumour since it is found that clumps of tumour cells, perhaps of the same clone, express the epitope whereas other clumps do not. This does not matter in principle for RIS since the binding of an antibody to one cell in every 100 tumour cells would still enable identification of the tumour, but it is a major problem for RIT.

Antigen modulation is the name given to the ability of certain cells to change their surface antigenic composition. Antigens can be 'up-regulated' particularly in the presence of biologically active cytokines such as the interferons and the interleukins. This is particularly a feature of lympho-

Table 68.1 Classification of tumour antigens with examples of monoclonal antibodies used for radioimmunoscintigraphy

	Abbreviation of monoclonal antibody	Full name	Usage
Normal epithelial surface antigens	HMFG1,2	human milk fat globule	gynaecological cancer
	SM3	stripped mucin protein 3	gynaecological cancer breast cancer
	PR1A3	anti colonic crypt surface antigen	colorectal cancer
	AUAI	Arklie's unknown antigen	colorectal & bladder cancer
Oncofetal antigens	anti-CEA e.g. C46, BW 431/26	anti carcinoembryonic antigen	colorectal cancer
	FOC 23C5		lung, breast, bladder and gut cancer
	anti-HCG	anti human choriogonadotrophin	choriocarcinoma
	anti α-FP	anti alpha fetoprotein	hepatoma
Receptor antigens	anti-EGFR	anti epidermal growth factor receptor	brain tumour
Enzymes	anti-PLAP e.g H17E2	anti placental alkaline phosphatase	testicular and ovarian cancer cervical cancer
Tumour derived antigens	B72.3	anti TAG72, a tumour associated glycoprotein	some colorectal and gynaecological cancers
	MOv18	malignant ovarian antigen	ovarian cancers
	225-28S	anti high-molecular-weight melanoma antigen	cutaneous and ocular melanomas
Lymphocyte antigens	CD3, CD4	anti T cell	leukaemia
	CD19,20,22	anti B cell	lymphoma
Viral antigens	various	anti hepatitis B	hepatoma
Synthetic antigens	H170	anti pan adenocarcinoma	breast cancer
Structural	various	anti-keratin	squamous cell cancer
		anti-tenascin	glioma
Oncogene products	various	anti c erb2	breast cancer

cytes and their related malignancies. For solid tumours increasing the antigenic expression by cytokines experimentally gives a less than two-fold response and so this approach is unlikely to benefit RIS. The high antigen expression of cancer cells for those antibodies used for RIS will never be saturated by the injected antibody when amounts of up to 2 mg per dose are used, as is conventional.

Another consideration is the relationship between the histological grading and antigen expression. Whereas well or moderately well differentiated cancers may have good antigenic expression and antibody uptake, some poorly differentiated tumours may have much less expression and this varies from antigen to antigen. For example, the monoclonal antibody C46 (anti-CEA) and PR1A3 have similar uptake in moderately well differentiated colorectal cancer but PR1A3 is taken up three times better than C46 by poorly differentiated tumours.[1]

The tumour environment

The blood supply to the tumour is most important. For each circulation time of 15–20 s, an amount of injected antibody is brought to the tumour in proportion to its blood supply and the plasma concentration of the antibody. It is evident that the greater the blood supply to the tumour and the longer the residence time of the antibody in the blood, the more will be delivered to the tumour. This statement needs qualification. The smaller the tumour the higher is the proportion of tumour cells to stromal cells so the greater is the relative density of antigen expressing cells to receive antibody and the better vascularized the tumour is for its weight. The tumour grows in volume cubically but its surface area grows by a power function of two so the blood supply becomes relatively decreased in larger tumours, e.g. over 3 cm diameter. This leads to central necrosis and cyst formation with reduction or loss of antigen expression.

There is also a complex relationship between binding affinity and blood level of antibody. A very high affinity binds more antibody per circulation and counteracts the effect of a more rapid blood clearance.

Tumour stimulated angio-neogenesis gives abnormal capillaries which are not under autonomic control and which are more leaky to large molecules than are normal capillaries. For a small tumour the malignant cells are closely apposed to these leaky capillaries and potential antibody delivery and uptake is good. Selectivity of uptake of antibody which is also dependent on its binding characteristics is good. As the tumour enlarges more extracellular fluid and stroma intervenes. Leaky capillaries are leaking non-specific proteins and the degree of selectivity is lost. Large tumours will take up in a non-specific way almost any large molecule that is presented to them. Indeed radiolabelled fibrinogen and albumin were used in the past for tumour imaging. As the tumour enlarges the properties of its intercellular stroma may become inimical to antibody diffusion through alteration of charge, composition, or viscosity. This appears to be one reason why breast cancer may be difficult for RIS.

It is evident from these considerations that if the selectivity of RIS is to be maintained then it is small tumours that it is best designed to image and such tumours are those least likely to be detected by clinical or radiological methods. Again it should be noted that, for imaging, only those surface cells close to the supplying capillaries need to take up the labelled antibody. Indeed this process reduces the availability of antibody to deeper parts of the tumour. Given a good signal remaining attached to the antibody, uptake at the tumour surface will be sufficient to identify the tumour by imaging. Penetration of the antibody or fragment is thus not a requirement for RIS, but is an essential requirement and major problem for RIT.

When imaging is considered, the vascularity of the tumour and its environment also has an effect on the quality of the image and the ease of tumour detection. A long persisting blood pool may obscure tumour uptake so a slow blood clearance of antibody is not necessarily an advantage. Conversely an antibody fragment or smaller antibody-like agent may be cleared rapidly from the blood which reduces this blood background activity; but where is it cleared to? Its smaller size increases its penetration not only to tumour but also the extracellular fluid of the tumour environment which increases the tissue background. Murine antibody with a typical blood clearance half-life of 24 h is about right for imaging, especially when a short lived radionuclide is used as the label.

Another factor affecting RIS is the extent to which the tumour-associated antigen is expressed in other diseases and normal tissues. For example, uptake of anti-CEA by Crohn's disease is well established. Staging of a tumour is usually related to the degree and extent of lymph node involvement. If the antigen is easily released from the tumour (as is required for a good serum marker) then the normal lymphatic drainage of the tumour will bring the antigen to the local nodes. Thus anti-CEA antibodies can be imaged in normal uninvolved nodes related to a colorectal cancer, for example.[2] The normal peri-hilar nodes in the porta hepatis may contain the diffusible antigen and interfere with preoperative probe assessment of node involvement.[3]

The monoclonal antibody

An antibody is a gamma globulin made naturally by the body in response to a foreign substance entering the body. Lymphocytes are activated by surface molecules on the foreign substance which are called antigens, and produce a range of antibodies in response. A part of each antibody called the complementarity determinant region (CDR) reacts with part of an antigen which is called the epitope. Each activated lymphocyte produces a single antibody. The hybridoma technique is a method of isolating and reproducing lymphocytes which produce a single antibody. Lymphocytes from the spleen of a mouse immunized against a chosen antigen are fused with myeloma lymphocytes to produce a potentially immortal strain of lymphocyte. These fused lymphocytes are separated in wells and are selected for the specificity and avidity of their particular antibody production. The appropriate lymphocyte hybridoma is cultured to produce a clone. This clone produces a single antibody – the monoclonal antibody – MAb for short. Murine MAb are harvested from the culture supernatant, purified and prepared to meet pharmaceutical standards. A range of MAbs each reacting with one or more of almost every known cancer are under experimental evaluation. Many of these are undergoing clinical trials in academic institutions. Very few MAb are commercially available. This is due to inappropriately unfavourable regulatory requirements, a concern about the patent situation, and the long time between development and profit which are adverse commercial features. Yet the potential and power of this selective approach to cancer imaging and therapy is unquestionable.

The gamma globulin exists in a number of classes such as IgM, where it is an aggregate; IgG1 which is a common class for RIS, and IgG2a which will fix complement and may be cytotoxic as a result. The structure is a combination of two short 'light' chains and two long 'heavy' chains in a Y-shaped configuration (Fig. 68.1). The tips of the branches of the Y contain the CDRs of which there are three on each branch. The stalk of the Y is called the Fc protein and may bind non-specifically to reticuloendothelial cells. Pepsin and other enzymes may be used to break up the Y. Removal of the Fc portion gives a fragment called an $F(ab')_2$ and one arm of the Y is called an Fab. Both still have specific binding properties, usually weaker than the whole MAb. Their smaller size means more rapid clearance from blood into extracellular fluid and kidneys. The smaller fragments are filtered and then reabsorbed and metabolized in the proximal tubules, depositing any attached metal radionuclide. Genetic engineering techniques are able to replace the Fc portion of the murine MAb with the human equivalent, which is called a chimeric antibody; or both the Fc portion and the frame leaving only the CDRs of murine origin. This is called a 'human reshaped' antibody or a CDR grafted antibody. The elements of the frame and the CDRs may be engineered further[4] into a frame and binding site called an Fv, a single chain antibody where two Fvs are linked, single domain antibodies, dabs, and a single binding site called a molecular recognition unit (mru) (Fig. 68.1). These engineered molecules may be combined, for example, with a binding site for ^{99m}Tc made of the amino acids LCTCCA (lysine, cysteine, threonine, cysteine, cysteine, arginine) from the metallothionein protein for imaging;[5] or for ^{32}P phosphorus from the kemptide sequence[6] for therapy. The development of these 'designer' molecules is the future direction of RIS and RIT.

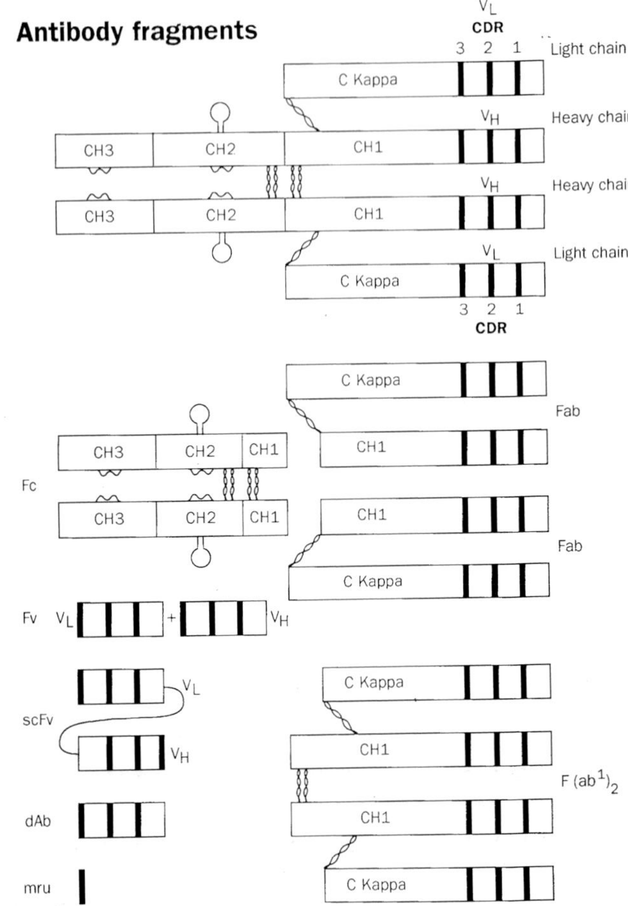

Fig. 68.1 The structure of the antibody and its fragments.
Top: Whole antibody
The light chain, C Kappa also called V_L.
The heavy chain also called V_H is made up of four components, CH3, CH2 with a carbohydrate side chain, CH1, and an Fv portion which contains the three complementarity determinant regions, CDR, the active binding sites.
The chains are connected to each other and internally by S–S bonds.
Centre: Enzyme digestion of the whole antibody can break it into two Fab fragments and an Fc portion, or an $F(ab')_2$
Fv is the name given to the combination of the binding sites of the V_L and V_H portions containing the frames holding the CDRs.
scFv is the single chain Fv where the V_L and V_H portions are attached together with a chemical linker.
dAb is a 'single domain antibody' made up of part of an Fv.
mru is the molecular recognition unit made up of one of the six CDRs.
Chimeric antibody: C Kappa, part of CH1, Fv, are murine. CH3, CH2 and part of CH1 are human.
Human reshaped antibody: Only the CDRs are murine. All the rest of the structure is human.

Murine antibodies, however, are quite acceptable for RIS. The human antimouse antibody (HAMA) response is an entity but not a problem. It is much decreased by avoiding skin testing and by using less than 1 mg of antibody, when it has about the same incidence as with fragments – about 30%.[7] It does not interfere with imaging but may make the blood clearance of whole antibody more rapid. It does not relate to clinical reactions which are rare, of the order of 1 in 1000 (if less than 1 mg is used) – similar to a ^{99m}Tc DTPA renal or ^{99m}Tc MDP bone study. The frequency of HAMA is related to the frequency of injection – 30% one dose, 50% two doses, 70% after three doses. In about 10% of the three dose schedule, diagnostic imaging will be impaired.[7] Two types of response occur: 'isotypic' against the Fc portion and frame region and 'idiotypic' against the CDR.

The radionuclide signal

The key to successful RIS is the choice of radiolabel given that the chosen monoclonal antibody binds to the tumour. Although ^{131}I was the original radiolabel for RIS, its evident disadvantages of low count rate and beta emission would exclude its choice for RIS now. Because of its low count rate, it was noted that small tumours would only be seen after several days when the blood and tissue background had fallen to very low levels. At the time this led to the belief that antibodies took several days to bind to the tumour. That this is not so was evident when a high-signal short-lived radionuclide such as ^{123}I was substituted. The same monoclonal antibody with the same administered activity of ^{123}I as ^{131}I was able to image the same tumour within 4 h as compared to 72 h in spite of a 'high' blood background.[8]

^{123}I iodine ^{123}I iodine has a half-life of 13 h and a gamma-ray energy of 159 keV, a fair amount of Auger electron production, which can be used for autoradiography and some think also for therapy, and a small amount of high energy gamma which is negligible in practice although some think otherwise.[9] A low 'technetium' energy collimator is generally used. Labelling with ^{123}I followed the established methods used for many years for radioimmunoassay. The first use of ^{123}I-labelled monoclonal antibodies was in 1982.[10] The labelling was via the tyrosine residue through the iodogen technique.[11] Planar and SPECT imaging[10,12] is easy to perform with the high count rate signal that ^{123}I provides, which is about 20 times that of ^{131}I for the same administered activity. This gives a reduction of Poisson noise from 14% (50 counts per pixel for ^{131}I) to 3% (1000 counts per pixel for ^{123}I) at sites of high uptake.[8] Imaging is undertaken at 10 min, 6 and 22 h, with SPECT at 7 and/or 22 h using 120 MBq ^{123}I MAb.

^{123}I is metabolized to give a high urinary output of ^{123}I. In spite of thyroid blockage with potassium iodide, 60 mg b.d. for 3 days; or potassium iodate, some stomach, salivary and thyroid uptake may be seen. However, the liver and the kidneys have low uptake because both contain deiodinases that prevent the retention of ^{123}I in these organs. Thus liver metastases may be identified using ^{123}I MAb.

^{123}I is expensive, not readily available and has to be ordered. It needs to be cyclotron produced in such a way that ^{125}I or ^{124}I are negligible contaminants.

^{111}In indium Indium-111, a metal, has gamma-ray energies of 171 and 247 keV and a half-life of 67 h. To label a monoclonal antibody, initially a bifunctional chelate was used, typically the cyclic anhydride of DTPA.[13–15] A number of precautions have to be taken. There must be meticulous exclusion of trace metals in the solutions and containers used for the radiolabelling, since the DTPA chelate has a higher affinity for other metals such as iron than for indium. Use of too much DTPA will cause cross linking of one antibody molecule to another leading to aggregation and loss of immunoreactivity. The indium-DTPA chelate is not particularly stable in vivo and the distribution of indium-labelled antibody as judged by the ^{111}In label is rather different than that of radioiodine. There is a high and persistent liver uptake which has a number of explanations. The transchelation of the indium followed by hepatocellular deposition is a conventional explanation but experimental work suggests that the deposition is sinusoidal rather than into hepatocytes.[16] ^{111}In-labelled antibodies also show very prominent marrow uptake probably related to the deposition of indium in phagocytes. There is also gut uptake and some renal uptake which may be related to free ^{111}In chloride. The marrow and bowel sites of 'normal' ^{111}In antibody uptake reduce the specificity of abdominal imaging since bowel activity may overlay, and marrow activity underlie, a suspect lesion. The reliable evaluation of liver metastases is not able to be undertaken using ^{111}In as the radiolabel for RIS. More stable chelates for ^{111}In are now available: benzyl DTPA and macrocycles for ^{111}In.[17]

^{111}In is the most expensive of radionuclides. It has to be ordered and its availability may be only once weekly. It gives a high absorbed radiation dose of the order of 24 mSv effective dose per administered dose of 100 MBq, which some national licensing authorities will not accept. The higher energy gamma emission requires that a low medium energy 'gallium' collimator is used with the gamma-camera. Apart from the inconvenience of changing collimators, the heavier collimation reduces sensitivity to some extent. For better spatial resolution, the count rates of the two photopeaks are summed although this may be difficult with some technetium-99m optimized automatic energy correction gamma-camera systems. Although the tendency is to perform RIS with ^{111}In-labelled antibody at 1–5 days after injection, tumour uptake may be visualized as early as 4 h and a baseline image at 10 min after injection is recommended.

^{99m}Tc technetium The twin advantages of on site availability and its optimal 140 keV energy for the gamma-camera, make ^{99m}Tc the radionuclide of choice for nuclear medicine studies. The ability to undertake planar imaging and SPECT up to 24 h after injection covers the key time of tumour uptake of MAb, for approximately 75% of tumour uptake is complete by 12 h.

The first labelling of MAb by ^{99m}Tc was by a pretinning method.[18,19] This approach was adapted to labelling an anti-high-molecular-weight melanoma antigen[20] which was successfully used. The optimal time for imaging with ^{99m}Tc MAb was shown to be between 6 and 24 h.[21] The problem with the pretinning method was that some pertechnetate was weakly bound to the antibody and eluted in vivo. The breakthrough came with the S-S bond reduction technique where 1:1000 2-mercapto ethanol is used to reduce the S-S bridges in the hinge region. The reduced MAb can be stored in this form at −20°C until needed. A normal bone scanning kit is added after thawing followed by ^{99m}Tc eluate. The bone kit provides tin to reduce the ^{99m}Tc and phosphate to prevent the non-specific binding of ^{99m}Tc to the protein.[22–24] This technique is excellent for radiolabelling whole MAb but less successful for fragments. Many other reducing agents are now available for ^{99m}Tc labelling of MAb. Two alternative approaches are used: prechelation of ^{99m}Tc by a chelator followed by attachment of this to the MAb;[25] and addition of ^{99m}Tc to a prechelated antibody.[26] These provide suitable methods for labelling peptides and MAb fragments.

No thyroid blockade is required. Imaging is undertaken at 10 min, 6 and 22 h after injection with SPECT at 6–7 and 22–24 h as required. Serial squat views are helpful for separation of tumour uptake from bladder activity. Circulating ^{99m}Tc MAb is broken down with time and ^{99m}Tc peptide fragments such as ^{99m}Tc cysteine dimer are excreted in the urine. Liver, marrow and bowel uptake is much less than with ^{111}In-labelled MAb, but renal uptake is higher since these fragments are filtered and reabsorbed at the proximal tubule. There is deposition and thus retention of ^{99m}Tc in the tubules. The use of ^{99m}Tc as a label brings RIS into routine use. The test may be completed and reported within 24 h of the request. The effective dose is about 4 mSv for 600 MBq ^{99m}Tc MAb administered. The high count signal gives the best imaging of tumour uptake. It meets the aphorism that the shorter the radionuclide half-life, the greater the activity administered, the higher the count rate achieved, the lower the Poisson noise, the earlier the detection and the smaller the lesion that is detected. The initial high blood and tissue activity is not a problem provided the rules of RIS are respected.

The rules of radioimmunoscintigraphy

1. Specific uptake increases with time. Non-specific uptake after an initial distribution decreases with time during the first 24 h.
2. A template with which to compare later images is essential. This is the set of images starting 10 min after injection. It shows the distribution of vascular and non-specific activity and provides the baseline with which later images may be compared.
3. Serial imaging e.g. 10 min, 6 h and 22 h shows increasing uptake in the tumour in the later set of images.
4. For good quality images, a minimum of 800 000 counts per view should be acquired.
5. SPECT and/or squat views are essential to evaluate the pelvis and SPECT is helpful for the liver.

The clinical protocol

Detailed explanation of the test to the patient, to medical and nursing colleagues is essential. We insist on informed signed consent since all initial RIS studies are under ethics committee control. No skin test is advised since this may sensitize the patient to produce human antimouse antibodies, HAMA. Patients with a history of allergy to foreign protein or with a severe atopic predisposition are excluded from RIS.

The patient receives the injection of ^{99m}Tc-labelled MAb, typically 600 MBq with 0.5 mg MAb. The patient is then positioned supine on the couch. The gamma-camera, which has previously been set up with a 20% window around the 140 keV photopeak and with a low energy 'technetium' parallel hole collimator, is placed over the lower abdomen and imaging is commenced. 800 000 counts are collected per view for a set of two anterior and two posterior images, e.g. for colorectal and gynaecological cancers. For image analysis, a separate set of images of radiolabelled markers, usually cobalt-57, set on ink marks on prominent bones are collected: for the abdomen xiphisternum, costal margins, iliac crests and symphysis pubis;[27] and for the breast, sternal notch, xiphisternum, point of the acromion and costal margin on the anterior view; anterior and posterior axillary folds with a nipple marker in addition for the lateral views. Prone views may be considered. A film of the marker sites is made and placed over the oscilloscope screen. On subsequent imaging, the patient with the ^{57}Co markers is moved until the markers' activity approximates to those previously imaged. This repositioning protocol is simple to perform. Accurate marker image repositioning is undertaken using a translation rotation programme. The recorded serial patient images are then realigned in the same way.[28]

The images

The normal anatomical features of serial images obtained with ^{99m}Tc-labelled MAb need to be recognized. The normal distribution of vascularity decreases with time on the series of images. There is a homogenous distribution of uptake in the liver which increases slightly during the series of images. Renal activity increases with time to a greater extent than the liver. Urinary activity, after an initial increase in the first 6 h, then decreases. Slight marrow and, occasionally, large bowel uptake in the region of the caecum, may be seen on the 22 h image. No evidence of thyroid uptake is seen during the 24 h without thyroid blocking medication.

A typical finding of malignancy is that the early image is normal. Then increased MAb uptake occurs at the sites of malignancy at 6 h, increasing further at 22 h (Fig. 68.2a). Using the 10 min image as the template for comparison, even small sites of abnormality may be recognized. Squat views (Fig. 68.3) and SPECT are important to distinguish between bladder activity and the site of a primary rectal tumour or a pelvic recurrence. For SPECT, orthogonal views should be examined and the combination of, at least two views, usually coronal and sagittal, showing a focal area of abnormal uptake posterior to the bladder in conjunction with the planar and squat views is taken as a positive finding.

In liver metastases a focal defect in the liver may be seen on the 10 min image which usually, depending on size, changes in one of four ways on the later images. In a very large metastasis, the defect persists unchanged. In a smaller metastasis the defect appears to become smaller as the edge shows uptake on the later images (Fig. 68.4) or else the uptake becomes homogenous with that of normal liver; alternatively the metastasis, which is usually very small, becomes a more active 'hot spot' than the initially normal liver. All these changes may be called positive for liver metastases on RIS, although it should be recognized that a defect that persisted unchanged could be due to a cyst or other benign space occupying lesion. SPECT enhances the detection of liver metastases.

After, for example, colorectal surgery, the tumour specimen may be imaged under the gamma-camera. The histopathologist dissects out the tumour and lymph nodes and records the presence and sites of these, any polyps, adenoma, previous surgery and other disease. A map of the specimen is drawn. Samples are obtained and weighed. These specimens are then counted in a gamma counter set up for ^{99m}Tc with appropriate background tubes and standards so that the activity in each sample could be determined. These values may then be related to the activity of the injection through the standards and expressed as a percentage of the injected dose, typically as 10^{-3} per g of specimen.

To assess the pharmacokinetics of a ^{99m}Tc MAb, serial blood samples should be taken into weighed tubes and re-weighed and counted as above. 4 h and 24 h urine volumes should be measured and aliquots taken into weighed tubes, re-weighed and counted. These activities should be decay corrected and related back to the initial injection. For blood clearance analysis, the activity in the 5 min sample is usually taken as 100%.

The images of the specimen may also be analysed by drawing regions of interest around the tumour and

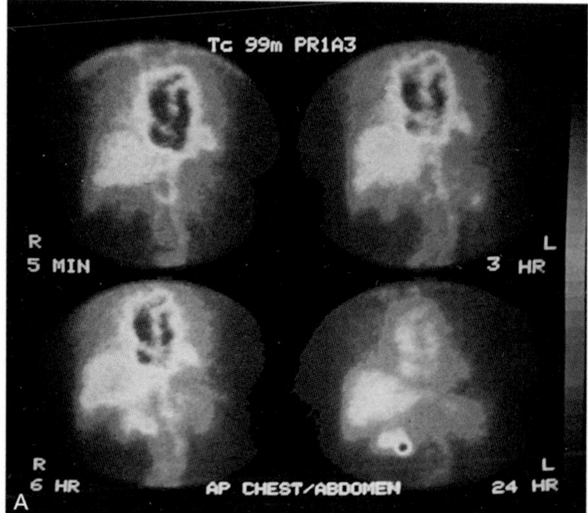

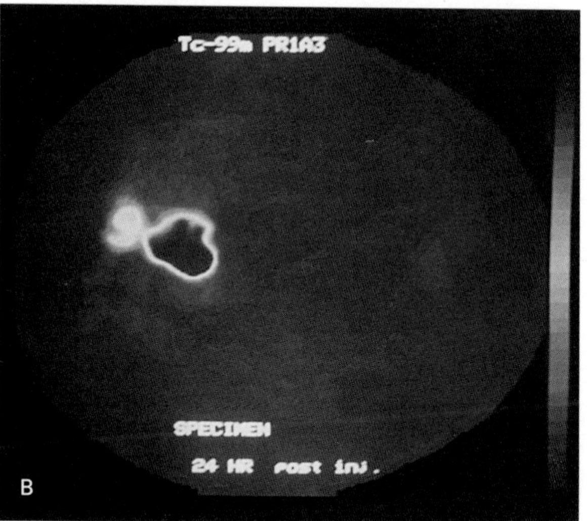

Fig. 68.2 Colon cancer: (A) RIS with ^{99m}Tc PR1A3 (ICRF) was undertaken in a man with carcinoma of the transverse colon starting the day before surgery. Anterior views of the upper abdomen are shown at 5 min top left, 3 h top right, 6 h bottom left and 24 h bottom right. The blood pool, initially red, decreases with time to yellow; the liver, yellow, stays much the same with time; an area of abnormal uptake inferior to the liver first appears at 6 h, yellow, and increases in uptake at 24 h, red, so that it is more active than the adjacent liver. This is specific uptake increasing with time in the colon carcinoma.
(B) Image of the surgical specimen on the same day as the 24 h image. The tumour, red and yellow, has high uptake compared to the mucosa, blue, tumour to mucosa ratio 63:1. 0.014% of the injected dose was in the tumour. Note no lymph nodes are seen in the specimen, none were involved with tumour, Duke's B. (Also shown in colour on Plate 18.)

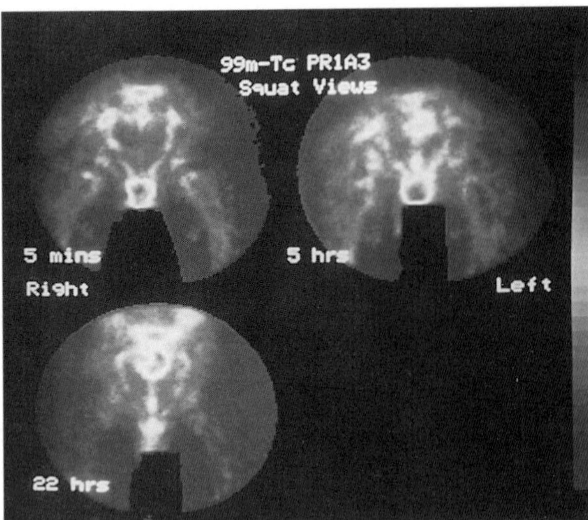

Fig. 68.3 Rectal cancer: RIS with ^{99m}Tc PR1A3. Squat views at 5 min top left, 5 h top right and 22 h bottom left. Uptake is seen in the scrotum at 5 min anteriorly but the pre-sacral area shows no uptake. At 5 h in addition to the scrotal and bladder activity, pre-sacral uptake is seen. At 22 h scrotal and bladder activity is reduced and pre-sacral uptake is further increased. A rectosigmoid adenocarcinoma, moderately differentiated, Dukes B, was resected. (Reproduced with permission from Eur J Nucl Med.) (Also shown in colour on Plate 18.)

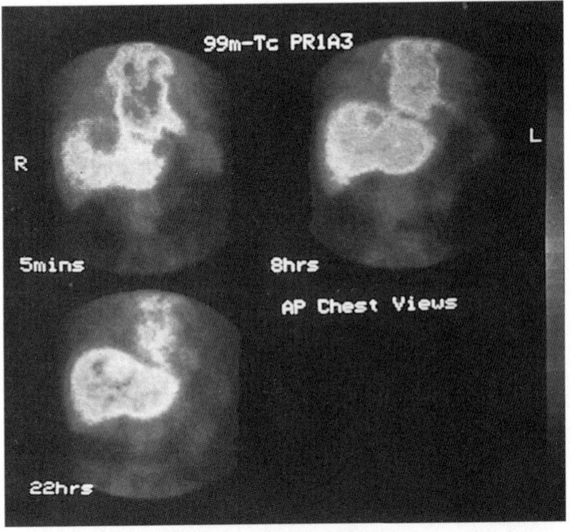

Fig. 68.4 Liver metastases: a 63-year-old man had rectal adenocarcinoma with a solitary hepatic metastasis 1 year previously. Anterior resection, chemotherapy and laser treatment of the liver metastasis was undertaken. X-ray CT of the liver metastasis showed complete necrosis and normal liver and abdomen elsewhere. It was thought that the laser treatment was a success. RIS with ^{99m}Tc-PR1A3 (ICRF) was performed. Anterior views of the upper abdomen top left 5 min, top right 8 h, bottom left 22 h. A large defect in the superior part of the right lobe and a small defect superiorly at the tip of the left lobe are seen on the 10 min image. Both show increasing uptake around the defects with time, indicating viable metastases. The defect of the right lobe appears to diminish in size with time and that in the left lobe becomes similar to the normal liver. (Reproduced with permission from Eur J Nucl Med). (Also shown in colour on Plate 19.)

adjacent normal tissue or surrounding mucosa. The counts per pixel for each region may be obtained and a tumour to normal tissue ratio calculated.

Image enhancement and analysis

The tumour signal is all important. The higher the count rate from the tumour, the easier its identification. This signal may be enhanced by a better antibody such as PR1A3 of which 0.01% injected dose per g of tumour is taken up as compared to an anti-CEA antibody where about 0.002% injected dose per g is bound. The signal advantage of ^{99m}Tc 600 MBq over ^{111}In 100–150 MBq, ^{123}I 120 MBq and ^{131}I 60 MBq injected is evident.[8] Once a high signal is established, then improvement in contrast may be obtained by reducing the tissue background. This may be by means of the more rapid clearance of a MAb fragment,[29,30] although part of this clearance is into the tumour environment; by SPECT;[10,12,31,32] by a second antimouse antibody injected to remove the unbound circulating primary murine antibody;[33] by a two or three stage technique[34–36] or by a subtraction technique.[27,37–39]

The more rapid the clearance, the greater the avidity of the MAb for tumour binding needs to be. Genetic engineering can increase the avidity of a 'designer' molecule based on a chosen highly selective antibody, but conventional Fab' and $F(ab')_2$ antibodies usually have lower affinity for tumour epitopes than the parent whole antibody.

The advantages of SPECT in reducing the effect of the tumour environment on the image is well known. The loss of familiar landmarks may be compensated for by using an arrow marker on one orthogonal view e.g. a transverse section, that automatically gives rise to the same site identified on the other planes e.g. coronal and sagittal; by three dimensional voxel rendering; or by superimposition of a transverse section on a corresponding X-ray CT or MRI image.[40] The problem of how to choose the correct contour as the cut-off to determine the volume of the lesion is not solved.[41] The use of a chaser system,[34,42] whether a second autoimmune antibody or a binding agent, has its main application to RIT. The three stage combination of an intravenous injection of a biotinylated tumour associated MAb, an injection of avidin (which has four potential binding sets for biotin) 3 days later to clear the blood of unbound biotin-MAb to the liver, and to link to the bound biotin-MAb on the tumour, and a day later injection of an ^{111}In-biotin complex, leads to background free tumour imaging within 1 h of the third stage.[35] Similar avidin–biotin dependent two stage approaches have been tried.[43] An alternative approach is to use a radiolabelled bifunctional antibody as a prelude to targeted RIT.[44–47]

Subtraction techniques have progressed. The early use of a ^{131}I MAb from which a ^{99m}Tc albumin distribution was subtracted[37] suffered from being subjective and from the inability to correct for the different attenuations of the differing radionuclides. Usually only large tumours were identified. A quantitative approach provided some improvement for colorectal cancer.[38] The method we

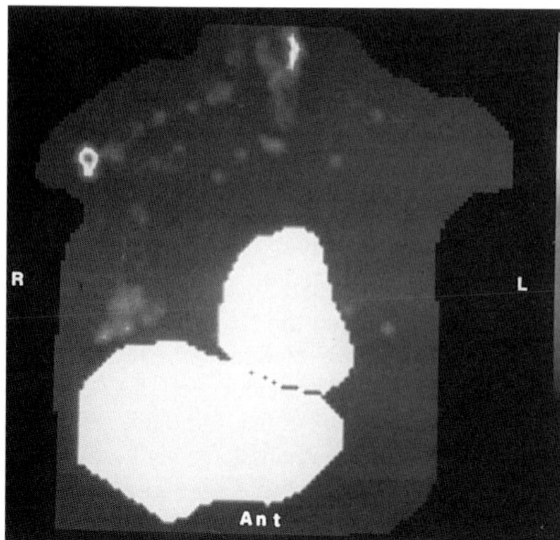

Fig. 68.5 Breast cancer: a woman with carcinoma evident clinically and on mammography in the right breast had RIS with ^{99m}Tc-SM3 (ICRF) before surgery to determine node involvement. Kinetic analysis with probability mapping was undertaken on the 10 min and 24 h anterior view images. The heart and liver are masked in yellow, the left breast and axilla are normal in dark blue ($P>0.05$ for change). The right breast shows significant uptake over an area ($P<0.05$ light blue) and the right axilla shows highly significant uptake ($P<0.001$ red). Changes in the neck and throat area are to be discounted because of movement. Involvement of right axillary nodes was confirmed at surgery. (Also shown in colour on Plate 19.)

adopted was to subtract the early (10 min) template image from the later images to show the sites of specific MAb uptake. This required the use of the repositioning protocol described before and was successful,[27] but also rather subjective. The development of a change detection algorithm called kinetic analysis with probability mapping overcame this problem. A simplified description is to say that the early image is plotted along one axis and the later image along the other axis so that no change between the two images is shown graphically as the 45° line of identity. A change between the images is shown as a deviation from this line. A chi square statistic is used to test the significance of the observed deviation from the expected line. Provided a cluster of five pixels shows significant differences, they are plotted as a probability value in the appropriate site in a new 'probability map' e.g. $P<0.05$ in green, $P<0.01$ in orange and $P<0.001$ in red with blue for the non-significant regions. In this way, in a prospective study, lesions down to 0.5 cm were identified in the abdomen.[28] The technique is applicable to demonstrating involved lymph nodes in breast cancer. Related approaches using change detection algorithms are being developed (Fig. 68.5).

THE ROLE OF RADIOIMMUNOSCINTIGRAPHY IN CANCER MANAGEMENT

The general approach has already been set out. This section describes applications of RIS in particular malignancies.

Melanoma

The increased desire for white races to expose their skin to the sun has led to a substantial increase in cutaneous melanoma. Extensive retrospective[20,21,48,49] and prospective multicentre studies[50] have been carried out in Italy using the Ferrone antibody against the high-molecular-weight antigen (supplied by Sorin Biomedica mainly as the 225.28S F(ab')$_2$ fragment). It has been labelled with the range of radionuclides. Sensitivity to melanoma detection was for ^{131}I 57%, for ^{111}In 77% and for ^{99m}Tc 86% when the data were analysed for stage II and stage III disease. Many unsuspected lesions were found but in stage IV disease many known lesions were not seen, probably because of loss of antigenic expression in the advanced disease. In the multicentre European study, the overall sensitivity was 78%, 501/728 positive lesions. In the prospective study using ^{99m}Tc 225.28S, the sensitivity was 78% and specificity 100%, an overall accuracy of 87%.[50]

The potential clinical benefits are less evident. Advanced stage melanoma has as yet no effective therapy so the identification of extra metastases above those already known is of marginal help to patient management. More important is the demonstration of lymph node involvement in relation to the primary tumour to identify the extent of primary surgery. This may be done by imaging after intralymphatic[51] or intravenous injection. Other anti-melanoma antibodies include P97,[52] 96.5[53] and anti GD$_2$, disialoganglioside, both murine and chimeric.[54]

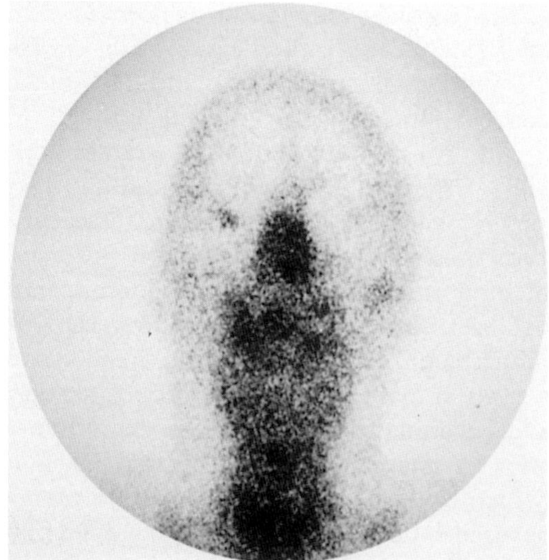

Fig. 68.6 Ocular melanoma: RIS with ^{99m}Tc-225.28S anti-melanoma fragments (Sorin) was performed at 10 min, 2, 4 and 6 h. There was increasing uptake with time in the superior part of the right orbit and not in the left orbit. The anterior 6 h view is shown. Malignant choroidal melanoma was confirmed at surgery.

Ocular melanoma has also been shown to react histologically and clinically with 225.28S. Imaging the eye helps to distinguish the pigmented melanoma from a benign naevus and melancytoma, and the amelanotic melanoma from the choroid haemangioma (Fig. 68.6). The sensitivity and specificity for melanoma are 95%.[55] Identification of neck glands or liver metastases helps to avoid unnecessary enucleation of the eye. Other metastases to the eye do not take up the anti-melanoma antibody but take up the appropriate tumour-associated MAb.[56]

Gastrointestinal cancers

Colorectal cancers

The survival of colorectal cancer is related to its staging at operation. The Dukes' classification[57] is as follows:

Dukes A: the tumour has spread into the tissue of the bowel wall but not beyond the muscularis propria

Dukes B: where the spread is beyond into perirectal or pericolonic tissue but no lymph nodes are involved

Dukes C: where lymph nodes are involved in addition.

X-ray CT has a poor record in determining lymph node involvement, for size, usually over 1 cm diameter, is taken as a criteria of malignancy. One survey showed 39 out of 59 nodes of less than 5 mm were in fact involved.[58] Another showed that CT had a sensitivity of 22% with 13 out of 20 involved nodes missed.[59] This is important since Dukes stage C1, less than four nodes involved, has a 50% 5 year survival whereas C2, four nodes or more, has a 25% 5 year survival.

This, the second commonest cancer in man, has attracted RIS from its earliest days. Early studies were with ^{131}I polyclonal antibodies[37] and ^{131}I monoclonal antibodies.[60,61] Imaging has evolved through ^{123}I[12,31], ^{111}In[2,62] and ^{99m}Tc radionuclides,[63–65] and through whole antibodies,[1] fragments,[29] including a multicentre study[66] and chimeric antibodies,[67] since then. Three types of antigen are used for making MAbs for RIS. First the dedifferentiation antigens such as carcinoma embryonic antigen (CEA). This is easily liberated from tumour tissue into venous blood and to lymphatics. In the blood it is used as a serum marker. It is in high concentration in the lymphatics draining the primary tumour and so normal nodes may be imaged[2] and porta hepatis nodes may be wrongly identified as being involved when a preoperative probe is used.[3] CEA is widely expressed in malignant tissues including lung, bladder and breast as well as gastrointestinal cancers. Good studies have been performed with ^{111}In anti-CEA[62] and with ^{99m}Tc anti-CEA.[63–65] There is an inverse relationship between tumour mass and tumour uptake of anti-CEA.[68]

Antigens may be extracted from malignant cells such as the tumour associated glycoprotein, TAG72, against which the B72.3 antibody is raised. This reacts with a number of malignancies because of its wide distribution. About 80% of colorectal cancers have this antigen. The antibody is commercially available with an ^{111}In label as Oncoscint[69–71] and may be available as a chimeric antibody[67] as is anti-CEA.[72]

An alternative approach is to use an epithelial surface antigen that is remote from the blood, but which the architectural disruption of the malignancy exposes in greater density to blood. PR1A3, also called 1A3, is such an antibody which reacts with a fixed antigen on the surface of colonic crypt cells.[73] It has a high specificity for colorectal cancer and due to the biological barriers, very little mucosal uptake. Normal lymph nodes do not show abnormal uptake since the antigen is fixed to the colorectal cancer cell surface (Fig. 68.2b).

Radioimmunoscintigraphy with ^{111}In anti-CEA[2,62] or ^{111}In B72.3[69,70] may identify primary cancer but excreted bowel and marrow activity may reduce specificity and liver metastases show poor contrast due to the high deposition of ^{111}In in the liver. Normal bowel activity is seen to move on serial images but inflammatory bowel disease, particularly Crohn's disease, will show a persistent site of abnormal bowel uptake with anti-CEA. Involved abdominal and extra-abdominal lymph nodes may be detected even when of normal size. Radioimmunoscintigraphy with ^{99m}Tc anti-CEA[63–65] or ^{99m}Tc 1A3[1,74,75] is generally positive for primary colorectal cancer (Fig. 68.2a and 68.3). It contributes to the management in the following circumstances. A second site of cancer may be identified and pelvic, abdominal or liver metastases may be demonstrated even when X-ray, CT or ultrasound may be normal. This change in staging alters management and prognosis and an unnecessary operation may be avoided.

The evaluation of recurrent colorectal cancer is no longer academic as second look surgery and radiotherapy are used to treat local recurrence. A direct attack on liver metastases may be made by surgery or laser treatment, and chemotherapy has become more effective. Intra-arterial radionuclide therapy is being evaluated. The identification of liver metastases is shown in Fig. 68.4.

Typically serum markers such as CEA are taken serially, and a rise is used to indicate recurrence. However, serum markers are not sensitive to small recurrences since a tumour has to be a certain size to liberate sufficient marker to reach a diagnostic level despite the dilution in the extracellular fluid volume, the normal biological variation and non-specific effects such as smoking. Serum markers may be normal in one third of patients who have a recurrence and do not localize the tumour or recurrence. Their most appropriate use is to follow the effects of therapy once they are elevated.

Dukes C colorectal cancers have a 50% chance of recurrence within 1 year. A policy of imaging patients using RIS at 1 year after primary surgery, even if symptom free and with a normal serum CEA, picks up a number of otherwise unsuspected recurrences, in 40% of patients in one small series.[75] After surgery symptoms may lead to ultrasound or X-ray CT of the abdomen or pelvis and a mass may be demonstrated. RIS has a number of advantages. The radiological techniques may not be able to distinguish whether it is due to post-surgical fibrosis or infection, or due to viable tumour. RIS shows specific uptake increasing with time only in the viable tumours. When serum markers are elevated, RIS can localize the recurrence which may be plaque-like and not seen on X-ray CT or ultrasound. The extent of disease shown by RIS may be greater than that shown radiographically and be an aid to local radiotherapy planning. These benefits of RIS make it an indispensable imaging technique in the management of patients with colorectal cancer after their primary surgery.

Preoperative radioimmunodetection (PROD) using a probe sensitive to ^{111}In or ^{99m}Tc may be helpful to the surgeon. Martin et al[76] undertook the original work with ^{125}I MAb injected 20–30 days before surgery and demonstrated the efficacy of this approach. Now the combination of RIS completed on the morning of surgery and PROD make for an efficient use of radiolabelled antibody. A typical protocol is to use a probe set for ^{99m}Tc such as the C-trak oncoprobe. This has a sensitivity of 22 counts/5s/kBq. It is covered with a sterile sheath. A series of three 5 s measurements are taken using a foot pedal and printer, first over the suspect tissue and then over the adjacent normal tissue. A ratio of 1.5 to 1 is considered significant and 2.3 to 1 highly significant. Highly vascular areas such as the aorta are shielded using a small sheet of tungsten in a sterile cover. The cut edge of a potential anastomotic site and the bed of the excised tumour are checked. Suspicious tissue is excised and counted again outside the operative field and compared with excised normal tissue.

Finally, specimens are re-weighed in weighed tubes, preserved, labelled, counted in a sample counter and sent for histology for final correlations to be made. In one series, 17 out of 19, 89% of patients had samples correctly identified by PROD with an average ratio of 2.3 ± 0.37 (1SEM) tumour to non-tumour tissue. The excised tissue had a mean ratio of 14 to 1 (uncorrected for weight) in the operating room. It is possible that this approach might become a form of 'instant frozen section'. The mean per cent injected dose per g for ^{99m}Tc 1A3 was 0.0094 ± 0.014 for the tumour tissue.[77] Preoperative probe studies, using ^{111}In or ^{99m}Tc MAb are still being generally evaluated.[3,78–80] There is a negligible radiation dose to the operators.[81]

In conclusion, imaging colorectal cancer by RIS with ^{99m}Tc MAb is successful in meeting the main clinical problems: the staging of primary colorectal cancer through the demonstration of involved intra- and extra-abdominal nodes, even when less than 1 cm, and the identification of small liver metastases; the early detection of recurrences; the separation of radiologically evident masses into those with viable tumour and those without, and assisting the surgeon at operation in demonstrating that a tumour bed is clear of disease.

Liver and pancreas cancer

Primary liver cancer, although rare in Europe and the United States is a major cancer worldwide. Only by early identification is it likely to be amenable to cure. Neither X-ray, CT or ultrasound are reliable for small tumours nor are they specific to primary liver tumours as compared to secondaries. The production of alphafetoprotein (AFP) by hepatoma has led to the development of MAbs against this antigen.[82–84] The Fc portion of whole antibody increases the non-specific liver uptake, so fragments are preferred. Addition of SPECT and the use of the radioiodine label which is deiodinated in the normal liver improves the image contrast. Alternative MAbs against hepatitis B antigen or hepatoma extracts are under consideration. The ^{99m}Tc label should help. Liver metastases are considered under colorectal cancer.

Stomach and pancreatic cancers may react with anti-CEA or anti-Ca19 MAbs.[85] RIS has made no clinical impact in their management as yet.

Insulinoma has been detected with ^{131}I radiolabelled anti-insulin antibodies.[86]

Gynaecological cancers

In recurrent gynaecological cancer RIS is particularly beneficial because the usual nature of spread is superficial and plaque-like. This spread is identified as positive on RIS but is often negative on ultrasound or X-ray CT, both of which have sensitivities of under 50% for recurrent ovarian cancer in the abdomen and pelvis.[87–89] The combination of serial imaging, squat views and SPECT, however, is necessary for the best results and this may be time-consuming. The same arguments apply in gynaecological recurrences as in colorectal cancer recurrences for serum markers and radiographically evident masses. The identification by RIS of recurrent disease after full chemotherapy is reducing the need for second look laparotomy. The demonstration of selective uptake in patients with malignant ascites strengthens the case for intra-abdominal RIT.

Ovarian cancer

Ovarian cancer is the second commonest cancer in women and often presents late. A range of antigens and antibodies are used and the generally vascular tumours give a good uptake.

The human milk fat globule (HMFG) glycoprotein antigens also called PEM (polymorphic epithelial mucin), were identified on the epithelial surface of the lactiferous duct of the breast, the lining of the ovarian follicle and at other sites, and led to the production of MAbs HMFG1 and HMFG2.[90] These are IgG1 class gamma globulins produced by the Imperial Cancer Research Fund Laboratories. The HMFG2 antigen has a 24 amino acid repeat sequence with Asp. Thr. Arg. in its epitope.[91] It was one of the first to be used for RIS of ovarian cancer. It was labelled initially with ^{123}I allowing SPECT to be undertaken as well as planar imaging,[10,11] and then with ^{99m}Tc.[1] It was successful in imaging cancer but reacted with many benign tumours.

SM3 (anti-stripped mucin 3) is a MAb against a core protein epitope of the polymorphic epithelial mucin antigen and was devised when it was shown that cancer cells have a reduced ability to glycosylate glycoprotein in their surface membrane. The mucin core protein was stripped of its glycosyl groups with hydrogen fluoride and used as an immunogen. SM3 was obtained and found to react with the epitope amino acid sequence: Pro. Asp. Thr. Arg. Pro., which includes the epitope with which HMFG2 reacts.[92,93] This is thought to be accessible in the cancer cell glycoprotein since there are fewer glycosyl branches concealing it from the antibody, whereas in the benign cell the more extensive branching tends to cover this larger sequence. SM3 has been shown to be more specific than HMFG for breast cancer as compared to benign breast tumours.[93] It has a high selectivity for breast, uterine and ovarian cancer, low selectivity for other cancers and for normal tissues. SM3 has a 17 times greater selectivity for malignant as compared to benign tumour on flow cytometric studies, whereas HMFG1 and HMFG2 have a selectivity of only 6 and 9 to 1 respectively.

At one extreme some gynaecological surgeons argue that any mass in the pelvis must be removed on the grounds that it may be malignant or that, if large and cystic, it may rupture. A screening study of 5000 well women led to 234 being operated for an ultrasound detected mass and nine malignancies were removed.[94] How many of the 225 women with benign disorders really needed operation? It may be reasonable to conclude that cysts over a certain size and cystadenoma should be removed although there is no convincing evidence that the cystadenoma is premalignant since their removal excludes the likelihood of recurrence. However, there is a histological spectrum from the benign adenoma through the 'borderline' malignant which does recur, to the definite ovarian cancer. A parallel may be drawn with the progression of a colorectal adenoma over a certain size to malignancy.[95] Clearly ultrasound is positive in the whole range of benign lesions and may be too non-specific. Corpus luteal cysts which are vascular on colour doppler ultrasound may be difficult to distinguish from malignancy. Is RIS with an agent such as ^{99m}Tc SM3 able to characterize not only the 'borderline malignancies' and cancers, but also to demonstrate those benign cystadenoma that 'need' operation? In such a case it would be reasonable to interpose ^{99m}Tc SM3 RIS between the ultrasound positive screen of well women and surgery. A study in a relatively unselected population would further validate or otherwise the efficacy of ^{99m}Tc RIS. This would be appropriate for the subgroup of well women with a higher risk of cancer.[96]

A wide range of MAb have been shown to be successful in imaging ovarian cancer. MOV18 is a MAb against an epitope extracted for ovarian cancer which appears to be related to folate reductase. It is labelled with ^{99m}Tc and used successfully for RIS.[97] OVTL3 is another well studied MAb for RIS of ovarian cancer,[30,98] as is OC125,[99] and Ovoscint.[100] The superiority of ^{111}In-OC125 over ultrasound and X-ray CT has been demonstrated in a correlative imaging study.[101]

The effectiveness of RIS in clinical management is increasing, both before primary surgery and after completion of chemotherapy.

Typical specificity in ovarian cancer for ^{99m}Tc MAb such as SM3 is 75%, sensitivity 100% and overall accuracy 93% with a positive predictive value of 92% and a negative predictive value of 100% at a prevalence of 76%,[102] (Figs 68.7 and 68.8).

Uterine and germ cell cancers

Many of the MAbs that react with ovarian cancer also act with endometrial cancers. An antibody against placental alkaline phosphatase H17E2 reacts both with endometrial and cervical cancers, as well as germ cell tumours of the ovary and testis.[103] H17E2 has been genetically engineered as a CDR grafted human reshaped antibody, labelled with ^{111}In[104] or with ^{99m}Tc[105] and used for RIS. Imaging choriocarcinoma using radiolabelled anti-HCG is well documented.[106,107]

Breast cancer

Breast cancer is the major cancer of women and small improvements in outcome mean a large number of women would benefit. The poor specificity of mammography has led to a large increase in breast biopsy.[108] It is said that for every 1000 mammographies 30 lesions are biopsied and three to five cancers found. Three in four impalpable mammography positive lesions are not malignant and five in six palpable mammography positive lesions are not malignant. MRI also has poor specificity.[109] Thallium-201 has a role in aiding the identification of malignancies in breasts whose mammography findings are difficult to interpret,[110] but ^{99m}Tc-MIBI, combined with mammog-

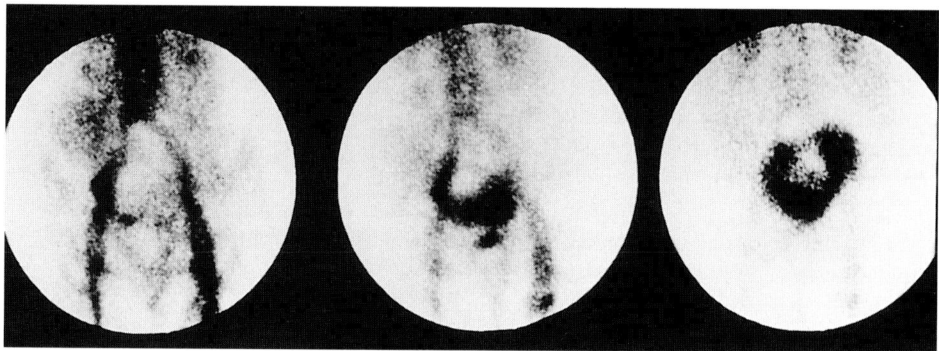

Fig. 68.7 Primary ovarian cancer: RIS with ^{99m}Tc-SM3 (ICRF) anterior views of the pelvis at 10 min left, 6 h centre and 22 h right. There is progressive uptake with time of the ^{99m}Tc-SM3 in the tumour mass which has a central defect; no abnormality is seen on the 10 min 'template' image, the first abnormality is seen at 22 h, due to an undifferentiated serous cystadenocarcinoma. (Reproduced with permission from Int J Biol Markers.)

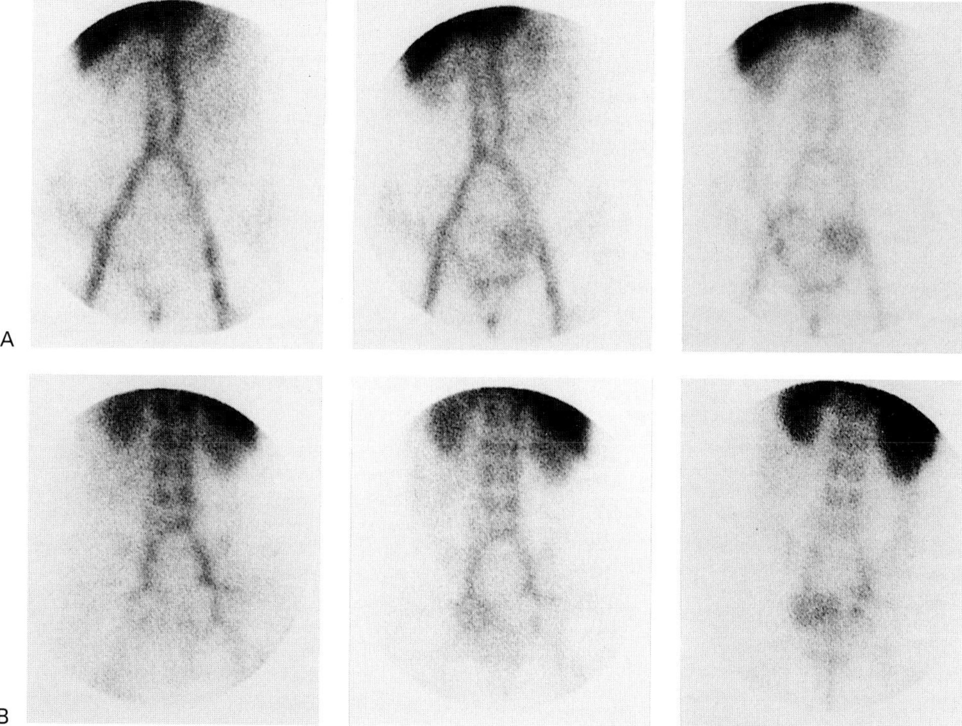

Fig. 68.8 Recurrent ovarian cancer: a 41-year-old woman had a left mesonephric ovarian cancer, FIGO stage 1c, removed 3 years previously followed by cisplatin. A recurrence last year was treated with radiotherapy. Left-sided abdominal pain led to examination showing a small left pelvic mass. CA125 was 21 units/ml, in the normal range.
(A) Radioimmunoscintigraphy with ^{99m}Tc-SM3 (ICRF), anterior views of the pelvis at 10 min (left), 4 h (centre) and 22 h (right) showed focal uptake increasing with time with a central defect situated in the left side of the pelvis. There is also a small focal area of uptake in the right side of the pelvis by the iliac vessels at 22 h.
(B) Posterior views of the pelvis at the same times. Focal uptake increasing with time is seen in the left side of the pelvis and the smaller site on the right side is evident. Left ovarian and right pararectal recurrences were confirmed at surgery.

raphy, is becoming the method of choice in improving the negative predictive value over the X-ray technique to 97%, and in reducing the number of unnecessary biopsies. It has a sensitivity of 96% and specificity of 75%.[111] The radical mastectomy, in which the breast cancer and the axillary nodes were all removed in one piece, has given way to the local lumpectomy and a variable degree of axillary sampling. The evidence from radical mastectomy showed that the presence and number of nodes involved is a major determinant of the prognosis of the patient. Since lumpectomy with local radiotherapy and/or adjuvant chemotherapy with tamoxifen is current treatment, so the determination, before surgery, of whether or not the local lymphatic nodes are involved before surgery has become of considerable importance. A reliable method of preoperative identification of involved nodes would help the surgeon to pursue lymph node sampling energetically.

The first approach was RIS after lymphangiography using anti-CEA initially labelled with ^{131}I,[112,113] and more recently ^{99m}Tc.[114] Although sensitivity and specificity are high, there are a number of problems with the intralymphatic approach. The MAb itself is a protein cleared intralymphatically to local nodes even in the absence of specific uptake. If the antigen, such as CEA, is shed from the tumour then it too will be in regional nodes even if malignant cells are not.

The intravenous route with a ^{99m}Tc radiolabel and a good MAb may be more efficacious. Lind et al have used ^{99m}Tc anti-CEA with SPECT,[115] for planar imaging is insufficient. 83% sensitivity was found in 45 patients, with nodes down to 7 mm being shown to be involved.

Distant metastases of breast cancer have been imaged. Problems include the effect of a high blood pool when ^{111}In-labelled MAb is used.[116] There is a feeling that the environment of breast cancer, whether due to charge or viscosity of the stroma, makes primary and metastatic breast cancer detection difficult. ^{111}In B72-3,[117] ^{111}In HMFG1,[118] ^{111}In-BrE-3 MAb[119] and ^{111}In human IgM MAb[120] have also been evaluated.

Other relatively specific antibodies include HMFG1 and two against the human milk fat globulin of the duct of the lactating breast[91] and SM3[93] against the mucin core protein of this polymorphic epithelial mucin.^{123}I HMFG2 was first used for breast RIS in 1982.[10] SM3 has a much more selective uptake by malignant than benign breast tumours. Studies with ^{99m}Tc SM3 are in progress,[121] (Fig. 68.5).

Since infection in the breast is a rare differential diagnosis for malignancy, non-specific tumour imaging techniques such as ^{18}F-deoxyglucose PET[122] and ^{99m}Tc-MIBI planar imaging and/or SPECT[111] are also effective in primary diagnosis. Their efficacy, and that of RIS, in the detection of involved axillary lymph nodes has to be better established with histopathological correlations before a definite clinical role can be established.[123,124]

Genitourinary cancer

Prostate cancer

Prostate cancer is common and approximately half prostate cancer patients present with disease which is not confined to the prostate (stages C and D). Such a finding at initial presentation considerably worsens the prognosis. In contrast to benign prostatic hypertrophy most carcinomas arise in the peripheral zone of tissue and the tumour often extends into and through the capsule of the gland to periprostatic tissues, to the seminal vesicles, to the bladder neck or rectum. Tumour invasion of perineural spaces and lymphatics as well as blood vessel invasion explains the tendency of prostate cancer to produce both lymphatic and distant metastases. The earliest lymph nodes to be involved are those in the periprostatic and obturator areas, next the external iliac and hypogastric lymph nodes and later the common iliac and para-aortic nodes. Lymph node involvement may be bilateral. Distant metastases usually involve the bony skeleton, less frequently liver, lungs and other sites. Five year survival in patients without pelvic lymph node involvement is 84% *vs.* 35% in patients with positive nodes.

The diagnostic evaluation of these patients includes CT scanning which has significant problems in detecting positive pelvic nodes. If the involved nodes are enlarged, that may either be due to involvement or due to the result of previous pelvic inflammatory disease. If the lymph nodes are normal, then involvement with prostate cancer cannot be excluded. CT is helpful, however, in determining whether other tissues are involved. Clearly, radioimmunoscintigraphy would be a useful adjunct to the staging of patients with prostate cancer and the selection of appropriate patients for radical prostatectomy.

Previous attempts to image prostate cancer have been with radiolabelled monoclonal antibodies against acid phosphatase which is not specific and against prostatic specific antigen which fails to work when, as often happens, the level of this antigen is raised in the blood.[125] The monoclonal antibody CYT356 reacts with a cytoplasmic membrane antigen of prostatic cancer cells. It is a murine IgG1 monoclonal antibody (Cytogen Corp). It has been labelled with ^{123}I and phase 3 clinical trials are underway with ^{111}In as the radiolabel.[126–128] It is also being labelled with ^{99m}Tc. Serial imaging is undertaken and squat views and SPECT are essential to aid the evaluation of the pelvis (Fig. 68.9).

The second main application is in patients who already present with metastatic disease. Bone scanning is well established but RIS can confirm that a lesion is due to metastases (Fig. 68.9). With the advent of radionuclide therapy for prostatic bone metastases, the need for demonstrating soft-tissue metastases becomes more important and RIS should have a role in this.

Carcinoma of the bladder

Bladder cancer has been imaged using ^{99m}Tc anti-CEA and involved lymph nodes have been successfully detected.[129] This has led to a trial of intravesical RIT.[130]

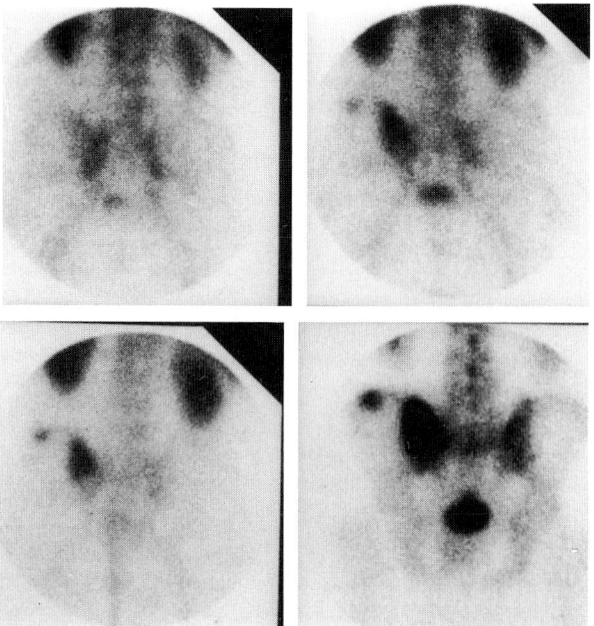

Fig. 68.9 Recurrent prostate cancer: RIS with ^{99m}Tc-CYT 351 (Cytogen), posterior views of the pelvis at 10 min top left, 6 h top right and 24 h bottom left. There is increasing uptake with time in two sites, the left sacroiliac region and the left iliac crest. Kidneys are evident superiorly and bladder activity inferiorly. ^{99m}Tc-MDP bone scan at 3 h bottom right was performed first and shows uptake only at these two sites. RIS confirmed that these sites are due to prostatic cancer.

Renal carcinoma

A number of investigators have tried RIS for renal carcinoma.[131–133] No clinical benefit has been reported as yet.

Lung cancer

Lung cancer is common and lethal. The clinical problems include the differentiation of a benign from a malignant lesion in a patient with a chest X-ray shadow; the evaluation of operability, particularly local hilar lymph node involvement; the presence of metastases; and the response to therapy. The range of lung cancers – small cell (SCLC) and non-small cell (NSCLC), including squamous cell, have a range of different tumour-associated antigens with some overlap. In SCLC and NSCLC there has been some success in imaging with anti-CEA MAb labelled with ^{111}In,[134] and ^{99m}Tc[135,136] and with HMFG1 labelled with ^{111}In.[137] Squamous cell cancer has been imaged with ^{131}I Po66.[138] Recently ^{99m}Tc-labelled antibodies, particularly NR-LU-10 Fab fragments have been used for RIS for staging the SCLC[139] and NSCLC.[140] Twenty-two out of 23 primary lung lesions were image positive correctly and the one negative image was a benign lesion. Sixteen out of the 21 patients who were mediastinal image positive were node positive confirmed at surgery. The RIS false-positives were less than those with X-ray CT.[141] Metastatic lung cancer was also well detected except for bone secondaries. Lung cancer, node involvement and metastatic lung disease are developing areas of RIS with potential clinical benefits.

Carcinoma of the head and neck

Squamous tumours

The clinical requirements are to detect local regional spread of nasopharyngeal buccal and lung cancers and identify involved nodes. When more than four lymph nodes are involved the risk of widespread metastases is 50%.

Because of the frequency of tonsillitis and other mouth infections, head and neck lymph nodes are often enlarged. Thus X-ray CT evidence of enlarged nodes does not in any way confirm that they are malignantly involved. Infection may also complicate the primary cause. Clinical assessment may be difficult due to induration of local tissues. Use of PET with ^{18}F-deoxyglucose is also non-specific as is MRI.[142] Conventional nuclear medicine techniques such as ^{99m}Tc DMSA(V) are not helpful.[143] Evidence of distant metastases together with knowledge of the extent of local involvement would be helpful in planning the surgical approach. It is also necessary to evaluate the completeness of resection after surgery and/or response to radiotherapy and give information on progression. MAbs reacting with squamous cell cancers have been made and used for RIS. MAb174 (H.64) from Biomira is used with 1.1 GBq ^{99m}Tc with planar and SPECT imaging at 6 and 18 h.[144] Successful demonstration of primary tongue, epiglottal and nasopharyngeal cancer has been achieved. The identification of lymph node involvement before surgery and recurrences after surgery have been demonstrated. A sensitivity of 96% and specificity of 97% is reported with lesions down to 1 cm confirmed.

^{99m}Tc E48-F(ab')$_2$ is another MAb used successfully for squamous carcinomas with similar results.[145]

Attempts have also been made to demonstrate parotid[146] and pharyngeal tumours[147] using RIS.

Thyroid carcinoma

Although the common thyroid cancers have been imaged with radiolabelled anti-thyroglobulin,[148,149] most attention has been paid to medullary carcinoma of the thyroid. RIS with radiolabelled anti-CEA has been successful[150,151] as has the bifunctional two stage approach[152] and probe localization of tumour during operation has been performed. Anti-calcitonin MAbs have also been used.[153]

Brain tumours

Disruption of the blood–brain barrier allows non-specific as well as specific antibodies to be taken up. As a prelude to the intrathecal therapy of malignant cerebral meningitis, Richardson et at[154] have demonstrated a range of brain tumours with radiolabelled UJ13A which also reacts with neuroblastoma. RIS has also been performed with MAbs against epidermal growth factor receptor and against placental alkaline phosphatase,[155] as a prelude to intra-arterial RIT; and with an anti-tenascin MAb as a prelude to intratumoral RIT of glioblastoma.[156,157]

Lymphoma

Hodgkins and non-Hodgkins lymphoma includes a diverse group of lymphoid neoplasms with a spectrum of clinical, morphological, immunological and molecular characteristics. Current treatment is curative for a proportion of patients with high grade lymphoma, but lymphomas of low grade malignancy are paradoxically much more difficult to cure. The majority are of B cell malignancy and appropriate characteristic surface antigens include CD19, 20, 21, 22, and 37. Unlabelled MAbs against such antigens have been used in serotherapy, but the problems include the low endogenous cytotoxicity of MAb, heterogeneity of antigen expression and the existence of antigen-negative tumour cells.

Lymphomas, because of their inherent radiosensitivity and easy access via the blood, appear good targets for RIT.[158–160] Uptake should first be confirmed by an imaging technique, although this principle is often ignored by oncologists who infuse large amounts of interferons and other biologically active cytokines unlabelled, without any check of their pharmacokinetics or tumour uptake using the radiolabelled equivalent. For example, interleukin 2 has been labelled with ^{123}I.[161] A number of studies of RIS and RIT have been performed using MAb Lym-1, an IgG2a, by the DeNardos.[162] A new ^{99m}Tc-labelled MAb LL2 has been successful in imaging lymphoma[163] and ^{131}I-LL2 for dosimetry for RIT.[160]

Cutaneous T cell lymphoma has been demonstrated by RIS with ^{131}I and ^{111}In radiolabelled MAb T101.[164,165] A new antibody reacting with Hodgkins disease, Ber-H2 against CD30 is being investigated. This, or the humanized CAMPATH II anti-CD4 antibody[166] are infused for direct immunotherapy but appear not to have been radiolabelled for RIS. Immunoscintigraphy of Hodgkins disease has been performed using ^{131}I antiferritin antibodies[159] and with MAbs derived from Hodgkins cell lines.[167] Anti-CD-33 MAb has been used in acute myeloid leukaemia mainly to evaluate marrow dosimetry for RIT.[168]

Sarcoma and neuroblastoma

Sarcoma in bone has been imaged with ^{131}I-791T/36,[169] a MAb that reacts with a number of adenocarcinomas as well. Rhabdomyosarcoma has been demonstrated using ^{111}In-labelled anti-myosin.[170]

RIS of neuroblastoma was keenly investigated with MAbs such as UJ13A (Fig. 68.10) before imaging and therapy with ^{123}I-MIBG and ^{131}I-MIBG became routine.[171] High affinity antibodies have been developed against ganglioside GD2 which give good results from RIS.[54] Dosimetry has been judged by using ^{124}I MAb with positron emission tomography.[172]

FUTURE DEVELOPMENTS

The future is 'designer molecules' for cancer targeting and therapy.[173,174]

Fear of the human antimouse antibody (HAMA) response, mainly by regulatory bodies, has led to the development of chimeric antibodies where the murine Fc portion is replaced by a human Fc, and human reshaped antibodies where all but the murine CDRs are genetically engineered to be human (Fig. 68.1). Whereas the HAMA response is unimportant for RIS where 0.5 mg MAb is typically sufficient, it becomes important for RIT where at least 10 mg of MAb are used in order to meet the therapeutic activity requirements and the need for tumour penetration. This is because a second injection of the MAb will be rapidly cleared by the HAMA in the form of immune complexes to the liver and reticuloendothelial system. This impairs its therapeutic efficiency. The HAMA response is two-fold. Antibodies are made against the Fc portion and frame which are called 'isotypic'; and antibodies are made against the CDRs which are called 'idiotypic'. Reshaped human MAb avoid the isotypic HAMA, but not the idiotypic response. Murine MAbs

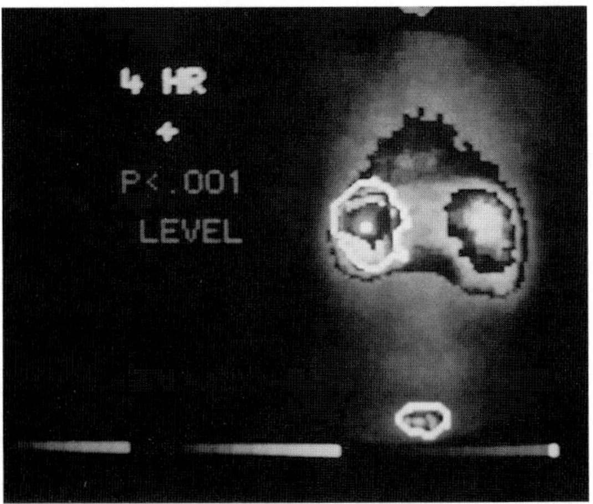

Fig. 68.10 Neuroblastoma: RIS with ^{99m}Tc-UJ13A (ICRF). Posterior view of a 4-year-old child at 4 h. Visual display shows the tumour superior to the spleen in red, the spleen, liver and bladder in yellow and green, and tissue background activity in blue. Kinetic analysis with probability mapping of the 10 min and 4 h images is displayed as a white contour at sites of significant change between the two images: the tumour site and urinary excretion of activity into the bladder. (Also shown in colour on Plate 19.)

generate both responses but HAMA is not related to clinical reactions which occur in about 1:1000 patients when less than 1 mg MAb is given intravenously.

The idiotypic response is complex. A human idiotype 1 is induced first and then a human idiotype 2 can be induced against the CDRs of the idiotype 1. The CDRs of idiotype 2 are now appropriate to react with the original tumour epitope. In this way, the idiotypic HAMA response actually induces human anti-tumour human antibodies, HAHA.[175] A survival advantage has been observed for patients with ovarian cancer having RIS in whom idiotype 2 antibodies have been demonstrated.[176] Thus HAMA and HAHA may have unexpected benefits. The development of such 'antigenized' antibodies is active.[177]

Genetic engineering is playing a major role in the development of RIS and RIT[178–180] and is progressing in two directions[4] (see Fig. 68.1): the development of single chain Fv and molecular recognition units, and the clinical application for RIS of chimeric and reshaped human antibodies. The new generation of humanized MAbs[181–183] include the Campath IH for lymphoma,[166] the 88BV59 anti-cytokeratin for colorectal cancer[184] and the humanized H17E2 for ovarian cancer.[104,105]

An alternative approach to the production of human MAb is through the culture of human stem cell lymphocytes extracted from patients with cancer and the selection of appropriate human MAb producing clones.[185] Clinical tests of such human MAb have been undertaken in colorectal cancer[186,187] and breast cancer.[120] The progress has been summarized by De Jaeger et al.[188] By comparison, the production of human MAb from human hybridomas has met some difficulties.[189]

There are several techniques for the 'pretargeting' tumours through a two or three stage approach to RIS: the use of the avidin–biotin system.[35,36,43,46,190] and the use of a bifunctional antibody. This has two different antigen binding sites, for example one against a cancer epitope and one against a radiolabelled diagnostic or therapeutic agent.[44,46,47,191–193] These are being tested through imaging but are designed for therapy.

CONCLUSION

The selectivity of an antibody for an antigen is the motivation for RIS and RIT. As a tumour enlarges the proportion of cancer to stromal cells decreases and there is a greater opportunity for the uptake of non-specific agents. Thus RIS is designed to image small tumours, particularly those not evident clinically or radiologically. For this task RIS requires the best imaging signal, technetium-99m, and the most avid and specific antibody. Spurred on by the needs of RIT, the specific binding sites of the antibody are being manipulated by genetic and chemical engineering to improve affinity, reduce antigenicity and increase delivery. This in turn leads to a convergence of receptor binding agents, biologically active molecules, enzymes and their substrates and antibody–antigen reactions to a common binder–bindee framework. The mimicking of the strategies of the immune system by engineering repertoires of human antibodies of high specificities and affinities is a major development.[194] The use of two or three stage targeting enables selective tumour uptake of such agents to be associated with very low non-target uptake. The search for the cancer-specific bindee, based on its genetic abnormalities and the interplay of oncogene and anti-oncogene determined growth control, has caught the imagination of the scientific community and the eye for a market of commercial companies.

By contrast, man the regulator[173,195] and man the seeker after patents[196] is having a generally negative effect on the development of this field by imposing heavy costs. Nevertheless, now that the first murine antibodies are licensed for imaging, new generations of antibodies, both murine and humanized, and new related designer molecules will benefit the diagnosis and management of patients with cancer in the future.

REFERENCES

1. Granowska M, Mather S J, Britton K E 1991 Diagnostic evaluation of ^{111}Tc and ^{99}Tc^{m} radiolabelled monoclonal antibodies in ovarian and colorectal cancer: correlations with surgery. Nucl Med Biol 18: 413–424
2. Granowska M, Jass J R, Britton K E, Northover J M A 1989 A prospective study of the use of ^{111}In-labelled monoclonal antibody against carcino-embryonic antigen in colorectal cancer and of some biological factors affecting its uptake. Int J Colorectal Dis 4: 97–108
3. Kuhn J A, Corbisiero R M, Buras R R et al 1991 Intraoperative gamma detection probe with presurgical antibody imaging in colon cancer. Arch Surg 126: 1398–1403
4. Winter G, Milstein C 1991 Man made antibodies. Nature 349: 293–299
5. Kulkarni P V, Constantinescu P, Das C, Antich P P, Tucker P 1991 Design and evaluation of recombinant antibody-like metallothionein labelled with ^{99m}Tc for radioimmunoimaging. J Nucl Med 21: 915
6. Foxwell B M J, Band H A, Long J et al 1988 Conjugation of monoclonal antibodies to a synthetic peptide substrate for protein kinase: a method of labelling antibodies with 32-P. Brit J Cancer 57: 489–503
7. Hertel A, Baum R P, Auerbach B, Herrmann A, Hör G 1990 Klinische Relevanz humaner Anti-Maus-Antikorper (HAMA) in der Immunszintigraphie. Nucl Med 29: 221–227
8. Britton K E, Granowska M 1987 Radioimmunoscintigraphy in tumour identification. Cancer Surveys 6: 247–267
9. Macey D J, DeNardo G L, DeNardo S J, Hines H H 1986 Comparison of low and medium energy collimaters for SPECT imaging with iodine-123-labelled antibodies. J Nucl Med 27: 1474–1476
10. Epenetos A A, Britton K E, Mather S et al 1982 Targeting of

iodine-123 labelled tumour-associated monoclonal antibodies to ovarian, breast and gastrointestinal tumours. Lancet ii: 999–1005
11. Granowska M, Shepherd J, Britton K E et al 1984 Ovarian cancer: diagnosis using I-123 monoclonal antibody in comparison with surgical findings. Nucl Med Commun 5: 485–499
12. Berche C, Mach J P, Lumbroso J D et al 1982 Tomoscintigraphy for detecting gastrointestinal and medullary thyroid cancers: first clinical result using radiolabelled monoclonal antibodies against carcino-embryonic antigen. Brit Med J 285: 1447–1451
13. Hnatowich D J, Childs R L, Lanteigne D, Najafi A 1983 The preparation of DTPA-coupled antibodies radiolabelled with metallic radionuclides: an improved method. J Immunol Methods 65: 147–157
14. Hnatowich D J 1990 Antibody radiolabelling, problems and promises. Nucl Med Biol 17: 49–55
15. Mather S J 1987 Labelling with Indium-111. In: Kristensen K, Norbygaard E, eds. Safety and efficacy of radiopharmaceuticals. Martinus Nijhoff, Amsterdam. pp 51–66
16. Boyle C C, Paine A J, Mather S J 1992 The mechanism of hepatic uptake of a radiolabelled monoclonal antibody. Int J Cancer 50: 912–917
17. Meares C F, Moi M K, Diril H et al 1990 Macrocyclic chelates of radiometals for diagnosis and therapy. Br J Cancer 62(Suppl X): 21–26
18. Rhodes B A, Zamora P A, Newell K D, Valdez E F 1986 Tc-99m labelling of murine monoclonal antibody fragments. J Nucl Med 27: 685–693
19. Rhodes B A, Burchiel S W 1982 Radiolabelling of antibodies with technetium-99m. In: Burchiel S W, Rhodes B A, eds. Radioimmunoimaging. Elsevier Science, New York. pp 207–222
20. Buraggi G L, Callegaro L, Turrin A et al 1984 Immunoscintigraphy with I-123, $^{99}Tc^{m}$ and In-111 F $(ab')_2$ fragments of monoclonal antibodies to a high molecular weight melanoma associated antigen. J Nucl Med Allied Sci 28: 283–295
21. Buraggi G L, Turrin A, Cascinelli N et al 1984 Immunoscintigraphy with antimelanoma monoclonal antibodies. In: Donato L, Britton K E, eds. Proceedings of the European Symposium on Immunoscintigraphy, Saariselka, Finland 1983. Monographs in nuclear medicine, Vol I Immunoscintigraphy. Gordon & Breach, New York. pp 215–253
22. Schwarz A, Steinstrasser A 1987 A novel approach to Tc-99m labelled monoclonal antibodies. J Nucl Med 28: 721 (Abstract)
23. Mather S J, Ellison D 1990 Reduction-mediated Tc-99m labelling of monoclonal antibodies. J Nucl Med 31: 692–697
24. Thakur M L, DeFulvio J, Richard M D, Park C H 1991 Technetium-99m labelled monoclonal antibodies: evaluation of reducing agents. Nucl Med Biol 18: 227–233
25. Fritzberg A R, Abrahams P G, Beaumier P L et al 1989 Specific and stable labelling of antibodies with technetium 99m with a diamide dithiolate chelating agent. Proc Nat Acad Sci USA 85: 4025–4029
26. Lanteigne D, Hnatowich D J 1984 The labelling of DTPA-coupled proteins with Tc99m. Int J Appl Radiat Isotopes 35: 617–621
27. Granowska M, Britton K E, Shepherd J 1983 The detection of ovarian cancer using 123-I monoclonal antibody. Radiobiol Radiother (Berlin) 25: 153–160
28. Granowska M, Nimmon C C, Britton K E et al 1988 Kinetic analysis and probability mapping applied to the detection of ovarian cancer by radioimmunoscintigraphy. J Nucl Med 29: 599–607
29. Wahl R L, Parker C W, Philpot G 1983 Improved radioimaging and tumour localisation with monoclonal $(Fab')_2$. J Nucl Med 24: 316–325
30. Tibben J G, Massuger L F A G, Claessens R A M J et al 1992 Tumour detection and localisation using $^{99}Tc^{m}$ labelled OVTL3 Fab' in patients suspected of ovarian cancer. Nucl Med Commun 13: 885–893
31. Delaloye B, Bischof-Delaloye A, Buchegger F et al 1986 Detection of colorectal carcinoma by Emission-Computerized Tomography after injection of ^{123}I-labelled F ab and F $(ab')_2$ fragments from monoclonal anti-CEA antibodies. J Clin Invest 77: 301–321
32. Perkins A C, Whalley D R, Ballantyne K C, Pimm M V 1988 Gamma camera emission tomography using radiolabelled antibodies. Eur J Nucl Med 14: 45–49
33. Begent R H J, Keep P A, Green A J et al 1983 Liposomally entrapped second antibody improves tumour imaging with radiolabelled (first) anti-tumour antibody. Lancet ii: 739–741
34. Goodwin D A, Meares C F, McCall M J, Chaovapong W, MeTique M, Diamanti C I 1989 Improved tumour uptake with In-111, Ga-67 and Ga-68 labelled bivalent haptens in pretargetted immunoscintigraphy. J Nucl Med 30: 762–764
35. Paganelli G, Malcovati M, Fazio F 1991 Monoclonal antibody pretargetting techniques for tumour localisation: the avidin biotin system. Nucl Med Commun 12: 211–234
36. Paganelli G, Magnani P, Zito F et al 1991 Three-step monoclonal antibody tumour targetting in carcinoembryonic antigen-positive patients. Cancer Res 51: 5960–5966
37. Goldenberg D M, Kim E, Deland F H, Benne H S, Primus F J 1980 Radio-immunodetection of cancer with radioactive antibodies to carcino-embryonic antigen. Cancer Res 40: 2984–2992
38. Green A J, Begent R H J, Keep P A, Bagshawe K D 1984 Analysis of radio-immunodetection of tumours by the subtraction technique. J Nucl Med 25: 96–100
39. Liehn J C, Hannequin P, Nasea S et al 1987 A new approach to image subtraction in immunoscintigraphy: preliminary results. Eur J Nucl Med 13: 391–396
40. Loboguerrero A, Perault C, Liehn J C 1992 Volume rendering and bicolour scale in double isotope studies: application to immunoscintigraphy and bone landmarking. Eur J Nucl Med 19: 201–204
41. Macey D J, DeNardo G L, DeNardo S J 1988 Comparison of three boundary detection methods for SPECT using computer scattered photons. J Nucl Med 29: 203–207
42. Goodwin D A, Mears C F, McCall M J, McTigue M, Choavapong W 1988 Pretargetted immunoscintigraphy of murine tumours with In-111 labelled bifunctional haptens. J Nucl Med 29: 226–234
43. Kalofonos H P, Rusckowski M, Siebecker D A et al 1990 Imaging of tumour in patients with Indium-111 biotin and streptavidin-conjugated antibodies: preliminary communication. J Nucl Med 31: 1791–1796
44. Bosslet K, Steinstrasser A, Hermentin P et al 1991 Generation of bispecific monoclonal antibodies for 2 phase radioimmunotherapy. Brit J Cancer 63: 681–686
45. Britton K E, Slevin M L, Mather M et al 1990 Radiolabelled antibodies in therapy. In: Baldwin R W, Byers V S, Mann R D, eds. Monoclonal antibodies and immunoconjugates. Cornforth Pathenon, pp 145–157
46. Britton K E, Mather S J, Granowska M 1991 Radioimmunolabelled monoclonal antibodies in oncology, III. Radioimmunotherapy. Nucl Med Commun 12: 333–347
47. Le Doussal J M, Martin M, Gautherot E et al 1989 In vitro and in vivo targeting of radiolabelled monovalent and divalent haptens with dual specificity antibody conjugates; enhanced divalent haptens affinity for cell-bound antibody conjugate. J Nucl Med 30: 1358–1366
48. Siccardi A G, Buraggi G L, Callegaro L et al 1986 Multicentre study of immunoscintigraphy with radiolabelled monoclonal antibodies in patients with melanoma. Cancer Res 46: 4817–4822
49. Feggi L, Indelli M, Pansini G C et al 1993 Immunoscintigraphy in malignant melanoma: a five year clinical experience. Nucl Med Commun 14: 145–148
50. Siccardi A G, Buraggi G L, Natali P G et al 1990 European multicentre study on melanoma immunoscintigraphy by means of ^{99m}Tc-labelled monoclonal antibody fragments. Eur J Nucl Med 16: 317–323
51. Weinstein J, Parker R, Holton O et al 1985 Lymphatic delivery of monoclonal antibodies: potential for detection and treatment of lymph node metastases. Cancer Invest 3: 85–95
52. Larson S M, Brown J P, Wright P W, Carrasquillo J A, Hellstrom I, Hellstrom K E 1983 Imaging of melanoma with I-131 labelled monoclonal antibodies. J Nucl Med 23: 123–129
53. Halpern S E, Dillman R O, Witztium K F 1985

Radioimmunodetection of melanoma utilizing ^{111}In-96.5 monoclonal antibody. Radiology 155: 493–499
54. Cheung N K V, Lazarus H, Miraldi F D et al 1987 Ganglioside GD2 specific monoclonal antibody 3F8: a phase 1 study in patients with melanoma and neuroblastoma. J Clin Oncol 5: 1430–1440
55. Bomanji J, Hungerford J L, Granowska M, Britton K E 1987 Radioimmunoscintigraphy of ocular melanoma with ^{99}Tc^{m} labelled cutaneous melanoma antibody fragments. Br J Ophthalmol 71: 651–658
56. Bomanji J, Glaholm J, Hungerford J L et al 1990 Radioimmunoscintigraphy of orbital metastases from ovarian cancer. Clin Nucl Med 15: 825–827
57. Dukes C E 1932 The classification of cancer of the rectum. J Path Bact 35: 323–332
58. Herrera-Ornelas L, Justiniano J, Castillo N et al 1987 Metastases in small lymph nodes from colon cancer. Arch Surg 122: 1253–1256
59. Thompson W M, Halvorsen R A, Foster W L, Roberts L, Gibbons R 1986 Preoperative and postoperative CT staging of rectosigmoid carcinoma. Am J Roentgenol 146: 703–710
60. Mach J P, Carrel S, Forni M et al 1980 Tumour localisation in patients by radiolabelled antibodies against carcinoembryonic antigen in patients with carcinoma. New Eng J Med 303: 5–10
61. Chatal J F, Saccavini J C, Furnoleau P et al 1984 Immunoscintigraphy of colon carcinoma. J Nucl Med 25: 307–314
62. Halpern S E, Dillman D O, Amox D et al 1992. Detection of occult tumour using indium-111 labelled anticarcinoembryonic antigen antibodies. Arch Surg 127: 1094–1100
63. Baum R P, Hertel A, Lorenz M et al 1989 ^{99}Tc^{m} labelled anti-CEA monoclonal antibody for tumour immunoscintigraphy: first clinical results. Nucl Med Commun 10: 345–348
64. Lind P, Langsteger W, Költringer P et al 1989 Tc^{99m}-labelled monoclonal anticarcinoembryonic antigen antibody (BW 431/26). Scand J Gastrenterol 24: 1205–1211
65. Muxi A, Sola M, Bassa P et al 1992 Radioimmunoscintigraphy of colorectal carcinoma with a ^{99m}Tc-labelled anti-CEA monoclonal antibody (BW 431/26). Nucl Med Commun 13: 261–270
66. Siccardi A G, Buraggi G L, Callegaro L et al 1989 Immunoscintigraphy of adenocarcinomas by means of radiolabelled F (ab')$_2$ fragments of anti-carcinoembryonic antigen monoclonal antibody: a multicenter study. Cancer Res 49: 3095–3103
67. LoBuglio A F, Wheeler R H, Trang J et al 1989 Mouse/human chimeric monoclonal antibody in man: kinetics and immune response. Proc Natl Acad Sci USA 86: 4220–4224
68. Williams L E, Barnes R B, Fass J et al 1993 Uptake of radiolabelled anti-CEA antibodies in human colorectal primary tumours as a function of tumour mass. Eur J Nucl Med 20: 345–347
69. Collier B D, Abdel-Nabi H, Doerr R J et al 1992 Immunoscintigraphy performed with In-111 labelled CYT-103 in the management of colorectal cancer; comparison with CT. Radiology 185: 179–186
70. Doerr R J, Abdel-Nabi H, Krag D, Mitchell E 1991 Radiolabelled antibody imaging in the management of colorectal cancer; results of a multicenter clinical study. Ann Surg 214: 118–124
71. Abdel-Nabi H, Doerr R J 1993 Clinical applications of indium-111-labelled monoclonal antibody imaging in colorectal cancer patients. Semin Nucl Med 23: 99–113
72. Bischof-Delaloye A, Delaloye B 1992 Diagnostic applications and therapeutic approaches with different preparations of anti-CEA antibodies. Int J Biol Mark 7: 193–197
73. Richman P I, Bodmer W F 1987 Monoclonal antibodies to human colorectal epithelium: markers for differentiation and tumour characterization. Int J Cancer 39: 317–328
74. Granowska M, Mather S J, Britton K E et al 1990 ^{99}Tc^{m} radioimmunoscintigraphy of colorectal cancer. Br J Cancer 62(Suppl X): 30–33
75. Granowska M, Britton K E, Mather S J et al 1993 Radioimmunoscintigraphy with technetium-99m labelled monoclonal antibody 1A3 in colorectal cancer. Eur J Nucl Med 20: 690–698
76. Martin E W, Mojzisik C M, Hinkle G H et al 1988 Radioimmunoguided surgery using monoclonal antibody. Am J Surg 156: 386–392
77. Granowska M, Britton K E, Morris G et al 1993 Peroperative radioimmunodetection with Tc-99m labelled monoclonal antibodies in colorectal and gynaecological surgery. J Nucl Med 34: 82P
78. Reuter M, Montz R, de Heer K et al 1992. Detection of colorectal carcinomas by investigative RIS in addition to preoperative RIS: surgical and immunohistochemical findings. Eur J Nucl Med 19: 102–109
79. Curtet C, Vuillez J P, Daniel G et al 1990 Feasibility study of radioimmunoguided surgery of colorectal carcinomas using indium-111 CEA specific monoclonal antibody. Eur J Nucl Med 17: 299–304
80. Aprile C, Prati U, Saponaro R, Roveda L, Carena M, Gastaldo L 1991 Radioimmunolocalization of pelvic recurrences from rectosigmoid cancer employing ^{111}In-anti CEA F (ab'$_2$). Nucl Med Biol 18: 51–52
81. Bares R, Muller B, Fass J, Buell V, Schumpelick V 1992 The radiation dose to surgical personnel during intraoperative radioimmunoscintigraphy. Eur J Nucl Med 19: 110–112
82. Kim E E, Deland F H, Nelson M D et al 1980 Radioimmunodetection of cancer with radiolabelled antibodies to alpha-fetoprotein. Cancer Res 40: 3008–3012
83. Nakata K, Furukawa R, Kono K et al 1984 Tumour-serum ratios of alpha-fetoprotein and radioimmunolocalization of primary liver cancer. Tumour Biol 5: 161–169
84. Bergman J F, Lambroso J D, Manil L et al 1987 Radiolabelled monoclonal antibodies against alpha-fetoprotein for in vivo localization of human hepatocellular carcinoma by immunotomoscintigraphy. Eur J Nucl Med 13: 385–390
85. Montz R, Klapdor R, Rothe B et al 1986 Immunoscintigraphy and radioimmunotherapy in patients with pancreatic carcinoma. Nucl Med 25: 239–244
86. Chapman C E, Fairweather D S, Keeling A A et al 1987 An evaluation of anti-insulin scanning in patients with suspected insulinoma. Clin Endocrinol 26: 433–440
87. Blaquire R M, Husband J E 1983 Conventional radiology and computed tomography in ovarian cancer. J Roy Soc Med 76: 574–579
88. Khan O, Cosgrove D O, Wiltshaw K et al 1983 Role of ultrasound in the management of ovarian carcinoma. J Roy Soc Med 76: 821–827
89. Calkins A R, Stehman F B, Wass J L, Smirz L R, Ellis J H 1987 Pitfalls in interpretation of computed tomography prior to second look laparatomy in patients with ovarian cancer. Br J Radiol 60: 975–979
90. Taylor-Papadimitrou J, Peterson J A, Arklie J et al 1981 Monoclonal antibodies to epithelium specific components of the human milk fat globule membrane, production and reaction with cells in culture. Int J Cancer 28: 17–21
91. Burchell J, Gendler S, Taylor-Papadimitrou J et al 1987 Development and characterisation of breast cancer reactive monoclonal antibodies directed to the core protein of the human milk mucin. Cancer Res 47: 5476–5482
92. Burchell J, Taylor-Papadimitrou J, Boshell M et al 1989 A short sequence, within the amino acid repeat of a cancer-associated mucin, contains immunodominant epitopes. Int J Cancer 44: 691–696
93. Girling A, Bartkora J, Burchell J et al 1989 A core protein epitope of the polymorphic epithelial mucin detected by monoclonal antibody SM3 is selectively exposed in a range of primary carcinomas. Int J Cancer 43: 1072–1076
94. Campbell S, Bhan V, Royston P et al 1989 Transabdominal ultrasound screening for early ovarian cancer. Brit Med J 76: 574–579
95. Day D W, Morson B C 1978 The adenoma carcinoma sequence. In: Morson B C, ed. The pathogenesis of colorectal cancer. W B Saunders & Co, Philadelphia. pp 48–61

96. Bourne T H, Whitehead M I, Campbell S et al 1991 Ultrasound screening for familial ovarian cancer. Gynaecol Oncol 43: 92–97
97. Crippa F, Buraggi G L, Di Re E et al 1991 Radioimmunoscintigraphy of ovarian cancer with the MOV-18 monoclonal antibody. Eur J Cancer 27: 724–729
98. Massuger L, Claessens R, Kenemans P et al 1991 Kinetics and biodistribution in relation to tumour detection with 111-In-labelled OV-TL3 F $(ab')_2$ in patients with ovarian cancer. Nucl Med Commun 12: 593–609
99. Maughan T S, Haylock B, Hayward M et al 1990 OC 125 immunoscintigraphy in ovarian carcinoma: a comparison with alternative methods of assessment. J Clin Oncol 2: 199–205
100. Jusko W J, Kung L P, Schmelter R F 1992 Immunopharmacokinetics of ^{111}In-CYT-103 in ovarian cancer patients. In: Maguire R T, Van Nostrand D, eds. Diagnosis of colorectal and ovarian carcinoma. Marcel Dekker, New York. Ch 10
101. Peltier P, Wiharto K, Dutin J P et al 1992 Correlative imaging study in the diagnosis of ovarian cancer recurrences. Eur J Nucl Med 19: 1006–1010
102. Granowska M, Britton K E, Mather S J et al 1993 Radioimmunoscintigraphy with technetium-99m labelled monoclonal antibody, SM3, in gynaecological cancer. Eur J Nucl Med 20: 483–489
103. Epenetos A A, Snook D, Hooker G et al 1985 Indium-111 labelled monoclonal antibody to placental alkaline phosphatase in the detection of neoplasms of testes, ovary and cervix. Lancet 2: 350–353
104. Snook D E, Verheoyen M, Kormas C et al 1993 A preliminary comparison of a tumour associated reshaped human monoclonal antibody (Hu2 PLAP) with its murine equivalent (H17E2). In: Epenetos A A, ed. Monoclonal antibodies 2: applications in clinical oncology. Chapman and Hall, London. pp 391–400
105. Granowska M, Mather S J, Britton K E 1993 ^{99m}Technetium-labelled antibodies for radioimmunoscintigraphy. In: Epenetos A A, ed. Monoclonal antibodies 2: applications in clinical oncology. Chapman and Hall, London. pp 375–382
106. Begent R H J, Stanway G, Jones B E et al 1980 Radioimmunolocalisation of tumours by external scintigraphy after administration of ^{131}I antibody to human gonadotrophin. Preliminary communication. J Roy Soc Med 73: 624–650
107. Morais J, Peltier P, Chatal J F, Fumoleau P, Chetanneau A, Bourguet P 1992 Anti-βHCG abdominopelvic immunoscintigraphy in patients with resistant gestational trophoblastic disease. Nucl Med Commun 13: 464–466
108. Hams J R, Lippman M E, Veronesi W, Willett W 1993 Breast cancer. New Eng J Med 327: 319–328, 390–398, 473–480
109. Harms S E, Flamig D P, Hesley K L et al 1993 MR imaging of the breast with rotating delivery of excitation of resonance; clinical experience with pathological correlation. Radiology 187: 493–501
110. Waxman A D, Ramanna L, Memscio L D et al 1993 Thallium scintigraphy in the evaluation of mass abnormalities of the breast. J Nucl Med 34: 18–23
111. Khalkhali I, Mena I, Jouanne E et al 1993 Tc-99m-sesta MIBI prone imaging in patients with suspicion of breast cancer. J Nucl Med 34: 140P
112. Deland F H, Goldenberg D M 1982 In vivo radioimmunological lymphoscintigraphy in cancer. The implication of positive findings. J Canad Assoc Radiol 33: 4–9
113. Tjandra J J, Sacks N P M, Thompson C H et al 1989 The detection of axillary lymph node metastases from breast cancer by radiolabelled monoclonal antibodies; a prospective study. Br J Cancer 59: 296–302
114. Kairemo K J A 1989 Immunolymphoscintigraphy for the detection of lymph node metastases from breast cancer. Cancer Res 49: 1600–1608
115. Lind P, Smola M G, Lechner P et al 1991 The immunoscintigraphic use of Tc-99m-labelled monoclonal anti-CEA antibodies (BW 431/26) in patients with suspected primary, recurrent and metastatic breast cancer. Int J Cancer 47: 865–869
116. Rainsbury R M, Ott R J, Westwood J H et al 1983 Location of metastatic breast carcinoma by a monoclonal antibody chelate labelled with In-111. Lancet 2: 934–938
117. Lamki M, Buzdar A V, Singletanj S E et al 1991 Indium-111 labelled B72-3 monoclonal antibody in the detection and staging of breast cancer. A phase 1 study. J Nucl Med 32: 1326–1332
118. Kalafonos N P, Sackier J M, Hatzistylianou M et al 1989 Kinetics, quantitative analysis and radioimmunolocalization using indium-111 HMFG1 monoclonal antibody in patients with breast cancer. Br J Cancer 59: 939–942
119. Kramer E L, DeNardo S J, Liebes L et al 1993 Radioimmunolocalization of metastic breast carcinoma using indium-111 methyl benzyl DTPA BrE-3 monoclonal antibody; phase 1 study. J Nucl Med 34: 1067–1074
120. Ryan K P, Dillman R O, DeNardo S J et al 1988 Breast cancer imaging with In-111 human IgM monoclonal antibodies; preliminary studies. Radiology 167: 71–75
121. Granowska M, Britton K E, Mather S J et al 1992 Radioimmunoscintigraphy with technetium-99m SM3 in breast cancer. Annual Report Imperial Cancer Research Fund London. p 515
122. Dehdashti F, Griffeth L K, Mortimer J E et al 1993 Positron tomographic assessment of breast lesions with FDG and FES. J Nucl Med 34: 56p
123. Al-Nahhas A M, McCready V R 1993 The role of radionuclide studies in breast cancer. Nucl Med Commun 14: 192–196
124. Allan S M 1992 The prospects for imaging lymph nodes in breast cancer. Eur J Nucl Med 19: 836–837
125. Boniface G R, McEwan A W, Baum R P et al 1992 The effect of circulating PSA on the localization and diagnostic ability of ^{99m}Tc-labelled anti-PSA MAb B80.3. Nucl Med Commun 13: 634
126. Babaian R J, Murray J L, Lamki L M et al 1987 Radioimmunological imaging of metastatic prostatic cancer with ^{111}Indium labelled monoclonal antibody PAY-276. J Urol 137: 439–443
127. Wynant G E, Murphy G P, Horoszewicz J S et al 1991 Immunoscintigraphy of prostate cancer: preliminary results with 7E11-C5.3 (CYT–356). Prostate 18: 229–241
128. Abdel-Nabi H, Wright G L, Gulfo J V et al 1992 Monoclonal antibodies and radioimmunoconjugates in the diagnosis and treatment of prostate cancer. Semin Urol 10: 45–84
129. Boechmann W, Baum R P, Schuldes H et al 1990 Tumour imaging of bladder carcinoma and metastases with radiolabelled monoclonal anti CEA antibodies. Br J Cancer 62(Suppl X): 81–84
130. Bamias A, Keane P, Krausz T et al 1991 Intravesical administration of radiolabelled anti-tumour monoclonal antibody in bladder carcinoma. Cancer Res 51: 724–728
131. Belitsky P, Ghose T, Aquino J et al 1978 Radionuclide imaging of metastases from renal cell carcinoma by 131-I labelled anti-tumour antibody. Radiology 126: 515–517
132. Baum R P, Fischer P, Taubert M et al 1991 Immunoscintigraphic evaluation of a new monoclonal antibody (138 H11) directed against renal cell carcinoma in an extra corpora perfusion model. Int J Biol Mark 6: 259–260
133. Oosterwijk E, Bander N H, Divgi C R et al 1993. Antibody localization in human renal cell carcinoma: a phase I study of monoclonal antibody G250. J Clin Oncol 11: 738–750
134. Krishnamurthy S, Morris J F, Antonovic R et al 1990. Evaluation of primary lung cancer with indium-111 anti carcinoembryonic antigen (type 2CE-025) monoclonal antibody scintigraphy. Cancer 65: 458–465
135. Vansant J P, Johnson D H, O'Donnell D M et al 1992 Staging lung carcinoma with a Tc-99m labelled monoclonal antibody. Clin Nucl Med 17: 431–438
136. Leitha T, Walter R, Schlick W, Dudczak R 1991 ^{99m}Tc-anti-CEA radioimmunoscintigraphy of lung adenocarcinoma. Chest 99: 14–19
137. Kalofonos H P, Sivolapenko G B, Courteney-Luck N S et al 1988 Antibody guided targetting of non-small lung cancer using ^{111}In-labelled HMFG1 $F(ab')_2$ fragments. Cancer Res 48: 1977–1984
138. Bourget P, Dazard L, Desrues B et al 1990 Immunoscintigraphy of human lung squamous cell carcinoma using an iodine-131 labelled monoclonal antibody (Po66). Br J Cancer 61: 230–234
139. Friedman S, Sullivan K, Salk D et al 1990 Staging non-small cell

carcinoma of the lung using technetium-99m-labelled monoclonal antibodies. Hematol Oncol Clin North Am 4: 1069–1078
140. Breitz H B, Sullivan K, Nelp W B 1993 Imaging lung cancer with radiolabelled antibodies. Semin Nucl Med 23: 127–132
141. Rusch V, Macapinlac H, Keelan R et al 1993 NR-LU-10 monoclonal antibody scanning: a helpful new adjunct to CT in evaluating non-small cell lung cancer. J Thorac Cardiovasc Surg 106: 300–304
142. Braams J W, Pruim J, Nikkels P et al 1993 Detection of lymph node metastases in squamous head-neck cancer with MRI and FDG-PET. J Nucl Med 34: 55P–56P
143. Watkinson J C, Lazarus C R, Mistry R, Maisey M N, Clarke S E M 1990 ^{99m}Tc (V) DMSA and ^{67}Ga-citrate imaging in patients with head and neck squamous carcinoma, a clinical and scintigraphy study. Nucl Med Commun 11: 111–120
144. Baum R P, Knecht R, Howaldt H P et al 1992 Staging head and neck cancer by SPECT immunoscintigraphy using the ^{99m}Tc^{m} labelled monoclonal antibody 174.H64 directed against a squamous cell carcinoma antigen. Nucl Med Commun 13: 629
145. van Dongen G A, Leverstein H, Roos J C et al 1992 Radioimmunoscintigraphy of head and neck cancer using ^{99m}Tc-labelled monoclonal antibody E48 F (ab')$_2$. Cancer Res 52: 2569–2574
146. Kareimo K J A, Hopsu E V M 1990 Imaging of tumours of the parotid region with indium-111-labelled monoclonal antibody reacting with carcinoembryonic antigen. Acta Oncologica 29: 539–543
147. Kareimo K J A, Hopsu E V M 1990 Imaging of pharyngeal and laryngeal carcinomas with indium-111-labelled monoclonal anti-CEA antibodies. Laryngoscope 100: 1077–1082
148. Fairweather D S, Bradwell A R, Watson-James S F et al 1983 Detection of thyroid tumours using radiolabelled anti-thyroglobulin. Clin Endocrinol 18: 563–570
149. Shepherd P S, Lazarus C R, Mistry R D, Maisey M N 1985 Detection of thyroid tumours using a monoclonal ^{123}I anti-human thyroglobulin antibody. Eur J Nucl Med 10: 291–295
150. Berche C, Mach J P, Lumbroso J D et al 1983 Tomoscintigraphy for detecting gastrointestinal and medullary thyroid cancers: first clinical results using carcinoembryonic antigen. Brit Med J 285: 1447–1451
151. O'Byrne K J, Hamilton D, Robinson I et al 1992 Imaging of medullary carcinoma of the thyroid using ^{111}In-labelled anti-CEA monoclonal antibody fragments. Nucl Med Commun 13: 142–148
152. Chatal J F, Le Doussal J M, Chetanneau A et al 1992 Pretargetting of colorectal and medullary thyroid carcinomas with bispecific immunoconjugates. Nucl Med Commun 13: 632–633
153. Manil L, Boudet F, Motte P et al 1989 Positive anticalcitonin immunoscintigraphy in patients with medullary thyroid carcinoma. Cancer Res 49: 5480–5485
154. Richardson R B, Davies A G, Bourne S P et al 1986 Radioimmunolocalization of human brain tumours: biodistribution of radiolabelled monoclonal antibody UJ13A. Eur J Nucl Med 12: 313–320
155. Kalofonos H P, Pawlikofska T R, Hemingway H et al 1989 Antibody guided diagnosis and therapy of brain glioblastomas using radiolabelled monoclonal antibodies against epidermal growth factor receptor and placental alkaline phosphatase. J Nucl Med 30: 1636–1645
156. Riva P, Marangolo M, Arista A et al 1993 Radioimmunotherapy of solid tumours; five years' experiences in the treatment of gastrointestinal cancers and preliminary results obtained in brain glioblastomas. In: Epenetos A A, ed. Monoclonal antibodies 2. Applications in clinical oncology. Chapman & Hall, London. pp 463–472
157. Zalutsky M R, Moseley R P, Coakham H B et al 1989 Pharmacokinetics and tumour localization of ^{131}I labelled antitenascin monoclonal antibody 81C6 in patients with gliomas and other intracranial malignancies. Cancer Res 49: 2807–2813
158. Eary J F, Press O W, Badger C C et al 1990 Imaging and treatment of B cell lymphoma. J Nucl Med 31: 1257–1268
159. Lenhard R E, Order S E, Spunberg J J, Asbell S O, Liebel S A 1985. Isotopic immunoglobulin: a new systemic therapy for advanced Hodgkin's disease. J Clin Oncol 3: 1296–1300
160. Goldenberg P M, Horowitz J A, Starkey R M et al 1991 Targetting, dosimetry and radioimmunotherapy of B cell lymphomas with iodine-131-labelled LL2 monoclonal antibody. J Clin Oncol 9: 548–564
161. Signore A, Chianelli M, Toscano A et al 1992 A radiopharmaceutical for imaging areas of lymphatic infiltration: ^{123}I-interleukin-2 labelling procedure and animal studies. Nucl Med Commun 10: 713–722
162. De Nardo G L, De Nardo S J, Levy N 1993 Treatment of B cell malignancies with ^{131}I-lym-1 and mechanisms for improvement. In: Epenetos A A, ed. Monoclonal antibodies 2. Chapman & Hall, London. pp 355–367
163. Murthy S, Sharkey R M, Goldenberg D M et al 1992 Lymphoma imaging with a new technetium-99m labelled antibody. LL2. Eur J Nucl Med 19: 394–401
164. Carrasquillo J A, Bunn P A, Keenan A M et al 1986 Radioimmunodetection of cutaneous T cell lymphomas with ^{111}In-labelled T101 monoclonal antibody. New Eng J Med 315: 673–680
165. Keenan A M, Weinstein J N, Mulshine J L et al 1987 Immunolymphoscintigraphy in patients with lymphoma after subcutaneous injection of indium-111 labelled T101 monoclonal antibody. J Nucl Med 28: 42–46
166. Hale G, Dyer M J, Clark M R et al 1988 Remission induction in Non-Hodgkins lymphoma with reshaped human monoclonal antibody CAMPATH-1H. Lancet 2: 1394–1399
167. Carde P, Da Costa L, Manil L et al 1990 Immunoscintigraphy of Hodgkins disease: in vivo use of radiolabelled monoclonal antibodies derived from Hodgkins cell lines. Eur J Cancer 26: 474–479
168. Sgouros J, Graham M C, Divgi C R, Larson S M, Scheinberg D A 1993 Modelling and dosimetry of monoclonal antibody M195 (Anti-CD33) in acute myelogenous leukaemia. J Nucl Med 34: 422–430
169. Farrands P A, Perkins A C, Sully L et al 1983 Localization of human osteosarcoma by antitumour monoclonal antibody. J Bone Joint Surg 65B: 638–640
170. Cox P H, Verweij J, Pillay M et al 1988 Indium anti myosin for the detection of rhabdo and leiomyosarcoma. Meeting IRIST group, Frankfurt. March 4
171. Goldman A, Vivian G, Gordon I, Pritchard J, Kemshead J T 1984 Immunolocalization of neuroblastoma using radiolabelled monoclonal antibody UJ13A. J Paediatr 105: 252–256
172. Larson S M, Pentlow K S, Volkow N D et al 1992 PET scanning of iodine-124-3F9 as an approach to tumour dosimetry during treatment planning for radioimmunotherapy in a child with neuroblastoma. J Nucl Med 33: 2020–2023
173. Britton K E 1990 The development of new radiopharmaceuticals. Eur J Nucl Med 16: 373–385
174. Britton K E, Granowska M 1993 The present and future of radiolabelled antibodies in oncology. Ann Nucl Med 7: 127–132
175. Courtenay-Luck N S, Epenetos A A, Sivolapenko G B et al 1988 Development of anti-idiotypic antibodies against tumour antigens and autoantigens in ovarian cancer patients treated intermittently with mouse monoclonal antibodies. Lancet 2: 894–899
176. Oehr P, Wagner V, Briele B et al 1991 Improved survival of patients with advanced ovarian cancer after repeated immunoscintigraphy and induction of anti-idiotypic antibodies. J Nucl Med 32: 1051
177. Zanetti M. 1992 Antigenised antibodies. Nature 355: 476–477
178. Jones P T, Dear P M, Foote J et al 1986 Replacing the complementarity-determining regions in the human antibody with those from a mouse. Nature 321: 522–525
179. Reichmann L, Clark M, Waldmann H, Winter G 1988 Reshaping human antibodies for therapy. Nature 332: 323–327
180. Rodwell J D 1989 Engineered monoclonal antibodies. Nature 342: 99–100
181. Bolt S, Routledge E, Lloyd L et al 1993 The generation of humanised non mitogenic CD3 monoclonal antibody which retains in vitro immunosuppressive properties. Eur J Immunol 23: 403–411

182. Greenwood J, Clark M, Waldmann H 1993 Structural motifs involved in human IgG antibody effector functions. Eur J Immunol 23: 1098–1104
183. Waldmann T A 1991 Monoclonal antibodies in diagnosis and therapy. Science 252: 1657–1662
184. De Jager R, Abdel-Nabi H, Serafini A et al 1994 Radioimmunoscintigraphy of colorectal cancer with human monoclonal antibody 88BV59. In: Epenetos A A, ed. Advances in the applications of monoclonal antibodies in clinical oncology. In press
185. Hanna M G, Haspel M V, McCabe R P et al 1991 Development and application of human monoclonal antibodies. Antibody Immunoconj Radiopharm 4: 67–75
186. Steis R G, Carrasquillo J A, McCabe R et al 1990 Toxicity, immunogenicity and tumour radioimmunodetecting ability of two human monoclonal antibodies in patients with metastatic colorectal cancer. J Clin Oncol 8: 476–490
187. Boven E, Haisma H, Bril H et al 1991 Tumour localization with ^{131}I-labelled human IgM antibody 16.88 in advanced colorectal cancer patients. Eur J Cancer 27: 1430–1436
188. De Jager R, Abdel-Nabi H, Serafini A et al 1993 Current status of cancer immunodetection with radiolabelled human monoclonal antibodies. Semin Nucl Med 23: 165–179
189. Erb K, Borup-Christensen P, Kitzel H et al 1990 Human hybridomas producing monoclonal antibodies against colorectal cancer associated antigens. APMIS 98: 674–684
190. Paganelli G, Belloni C, Magnani P et al 1992 Two step targetting in ovarian cancer patients using biotinylated monoclonal antibodies and radioactive streptavidin. Eur J Nucl Med 19: 322–329
191. Stickney D R, Slater J B, Kirk G A et al 1989 Bifunctional antibody: 2CH/CHA indium-111 BLEDTA-IV clinical imaging in colorectal cancer. Antibody Immunoconj Radiopharm 2: 1–14
192. Stickney D R, Anderson L D, Slater J B et al 1991 Bifunctional antibody: a binary radiopharmaceutical delivery system for imaging colorectal carcinoma. Cancer Res 51: 6650–6655
193. Bos E S, Kuijpus W H A, Kaspersen F H 1994 DNA-DNA hybridisation; a novel two-step approach in radioimmunotherapy. In: Epenetos A A, ed. Advances in the applications of monoclonal antibodies in clinical oncology. In press
194. Koogenboom H R, Marks J D, Griffiths A D, Winter G 1992 Building antibodies from their genes. Immunol Rev 130: 41–68
195. Britton K E 1991 Potential clinical applications of monoclonal antibodies. In: Bringing biotechnology to the market. British Institute of Regulatory Affairs, London. pp 3–26
196. Abbott A, Klaffke O 1993 Europeans protest against patent for Harvard mouse. Nature 361: 574

69. Positron emission tomography: applications in oncology

Richard L. Wahl

While the method of positron emission tomography (PET) has been in existence for nearly two decades, much of the work with this method has been focused on the brain, with some emphasis on the heart. In the past decade, and particularly in the past 5 years, it has been increasingly recognized that PET has considerable current clinical value and substantial potential for applications in the management of patients with cancer. Like all nuclear medicine tests, PET demonstrates physiology in addition to anatomy and does so more quantitatively than do other nuclear medicine procedures. When applied to cancer, the PET scintigraphic representation of tumour physiology and anatomy represents the unique advantage of PET over other cross-sectional imaging methods such as computerized tomography (CT). Despite resolution superior to that of PET, both CT and magnetic resonance imaging (MRI) still remain limited in their ability to characterize mass lesions as viable tumour or scar, in determining whether mildly enlarged lymph nodes represent tumour or a non-malignant process, and in detecting cancer foci <1 cm in diameter. Similarly, CT and MRI are unable to predict whether cancers will respond to therapy. PET appears to offer answers to some of these difficult diagnostic problems by supplying a quantitative metabolic characterization to masses identified by CT, and appears to allow more accurate detection of small tumour foci than standard cross-sectional methods. The 'fusion' of PET metabolic images and CT or MRI anatomy into 'anatometabolic' images provides a unique mode for displaying complex anatomic and physiological information in a single 'anatometabolic' image. This chapter surveys the current state of the rapidly evolving field of PET applications in oncological imaging.

TUMOUR PHYSIOLOGY AND PET

Fundamental to tumour imaging with PET or any nuclear medicine procedure is the need for a specific uptake mechanism for the radiopharmaceutical chosen. Potential radiopharmaceuticals can be chosen based on known differences in physiology or metabolism between tumours and normal tissues. These differences in physiology can be fairly wide in their spectrum, including (as was discussed in the chapter on antibody imaging) differences in the tumour cell surface antigenic phenotype *vs.* normal tissues (Ch. 68). Other differences can include the avidity of ^{67}Ga for the tumour *vs.* normal tissues. As is discussed elsewhere in this chapter (along with the physics of PET imaging), the use of a cyclotron to produce short-lived positron-emitting isotopes such as ^{11}C, ^{15}O, ^{13}N, and ^{18}F has allowed a wide array of compounds to be labelled, something less easy to do in the case of SPECT.

Several relatively common alterations in physiology are seen in tumours which have been used for PET imaging. Tumours have increased rates of growth, in many circumstances, than normal tissues. This means that the use of DNA precursors such as thymidine are often increased *vs.* most normal tissues.[1] Similarly, tumours often have increased rates of protein synthesis *vs.* normal tissues.[2] This means that the transport and incorporation of many different types of amino acids are increased in cancers *vs.* normal tissues. Thus [^{11}C]methionine and [^{11}C]tyrosine have been applied to PET imaging of cancers.[3,4] Perhaps of greatest practical application, to date, has been the observation that tumours have greater rates of anaerobic and aerobic glycolysis than most normal tissues,[5] and thus greater rates of glucose utilization. These alterations are quite common across a wide range of tumour types. The quantitative level of alterations in these pathways will often be greater in the more aggressive than the less aggressive tumours.

Other alterations in tumour physiology may be more restricted than general, allowing for the development of very specific PET radiopharmaceuticals. As an example, radioligands with specificity for the oestrogen receptor expressed on many well-differentiated breast cancers are quite specific for their uptake into oestrogen receptor rich tissues.[6] Similarly, PET tracers specific for monoamine

Table 69.1 Some alterations in physiology which may be used to distinguish tumour from normal tissues

Physiologic alteration	Tracer(s)
Increased glucose utilization	FDG, [^{11}C]glucose
Increased amino acid transport/ protein synthesis	[^{11}C]methionine, [^{11}C]ACHC, [^{11}C]tyrosine
Increased DNA synthesis	[^{11}C]thymidine
Increased estrogen receptor levels	[^{18}F]β-oestradiol
Increased blood flow	[^{15}O]H_2O, [^{62}Cu]PTSM
Increased antigen density	[^{18}F]-labelled anti-tumor monoclonal antibodies
Increased D-2 receptor density	[^{11}C]spiperone
Increased retention of chemotherapeutic agents	5-[^{18}F]fluorouracil

These represent a few of the alterations which can distinguish malignant from normal tissues ; and some examples of tracers which can be utilized to image these alterations.
FDG = 2-[^{18}F] fluoro-2-deoxy-D-glucose; ACHC = 1-[11C] Aminocyclohexanecarboxylate;
PTSM = Pyruvaldehyde bis-(N4-thiosemicarbazone)

uptake pathways are quite specific for adrenergic tissues, phaeochromocytomas.[7] Monoclonal antibodies labelled with positron emitters with specificity for tumour antigens may be quite specific in their targeting a tumour of a given histology.[8] Thus, tumours commonly have altered metabolism which potentially can be detected using specific tracers labelled with positron emitters. Some of the alterations in tumour physiology which may be targeted by PET tracers are shown in Table 69.1.

PET tracers for cancer imaging

2-[^{18}F]fluoro-2-deoxy-D-glucose (FDG) and labelled glucose analogues

While a wide array of biochemical alterations are present in cancer cells, the one most useful for PET imaging has been the situation of increased use of glucose by the tumour cell. FDG is a structural analogue of 2-deoxyglucose. 2-Deoxyglucose is, as is obvious by its name, D-glucose without an OH group in the 2-position. Because of this structural alteration, 2-deoxyglucose is transported into the cancer cell like glucose, and is phosphorylated by hexokinase. This phosphorylation to 2-DG-6-phosphate results in a polar intermediate which does not cross cell membranes well, i.e. it is trapped in cancer cells. 2-DG can be dephosphorylated to 2DG by glucose-6-phosphatase, but this reaction occurs relatively slowly, particularly in cancer cells, which commonly lack glucose-6-phosphatase. ^{18}F attached to the 2-position of this molecule results in FDG, which behaves in a similar fashion to 2-DG, but the ^{18}F emits positrons, the decay of which can be imaged. FDG was first used in humans for brain imaging in the mid 1970s.[9] In 1980 Som et al[10] demonstrated that FDG accumulated in rodent tumours following i.v. administration, apparently due to metabolic trapping. In 1982, the first imaging of human tumours was reported, both in brain tumours and colorectal cancer metastatic to the liver.[11,12]

In the past decade, and particularly in the past 5 years, the uptake of FDG into a wide variety of human cancers has been shown to occur, with high tumour/background uptake ratios at just 1–2 h post i.v. injection.[13,14] The mechanisms for this increased FDG-6-phosphate accumulation in many cancer cells has been shown to be due to:

- increased expression of glucose transporter molecules at the tumour cell surface
- increased levels/activity of hexokinase
- reduced levels of glucose-6-phosphatase *vs.* most normal tissues.[15]

Autoradiographic studies have shown that there is much more FDG uptake into areas of viable tumour than areas of frank necrosis. In some rodent tumour models and in man, it has been shown that the uptake of FDG can be into areas where inflammatory cells are present or into areas of infection, though the bulk of activity generally is into tumours.[16,17]

The normal in vivo distribution of FDG includes the brain, heart, kidneys and urinary tract, at 1 h after tracer injection. Myocardial uptake is variable and highly dependent on the fast or fed state of the patient, as the heart has an insulin-sensitive glucose transporter and myocardial uptake is enhanced in the presence of insulin. Similarly, skeletal muscle has increased uptake of FDG in the presence of insulin. In general, fasting is recommended by FDG PET studies for cancer, as this lowers insulin levels and also generally reduces blood sugar levels.[18] High blood glucose levels can interfere with tumour targeting due to competitive inhibition of FDG uptake by D-glucose.[18] The latter phenomenon has been shown in preclinical and clinical series, although diabetes does not preclude the possibility of PET imaging of cancer in certain patients. At present, the optimal method for handling diabetic patients is uncertain, but many centres fast the patients and do not administer additional insulin, despite serum glucose level elevations.

While initial studies in brain tumours suggested that FDG uptake was strongly related to the proliferative activity of tumour cells, this has been questioned in vitro, a strong correlation has since also been seen in vitro between the number of viable cancer cells and the extent of FDG uptake, though this area has only had limited careful evaluation.[19] This area remains under intense study, but there seems little question that high levels of FDG uptake are most consistent with a substantial number of viable cancer cells being present, particularly in the absence of an overt infectious/inflammatory process. It should be noted that preliminary clinical data from several centres suggests that some tumours are less well seen with FDG PET than others, and the reasons for these disparities are under evaluation.

[^{11}C]Methionine and labelled amino acid analogues

[^{11}C]L-Methionine represents the amino acid with which there is the greatest clinical experience in PET imaging. As indicated above, increased transport and use of amino acids is common in cancers. Use of L-methionine in cancer imaging is based on this observation and the increased activity of the transmethylation pathways in some cancers. There is normally substantial uptake of this tracer in the pancreas, salivary glands, liver and kidneys. As a natural amino acid, there is some metabolism of L-methionine in the blood stream. This tracer has been used in brain tumour imaging (including pituitary adenomas), in head and neck cancer imaging, in lymphomas and in lung cancers.[20–22] The clinical results will be discussed separately. Early clinical studies demonstrated the stereospecificity of tumour uptake, with L-methioinine uptake much greater in brain tumours than that of D-methionine, when an intact blood–brain barrier was present.[23]

Other amino acids have been used in cancer imaging with PET including L-tyrosine and non-natural amino acids such as ACHC, ACPC etc.[24] These latter agents are not substantially metabolized in vivo, and thus represent attractive choices to examine the transport of amino acids into tumours. This study of amino acid transport may be all that is possible if ^{11}C is chosen as the tracer, as even with methionine, much of the early imaging done is of the transport, with relatively less of the phosphorylation process.

[^{11}C]Thymidine and other DNA precursors

Increased rates of DNA synthesis are typical of many fast-growing tumours and rapidly proliferating normal tissues. For this reason, some human tumours can be imaged with [^{11}C]thymidine and its structural analogues. Thymidine is appealing in that it targets only tissues with ongoing DNA synthesis. Its use is made complicated by the fact that it is rapidly metabolized in the blood, meaning that only a small fraction of the labelled material in the blood is [^{11}C]-thymidine.[1] The location of the radioactive label is important to the use of [^{11}C]thymidine. For example, if it is labelled in the ring *vs.* the C-1 position, different metabolites will be seen, making exact quantitation more difficult.[25] Other compounds such as [^{18}F]fluorodeoxyuridine also represent potential tumour imaging agents.[26] ^{18}F structural analogues of thymidine are under development, but have not been extensively studied in vivo in patients.

Labelled chemotherapeutic agents

Positron emitter-labelled chemotherapeutic agents have been synthesized and applied to patient care to a limited extent. The rationale for such studies is that delivery and accumulation of a chemotherapeutic agent within a cancer would seem obligatory for the successful treatment of the cancer. This attractive concept has not been extensively studied to date, but has been applied with [^{18}F]fluorodeoxyuridine.[27] This chemotherapeutic agent has been used in the therapy of colorectal and other cancers and preliminary studies have suggested that it has potential in the prediction of cancer response based on an initial PET scan. It is possible that the use of labelled chemotherapeutic agents may represent a broad new area for PET imaging research in the next decade.

Tumour flow/volume/volume of distribution

A variety of fundamental physical properties of tumour physiology can be defined by PET imaging. Tumour blood flow can be measured using [^{15}O]H^2O or [^{15}O]-CO^2 inhalation with image quantification. Tumour blood volume can be estimated by using [^{15}C]CO_2 inhalation. Tumour volume of distribution (i.e. that portion of the tumour that freely communicates with the blood) can be imaged using [^{15}O]H_2O. These parameters can be determined quantitatively using mathematical modelling techniques.[28] In some instances, though this is quite variable, the increased blood flow in a tumour may be sufficient to allow it to be defined as cancer.

Tumour receptor status

Tumours can express a variety of markers on their surface including tumour-associated antigens or receptors, such as the oestrogen or progesterone receptor. Ligands with specificity for these receptors have been synthesized and can be imaged if labelled with PET emitters. Perhaps the best known ligand is [^{18}F]17β-oestradiol (FES), which has been used in breast cancer imaging studies. Recently, tumour imaging with antibodies labelled with ^{18}F and ^{124}I has been reported, and the potential for labelled peptide imaging is also substantial.[6]

METHODOLOGICAL ISSUES IN PET CANCER IMAGING

PET scanning of cancer can be performed in several ways with several tracers. An important consideration in PET tumour imaging is that the field of view of the PET camera is generally quite limited, with the largest *z*-axis field of view for a single acquisition of only about 15–16 cm, at present.[29] This limitation can be overcome by obtaining multiple scanning levels, but the number of levels that can be obtained is limited by the half-life of the tracer and its time to optimal tumour localization. Indeed, with ^{11}C-labelled tracers, a single level of imaging is generally acquired, with a second level sometimes possible.

For tracers with an ^{18}F label, there can be sufficient

time to acquire multiple imaging levels. Indeed, methods which allow for imaging of the entire body, or at least most of it, have been developed recently. These methods are possible as ^{18}F has a 110 min half-life, which is sufficient for tumour visualization following localization.[30,31]

For true quantitation of tracer uptake, transmission images are generally obtained. These images can be obtained before any tracer has been injected, or can be obtained after the tracer has been injected and has a reasonably stable distribution. The highest quality PET images are made after correction for attenuation by the body for 511 KeV photon absorption. It should be noted that the whole body and static images are not necessarily exclusive of one another. It is possible to perform a detailed dynamic or static acquisition with transmission correction for attenuation, followed by a dynamic acquisition, as well as a static image of a given area in question following a whole body image. There is a lengthening of the procedure, however, with a prolonged imaging sequence being utilized. At present, the optimal PET imaging algorithm may depend on the type of cancer being studied. For the assessment of regional disease, detailed imaging of a region of the body is recommended. To screen for metastatic disease, whole body imaging may be most appropriate.

An issue that needs to be resolved is whether dynamic or static image acquisition needs to be routinely performed. Dynamic acquisition requires the patient to be in the PET scanner for a fairly long time period while multiple images are obtained over the period of tracer accumulation in the tumour. This allows for the determination of a direct quantitation of the rate of tracer uptake over time. These data, along with a measurement of the tracer quantity in the blood over time (either determined by arterial sampling or by direct imaging of a blood vessel), can be used to model mathematically the kinetics of tracer uptake into a tissue.[32] Such data may provide more information than simple static imaging, but the clinical necessity for modelling using FDG has not been convincingly demonstrated to date. The approach chosen depends on the tracer utilized and its in vivo behaviour. Thus simple (one-compartment) or more complex models can be used. For FDG, a three-compartment modelling approach is generally used. Whether or not modelling is performed, standardization of the patient's diet is generally recommended prior to imaging.

For FDG studies, patients are generally fasted for 4 h or longer prior to imaging, in an effort to reduce serum insulin levels to near basal quantities. This is important, as insulin can direct FDG away from the blood. Following this, patients are injected with about 10 mCi i.v. of FDG. Imaging can be done dynamically or be initiated at 40–60 min after tracer injection.

Images are reconstructed by vendor-supplied algorithms, with the most commonly applied method being filtered back-projection. The images can be displayed as cross-sectional images in the transverse, coronal or sagittal planes. Interpretation is based on experience in examining many images, but is generally a form of 'hot spot' imaging for most PET tracers. Simple quantification can be performed by measuring tumour/non-tumour uptake ratios using a digital computer, but can also be performed by determining the 'standardized uptake value' (SUV). This latter value is often used to reflect the uptake of the tracer in tumour or normal tissues. Generally, the higher the value, the more likely it is that tumour is present.

$$\text{SUV} = \frac{\text{decay-corrected dose/cc tumour}}{\text{injected dose/patient weight (g)}}$$

Recently, it has been shown that SUV, at least for FDG, is not weight independent. Rather, for patients of high body weights, SUV substantially increases in blood and several other normal tissues compared with patients of lower body weights (see Fig. 69.1). This weight-related increase in the SUV of normal tissues is largely eliminated by using the lean body mass in the denominator of the equation, rather than the total body weight. This weight-corrected parameter is referred to as the 'SUV lean'.[33]

$$\text{SUV lean} = \frac{\text{decay-corrected dose/cc of tumour}}{\text{injected dose/patient lean body mass (g)}}$$

It should be noted that there is some variation in SUV with the time following tracer injection, rising over time in most untreated tumours. Thus, standardization of imaging time for SUV determination is important in these studies. Most investigators use a small region of interest (relative to the tumour size) and attempt to quantify activity in the most metabolically active portion of the tumour, but there is some variability in practice, and SUVs from institutions with different types of scanning device cannot necessarily be directly compared.

SUV lean can be determined from static images, but determination of the influx constant or formal kinetic modelling requires several dynamic frames. While a description of kinetic modelling is beyond the scope of this discussion, it should be realized that the Patlak–Gjedde plot described in Chapter 110 can also be applied to tumour imaging to produce a rate of influx for FDG or other tracers (where there is little efflux).[33] Similarly, compartmental analysis ranging from a one- to a three-compartment model (or even more with thymidine) can be applied. Such applications require more complex data acquisition and more analytical labour.

At present, most PET centres performing frequent clinical studies apply the SUV or SUV lean in their imaging analysis to assist in lesion characterization. Whether more complex analyses will be necessary depends on the incremental clinical value they provide, an issue still under study.

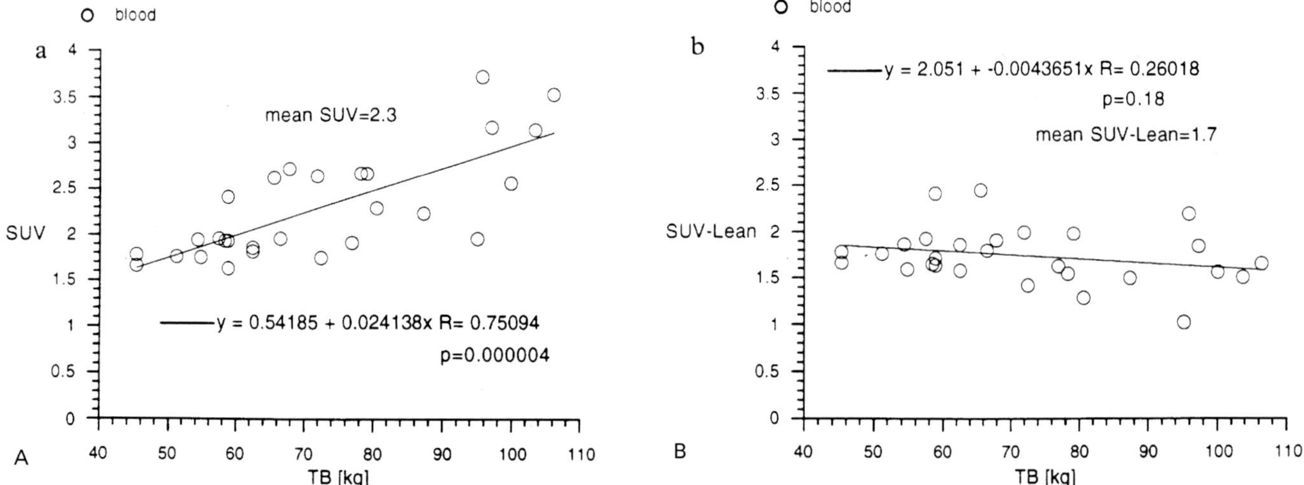

Fig. 69.1 Graph of standardized uptake value (SUV) for FDG in blood *vs.* body weight. Note that the SUV rises in heavier patients (A). This is corrected for by the use of the 'SUV-lean' (B).

DISEASE-SPECIFIC APPLICATIONS OF PET

Brain tumours

While brain tumours are discussed elsewhere they have been the most extensively studied of any tumour type using PET, particularly because many of the first PET scanners were designed in size and shape to be well suited to brain imaging. Indeed, in several countries, the use of FDG and PET have been sufficiently validated that these are routine clinical procedures and reimbursed by insurance carriers.

Di Chiro et al recognized the potential of FDG for imaging brain tumours and reported on this approach in 1982.[11,34] Since their initial report, many subsequent studies have examined the ability of FDG and PET to separate between histologically aggressive and less aggressive brain tumours, as well as to separate viable tumour from scar or necrosis.[35] In addition, determining if a low grade glioma is progressing is also possible.[36] It appears, from the data available, that in large series higher grade tumours generally have higher FDG uptake and utilization than lower grade tumours. It is also clear that there is overlap between the extent of FDG uptake in low *vs.* high grade brain tumours.[35] Similarly, elevated FDG uptake in a brain tumour is generally associated with a poorer prognosis than lower levels of FDG uptake.

Following the completion of radiation therapy, FDG uptake into a contrast-enhancing lesion suggests the presence of viable tumour, while absent FDG uptake suggests that necrosis is present (at least if the tumour was visible on PET before the treatment).[37] To date, qualitative visual analysis, in which FDG uptake is compared to normal white or grey matter, is generally used for analysis, in preference to quantitative analysis. This approach generally means that any focus of activity which is more intense in tracer uptake than normal brain white matter is considered to represent viable tumour. It is generally recognized that FDG PET has substantial difficulty in detecting low grade gliomas as well as in some intermediate grade gliomas, as their FDG uptake can be quite low.[37,39] The reason FDG uptake appears to correlate with survival and tumour grade is not yet fully clear, but may be related to the increased cellular density seen in high grade tumours or may be related to increased FDG uptake in the more rapidly proliferating tumour cells. Since in vitro studies available to date have suggested that viable cancer cell numbers and not proliferative rate are best correlated with FDG uptake, the increased uptake in high grade brain tumours may be associated with the quantity of viable tumour cells, i.e. a high signal may mean more living tumour cells and thus a poorer prognosis.[19]

It should be noted that there has been some controversy related to the extent of FDG uptake in brain tumours of a variety of grades. Clearly, uptake of FDG in some low grade tumours is inadequate for reliable detection.[37,38] In other cases, high uptake of FDG can be seen in tumours which have evidence of contrast enhancement on CT, but which are associated with a reasonably good prognosis – this has been seen in juvenile pilocytic astrocytomas.[39] In the situation of low grade gliomas, other tracers, such as [^{11}C]methionine, [^{11}C]thymidine may represent reasonable alternatives to FDG.[23,43] These latter tracers have only a low level of uptake into normal brain, and for this reason often allow for higher tumour/background uptake ratios than FDG. [^{11}C]Methionine has been shown not to accumulate into focal radiation necrosis in the relatively small number of patients so far studied and to accumulate into many low grade gliomas. Bergstrom et al[43] reported that 7/11 low grade gliomas had increased uptake of [^{11}C]methionine *vs.* normal brain. Similarly, Bergstrom et al[21] reported a difference in the intratumour deposition of radiolabelled glucose *vs.* FDG in a case in which careful histological correlation was performed. In low grade tumour assessment, it must be noted that with FDG, investigators at the National Institutes of Health have described instances in which areas of low FDG uptake in low grade gliomas have, on sequential studies, developed foci of increased FDG uptake.[36] These changes of increasing uptake were seen when transformation of a low grade to a higher grade glioma occurred. Thus, it might be possible to 'follow' low grade gliomas with FDG PET and only operate when there is scintigraphic evidence suggesting malignant change. This aspect of patient management needs more study, as surgical resection of low grade gliomas can be curative. Such an approach to management could conceivably be undertaken if the tumour were located in an area where surgery would result in a severe functional impairment, and thus waiting on treatment might be considered a reasonable alternative.[36]

While experience is limited in terms of absolute numbers of patients, it seems clear that alternative tracers to FDG may play an increasingly important role in intra-axial brain tumour imaging, at least for low grade tumours, although FDG has already been established to be very useful. It should be noted that ^{201}Tl, a SPECT agent, also can be used to image brain tumours, and that direct comparative studies between ^{201}Tl and PET tracers are ongoing. In some instances, ^{201}Tl, and perhaps other SPECT tracers, may also be valuable for brain tumour imaging and may compare favourably in cost to PET.

Pituitary adenomas have been successfully imaged using PET with FDG, [^{11}C]methionine and, for functioning prolactinomas, with the dopamine D-2 receptor binding ligand, [^{11}C]deprenyl. While there is some level of methionine accumulation in the normal pituitary, this should not be confused with an adenoma.[43,44] The response of pituitary adenomas to therapy has also been evaluated by PET. The differential diagnosis of pituitary disease has been made much easier in the past decade through the availability of CT and MRI, but PET may have a role in selected instances.

While FDG has clear utility in imaging primary brain tumours, especially high grade tumours, data on imaging intra-axial metastases to brain is more limited. Griffeth et al[45] reported that FDG uptake into untreated metastases from a variety of cancers can, in a significant fraction of cases (up to 1/3 of patients in his study), be insufficient to produce satisfactory images of the metastases. This is particularly the case when small lesions are located in very close proximity to grey matter folds in the brain. Increased FDG uptake in brain metastases is commonly seen, however, and the demonstration of increased FDG uptake in treated metastatic brain tumours should suggest the presence of residual or recurrent viable cancer. An example of successful FDG PET imaging of a recurrent brain tumour metastasis from lung cancer is shown in Fig. 69.2.

It should be noted that CNS lymphomas, both intra- and extra-axial, have been reported to be well visualized by PET using FDG. The intensity of FDG uptake into lymphomas has been reported to be comparable to that seen in high grade gliomas and is significantly more than that reported in low grade gliomas ($P<0.001$).[46] Recently, FDG PET was shown to be capable of accurately detecting the presence of CNS lymphoma in patients with AIDS, and in differentiating this pattern from that seen in CNS infectious processes.[47]

As regards extra-axial tumours, meningiomas can be imaged using FDG PET. Di Chiro et al[48] reported on a series of 17 patients, and observed generally similar findings to those he had seen with brain tumours, in that those with the highest FDG uptake appeared to have the most aggressive histological appearance, while those with low FDG uptake appeared to have a less aggressive histology. In this series, FDG uptake appeared to be correlated with the growth rate of the meningiomas, and the tumours with the lowest FDG uptake were found to have the greatest long term likelihood for survival. It is uncertain if low FDG uptake in a meningioma would suggest that surgery could be delayed, but such metabolic information may be a useful adjunct in challenging cases.

Lung carcinoma

In much of the industrialized world, lung cancer represents the malignancy with the greatest level of lethality. This tumour is increasing in frequency worldwide, deaths in women from lung cancer now exceeding those seen from breast carcinoma. Lung cancer has been imaged in several trials using PET with both [^{11}C]methionine and FDG. Kubota[20] first reported successful imaging of lung cancer in 8/8 patients with primary lung cancers, with substantially more [^{11}C]methionine uptake in tumour than in normal lung tissue. In a follow-up series of 16 patients, the same team showed increased [^{11}C]methionine uptake in each case of primary lung cancer, with somewhat more uptake in the large cell than in the squamous cell carcinomas.[49]

Nolop et al[50] showed that FDG accumulated in 12/12 lung carcinomas studied with FDG, with all histologies imaging in the study. Mean tumour/non-tumour ratios of >6/1 were seen, and no obvious correlation was observed between tumour grade and FDG uptake, in this small series. It has been shown[51] that about 85–90% of solitary pulmonary nodules are detected by PET with either FDG or methionine. This study observed an elevated SUV with FDG and methionine in patients with lung cancer, while in benign lesions, the SUV was significantly lower.[51] Similar results were recently reported by Gupta et al[52] who showed that FDG uptake by primary

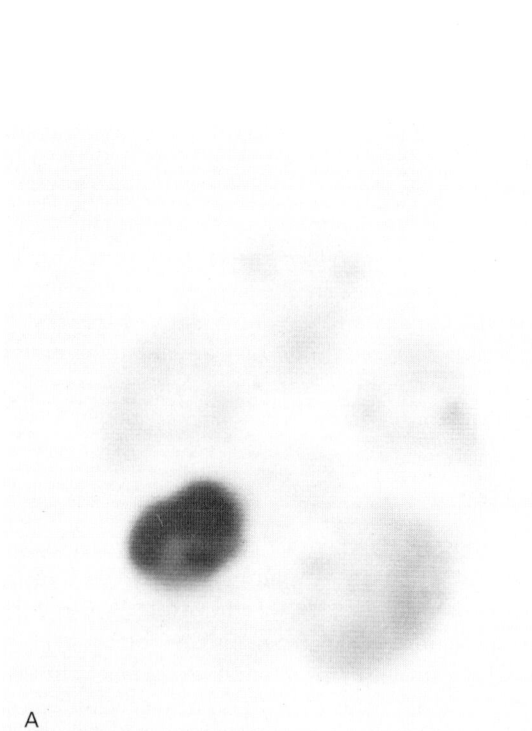

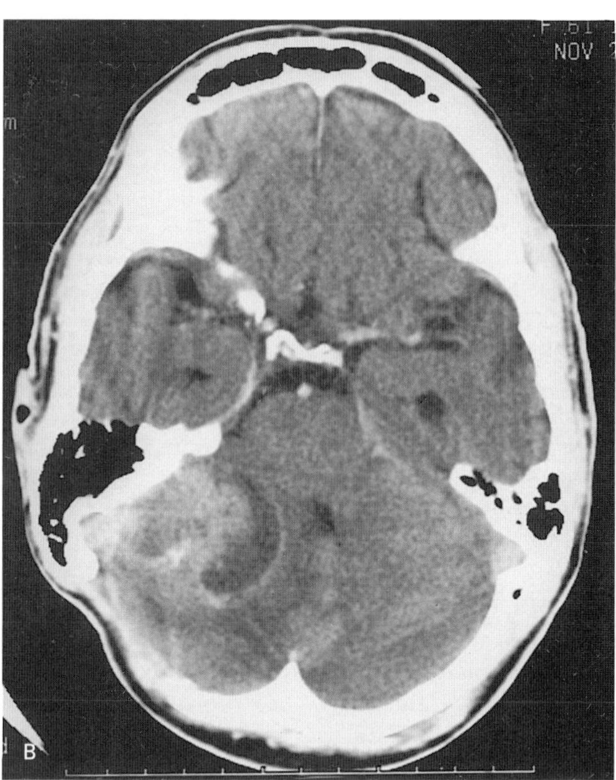

Fig. 69.2 Transverse FDG PET image of the brain at 50 min after tracer injection (A). This demonstrates a marked increase in uptake in the posterior aspect of the brain, corresponding to a focus of recurrent adenocarcinoma of the lung. Compare with CT (B) which shows only a contrast-enhancing area, the differential diagnosis for which included tumour or radiation necrosis prior to PET.

lung cancers was significantly greater than that seen by benign pulmonary lesions, with SUV of 5.63 ± 2.38 (1 SD) in malignant and 0.56 ± 0.27 in benign lesions ($P<0.001$). Patz et al[53] recently demonstrated that FDG PET is very effective at separating primary lung cancers from inflammatory processes in the lung based on the lesion SUV. In a series of 51 patients with focal pulmonary abnormalities (of which 38 were solitary pulmonary nodules), it was noted that the 33 malignant lesions had an SUV of 6.5 ± 2.9, while benign lesions had an SUV of 1.7 ± 1.2. Thus, an excellent, but not complete, separation was possible between benign and malignant lesions.

Kubota et al[51] also compared the accuracy of FDG and methionine PET in assessing pulmonary nodules. Both PET and FDG were comparable in their imaging accuracies, with a 93% sensitivity, 60% specificity and 79% accuracy for methionine, and an 83% sensitivity, 90% specificity and 86% accuracy for FDG. Tumours <1 cm in diameter were noted to be particularly difficult to evaluate because of their small size relative to the resolution of the PET scanner.

The ability of PET to separate malignant from benign lesions is high, but not perfect. Thus, a high SUV can sometimes be seen in an inflammatory or infectious process, such as aspergillosis, tuberculosis, or (according to preliminary reports), lymph nodes affected with sarcoidosis. Preliminary reports suggest that the smallest of pulmonary nodules may not be as well characterized by PET as larger nodules, possibly due to their motion in the PET scanner field of view and the incomplete signal recovery from small lesions, which results in underestimation of their SUV, unless a correction for scanner resolution is applied. The whole body PET technique has also been applied to the detection of intrathoracic masses, and in eight patients with bronchogenic carcinoma, there was clear visualization of the tumours by PET, as areas of increased focal tracer accumulation.[54] Several metastatic lung nodules could also be detected by this approach, though it must be realized that quantification is not possible with this method.

Another issue in lung cancer management is whether the tumour has spread to the mediastinal lymph nodes. This question is of substantial importance in non-small cell lung cancer, where cure is generally possible only with complete excision of viable tumour from the thorax. By contrast, small cell lung cancer is more commonly treated non-surgically by chemotherapy or irradiation. With non-small cell lung cancer, it has been recognized that if there is tumour involvement of the mediastinum at the time of initial diagnosis, the patient's probability of survival for

5 years is reduced to just 5–10%. By contrast, if there is no mediastinal lymph node involvement, 5 year survival is increased to a 40–50% probability. This can alter the approach to management, as in high risk patients for surgery, thoracotomy may become too risky. There are only limited data published so far on this topic. A report on 25 patients studied with [^{11}C]methionine PET showed that there was higher ^{11}C uptake in the tumour-involved lymph nodes than in the tumour negative, at 3.89 *vs* 2.38 mean SUV ($P<0.001$) and that with threshold setting post hoc, a nearly 90% accuracy in detecting mediastinal metastases could be defined.

Preliminary data from the University of Michigan have shown PET to be substantially more accurate than CT in staging presumed non-small cell lung cancer. In a prospective study of 23 patients, PET was about 82% accurate, CT about 52% ($P<0.05$).[56] It should be noted that neither CT nor PET was perfect in this clinical setting, but PET often had the capability to detect tumour in some normal sized lymph nodes and to exclude tumour involvement in enlarged lymph node (Fig. 69.3). A preliminary report from Heidelberg[57] has shown even better accuracy for FDG PET, but was performed with a PET scanner which had a limited field of view, and thus which was not able to evaluate the entire mediastinum at risk for metastases. Application of strict quantification to the PET data may be of utility in additionally refining the accuracy of PET. It should be noted that accurately determining tracer uptake in mediastinal lymph nodes is difficult with PET, because count recovery is somewhat limited when the lymph nodes are small. Thus, systematic underestimation of SUV can occur in small nodes without a correction for count recover. The role of PET in assessing the response of lung cancers to treatment will be discussed later in this chapter.

Only limited published data exist regarding the ability of PET to detect visceral metastases of lung cancer, but anecdotal experiences in the literature support the feasibility of the approach. The comparative accuracy of PET to more standard methods of assessment of metastases, such as CT or bone scan, is not known at present and awaits comparative trials.

Breast carcinoma

Breast carcinoma is the most common visceral malignancy in North America and much of Europe. Its frequency is increasing in the industrialized world. While curable if diagnosed in its earliest form, this neoplasm represents a diagnostic problem in several specific settings. For example, the detection of the primary cancers can be particularly challenging in younger women with dense breasts, as mammograms which show dense glandular tissue can obscure the tumours. Similarly, the specificity of mammography is relatively low, with a larger fraction of mammographic abnormalities being found, on biopsy, to

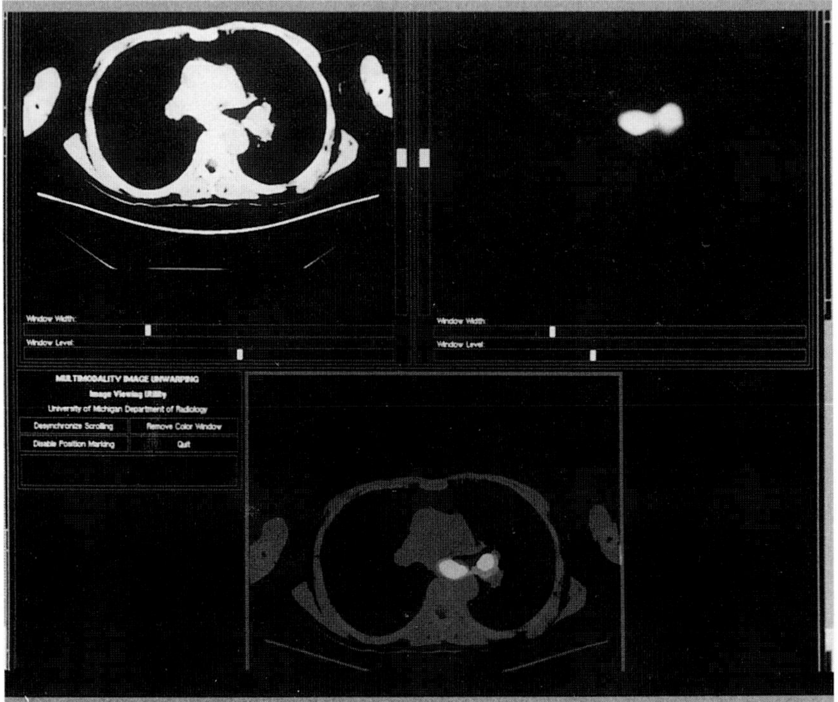

Fig. 69.3 Intense FDG uptake is seen into enlarged lymph nodes in a patient with non-small cell lung carcinoma. These lymph nodes were proven to be involved with cancer at surgery. The method of display here is that of an 'anatometabolic' image (see text). **Top left**: CT. **Top right:** FDG PET. **Bottom centre**: anatometabolic image. (Also shown in colour on Plate 20.)

represent non-malignant processes than cancer in most series. Once breast cancer is identified, the only method to determine reliably whether the tumour has spread to regional lymph nodes is to remove the nodes surgically and examine them pathologically. Similarly, detecting some foci of tumour involvement, such as in some soft tissues, can be difficult with current methods. PET offers the potential to evaluate primary, regionally metastatic and systemic metastases of breast cancer.

The first imaging of breast cancer with PET involved studies of tumour blood flow, oxygen extraction and oxygen utilization in nine patients using ^{11}C-labelled tracers. Beaney et al[58] reported that regional blood flow was higher in the viable tumour than in surrounding normal breast and that while the oxygen utilization was slightly more in tumour than normal breast, the oxygen extraction ratio was significantly lower in tumour than normal breast tissues. A follow-up study on 20 patients showed mean tumour flow to be 29.8 ± 17.0 (SE) ml/dl/min of tissue, while normal breast flow was 5.6 ± 1.4 ml/dl/min of tissue.[60] These studies provided interesting fundamental data regarding breast cancer physiology.

An alternative approach with a radiopharmaceutical with specificity for the oestrogen receptor expressed on many breast cancers was developed and then applied to PET imaging. In the initial report,[6] 13 women with primary breast masses were imaged with 16-α-[^{18}F]-fluoroestradiol (FES).[6] PET demonstrated uptake of the radiotracer in the primary breast mass and the axillary nodes in several instances. There was an excellent correlation (0.96) between the oestrogen receptor concentration measured in the tumours and the extent of FES uptake into the tumours in this study. A follow-up study by the same group[58] evaluated 16 patients with 57 known foci of metastatic disease and demonstrated an approximately 93% lesion detection sensitivity. Patients who received antioestrogen therapy had declines in the fraction of FES reaching the tumours after treatment. Obviously, imaging tumours which are oestrogen receptor negative would generally be expected to be unsuccessful with this method, which is associated with moderate hepatic uptake of the tracer, limiting the utility of scans of the upper abdomen.

The feasibility of imaging advanced breast cancers with the glucose analogue FDG and planar imaging (non-PET) was shown by Minn et al[60] in 1989. Using a specially collimated planar gamma-camera, they studied 17 patients. They were able to detect tumour in 14/17 patients (82%), including 6/8 known lymph node metastases. FDG was also able to detect bone metastases, but more effectively in lytic or mixed lesions than in purely sclerotic lesions. The authors speculated that superior imaging sensitivity would be achieved by using PET rather than planar imaging. In assessing treatment response in 10 patients, increases in FDG uptake were consistently associated with disease progression, while declines in FDG uptake were commonly, but not invariably, associated with resolving or stable disease.

In preliminary reports in 1989, Wahl et al[61] and Kubota et al[62] separately reported on the feasibility of imaging breast cancer using PET with FDG in several patients. Subsequently, the feasibility of imaging primary, regional and systemic metastases of breast cancer using FDG PET was shown in a larger series of patients.[63] The FDG PET technique allowed for the detection of 25/25 known foci of breast cancer including primary lesions (10/10), soft-tissue lesions (5/5) and bone metastases (10/10). The PET method allowed for detection of four additional lesions which were nodal, and not previously identified. Of note was that several of the primary cancers detected were in women with radiographically dense breasts.

Preclinical studies of FDG uptake into several tumour systems in rodents suggested that FDG would be able to detect lymph node metastases of cancer as tumour/background (normal node) ratios were quite high. It was noted that if FDG was injected s.c., there would be intense tracer uptake in the lymph nodes proximal to the injection site.[64] Preliminary studies of FDG PET in staging for the presence or absence of axillary nodal metastases have recently appeared. Wahl et al[65] were able to characterize 8/9 axillae correctly with FDG PET in the preoperative setting, with injections in the arm opposite the tumour. In that prelimary report, no false positive uptake occurred, but there was one false negative result.

Several other reports of imaging breast cancer with PET have now appeared. Using a whole body imaging technique, Hoh et al[31] were able to detect 15/17 foci primary breast carcinomas, as well as regionally metastatic and systemic metastases of breast cancer. In a closely related initial report by Tse et al,[66] using the whole body technique, 11/14 axillae were properly characterized as to the presence or absence of tumour involvement. In a study of transverse PET with attenuation correction in 11 patients with primary breast cancer,[67] 10/11 primary lesions were identified by FDG PET. In five cases there was uptake of FDG in the axillary nodal region, and in each instance there was tumour involvement in the axilla. Only modest uptake was seen in patients with fibrocystic disease. Tumour/normal tissue uptake ratios were 4.9/1.

In a somewhat larger prospective study, Adler et al[68] reported FDG PET results (using attenuation correction) from 28 patients with 35 suspicious breast masses. 26/27 malignant lesions were identified (sensitivity of 96%) and separated (in retrospect) from the eight benign breast lesions; the separation was based on FDG uptake levels into the primary lesions. There was a general correlation between the nuclear grade of the tumours and the quantity of FDG uptake. 20 of the patients had lymph node dissections following the PET scans, 9/10 with nodal metastases were detected, while 10/10 disease negative axillae were found not to have increased FDG uptake. It should be noted that overexpression of the GLUT1 glucose transporter is very commonly seen in breast cancers, which no doubt contributes to their increased uptake of FDG.[69]

L-Methyl[^{11}C]methionine PET has also been used in the imaging of breast cancer. In a pilot study of 11 breast cancers (eight in the breast), the mean (± SD) SUV for breast cancer was 8.5 ± 3.3, while the maximal uptake in the liver was 12.4 ±1.6, in the bone marrow 5.8 ± 0.7, and in the myocardium 3.4 ± 0.6. Tumours larger than 3 cm diameter accumulated [^{11}C]methionine, while none of the three smaller cancers (12–15 mm in diameter) were visualized. A strong uptake of [^{11}C]methionine was associated with a large S-phase fraction (SPF) measured by flow cytometry (r=0.77, P=0.01), and the non-visualized cancers had all a small SPF (< 5.5%). One benign tumour (an abscess) accumulated a small amount of [^{11}C]methionine. These data indicate that [^{11}C]methionine can image breast cancer, but suggest that it may not be useful in small lesions or in the liver, due to high background uptake.[70]

These studies of PET imaging of breast carcinoma are encouraging, but it must be realized that the technique is in its infancy. Since most of the studies have examined breast masses of >1.0 cm in diameter, the sensitivity of PET in smaller breast cancers has yet to be defined. Much more study needs to be done to determine the specificity of the method and the sensitivity in small lesions. Similarly, the specificity of PET has not been fully determined in benign lesions, as few were included in the studies reported to date. PET is also able to assess the response of breast cancers to treatment, as is discussed. Examples of PET studies of imaging breast cancer with PET are shown in Figs. 69.4 and 69.9.

Colorectal carcinoma (Fig. 69.5)

Colorectal carcinoma is one of the most frequent neoplasms in the industrialized world, representing a problem for initial diagnosis, staging and assessment of recurrence following therapy. FDG was first reported to image liver metastases of colorectal cancer in 1982 in a feasibility study using PET:[12] three patients with liver metastases had tumour/normal liver uptake ratios of about 4/1 at less than 1 h after tracer injection. Subsequently, the ability of FDG PET to separate recurrent colorectal carcinoma from scar was shown by two research groups.[71,72] More recently, PET has been used to image the recurrence of colorectal cancer in patients following radiotherapy. Relatively few data exist regarding the comparative sensitivity of FDG PET *vs* CT in detecting colorectal cancer, but it is clear that PET is at least reasonably sensitive for this purpose in the abdomen. Gupta et al[73] reported on 16 patients with colorectal cancer: accuracy with PET was 87%, compared with 65% for CT. Microscopic tumour foci were not identified by PET, but PET could detect primary tumours, nodal metastases and liver metastases.[73] Additional studies with histological correlation will be necessary to determine more completely the role of PET in evaluating colorectal cancers. The role of PET in treatment assessment is discussed on p. 811.

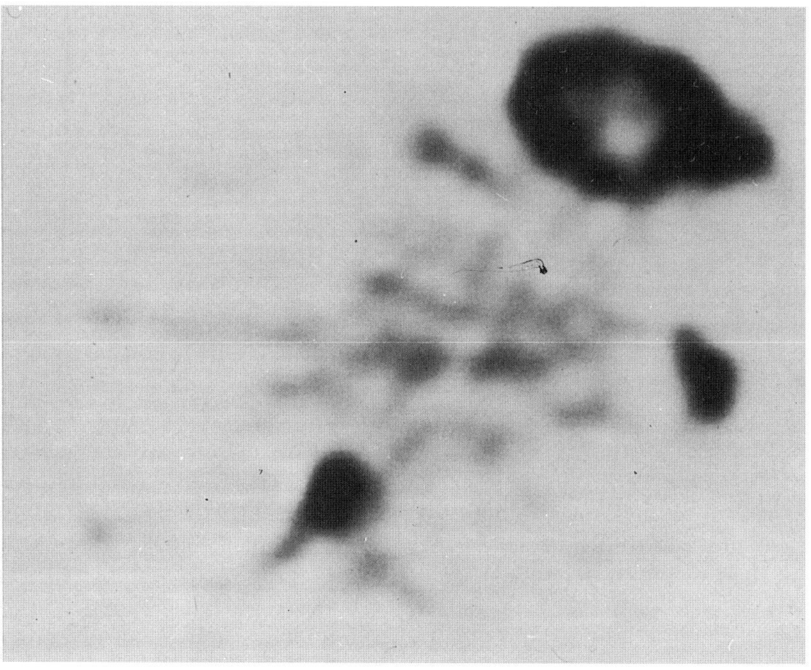

Fig. 69.4 Intense FDG uptake is seen into foci of primary breast cancer (cold in centre), as well as into an axillary nodal metastasis and a spinal metastasis with images obtained at between 50 and 70 min post injection.

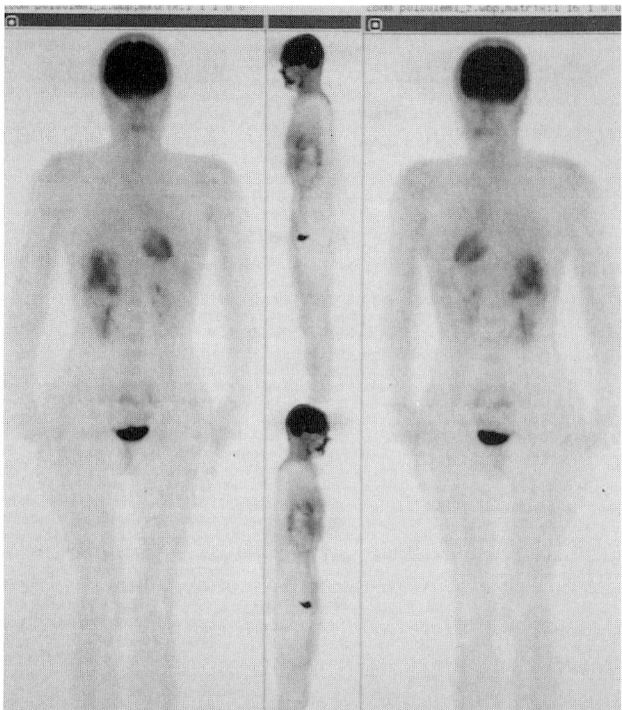

Fig. 69.5 Anterior (**left**) and posterior (**right**) whole body FDG PET images of a woman with a rising CEA level following surgery for colorectal cancer. Increased uptake is noted in the normal brain, heart and bladder, along with faint bilateral renal uptake. Intense right upper quadrant activity is seen in liver metastases, while faint activity above the bladder is in the pelvic recurrence. Normal uptake in vertebral bone marrow is noted.

Pancreatic carcinoma

Pancreatic carcinoma was one of the first neoplasms imaged with PET. Since the pancreas is known to use amino acids in excess of most normal tissues, [^{11}C]tryptophan has been used.[74] The normal pancreas showed intense tracer uptake when using a non-PET imaging device, the 'Pho Con' focused probe scanner. Decreased tracer uptake was identified in patients with chronic pancreatitis or pancreatic carcinoma relative to the normal pancreas.[74] [^{11}C]Methionine was then used in 100 patients with possible pancreatic disease with PET.[75] [^{11}C]Methionine, like [^{11}C]tryptophan, showed a lack of specificity in separating between pancreatic cancer and pancreatitis using this 'cold spot' imaging approach.[75] Pancreatic blood flow has also been examined by PET, in normal pancreas and in pancreatic carcinomas. The normal pancreas is quite metabolically active and its flow, as assessed by [^{15}O]H_2O PET, is roughly twice that seen in pancreatic cancers.[76] If the cancer obstructs the pancreatic duct, the pancreas whose drainage is obstructed by the tumour has diminished flow, while the non-obstructed pancreas has normal tracer accumulation, using [^{15}O]-H_2O.[76] Thus, other tracers needed evaluation, at least for tumour imaging, as 'cold spot' imaging of pancreatic cancer was not particularly successful.

Pancreatic adenocarcinoma is also imaged well using FDG. A recent report from Bares et al[77] indicated that in 15 patients with pancreatic masses on CT, PET images begun at 45 min after tracer injection were able to identify pancreatic adenocarcinoma in 12 of 13 patients with the neoplasm, failing to detect the tumour only in one patient who was hyperglycaemic due to insulin dependent diabetes. In addition to detecting primary tumours, 8/9 nodal metastases and 4/5 liver metastases were detected as foci of increased tracer accumulation. Two patients with chronic pancreatitis were noted to have low uptake of FDG. These data suggest that FDG PET may be very useful in characterizing pancreatic carcinoma and pancreatic masses, though more study is certainly necessary to determine the precise role of PET in managing this highly lethal cancer.

Hepatoma

Hepatoma is an extremely common and lethal neoplasm in the Pacific Rim countries and China. Diagnostic issues in detecting hepatoma with conventional imaging methods include separating hepatoma from cirrhosis and in assessing the response of hepatomas to treatment. CT alone can be inadequate for such assessments.

Early imaging studies of human hepatomas involved the use of [^{13}N]ammonia. Rapid uptake of the tracer in the hepatomas was reportedly present, with an uptake slope more rapid than seen in the normal liver tissues. Tumours <2 cm in size were identified using a relatively low resolution PET scanning device.[77] A follow-up report in 16 patients with hepatocellular carcinoma showed that 12/16 such tumours had markedly increased [^{13}N]ammonia uptake *vs.* normal liver, with a tumour/liver ratio of $>2.6/1$ (median), though in a few poorly vascularized tumours it was not possible to distinguish the tumour from the normal liver. On occasion however a 'cold' defect could be present.[79] Patients with metastastic liver cancer were also noted to have low ^{13}N uptake *vs.* normal liver.[79]

Imaging of hepatomas with FDG was initially performed in nine patients who then went on to therapy. In these patients, the uptake rate of FDG declined with treatment.[80] In three cases, it was suggested that the FDG PET was substantially more useful than CT in assessing the response of liver tumours to therapy.[81] It is clear that while a large fraction of hepatomas are well imaged by PET using FDG as hot spots relative to liver, up to half of the tumours cannot be detected as regions of increased tracer uptake compared with normal liver. Apparently this is not due to a low K3 rate constant but is due to a high K4 or dephosphorylation rate, at least based on results in 23 patients studied by Enomoto et al.[82] They suggested that kinetic modelling could be used to better characterize hepatomas than a single delayed image of hepatic and tumour FDG uptake. Of interest was that there was a patient group identified with a high K4/K3 ratio, and this group had the best survival. These investigators went on to expand their study to 35 patients with liver lesions who underwent surgery after their PET scans. They found K3 to be correlated with tumour hexokinase content and that a K3 > 0.25 was consistently associated with the presence of cancer.[83] It remains to be seen how reliable this determination is in predicting outcome. In another large series, a relatively substantial percentage of hepatic lesions showing low tracer uptake (in the range of normal liver) were hepatomas.[84] Thus, it is clear that the diagnosis of hepatoma is more challenging than the diagnosis of several other cancers in man, as the target/background ratios can be quite low in many cases. None the less, the metabolic information provided by PET about the liver tumours appears to be clinically useful in many instances.

Head and neck carcinomas

Cancers of the head and neck are increasing in frequency and are commonly associated with the use/abuse of alcohol and/or tobacco. Successful imaging of these tumours has been achieved with FDG using planar and PET methods, as well as with using several other tracers. Using a specially collimated gamma-camera, investigators in Turku, Finland, were able to image 13/13 head and neck cancers using FDG. There was not a reliable correlation between tumour grade and FDG uptake, but FDG uptake appeared to be well correlated with the proliferative rate of the tumours.[85]

Follow-up studies using PET have shown excellent imaging of head and neck tumours using FDG.[86] Haberkorn et al[86] reported on 46 patients with tumours in the head and neck region (42 primary tumours); flow cytometry was performed in 35 patients and $[^{15}O]H_2O$ studies done in 17 cases. Perfusion was not correlated with the proliferative rate. It was suggested that two groups of tumours, one with high SUVs and one with low SUVs, were present and that within the two groups, the SUV was correlated with the proliferative rate. Another possible explanation would be that no correlation between FDG uptake and tumour proliferative rate was present across the entire group. In any case, the head and neck tumours were successfully imaged with FDG and PET.

Bailet et al[87] were able to image 16/16 foci of primary head and neck cancer using PET, detecting one lesion not well delineated on MRI or CT. In addition, they were able to detect 12 foci of lymph node metastases, a result which compared very favourably with the 10 foci defined by MRI. A follow-up study[88] in 12 patients from the same institution showed that 25/34 lymph nodes proven to be involved with cancer were detected by PET, while only 24 were positive by MRI. PET allowed detection of tumour in three normal size nodes.

Data from Reisser et al[89] suggest that the FDG uptake of the primary lesion is correlated inversely with prognosis, i.e. high FDG uptake tumours did poorly. Following the FDG uptake, treatment of these tumours has also been undertaken.

$[^{11}C]$Thymidine (methyl) has been applied in imaging head and neck cancers in a small series ($n = 13$ patients):[90] all primary tumours had some increased ^{11}C activity compared with background, suggesting considerable potential of this tracer in following tumour DNA synthesis. $[^{11}C]$Methionine has also been used to image head and neck cancers in pilot studies from Finland. Since methionine traffics to the normal parotid gland, it is clear that it will have difficulty in detecting tumours in the region of the parotid. It is clear that not all foci of head and neck cancer metastatic to lymph nodes are identified with PET, however.

Additional, carefully performed prospective studies will be necessary to determine the extent of correlation and accuracy of PET in staging head and neck cancer.

Melanoma

Melanoma is, like so many cancers, increasing in frequency, particularly in Caucasians in areas of high sun exposure. In animals, melanoma is one of the cancers which has the most avid levels of FDG uptake and glycolytic metabolism.[14] Initial clinical evaluation was in suspected uveal melanoma. In this setting, only 3/12 lesions were detected by PET, a disappointing result.[91] By contrast, Gritters et al[92] recently demonstrated that melanoma could be imaged using PET with FDG in 12 cases. In this small study, 15/15 intra-abdominal and lymph node metastases were detected by PET. PET also identified three additional metastastic foci only noted retrospectively on CT. PET correctly identified tumour in 7/7 lymph nodes, including three cases where the nodes were of normal size, and excluded tumour in 6/6 nodal regions for a 13/13 accuracy in nodal disease characterization. PET was not as sensitive as CT for small lesions in the lungs, however.[92] Of particular interest was that small bowel metastases, which are extremely difficult to identify by any method other than autopsy, were detected in several instances in this study. FDG appears to be an excellent imaging agent for melanomas, but more study is needed to define its optimal place in the patient management scheme.

Lymphomas

Non-Hodgkin's lymphoma and Hodgkin's lymphoma commonly present challenges in diagnostic imaging. Determining where tumour is located at the time of diagnosis (staging) and assessing whether the tumour has responded to therapy are examples of the difficulties faced. Several reports have shown the feasibility of

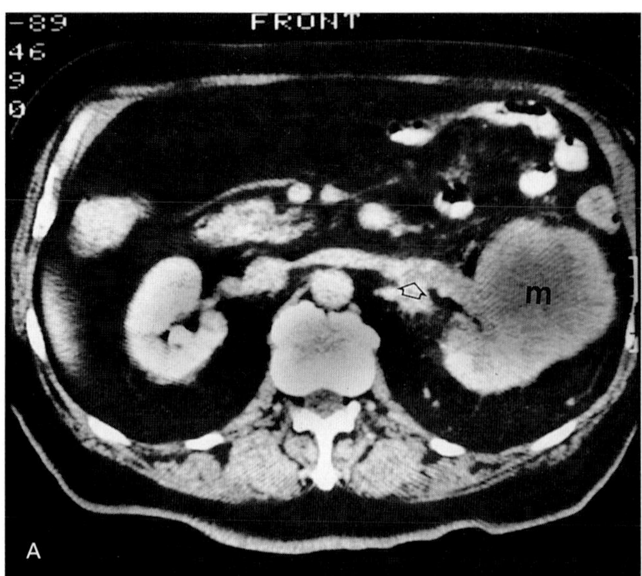

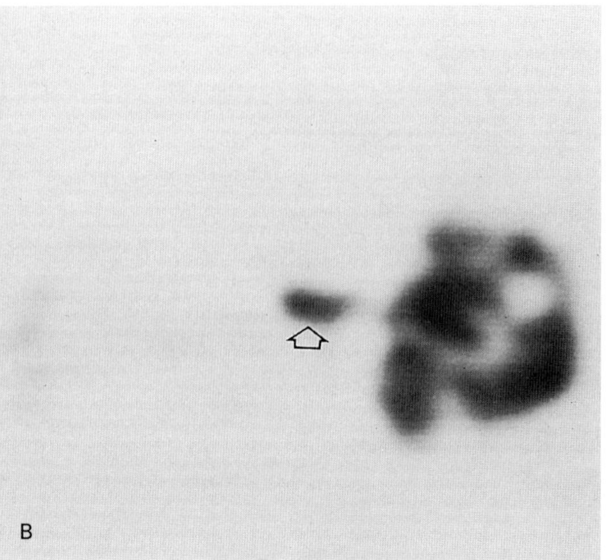

Fig. 69.6 CT scan (A) of a patient with melanoma shows subtle abnormality of left kidney. FDG PET (B) demonstrates intense focal tracer uptake in three lesions, two associated with left kidney, one near duodenal bulb. All represented metastatic melanoma.

imaging lymphomas using FDG; one of the earliest was a comparison with ^{67}Ga in five patients with non-Hodgkin's lymphoma using planar imaging.[94] FDG was found to detect 4/5 lymphomas, while ^{67}Ga detected only 2/5. Subsequent studies have shown that both Hodgkin's lymphoma and non-Hodgkin's lymphoma can be imaged with PET. As was indicated in the section on brain tumours, CNS lymphomas are generally well visualized by PET, particularly relative to normal brain in the untreated state.[46] At least one report[94] suggests that low grade lymphomas have less uptake of FDG than higher grade lymphomas. Additionally, it has been suggested that increased FDG uptake is associated with a less favourable prognosis for the lymphoma patient. These data are from patients with lymphomas of the head and neck region and are based on relatively limited numbers of patients.[94]

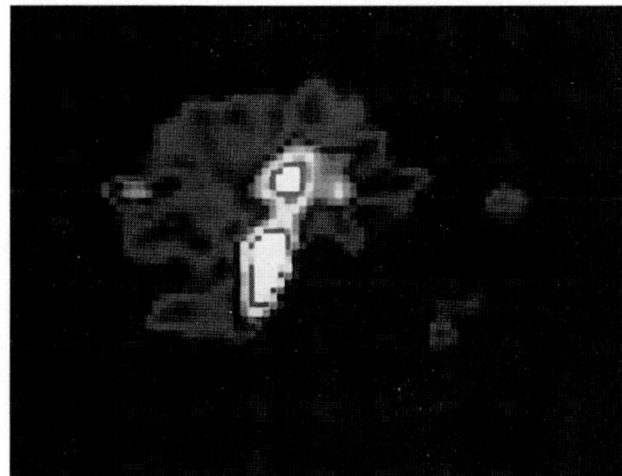

Fig. 69.7 Transverse FDG PET image demonstrates intense uptake immediately posterior to the liver and just above the right kidney. Intense uptake was seen, despite the fact that this represents a low grade lymphoma. (Also shown in colour on Plate 20.)

None the less, the results are provocative and suggest that FDG PET may have prognostic value when assessing a lymphoma.

FDG and [^{11}C]methionine were directly compared in 14 patients with non-Hodgkin's lymphoma.[22] It was noted that the influx rate of [^{11}C]methionine was substantially higher than that of FDG into this type of tumour; 13/14 lymphomas accumulated [^{11}C]methionine, but two intermediate and three low grade lymphomas had relatively poor tracer uptake compared with surrounding normal tissues. With both tracers there was more rapid tracer uptake into the higher grade tumours than into the low grade tumours, but there was considerable overlap. The author of this study concluded that [^{11}C]methionine might be superior to FDG in detecting lymphomas, but that FDG was better at distinguishing tumour grade.

A very recent study[95] has been reported which compared the lesion detection efficacy of CT and PET with FDG in the same patients. It was found that PET could detect all of the approximately 50 lesions identified at CT and could find additional tumour foci in lymph nodes of normal size. No clear relationship was found between tumour size or grade and the extent of FDG uptake, and all tumours were identified. In that study, PET was able to detect intrasplenic lymphoma, in addition to lymphoma in a wide variety of other locations in several instances.[95]

It is clear that PET imaging of lymphomas will be more extensively studied in the next several years. The ability to acquire images in just 1 h following tracer injection, and the modest quantity of activity in the gut, make FDG compare quite favourably with ^{67}Ga as a tumour-seeking agent. It will be of interest to see if methionine, thymidine or FDG prevail as the PET imaging agent of choice in lymphoma, but current data suggest that FDG will be very useful in many circumstances. Following the response of lymphomas to therapy is also possible, and will be discussed later in this chapter.

Musculoskeletal neoplasms

Sarcomas and primary musculoskeletal tumours can be imaged using PET. At least three separate reports have shown the feasibility of this approach. In a first small report,[96] five patients with musculoskeletal tumours were studied, four with soft-tissue tumours, one with an osteogenic sarcoma; the extent of FDG uptake appeared to correlate with the grade of the sarcoma. In similar reports, this has been substantiated, and malignant tumours of the musculoskeletal system have been shown generally to have increased levels of FDG uptake in comparison to benign tumors.[97] A study of twenty-five patients with musculoskeletal lesions included six benign and malignant lesions. All lesions with an SUV>1.6 were high grade while those with an SUV of <1.6 were benign or of low grade. In addition, the grade of the tumours was correlated with the FDG uptake.[98] In a report by Griffeth,[99] using FDG PET it was demonstrated in 19 patients with 20 lesions that, by using the DUR or SUV, a complete separation of the 10 benign from the 10 malignant lesions was possible. By contrast, tumour/background ratios were inadequate, with overlap between malignant and benign uptake in over half of the cases.[99] Taken together, these studies suggest that FDG PET can be a useful method to help characterize soft-tissue masses non-invasively.

Genitourinary neoplasms

Cancers of the kidney can be imaged by PET using FDG. While FDG is excreted by the kidneys, delays from injection of the tracer until imaging allow the renal neoplasms to develop sufficiently high tumour/kidney ratios in many instances to allow for successful imaging. Initial reports[100,101] have shown that with sufficient delays following FDG injection, satisfactory tumour imaging may be achieved. Both adenocarcinomas of the kidney and transitional cell carcinomas have been imaged. It remains to be seen if PET will provide information beyond that provided by CT, but it must be recognized that CT is not able to characterize all renal masses as benign or malignant, nor is it able to identify renal lymph node involvement with this tumour consistently.

Bladder cancer can be imaged with PET, although the experience with the technique is quite limited, to date. Primary tumours, regional nodal metastases and pulmonary metastases can be imaged, but too few cases have been studied to identify confidently the accuracy of the PET method in this disease.[102] One of the limitations of PET with FDG in patients with bladder carcinoma is dealing with the issue of excreted FDG activity in the urine. The intense FDG activity in the bladder can substantially degrade the visualization of lymph nodes in the anatomic pelvis, though this can be partly addressed through the use of a Foley catheter to drain the bladder during the conduct of the study.[102]

Published data on PET imaging of prostate cancer is limited. While anecdotal accounts have suggested the feasibility of the technique, recent reports have indicated that PET with FDG is not particularly sensitive in the

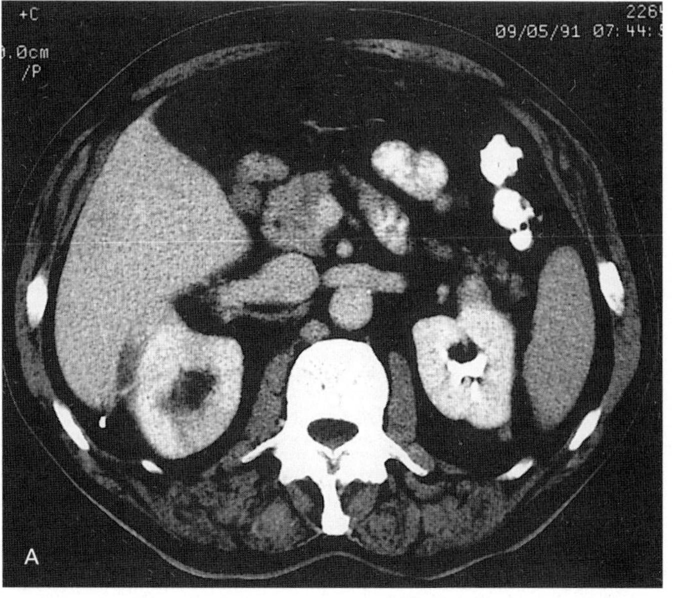

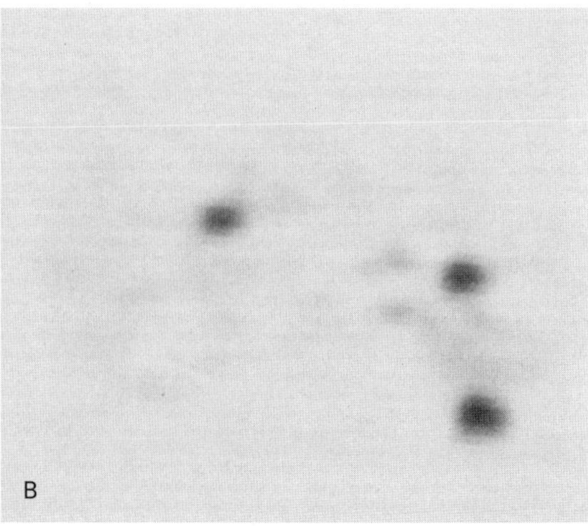

Fig. 69.8 Renal cancer. CT (A) shows left renal mass. PET (B) shows primary tumour and uptake in the left renal vein consistent with renal vein tumour involvement. Distinguishing FDG uptake in tumour from normal excreted activity can be challenging, however.

detection of bone metastases of prostate carcinoma.[31] While this needs additional study, a preliminary communication by Shreve et al[103] suggested that nearly 50% of patients with prostate carcinoma metastatic to bone do not have successful imaging of their bone tumours with PET. The sensitivity of PET for detecting the primary lesion of prostate cancer or nodal metastases has not yet been determined. Whether FDG PET of prostate cancer will be clinically valuable remains an open question.

Few complete reports exist regarding the ability of PET to image ovarian and germ cell neoplasms; however, data from preclinical trials strongly support this approach.[114,104–106] Preliminary communications from several groups have indicated that these tumours can be well imaged with FDG, though again more studies are necessary[31,105,106]

Endocrine neoplasms

Some of the earliest work with FDG was performed in patients with thyroid cancer. In these studies, tumours which were FDG avid, but not iodine avid, were suggested to be the most aggressive.[107] In addition, tumours which were iodine avid and FDG negative, and those which were negative for both tracers, were both identified. Fourteen thyroid tumours were studied using FDG and planar imaging. In that study, none of the papillary carcinomas were seen to accumulate FDG, though some of the more aggressive thyroid tumours, such as anaplastic carcinoma, had FDG accumulation.[108] In addition, several benign tumours were shown to accumulate FDG, notably cancers with an elevated proliferative index as assessed by DNA flow cytometry.[108] Subsequent reports using PET have shown that thyroid cancer can be imaged using PET with FDG and have indicated that the quantity of FDG uptake, into the tumour may be related to the level of thyroid-stimulating hormone stimulation of the thyroid cancer.[109] FDG uptake is clearly not specific for malignancy in the case of the thyroid gland and FDG appears to fail to image some well-differentiated, and perhaps other, thyroid malignancies.

Fewer data exist regarding the uptake of FDG into other endocrine neoplasms, although it is clear that the neuroendocrine tumour, phaeochromoctyoma, accumulates FDG and can be imaged by the PET method. Indeed, two phaeochromocytomas which did not accumulate metaiodobenzylguanidine were successfully imaged with FDG in a recent case study.[7]

Treatment response monitoring

The quantitative character of PET suggests that it has an important potential role as a non-invasive method to assess tumour response. This matter has been touched upon previously. Indeed, the first published report of FDG PET imaging of brain tumours included five patients who had received radiation therapy.[11] In three of the patients, increased FDG uptake was present and they had recurrent brain tumour. In two patients, FDG uptake was low, and there was evidence of radiation

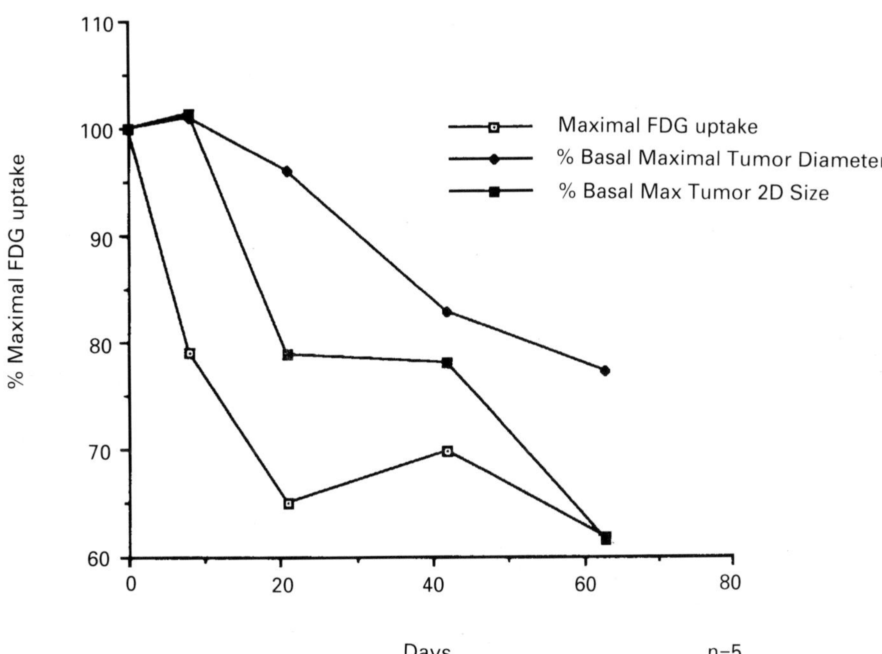

Fig. 69.9 Tumour diameter *vs.* maximal FDG uptake in a group of patients being treated for breast cancer. Note that there is a prompt decline in FDG uptake before the tumour begins to shrink. In most PET studies of treatment response, metabolic changes antedate those in anatomy.

necrosis. This experience in brain tumours has generally been replicated in subsequent larger series assessing the long term effects of radiotherapy. While many studies have been published concerning the CNS and more recently about the rest of the body, it is generally the case that tumours that have responded to treatment of a variety of types have much lower FDG or other tracer uptake than they did at the outset of therapy. With radiation therapy or chemotherapy, eventual success is generally associated with a decline in tracer uptake *vs.* starting levels.

Most PET studies of brain tumours have evaluated the appearance of the tumour before and after the completion of chemotherapy. Low uptake of FDG after treatment has generally correlated with a good response to treatment, while high uptake of the tracer has suggested recurrent or residual tumour. The ability of PET to separate post-radiation necrosis from residual tumour relatively accurately has been shown in several series, where accuracies of about 85% are common. It must be noted that PET cannot detect microscopic foci of cancer, and that low grade gliomas can be very difficult to detect with FDG and, in some cases, with [^{11}C]methionine. In the brain, uptake of FDG or [^{11}C]methionine into pure radiation necrosis would not be an expected nor an observed finding, to date.

There is substantially less information on the response of brain tumours to treatment during the course of therapy. The available data are somewhat confusing, but, for example, indicate that at one day after radiotherapy is initiated, it is possible to observe an increase, not a decrease, in tracer uptake (for FDG).[110] Some data suggest that such an increase may be associated with a relatively good prognosis; other data that tumour FDG uptake which declines shortly after treatment gives the best prognosis.

In brain tumours, it seems clear that a decline in FDG uptake in a tumour at several weeks to months after the conclusion of therapy suggests a good response.

By contrast, increased FDG uptake *vs.* the basal level, or persistent FDG uptake, would strongly suggest residual tumour being present despite treatment. It is clear that microscopic foci of tumour would not be expected to be detected by PET, so that a negative scan does not completely exclude the possibility of residual tumour being present. It should be noted that in the assessment of 48 patients who underwent FDG PET, there was no complete concordance between a good prognosis and the absence of FDG uptake by tumours. This was particularly the case in patients studied following intensive radiotherapy, where declines in FDG uptake could be seen, even if viable tumour was present.[38] Thus, while FDG PET is very useful, it is not a perfect test in assessing the post-treatment brain.

There are limited data on the response of other tumours to treatment. Minn et al[111] examined the response of patients with head and neck carcinoma to radiation treatment using a planar gamma-camera device. There were declines in FDG uptake in nearly all patients, but they appeared to be greatest in the responding patients. FDG uptake midway through the treatment programme was not consistently able to separate the responding from the non-responding patients, however. Minn et al also examined women with breast carcinoma during therapy using a planar gamma-camera, and found that a decline in FDG uptake was consistently seen in responding patients, but that some patients who failed therapy did have transient declines in FDG uptake. An increase in FDG uptake was consistently associated with treatment failure, however.

Strauss et al[71] have reported on the appearance of PET scans of the pre-sacral area in patients with a history of colorectal carcinoma who have received external beam radiation therapy. A similar report has appeared from Ito el al.[72] In both of these studies, pre-sacral masses with avid FDG accumulation were generally found to represent recurrences of colorectal carcinoma, while areas with low FDG uptake were generally found to represent scarring. In a follow up paper, Haberkorn et al[112] showed that increased FDG uptake in the immediate post-irradiation period was not as reliably associated with tumour involvement as had been suspected initially. It remains unclear as to how long one has to wait following radiotherapy to perform PET, in order to achieve satisfactory results, but waiting 6 months is probably appropriate for colorectal cancer.[112]

Recent in vitro data presented by Higashi et al have indicated that tumour cells in culture have increases in FDG, methionine and thymidine uptake in the period of a few days to a few weeks following external beam therapy.[113] These data must be contrasted with in vivo data from animal models in which it has been shown that there is a rapid decline in the uptake of FDG, methionine and thymidine following effective external beam therapy.

With external beam radiation, it is quite typical that, once a decision is made to perform the treatment, a full course of radiation be given. This implies that there is no need to perform assessments of tracer uptake in the period immediately after therapy is initiated. Thus, with radiation therapy, the key issue at present is whether there is any reproductively viable tumour present at the conclusion of a 'full course' of radiation treatment. At present, it is unclear how long one has to wait to make such a determination, but it is suggested that PET scans in the first month or two after treatment may be misleading if persistent signal is seen in the tumour. This might occur if a tumour is reproductively dead, but histologically still viable. Indeed, pathologists are reluctant even to assess whether residual tissue from a tumour bed is alive or dead in the first few months following the conclusion of radiation therapy.

Ichiya et al[114] studied the FDG uptake of a variety of

tumours before and after treatment. A variety of treatment methods were used, but mainly radiotherapy. Declines in FDG uptake were common, but only one patient in the study had a complete remission, so assessment of patterns of scans in the complete remission population is not possible. In a single patient in whom kinetic modelling was performed, a decline in K3 was seen with successful treatment (embolotherapy of a liver lesion).[114] Similarly, declines in SUV were seen with effective therapy of head and neck cancer, when FDG was used as the tracer.[115]

A recent prospective evaluation of PET during breast cancer chemohormonotherapy[32] demonstrated that in women treated with a multi-agent regimen, there was a rapid and significant decline in the tumour FDG uptake, K3 kinetic rate constant, and K_i (or influx constant for FDG) by just 8 days after treatment was initiated. Further declines in FDG uptake were apparent in the patients who went on to complete or partial responses at 21, 42 and 63 days of treatment, while no significant decline in FDG uptake was seen in the non-responding patients (n=3) when examined at 63 days post-initiation of treatment. The metabolic changes antedated the anatomic changes, and substantial declines in tumour glucose metabolism were apparent, despite no change in the tumour size in the responding patient population.

While FDG has been used most in treatment monitoring, it should be noted that other tracers such as [^{11}C]methionine have been employed. For example, in lung and breast cancer treatment monitoring, declines in [^{11}C]methionine uptake into tumours were commonly seen with effective therapy. In some instances, such decline was more predictive of the long term patient survival than was the change in tumour size. [^{11}C]Methionine uptake into pituitary tumours has been shown to be very sensitive to treatment, and rapid declines (in < 1 day) have been reported in response to specific inhibitors of pituitary secretion.

Agents other than substrates for cellular metabolism have been applied to PET imaging in an effort to characterize or predict tumour response to treatment. One of the most interesting approaches is the use of positron emitter-labelled chemotherapeutic agents, such as 5-[^{18}F]-fluorouracil (FU). Fifty patients with 78 liver metastases were evaluated. Lesions with high and low FU concentration were observed. Preliminary data suggest that lesions with higher uptake may respond better to this type of treatment, but more study is essential to confirm this.[27] Labelled chemotherapeutic agents warrant further study, but if validatd with FU and other agents, could be a most valuable predictor of tumour response to therapy.

Much more needs to be learned regarding tumour response assessment with PET tracers. Whether FDG, methionine, thymidine or some other tracer will be best, will require substantial long-term study in patients, as only clinical trials will define the clinical relevance of radiopharmaceuticals for treatment.

Future of PET in oncology

The use of PET in cancer imaging and treatment planning is increasing at a very rapid rate, so that this chapter could well be out of date soon after it is published. It seems clear that PET will not replace CT, which is a well established technology capable of high levels of patient throughput. Rather, PET will be used to approach and hopefully answer the difficult diagnostic problems which CT and other imaging tests cannot adequately address at present. These problems include assessment of residual masses following treatment, assessment of the patient with residual clips or postoperative deformity, in detecting the presence or absence of cancer in lymph nodes, and in determining whether cancer is present in the normal breast, etc.

In some parts of the world, socioeconomic and political issues regarding health care are slowing the dissemination and approval of many new technologies, including PET. As the number of useful clinical applications continues to increase, it is clear that PET will have an important and growing role in tumour imaging and cancer therapy planning in clinical practice.

REFERENCES

1. Larson S M, Grunbaum Z, Rasey J S 1980 Positron* imaging feasibility studies: selective tumor concentration of 3H-thymidine, 3H-uridine, and 14C-2-deoxyglucose. Radiology 134: 771–773
2. d'Argy R, Paul R, Frankenberg L et al. Comparative double tracer whole body autoradiography: uptake of 11C, 18F and 3H labeled compounds in rat tumors. Int J Rad Appl Ins B 15: 577–585
3. Shiba K, Mori H, Hisada K 1984 Comparative distribution study of 14C labeled amino acids, glucose-analogue and precursor of nuclei acid, as tumor seeking agents. Radioisotopes 33(8): 526–532
4. Ishiwata K, Vaalburg W, Elsinga P H, Paans A M, Woldring M G 1988 Metabolic studies with L-[1–14C]tyrosine for the investigation of a kinetic model to measure protein synthesis rates with PET. J Nucl Med 29(4): 524–529
5. Warburg O 1931 The metabolism of tumors. Richard R. Smith, Inc., New York, pp 129–169
6. Mintun M A, Welch M J, Siegel B A, Mathias C J, Brodack J W, McGuire A H, Katzenellenbogen J A 1988 Breast cancer: PET imaging of estrogen receptors. Radiology 169(1): 45–48
7. Shulkin B L, Koeppe R A, Francis I R, Deeb G M, Lloyd R V, Thompson N W 1993 Pheochromocytomas that do not accumulate metaiodobenzylguanidine: localization with PET and administration of FDG. Radiology 186(3): 11–15
8. Snook D E, Rowlinson Busza G, Sharma H L, Epenetos A A 1990 Preparation and in vivo study of 124I-labelled monoclonal antibody H17E2 in a human tumour xenograft model. A prelude to positron emission tomography (PET). Br J Cancer 10 (suppl): 89–91
9. Phelps M E, Huang S C, Hoffman E J, Selin C, Sokoloff L, Kuhl D E 1979 Tomographic measurement of local cerebral glucose metabolic rate in humans with (F-18)2-fluoro-2-deoxy-D-glucose: validation of method. Ann Neurol 6(5): 371–388

10. Som P, Atkins H L, Bandoypadhyay D, Fowler J S, MacGregor R R, Matsui K, Oster Z H, Sacker D F, Shiue C Y, Turner H, Wan C N, Wolf A P, Zabinski S V A fluorinated glucose analog, 2-fluoro-2-deoxy-D-glucose (F-18): nontoxic tracer for rapid tumor detection.
11. Patronas N J, Di Chiro G, Brooks R A, DeLaPaz R L, Kornblith P L, Smith B H, Rizzoli H V, Kessler R M, Manning R G, Channing M, Wolf A P, OConnor C M 1982 Work in progress: [18F]fluorodeoxyglucose and positron emission tomography in the evaluation of radiation necrosis of the brain. Radiology
12. Yonekura Y, Benua R S, Brill A B, Som P, Yeh S D, Kemeny N E, Fowler J S, MacGregor R R, Stamm R, Christman D R, Wolf A P 1982 Increased accumulation of 2-deoxy-2-[18F]fluoro-D-glucose in liver metastases from colon carcinoma. J Nucl Med 23(12): 1133–1137
13. Larson S M, Weiden P L, Grunbaum Z, Kaplan H G, Rasey J S, Graham M M, Sale G E, Harp G D, Williams D L 1981 Positron imaging feasibility studies. II: Characteristics of 2-deoxyglucose uptake in rodent and canine neoplasms: concise communication. J Nucl Med. 22(10): 875–879
14. Wahl R L, Hutchins G D, Buchsbaum D J, Liebert M, Grossman H B, Fisher S 1991 18F-2-deoxy-2-fluoro-D-glucose uptake into human tumor xenografts. Feasibility studies for cancer imaging with positron-emission tomography. Cancer 67: 1544–1550
15. Wahl R L, Cody R, Hutchins G D, Mudgett E 1991 Primary and metastatic breast carcinoma: initial clinical evaluation with PET with the radiolabeled glucose analog 2-[F-18]-fluorodeoxy-2-D-glucose (FDG). Radiology 179: 765–770
16. Brown R S, Fisher S J, Wahl R L 1993 Autoradiographic evaluation of the intra-tumoral distribution of 2-deoxy-D-glucose and monoclonal antibodies in xenografts of human ovarian adenocarcinoma. J Nucl Med 34(1): 75–82
17. Kubota R, Yamada S, Kubota K, Ishiwata K, Tamahashi N, Ido T 1992 Intratumoral distribution of fluorine-18-fluorodeoxyglucose in vivo: high accumulation in macrophages and granulation tissues studied by microautoradiography. J Nucl Med 33(11): 1972–1980
18. Wahl R L, Henry C A, Ethier S P 1992 Serum glucose: effects on tumor and normal tissue accumulation of 2-[F-18]-fluoro-2-deoxy-D-glucose in rodents with mammary carcinoma. Radiology 183(3): 643–647
19. Higashi K, Clavo A C, Wahl R L 1993 Does FDG uptake measure proliferative activity of human cancer cells? In vitro comparison with DNA flow cytometry and tritiated thymidine uptake. J Nucl Med 34: 414–419
20. Kubota K, Matsuzawa T, Ito M, Ito K, Fujiwara T, Abe Y, Yoshioka S, Fukuda H, Hatazawa J, Iwata R et al 1985 Lung tumor imaging by positron emission tomography using C-11 L-methionine. J Nucl Med 26: 37–42
21. Bergstrom M, Collins V P, Ehrin E, Ericson K, Eriksson L, Greitz T, Halldin C, von-Holst H, Langstrom B, Lilja A et al 1983 Discrepancies in brain tumor extent as shown by computed tomography and positron emission tomography using [68Ga]EDTA, [11C]glucose, and [11C]methionine. J Comput Assist Tomogr 7(6): 1062–1066
22. Meyer G J, Schober O, Hundeshagen H 1985 Uptake of 11C- L- and D-methionine in brain tumors. Eur J Nucl Med 10(7–8): 373–376
23. Bergstrom-M, Lundqvist H, Ericson K, Lilja A, Johnstrom P, Langstrom B, von Holst H, Eriksson L, Blomqvist G 1987 Comparison of the accumulation kinetics of L-(methyl-11C)-methionine and D-(methyl-11C)-methionine in brain tumors studied with positron emission tomography. Acta Radiol 28(3): 225–229
24. Kubota K, Yamada K, Fukada H, Endo S, Ito M, Abe Y, Yamaguchi T, Fujiwara T, Sato T, Ito K et al 1984 Tumor detection with carbon-11-labelled amino acids. Eur J Nucl Med 9(3): 136–140
25. Shields A F, Lim K, Grierson J, Link J, Krohn K A 1990 Utilization of labeled thymidine in DNA synthesis: studies for PET. J Nucl Med 31(3): 337–342
26. Ishiwata K, Ido T, Abe Y, Matsuzawa T, Murakami M 1985 Studies on 18F-labeled pyrimidines III. Biochemical investigation of 18F-labeled pyrimidines and comparison with 3H-deoxythymidine in tumor-bearing rats and mice. Eur J Nucl Med 10(1–2): 39–44
27. Dimitrakopoulou A, Strauss L G, Clorius J H, Ostertag H, Schlag P, Heim M, Oberdorfer F, Helus F, Haberkorn U, van-Kaick G 1993 Studies with positron emission tomography after systemic administration of fluorine-18-uracil in patients with liver metastases from colorectal carcinoma. J Nucl Med 34(7): 1075–1081
28. Ito M, Lammertsma A A, Wise R J, Bernardi S, Frackowiak R S, Heather J D, McKenzie C G, Thomas D G, Jones T 1982 Measurement of regional cerebral blood flow and oxygen utilisation in patients with cerebral tumours using 15O and positron emission tomography: analytical techniques and preliminary results. Neuroradiology 23: 63–74
29. Wahl R L Quint L E, Cieslak R D, Aisen A M, Koeppe R A, Meyer C R 1993 'Anatometabolic' tumor imaging: fusion of FDG PET with CT or MRI to localize foci of increased activity. J Nucl Med 34(7): 1190–1197
30. Dahlbom M, Hoffman E J, Hoh C K, Schiepers C, Rosenqvist G, Hawkins R A, Phelps M E 1992 Whole-body positron emission tomography: Part I. Methods and performance characteristics. J Nucl Med 33: 1191–1199
31. Hoh C K, Hawkins R A, Glaspy J A, Dahlbom M, Tse N Y, Hoffman E J, Schiepers C, Choi Y, Rege S, Nitzsche E et al 1993 Cancer detection with whole-body PET using 2-[18F]fluoro-2-deoxy-D-glucose. J Comput Assist Tomogr 17(4): 582–589
32. Wahl R L, Zasadny K R, Hutchins G D, Helvie M, Cody R 1993 Metabolic monitoring of breast cancer chemohormonotherapy using positron emission tomography (PET): initial evaluation. J Clin Oncol 11(11): 2101–2111
33. Zasadny K, Wahl R 1993 Standardized uptake values of normal tissues in FDG/PET: Variations with body weight and a method for correction: SUV-lean. Radiology 189: 847–850
34. Di Chiro G, DeLaPaz R L, Brooks R A, Sokoloff L, Kornblith P L, Smith B H, Patronas N J, Kufta C V, Kessler R M, Johnston G S, Manning R G, Wolf A P 1982 Glucose utilization of cerebral gliomas measured by [18F]fluorodeoxyglucose and positron emission tomography. Neurology 32(12): 1323–1329
35. Schifter T, Hoffman J M, Hanson M W, Boyko O B, Beam C, Paine S, Schold S C, Burger P C, Coleman R E 1993 Serial FDG-PET studies in the prediction of survival in patients with primary brain tumors. J Comput Assist Tomogr 17(4): 509–561
36. Francavilla T L, Miletich R S, Di Chiro G, Patronas N J, Rizzoli H V, Wright D C 1989 Positron emission tomography in the detection of malignant degeneration of low-grade gliomas. Neurosurgery 24(1): 1–5
37. Ishikawa M, Kikuchi H, Miyatake S, Oda Y, Yonekura Y, Nishizawa S 1993 Glucose consumption in recurrent gliomas. Neurosurgery 33(1): 28–33
38. Janus T J, Kim E E, Tilbury R, Bruner J M, Yung W K 1993 Use of [18F]fluorodeoxyglucose positron emission tomography in patients with primary malignant brain tumors. Ann Neurol 33: 540–548
39. Fulham M J, Melisi J W, Nishimiya J, Dwyer A J, Di Chiro G 1993 Neuroimaging of juvenile pilocytic astrocytomas: an enigma. Radiology 189(1): 221–225
40. Tyler J L, Diksic M, Villemure J G, Evans A C, Meyer E, Yamamoto Y L, Feindel W 1987 Metabolic and hemodynamic evaluation of gliomas using positron emission tomography. J Nucl Med 28(7): 1123–1133
41. Kim C K, Alavi J B, Alavi A, Reivich M 1991 New grading system of cerebral gliomas using positron emission tomography with F-18 fluorodeoxyglucose. J Neurooncol 10(1): 85–91
42. Doyle W K, Budinger T F, Valk P E, Levin V A, Gutin P H 1987 Tl Differentiation of cerebral radiation necrosis from tumor recurrence by [18F]FDG and 82Rb positron emission tomography. J Comput Assist Tomogr 11 (4): 563–570
43. Bergstrom M, Muhr C, Lundberg P O, Bergstrom K, Gee A D, Fasth K J, Langstrom B 1987 Rapid decrease in amino acid metabolism in prolactin secreting pituitary adenomas after bromocriptine treatment: a PET study. J Comput Assist Tomogr 11 (5): 815–819

44. Ericson K, Blomqvist G, Bergstrom M, Eriksson L, Stone Elander S 1987 Application of a kinetic model on the methionine accumulation in intracranial tumours studied with positron emission tomography. Acta Radiol 28(5): 505–509
45. Griffeth L K, Rich K M, Dehdashti F, Simpson J R, Fusselman M J, McGuire A H, Siegel B A 1993 Brain metastases from non-central nervous system tumors: evaluation with PET Radiology 186(1): 37–44
46. Rosenfeld S S, Hoffman J M, Coleman R E, Glantz M J, Hanson M W, Schold S C 1992 Studies of primary central nervous system lymphoma with fluorine 18 fluorodeoxyglucose positron emission tomography. J Nucl Med 33(4): 532–536
47. Hoffman J M, Waskin H A, Schifter T, Hanson M W, Gray L, Rosenfeld S, Coleman R E 1993 FDG-PET* in differentiating lymphoma from nonmalignant central nervous system lesions in patients with AIDS. J Nucl Med 34: 567–575
48. Di Chiro G, Hatazawa J, Katz D A, Rizzoli H V, De Michele D J 1987 Glucose utilization by intracranial meningiomas as an index of tumor aggressivity and probability of recurrence: a PET study. Radiology 164: 521–526
49. Fujiwara T, Matsuzawa T, Kubota K, Abe Y, Itoh M, Fukuda H, Hatazawa J, Yoshioka S, Yamaguchi K, Ito K 1989 Relationship between histologic type of primary lung cancer and carbon-11-L-methionine uptake with positron emission tomography. J Nucl Med 30(1): 33–37
50. Nolop K B, Rhodes C G, Brudin L H, Beaney R P, Krausz T, Jones T, Hughes J M 1987 Glucose utilization in vivo by human pulmonary neoplasms. Cancer 60(11): 2682–2689
51. Kubota K, Matsuzawa T, Fujiwara T, Ito M, Hatazawa J, Ishiwata K, Iwata R, Ido T 1990 Differential diagnosis of lung tumor with positron emission tomography: a prospective study. J Nucl Med 31 (12): 1927–1932
52. Gupta N C, Frank AR, Dewan N A, Redepenning L S, Rothberg M L, Mailliard J A, Phalen J J, Sunderland J J, Frick M P 1992 Solitary pulmonary nodules: detection of malignancy with PET with 2-[F-18]-fluoro-2-deoxy-D-glucose. Radiology 184(2): 441–444
53. Patz E F Jr, Lowe V J, Hoffman J M, Paine S S, Burrowes P, Coleman R E, Goodman P C 1993 Focal pulmonary abnormalities: evaluation with F-18 fluorodeoxyglucose PET scanning. Radiology 188(2): 487–490
54. Rege S D, Hoh C K, Glaspy J A, Aberle D R, Dahlbom M, Razavi M K, Phelps M E, Hawkins R A 1993 Imaging of pulmonary mass lesions with whole-body positron emission tomography and fluorodeoxyglucose. Cancer 72(1): 82–90
55. Miyazawa H, Arai T, Inagaki K, Morita T, Yano M, Hara T 1992 Detection of mediastinal lymph node metastasis from lung cancer with positron emission tomography (PET) using 11C-methionine. Nippon Kyobu Geka Gakkai Zasshi 40(12): 2125–2130 (in Japanese)
56. Wahl R L, Quint L E, Orringer M and Meyer C 1992 Staging non-small cell lung cancer: comparison of FDG-PET, CT and hybrid 'anatometabolic' fusion images with pathology. Radiological Society of North America 78th Scientific Assembly and Annual Meeting, December 4, 1992
57. Knopp M V, Bischoff H, Oberdorfer F, van-Kaick G 1992 Positronenemissionstomographie des Thorax. Derzeitiger klinischer Stellenwert. [Positron emission tomography of the thorax. The current clinical status.] Radiologe 32 (6): 290–295
58. Beaney R P, Lammertsma A A, Jones T, McKenzie C G, Halnan K E 1984 Positron emission tomography for in vivo measurement of regional blood flow, oxygen utilisation, and blood volume in patients with breast carcinoma. Lancet 1(8369): 131–134
59. McGuire A H, Dehdashti F, Siegel B A, Lyss A P, Brodack J W, Mathias C J, Mintun M A, Katzenellenbogen J A, Welch M J 1991 Positron tomographic assessment of 16 alpha-[18F]-fluoro-17 beta-estradiol uptake in metastatic breast carcinoma. J Nucl Med 32 (8): 1526–1531
60. Minn H, Soini I, 1989 [18 F]Fluorodeoxyglucose scintigraphy in diagnosis and follow up of treatment in advanced breast cancer. Eur J Nucl Med 15(2): 61–66
61. Wahl R L, Cody R L, Hutchins G D, Kuhl D E 1989 PET imaging of breast cancer with 18FDG. Radiology 173: 419
62. Kubota K, Matsuzawa T, Amemiya A, Kondo M, Fujiwara T, Watanuki S, Ito M, Ido T 1989 Imaging of breast cancer with [18 F]fluorodeoxyglucose and positron emission tomography. J Comput Assist Tomogr 13 (6): 1097–1098
63. Wahl R L, Cody R, Hutchins G D, Mudgett E 1991 Primary and metastatic breast carcinoma: initial clinical evaluation with PET with the radiolabeled glucose analog 2-[F-18]-fluorodeoxy-2-D-glucose (FDG). Radiology 179: 765–770
64. Wahl R L, Kaminski M S, Ethier S P, Hutchins G D 1990 The potential of 2-deoxy-2[18F]fluoro-D-glucose (FDG) for the detection of tumor involvement in lymph nodes. J Nucl Med 31 (11): 1831–1835
65. Wahl R L, Cody R L, August D 1991 Initial evaluation of FDG PET for the staging of the axilla in newly-diagnosed breast carcinoma patients. J Nucl Med 32 (5): 981
66. Tse N Y, Hoh C K, Hawkins R A, Zinner M J, Dahlbom M, Choi Y, Maddahi J, Brunicardi F C, Phelps M E, Glaspy J A 1992 The application of positron emission tomographic imaging with fluorodeoxyglucose to the evaluation of breast disease. Ann Surg 216(1): 27–34
67. Nieweg O E, Kim E E, Wong W H, Broussard W F, Singletary S E, Hortobagyi G N, Tilbury R S 1993 Positron emission tomography with fluorine-18-deoxyglucose in the detection and staging of breast cancer. Cancer 71(12): 3920–3925
68. Adler L P, Crowe J P, al-Kaisi N K, Sunshine J L 1993 Evaluation of breast masses and axillary lymph nodes with [F-18] 2-deoxy-2-fluoro-D-glucose PET 1993 Radiology 187(3): 743–750
69. Brown R S, Wahl R L 1993 Over expression of Glut-1 glucose transporter in human breast cancer: an immunohistochemical study. Cancer 72(10): 2979–2985
70. Leskinen-Kallio S, Nagren K, Lehikoinen P, Ruotsalainen U, Joensuu H 1991 Uptake of 11C-methionine in breast cancer studied by PET. An association with the size of S-phase fraction. Br J Cancer 64(6): 1121–1124
71. Strauss L G, Clorius J H, Schlag P, Lehner B, Kimmig B, Engenhart R, Marin Grez M, Helus F, Oberdorfer F, Schmidlin P et al 1989 Recurrence of colorectal tumors: PET evaluation. Radiology 170(2): 329–332
72. Ito K, Kato T, Tadokoro M, Ishiguchi T, Oshima M, Ishigaki T, Sakuma S 1992 Recurrent rectal cancer and scar: differentiation with PET and MR imaging. Radiology 182(2): 549–552
73. Gupta N C, Falk P M, Frank A L, Thorson A M, Frick M P, Bowman B 1993 Pre-operative staging of colorectal carcinoma using positron emission tomography. Nebr Med J 78(2): 30–35
74. Kirchner P T, Ryan J, Zalutsky M, Harper P V 1980 Positron emission tomography for the evaluation of pancreatic disease. Semin Nucl Med 10(4): 374–391
75. Syrota A, Duquesnoy N, Paraf A, Kellershohn C 1982 The role of positron emission tomography in the detection of pancreatic disease. Radiology 143(1): 249–253
76. Kubo S, Yamamoto K, Magata Y, Iwasaki Y, Tamaki N, Yonekura Y, Konishi J Assessment of pancreatic blood flow with positron emission tomography and oxygen-15 water.
77. Bares R, Klever P, Hellwig D, Hauptmann S, Fass J, Hambuechen U, Zopp L, Mueller B, Buell U, Schumpelick V 1993 Pancreatic cancer detected by positron emission tomography with 18F-labelled deoxyglucose: method and first results. Nucl Med Commun 14(7): 596–601
78. Hayashi N, Tamaki N, Yonekura Y, Senda M, Saji H, Yamamoto K, Konishi J, Torizuka K 1985 Imaging of the hepatocellular carcinoma using dynamic positron emission tomography with nitrogen-13 ammonia. J Nucl Med 26(3): 254–257
79. Shibata T, Yamamoto K, Hayashi N, Yonekura Y, Nagara T, Saji H, Mukai T, Konishi J 1988 Dynamic positron emission tomography with 13N-ammonia in liver tumors. Eur J Nucl Med 14(12): 607–611
80. Okazumi S, Enomoto K, Ozaki M, Yamamoto H, Yoshida M, Abe Y, Takayama W, Yamada S, Isono K, Imazeki K et al 1989 Evaluation of the effect of treatment in patients with liver tumors using 18F-fluorodeoxyglucose PET. Kaku-Igaku. 26(6): 793–797 (in Japanese)
81. Nagata Y, Yamamoto K, Hiraoka M, Abe M, Takahashi M,

Akuta K, Nishimura Y, Jo S, Masunaga S, Kubo S, et al 1990 Monitoring liver tumor therapy with [18F]FDG positron emission tomography. J Comput Assist Tomogr 14(3): 370–374
82. Enomoto K, Fukunaga T, Okazumi S, Asano T, Kikuchi T, Yamamoto H, Nagashima T, Isono K, Itoh H, Imazeki K et al 1991 Can fluorodeoxyglucose-positron emission tomography evaluate the functional differentiation of hepatocellular carcinoma? Kaku Igaku 28(11): 1353–1356 (in Japanese)
83. Okazumi S, Isono K, Enomoto K, Kikuchi T, Ozaki M, Yamamoto H, Hayashi H, Asano T, Ryu M 1992 Evaluation of liver tumors using fluorine-18-fluorodeoxyglucose PET: characterization of tumor and assessment of effect of treatment. J Nucl Med 33(3): 333–339
84. Fukunaga T, Enomoto K, Okazumi S, Kikuchi T, Yamamoto H, Asano T, Isono K, Arimizu N, Imazeki K, Itoh Y 1992 Evaluation of gastroenterological disease by using 18F-FDG PET–differential diagnosis of malignancy from benignity. Kaku-Igaku 29(6): 687–690 (in Japanese)
85. Minn H, Joensuu H, Ahonen A, Klemi P I 1988 Fluorodeoxyglucose imaging: a method to assess the proliferative activity of human cancer in vivo. Comparison with DNA flow cytometry in head and neck tumors. Cancer 61(9): 1776–1781
86. Haberkorn U, Strauss L G, Reisser C, Haag D, Dimitrakopoulou A, Ziegler S, Oberdorfer F, Rudat V, van Kaick G 1991 Glucose uptake, perfusion, and cell proliferation in head and neck tumors: relation of positron emission tomography to flow cytometry. J Nucl Med 32(8): 1548–1555
87. Bailet J W, Abemayor E, Jabour B A, Hawkins R A, Ho C, Ward P H 1992 Positron emission tomography: a new, precise imaging modality for detection of primary head and neck tumours and assessment of cervical adenopathy. Laryngoscope 102(3): 281–288
88. Jabour B A, Choi Y, Hoh C K, Rege S D, Soong J C, Lufkin R B, Hanafee W N, Maddahi J, Chaiken L, Bailet J et al 1993 Extracranial head and neck: PET imaging with 2-[F-18]fluoro-2-deoxy-D glucose and MR imaging correlation. Radiology 186(1): 27–35
89. Reisser-C, Haberkorn U, Strauss L G 1992 Stoffwechseldiagnostik bei HNO-Tumoren – eine PET-Studie. [Diagnosis of energy metabolism in ENT tumors – a PET study.] HNO 40(6): 225–231
90. van-Eijkeren M E, De Schryver A, Goethals P, Poupeye E, Schelstraete K, Lemahieu I, De Potter C R 1992 Measurement of short-term 11C-thymidine activity in human head and neck tumours using positron emission tomography (PET). Acta Oncol 31(5): 539–543
91. Lucignani G, Paganelli G, Modorati G, Pieralli S, Rizzo G, Magnani P, Colombo F, Zito F, Landoni C, Scotti G et al 1992 MRI, antibody-guided scintigraphy, and glucose metabolism in uveal melanoma. J Comput Assist Tomogr 16(1): 77–83
92. Gritters L S, Francis I R, Zasadny K R, Wahl R L 1993 Initial assessment of positron emission tomography using 2-fluorine-18-fluoro-2-deoxy-D-glucose in the imaging of malignant melanoma. J Nucl Med 34(9): 1420–1427
93. Paul R 1987 Comparison of fluorine-18-2-fluorodeoxyglucose and gallium-67 citrate imaging for detection of lymphoma. J Nucl Med 28(3): 288–292
94. Okada J, Yoshikawa K, Imazeki K, Minoshima S, Uno K, Itami J, Kuyama J, Maruno H, Arimizu N 1991 The use of FDG-PET in the detection and management of malignant lymphoma: correlation of uptake with prognosis. J Nucl Med 32(4): 686–691
95. Newman J S, Francis I R, Kaminski M S, Wahl R L FDG-PET imaging in lymphoma: correlation with CT. Radiology (in press)
96. Kern K A, Brunetti A, Norton J A, Chang A E, Malawer M, Lack E, Finn R D, Rosenberg S A, Larson S M 1988 Metabolic imaging of human extremity musculoskeletal tumors by PET. J Nucl Med 29(2): 181–186
97. Adler L P, Blair H F, Williams R P, Pathria M N, Makley J T, Joyce M J, al Kaisi N, Miraldi F 1990 Grading liposarcomas with PET using [18F]FDG. J Comput Assist Tomogr 14(6): 960–962
98. Adler L P, Blair H F, Makley J T, Williams R P, Joyce M J, Leisure G, al-Kaisi N, Miraldi F 1991 Noninvasive grading of musculoskeletal tumours using PET. J Nucl Med 32(8): 1508–1512
99. Griffeth L K, Dehdashti F, McGuire A H, McGuire D J, Perry D J, Moerlein S M, Siegel B A 1992 PET evaluation of soft-tissue masses with fluorine-18 fluoro-2-deoxy-D-glucose. Radiology 182(1): 185–194
100. Kawamura J, Hida S, Yoshida O, Yonekura Y, Senda M, Yamamoto K, Saji H, Fujita T, Konishi J 1988 Validity of positron emission tomography (PET) using 2-deoxy-2-[18F]fluoro-D-glucose (FDG) in patients with renal cell carcinoma (preliminary report). Kaku-Igaku 25(10): 1143–1148 (in Japanese)
101. Wahl R L, Harney J, Hutchins G, Grossman H B 1991 Imaging of renal cancer using positron emission tomography with 2-deoxy-2-(18F)-fluoro-D-glucose: pilot animal and human studies. J Urol 146(6): 1470–1474
102. Harney J V, Wahl R L, Liebert M, Kuhl D E, Hutchins G D, Wedemeyer G, Grossman H B 1991 Uptake of 2-deoxy, 2-(18F) fluoro-D-glucose in bladder cancer: animal localization and initial patient positron emission tomography. J Urol 145(2): 279–283
103. Shreve P, Grossman H B, Wahl R L 1993 Initial assessment of FDG/PET detection of skeletal metastatic prostate carcinoma. J Nucl Med 34(5): 223P (abstract)
104. Brown R S, Fisher S J, Wahl R L 1993 Autoradiographic evaluation of the intra-tumoral distribution of 2-deoxy-D-glucose and monoclonal antibodies in xenografts of human ovarian adenocarcinoma. J Nucl Med 34(1): 75–82
105. Wahl R L, Greenough R, Clark M F, Grossman H B 1993 Initial evaluation of FDG/PET imaging of metastatic testicular neoplasms. J Nucl Med 34(5): 6P (abstract)
106. Wahl R L, Hutchins G D, Roberts J 1991 FDG PET imaging of ovarian cancer: Initial evaluation in patients. J Nucl Med 32(5): 982
107. Joensuu H, Ahonen A 1987 Imaging of metastases of thyroid carcinoma with fluorine-18 fluorodeoxyglucose. J Nucl Med 28(5): 910–914
108. Joensuu H, Ahonen A, Klemi P J, 1988 18F-fluorodeoxyglucose imaging in preoperative diagnosis of thyroid malignancy. Eur J Nucl Med 13(10): 502–506
109. Sisson J C, Ackermann R, Meyer M A, Wahl R L 1993 Uptake of FDG by thyroid cancer: implications for diagnosis and therapy. J Clin Endocrinol Metab 77: 1090–1094
110. Rozental J M, Levine R L, Nickles R J, 1991 Changes in glucose uptake by malignant gliomas: preliminary study of prognostic significance. J Neurooncol 10(1): 75–83
111. Minn H, Paul R, Ahonen A 1988 Evaluation of treatment response to radiotherapy in head and neck cancer with fluorine-18 fluorodeoxyglucose. J Nucl Med 29(9): 1521–1525
112. Haberkorn U, Strauss L G, Dimitrakopoulou A, Engenhart R, Oberdorfer F, Ostertag H, Romahn J, van Kaick G 1991 PET studies of fluorodeoxyglucose metabolism in patients with recurrent colorectal tumors receiving radiotherapy. J Nucl Med 32(8): 1485–1490
113. Higashi K, Clavo A C, Wahl R L 1993 In vitro assessment of 2-fluoro-2-deoxy-D-glucose, L-methionine and thymidine as agents to monitor the early response of a human adenocarcinoma cell line to radiotherapy. J Nucl Med 34(5): 773–779
114. Ichiya Y, Kuwabara Y, Otsuka M, Tahara T, Yoshikai T, Fukumura T, Jingu K, Masuda K 1991 Assessment of response to cancer therapy using fluorine-18-fluorodeoxyglucose and positron emission tomography. J Nucl Med 32(9): 1655–1660
115. Haberkorn U, Strauss L G, Dimitrakopoulou A, Seiffert E, Oberdorfer F, Ziegler S, Reisser C, Doll J, Helus F, van Kaick G 1993 Fluorodeoxyglucose imaging of advanced head and neck cancer after chemotherapy. J Nucl Med 34(1): 12–17
116. Kubota K, Yamada S, Ishiwata K, Ito M, Fujiwara T, Fukuda H, Tada M, Ido T 1993 Evaluation of the treatment response of lung cancer with positron emission tomography and L-[methyl-11C]methionine: a preliminary study. Eur J Nucl Med 20(6): 495–501

PART B

Radionuclide therapy

70. Principles of radionuclide therapy

Duncan Ackery

The concept of carrying a cytotoxic agent, such as a radionuclide, direct to an aberrant cell remains an attractive alternative to conventional forms of radiation treatment. In theory, the intimate contact between a radioactive conjugate and a cell enables the absorbed radiation dose to be concentrated at the site of abnormality with minimal injury to normal tissues.[1] A variety of approaches to this problem is possible (Table 70.1). Some of the principles underlying radionuclide therapy will be discussed here. Clinical experience is described in subsequent chapters in this section.

TISSUE FACTORS AFFECTING RADIOPHARMACEUTICAL UPTAKE

Several factors affect the uptake of radiopharmaceuticals into diseased tissue, in particular malignant tumours.[2] They include changes in blood perfusion, increases in extravascular space and changes in interstitial pressure and permeability.

A malignant tumour derives its perfusion from the blood vessels of the tissue in which it is located. As the tumour grows, increasing pressure is put upon these vessels, and this leads to dramatic changes in blood perfusion.[3] Blood flow decreases exponentially in relation to tumour mass (Fig. 70.1). In addition, vascular stasis leads to thrombosis and occlusion. Tumour cells become hypoxic[4] and nutritionally deficient, and eventually die, giving regions of local necrosis. This occurs in tumours of a diameter of only a few millimetres. Animal tumours, and some of those in man, have been shown to have no adrenergic innervation, although alpha-receptors may be present and be able to respond to vasoactive drugs. Vasomotor tone can be modulated in the afferent vessels which supply the tumour vascular network.[5]

Table 70.1 Types of radionuclide therapy

Elemental e.g. ^{131}I, ^{32}P, ^{89}Sr
Metabolic agents, e.g. ^{131}I-MIBG
Antibodies
Bone-seeking chelates
Bioreductive agents
Labelled cells
Liposomes
Vascular blockade, e.g. labelled lipiodol or microspheres
Direct administration into body cavities

A reduction in blood flow may lower the efficacy of radionuclide treatment in three ways: less radiopharmaceutical is supplied to viable cells; the functional integrity of tumour cells declines so that demand for metabolic substrates is less; and the hypoxic state of the cells reduces the sensitivity of the tissue to the effects of radiation.

RADIOPHARMACEUTICAL UPTAKE AND RETENTION

The cumulative absorbed radiation dose to tissues under-

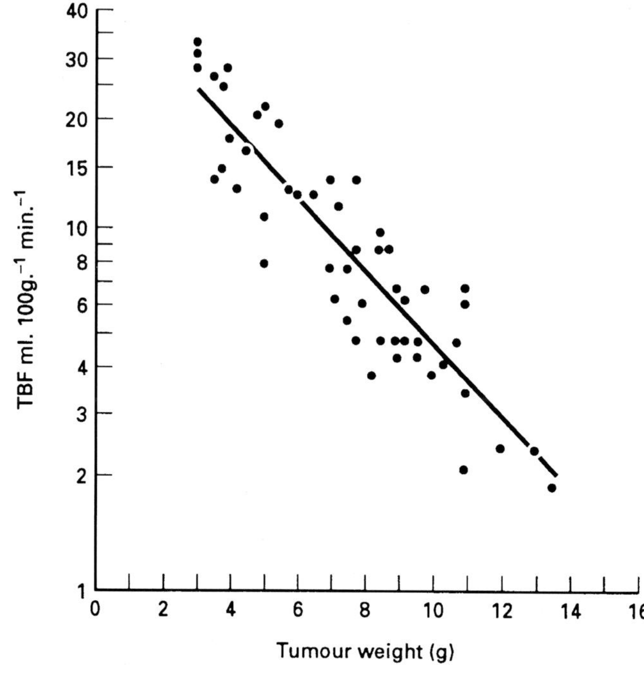

Fig. 70.1 Exponential decrease in total blood flow with increasing tumour weight. (Reproduced with permission from Vaupel.[4])

going radionuclide treatment is a function both of the quantity of radiopharmaceutical taken up at a cellular site and its subsequent retention at that site.

When planning radionuclide therapy the physical half-life of the radionuclide label should be chosen, if possible, to match the biological half-life of the radiopharmaceutical in the tissue to be treated. Although some compromise on this is usually necessary, in general a physical half-life that is too short will not take full advantage of the residence time in the tissue, whereas a long physical half-life gives unnecessarily protracted doses to normal tissues. The physical half-life also influences the dose rate at which the radiation is given, which may bring about a different response because of an enhanced radiobiological effect at higher dose rate. Uptake that is non-homogeneous because of uneven blood flow or non-uniform trapping of radiopharmaceutical reduces local absorbed doses when radiation of low penetration is used.

No radiopharmaceutical is entirely selective, and other tissues will compete for its uptake, reducing the final concentration at the treatment site. For example, in the case of differentiated thyroid malignancy the amount of radioiodine taken up by metastases is usually negligible if normally functioning thyroid tissue is present.

Pharmacological intervention may enhance uptake by altering the biokinetics of the radiopharmaceutical in favour of the tissue to be treated. An increase in concentration of labelled monoclonal antibody is possible with beta-adrenergic blocking agents, which decrease the cardiac output to normal tissues, e.g. the liver, without affecting the poorly innervated tumour vessels.[6] Alternatively, local tumour blood flow might be relatively increased by vasodilation. Another approach is to use calcium channel blocking drugs which can enhance the retention of metaiodobenzylguanidine in malignant phaeochromocytoma.[7] The potential of other pharmaceuticals for enhancing radiopharmaceutical uptake requires further investigation.

Drug intervention can also be used by the prior administration of chemotherapeutic agents which inhibit DNA synthesis in normal cells but not in those of the tumour.[8]

CHOICE OF RADIOLABEL

It has been suggested[9] that radionuclides be classified into five groups according to the range of principal radiation emitted (Table 70.2). The first group comprises alpha-emitters. Alpha-particles have a relatively short range (around 50–90 μm) and traverse up to about 10 cell diameters from the point of radioactive decay. The great therapeutic potential of alpha-emitters lies in the high energy loss within this short track; about 400 times more energy is deposited per unit distance than for beta-radiation, and the high linear energy transfer (80–100 keV/μm) deposits approximately 1.0 MeV upon traversing the

Table 70.2 Potential radionuclides for targeting radiotherapy (Modified from Humm.[9])

Alpha	Beta mean range <200 μm	Beta mean range >200 μm<1 mm	Beta mean range >1 mm	Electron capture/ internal conversion
^{211}At	^{33}P	^{47}Sc	^{32}P	^{67}Ga
$^{212}Bi(^{212}Pb)$	^{121}Sn	^{67}Cu	^{89}Sr	^{71}Ge
^{223}Ra	^{177}Lu	^{77}As	^{90}Y	^{77}Br
	^{191}Os	^{105}Rh	^{114m}In	^{103}Pd
^{225}Ac	^{199}Au	^{109}Pd	^{188}Re	^{119}Sb
		^{111}Ag		^{123}I
		^{131}I		^{125}I
		^{143}Pr		^{131}Cs
		^{153}Sm		^{193m}Pt
		^{161}Te		^{197}Hg
		^{186}Re		

diameter of a cell nucleus. This is sufficient to give multiple double strand breaks of DNA from a single traversal. Cell survival studies with alpha-emitters show no oxygen enhancement and little subsequent repair of radiation damage. The alpha-emitters of most interest for radionuclide therapy have been ^{211}At and ^{212}Bi. Both have rather short physical half-lives, 7.2 h and 60.6 min respectively, although by conjugating the lead parent of ^{212}Bi the peak energy loss of this nuclide can be extended to 3.8 h. ^{211}At, as astatide or as a chemical conjugate, has been tested in experimental animal models, but its use has been reported only anecdotally in man.[10] Other possible alpha-emitters are ^{223}Ra and ^{225}Ac, which has a half-life of 10 days with a daughter radionuclide, ^{213}Bi, that could possibly be supplied from a bedside generator.[11]

The next three groups of radionuclides which have potential for therapy are the beta-emitters. These may be classified into those of short range (less than 200 μm), of medium range (>200 μm and <1 mm) and of long range (>1 mm). A number of possible candidates exist in these categories and some (e.g. ^{131}I, ^{32}P, ^{89}Sr, ^{90}Y) have been in clinical use for many years. Iodine has been the first choice for ligand labelling; it is easily conjugated to organic compounds and biochemical macromolecules. As ^{131}I it is available with high radionuclidic purity, enabling high specific activity labelling, an important consideration when the number of binding sites in the target tissue is limited. Its use also permits measurements of the biokinetics and tissue retention of its labelled conjugates.

The final group contains radionuclides which decay by electron capture and/or internal conversion. These transitions bring about a series of vacancies in the electron shells of the disintegrating atom, which in turn result in the emission of a cascade of Auger and Coster–Kronig conversion electrons of low energy. Many of these have a very short range (less than 10 Å), and significant radiobiological damage will only result if the emission takes place very close to the cellular DNA. For example for ^{125}I, cell killing is more than 300 times more effective if the electron emission occurs close to the genome compared with decay at the level of the cell membrane (Fig. 70.2).[12] It is essential therefore that the precise location of the radiopharmaceutical in the cell is determined if an optimal choice of radiolabel is to be administered. Quantitative autoradiography or other methods of defining this are required. Different Auger emitters have been compared for their potential for radionuclide therapy.[13]

Although ^{125}I as iodide has been shown to be effective for the treatment of thyrotoxicosis,[14] few conjugated radiopharmaceuticals are available as DNA ligands. One of the few is ^{125}I-labelled deoxyuridine, which may break DNA both by Auger deposition of energy and by charge-induced molecular fragmentation.[12] When the decay of ^{125}I occurs in the cytoplasm the energy loss within DNA is calculated to be much less, which could be a limitation in its value as a radiolabel for metaiodobenzylguanidine, which is concentrated mainly in the cytoplasm of neuroectodermal tumour cells.

^{123}I also emits Auger electrons and an energetic (125–155 keV) internal conversion electron which gives a similar dose at approximately one cell diameter as ^{131}I.[15] The cell killing effect of ^{123}I has been confirmed when conjugated to deoxyuridine.[16] If problems of production and cost could be overcome the use of ^{123}I might avoid some of the radiotoxicity due to protracted doses given by ^{131}I.

The size of tumour masses and the potential inhomogeneity of uptake of radiopharmaceutical also affect the choice of a radionuclide label. Using model systems the energy absorbed fraction can be calculated for different beta emissions. When deposition is not uniform the energy loss in 'cold' regions is a function of both the diameter of the unlabelled region and of the emitted beta-energy.[17]

Availability and cost are important considerations in the choice of radionuclide for therapy. Cyclotron production is expensive for therapeutic quantities of material, and a short physical half-life means loss of radioactivity during transit. Clinical use becomes feasible if delivery can be made within the period of one physical half-life. Generator systems are available for some radionuclides, but few hospitals have the hot cell facilities necessary for the handling and chemistry of therapeutic radiopharmaceutical doses.

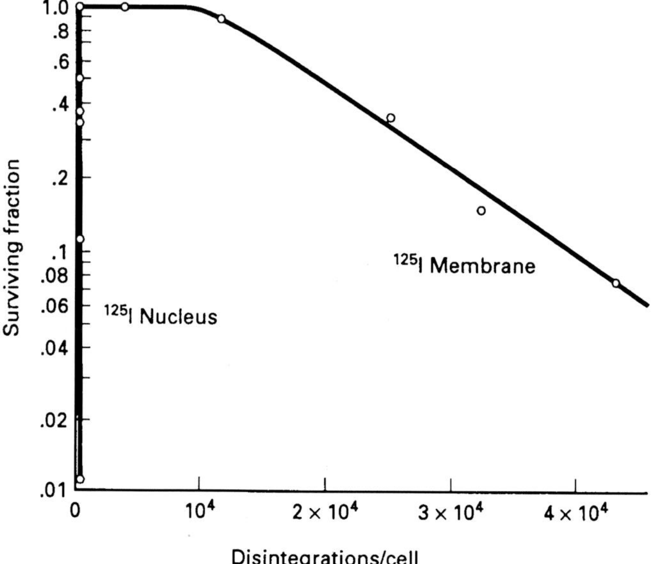

Fig. 70.2 Fraction of cells surviving various doses of ^{125}I deoxyuridine (DNA) or ^{125}I-labelled concanavalin (membrane). (Reproduced with permission from Hofer.[12])

CHEMICAL CONJUGATION

Chemical combination of a radionuclide with a tissue-selective pharmaceutical is often complex, particularly in the case of radiometals. In limited circumstances direct labelling may be possible, but more usually a conjugating molecule (usually a chelate) needs to be attached to the pharmaceutical. Chelate molecules are usually large and their attachment may adversely influence the behaviour of the radiopharmaceutical with reduction in the final tissue concentration. Simple chelates which bind radiometals in vitro may release them subsequently in vivo, giving an increase in radiation burden from free radionuclide, the ultimate whole-body dose depending on whether it is excreted, stored or re-utilized.

After preparation radioconjugates are subject to high radiation fluxes and may undergo self-irradiation autoradiolysis. Decomposition into a variety of radiolabelled subspecies may occur with release of free radionuclide.[18] This can be minimized by dilution or by freezing the radiopharmaceutical solution[19] or by the addition of non-toxic radical scavenging compounds. In spite of these precautions it is advisable to minimize the time between synthesis of the radiopharmaceutical and delivery to the patient.

ASSESSMENT OF RADIATION TOXICITY

As no radiopharmaceutical is entirely tissue specific, some administered radioactivity will inevitably concentrate in other parts of the body. In most cases the stem cells of bone marrow are the critical site and show slow recovery after evidence of initial injury at about 4–6 weeks. Radioactivity is taken up by other tissues, such as the liver or thyroid, and the urinary tract is subject to irradiation from excreted radiopharmaceutical. Radiation doses to these tissues are greater with long-lived radionuclidic impurities or when free radionuclide is released into the circulation. Normal tissue may also be at risk if it lies adjacent to the treatment site or if it contains foci of malignant cells, e.g. in bone marrow.[20] In spite of predicted high radiation doses to the liver, urinary tract or other organs, it is unusual to observe functional changes in these organs following treatment. Radiation doses to the thyroid when radioiodine-labelled compounds are used are minimized by the use of drugs which block uptake of iodide.

When irreversible marrow injury is anticipated it is common practice to harvest and store autologous marrow cells from the patient prior to the onset of chemotherapy.[21] This should also be the practice with radionuclide therapy, particularly when repeated infusions of several gigabecquerels of radioactivity over a long period are planned.

REFERENCES

1. Sisson J C 1986 Radionuclide therapy for malignancy: influences of physical characteristics of radionuclides and experience with meta-iodobenzylguanidine. Clin Oncol 5: 1–21
2. Cobb L M 1989 Intratumour factors influencing the access of antibody to tumour cells. Cancer Immunol Immunother 28: 235–240
3. Reinhold H S 1979 In vivo observations of tumor blood flow. In: Petersen H-I (ed) Tumor blood circulation: angiogenesis, vascular morphology and blood flow of experimental and human tumors. CRC Press, Boca Raton, p 115
4. Vaupel P 1979 Oxygen supply to malignant tumors. In: Petersen H-I (ed) Tumor blood circulation: angiogenesis, vascular morphology and blood flow of experimental and human tumors. CRC Press, Boca Raton, p 143
5. Mattson J, Appelgren L, Hamberger B, Petersen H-I 1979 Tumor vessel innervation and influence of vasoactive drugs on tumor blood flow. In: Petersen H-I (ed). Tumor blood circulation: angiogenesis, vascular morphology and blood flow of experimental and human tumors. CRC Press, Boca Raton, p 129
6. Smyth M J, Pietersz G A, McKenzie I F C 1987 Use of vasoactive agents to increase tumor perfusion and the antitumor efficacy of drug–monoclonal antibody conjugates. J Natl Cancer Inst 79: 1367–1373
7. Blake G M, Lewington V J, Fleming J S, Zivanovic M A, Ackery D M 1988 Modification by nifedipine of I-131 metaiodobenzylguanidine kinetics in malignant phaeochromocytoma. Eur J Nucl Med 14: 345–348
8. Bagshawe K D 1986 Reversed-role chemotherapy for resistant cancer. Lancet 2: 778–781
9. Humm J L 1986 Dosimetric aspects of radiolabeled antibodies for tumor therapy. J Nucl Med 27: 1490–1497
10. Brown I 1986 Astatine-211: its possible applications in cancer therapy. Appl Radiat Isot 37: 789–798
11. Geerlings M W, Kaspersen F M, Apostolidis C, van der Hout R 1993 The feasibility of 225Ac as a source of alpha-particles in radioimmunotherapy. Nucl Med Commun 14: 121–125
12. Hofer K G 1980 Radiation biology and potential, therapeutic applications of radionuclides. Bull Cancer 67: 343–353
13. Humm J L, Charlton D E 1989 A new calculational method to assess the therapeutic potential of Auger electron emission. Int J Radiat Oncol Biol Phys 17: 351–360
14. McDougall I R, Greig W R, Gillespie F C 1971 Radioactive iodine (125I) therapy for thyrotoxicosis. N Engl J Med 285: 1099–1104
15. Jungerman J A, Kin-Hung P Y, Zanelli C I 1984 Radiation absorbed dose estimates at the cellular level for some electron-emitting radionuclides for radioimmunotherapy. Int J Appl Radiat Isot 9: 883–888
16. Makrigiorgos G M, Kassis A I, Baranowska-Kortylewicz J, McElvany K D, Welch M J, Sastry K S R, Adelstein S J 1989 Radiotoxicity of 5-[123I]iodo-2′-deoxyuridine in V79 cells: a comparison with 5-[125I]iodo-2′-deoxyuridine. Rad Res 118: 532–544
17. Humm J L, Cobb L M 1990 Nonuniformity of tumor dose in radioimmunotherapy. J Nucl Med 31: 75–83
18. Kishore R, Eary J F, Krohn K A et al 1986 Autoradiolysis of iodinated monoclonal antibody preparations. Nucl Med Biol 13: 457–459
19. Wahl R L, Wissing J, del Rosario R, Zasadny K R 1990 Inhibition of autoradiolysis of radiolabeled monoclonal antibodies by cryopreservation. J Nucl Med 31: 84–89
20. Hoefnagel C A, Voûte J, de Kraker J, Marcuse H R 1987 Radionuclide diagnosis and therapy of neural crest tumors using iodine-131 metaiodobenzylguanidine. J Nucl Med 28: 308–314
21. Pritchard J, McElwain T J, Graham-Pole J 1982 High dose melphalan with autologous bone marrow for treatment of advanced neuroblastoma. Br J Cancer 45: 86–94

71. Dosimetric considerations

Maggie A. Flower

Radionuclide therapy offers a wide variety of new approaches in the treatment of malignancy and other diseases,[1] but toxicity and dose–response studies are essential in order to evaluate the efficacy of new treatments. The assessment of radiation dose delivered internally during systemic radionuclide therapy is difficult and challenging. This chapter covers the dosimetric considerations of radionuclide therapy and will review both conventional and new approaches to internal dosimetry. Whatever the mechanism used to target radionuclides for therapy, the dose distribution, and hence the therapeutic effect, will depend on the properties of the specific radionuclides employed.

CHOICE OF RADIONUCLIDE

There are two basic considerations in choosing a radiopharmaceutical for radionuclide therapy:

1. physical properties of the radionuclide (i.e. type, energy and abundance of emissions and physical half-life);
2. chemical properties required for localization and retention in the tumour (i.e. stability, specific activity, pH).

The types of radionuclide decay which are of greatest potential use in radionuclide therapy are those which involve the emission of beta-particles, Auger electrons and alpha-particles, with few or no accompanying gamma-rays. ^{131}I and ^{32}P have been the most commonly used radionuclides, but their physical properties are not necessarily ideal. Other radionuclides together with new pharmaceuticals have been considered.[1–4]

Beta-emitters

Although pure beta-emitters (e.g. ^{32}P) may be considered as ideal, since they deliver a high local dose while sparing tissues at a distance, radionuclides that emit gamma-rays in addition to beta-particles (e.g. ^{131}I) have the advantage that external counting and imaging techniques can be used to assess the uptake and distribution of the therapy agent. However, these gamma-rays cause increased dose to the normal tissues. The values of Δ_p and Δ_{np} (the total equilibrium dose constants for penetrating and non-penetrating radiations respectively) are useful indicators of the gamma dose relative to the beta dose for each beta-emitting therapy radionuclide (Table 71.1).

The beta range is important in relation to the size of

Table 71.1 Physical properties of beta-emitting radionuclides with half-lives greater than 2 days, which are of potential use or have been used for radionuclide therapy (Data from International Commission on Radiological Protection.[5])

Radio nuclide	$t_{1/2}$	$n_{i,np}$	$\bar{E}_{i,np}$	$n_{i,p}$	$\bar{E}_{i,p}$	Δ_{np}	Δ_p
	(days)		(MeV)		(MeV)	($\times 10^{-14}$Gy kg/Bq/s)	
^{191}Os	15.4	1.00	0.038	0.26	0.129	2.17	1.28
^{35}S	87.4	1.00	0.049	–	–	0.78	–
^{33}P	25.4	1.00	0.077	–	–	1.22	–
^{45}Ca	163.	1.00	0.077	–	–	1.22	–
^{199}Au	3.2	0.66	0.082	0.37	0.158	2.28	1.42
^{169}Er	9.3	0.55	0.101	–	–	1.67	–
^{67}Cu	2.6	0.57	0.121	0.49	0.185	2.47	1.83
^{47}Sc	3.4	0.68	0.143	0.68	0.159	2.59	1.72
^{177}Lu	6.7	0.79	0.149	0.11	0.208	2.36	0.56
^{161}Tb	6.9	0.67	0.154	0.22	0.025	3.14	0.56
^{131}I	8.0	0.89	0.192	0.81	0.364	3.03	6.09
^{153}Sm	2.0	0.43	0.229	0.28	0.103	4.34	0.97
^{143}Pr	13.6	1.00	0.314	–	–	5.03	–
^{198}Au	2.7	0.99	0.315	0.96	0.412	5.23	6.48
^{186}Re	3.8	0.73	0.362	0.09	0.137	5.50	0.33
^{111}Ag	7.5	0.93	0.363	0.07	0.342	5.67	0.42
^{89}Sr	50.5	1.00	0.583	–	–	9.34	–
^{32}P	14.3	1.00	0.695	–	–	11.12	–
^{124}I	4.2	0.22	0.830	0.61*	0.603*	3.09	17.29
^{90}Y	2.7	1.00	0.935	–	–	14.98	–

n_i and $\bar{E}_i$ are the mean number and mean energy for the most abundant radiations

Δ_{np} and Δ_p are the total equilibrium dose constants (i.e. total energy emitted per nuclear disintegration) for non-penetrating and penetrating radiations respectively.

*^{124}I decays via electron capture and positron emission. In addition to the photons listed, photons with $n_i = 0.451$, $E_i = 0.511$ are emitted following positron annihilation.

tumour to be treated. There is a wide choice of beta-emitting radionuclides (Table 71.1) for radionuclide therapy and hence a flexibility in the choice of beta range in tissue. The relationship between the specific ionization and the range of beta-particles in soft tissue with respect to beta-energy is shown in Figure 71.1. The average energy of an emitted beta-particle is approximately one-third of its maximum energy, and the maximum range in soft tissue (in mm) is approximately equal to the maximum energy (in MeV) multiplied by 5.[2] High-energy beta-particles with their longer range are better suited to the treatment of larger volumes. If the tumour is large compared with the beta range, and the beta-emitter is uniformly distributed throughout the tumour volume, the dose rate is uniform throughout this volume except for a reduction near the outer edge. For tumours which are small compared with the beta range, a large fraction of the total energy from beta-particles emitted within the tumour will be deposited in surrounding tissues (Fig. 71.2). Hence, for the treatment of micrometastases, short-range electrons and alpha emitters would be more appropriate.

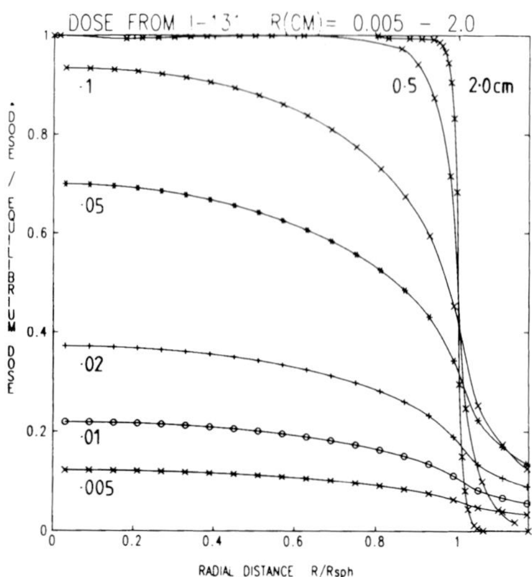

Fig. 71.2 Graphs of beta dose (expressed as a fraction of the equilibrium dose) versus radial distance (R) expressed as a fraction of the sphere radius, R_{sph} for a sphere uniformly filled with ^{131}I (maximum range = 1.5 mm). (Reproduced with permission from Nahum & Babich.[7])

Auger electrons

Radionuclides (e.g. ^{125}I) that decay by electron capture or internal conversion emit low-energy characteristic X-rays and Auger electrons. Most of these electrons have very short range (< 1 μm) and therefore are only of use in therapy if the source is attached, or very close, to the cell nucleus. The potential use of Auger emitters specifically for radioimmunotherapy has been discussed elsewhere.[3]

Alpha-emitters

The advantages of alpha-emitters (e.g. ^{211}At, ^{212}Bi) for radionuclide therapy are their short range (typically 50–90 μm, i.e. several cell diameters) and high linear energy transfer (LET). A single alpha-particle can deposit approximately 0.25 Gy in a 10-μm-diameter cell nucleus.[3] However, alpha-emitters have several disadvantages. Most of the tumour cells or their nearest neighbours need to be labelled with the alpha-emitting radionuclide in order to irradiate all tumours cells. Also, any energy deposition in normal cells, being of high LET, increases the possibility of normal tissue damage and second cancers.[2] Finally, the handling of alpha-emitters is a more hazardous procedure compared with handling beta-emitters. Examples of experimental studies using alpha-emitters include ^{211}At-conjugated antibodies for the treatment of lymphoma[3] and ^{211}At-methylene blue targeted radiotherapy of pigmented melanomas.[8]

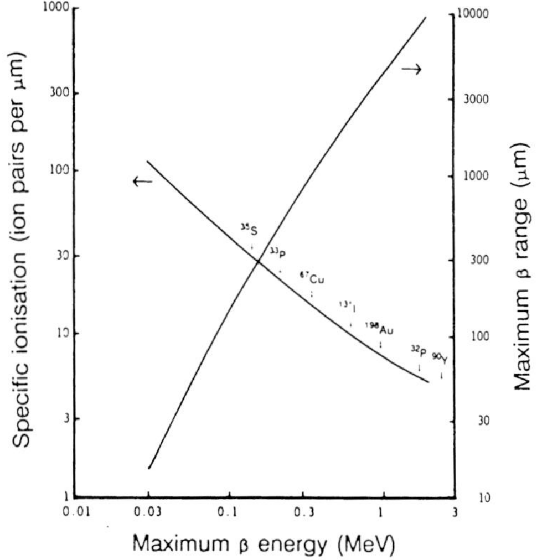

Fig. 71.1 The relationships between the specific ionization and the range of beta-rays in soft tissue with respect to the beta-energy. (Reproduced with permission from Flower & Chittenden.[6])

DOSE-LIMITING ORGANS

The dose which can be delivered to the tumour is limited by the maximum dose which can be tolerated by normal tissues. The dose-limiting organs for radionuclide therapy depend on the route of administration and on the radiopharmaceutical. In systemic therapy the dose-limiting organ is often the bone-marrow: if there is a risk of bone marrow ablation, a bone marrow harvest may be performed prior to therapy, for subsequent regrafting if necessary. For intrathecal administrations the dose-limiting organ is the spinal cord. The bladder is at risk from radioactivity in the urine, and patients should be hydrated to reduce the dose to the bladder wall: guidance for establishing protocols for bladder dose reduction is provided in a recent MIRD pamphlet.[9] If there is high uptake in the liver, this could lead to radiation hepatitis and chronic veno-occlusive liver disease.

The dose-limiting organs for new agents are not necessarily known in advance, and it is important that detailed dosimetry estimates and toxicity studies are performed for each new agent considered for radionuclide therapy.

DOSIMETRY CALCULATIONS

It is difficult to achieve precise estimates of the magnitude and distribution of internal dose delivered from unsealed sources. As a result of the inherent large uncertainties, dosimetry calculations are often not performed on individual patients. However, with the advent of improved imaging and counting techniques, estimates of internal dose are becoming more commonplace.[10] Even then, these are often retrospective dosimetry calculations performed using data acquired during therapy, rather than pretreatment planning. However, a method of three-dimensional treatment planning for internal radionuclide therapy has been described.[11]

The MIRD schema

The conventional method of calculating absorbed dose delivered internally is known as the MIRD schema,[12] which has been described briefly in the Basic Sciences Section of this book (Section 8). The first step in applying the MIRD schema is to identify all the source and target organs. In the treatment of tumours, the source organs are ideally just the tumours, although in practice other organs and tissues are involved and have to be considered; the target organs (using MIRD terminology) and both the tumours and the dose-limiting organs. For each pair of source and target organs, the following equation is used to calculate the absorbed dose, $D_{t \leftarrow s}$ (in Gy), to a target organ from activity in a source organ:

$$D_{t \leftarrow s} = \tilde{A}_s \left[\frac{1}{m_t} \sum_i \Delta_i \, \phi_i \right] \qquad (1)$$

where $\tilde{A}_s$ is the cumulated activity in the source (in Bq s); m_t is the mass of the target organ (in kg); Δ_i is the equilibrium absorbed dose constant for radiation of type i, or the mean energy per nuclear disintegration (in Gy kg/Bq/s); and ϕ_i is the absorbed fraction, defined as the fraction of the radiation of type i emitted from the source and absorbed by the target.

Applying MIRD in practice

Chapter 000 provides more details of the parameters in equation (1) and how each parameter is determined in practice. If sequential gamma camera imaging is used to determine the cumulated activity, $\tilde{A}_s$, in each source organ, deadtime corrections[13] may be necessary during the first few days after a therapy administration. Alternatively, lead sheets can be attached to the front face of the camera in order to reduce the count rate.[14]

None of the currently used therapy radionuclides is ideal for imaging with a gamma-camera as they are either pure beta-emitters (e.g. ^{32}P) or the energies of the gamma-rays emitted (e.g. from ^{131}I) are such that poor-quality images are obtained (owing to penetration of and scattering in the collimator). Hence, alternatives to the gamma-camera (e.g. stationary probe or whole-body scanner) are recommended for quantitative measurements of tumour or organ uptake when dealing with therapy radionuclides. Other options are:

1. to perform a tracer study prior to therapy using a radioisotope more suited to gamma-camera imaging (e.g. ^{123}I instead of ^{131}I, although the advantages offered by the lower energy photons (159 keV) are offset by the shorter half-life (13 h), which limits its usefulness in the determination of $A_s(t)$ at $t > 24$ h);
2. to use dual radionuclides, using a simultaneous injection of both imaging and therapy radionuclides (e.g. $^{51}Cr/^{32}P$ [15] or $^{85}Sr/^{89}Sr$ [16] for imaging/therapy respectively);
3. to image the bremsstrahlung radiation from beta-emitters;[17]
4. to use tomographic imaging (SPECT[18,19] or PET[20,21]) as an alternative to planar imaging.

Radiation protection problems and count rate limitations of the gamma-camera make data acquisition at early time points difficult. A combination of early measurements during a tracer study and late measurements following therapy administration is a reasonable compromise. However, the kinetics of the radiopharmaceutical may not be identical in the tracer and therapy studies, so extrapolation of data can also be subject to error. Sequential quantitative tomographic imaging can be used to assess the cumulated radioactive concentration, $\tilde{A}_s/m_t$. If ^{131}I is the therapy radionuclide, the various ways of determining the radioactive concentration are (in order of increasing accuracy):

1. ^{131}I SPECT (using ultra-high resolution, high-energy collimators);
2. ^{123}I SPECT tracer study prior to therapy;
3. ^{124}I positron emission tomography (PET) tracer study prior to therapy.

In addition to using ^{124}I for pretherapy tracer studies,[21,22] it is also a potential therapy radionuclide [since the values of Δ_{np} (Table 71.1) for ^{124}I and ^{131}I are virtually identical]. However, the problem of production in sufficient quantities needs to be solved, for example using internal targetry in a cyclotron[22] or using the $^{124}Xe(n,p)^{124}I$ reaction in a reactor with a high neutron flux. As PET usually offers the best spatial resolution, other positron emitters are being considered for tracer studies prior to unsealed source therapy (e.g. ^{64}Cu, ^{83}Sr and ^{86}Y tracer studies prior to ^{67}Cu, ^{89}Sr and ^{90}Y therapy respectively).[23]

Bone marrow dosimetry

As the bone marrow is the dose-limiting organ in systemic radionuclide treatments, bone marrow dosimetry is worthy of special attention. Various methods[24] have been used to calculate the marrow dose. Inaccuracies in bone marrow dose in radioimmunotherapy (RIT) are caused by:

1. inadequate knowledge of the distribution of antibody within the marrow;
2. treating the beta-rays as non-penetrating (i.e. ignoring the implications of Fig. 71.2);
3. ignoring the photon dose to the marrow from source organs other than the bone marrow;
4. ignoring the effects of backscattering of electrons at the marrow–bone interface.

In the estimation of absorbed dose to red marrow from non-specific uptake of radiolabelled antibodies, it is recommended[24] that the following assumptions be made:

1. marrow specific activity is one-third of blood specific activity;
2. clearance of activity from bone marrow is equal to that from blood;
3. marrow activity is uniformly distributed.

Given the uncertainties associated with marrow dose estimates, the current method of choice for the assessment of bone marrow toxicity from radioimmunotherapy (RIT) is the radiobiological end-point method whereby the activity administered is slowly escalated until critical haematopoietic depression is reached.

Alternative dosimetry methods

The alternative methods of in vivo dosimetry are autoradiography and the use of miniature thermoluminescent dosimeters (TLDs). These techniques have been developed and evaluated in tumour models but provide valuable insight into the optimal properties of therapy agents.

Autoradiography

Autoradiography provides high-resolution images of radionuclide distributions at the subcellular level and has been particularly useful in providing an understanding of the dose delivered to tumour during RIT.[25] However, autoradiography only provides a single time point on the activity–time curve and in only a thin two-dimensional section of the tumour (unless multiple sections are obtained). The use of single sections is a particular disadvantage for long-range beta-emitters.[26] The information provided by autoradiography is often used as the input to theoretical microdosimetric calculations.

Thermoluminescent dosimetry

A direct measurement of the integrated absorbed dose can be achieved via the use of implanted dosimeters. TLD measurements in a tumour phantom model[27] have confirmed that the absorbed dose at the outer tumour boundary depends on the specific activity in the tumour, the beta range and tumour size. The local absorbed dose can be determined from micro-TLDs recovered from tissue sections cut with a microtome. Unfortunately, in vivo signal fading occurs, in which the signal loss is proportional to the length of time the TLD remains in vivo. However, provided individual sensitivity factors were used, micro-TLDs (82 μm thick) have been used in vivo to determine doses to within ± 12%.[28]

Theoretical dosimetry studies

Dose distributions can be calculated using Monte Carlo techniques[29] or by integrating theoretically derived dose point kernels over the radionuclide distribution.[7,30] Theoretical calculations of dose distributions can be performed at both the macroscopic and microscopic level, since the kernel can describe the dose deposition over centimetres or microns respectively.[31]

Theoretical studies of the microscopic distribution of radionuclides provide an insight into the dose distribution at the cellular and subcellular level. Microdosimetry is particularly valuable in assessing the dose distribution from inhomogeneous depositions of short-range emitters.

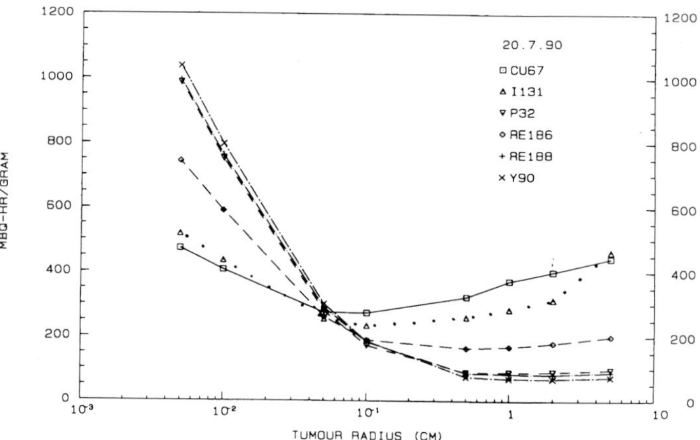

Fig. 71.3 The cumulated activity per unit mass required for a tumour control probability of 0.5 as a function of tumour radius for a range of radionuclides and for neuroblastoma tumour cells. The model assumes uniform uptake and uniform radiosensitivity, and the effect of the gamma dose was ignored. (Reproduced with permission from Nahum & Babich.[7])

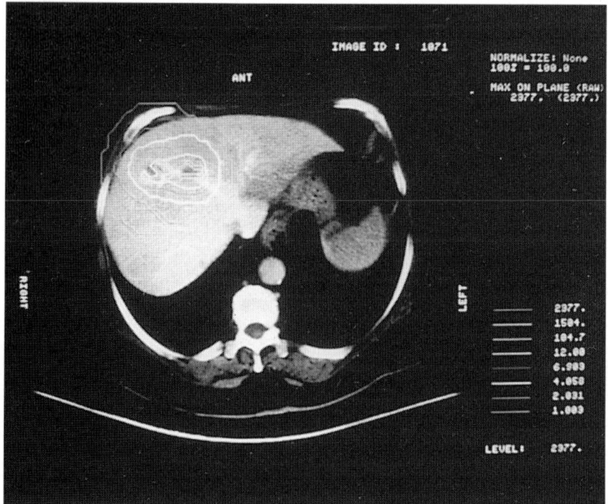

Fig. 71.4 Isodose contours superimposed on a CT image through the liver. The dose values (in cGy) assigned to each isodose contour arise from a cumulated activity concentration of 740 GBq s/ml in the two tumours seen in the anterior portion of the liver and in a third tumour seen in a different slice. (Reproduced with permission from Sgouros et al.[11]) (Also shown in colour on Plate 21.)

For example, in RIT cell killing will depend on whether or not the antibody binds to the cell-surface membrane or is internalized by the tumour cells.[29]

A theoretical model used to study the effect of beta range on tumour dose (Fig. 71.2) has been extended to predict tumour control probability (TCP) for spherical neuroblastoma tumours of different size.[7] Figure 71.3 shows that the cumulated activity per unit mass required for a given TCP (=0.5) passes through a minimum at a tumour radius approximately equal to the maximum beta range. The increase at small radii demonstrates that the reduction in dose due to lack of electronic equilibrium dominates over the reduction in cell numbers. Similar results have been reported by other authors.[32]

SUMMARY

While the MIRD technique can provide reasonable estimates of the absorbed dose to large tumours containing uniformly distributed beta-emitters, it is less useful when considering small tumours (<10 mm) and non-uniform source distributions. Evidence from microautoradiography and from miniature dosimeters suggests that the assumption of a uniform distribution of beta-emitters and hence uniform irradiation of tissue is incorrect. There may be significant heterogeneity at the 10–100 μm level. Studies involving tumour models, microdosimetry using information from autoradiography or TLD measurements and computer modelling of pharmacokinetics will aid in achieving a better assessment of tumour and normal tissue doses delivered internally via radionuclide therapy.

Conventional methods of dosimetry need to be replaced with more accurate methods. Instead of quoting average doses to large critical organs, information is required on the spatial variation of dose to both normal and tumour-containing tissues. In the future it should be possible for computerized radiotherapy treatment-planning systems to incorporate radionuclide therapy plans in three dimensions. One such approach has been described[11] in which the three-dimensional dose distribution is displayed as a set of colour-coded isodose contours superimposed on CT images (Fig. 71.4).

REFERENCES

1. Hoefnagel C A 1991 Radionuclide therapy revisited. Eur J Nucl Med 18: 408–431
2. Adelstein S J, Kassis A I 1987 Radiobiologic implications of the microscopic distribution of energy from radionuclides. Int J Radiat Appl Instrum Part B Nucl Med Biol 14: 165–169
3. Humm J L 1986 Dosimetric aspects of radiolabeled antibodies for tumor therapy. J Nucl Med 27: 1490–1497
4. Wessels B W, Rogus R D 1984 Radionuclide selection and model absorbed dose calculations for radiolabeled tumour associated antibodies. Med Phys 11: 638–645
5. International Commission of Radiological Protection (ICRP) 1983 Radionuclide transformations. Energy and intensity of emissions. IRCP Publication 38. Ann ICRP 11–13 Pergamon Press, Oxford
6. Flower M A, Chittenden S J 1993 Unsealed source therapy. In: Williams J R, Thwaites D I (eds) Radiotherapy physics: in practice. Oxford University Press, Oxford, p 258
7. Nahum A E, Babich J W 1990 The effect of β-ray range on tumour control probability in targetted radionuclide therapy. In: Programme and Abstracts of the Ninth Annual Meeting of the European Society of Therapeutic Radiology and Oncology, Montecatini Terme, Italy, p 131
8. Link E M, Brown I, Carpenter R N, Mitchell J S 1989 Uptake and therapeutic effectiveness of ^{125}I- and ^{211}At-methylene blue for pigmented melanoma in an animal model system. Cancer Res 49: 4332–4337
9. Thomas S R, Stabin M G, Chen C-T, Samaratunga R C 1992 MIRD pamphlet no. 14: a dynamic urinary bladder model for radiation dose calculations. J Nucl Med 33: 738–802
10. Maxon III H R, Englaro E E, Thomas S R et al 1992 Radioiodine-131 therapy for well-differentiated thyroid cancer – a quantitative radiation dosimetric approach: outcome and validation in 85 patients. J Nucl Med 33: 1132–1136
11. Sgouros G, Barest G, Thekkumthala J et al 1990 Treatment planning for internal radionuclide therapy: three-dimensional dosimetry for non-uniformly distributed radionuclides. J Nucl Med 31: 1884–1891
12. Loevinger R, Budinger T F, Watson E E et al (eds) 1989 MIRD primer for absorbed dose calculations. Society of Nuclear Medicine, New York
13. Fielding S L, Flower M A, Ackery D, Kemshead J T, Lashford L S, Lewis I 1991 Dosimetry of iodine 131 metaiodobenzylguanidine for treatment of resistant neuroblastoma: results of a UK study. Eur J Nucl Med 18: 308–316
14. Pollard K R, Bice A N, Eary J K, Durack L D, Lewellen T K 1992 A method for imaging therapeutic doses of iodine-131 with a clinical gamma camera. J Nucl Med 33: 771–776
15. Ott R J, Flower M A, Jones A, McCready V R 1985 The measurement of radiation doses from P32 chromic phosphate therapy of the peritoneum using SPECT. Eur J Nucl Med 11: 305–308

16. Blake G M, Zivanovic M A, McEwan A J, Ackery D M 1986 Sr-89 therapy: strontium kinetics in disseminated carcinoma of the prostate. Eur J Nucl Med 12: 447–454
17. Smith T, Crawley J C W, Shawe D J, Gumpel J M 1988 SPECT using Bremsstrahlung to quantify ^{90}Y uptake in Baker's cysts: Its application in radiation synovectomy of the knee. Eur J Nucl Med 14: 498–503
18. Zanzonico P B, Bigler R E, Sgouros G, Strauss A 1989 Quantitative SPECT in radiation dosimetry. Semin Nucl Med 19: 47–61
19. Strand S E, Ljungberg M 1991 Absorbed dose planning in radionuclide therapy based on quantitative SPECT. Antibody immunoconjugates and radiopharmaceuticals 4: 673–680
20. Flower M A, Schlesinger T, Hinton P J et al 1989 Radiation dose assessment in radioiodine therapy. 2. Practical implementation using quantitative scanning and PET, with initial results on thyroid carcinoma. Radiother Oncol 15: 345–357
21. Ott R J, Tait D, Flower M A, Babich J W, Lambrecht R M 1992 Treatment planning for ^{131}I-mIBG radiotherapy of neural crest tumours using ^{124}I-mIBG positron emission tomography. Br J Radiol 65: 787–791
22. Zweit J, Bakir M A, Ott R J, Sharma H, Cox M, Goodall R 1992 Excitation functions of proton induced reactions in natural tellurium: production of no-carrier added iodine-124 for PET applications. In: Weinreich R (ed) Targetry '91. (Proceedings of the Fourth International Workshop on Targetry and Target Chemistry.) Paul Scherrer Institut, Villigen, Switerland, pp 76–78
23. Zweit J, Flower M A, Ott R J 1994 Positron-emitting radionuclides and their beta emitting analogues for imaging and therapy: decay properties, chemical aspects and production methods. Appl Radiat Isot Int J Appl Radiat Instrum Part A. (submitted)
24. Siegel J A, Wessels B W, Watson E E et al 1990 Bone marrow dosimetry and toxicity for radioimmunotherapy. Antibody, immunoconjugates, and radiopharmaceuticals 3: 213–233
25. Esteban J M, Schlom J, Mornex F et al 1987 Radioimmunotherapy of athymic mice bearing human colon carcinomas with monoclonal antibody B72.3: histological and autoradiographic study of effects on tumors, and normal organs. Eur J Cancer Clin Oncol 23: 643–655
26. Van Dieren E B, Van Lingen A, Roos J C, Teule G J J 1992 Validation of the histogram technique for three-dimensional and two-dimensional dosimetric calculations. Appl Radiat Isot 43: 1211–1221
27. Wessels B W, Griffith M H 1986 Miniature thermoluminescent dosimeter absorbed dose measurements in tumor phantom models. J Nucl Med 27: 1308–1314
28. Heidorn D B, Ten Haken R K, Roberson P L, Buchsbaum D J 1991 A sensitivity study of micro-TLDs for in vivo dosimetry of radioimmunotherapy. Med Phys 18: 1195–1199
29. Humm J L, Cobb L M 1990 Nonuniformity of tumour dose in radioimmunotherapy. J Nucl Med 31: 75–83
30. Prestwich W V, Nunes J, Kwok C S 1989 Beta dose point kernels for radionuclides of potential use in radioimmunotherapy. J Nucl Med 30: 1036–1046
31. Roberson P L, Ten Haken R K, McShan D L, McKeever P E, Ensminger W D 1992 Three-dimensional tumor dosimetry for hepatic yttrium-90-microsphere therapy. J Nucl Med 33: 735–738
32. Wheldon T E, O'Donoghue J A, Barrett A, Michalowski A S 1991 The curability of tumours of differing size by targeted radiotherapy using ^{131}I or ^{90}Y. Radiother Oncol 21: 91–99

72. Radioiodine therapy of the thyroid

S. E. M. Clarke

Although there have been very significant developments in the field of radionuclide therapy within the past 10 years, it is important to remember that radionuclide therapy in the form of iodine-131 has been in use for over 46 years.[1]

The early reports of radioiodine usage were for the treatment of thyrotoxicosis and utilized iodine-130.[2] ^{131}I, however, became the radioisotope of choice within a few years with a more useful half-life and more energetic beta-particles (Table 72.1). Again, the early use of this radioisotope was in the treatment of thyrotoxicosis,[3] but within a few years reports appeared in the literature exploring its use in the treatment of differentiated thyroid cancer.[4] In the past 40 years, many patients throughout the world have received treatment for both thyrotoxicosis and thyroid carcinoma, and the cumulative experience with this form of radionuclide therapy has confirmed its safety and efficacy.

Despite this breadth of experience, however, controversies still exist as to which patients should receive treatment for thyrotoxicosis and with what administered dose of radioiodine. In the management of differentiated thyroid cancer, the relative roles of ^{131}I diagnostic imaging, whole-body retention studies and thyroglobulin estimations remain a subject of debate.

This chapter will outline the accepted protocols for the usage of ^{131}I in the treatment of thyrotoxicosis and differentiated thyroid cancer, will discuss the issues associated with treatment, including radioprotection, and explore the controversies that still exist with this oldest form of radionuclide therapy.

Table 72.1 Physical properties of ^{131}I

Half-life	8.04 days
Principal gamma-energies	80 keV
	284 keV
	364 keV
	637 keV
Prinicpal beta E_{max}	0.61 MeV

IODINE-131

A summary of the properties of ^{131}I is contained in Table 72.1. As can be seen, ^{131}I has a half life of 8.04 days and medium-energy beta emissions (E_{max} = 0.61 MeV). It is essential, when selecting a therapy radionuclide, to match the physical half-life of the radionuclide with its biological half-life in vivo.

Iodine is a precursor of thyroxine and is taken up into the follicular cells of the thyroid. Its retention in the follicular cell is dependent on the metabolic activity of the cell, and in the thyrotoxic patient the biological half-life of iodine will be shorter than in the euthyroid patient. In patients with differentiated thyroid cancer, the retention of iodine is variable but activity may still be visualized at the site of thyroid tumour a month after treatment has taken place. As the path length of the beta-particle is about 0.5 mm, the toxic effects are limited to the thyroid, with sparing of adjacent tissues. The normal biodistribution of iodine, however, includes salivary glands, stomach and renal tract including the bladder. These organs also receive a radiation dose during therapy with ^{131}I, although this dose may be reduced by stimulating salivary flow and maintaining a high urine output during the early treatment period. The high-energy gamma emissions also contribute to an unwanted whole-body radiation dose and also to the radiation protection problems associated with radioiodine therapy. These issues will be discussed later.

Although the main uses of ^{131}I are for the treatment of thyrotoxicosis and differentiated thyroid cancer, the use of radioiodine in the treatment of euthyroid goitre will also be discussed.

THYROTOXICOSIS

Clinical features

Thyrotoxicosis is a term used to describe the clinical condition that results from high levels of circulating thyroxine (T_4) and triiodothyronine (T_3). The clinical picture results from the effects of free thyroxine and T_3 on the metabolic rate, with palpitations, sweating, weight loss and nervousness being the most common presenting symptoms. On examination, the classical features of tremor, tachycardia and goitre are usually present. In the elderly, however, many or all of the classical features are frequently absent with atrial fibrillation being the only discernible sign of the disease.

Less commonly, features of proptosis and exophthalmos, muscle wasting, pretibial myxoedema and thyroid acropachy may be evident. The severity of the clinical syndrome is generally proportional to the degree of elevation of thyroid hormones but is often unrelated to the duration of the disease.

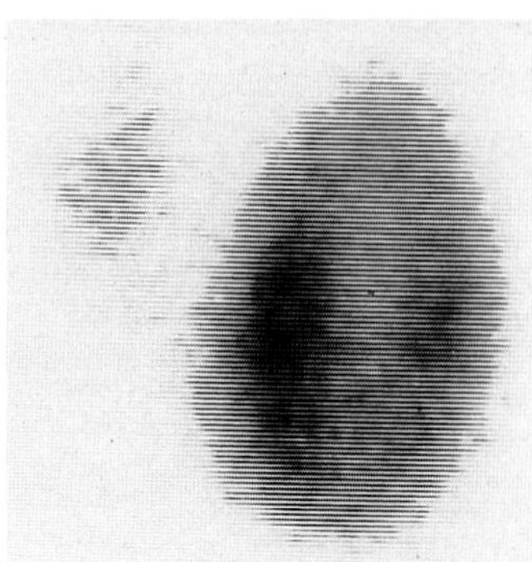

Fig. 72.2 ^{99m}Tc pertechnetate thyroid scan in a patient with a single toxic nodule. Note the suppression of the remainder of the gland.

Pathology

There are two main pathological causes of thyrotoxicosis. Graves' disease is an autoimmune condition caused by overproduction of an antibody to the TSH receptor, thyroid-stimulating immunoglobulin (TSI).[5] The disease may well be familial, although the pattern of inheritance is unclear (Fig. 72.1). As well as affecting the function of the thyroid gland, the autoimmune process variably affects the eyes of patients with Graves' disease with resulting lymphocytic infiltration of the orbital muscles and deposition in the orbit of fatty tissues, leading to proptosis and ophthalmoplegia.

The second main cause of thyrotoxicosis is the development of one or more autonomous nodules that hypersecrete thyroxine and T_3, having escaped the normal feedback control mechanisms. Unlike Graves' disease, which affects the whole of the thyroid gland, toxic nodular goitre is a focal disease (Figs 72.2 and 72.3). These differences in the two disease processes have implications when dosimetric calculations are made prior to therapy and in the incidence of hypothyroidism following treatment with ^{131}I.

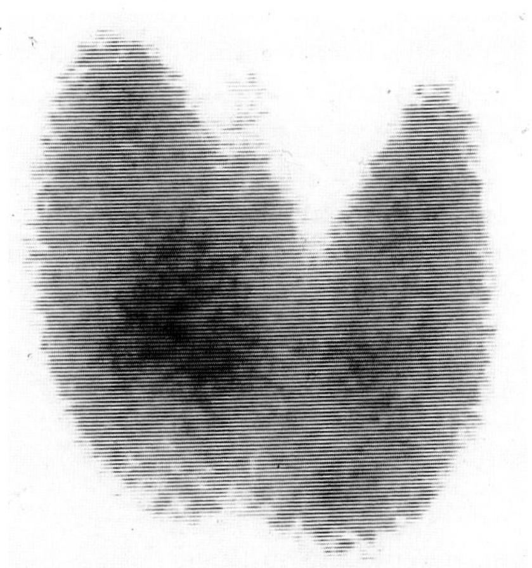

Fig. 72.1 ^{99m}Tc pertechnetate scan in a patient with toxic diffuse goitre (Graves' disease).

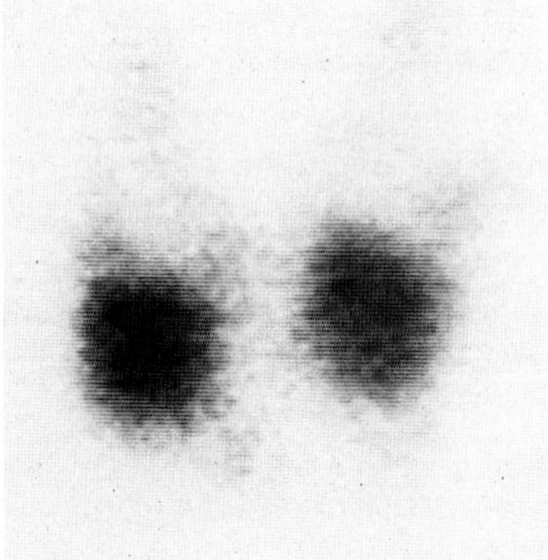

Fig. 72.3 ^{99m}Tc pertechnetate scan in a patient with two toxic nodules.

Other causes of thyrotoxicosis are subacute viral thyroiditis, iodine-induced thyrotoxicosis and thyrotoxicosis factitia. ^{131}I has no role in the treatment of these conditions.

Selection of patients

While little doubt remains about the efficacy of ^{131}I therapy in the treatment of thyrotoxicosis, significant debate takes place as to which patients should be submitted for radioiodine therapy. There is a general consensus that radioiodine is an appropriate treatment for men and women of middle age upwards. There is still concern expressed by some clinical groups about treating women of child-bearing years. Since the publication of the Gardner Report, the use of radioiodine in young men has also been questioned. The use of radioiodine in children is a further subject of debate. These concerns over the safety of ^{131}I in some age groups has led to variations in practice throughout Europe and North America. A recent survey of practice in Europe, Japan and USA found that a third of doctors in the USA believed ^{131}I to be an appropriate treatment for a woman of 19. Only 4% of European doctors thought that ^{131}I was appropriate in such a case, although this does not reflect general European practice.[6]

The rationale for restricting treatment to certain groups of patients is the potential risk of carcinogenesis and leukaemia in patients and the risk of congenital abnormality in their offspring. Since radioiodine therapy has now been extensively used for over 40 years, data are available to confirm that there is no demonstrable risk associated with ^{131}I administration. The risk of developing leukaemia or thyroid malignancy has been assessed in large follow-up studies in the USA with no increased incidence of either detected.[7–11] Similar long-term studies in the UK have also been reported as showing no increased incidence of leukaemia or thyroid malignancy.[12,13]

The theoretical risks of radionuclide therapy must be offset against the known risk of surgery in both children and adults. In children, acute complications in between 16 and 35% of children treated with subtotal thyroidectomy have been reported, with permanent complication occurring in up to 8% of children.[7,14,15]

The risks of genetic abnormality induction have been assessed by Hayak et al[16] and Safa et al.[17] Although data are limited, no increased incidence of genetic defects in children born to women who have been treated with radioiodine for hyperthyroidism has been demonstrated. The dose to the ovaries has been estimated by Robertson & Gorman[18] to be less than 3 rads per 370 MBq, which is similar to the ovarian dose from a barium enema study.

Radioiodine would appear, from all available data, to be a safe form of treatment in all patient groups, including women of child-bearing years and children but excluding women who are pregnant or breastfeeding.

Practical aspects of therapy

Before radioiodine therapy is instigated it is essential that the diagnosis of thyrotoxicosis has been confirmed both clinically and biochemically. The nature of the thyrotoxicosis should also be determined as the dose of ^{131}I to be administered and the follow-up protocol will vary depending on whether the cause of the thyrotoxicosis is toxic diffuse goitre (Graves' disease) or toxic nodular goitre (Plummer's disease). Self-limiting causes of thyrotoxicosis such as viral subacute thyrotoxicosis and iodine-induced thyrotoxicosis (Jod–Basedow) should not be treated with radioiodine.

The use of a radionuclide scan using ^{99m}Tc pertechnetate or ^{123}I as part of the diagnostic protocol in the diagnosis of patients with thyrotoxicosis is vital. The scan will usually confirm the nature of the thyrotoxicosis if this is in doubt clinically. This is particularly valuable in patients who have developed Graves' disease in a multinodular goitre, as a mistaken diagnosis of Plummer's disease may be made if clinical examination alone is used (Fig. 72.4). The presence of unsuspected coexistent non-

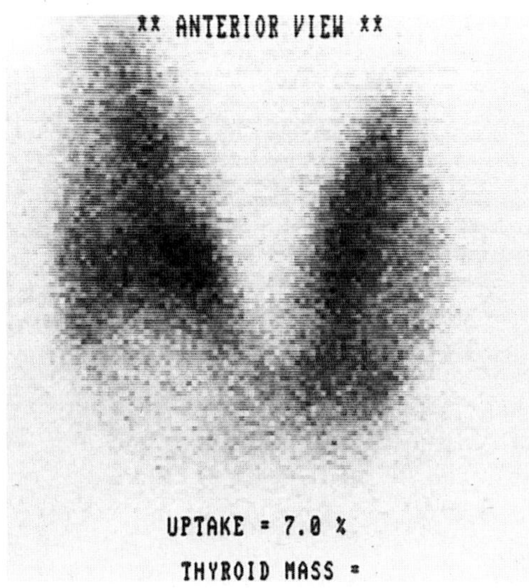

Fig. 72.4 ^{99m}Tc pertechnetate scan in a thyrotoxic patient. The thyroid felt nodular on palpation. The scan confirms non-homogeneity of tracer uptake consistent with a multinodular goitre, but the overall uptake is diffusely increased at 7% (normal range 0.4–4%), confirming a diagnosis of Graves' disease in a multinodular goitre.

functioning nodules will also be demonstrated with a radionuclide scan (Fig. 72.5). If such a nodule is demonstrated, aspiration cytology should be performed to evaluate the lesion and the patient referred for surgery rather than radioiodine if there is any suspicion of malignancy. In Graves' disease, the Marie–Lenhart syndrome of a non-functioning nodule that normalizes following radioiodine therapy may also be demonstrated. A radionuclide scan will confirm the trapping capabilities of the thyroid prior to treatment of patients with a 'blocked uptake' pattern.

It is generally accepted that it is advisable to render patients euthyroid prior to therapy with radioiodine to avoid unpleasant exacerbations of thyrotoxic symptoms that may occur at 1 week after therapy in patiens who are

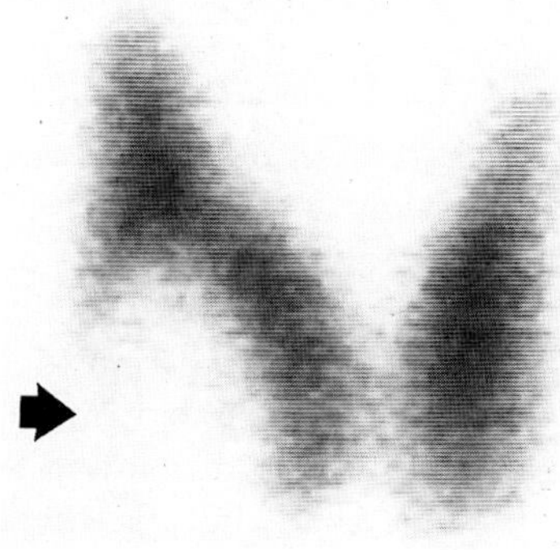

Fig. 72.5 ^{99m}Tc pertechnetate thyroid scan in a patient with Graves' disease. The scan confirms diffusely increased uptake but also identifies an unsuspected cold nodule in the right lobe. This nodule was solid on ultrasound but was revealed on FNA (fine needle aspiration) to be a colloid cyst.

clinically toxic at the time of treatment. Carbimazole or propylthiouracil may be used for this purpose. This pretreatment is particularly important in the elderly, as atrial fibrillation may occasionally occur in the early post-treatment period with the discharge of thyroxine from the gland. Patients may be spared pretreatment if they are young or their clinical symptoms are mild. In patients with severe symptoms, a beta-blocker may be added to the pretreatment regimen. Digoxin should also be used in those patients who present in atrial fibrillation.

It is important to ensure that patients who have received pretreatment have not been rendered hypothyroid before treatment, as the uptake of radioiodine may be significantly reduced. It is usual policy, therefore, to discontinue carbimazole or propylthiouracil for several days before the ^{131}I is given to ensure adequate trapping and binding of the therapeutic dose. Discontinuing tablet treatment in patients with toxic nodular goitre is also advisable to ensure that the normal tissue within the gland is suppressed and thereby spared an unnecessary radiation dose, although this varies.

All patients should be seen by a clinician within the week before therapy is to be undertaken to ensure that the patient is euthyroid, not pregnant (if female) and to answer any final questions that the patient may have. It is important that the patients understand the nature of radioiodine treatment, the precautions that should be observed immediately after treatment and the requirement for follow-up. In several countries it is a legal requirement to give the patient written as well as verbal information and to ask the patient to sign a written consent form before treatment, confirming that the patient understands the implications of treatment.

The dose administered ranges from 74 MBq (2 mCi) to a usual maximum of 550 MBq (15 mCi), although larger doses may be given to inpatients, particularly if ablation is the intention of treatment.

In most countries, therapeutic doses of radioiodine for thyrotoxicosis may be administered as an outpatient provided the patient discontinues work for a period of approximately 1 week after treatment and avoids pregnant women and small children. The maximum dose of ^{131}I that can be administered as an outpatient varies between countries and may be as low as 185 MBq (5 mCi) in some. Certain patients will require admission on logistical grounds, particularly young women with small children, in order to prevent unnecessary radiation doses to the growing thyroid. Patients who are elderly may also require admission on medical grounds if they are in heart failure as this may be exacerbated in the post-therapy period. Admission in this situation should be for at least 1 week as the peak release of thyroxine occurs between 7 and 10 days after treatment. In most patients with adequate pretreatment, admission should not be necessary.

The instructions given to patients should be clear and worded in non-medical language. Instructions on contact with small children should be specific and identify the amount of time that may be spent in close contact and the nature of that contact. Evidence is now available that confirms that the radiation dose received by family members is low but is proportional to the close contact time such as meal times, car travel and sleeping in a double bed. This should be explained clearly to the patient before treatment is undertaken.[19–22]

Iodine administration should be undertaken in an approved environment by adequately trained and authorized staff. Decontamination facilities must be available to deal with ^{131}I spillage or patient vomit.

The use of liquid ^{131}I or capsules is a subject of some debate. The radiation dose to staff drawing up and administering the liquid form will be higher than that received if a capsule is used. Many patients will find swallowing a capsule less difficult and less worrying than sucking up liquid through a straw. Capsules are, however, significantly more expensive than liquid radioiodine and there is no possibility of adjusting the dose immediately before administration. If the patient has been rendered euthyroid prior to radioiodine treatment there is no requirement to recommence carbimazole after treatment. In those patients with hyperthyroid symptoms persisting after radioiodine, carbimazole treatment may be necessary for a short interval but careful monitoring of thyroid function tests is essential to avoid early hypothyroidism as the patient responds to the radioiodine dose.

Dose considerations

The theoretical goal of radioiodine therapy in patients with thyrotoxicosis is to render the patient rapidly euthyroid and to avoid subsequent hyper- or hypothyroidism. To this end, much time has been spent attempting to devise formulae which will permit precise calculations of the dose of radioiodine that is required. Dosimetric calculations must take into account all the factors that are included in Table 72.2. These include an accurate measurement of the functioning mass of the thyroid, an assessment of the percentage uptake of the administered dose into the gland, the rate of clearance of radioiodine from the gland and the radiosensitivity of the gland. A precise calculation of the dose to be administered is also to be commended on the grounds of keeping the amount of administered activity to the effective minimum.

Table 72.2 Factors to be considered in dosimetric calculations

Functioning thyroid mass
^{131}I uptake
^{131}I retention
Radiosensitivity

Unfortunately, all attempts at dosimetry have thus far failed to reliably deliver a dose to the thyroid that avoids recurrence and does not ultimately lead to hypothyroidism. The reason for this failure is complex. Measurements of functioning thyroid mass must be undertaken using tracer studies since measurements of thyroid size alone take no account of the variable distribution of radioiodine throughout the gland. This is a particular problem in patients with toxic nodular goitre in whom radioiodine distribution is particularly non-homogeneous. Sophisticated studies have been undertaken by Flowers et al[68] using ^{124}I, a positron-emitting radionuclide of iodine. Using tomographic imaging they have attempted to define the functioning thyroid mass. Despite these complex imaging techniques, follow-up of patients treated using these functioning volume calculations shows a persistent development of post-treatment hypothyroidism.

The measurement of iodine uptake into the gland may be determined from a tracer study prior to the diagnostic dose.[23,24] This tracer study should be performed as close as possible to the diagnostic dose since there is a daily variation in iodine uptake which may relate to the dietary intake of iodine. Concern has also been expressed that the tracer dose of ^{131}I may itself affect subsequent uptake of ^{131}I by the follicular cells.

The retention of ^{131}I within the thyroid may also be determined from a tracer study. It should be remembered, however, that certain drugs such as lithium will modify the retention of iodine within the gland.[23,25]

The variability of radiosensitivity is well recognized. The same calculated dose administered will render one patient rapidly hypothyroid while another patient may require up to five doses before being rendered euthyroid.

However complex the formula used to calculate the dose of ^{131}I to be administered, long-term hypothyroidism appears inevitable since no published dosimetric method has yet avoided a percentage of patients becoming hypothyroid. The published incidence of hypothyroidism in the first year ranges between 7% and 25% with an annual increment of 2–4% depending on the size of the administered dose.[23,26–28] A low-dose treatment regimen aiming to deliver 35 Gy to the thyroid may have a low incidence of hypothyroidism in the first year but still have a significant incidence of hypothyroidism at 15 years of 35–40% compared with a 50–70% incidence using a high-dose regimen.[15]

Those studies that utilized a low administered dose of radioiodine also show that many of the patients thus treated remain hyperthyroid after treatment and require further treatments. It should be remembered that many patients find the symptoms of hyperthyroidism unpleasant, and in the elderly failure to render the patient euthyroid may result in the patient subsequently developing atrial fibrillation.

Some authors have advocated that a dose of radioiodine should be chosen that will effectively ablate the thyroid. This philosophy has the advantage of rendering the patient euthyroid during the first year after treatment, following which thyroxine therapy may be instigated and the euthyroid state restored with no subsequent risk of relapse. Some patients, however, are not rendered hypothyroid by these doses of 550 MBq and still require further treatments to gain control. Kendal-Taylor et al[29] using this regimen found that 36% of patients were not ablated by this dose. This philosophy may also be challenged since those patients in whom ablation is achieved have one disease state replaced by another and will require medication and monitoring for life. The main advantage for the patient, in addition to the lower risk of relapse, is the release from hospital follow-up with the attendant constraints of time and loss of earnings. Hardisty et al[26] have clearly shown that the total cost of care for patients treated with a low-dose regimen is higher than that for patients treated with a high-dose regimen.

Unlike Graves' disease, treatment of patients with toxic nodular goitre is significantly less likely to result in hypothyroidism. This is explained by the localization of ^{131}I in the thyroid with the sparing of the suppressed parts of the gland.[15] Patients with toxic nodular goitre will therefore tolerate higher doses of ^{131}I with a progressive incidence of hypothyroidism of about 2% per year reported[27] (Fig. 72.6). Radioiodine may also be used to treat patients with autonomous nodules suppressed before biochemical thyrotoxicosis ensues. The incidence of hypothyroidism subsequently will be low provided that suppression of normal thyroid tissue has been confirmed before treatment using a radionuclide scan.

After treatment

Whichever dose regimen is chosen, the patient will require follow-up after treatment. As the patient may become rapidly hypothyroid after treatment, particularly when high-dose regimens are used, a blood test should be performed as early as 6 weeks post treatment. Thyroid functions tests should then be performed at frequent intervals over the first 6 months to detect those patients with rising TSH levels. Occasionally the thyroid gland may be transiently damaged with a fall in function that subsequently recovers. It is important to demonstrate clearly that a patient has non-recoverable hypothyroidism before committing the patient to lifelong thyroxine treatment. The clinical features of weight gain, cool peripheries and bradycardia are useful indicators of developing hypothyroidism.

Opinions as to whether carbimazole should be used in the early post-treatment period are varied. Provided the patient had been adequately pretreated, post-radioiodine carbimazole therapy is usually unnecessary. In a few

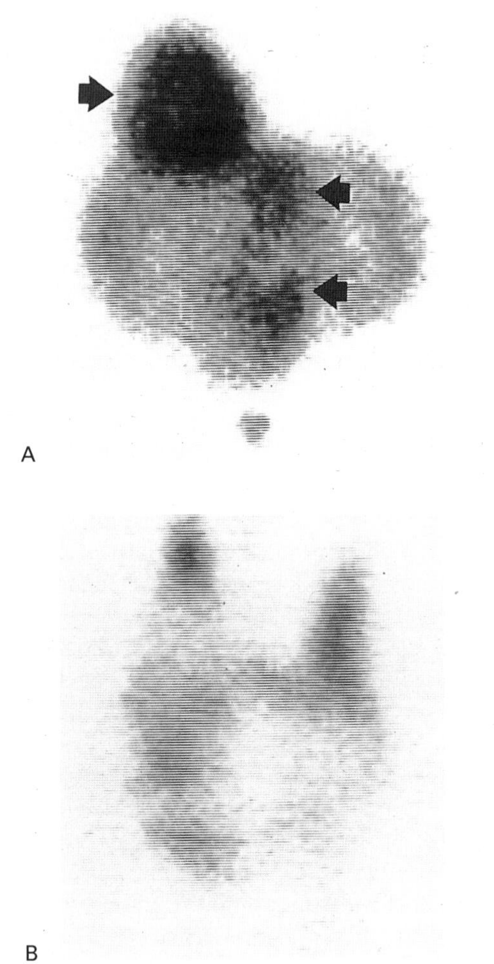

Fig. 72.6 ^{99m}Tc pertechnetate scans in a patient before (A) and after (B) treatment with radioiodine. The initial scan (A) shows non-homogeneous tracer uptake with several foci of increased uptake seen. When the patient became thyrotoxic radioiodine was given and a subsequent scan (B) demonstrates good resolution of the toxic nodules with preservation of function in the remainder of the gland.

patients, exacerbation of hyperthyroid symptoms in the early post-treatment period will necessitate carbimazole usage. It is far more likely that carbimazole will be required in those patients who have been treated with a low dose of radioiodine.

All patients who are rendered euthyroid after iodine will require long-term follow-up as the risk of hypothyroidism persists for life. This follow-up has been traditionally undertaken by a hospital clinician, but increasingly the follow-up of these patients is being undertaken by primary care clinicians with the aid of computerized databases. Others have opted for a shared care policy.

In the elderly, follow-up becomes more difficult, and again an effective database is essential to ensure that follow-up is maintained. In those elderly patients who become hypothyroid and are commenced on thyroxine, follow-up is equally important to ensure that the patient is remembering medication. In a study by Kendall-Taylor et al[29] it was shown that 2% of patients were not taking their thyroxine and a further 3% were poorly compliant.

Side-effects

In addition to the recognized side-effect of hypothyroidism, other side-effects may be experienced by patients following ^{131}I therapy. Exacerbations of thyrotoxicosis at 7–10 days following radioiodine administration have been mentioned. The incidence of this side-effect is significantly reduced by adequate pretreatment with carbimazole or propylthiouracil before treatment is undertaken.

Sialitis may be experienced by some patients in the post-treatment period. This presents as discomfort and swelling in the region of the salivary glands and may be accompanied by alterations in taste. These symptoms are usually short-lived, although some patients may experience long-term problems with taste after radioiodine therapy. The radiation dose to the salivary glands may be reduced by increasing salivary flow in the immediate post-treatment period using sweets.

Occasionally patients with large goitres and high uptake values experience some discomfort in the region of the thyroid gland in the first weeks after treatment. Again this symptom is generally self-limiting and requires no treatment apart from mild analgesia if the discomfort is disturbing.

In patients with significant retrosternal extension there is a theoretical risk of tracheal or oesophageal compression in the early post-iodine period. In clinical practice this is extremely rarely observed. Compressive symptoms may be alleviated by oral steroids in the few patients who develop compressive symptoms.

It has been suggested by some workers that Graves' ophthalmology may worsen after radioiodine. Tallstedt et al[30] showed significant worsening of the ophthalmology after radioiodine for Graves' disease when the patient group was compared with one treated by tablet medication alone with 33% of patients treated with radioiodine developing dysthyroid disease compared with 10% treated with tablets. Hashizume et al,[31] however, showed no difference in the development or worsening of dysthyroid eye disease when compared with patients treated medically or surgically. Hashizume et al[31] demonstrated that 5–7% of patients with Graves' disease develop dysthyroid eye disease irrespective of the mode of treatment. Some workers have suggested that Graves' ophthalmopathy improves following radioiodine ablation on the basis that the antigenic stimulus for the production of the antibody to the occular muscles has been destroyed.[32,33] Perequat et al[34] showed that with non-ablative doses of radioiodine the response was variable, with 40% of patients showing some improvement and 25% showing a deterioration.

One of the main problems in assessing the effect of radioiodine on dysthyroid eye disease is the natural history of the condition with fluctuations in severity of the eye signs in patients in whom there is no alteration in medication. This phenomenon makes interpretation of post-radioiodine data difficult to assess. As no consensus exists, radioiodine is not contraindicated at the present time in patients with dysthyroid eye disease.

NON-TOXIC GOITRE

Since a radiation dose will be delivered to the thyroid if there is an accumulation of ^{131}I, it is logical to suppose that some reduction in goitre size may be achieved in patients with euthyroid goitres. Several studies have now been performed both in patients with primary goitres and in those patients with multinodular goitres that have recurred after surgery. In this particular group, repeat surgery has an increased morbidity since the post-operative fibrosis affects definition of tissue planes and makes identification of the recurrent laryngeal nerves more difficult. Numerous workers[35–38] have demonstrated the efficacy of ^{131}I in reducing goitre size significantly in the majority of patients treated. The incidence of hypothyroidism after treatment varied depending on whether the patient had undergone previous surgery. Although there is a theoretical risk of pressure symptoms developing in those patients with retrosternal extensions of their multinodular goitre, this was not reported as occurring in any of the studies.

THYROID CARCINOMA

Clinical features

Most patients with carcinoma of the thyroid present with a painless swelling in one lobe of the thyroid. The swelling is commonly reported as gradually increasing in size, although many patients may claim that it has been present in an unchanged state for many years. In some patients the nodule may be noticed incidentally during a medical examination. Pressure symptoms of dysphagia and stridor are relatively rare, as are symptoms of infiltration such as hoarseness of the voice due to laryngeal nerve involvement. Patients are generally well systemically, with weight loss being an unusual problem.

Pathology

The various histological types of cancer of the thyroid are listed in Table 72.3. As can be seen, the most common form of thyroid malignancy is the papillary carcinoma of the thyroid. Most of these papillary tumours demonstrate some evidence of follicle formation with the production of colloid. These tumours are highly likely to take up radioiodine. Pure papillary tumours, however, with significant formation of papillae and no colloid visible on histology are unlikely to take up radioiodine. Papillary carcinomas of the thyroid commonly metastasize to local lymph nodes, but distant metastases are less common.

Table 72.3 Histological types of thyroid cancer

Papillary	65%
Follicular	25%
Medullary	10%
Anaplastic	5%
(Lymphoma)	

Follicular carcinomas of the thyroid are generally well differentiated with good colloid production. These tumours in general take up radioiodine. They metastasize to bone, lungs and brains as well as local lymph nodes. The Hurthle cell variant of follicular carcinoma of the thyroid is a less common form of thyroid cancer, and only 10% of these tumours take up radioiodine.

Other types of thyroid malignancy do not take up radioiodine, although radioiodine may be used to ablate residual normal thyroid tissue in the period following total thyroidectomy.

The role of radioiodine

Following surgical removal of the tumour with a total thyroidectomy and extirpation of any evident nodal disease, radioiodine has a major role in achieving a complete cure[39,40] A strict therapeutic protocol is essential to ensure eradication of possible metastatic disease. A review by Maxon & Smith[41] of major series showed that nodal metastases were present at diagnosis in 36% of patients with papillary carcinoma and in 13% of those with follicular carcinoma, while distant deposits were associated with 4% of papillary carcinomas and 16% of follicular carcinomas. Further evaluation of published series clearly demonstrated the development of metastases in patients who had been considered disease free at the time of their initial treatment.

Radioiodine has three major roles: diagnosis, ablation and treatment. The initial diagnostic approach is the demonstration of residual normal thyroid tissue following the removal of the tumour. It is essential that the patient has a high TSH level when this study is performed in order to permit maximum stimulation of any thyroid tissue. Several weeks should elapse prior to the scintigraphic evaluation. The scan may show small fragments in the thyroid bed or 'rests' of normal tissue in the thyroglossal tract, only demonstrable after removal of the gland and often seen as a chain of small foci high in the midline of the neck. If any thyroid tissue is visualized, ablation with radioiodine should be undertaken (Fig. 72.7).

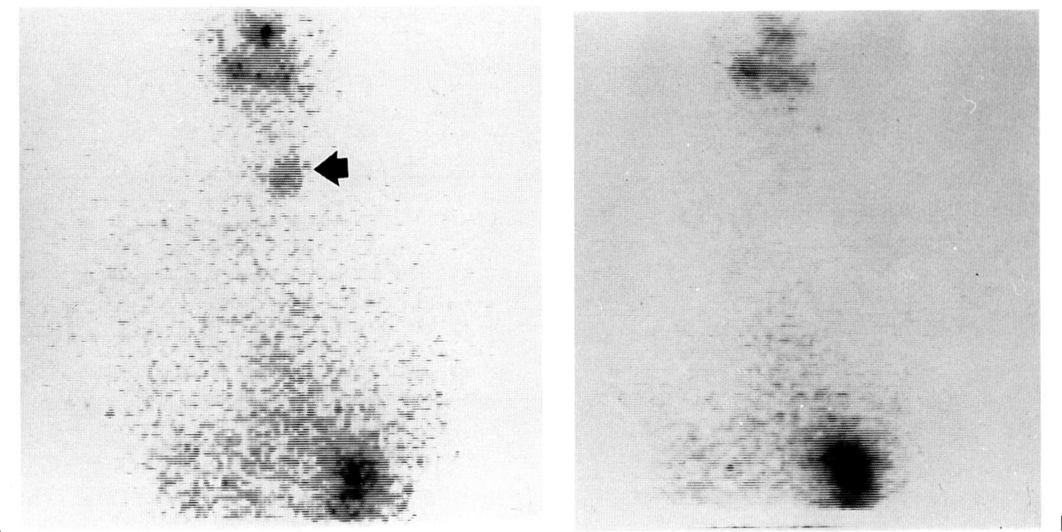

Fig. 72.7 ^{131}I scans in a patient with a thyroid remnant (A) successfully destroyed following 3000 MBq of radioiodine (B).

Thyroid remnant ablation

The rationale for ablating residual thyroid tissue following surgery for thyroid carcinoma is threefold. After successful thyroid ablation interpretation of subsequent whole-body iodine scans is simplified since activity in the neck must relate to recurrent tumour. Interpretation of thyroglobulin levels is also aided. Remnant thyroid tissue will continue to secrete thyroglobulin into the circulation and a raised thyroglobulin level will be non-specific. Following successful thyroid ablation with a negative whole-body study, subsequent elevations in thyroglobulin may be attributed to recurrent thyroid tumour (Fig. 72.8).[42] Finally, the subsequent administration of therapy doses will be more effective if all normal thyroid tissue is ablated since normal thyroid tissue is significantly more avid for iodine than malignant tissue and most of an administered dose of ^{131}I will be to the normal thyroid tissue rather than the sites of tumour.[43,44]

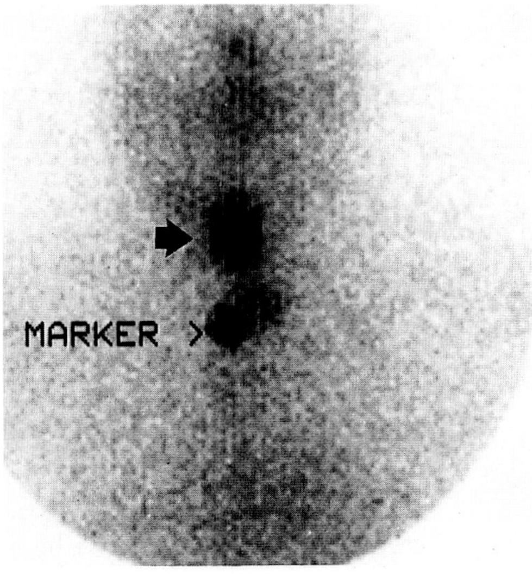

Fig. 72.8 ^{131}I scan in a patient with a successfully ablated thyroid gland who subsequently developed a raised thyroglobulin level. An ^{131}I scan demonstrates uptake in locally recurrent tumour.

The concept of 'stunned' thyroid function has raised controversy as to the dose of ^{131}I to be used for these diagnostic studies. Many believe that a large dose is essential, Waxman et al,[45] for example, having shown that identification of an increasing number of remnants was associated with increasing the dose up to 30 mCi or more (1100 MBq). However, several authors have observed that the uptake of a therapeutic dose may be less than that of a preceding diagnostic dose. Even a 5 mCi dose was found sufficient to reduce the uptake of a therapeutic dose by 54%.[46] Reporting the induction of the 'stunned' thyroid by a 10 mCi dose which invalidated a 100 mCi dose, Park[47] recommended that pretherapy scanning should be undertaken with ^{123}I. If only an estimate of the amount of remaining normal tissue is required, ^{99m}Tc can be used, but when, in follow-up studies, identification of possible metastases is sought, an iodine isotope is essential because of the relatively poor trapping avidity of neoplastic tissue. Certainly the dose to be used for thyroid ablation is also a subject of debate. Some authors advocate using a low ablation dose (1100 MBq, 30 mCi) on the grounds of environmental considerations and radiation protection.[48] However, since the purpose of the ablation dose is to destroy any thyroid remnant efficiently and effectively, doses of up to 7400 MBq (200 mCi) have been advocated as a more reliable dose for destroying the residual thyroid.[49] Maxon et al[50] reported that successful ablation of thyroid remnants by a single initial ^{131}I dose was achieved in 248/287 (86%) with a single initial dose of ^{131}I of 100 mCi (3700 MBq) or more, whereas it occurred in only 104/195 (53%) when the dose was up to 30 mCi (1100 MBq).

It will be necessary to admit patients for ablation doses since they will represent a radiation hazard for a number of days following treatment. Admission should be into a dedicated room with en-suite bathroom. Special precautions should be taken to protect the floor around the lavatory as the urine will be particularly radioactive for the first 24 h during which, on average, 50% of the administered dose is excreted. Nursing care should be kept to a minimum and visitors restricted to a single short visit each day as a maximum. Using counting equipment, the activity retained within the patient should be measured daily until the level of activity falls below that permitted for discharge. During the inpatient stay, the patient should keep a set of cutlery and crockery in the room and wash them personally since saliva is another significant source of contamination. Following discharge, the room should be monitored for sites of contamination. It is essential that patients should not be taking thyroxine at the time of radioiodine ablation, and this should therefore be undertaken after surgery before commencing thyroxine or a few months after surgery after a 1 month discontinuation of thyroxine. The use of a low-iodine diet in the month before treatment will enhance remnant uptake of radioiodine.

In order to avoid admission, Arad et al[51] have attempted to achieve thyroid ablation using a fractionated dose regimen of 30–50 mCi per week to a dose of 111 mCi. 5% of patients were successfully ablated using this regimen as compared with 80% of patients with a standard regimen.

Follow-up

Following ablation of the thyroid remnant, the patient should be maintained on TSH-suppressive doses of thyroxine. Some adjustment to the dose may be necessary to avoid symptoms of overtreatment while maintaining a suppressed TSH.

Six months after the thyroid ablation, thyroxine should be discontinued to allow the TSH levels to rise prior to a tracer ^{131}I whole-body scan. Some groups advocate that the use of T_3 to maintain TSH suppression as therapy need only be discontinued for 2 weeks before the TSH level rises because of the shorter half-life of T_3. Many patients find the thrice-daily regimen of T_3 less satisfactory than the once-daily regimen of thyroxine. However, again, a low-iodine diet while the patient is off thyroxine is recommended to enhance tumour uptake.

If recurrent disease is demonstrated on the whole-body scan, or if the whole-body retention of ^{131}I assessed by a whole-body counter is increased, the patient should be admitted for a therapy dose of ^{131}I. The therapy dose will usually vary from 1800 to 5500 MBq (50–150 mCi) (Fig. 72.9).

Using ^{131}I, extremely high radiation doses to tumour sites may be achieved, with the radiation dose depending on the degree of uptake of radioiodine and the retention of

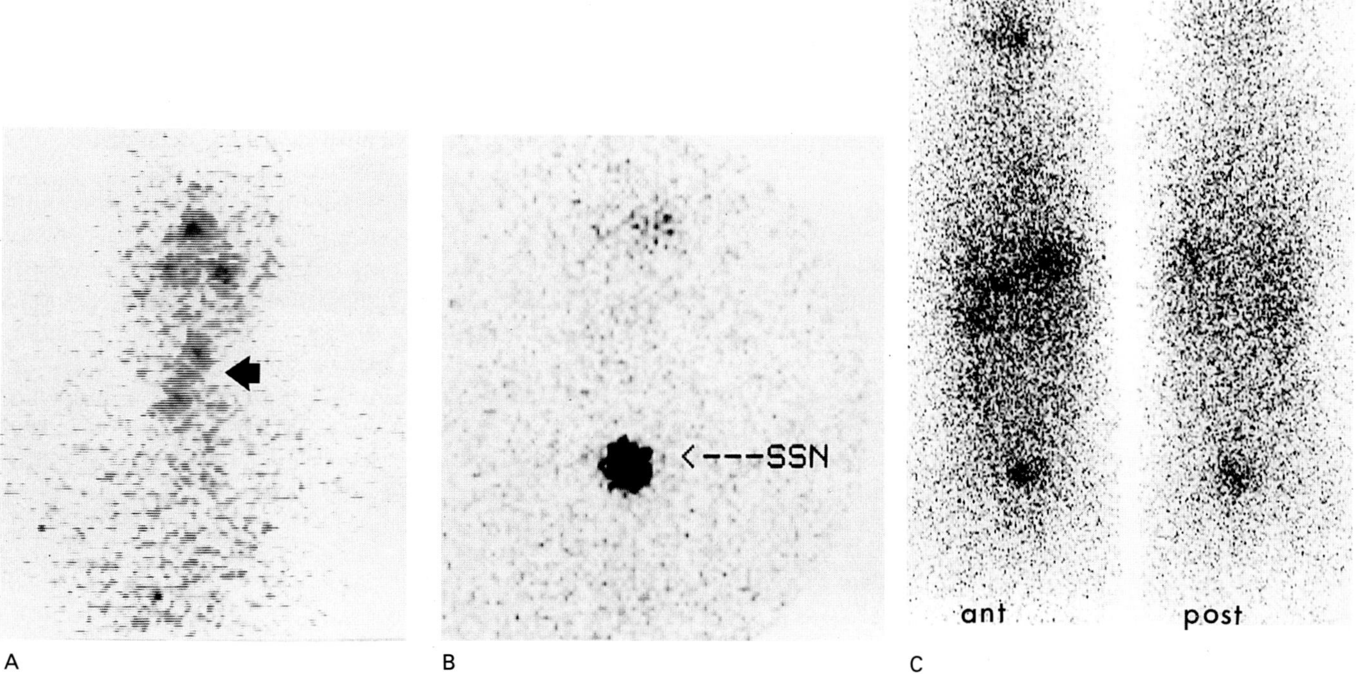

Fig. 72.9 ^{131}I scan (A) in a patient with locally recurrent thyroid cancer. Following 5500 MBq of ^{131}I a radioiodine scan of the neck (B) 6 months later confirms successful treatment of the recurrence. The whole-body ^{131}I scan (C) is also negative, showing only the normal biodistribution of ^{131}I in the salivary glands, stomach and bladder.

tracer within the tumour. The size of the tumour is also critical. When the mass of papillary carcinoma was less than 50 g, Glanzmann & Horst[52] found it reacted positively to treatment, whereas none of seven patients with a tumour mass greater than 200 g responded. In patients with follicular carcinoma a response was induced in 18/29 in whom the tumour mass was less than 10 g but in none when it was greater than 100 g. The role of surgical intervention to achieve mass reduction must be borne in mind. Some authors have suggested the use of lithium to prolong the retention of ^{131}I within the tumour site and thereby increase the dose received by the tumour.[53,54]

The decision on the dose to be used for therapy is frequently chosen empirically, with administered doses of between 3700 and 5500 MBq (100–150 mCi) being standard. This regimen appears simple and effective. Some centres, however, advocate a dosimetric calculation to determine the dose to be administered. Maxon et al[55] based their calculation on whole-body counting measurements and blood and urine collections. This group[50] have also used an alternative quantitative radiation approach aimed at delivering at least 8500 rads to nodal metastases, the dose being calculated on the basis of an estimation of the mass size from a rectilinear scan and by sequential measurements of uptake in lesions. An alternative dosimetric approach is to calculate the beta dose to the blood based on tracer measurements. Doses are selected to give a maximum of 2 Gy (200 rads) to the blood with no more than 4.44 GBq retained in the whole body at 48 h.[36,56]

Doses of up to 450 mCi of ^{131}I have been administered with no permanent damage to bone marrow observed. Benua et al[56] have shown that average values of radiation delivered to the body are significantly less than those calculated from dosimetric tracer studies. This suggests that there is little value in complex dosimetric studies.

The dose delivered to tumour sites may be estimated retrospectively.[57] Using this study it has been found that doses of between 150 and 170 mCi deliver to the tumour radiation doses ranging from 400 to 2900 rads.

After treatment the patient recommences thyroxine. A repeat scan will be performed following an interval of 6–12 months and further therapy is given when necessary. When a negative tracer scan has been acquired, follow-up can continue using thyroglobulin measurements. An elevated value will indicate the need for the patient to be rescanned to assess the possible metastatic site.

Some discrepancies between whole-body ^{131}I scans and thyroglobulin estimations have been reported. One common problem appears to be that of persistent thyroid remnant, which may be visualized on the scan of the neck, while the thyroglobulin level is not elevated.[58] Such false-negative thyroglobulin estimations occurred in 12/284 (4%) patients studied by Ashcraft & Van Herle.[59]

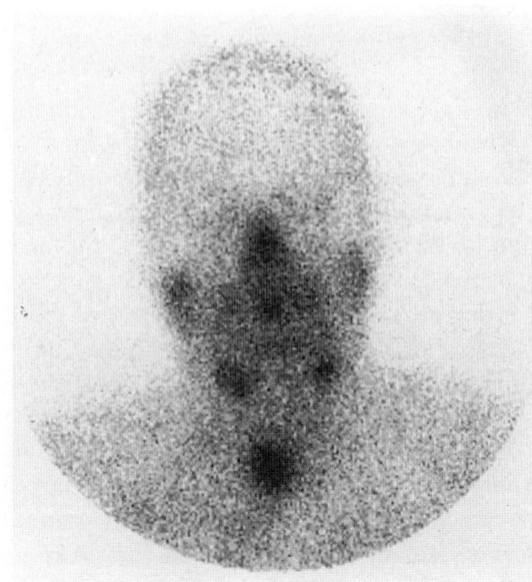

Fig. 72.10 ^{201}Tl scan in an asymptomatic patient with a persistently elevated serum thyroglobulin but repeatedly negative ^{131}I scans. The area of uptake was later demonstrated by fine-needle aspiration to be recurrence of follicular carcinoma.

However, false-negative ^{131}I scans were found in 37 (13%) of these 284 patients. This finding of an abnormal thyroglobulin level as the only indicator of residual or persistent disease poses a therapeutic dilemma. Several groups have accepted that further ^{131}I treatment is required and in subsequent post-therapy scans have identified the lesions not visualized previously. Pineda et al[60] for example, treated 14 patients with elevated thyroglobulin levels and negative scans after 5 mCi of ^{131}I. After therapeutic doses of 150–300 mCi, the scans were positive in 13 of these patients. One solution to the problem of unexplained thyroglobulin elevation may also be provided by scanning with ^{201}Tl (Ch. 63) since, in some patients, this may provide localization of the abnormal tissue.[61,62] (Figs 72.10 and 72.11). ^{99m}Tc diphosphonate scanning cannot be relied upon to identify all deposits of thyroid carcinoma in bone as its sensitivity is less than that in detecting osseous metastases from most other carcinomas. Skeletal metastases generally respond less well to radioiodine therapy,[41] and external radiation or surgical intervention may be required.

The patient should be aware of the need for, and value of, prolonged follow-up. Although Hoie et al[63] found that 43% of distant metastases developed in the first year after diagnosis, they showed that these developed between 1 and 5 years in 23%, and that it was more than 10 years in 9% of patients before the metastases were identified.

Papillary tumours

In patients with papillary carcinoma of the thyroid, radioiodine plays a variable role. Radiation may be used to diagnose the presence of remnant thyroid tissue and ablate

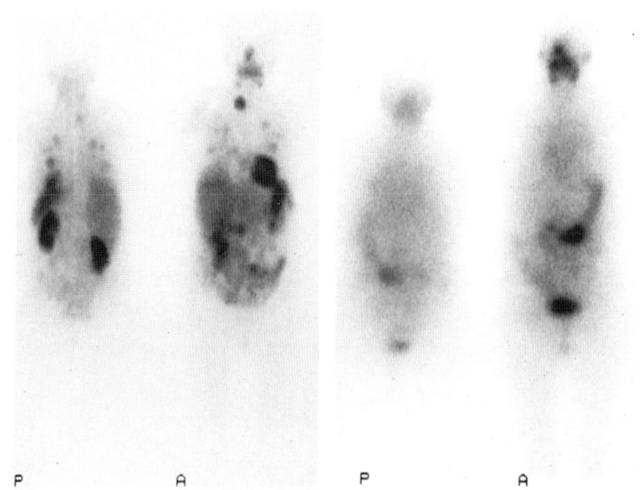

Fig. 72.11 Scans in a patient presenting with a local recurrence of a right neck mass 3 years after treatment of follicular thyroid carcinoma. A ^{201}Tl scan (A) shows uptake in this mass and multiple pulmonary metastases. Scans following 120 MBq of ^{131}I (B) showed no accumulation in any of these areas.

the remnant. Its use subsequently will depend on the presence of follicular elements. Pure papillary tumours will not concentrate radioiodine and recurrent pure papillary lesion will require surgical intervention or external beam radiotherapy. Papillary lesions with follicular elements will continue to concentrate radioiodine, and this therefore remains a therapeutic option for recurrences.

The management of small foci of papillary carcinoma found incidentally at partial or total thyroidectomy is a subject of debate. In the elderly patient a conservative approach can be adopted given the slow-growing, indolent nature of these tumours. Thyroxine replacement should be instigated if required post-operatively and monitoring of thyroglobulin at 6 monthly intervals. In young patients with long life expectancy, a total thyroidectomy with radioiodine ablation followed by thyroxine therapy and thyroglobulin monitoring is a common management strategy.

Side-effects of radioiodine therapy

Following a therapy dose of ^{131}I patients frequently complain of discomfort in the region of the salivary glands. This radiation sialitis is in general short-lived although some patients may notice a long-term alteration in taste. A sialogue in the form of an acid drop sweet will stimulate salivary flow and reduce the incidence of this side-effect.

Occasionally some patients complain of nausea, especially when higher therapeutic doses are used. This usually only lasts for the first or second day post therapy. Similarly, pain in the thyroid remnant is usually transient, but such radiation thyroiditis may be accompanied by perithyroidal swelling which, if severe and inducing symptoms, may require steroid therapy. Rarely, falls in the white blood cell and platelet count may be noted, particularly in those patients with widespread bone disease. A transfusion is rarely required, but low counts may persist for up to a year in 10%. Oligospermia or azoospermia may be present for up to 4 years in 70% of males.[41]

Long-term problems following radioiodine are the concerns regarding the risk of leukaemia and other neoplasia. Most of the deaths from leukaemia have been reported a few years following therapy, and it is often difficult to determine the cause. While a common factor in those patients who have developed leukaemia is that they had received a high cumulative dose of radioiodine over a short period,[56,64] recent surveys have not identified any clear-cut risk of leukaemia in patients following ^{131}I therapy.[65,66] These studies also found no increase in the risk for breast or bladder cancer, although the latter has been noted 14–20 years after treatment in a number of patients, all of whom had received a cumulative dose over 1 Ci.[64] An increased risk for salivary, kidney, stomach and female genital malignancies did appear to exist.[66]

Widespread diffuse pulmonary metastases with high radioiodine uptake on the tracer scans should be treated with caution as these patients may develop pulmonary fibrosis.[64]

As in the treatment of thyrotoxicosis, there are no reports in the literature of infertility, miscarriage prematurity or congenital abnormalities in children treated with radioiodine for thyroid carcinoma.[67]

CONCLUSION

^{131}I is a well-used radionuclide for the treatment of both thyrotoxicosis and differentiated thyroid cancer. It is well tolerated, simple to administer and has been proved in multiple follow-up studies to be safe and effective. It should now be the treatment of choice in all patients with Graves' disease in whom carbimazole therapy has failed and as first-line treatment for patients with toxic nodular goitre.

Radioiodine remains a pivotal part of the therapy of differentiated thyroid cancer, and the good survival rates for this disease confirm its efficacy.

Regulations for the use of radioiodine remain extremely variable throughout the world, although there is general acceptance of the basic radiation protection measures.

^{131}I demonstrates the potential of targeted radiotherapy and it is on the basis of experience gained with this therapy agent that work with new therapy radionuclides continues.

REFERENCES

1. Chapman E M, Maloof F 1955 The use of radioactive iodine in the diagnosis and treatment of hyperthyroidism: ten years' experience. Medicine 34: 261–270
2. Williams R H, Tovery B T, Jaffe H 1949 Radiotherapies. Am J Med 7: 702
3. Varma V M, Beierwaltes W H, Notal, Nishiyama R, Copp J E 1970 Treatment of thyroid cancer. JAMA 214: 1437–1442
4. Coliez R, Tubiana M, Sung J 1951 Disparition des metastases pulmonaires d'un cancer thyroiden sous l'influence d'iode radioactif. J Radiol Electrol 32: 396–398
5. Doniach D, Roitt I M 1976 Autoimmune thyroid disease. In: Miescher P A, Muller Eberhard H J (eds). Textbook of immunopathology, 2nd edn, Grune & Stratton, London, pp 715–735
6. Wartofsky L, Ransil B J, Ingbar S H 1970 Inhibition by iodine of the release of thyroxine from the thyroid glands of patients with thyrotoxicosis. J Clin Invest 49: 78–86
7. Reeve T S, Hales I B, White B, Thomas I D, Hunt P S 1969 Thyroidectomy in the management of thyrotoxicosis in the adolescent. Surgery 65: 694–699
8. Wieland D M, Win J L, Brown L E 1980 Radiolabelled adrenergic neuroblocking agents: adrenomedullary imaging with 131I MIBG. J Nucl Med 21: 349–353
9. Dobyns B M, Sheline G E, Workman J B, Tompkins E A, McConahey W M, Becker D V 1974 Malignant and benign neoplasms of the thyroid in patients treated for hyperthyroidism. A report of the Cooperative Thyrotoxicosis Follow-Up Study. J Clin Endocrinol Metab 38: 976–998
10. Hoffman D A 1984 Late effects of 131I therapy in the United States. In: Boice J D, Fraumeni J R (eds). Progress in cancer research and therapy, radiation carcinogenesis, epidemiology, and biological significance, Vol 26. Raven Press, New York, pp 273–280
11. Holm L E 1984 Malignant disease following 131I in Sweden. In: Boice J D, Fraumeni J R (eds) Progress in cancer research and therapy, radiation carcinogenesis, epidemiology and biological significance, Vol 26. Raven Press, New York, pp 263–271
12. Sheppard M C 1988 Radiation therapy for thyrotoxicosis and risk of malignancy. In: Rubery E, Smales E (eds). Iodine prophylaxis following nuclear accident. Pergamon, London, pp 111–118
13. Hall P, Boice J D, Berg G et al 1992 Leukaemia incidence after iodine-131 exposure. Lancet 340: 1–4
14. Bacon G E, Laury G H 1965 Experience with surgical treatment of thyrotoxicosis in children. J Paediatr 67: 1–5
15. Ching T, Warden M J, Fefferman R A 1977 Thyroid surgery in children and teenagers. Arch Otolaryngol 103: 544–546
16. Hayek A, Chapman E M, Crawford J D 1970 Long term results of treatment of thyrotoxicosis in children and adolescents with radioactive iodine. N Engl J Med 283: 949–953
17. Safa A N, Schumacher O P, Rodriquez-Antunez A 1975 Long term follow up results in children and adolescents treated with radioactive iodine for hyperthyroidism. N Engl J Med 292: 167–171
18. Robertson J S, Gorman C A 1976 Gonadal radiation dose and its genetic significance in radiation therapy of hyperthyroidism. J Nucl Med 17: 826–835
19. Culver C M, Dworkin H J 1991 Radiation safety consideration for post-iodine-131 hyperthyroid therapy. J Nucl Med 32: 169–173
20. Buchan R C T, Brindle J M 1970 Radioiodine therapy to outpatients – contamination hazard. Br J Radiol 43: 479–482
21. Jacobson A P, Plato P M, Toeroek D 1978 Contamination of the home environment by patients treated with iodine-131: initial results. Am J Public Health 68: 225–230
22. Harbert J C, Wells N 1974 Radiation exposures to the family of radioactive patients. J Nucl Med 15: 887–888
23. Becker D R 1982 Radioactive iodine (131I) in the treatment of hyperthyroidism. In: Beckers C (ed). Thyroid diseases. Pergamon Press, Paris, pp 145–158
24. Hayes A A, Akre C M, Gorman C A 1990 131 Iodine treatment of Graves' disease using modified early 131iodine uptake measurements in therapy dose calculations. J Nucl Med 31: 519–522
25. Turner J G, Brownlie B E W, Rogers T G H 1976 Lithium as an adjunct to radioiodine therapy for thyrotoxicosis. Lancet 1: 614–615
26. Hardistry C A, Jones S J, Hedley A J, Munro D S, Bewsher P D, Weir R D 1990 Clinical outcome and costs of care in radioiodine treatment of hyperthyroidism. J R Coll Physicians 24: 36–42
27. Kinser J A, Roesler H, Furrer T, Grutter D, Zimmerman H 1989 Non-immunogenic hyperthyroidism: cumulative hyperthyroidism incidence after radioiodine and surgical treatment. J Nucl Med 30: 1960–1965
28. Staffurth J S 1987 Hypothyroidism following radioiodine treatment of thyrotoxicosis. J R Coll Phys 21: 55–57
29. Kendall-Taylor P, Keir M, Ross W M 1984 Ablative radioiodine therapy for hyperthyroidism: long term follow up study. Br Med J 289: 361–363
30. Tallstedt L, Lundell G, Torring O et al 1992 Occurence of ophthalmopathy after treatment of Graves' hyperthyroidism. N Engl J Med 326: 1733–1738
31. Hamilton R, Mayberry W, McConnicky W, Hanson K 1967 Ophthalmology of Graves' disease: a comparison between patients treated surgically and patients treated with radio-iodine. Mayo Clinic Proceedings 42: 812–818
32. Catz B, Tsao J 1965 Total 131I thyroid ablation for pretibial myxoedema. Clin Res 13: 130
33. Hamilton R, Mayberry W, McConahey W, Hanson K 1967 Ophthalmopathy of Graves' disease: a comparison between patients treated surgically and patients treated with radioiodine. Mayo Clin Proc 42: 812–818
34. Pequegnat E, Mayberry W, McConahey W, Wyse E 1967 Large doses of radioiodine in Graves' disease: effect on ophthalmopathy and long acting thyroid stimulator. Mayo Clin Proc 42: 802–811
35. Keiderling W, Emrich D, Hanzwaldi C, Hoffman G 1964 Ergebnisse der Radiojod-Verleinerungs Therapie euthyreoter Strumen. Dtsch Med Wochenschr. 89: 453–457
36. Leeper R D, Shimaoka K 1980 Treatment of metastatic thyroid cancer (abstract). Clin Endocrinol Metab 9: 383–404
37. Kay T W H, d'Emden M C, Andrews J T, Martin F I R 1988 Treatment of non-toxic multinodular goitre with radioactive iodine. Am J Med 84: 19–22
38. Hegedus L, Hansen B M, Knudsen N, Hansen J M 1988 Reduction in the size of thyroid with radioactive iodine in multinodular non-toxic goitre. Br Med J 297: 661
39. DeGroot L J, Kaplan E L, McCormick M, Straus F H 1990 Natural history, treatment, and course of papillary thyroid carcinoma. J Clin Endocrinol Metab 7: 414–424
40. Mazzaferri E L 1991 Treating differentiated thyroid carcinoma: where do we draw the line? Mayo Clin Proc 66: 105–111
41. Maxon III H R, Smith H S 1990 Radioiodine-131 in the diagnosis and treatment of metastatic well differentiated thyroid cancer. Endocrinol Metab Clin N Am 19: 685–718
42. Schlumberger M, Fragu P, Parmentier C, Tubiana M 1981 Thyroglobulin assay in the follow-up of patients with differentiated thyroid carcinoma: comparison of its value in patients with or without normal residual tissue. Acta Endocrinol 98: 215–221
43. Beierwaltes W H 1978 The treatment of thyroid carcinoma with radioactive iodine. Semin Nucl Med 8: 79–84
44. Mazzaferri E 1981 Papillary and follicular thyroid cancer. Annu Rev Med 32: 171–196
45. Waxman A, Ramanna L, Chapman N et al 1981 The significance of I-131 scan dose in patients with thyroid cancer: determination of ablation (concise communication). J Nucl Med 22: 861–865
46. Jeevanram R K, Shah D H, Sharma S M, Ganatra R D 1986 Influence of initial large dose on subsequent uptake of therapeutic radioiodine in thyroid cancer patients. Nucl Med Biol 13: 277–279
47. Park H 1992 Stunned thyroid after high-dose I-131 imaging. Clin Nucl Med 17: 501–502
48. DeGroot L J, Reilly M 1982 Comparison of 30 and 50 mCi doses of ^{131}I for thyroid ablation. Ann Intern Med 96: 51
49. Sisson J C 1983 Applying the radioactive eraser: ^{131}I to ablate normal thyroid tissue in patients for whom thyroid cancer has been resected. J Nucl Med 24: 743–748
50. Maxon H R III, Englaro E E, Thomas S R et al 1992 Radioiodine-

131 therapy for well differentiated thyroid cancer – a quantitative radiation dosimetric approach: Outcome and validation in 85 patients. J Nucl Med 33: 1132–1136
51. Arad E, Flannery K, Wilson G, O'Mara R 1990 Fractionated doses of radio-iodine for ablation of past surgical thyroid tissue remnants. Clin Nucl Med 16: 676–677
52. Glanzmann C, Horst W 1979 Therapie des metastasierenden schilddrüsenadenokarzinomas mit 131-Jod. Erfahrungen bei 103 patienten aus dem zeitraum 1963 bis 1977. Strahlentherapie 155: 223–229
53. Briere J, Pousset G, Darcey P 1974 The advantage of lithium in association with iodine 131 in the treatment of functioning metastases of thyroid cancer. Ann Endocrinol 35: 281
54. Gershengorn M C, Izumi M, Robbins J 1976 Use of lithium as an adjunct to radioiodine therapy of thyroid carcinoma. J Clin Endocrinol Metab 12: 105–111
55. Maxon H R, Thomas S R, Hertzberg V S 1983 Relationship between effective radiation dose and outcome of radioiodine therapy for thyroid cancer (abstract). N Engl J Med 309: 937–941
56. Benua R S, Cicale N R, Sonenberg M 1962 The relation of radioiodine dosimetry to results and complications in the treatment of metastatic thyroid cancer. Am J Roent Radiat Ther Nucl Med 87: 171–182
57. Koral K F, Adler S F, Carey J, Beierwaltes W H 1986 Iodine 131 treatment of thyroid cancer: absorbed dose calculated from post therapy scans. J Nucl Med 27: 1207–1211
58. Clarke S E M, Coakley A J, Page C, Gaunt J, Croft D N R 1985 The significance of discordant thyroglobulin/scan findings in patients with CA thyroid. Eur J Nucl Med 11: A19
59. Ashcraft M W, Van Herle A J 1981 The comparative value of serum thyroglobulin measurements and iodine-131 total body scans in the follow-up study of patients with treated differentiated thyroid cancer. Am J Med 71: 806–814
60. Pineda J D, Lee T, Reynolds J, Robbins J 1991 ^{131}I therapy for thyroid cancer with elevated thyroglobulin and negative diagnostic scan (abstract). Thyroid 2: S16
61. Iida Y, Hidaka A, Hatabu H, Kasagi K, Konishi J 1991 Follow-up study of postoperative patients with thyroid cancer by thallium-201 scintigraphy and serum thyroglobulin measurement. J Nucl Med 32: 2098–2100.
62. Tonami N, Hisada K 1980 ^{201}Tl scintigraphy in postoperative detection of thyroid cancer: a comparative study with ^{131}I. Radiology 136: 461–464
63. Hoie J, Stenwig A E, Kullman G, Lindegaard M 1988 Distant metastases in papillary thyroid cancer: a review of 91 patients. Cancer 61: 1–6
64. Edmonds C J, Smith T 1986 The long-term hazards of the treatment of thyroid cancer with radioiodine. Br J Radiol 59: 45–51
65. Hall P, Boice Jr J D, Bjelkengren G et al 1992 Leukaemia incidence after iodine-131 exposure. Lancet 340 (8810): 1–4
66. Hall P, Holm L E, Lundell G et al 1991 Cancer risks in thyroid cancer patients. Br J Cancer 64: 159–163
67. Sarker S D, Beierwaltes W H, Gill S P, Contey B J 1976 Subsequent fertility and birth histories of children and adolescents treated with 131 iodine for thyroid cancer. J Nucl Med 17: 460–464
68. Flower M A, Al-Saadi A, McCready V R et al 1990 The measurement of in-vivo dose response relationships in radionuclide therapy for thyrotoxicosis using PET. Eur J Nucl Med 16 (S70): 277

73. Phosphorus-32 therapy in myeloproliferative diseases

Sten Nilsson

POLYCYTHAEMIA VERA

Characteristics and diagnosis of the disease

Polycythaemia vera (PV), Vaquez–Osler disease, was originally described by Vaquez over 100 years ago.[1] The disease is a clonal, chronic progressive myeloproliferative disorder which is characterized by an absolute increase in the red blood cell mass. Leucocytosis, thrombocytosis and splenomegaly usually occur.[2] PV is thought to arise from a neoplastic clone of a pluripotent haematopoietic stem cell[3] and to be dependent upon both genetic and environmental factors.[4–6] The median age at diagnosis is 60 years.[7] The disease, which is extraordinarily rare in childhood and adolescence, is an uncommon disorder with an annual incidence of about five new cases per million population and a 1.2 : 1 male–female ratio. PV is characterized by an increased production of blood cells but not an increased blood cell survival.[8] The production of red blood cells can be as high as 2–3 times the normal production rate.

Transitions from PV to post-polycythaemic myeloid metaplasia and acute leukaemia are common. Post-polycythaemic myeloid metaplasia develops in 5–15% of patients 10 years after the diagnosis of PV.[9–11] This stage of the disease is characterized by increasing splenomegaly, changes in red blood cell morphology, extensive bone marrow fibrosis, a leucoerythroblastic blood picture and a normal or decreasing blood cell mass.[11–13] The anaemia seen in this phase of the disease is primarily due to splenic pooling, ineffective erythropoiesis and reduced survival of the red blood cells.[11,13] Especially common during this phase of the disease are bleeding abnormalities.[13]

Between 25 and 50% of patients that enter the post-polycythaemic myeloid metaplasia phase will eventually undergo leukaemic transformation.[11–15] By far the most common phenotype of the leukaemia is myeloid.[14] About 50% of patients who develop acute leukaemia do so by progression directly from the erythrocytic phase.[14] The development of acute leukaemia rarely occurs before 8 years after the diagnosis of PV.

^{32}P therapy

From historical material it is well known that the median survival of patients with an untreated PV is short, approximately 1.5 years.[9,18] With existing treatment strategies, the median survival time exceeds 10 years.[19] Several treatment modalities and combinations, such as chemotherapy utilizing busulphan or hydroxyurea, radiophosphorus, phlebotomy and biological response modifiers, are available.[20] Nevertheless, knowledge concerning optimal treatment is lacking.[20–22] This chapter deals mainly with ^{32}P therapy and will also highlight some of its advantages and disadvantages in comparison with other treatment modalities. ^{32}P is a pure beta-emitter with a mean range in tissue of about 3 mm and a maximum of 8 mm. The biological half-life in bone marrow is 7–9 days, which corresponds to an effective dose equivalent of 2.2 mSv/MBq.[23] The radionuclide is utilized mainly to suppress hyperproliferative cell lines rather than to eradicate them. It is usually administered intravenously but may also be taken orally. ^{32}P is actively incorporated into proliferating cells and taken up primarily in the bone, spleen and liver. The high radiation dose delivered to the bone marrow accounts for the treatment effect in PV.[24] The treatment efficacy of ^{32}P in PV has been investigated in prospective randomized trials. Major studies have been performed by the Polycythaemia Vera Study Group (PVSG) and the European Organization for Research and Treatment of Cancer (EORTC). In an initial PVSG trial, ^{32}P was compared with phlebotomy alone and chlorambucil.[18,25] It has been clearly concluded from this study that chlorambucil leads to a reduction in survival in comparison with the other two treatment modalities, mainly because of the rapid appearance of acute leukaemia.[26] No statistical difference with respect to 10 year survival was seen between the phlebotomy arm and the ^{32}P arm. However, the morbidity of the disease and the complications arising from each treatment were different. The phlebotomy-treated patients developed a higher percentage of fatal thromboembolic complications, whereas close to 10% of the ^{32}P-treated patients developed malignant diseases, especially acute myeloid leukaemia, during the first 10 year period. Among these malignancies was also found a statistically increased percentage of non-haematological diseases such as gastrointestinal and skin cancers. This also held true for the chlorambucil-treated patients. In a subsequent PVSG trial, PV patients were randomized between ^{32}P and phlebotomy coupled with antiaggregating agents.[27] The results obtained showed an inferior outcome for the patients treated with phlebotomy/antiaggregating agents than with ^{32}P, with a significantly higher incidence of thrombosis as well as gastrointestinal haemorrhages.[27] In an EORTC trial comparing ^{32}P and busulphan in the treatment of PV, the latter treatment produced a survival advantage.[19] However, the difference in survival was, unexpectedly, found to be due to a three-fold higher prevalence of thrombotic events in the ^{32}P-treated group. The prevalence of acute myeloic leukaemia was less than 2% in both the treatment arms of this study.[19]

Treatment recommendations

Phosphorus-32 therapy should be preceded by repeated phlebotomies in order to reduce the haematocrit to 42–47%. The treatment regimen suggested by PVSG[10] is based on an intravenous initial dose of 74–111 MBq per m^2 body surface area with an upper limit of 185 MBq. An alternative approach is to administer a standard dose of 111 MBq. In the absence of treatment response a second treatment is given after 3 months, this time with a 25% increase in dose. This procedure, with dose augmentation, should be repeated every 3 months until an adequate response is obtained. The upper limit of a single treatment dose is, however, restricted to 260 MBq. The treatment response is considered inadequate if the haematocrit has risen above 47% or if the platelet count or white blood cell count has not fallen by at least 25%.[10] Remissions may last from several months to several years after this treatment. The average interval between repeated doses of 85 MBq/m^2 is about 2 years (see ref. 21 for a review).

The prevalence of acute leukaemia with phlebotomy alone is about 1%. With ^{32}P it varies between 2%, a rate that has little impact on the overall survival, and 15% at 10 years.[19,21,25,28] The discrepancy is probably related to the cumulative dose given and the stage of the disease at treatment (see ref. 21 for a review).

The optimal treatment strategy in PV is still a matter of debate. The choice of cytoreductive therapy lies mainly between ^{32}P, busulphan or hydroxyurea. Of these, hydroxyurea has, so far, showed very little evidence of carcinogenicity. However, since it is a ribonucleoside reductase inhibitor, it requires continuous treatment. This can be a disadvantage in elderly patients, who may have problems with treatment instructions and compliance.

It seems logical to state that, especially in elderly patients, who have a more limited survival because of their age, ^{32}P stands out as an easily administered and effective cytoreductive agent in the management of polycythaemia vera.

ESSENTIAL THROMBOCYTHAEMIA

Characteristics and diagnosis of the disease

Essential thrombocythaemia (ET) is an idiopathic myeloproliferative disorder which is characterized by an unremitting elevation of circulating thrombocytes (for review see ref. 22). Platelet count levels of 5000×10^9/l or even higher occur. The disease is rare and its exact prevalence is not known. Most patients present with recurrent spontaneous bleeding. Thromboembolic episodes are less frequent. Other symptoms include headache, paraesthesia, dizziness and generalized weakness. When coexisting vascular disease is present thrombohaemorrhagic complications occur. The use of platelet antiaggregating drugs leads to an increased risk of haemorrhagic complications. The exclusion of secondary thrombocytosis, which is by far the most common cause of elevated levels of platelets, is of utmost importance when considering ^{32}P therapy.

^{32}P therapy

The cytoreductive treatment strategies that can be used are ^{32}P, busulphan, hydroxyurea or melphalan. As in the case of the treatment of PV, ^{32}P and alkylating agents are associated with an increased risk of secondary malignancies. The use of ^{32}P in the management of ET should be considered especially in patients over the age of 50 years. The protocol recommended by PVSG entails an intravenous administration of 110 MBq of ^{32}P per m^2 body surface. The initial dose should not exceed 185 MBq. The platelet counts are checked every 4–6 weeks. Repeated doses of ^{32}P are administered every 3 months until an adequate response is obtained, i.e. a drop in the platelet count to below 450×10^9/l. The therapeutic dose should be 25% higher than the previously administered one, with the upper limit of 260 MBq. If the patient fails to respond after three ^{32}P doses, i.e. after 6 months, a change to chemotherapy should be considered. The ^{32}P treatment regimen has resulted in a 63% complete remission rate and a 37% partial remission rate at the end of the first year of therapy.[22]

REFERENCES

1. Vaquez H M 1892 Sur une forme speciale de cyanoses sáccompagnant d'hyperglobulie excessive et persistente. CR Soc Biol 44: 384–388
2. Berlin N 1975 Diagnosis and classification of the polycythemias. Semin Hematol 12: 339–351
3. Adamsom J W, Fialkow P J, Murphy S et al 1976 Polycythemia vera: Stem cell and probable clone origin of the disease. N Engl J Med 295: 913–916
4. Lawrence J H, Goetsch A T 1950 Familial occurrence of polycythemia and leukemia. California Med 73: 361–364
5. Brubaker L H, Wasserman L R, Goldberg J D et al 1984 Increased prevalence of polycythemia vera in parents of patients on Polycythemia Vera Study Group protocols. Am J Hematol 16: 367–373
6. Gurney C W 1965 Polycythemia vera and some possible pathogenetic mechanisms. Annu Rev Med 16: 169–186
7. Modan B 1965 An epidemiological study of the polycythemia vera. Blood 26: 657–667
8. London I M, Shemin D, West R, Rittenberg D 1943 Heme synthesis and red blood cell dynamics in normal humans and in subjects with polycythemia vera, sickle cell anemia and pernicious anemia. J Biol Chem 179: 463–484
9. Chievitz E, Thiede T 1962 Complications and causes of death in polycythemia vera. Acta Med Scand 172: 513–523
10. Wasserman L R 1976 The treatment of polycythemia vera. Semin Hematol 13: 57–78
11. Silverstein M H 1974 Postpolycythemia myeloid metaplasia. Arch Intern Med 134: 113–117
12. Najean Y, Aarago J P, Rain J D, Dresch C 1984 The spent phase of polycythemia vera: hypersplenism in the absence of myelofibrosis. Br J Haematol 56: 163–170
13. Silverstein M N 1976 The evolution into and treatment of late stage polycythemia vera. Semin Haematol 13: 79–84
14. Landaw S A 1986 Acute leukemia in polycythemia vera. Semin Hematol 23: 156–165
15. Najean Y, Deschamps A, Dresch C et al 1988 Acute leukemia and myelodysplasia in polycythemia vera: a clinical study with long-term follow up. Cancer 61: 89–95
16. Lawrence J H, Winchell H S, Donall W G 1969 Leukemia in polycythemia vera: relationship to splenic myeloid metaplasia and therapeutic radiation dose. Ann Intern Med 70: 763–771
17. Modan B 1975 Inter-relationship between polycythemia vera, leukemia and myeloid metaplasia. Clin Haematol 4: 427–439
18. Wasserman L R 1971 The management of polycythemia vera. Br J Haematol 21: 371–376
19. Haanen C, Mathe G, Hayat M (European Organization for Research and Treatment of Cancer, Leukemia/Hematosarcoma Cooperative Group) 1981 Treatment polycythaemia vera by radiophosphorus or busulphan: a randomised trial. Br J Cancer 44: 75–80
20. Hoffman R, Boswell H S 1990 Polycythemia vera. In: Hoffman R, Benz E J, Shattil S J, Furie B, Cohen H J eds. Hematology: basic principles and practices. Churchill Livingstone, New York, pp 834–854
21. Bareford D 1991 The role of ^{32}P in the management of haematological disorders. Nucl Med Comm 12: 751–755
22. Harbert J C 1986 Phosphorous-32 therapy in the myeloproliferative diseases. In: Harbert J C (ed) Nuclear medicine therapy. Thieme Medical Publishers, New York, pp 193–205
23. Silberstein E B 1979 Radionuclide therapy of hematologic disorders. Sem Nucl Med 100–107
24. Spiers F W, Beddoe A H, King S D 1976 The absorbed dose to bone marrow in the treatment of polycythaemia by ^{32}P. Br J Radiol 49(578): 133–140
25. Berk P D, Goldberg J, Donovan P B et al 1986 Therapeutic recommendations in polycythemia vera based on Polycythemia Vera Study Group protocols. Semin Hematol 23: 132–143
26. Berk P D, Goldberg J D, Silverstein M et al 1981 Increased incidence of acute leukemia in polycythemia vera associated with chlorambucil. N Engl J Med 304: 441–447
27. Tartaglia A P, Goldberg T D, Berk P D, Wasserman L R 1986 Adverse effects of antiaggregating platelet therapy in the treatment of polycythemia vera. Semin Hematol 23: 172–176
28. Modan B, Lilienfeld A N 1965 Polycythemia vera and leukemia: role of radiation. Treatment study of 1222 patients. Medicine 44: 305–344

74. MIBG therapy

C. A. Hoefnagel V. J. Lewington

INTRODUCTION

Since its clinical introduction in 1981,[1] radioiodinated metaiodobenzylguanidine (MIBG) has established its place in the diagnosis and treatment of tumours which are derived from the neural crest and present the characteristic features of an active uptake-1 mechanism at the cell membrane and storage granules in the cytoplasm, responsible for the uptake and retention of this radiopharmaceutical.

The high sensitivity (81–96%) and specificity (95%–100%) of this test in phaeochromocytoma and neuroblastoma led to the therapeutic use of the agent in these conditions.[2,3] In carcinoid and medullary thyroid carcinoma the sensitivities tend to be lower, 70% and 35% respectively. Fewer patients with the latter conditions will therefore be amenable to therapy.

High selective tumour uptake and a retention of MIBG is a prerequisite for successful treatment (Fig. 74.1). Used as a systemic treatment, ^{131}I MIBG will target the primary tumour and distant metastases.

Worldwide, more than 500 patients have been reported to have received ^{131}I MIBG therapy for phaeochromocytoma, neuroblastoma, paraganglioma, carcinoid and medullary thyroid carcinoma.

The decision to carry out ^{131}I MIBG therapy should be based on a tracer study, performed 1, 2 and 3 days after administration of 18.5–37 MBq (0.5–1 mCi) ^{131}I MIBG, in order to assess the tumour uptake and retention in view of the other therapeutic possibilities, as well as on the clinical condition of the patient.

Before scheduling ^{131}I MIBG therapy, one must be aware of the medication the patient is using, as many drugs are known or may be expected to interfere with the uptake and/or retention of ^{131}I MIBG by the tumour cell.[4,5] A list of these drugs is presented in Table 65.1. An example of this phenomenon is demonstrated in Fig. 74.2. Patients should be taken off these drugs for at least 1 week prior to diagnostic scintigraphy or therapy using MIBG, and, if necessary, may be put on propanolol and dibenilene (phenoxybenzamide) to control hypertension.

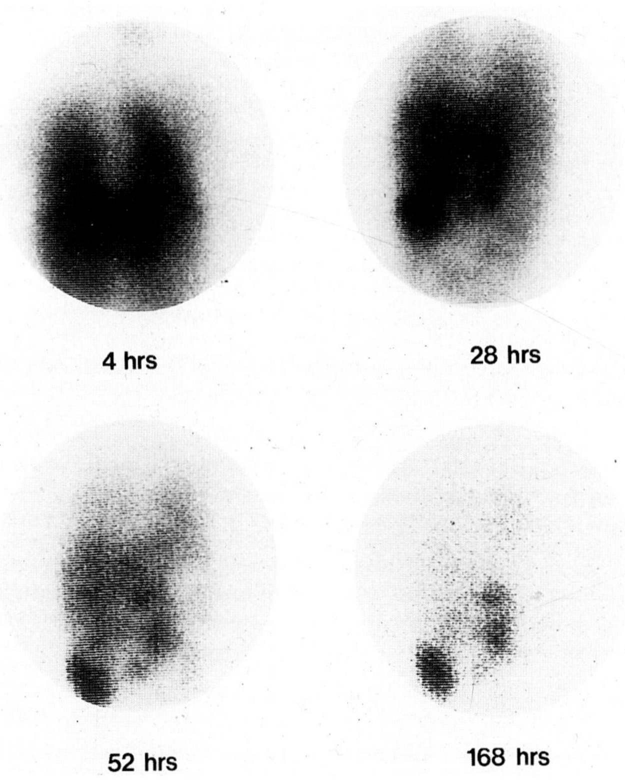

Fig. 74.1 Post-therapy scintigraphy at different intervals after administration of ^{131}I MIBG, demonstrating good concentration and persisting retention of the radiopharmaceutical in a neuroblastoma and the rapid clearance from the normal tissues. (From Hoefnagel,[86] with permission.)

As ^{131}I MIBG concentrates are usually shipped in frozen condition, upon arrival in the hospital defrosting is achieved by placing the vial within its lead container in a 37°C water bath for 45 min. The total activity is measured using a dose calibrator. Subsequently the concentrate is diluted into an infusion bottle or large syringe containing 0.9% NaCl or 5% glucose solution (dependent on the manufacturer's instructions). A sample is withdrawn for quality control. All these procedures are carried out in a

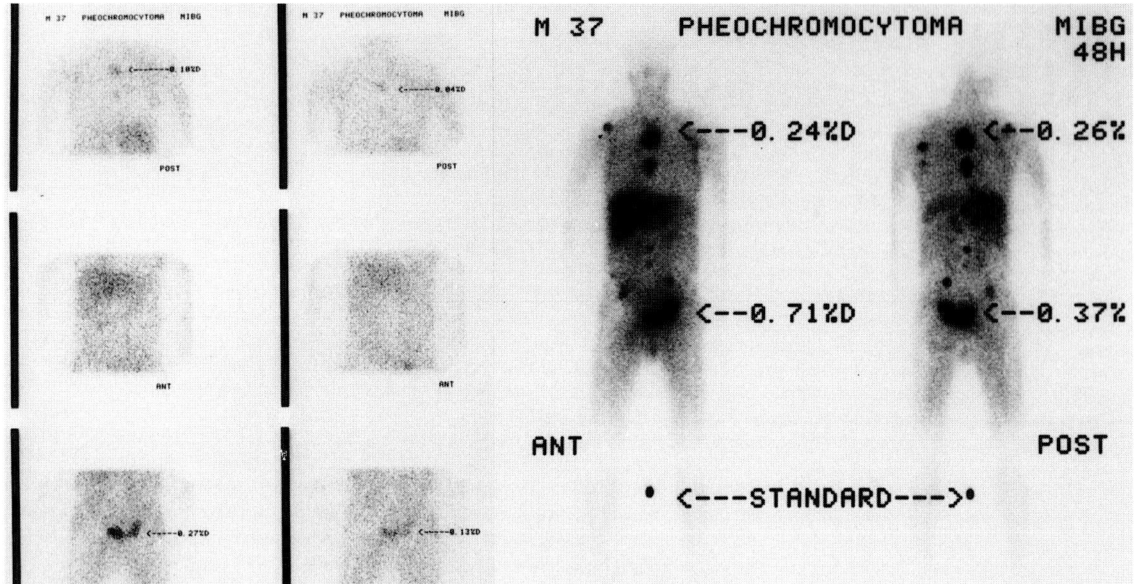

Fig. 74.2 **Left**: diagnostic ^{131}I MIBG scintigram of a patient with malignant phaeochromocytoma metastatic to bone, showing reduced tumour uptake due to concomitant Labetalol medication. **Right**: 2 weeks after the discontinuation of Labetalol, the tumour uptake is significantly increased and additional tumour sites are detected.

shielded laminar flow cabinet to reduce the radiation dose to personnel and to ensure sterility of the preparation to be infused.

Before the administration of a therapeutic dose, quality control, checking both the radionuclide and radiochemical purity, may be desirable, as impurities may add to the side-effects of the treatment. High doses of ^{131}I MIBG with a high specific activity are liable to autoradiolysis, which is dependent on the temperature, the volume, and the presence of stabilizers and scavengers in the formulation.[6] Although oral KI medication is an important aid to reduce the radiation dose to the thyroid, too much free ^{131}I will nevertheless result in uptake of some radioiodine in the thyroid.

In general, a fixed dose of 3.7–11.1 GBq (100–300 mCi) of ^{131}I MIBG with a high specific activity (up to 1.48 GBq/mg) is administered i.v. over a 1–4 h period through a lead-shielded infusion system. An alternative approach is to administer a varying, calculated dose, as assessed by a prior tracer study, aiming for the maximal acceptable 2 Gy bone marrow dose.[7]

Patients need to be isolated for 4–6 days, dependent on local legislation, and to use oral KI to protect the thyroid from free ^{131}I. Perchlorate may be added to the thyroid blockade. In the case of isolation of a child, the parents or grandparents may participate in the patient care.

Dependent on local legislation, the following criteria for discharge of a patient from isolation are considered. The period of rapid excretion of more than 50% of the radiopharmaceutical per day must have passed; the body burden of the patient must be such that the dose equivalent by internal contamination to the parent is negligible; and the product of exposure rate (μSv/h) at 1 m distance and effective half-life (h).

NEUROBLASTOMA

Neuroblastoma is a malignant tumour of the sympathetic nervous system, occurring most frequently in early childhood. The prognosis and the choice of treatment depends on the stage of disease: localized disease without distant metastases (TNM stages I and II) is treated by complete surgical excision and has a good prognosis (2 year survival rates of 90%); metastasis to lymph nodes and other organs (TNM stages III–V) is correlated with a poor prognosis and is treated by combination chemotherapy preceding surgery for the primary tumour; this is followed by post-operative chemotherapy, sometimes including high dose chemotherapy requiring allogenic or autologous bone marrow transplantation. Radiation therapy may be added.[8]

Although this treatment is characterized by a high initial response rate (up to 80% complete or partial response),[9] most of these children will relapse following completion of treatment. This is likely to reflect drug resistance. Despite combining chemotherapy, surgery and conventional radiotherapy the 5 year survival remains only 10–20%.[10]

Other prognostic factors are the patient's age, the site of the primary tumour, the pattern and rate of catecholamine excretion, the serum ferritin level at diagnosis, the tumour histology and the amplification of the *myc*-N oncogene.[8,11]

New approaches to the diagnosis and therapy of neuroblastoma include targeting of radionuclides via the immunological (monoclonal antibodies)[12] and metabolic (MIBG) route.[3]

^{131}I MIBG therapy after conventional treatment

After initial reports had indicated the feasibility and a certain degree of success of ^{131}I MIBG therapy in children with neuroblastoma,[3,13–23] greater numbers of patients were studied.

In general the following response criteria are used: complete remission (no more evidence of disease), partial remission (>50% reduction of tumour volume), stable disease (<50% reduction of volume or no change). Some groups score a near-total reduction of disease (e.g. by 90%) as a very good partial remission.

Between 1984 and 1991 a phase II study was carried out in 53 patients with progressive recurrent disease after conventional therapy had failed;[24] 49 were children with ages ranging 1–12 years; 10 had stage III and 43 stage IV disease. A fixed dose of 3.7–7.4 GBq (100–200 mCi) of ^{131}IMIBG was infused over 4 h.

Despite the unfavourable baseline for treatment with ^{131}I MIBG in these patients, the following response was observed:

- seven complete remissions: six of these patients had recurrence of disease 3–12 months after the end of therapy, two of whom could again be treated with ^{131}I MIBG; Fig. 74.3 demonstrates an example of a complete remission by ^{131}I MIBG therapy;
- 23 partial remissions: i.e. >50% reduction in tumour volume in 14 patients or significant scintigraphic improvement in nine patients with non-measurable lesions; Fig. 74.4 shows a good partial response after a single therapeutic dose of ^{131}I MIBG;
- arrest of disease (stable disease/no change) in 10 patients; Fig. 74.5 demonstrates an example of widespread neuroblastoma metastases, which had been progressive during multiple combination chemotherapy regimens but, after an initial reduction of some tumour masses by ^{131}I MIBG, continue to be stable for more than 60 months;
- nine patients had progressive disease and one patient was lost to follow-up.

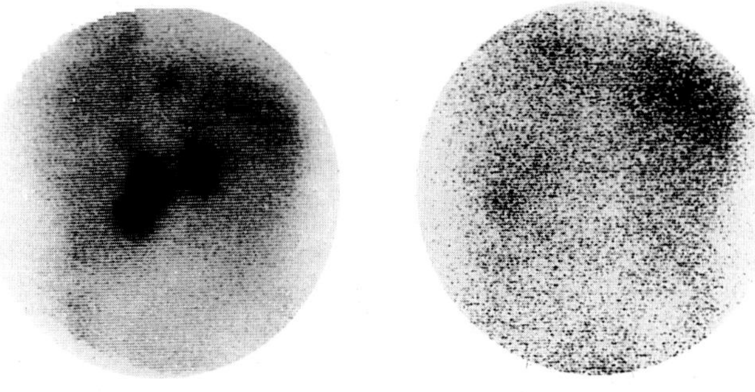

Fig. 74.3 Example of a complete remission of recurrent neuroblastoma.

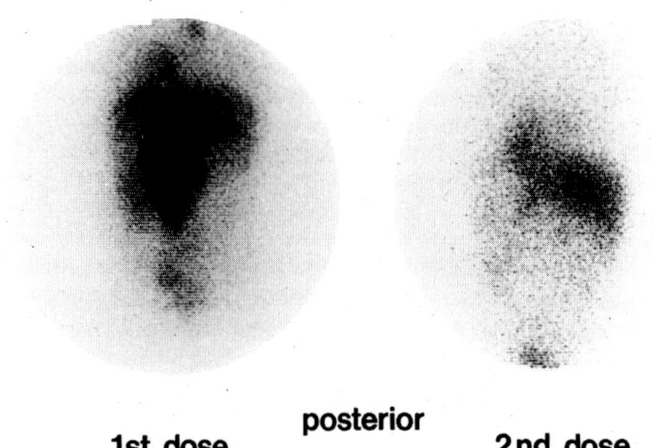

Fig. 74.4 Good partial remission after a single therapeutic dose of ^{131}I MIBG in a 4-year-old girl with an abdominal recurrence of neuroblastoma.

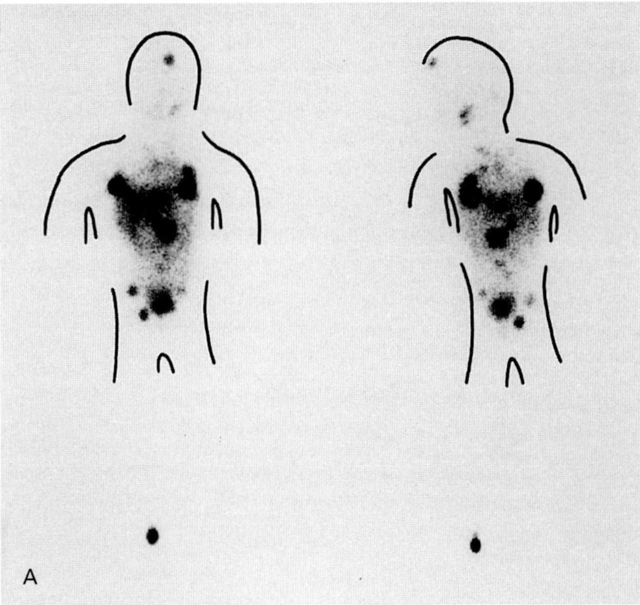

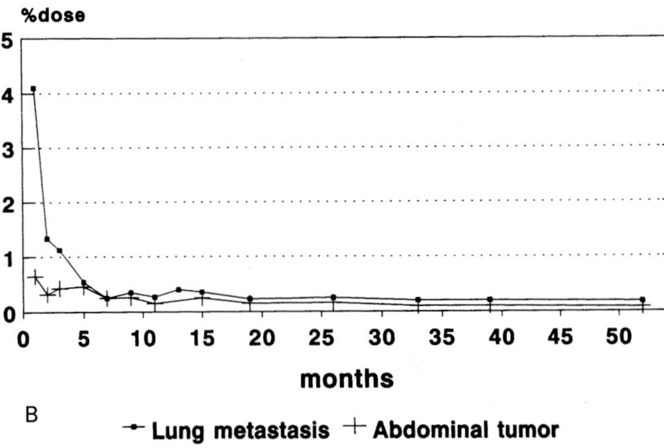

Fig. 74.5 **A** Post-therapy ^{131}I MIBG scintigram of a 3-year-old girl with stage IV neuroblastoma, refractory to combination chemotherapy: due to ^{131}I MIBG therapy the disease was arrested and continues to be stable after more than 5 years. **B** The curves demonstrate the ^{131}I MIBG uptake in the pulmonary and abdominal metastases during follow-up.

Apart from objective response, the palliative effect of the treatment under these conditions was impressive. The duration of remissions varied from two to 38 months and the best results were obtained in patients with bulky soft-tissue disease.

Similar results of ^{131}I MIBG treatment were recorded by Troncone et al[25] and in a German multicentre study involving 47 patients with stage III or IV neuroblastoma:[26] in this study nine children reached a complete or very good partial remission and 13 a partial remission (together giving a 47% objective response). Less favourable results (an objective response rate of 19%) were reported by Garaventa et al,[27] using lower doses of ^{131}I MIBG than the studies mentioned above and adjusting the administered dose to the body weight of the child.

In September 1991 the experience of the major centres in a total of 276 neuroblastoma patients (predominantly children) was collected.[24,28–36] The cumulative results indicate an overall objective response rate of 35% (Table 74.1). This is encouraging, taking into account that most of these patients had stage IV, progressive and intensely pretreated disease, and were only treated with ^{131}I MIBG after other treatment modalities had failed. In addition, MIBG therapy provided valuable palliation and improved quality of life for many children and was well tolerated in comparison with chemotherapy.

^{131}I MIBG therapy at diagnosis

The observed response to ^{131}I MIBG therapy in advanced neuroblastoma after conventional therapy, the non-invasiveness of the procedure, and the high metabolic activity which is frequently observed in untreated tumours, led to the concept of substituting ^{131}I MIBG therapy for combination chemotherapy at diagnosis prior to surgery.[37]

The objective of introducing ^{131}I MIBG therapy as the first therapy in the treatment schedule is to reduce the tumour volume, enabling adequate (>95%) surgical resection of the tumour and to avoid toxicity and the induction of early drug resistance. The advantages of this approach are that the child's general condition is unaffected or improved before it undergoes surgical resection and that chemotherapy is reserved to treat minimal residual disease postoperatively.

So far 22 patients (11 female, 11 male) who presented with inoperable neuroblastoma have been treated according to this protocol. Their age varied from 7 months to 13 years. Eight patients had stage III, 14 stage IV disease. A minimum of two cycles of ^{131}I MIBG therapy was given to all patients, after which the operability was re-evaluated; patients were then submitted to surgery, or, if still inoperable, received additional ^{131}I MIBG therapy or were crossed over to combination chemotherapy (Vincristine/Etoposide/Carboplatin/Ifosfamide: VECI). After surgery bone marrow was harvested for high dose chemotherapy with autologous bone marrow reinfusion. The following results had been obtained by March 1993:[38]

- 14 patients attained a partial remission: 12 have been successfully operated, with complete resection in three and more than 95% resection in nine patients; one had only minimal residual disease not requiring surgery and was moved on to chemotherapy, and after excellent response to ^{131}I MIBG therapy in another patient disease recurred just prior to surgery; Fig. 74.6 shows a clinical example of response to preoperative ^{131}I MIBG therapy;
- one patient showed a minimal response, which was associated with relatively little ^{131}I MIBG uptake; at surgery only 80% of the tumour could be resected;
- three patients showed stable disease and were still considered to be inoperable after ^{131}I MIBG therapy: they were crossed over to chemotherapy (VECI), after

Table 74.1 Cumulative results of ^{131}IMIBG therapy in neuroblastoma patients (Rome, September 1991)

Centre	Patients	CR	PR	SD	PD	NE	Objective response %	Ref.
NKI Amsterdam	66	7	29	18	9	3	57.1	24,37
Univ. Frankfurt	15	–	9	1	5	–	60.0	28
Univ. Tübingen	25	4	6	6	–	9	62.5	29
Germany, others	20	1	3	8	–	8	33.3	
France, multicentre	26	–	–	10	16	–	0.0	30
Genova and Brescia	43	2	5	23	12	1	16.7	31
Royal Marsden, Sutton	5	1	1	–	–	3	100	32
UKCCSG multicentre	25	–	8	9	7	1	33.3	
Gemelli, Rome	14	2	3	5	2	2	41.7	33
Univ. Michigan	14	–	1	3	10	–	7.1	34
INT Milan	7	–	2	2	3	–	28.6	35
UCSF, San Francisco	11	–	2	2	7	–	18.2	36
Univ. Turin	5	–	1	1	3	–	20.0	
Total	276	17	70	88	74	27	34.9%	

CR=complete remission; PR=partial remission; SD=stable disease/no change; PD=progressive disease; NE=not evaluable.

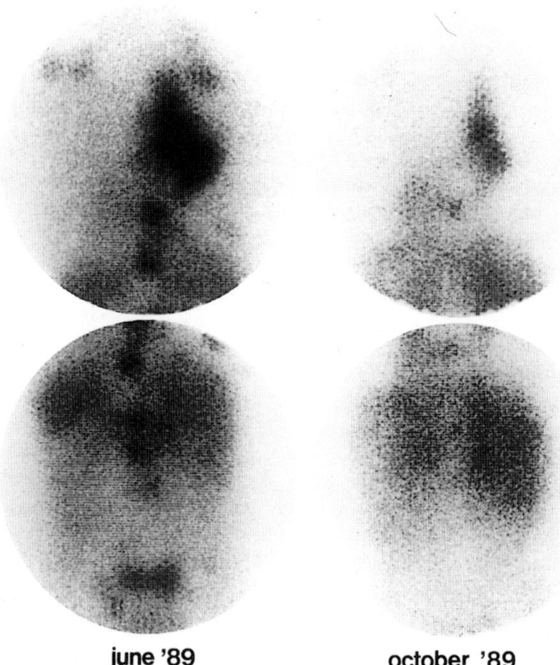

Fig. 74.6 **Left**: Preoperative ^{131}I MIBG therapy in a 13-year-old girl with a large, inoperable thoracic neuroblastoma, metastatic to the lymph nodes and bone. **Right**: after four cycles of ^{131}I MIBG there is no evidence of metastases and the primary tumour has been reduced to 30% of its original volume, enabling successful surgical resection. (From Hoefnagel,[86] with permission.)

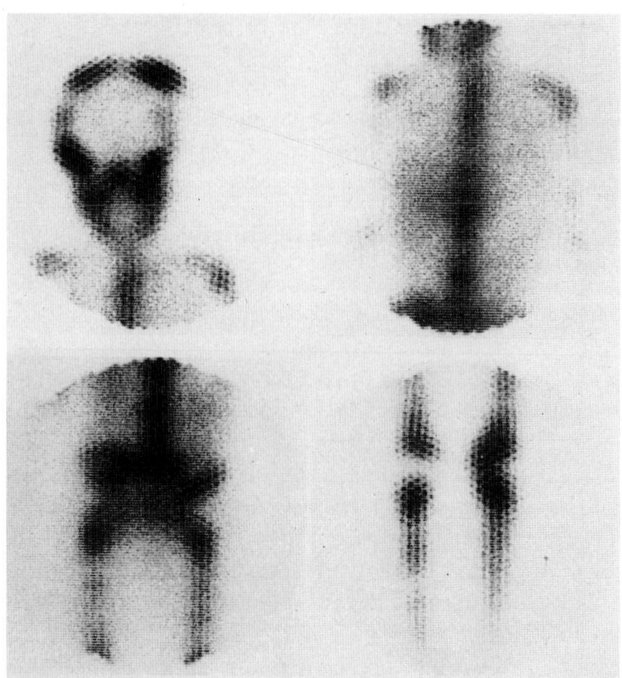

Fig. 74.7 Diffuse bone marrow invasion by neuroblastoma, as shown by post-therapy scintigraphy: ^{131}I MIBG therapy under such conditions may lead to severe myelosuppression.

which the tumour was still inoperable in two patients and progressive in the other;

- the remaining four patients are still undergoing ^{131}I MIBG treatment.

Mastrangelo et al,[39,40] treating three patients with ^{131}I MIBG at diagnosis, demonstrated complete disappearance of the tumour in one patient, persisting for 4 years, and a significant reduction of tumour masses in the other two.

Toxicity

In general both the ^{131}I MIBG treatment and the isolation are well tolerated by children but the following side-effects may be observed. Haematological effects occur most frequently, predominantly as an isolated thrombocytopenia;[24] this may be partly due to the radiation dose to the bone marrow,[41] but may also be explained by selective uptake of ^{131}I MIBG into the thrombocytes and megakaryocytes.[42] Severe bone marrow depression may occur in patients who have bone marrow involvement at the time of MIBG therapy (Fig. 74.7), and due to a high whole body radiation dose, in patients with delayed renal clearance of ^{131}I MIBG. Table 74.2 demonstrates the relation of the haematological toxicity to the status of the bone marrow.

Deterioration of renal function is occasionally observed in patients whose kidneys have been compromised by intensive pretreatment with Cisplatin and Ifosfamide.[43] Troncone et al[25] described one patient who acquired hypertensive crises shortly after ^{131}I MIBG therapy requiring alpha-blocking medication.

The toxicity of ^{131}I MIBG therapy at diagnosis is in contrast with the experience of ^{131}I MIBG therapy after conventional therapy: in the preoperative study[37] only six of 22 patients developed isolated thrombocytopenia and only two cases of moderate bone marrow depression occurred, despite the fact that the bone marrow was invaded in nine patients. In addition, the general condition of these children improved dramatically, as was demonstrated by a 10–15% increase in body weight during ^{131}I MIBG treatment. Both the improvement of the patient's general condition and the minimal toxicity are in contrast with the effects of preoperative combination

Table 74.2 ^{131}I MIBG therapy in children: toxicity *vs.* bone marrow status in 53 neuroblastoma patients after conventional therapy[24]

Bone marrow status	No effect	Thrombocytopenia	BM depression
Always negative	4	14 (7 mild)	2*
Previously positive, negative at therapy	4	13 (3 mild)	1
Positive at therapy	0	4 (1 mild)	11
Total	8	31 (11 mild)	14

BM=bone marrow; mild thrombocytopenia = at all times >100 000 × 10^9/l.
*Associated with impaired renal function.

chemotherapy; the relative lack of toxicity of ^{131}I MIBG therapy at diagnosis indicates that the previously observed more serious side-effects of ^{131}I MIBG therapy after combination therapy were partly due to the pretreatment, in particular with Cisplatin.

Special considerations in radionuclide therapy of children

Isolation presents major practical difficulties when treating young children. Problems can be minimized by inviting parents or other relatives to become actively involved in their child's care. This was found to be both feasible and safe, provided that a number of precautions were taken.[44]

Parents stay in an adjacent room, linked to the isolation unit by closed circuit television and intercom. When entering the isolation room they must wear disposable gown, gloves and shoes which are left in the locker when they leave the room. They need to be instructed to restrict the time of exposure to a minimum, to keep as much distance as possible, not to drink or eat in the isolation room and how to handle radioactive waste. Throughout the isolation period they receive an oral dose of 200 mg KI daily, starting the day before treatment, to protect the thyroid from inadvertent ^{131}I contamination. Pregnant women and children are excluded from patient care and visiting. The external radiation dose to the parent can be measured continuously by a pocket dosemeter and internal contamination may be monitored by measuring a urine sample in a gamma-counter. By adding up the measured external radiation dose, the (negligible) internal contamination and the calculated dose received at home assuming a 'mean distance factor', the overall radiation dose to which these parents theoretically may be exposed was estimated to vary between 0.4 and 3 mSv.[45] It can therefore be concluded that the participation of parents in patient care during ^{131}I MIBG therapy under the conditions mentioned above is safe.

As the isolation rather than the treatment will affect children most, they need to be kept busy and amused, e.g. by drawing and reading material, toys, games and video films (Fig. 74.8). It must be emphasized to both parents and child that personal belongings which become contaminated with ^{131}I may have to be stored temporarily and that it may therefore not be advisable to bring favourite clothes, toys or other items which the child cannot be without, into the isolation room.

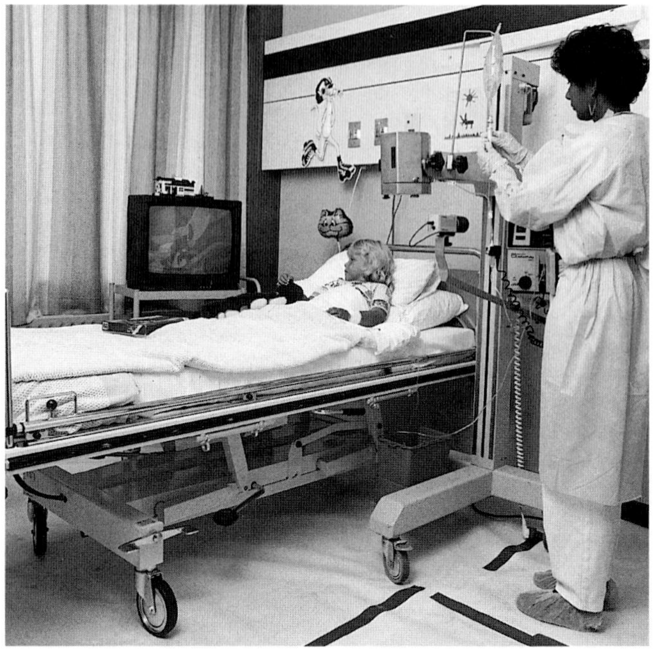

Fig. 74.8 A child in the isolation unit for radionuclide therapy. (Reproduced with permission of the Audiovisual Dept of The Netherlands Cancer Institute.)

[^{125}I]MIBG for therapy

An alternative approach to the management of neuroblastoma is the use of [^{125}I]MIBG for therapy. This may have a role in the treatment of micrometastases and bone marrow infiltration, particularly as the results of ^{131}I MIBG therapy under these circumstances are poor. Although the range of the ^{125}I Auger electrons in the storage vesicles would seem to be inadequate to deliver a lethal radiation dose to the nucleus, the finding of a considerable degree of extragranular storage in neuroblastoma[46] may provide a basis for this treatment. Preliminary experience in five patients with neuroblastoma[45,47,48] demonstrated tumour arrest and minor disease regression (Fig. 74.9), but the efficacy of this treatment needs to be confirmed in a greater number of patients. In a phase-1

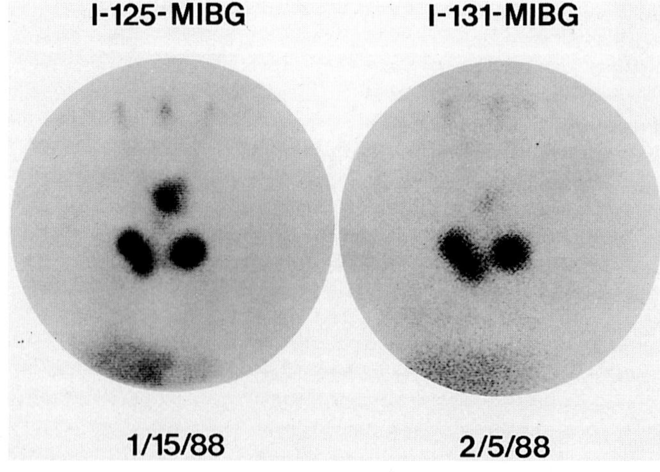

Fig. 74.9 [^{125}I]MIBG therapy of recurrent neuroblastoma in the neck and mediastinum: 3 weeks after 7.4 GBq [^{125}I]MIBG (**left**) the ^{131}I MIBG scintigram (**right**) shows a mixed response: objective regression of the lesion in the neck, but slight progression of disease in the mediastinum. (From Hoefnagel,[86] with permission.)

dose-escalating study it was shown that, as the whole body dose per MBq of [^{125}I]MIBG is about four times lower than that of ^{131}I MIBG, higher doses may be administered without causing serious toxicity,[49] although the problem of radioactive waste would require extra attention.

PHAEOCHROMOCYTOMA

Phaeochromocytomas arise from the chromaffin cells of the adrenal medulla or paraganglia. The incidence of malignancy at presentation is widely quoted as 10% but increases in tumours arising in childhood and from extra-adrenal primary sites.[50]

The diagnosis of malignancy is difficult on histological grounds and relies upon the demonstration of local tissue infiltration or distant metastasis, commonly to the skeleton, regional lymph nodes, liver and lung. The introduction of radiolabelled MIBG scintigraphy in the early 1980s offered a sensitive, non-invasive technique for detecting metastases.[51] Repeated ^{131}I MIBG tracer imaging after adrenalectomy or solitary intra-adrenal tumours indicates rates of local recurrence and subsequent dissemination approaching 50%,[52] suggesting that the malignant potential of phaeochromocytomas has been underestimated. Regular post-operative review is therefore mandatory following adrenal resection.

Malignant phaeochromocytomas secrete catecholamines, particularly noradrenaline, which lead to the clinical manifestations of hypertension, headaches, tachycardia and sweating. Dopamine excretion is a sensitive indicator of tumour aggressiveness and a rising plasma or urinary dopamine level is regarded as a poor prognostic indicator.[53,56,57]

Malignant phaeochromocytomas are associated with a broad spectrum of disease. At one extreme are indolent tumours which may be locally invasive but have low metastatic potential. At the opposite end of the spectrum are highly aggressive malignancies that behave as neuroblastomas.[54] The overall 5 year survival is 44%.[55] The variable natural history and rarity of the tumour present considerable difficulties when attempting to evaluate new treatments.

Management

Management is surgical in the first instance, and ideally includes resection of the primary tumour with debulking of soft-tissue metastases. Until recently, the management of inoperable or disseminated tumours was entirely symptomatic and relied upon combined alpha- and beta-adrenergic blockade and alpha-methyltyrosine to inhibit catecholamine synthesis.

In comparison with other solid tumours, phaeochromocytomas are relatively radioresistant. External beam radiotherapy has been used to control painful bone metastases but is of little or no value for the treatment of soft-tissue disease. In general, combination chemotherapy is also ineffective, although objective responses have been reported in 57% of patients treated using vincristine, decarbazine and cyclophosphamide.[58] The majority of patients treated using this regime had MIBG negative disease.

^{131}IMIBG therapy

Over 95% of phaeochromocytomas concentrate MIBG, which can therefore be used for targeted radiotherapy. The objectives of ^{131}I MIBG therapy and methods of response assessment were agreed at a consensus meeting in Rome in 1991.[59] Four treatment aims were identified.

1. Symptom palliation. Many patients may survive for several years with slow tumour progression. The quality of life may be severely limited by hypertension, bone pain, sweats or intractable constipation. Symptom relief should, therefore, be regarded as the primary objective of ^{131}I MIBG therapy.
2. Reduced tumour function. Prognosis in phaeochromocytoma is frequently governed more by the long term consequences of sustained or paroxysmal catecholamine hypersecretion than by the physical presence of a tumour.[58] Reducing tumour function might therefore be expected to prolong survival.
3. Tumour arrest. Accepted criteria for evaluating the efficacy of anti-cancer therapy may underestimate the value of halting tumour progression. This is particularly relevant in malignant phaeochromocytoma as patients may survive for many years with static, metabolically inactive tumours.
4. Tumour regression. Having gained tumour control, continued treatment may result in tumour regression. The benefit of reduced tumour volume must be balanced against the potential toxicity of repeated treatments and, on present evidence, is probably not justified.

The agreed treatment protocol is shown in Table 74.3. The pooled results from 99 patients are shown in Table 74.4. The aim of treatment is tumour eradication, although disease arrest is a more realistic goal for many patients. MIBG uptake frequently decreases after treatment, indicating a reduced functioning tumour mass. This change may not correlate with anatomical size and it is essential that apparent shrinkage demonstrated by gamma-camera imaging is confirmed by computerized tomography (CT) or magnetic resonance imaging (MRI).

Toxicity

Toxicity is limited to temporary myelosuppression, which typically occurs 4–6 weeks post-therapy. This is rarely of

Table 74.3 Malignant phaeochromocytoma: ^{131}I MIBG therapy protocol

1. Quantitative [^{123}I]- or ^{131}I MIBG tracer imaging; proceed to MIBG therapy if tumour uptake is demonstrated at all known tumour sites (ideally >1% administered activity, depending on tumour volume)
2. Stop drugs known to impair MIBG uptake 7 days prior to treatment
3. Block thyroid 24 h before treatment and continue for 3 weeks
4. Infuse ^{131}I MIBG for 60–90 min with continuous blood pressure monitoring
5. Quantitative post-therapy gamma-camera imaging, where feasible
6. Weekly full blood count for at least 6 weeks
7. Repeat treatment at approximately 6–8 weeks if platelet count >100 × 10^9/l
8. Assess response after 2–4 courses of treatment: CT; MRI; [^{123}I]MIBG tracer imaging; catecholamine excretion. Continue treatment if necessary

Table 74.4 Results of ^{131}I MIBG therapy: malignant phaeochromocytoma

Centre	Patients	CR	PR	SD	BR	PD	NE
Michigan	28	0	2	16	5	9	1
Brescia	6	0	2	3	2	1	0
Southampton	23	0	2	11	8	0	10
France (multicentre)	15	0	5	7		3	0
Kassel	14	0	2	8		4	0
Rome	5	1	1	2	2	1	0
Varese	4	0	0	3	1	1	0
Amsterdam	4	0	1	3	3	0	0
Total	99	1	15	53	21	19	11

LCR=complete remission; PR=partial response >50% tumour reduction; SD= stable disease (includes tumour reduction <50%); BR=biochemical response (>50% reduction catecholamines/metabolites); PD=progressive disease; NE=not evaluable.

clinical significance, but is cumulative with the result that the interval between treatments may be dictated by the rate of platelet recovery. The risk of myelosuppression rises in patients who have extensive osseous metastases.[59] Bone marrow harvesting is now recommended for all patients who are likely to undergo repeated ^{131}I MIBG treatments. The increased margin of safety this offers ensures that high activites can be administered at frequent intervals, as described above.

^{131}I MIBG therapy is otherwise well tolerated apart from nausea 48–72 h post-infusion. This responds well to ondansetron, which should be administered prophylactically. No neurological or genitourinary toxicity has been reported. Three cases of hypothyroidism have been recorded.[59]

Dosimetry

Numerous papers have drawn attention to the problem of dosimetry in targeted radiotherapy.[60] Calculations based on tracer studies rarely correlate with estimates derived from post-therapy imaging. Phaeochromocytoma presents specific difficulties due to the heterogeneous distribution of MIBG within the tumour. It is essential that dosimetry calculations are based upon functioning tumour mass rather than anatomical dimensions. Combined imaging, using CT to provide a map of attenuation coefficients for [^{123}I]MIBG single photon emission tomography has been developed for this purpose.[61] An example of this is given in Fig. 74.10.

Current status

Published data suggest that ^{131}I MIBG has not been as useful for the treatment of malignant phaeochromocytoma as was originally anticipated. There are several explanations for this.

^{131}I MIBG therapy was introduced with caution in all treatment centres and the cumulative activity received by many patients was <3.7 GBq. The majority of individuals referred for treatment had advanced malignancy and their general condition was often poor. The combination of large tumour volume and low administered activity inevitably led to such patients being undertreated. It is, therefore, not surprising that significant tumour regression was rarely observed. The efficacy of ^{131}I MIBG in reducing catecholamine secretion is more encouraging, as this would be expected to have a major influence on prognosis.

The most impressive results relate to symptomatic response, and ^{131}I MIBG therapy is undoubtedly an effective palliative treatment for disseminated phaeochromocytoma.

When ^{131}I MIBG therapy for malignant phaeochromocytoma was first introduced in the early 1980s, there were no effective alternative treatments. The results of ^{131}I MIBG therapy and its place in routine management must now be compared with the combination chemotherapy regimen reported by Averbuch et al.[58] Chemotherapy lacks tumour specificity and the toxicity of treatment is therefore significantly higher than that of ^{131}I MIBG. It has been suggested that ^{131}I MIBG therapy should be the treatment of choice for patients with malignant phaeochromocytoma who demonstrate high MIBG uptake and retention. Chemotherapy could then be reserved for patients who have MIBG negative tumours or who fail ^{131}I MIBG treatment. It has been observed that MIBG negative tumours may become MIBG positive after chemotherapy. An integrated protocol, combining both chemotherapy and ^{131}I MIBG treatment should therefore be considered.

The future

Several methods have been proposed to enhance the efficacy of ^{131}I MIBG targeted radiotherapy. Experience to data indicates that response is related to the cumulative absorbed radiation dose delivered to tumour.

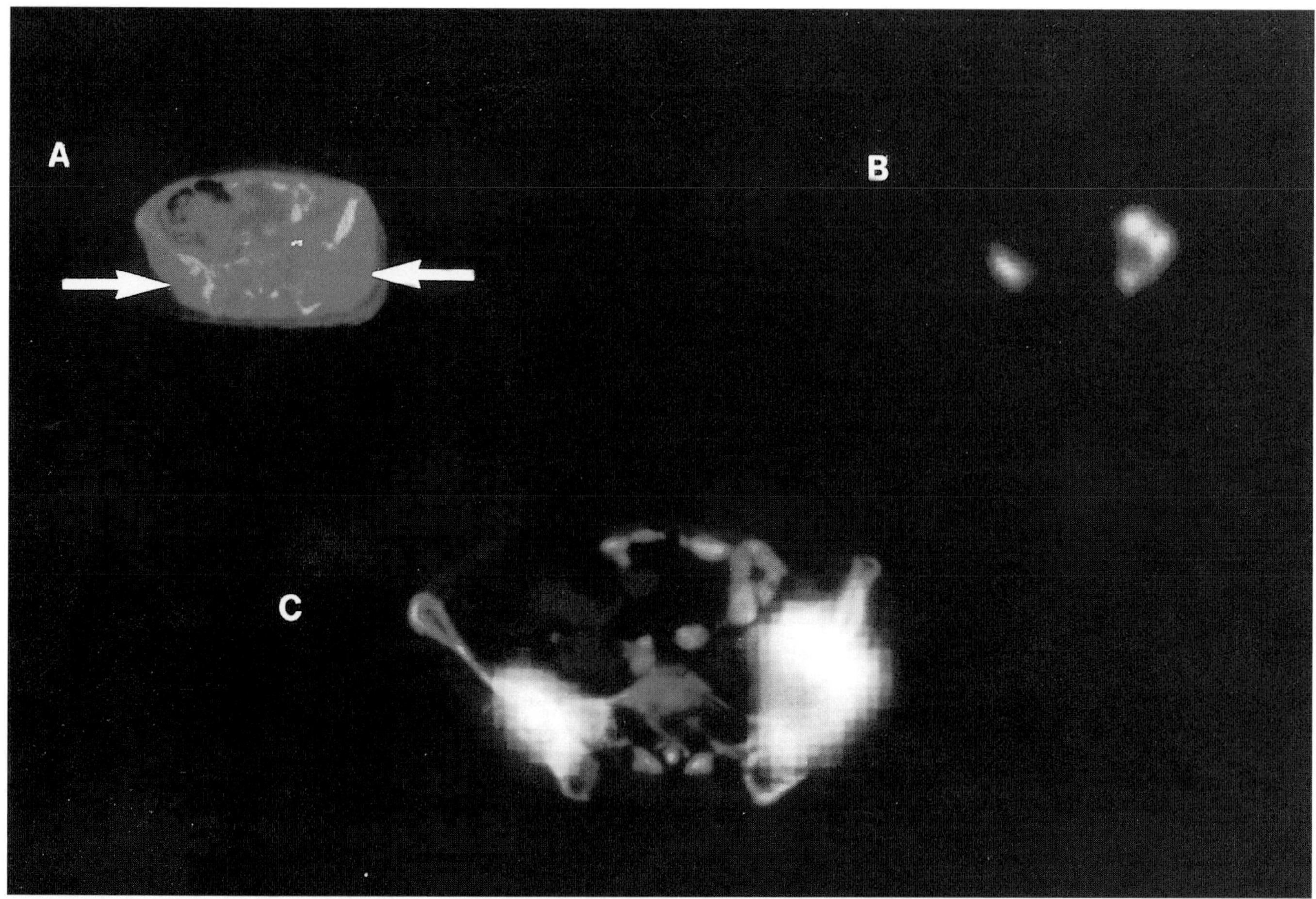

Fig. 74.10 The use of combined imaging, using computerized tomography (CT) to provide a map of attenuation coefficients for [^{123}I]MIBG single photon emission tomography (SPECT). **A** CT scan of pelvis showing tumour infiltration of the right acetabulum and left ilium (arrowed). **B** Corresponding SPECT [^{123}I]MIBG image. **C** CT/SPECT overlay confirming functioning phaeochromocytoma at tumour sites shown on CT. (Also shown in colour on Plate 21.)

Pharmacological intervention to enhance uptake and retention of MIBG has, therefore, been considered. Preliminary reports suggest that calcium channel antagonists may be of value in some patients. Concomitant use of vasodilators may also be of benefit. Phaeochromocytomas frequently comprise areas of central necrosis, which contribute to problems of radioresistance. Concomitant administration of radiosensitizers might be expected to improve radiopharmaceutical delivery, tumour uptake and sensitivity to MIBG.

The substitution of alternative radiolabels has also been considered. High energy beta-emitters or alpha-emitters, for example, might offer advantages in a hypoxic environment.

PARAGANGLIOMA

There are few reports in the literature of ^{131}I MIBG therapy of paraganglioma. Khafagi et al[62] treated a patient with widespread bone metastases from paraganglioma, non-responsive to radiotherapy and chemotherapy, with 3.85 GBq ^{131}I MIBG: no objective remission of the tumour was observed, but the patient was relieved of bone pain. Baulieu et al[63] described successful ^{131}I MIBG therapy in a patient with malignant, non-functioning paraganglioma, metastatic to the bone: an objective partial remission, together with pain relief, was attained and maintained for a period of 3 years. Thereafter a recurrence could again be treated with ^{131}I MIBG.[64]

More recently additional reports of paraganglioma patients treated with ^{131}I MIBG raised the total number to eight, among whom two were children.[65–69] Overall partial response was observed in six, complete remission in one and palliation, with sometimes dramatic improvement in the quality of life, in all patients. Although the numbers are small, these results are remarkable. Figure 74.11 shows an example of a partial remission of paraganglioma by two therapeutic doses of ^{131}I MIBG.

MEDULLARY THYROID CARCINOMA

Medullary thyroid carcinoma (MTC) arises from the

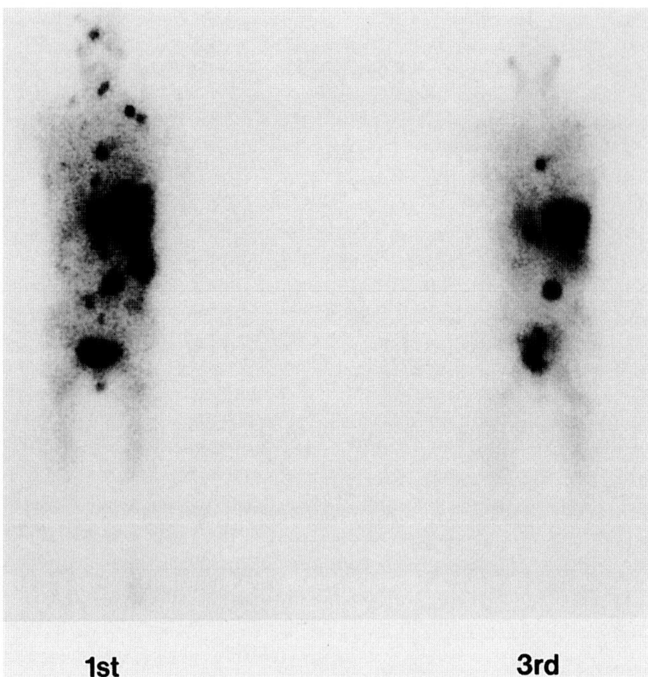

Fig. 74.11 ^{131}I MIBG therapy of multiple localizations of malignant paraganglioma (**left**): after two therapeutic doses a partial remission is attained (three of approximately 15 lesions remaining), which was accompanied by normalization of the catecholamine levels in serum and urine, as well as by a dramatic improvement in the quality of life.

parafollicular cells and accounts for 8–10% of all thyroid malignancy. 75% of cases arise sporadically but 25% occur as part of the hereditary multiple endocrine neoplasia type 2 syndrome. The tumour metastasizes by direct invasion and lymphatic spread to the cervical nodes and mediastinum. Distant metastases occur by haematogenous spread to lung, liver and bone. Ten year survival ranges from 90% for disease confined to the thyroid gland to 20% in patients with distant metastases.[70]

The majority of familial cases are now diagnosed by screening and are therefore detected at an earlier stage than non-hereditary tumours which commonly present as a painless mass in the neck. MTC may secrete a number of polypeptide hormones including calcitonin and bioactive peptides which may lead to profuse diarrhoea.

In both forms of the disease, surgery offers the only chance of cure. Radical surgery is the most important single factor influencing disease-free survival and most centres advocate total thyroidectomy, with neck dissection. The results of combination chemotherapy are disappointing, with partial response in a minority of patients.[71] Somatostatin inhibits calcitonin secretion, and may therefore relieve symptoms but has not been shown to induce tumour regression. External beam radiotherapy is of value for the treatment of painful bone metastases but is less successful in controlling local recurrence of soft-tissue deposits.

^{131}I MIBG therapy

Experience using ^{131}I MIBG in MTC has been limited both by the rarity of the tumour and by the small percentage of tumours that concentrate MIBG sufficiently to make targeted therapy a feasible option. 30–40% of MTC concentrate MIBG[72,73] although the mechanism of uptake is not understood.[74]

Treatment protocols are similar to that described for malignant phaeochromocytomas, and involve repeated high activity ^{131}I MIBG infusions at 2–8 month intervals. The results of 22 patients treated using ^{131}I MIBG are summarized in Table 74.5. Response, measured by symptom palliation, reduced calcitonin secretion and tumour regression, is variable. 50–100% of patients derive symptom relief from treatment. Complete remission is rare, although partial response with disease stabilization is reported in 30–80% (these data are derived from small series[74–77]). Treatment is well tolerated with toxicity limited to myelosuppression.

Table 74.5 Cumulative results of ^{131}I-MIBG therapy in carcinoid and medullary thyroid carcinoma (Rome, September 1991)

Centre	Patients	CR	PR	SD	PD	Objective response	Palliation	Ref.
Medullary thyroid carcinoma								
Guy's, London	7	–	2	5	–	2/7	6	74
Gemelli, Rome	5	1	2	1	1	3/5	2	75
CHU, Reims	2	–	–	2	–	0/2	–	76
NKI, Amsterdam	4	–	1	3	–	1/4	3	77
Brescia	4	–	1	1	2	1/4	–	
Total	22	1	6	12	3	31.8%	50%	
Carcinoid								
CCC, Edmonton	19	2	5	12	–	7/19	11	
Brescia	6	–	–	3	3	0/6	3	88
NKI, Amsterdam	20	–	–	18	2	0/20	13	89
INT, Milan	2	–	1	1	–	1/2	2	90
Busto Arsizio	5	–	–	2	3	0/5	5	91
Total	52	2	6	36	8	15.4%	65.4%	

CR=complete remission; PR=partial remission; SD=stable disease/no change; PD=progressive disease.

In conclusion, ^{131}I MIBG therapy is an effective palliative treatment for MTC, although objective response is low. From limited data, it seems that the best response is obtained after the first treatment and that benefit is dose-related.[75]

As with phaeochromocytoma, the majority of patients treated to date have had advanced malignancy. Attention should, therefore, be directed towards introducing MIBG therapy earlier, to treat smaller tumour volumes. The potential of ^{131}I MIBG as an adjuvant treatment at the time of primary surgery should also be considered, with the intention of prolonging the disease-free interval.

CARCINOID

Carcinoid tumours are derived from the 'APUD' (amine precursor uptake and decarboxylation) cells of the diffuse endocrine system and comprise 2% of all malignant tumours of the gastrointestinal tract. Their tumour categories are recognized according to embryonic origin and histochemical features: foregut (thymus, bronchial, gastric, duodenal and pancreatic), midgut (jejunum, ileum and proximal colon) and hindgut (distal colon and rectum). 85% of carcinoid tumours arise from the gastrointestinal tract, the most frequent sites being the appendix, small intestine and rectum. 10% are of bronchial origin.[78]

Carcinoid tumours contain and secrete a number of neuropeptides, although only a minority of patients present with hormone-related symptoms. Serotonin (5-hydroxytryptamine) and its metabolite 5-hydroxyindolacetic acid (5-HIAA) are used for tumour diagnosis and as markers of disease activity.[79] The classic carcinoid syndrome of diarrhoea, flushing, bronchoconstriction and right heart failure is associated almost exclusively with metastatic midgut tumours but occasionally with bronchogenic tumours that have venous anastomoses with the systemic circulation. The majority of patients present with abdominal pain, intestinal obstruction, gastrointestinal haemorrhage or hepatomegaly.

The 5 year survival for patients with localized carcinoid tumours from all sites is 70% but falls significantly in the presence of hepatic metastases, with a median survival of 23 months following diagnosis.[80]

Management

Surgery is the first-line treatment for both localized and metastatic tumour and may be curative for small appendiceal tumours. Segmental liver resection is of value if metastases are confined to one lobe but is impractical for symptomatic patients who have multiple hepatic metastases arising from midgut tumours. Hepatic artery embolization is of palliative value for this group of patients but, due to the development of collateral circulation, is rarely curative.[81] Radiotherapy is of little benefit for the control of soft-tissue disease but is an effective option for the relief of metastatic bone pain. The results of combination chemotherapy have been disappointing with poor, short-lived responses in most series.[82,83]

Objective response has been reported in 70% of patients treated with the somatostatin analogue octreotide.[84] Symptom control is achieved by reducing circulating neuropeptide levels and blocking the peripheral effects of circulating hormones, but there is no evidence for tumour regression. Other new developments include alpha-interferon which exerts a direct cytotoxic effect and inhibits peptide hormone production.[85,86] Increasing experience indicates that low dose maintenance therapy can be continued for up to 6 years and can give excellent symptom control with little risk of tumour resistance.

^{131}I MIBG

60% of carcinoid tumours concentrate MIBG,[87] although the degree of uptake expressed as a percentage of the administered activity is frequently too low for targeted therapy. Treatment protocols are similar to that described for malignant phaeochromocytoma and involve repeated infusions of high activity ^{131}I MIBG. Response is assessed in terms of subjective improvement, tumour stabilization and regression and reduced urinary 5-HIAA excretion.

The results of 52 patients treated using repeated high activity infusions are summarized in Table 74.5. As with phaeochromocytoma, the majority of patients derive significant symptom relief from ^{131}I MIBG therapy, but objective response, assessed by 5-HIAA excretion and tumour regression, is poor.[88–92]

Many patients exhibit both MIBG positive and negative tumour at different sites. Variable radiopharmaceutical uptake, with relative sparing of some metastases, may explain the poor objective responses observed to date. The consensus of opinion is that ^{131}I MIBG therapy should only be considered for patients in whom every known tumour site concentrates MIBG.

Treatment is well tolerated with toxicity limited to temporary myelosuppression.

Future developments

At best, ^{131}I MIBG is a palliative treatment for the carcinoid syndrome and must therefore compete with the newer, more convenient medical alternatives. The effects of octreotide or alpha-interferon on MIBG uptake and retention have not been investigated. The therapeutic potential of combining ^{131}I MIBG with medical treatment might be worth consideration.

CONCLUSION

^{131}I MIBG therapy is an effective treatment for several neural crest tumours, and can be safely applied, even in children, provided that the bone marrow is free of tumour cells; in patients with invaded bone marrow ^{131}I MIBG therapy should be considered with care, preferably having bone marrow salvage methods available. ^{131}I MIBG therapy is probably the best palliative treatment for patients with advanced disease, as the invasiveness and toxicity of this therapy compare favourably with that of chemotherapy, immunotherapy and external beam radiotherapy. Dosimetry in clinical practice remains difficult, with calculated absorbed radiation doses to the tumour not always matching the observed response. Dosimetric studies of ^{131}I MIBG therapy of human neuroblastoma xenografts in the nude mouse, however, did demonstrate a clear dose–response relationship.[93] The use of animal models enables study of the pharmacokinetics, dose-scheduling and pharmacological intervention, and may accelerate the rate of progress.

^{131}I MIBG therapy is of proven value in the treatment of neuroblastoma. The results call for incorporating ^{131}I MIBG treatment at an earlier, more favourable moment in the treatment protocol. ^{131}I MIBG therapy of neuroblastoma at diagnosis may be used instead of combination chemotherapy to attain operability of the primary tumour.

^{131}I MIBG therapy has a place in the management of malignant pheochromocytoma. Its value in the carcinoid syndrome and medullary thyroid carcinoma is less well established.

Clinical experience remains limited, governed, with the exception of carcinoid tumours, by the rarity of the individual tumours concerned. It is essential that ^{131}I MIBG therapy data are pooled from individual centres and that patients are treated using agreed protocols, so that results can be compared.

REFERENCES

1. Sisson J C, Frager M S, Valk T W et al 1981 Scintigraphic localization of pheochromocytoma. N Eng J Med 305: 12–17
2. Sisson J C, Shapiro B, Beierwaltes W H et al 1984 Radiopharmaceutical treatment of malignant pheochromocytoma. J Nucl Med 24: 197–206
3. Hoefnagel C A, Voûte P A, de Kraker J, Marcuse H R 1987 Radionuclide diagnosis and therapy of neural crest tumors using iodine-131 metaiodobenzylguanidine. J Nucl Med 28: 308–314
4. Khafagi F A, Shapiro B, Fig L M, Mallette S, Sisson J C 1989 Labetalol reduces iodine-131 MIBG uptake by pheochromocytoma and normal tissues. J Nucl Med 30: 481–489
5. Corbett R P, Peacock J, Meller S T 1991 Inhibition of ^{125}I-metaiodobenzylguanidine (MIBG) uptake into neuroblastoma monolayers by antiemetic agents. Eur J Nucl Med 18: 678
6. Wafelman A R, Suchi R, Hoefnagel C A, Beijnen J H 1993 Radiochemical purity of ^{131}I MIBG infusion fluids; a report from the clinical practice. Eur J Nucl Med 20: 614–616
7. Fielding S L, Flower M A, Ackery D M, Kemshead J T, Lashford L S, Lewis I 1991 The dosimetry of ^{131}I MIBG for treatment of resistant neuroblastoma – results of a UK study. Eur J Nucl Med 18: 308–316
8. Voûte P A, de Kraker J, Hoefnagel C A 1992 Tumours of the sympathetic nervous system. Neuroblastoma, ganglioneuroma and phaeochromocytoma. In: Voûte P A, Barrett A, Lemerle J (eds) Cancer in children: clinical management. Springer, Berlin, pp 226–243
9. Pinkerton C R, Pritchard J, de Kraker J et al 1987 ENSG 1-randomized study of high-dose melphalan in neuroblastoma. In: Dicke K A, Spitzer G, Jagannath S (eds) Autologous bone marrow transplantation – Proceedings of the third international symposium. University of Texas, MD Anderson Hospital and Tumor Institute, Houston, pp 401–405
10. Pinkerton C R, Philip T, Biron P, Frapazz D et al 1987 High-dose melphalan, vincristine, and total-body-irradiation with autologous bone marrow transplantation in children with relapsed neuroblastoma: a phase II study. Med Pediatr Oncol 15: 236–240
11. Seeger R C, Brodeur G M, Sather H et al 1985 Association of multiple copies of the N-myc oncogene with rapid progression of neuroblastomas. N Eng J Med 313: 1111–1116
12. Miraldi F 1989 Monoclonal antibodies and neuroblastoma. Seminars in Nuclear Medicine 19: 282–294
13. Edeling C J, Büchler Frederiksen P, Kamper J, Jeppesen P 1986 Diagnosis and treatment of neuroblastoma using ^{131}I-metaiodobenzylguanidine. J Nucl Med 25: 172–175
14. Gerrard M, Eden O B, Merrick M V 1986 Imaging and treatment of disseminated neuroblastoma with ^{131}I-metaiodobenzylguanidine. Br J Radiol 60: 393–395
15. Treuner J et al 1986 Clinical experiences in the treatment of neuroblastoma with ^{131}I-MIBG. Pediatr Hematol Oncol 3: 205–216
16. Bestagno M, Guerra P, Puricelli G P, Colombo L, Calculli G 1987 Treatment of neuroblastoma with ^{131}I-metaiodobenzylguanidine: the experience of an Italian study group. Med Pediatr Oncol 15: 203–205
17. Cottino F, Mussa G C, Madon E, Favero A, Silvestro L, Grazia G 1987 ^{131}I-metaiodobenzylguanidine treatment in neuroblastoma: report of two cases. Med Pediatr Oncol 15: 216–219
18. Fischer M, Wehinger H, Kraus C, Ritter J, Schröter W 1987 Treatment of neuroblastoma with ^{131}I-metaiodobenzylguanidine: experience of the Münster/Kassel group. Med Pediatr Oncol 15: 196–199
19. Hartmann O, Lumbroso J, Lemerle J et al 1987 Therapeutic use of ^{131}I-metaiodobenzylguanidine (MIBG) in neuroblastoma: a phase II study in nine patients. Med Pediatr Oncol 15: 205–211
20. Sanguinetti M 1987 Considerations on ^{131}I-metaiodobenzylguanidine therapy of six children with neuroblastoma. Med Pediatr Oncol 15: 212–215
21. Treuner J, Klingebiel Th, Bruchelt G, Feine U, Niethammer D 1987 Treatment of neuroblastoma with ^{131}I-Metaiodobenzylguanidine: results and side effects. Med Pediatr Oncol 15: 199–202
22. Troncone L, Riccardi R, Montemaggi P, Rufini V, Lasorella A, Mastrangelo R 1987 Treatment of neuroblastoma with ^{131}I-metaiodobenzylguanidine. Med Pediatr Oncol 15: 220–223
23. Voûte P A, Hoefnagel C A, de Kraker J, Evans A E, Hayes A, Green A 1987 Radionuclide therapy of neural crest tumors. Med Pediatr Oncol 15: 192–195
24. Hoefnagel C A, Voûte P A, de Kraker J, Valdés Olmos R A 1991 ^{131}I Metaiodobenzylguanidine therapy after conventional therapy for neuroblastoma. J Nucl Biol Med 35: 202–206
25. Troncone L, Rufini V, Montemaggi P, Danza F M, Lasorella A, Mastrangelo R 1990 The diagnostic and therapeutic utility of radioiodinated metaiodobenzylguanidine (MIBG). 5 years experience. Eur J Nucl Med 16: 325–335
26. Klingebiel T, Berthold F, Treuner J et al 1991 Metaiodobenzyl-

guanidine (mIBG) in treatment of 47 patients with neuroblastoma: results of the German neuroblastoma trial. Medical and Pediatric Oncology 19: 84–88
27. Garaventa A, Guerra P, Arrighini A et al 1991 Treatment of advanced neuroblastoma with I-131 metaiodobenzylguanidine. Cancer 67: 922–928
28. Hör G, Maul F D, Kornhuber B et al 1991 Outcome of ^{131}I metaiodobenzylguanidine therapy of neuroblastoma: seven years after. J Nucl Biol Med 35: 207–215
29. Klingebiel T, Feine U, Treuner J, Reuland P, Handgretinger R, Niethammer D 1991 Treatment of neuroblastoma with ^{131}I metaiodobenzylguanidine: long-term results in 25 patients. J Nucl Biol Med 35: 216–219
30. Lumbroso J, Hartmann O, Schlumberger M 1991 Therapeutic use of ^{131}I metaiodobenzylguanidine in neuroblastoma: a phase II study in 26 patients. J Nucl Biol Med 35: 220–223
31. Claudiani F, Garaventa A, Bertolazzi L et al 1991 ^{131}I metaiodobenzylguanidine therapy in advanced neuroblastoma. J Nucl Biol Med 35: 224–227
32. Corbett R P, Pinkerton R, Tait D, Meller S 1991 ^{131}I Metaiodobenzylguanidine and high-dose chemotherapy with bone marrow rescue in advanced neuroblastoma. J Nucl Biol Med 35: 228–231
33. Troncone L, Rufini V, Riccardi R, Lasorella A, Mastrangelo R 1991 The use of ^{131}I metaiodobenzylguanidine in the treatment of neuroblastoma after conventional therapy. J Nucl Biol Med 35: 232–236
34. Hutchinson R J, Sisson J C, Miser J S et al 1991 Long-term results of ^{131}I metaiodobenzylguanidine treatment of refractory advanced neuroblastoma. J Nucl Biol Med 35: 237–240
35. Castellani M R, Rottoli L, Maffioli L, Massimino M, Gasparini M, Buraggi G L 1991 Experience with palliative ^{131}I metaiodobenzylguanidine therapy in advanced neuroblastoma. J Nucl Biol Med 35: 241–243
36. Matthay K K, Huberty J P, Hattner R S et al 1991 Efficacy and safety of ^{131}I metaiodobenzylguanidine therapy for patients with refractory neuroblastoma. J Nucl Biol Med 35: 244–247
37. Hoefnagel C A, de Kraker J, Voûte P A, Valdés Olmos R A 1991 Preoperative ^{131}I metaiodobenzylguanidine therapy of neuroblastoma at diagnosis ('MIBG de novo'). J Nucl Biol Med 35: 248–251
38. De Kraker J, Hoefnagel C A, Voûte P A, Caron H 1994 ^{131}I-MIBG as first line treatment in high risk neuroblastoma patients. Proc Am Soc Clin Onc (in press)
39. Mastrangelo R, Troncone L, Lasorella A et al 1989 ^{131}I-Metaiodobenzylguanidine in the treatment of neuroblastoma at diagnosis. Am J Pediatr Hematol Oncol 11: 28–31
40. Mastrangelo R, Lasorella A, Troncone L, Rufini V, Iavarone A, Riccardi R 1991 ^{131}I metaiodobenzylguanidine in neuroblastoma patients at diagnosis. J Nucl Biol Med 35: 252–254
41. Sisson J C, Hutchinson R J, Carey J E et al 1988 Toxicity from treatment of neuroblastoma with ^{131}I-meta-iodobenzylguanidine. Eur J Nucl Med 14: 337–340
42. Rutgers M, Tytgat G A M, Verwijs-Janssen M, Buitenhuis C, Voûte P A, Smets L A 1993 Uptake of the neuro-blocking agent meta-iodobenzylguanidine and serotonin by human platelets and neuroadrenergic tumour cells. Int J Cancer 54: 290–295
43. Voûte P A, Hoefnagel C A, de Kraker J, Majoor M 1988 Side effects of treatment with ^{131}I-meta-iodobenzylguanidine (^{131}I-MIBG) in neuroblastoma patients. In: Evans A E (ed) Advances in Neuroblastoma Research 2. Alan R Liss, New York, pp 679–687
44. Van der Steen J, Maessen H J M, Hoefnagel C A, Marcuse H R 1986 Radiation protection during treatment of children with ^{131}I-metaiodobenzylguanidine. Health Physics 50: 515–522
45. Hoefnagel C A 1989 The clinical use of ^{131}I-metaiodobenzylguanidine (MIBG) for the diagnosis and treatment of neural crest tumors. Thesis, University of Amsterdam, ISBN 90-9003051-4
46. Smets L, Loesberg L, Janssen M, Metwally E, Huiskamp R 1989 Active uptake and extravesicular storage of metaiodobenzylguanidine in human SK-N-SH cells. Cancer Res 49: 2941–2944
47. Sisson J C, Hutchinson R J, Shapiro B et al 1990 Iodine-125-MIBG to treat neuroblastoma: preliminary report. J Nucl Med 31: 1479–1485
48. Hoefnagel C A, Smets L, Voûte P A, de Kraker J 1991 Iodine-125-MIBG therapy for neuroblastoma. J Nucl Med 31: 361–362
49. Sisson J C, Shapiro B, Hutchison R J et al 1991 Treatment of neuroblastoma with [^{125}I]metaiodobenzylguanidine. J Nucl Biol Med 35: 255–259
50. Manger W M, Gifford R W Jr 1977 Phaeochromocytoma. New York Springer, p 63
51. Ackery D M, Tippett R A, Condon B R, Sutton H E, Wyeth P 1984 New approach to the localisation of phaeochromocytoma; imaging with I-131 metaiodobenzylguanidine. Br Med J 288: 1587–1591
52. Lewington V J, Zivanovic M A, Tristam M, McEwan A J B, Ackery D M 1991 Radiolabelled metaiodobenzylguanidine targeted radiotherapy for malignant phaeochromocytoma. J Nucl Biol Med 35: 280–283
53. Shapiro B, Sisson J C, Lloyd R V et al 1984 Malignant phaeochromocytoma: clinical, biochemical and scintigraphic characterisation. Clin Endocrinol 20: 189–203
54. Scott H W Jr, Reynold V, Green N, Page D, Oates J A, Robertson D 1982 Clinical experience with malignant phaeochromocytoma. Surg Gynaecol Obstet 154: 801–818
55. Beierwaltes W H, Sisson J C, Shapiro B, Lloyd R V 1986 Malignant potential of phaeochromocytoma: implications for follow-up. Clin Res 34: 713A.
56. Weincove C 1988 Catecholamines: tumour markers more dangerous than the tumour. Ann Clin Biochem 25 (Suppl): 23S–26S
57. Tippett P A, West R S, McEwan A J, Middleton J E, Ackery D M 1987 A comparison of dopamine and homovanillic acid secretion as prognostic indicators in malignant phaeochromocytoma. Clin Chim Acta 166: 123–133
58. Averbuch S D, Steakley C S, Young R C, Gelmann E P, Goldstein D S, Stull R, Keiser H R 1988 Malignant phaeochromocytoma: effective treatment with a combination of cyclophosphamide, vincristine and decarbazine. Ann Intern Med 109: 267–273
59. Ackery D M, Troncone L 1991 Chairman's report: the role of ^{131}I metaiodobenzylguanidine in the treatment of malignant phaeochromocytoma. J Nucl Biol Med 34: 318–320
60. Blake G M, Lewington V J, Fleming J S, Zivanovic M A, Ackery D M 1988 Modification by nifedipine of ^{131}I metaiodobenzylguanidine kinetics in malignant phaeochromoctyoma. Eur J Nucl Med 14: 345–348
61. Fleming J S 1989 A technique for using CT images in attenuation correction and quantification in SPECT. Nucl Med Commun 10: 83–89
62. Khafagi F, Egerton-Vernon J, van Doorn T, Foster W, McPhee I B, Allison R W G 1987 Localization and treatment of familial malignant nonfunctional paraganglioma with Iodine-131 MIBG: report of two cases. J Nucl Med 28: 528–531
63. Baulieu J-L, Guilloteau D, Baulieu F et al 1988 Therapeutic effectiveness of Iodine-131 MIBG metastases of a nonsecreting paraganglioma. J Nucl Med 29: 2008–2013
64. Baulieu J L, Guilloteau D, Calais G, Lefloch O, Besnard J C 1991 ^{131}I metaiodobenzylguanidine treatment of a malignant paraganglioma. J Nucl Biol Med 35: 313–314
65. Castellani M R, Rottoli L, Maffioli L, Massimino M, Crippa F, Buraggi G L 1991 ^{131}I Metaiodobenzylguanidine therapy in paraganglioma. J Nucl Biol Med 35: 315–317
66. Ball A B S, Tait D M, Fisher C, Sinnett H D, Harmer C L 1991 Treatment of metastatic para-aortic paraganglioma by surgery, radiotherapy and ^{131}I mIBG. Eur J Surg Oncol 17: 543–546
67. Cornford E J, Wastie M L, Morgan D A L 1992 Malignant paraganglioma of the mediastinum: a further diagnostic and therapeutic use of radiolabelled mIBG. Br J Radiol 65: 75–78
68. Claessens R A M, Corstens F M 1992 Personal communication
69. Hoefnagel C A and Schornagel J 1992 Personal communication
70. Ponder B A J 1992 In: Grossman A (ed) Clinical Endocrinology. Blackwell, Oxford, pp 608–623
71. Hoskin P J, Harmer C L 1987 Chemotherapy for thyroid cancer. Radiother Oncology 10: 187–194

72. Baulieu J L, Guilloteau D, Delisle M J 1987 Radioiodinated metaiodobenzylguanidine uptake in medullary thyroid cancer. Cancer 60: 2189–2194
73. Troncone L, Rufini V, Montemaggi P, Danza F M, Lasorella A, Mastrangelo R 1990 The diagnostic and therapeutic utility of radioiodinated metaiodobenzylguanidine: 5 years of experience. Eur J Nucl Med 16: 325–335
74. Clarke S E M 1991 ^{131}I metaiodobenzylguanidine therapy in medullary thyroid cancer: Guy's Hospital experience. J Nucl Biol Med 35: 323–326
75. Troncone L, Rufini V, Maussier M L, Valenza V, Daidone M S, Luzi S, De Santis M 1991 The role of ^{131}I-mIBG in the treatment of medullary thyroid carcinoma: Results in five cases. J Nucl Biol Med 327–331
76. Schwartz C, Delisle M-J 1991 Results of ^{131}I metaiodobenzylguanidine therapy administered to two patients with medullary carcinoma of the thyroid J Nucl Biol Med 35: 332–333
77. Hoefnagel C A, Delprat C C, Valdes Olmos R A 1991 Role of ^{131}I-MIBG therapy in medullary carcinoma. J Nucl Med Biol 35: 334–336
78. Godwin D J 1975 Carcinoid tumours; an analysis of 2837 cases. Cancer 36: 56–69
79. Grahame-Smith D G 1979 The carcinoid syndrome. In: de Groot L J (ed) Endocrinology, Vol 3. Grune & Stratton, New York, pp 1721–1731
80. Moertel C G, Sauer W G, Dockerty M B, Baggentoss A M 1961 Life history of the carcinoid tumour of the small intestine. Cancer 14: 901–912
81. Carrasco C H, Chuang V P, Wallace S 1983 Apudomas metastatic to the liver: treatment by hepatic artery embolisation. Radiol 149: 79–83
82. Kvols L K, Buch M 1987 Chemotherapy of metastatic carcinoid and islet cell tumours; a review. Am J Med 82 (Suppl 5B): 77–83
83. Harris P E, Bouloux P M G, Wass H A N, Besser G M 1990 Successful treatment by chemotherapy for acromegaly associated with ectopic growth hormone releasing hormone secretion from a carcinoid tumour. Clin Encocrinol 32: 315–321
84. Kvols L K, Moertel C G, O'Connell M J, Schutt A J, Rubin J, Hahn R G 1986 Treatment of the malignant carcinoid syndrome: evaluation of a long acting somatostatin analogue. N Eng J Med 315: 663–666
85. Oberg K, Norheim I, Lind E et al 1986 Treatment of malignant carcinoid tumours with human leukocyte interfergon. Long term results. Cancer Treat Rep 70: 1297–1304
86. Hanssen L E, Schrumpf E, Kolbenstvedt A N, Tausio J, Dolva L O 1989 Recombinant alpha-2 interferon with or without hepatic artery embolisation in the treatment of midgut carcinoid tumours. Acta Oncol 28: 439–443
87. Hoefnagel C A 1991 Radionuclide therapy revisited. Eur J Nucl Med 18: 408–431
88. Bestagno M, Pizzocaro C, Pagliani R, Rossini P L, Guerra P 1991 Results of ^{131}I metaiodobenzylguanidine treatment in metastatic carcinoid. J Nucl Biol Med 35: 343–345
89. Hoefnagel C A, Taal B G, Valdés Olmos R A 1991 Role of ^{131}I metaiodobenzylguanidine therapy in carcinoids. J Nucl Biol Med 35: 346–348
90. Castellani M R, Di Bartolomeo M, Maffioli L, Zilembo N, Gasparini M, Buraggi G L 1991 ^{131}I metaiodobenzylguanidine therapy in carcinoid tumors. J Nucl Biol Med 35: 349–351
91. Colombo L, Vignati A, Lomuscio G, Dottorini M E 1991 Preliminary results of ^{131}I metaiodobenzylguanidine treatment in metastatic carcinoid tumors. J Nucl Biol Med 35: 352–354
92. Bestagno M 1991 Has ^{131}I-metaiodobenzylguanidine a role in the treatment of medullary thyroid cancer and carcinoid tumours? Chairman's report. J Nucl Med Biol 35: 355–356
93. Rutgers M, Gubbels A A T, Hoefnagel C A, Voûte P A, Smets L A 1991 A human neuroblastoma xenograft model for ^{131}I metaiodobenzylguanidine (MIBG) biodistribution and targeted radiotherapy. In: Evans A E, D'Angio G J, Knudson A G, Seeger R C (eds) Advances in Neuroblastoma Research 3. Wiley-Liss, New York, pp 471–478

75. Therapeutic use of radiolabelled antibodies

J. F. Chatal M. Mahé

Although the combined effects of surgery, radiotherapy, chemotherapy and biotherapy have led to substantial progress in the treatment of various cancers, results are not yet satisfactory and alternative therapy is required, particularly to eradicate residual microscopic disease which often influences prognosis. The objective is to employ a suitable therapeutic agent to target small tumour foci disseminated throughout the body. Such targeting requires an agent capable of selective recognition and efficient destruction of these tumour cell clusters. Monoclonal antibodies or their fragments have the capacity to select tumoral antigenic targets, although such selectivity is most often relative. Labelled with a suitable radionuclide, these antibodies can irradiate tumour cells over a distance of some fractions of a millimetre to several millimetres, corresponding to the maximum range of non-penetrating radiations. This is the principle of radioimmunotherapy (RIT), a special form of internal radiotherapy which, in oncology, has been used most often in recent decades for iodine-131 irradiation of metastases of differentiated carcinoma of the thyroid.

Numerous phase I–II clinical trials have evaluated the toxicity and efficacy of RIT. Analysis of results has determined the most suitable indications and the limitations of the methodology. However, these results should be considered with due caution since the trials were performed with various antibodies in different forms and labelled with different radionuclides.

Radioimmunotherapy is a multidisciplinary approach requiring complementary expertise covering the areas of antibody engineering, chemistry, radiochemistry, immunochemistry, radiobiology and radiophysics (dosimetry). Solid progress is being made or is forthcoming in each of these disciplines, and the ultimate success of RIT and its inclusion in clinical practice depend on coordinated activity among all of them.

RATIONALE OF RADIOIMMUNOTHERAPY

Despite a high percentage of complete remissions after first-line multimodality treatment, the main limitation accounting for the poor prognosis of many cancers is tumour cell resistance to chemotherapy, generally resulting from previous exposure to this therapeutic modality.[1] As RIT is characterized by non-cross-resistance and non-overlapping toxicity, it could be effective on tumour cells which have become resistant to chemotherapy. This potential efficacy is dependent on the delivery to tumour targets of tumoricidal absorbed doses. These doses are based on various parameters, including high cumulative tumour activity, which must be significantly greater than the cumulative activity of normal tissues, i.e. achieve a high therapeutic ratio for tumour and an acceptable level of toxicity for other adjacent tissues (Table 75.1).

Biodistribution studies involving systemic injection of radiolabelled antibodies into patients with bulky tumours have shown tumour uptake values generally lower than 0.02% injected dose per gram (% ID/g), providing absorbed tumour doses of less than 30–40 Gy, i.e. inadequate for tumoricidal action.[2] In these conditions, the potential utility of RIT has been regarded with scepticism.[3] Thus, bulky tumours are obviously unsuitable targets for RIT, an observation generally valid for applications of internal radiotherapy. In fact, the treatment of

Table 75.1 Parameters influencing RIT efficacy

Enhancement of tumour uptake	
Cytokines (increase of antigen expression)	
Irradiation	Vascular effects
hyperthermia	Vascular effects
Lymphokines	Vascular effects
Vasoactive drugs	Vascular effects
Intracavitary route (increase of tumour cell accessibility)	
Decrease of normal tissue activity	
Two-step pretargeting techniques	
Immunophoresis	
Control of haematologic radiotoxicity	
Growth factors	
Bone marrow transplantation	

macroscopic tumours, phaeochromocytomas and neuroblastomas with ^{131}I-metaiodobenzylguanidine (^{131}I-MIBG) can only have a palliative effect, despite the fact that tumour uptake values are sometimes elevated.[4] This unfavourable situation results mainly from the very heterogeneous distribution of radiopharmaceutical agents, including ^{131}I-MIBG and radiolabelled antibodies, in tumour. Consequently, certain tumour zones are too weakly irradiated to allow efficient cell destruction.

It would appear that small subclinical tumours or even microscopic tumours are more promising targets for internal radiotherapy since they are presumably less necrotic and thus more accessible to radiopharmaceutical agents. In iodine-131 treatment of well-differentiated thyroid cancer, the best (and probably curative) results have been obtained for disseminated pulmonary micrometastases, with a high percentage of complete remission over periods of more than 15 years.[5,6]

It is difficult to determine the radioactivity of radiolabelled antibody taken up by microscopic tumour targets not visible during surgery. However, targets can be isolated in particular circumstances, e.g. when they are in a cavity and immediately accessible to radiolabelled antibody injected directly into the cavity. After intraperitoneal injection in patients who underwent surgery for ovarian carcinoma, tumour uptake was low for bulky tumours (differing little from that obtained after injection of non-specific immunoglobin), moderately elevated for small tumour nodules several millimetres in diameter and elevated or even quite elevated (>1% ID/g) for clusters of malignant cells corresponding to micrometastases less than a millimetre in diameter[7] (Fig. 75.1). In an in vitro study, multicell spheroids were used to simulate the in vivo behaviour of microtumours. After incubation with concentrations of radiolabelled antibody compatible with clinical application, absorbed doses greater than 100 Gy (probably tumoricidal) were obtained using beta-emitting radionuclides of variable energy.[8]

RIT doses deliverable to tumour targets range between 20 and 150 Gy depending on administration route and tumour size. An important parameter in evaluating RIT efficiency is the low dose rate compared with that of external radiotherapy. Fowler[9] has demonstrated that in order to compensate for the effect of this low dose rate, which allows more time for repair of sublethal damage, absorbed doses must be increased by 20% to produce the same effect as with the high dose rate delivered by external radiotherapy (Table 75.2).

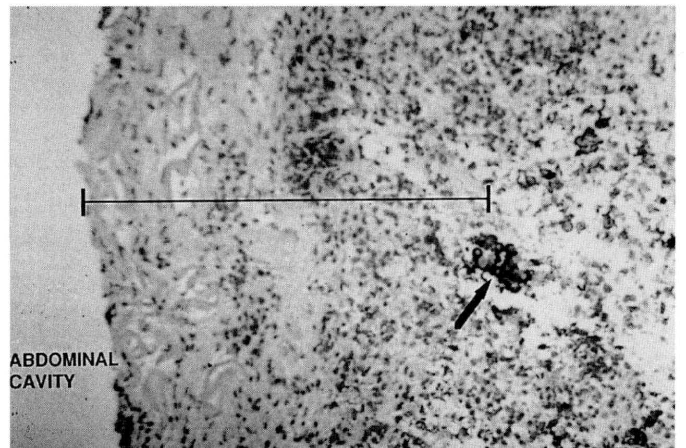

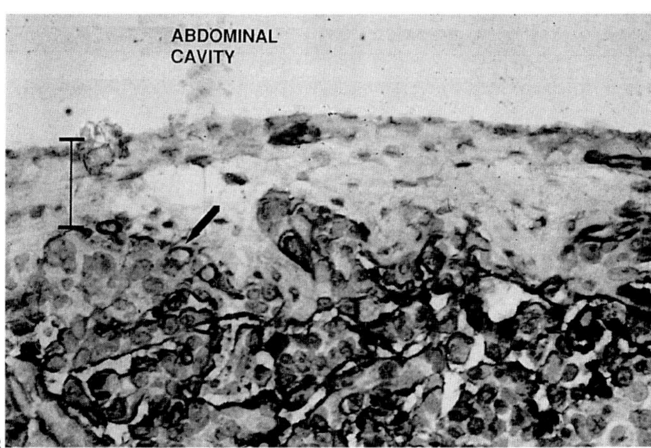

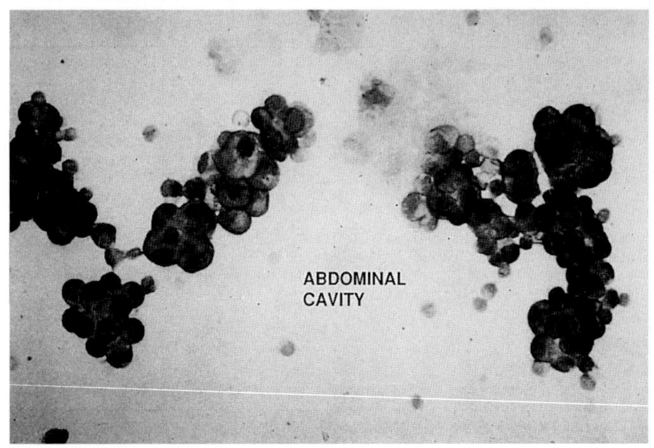

Fig. 75.1 Immunohistochemical pattern of CA 125 antigenic expression in large (>1 cm diameter) serous ovarian carcinomas (A), macroscopic (<0.5 cm diameter) tumours (B) and in microscopic (<0.5 mm diameter) clusters of malignant cells (C). For macroscopic tumours the accessibility of antibody fragments to tumour cells (brown colour) is limited by the thickness of connective tissue located between the abdominal cavity (in which the radioantibody is infused) and the tumour cells expressing the antigen (as indicated by solid line). (Reproduced with permission from Chatal et al.[7]) (Also shown in colour on Plate 22.)

Table 75.2 Tumoricidal absorbed doses (Gy) in radioimmunotherapy and external beam radiotherapy

	(10^9 cells) 1 cm	(10^6 cells) 1 mm	(10^3 cells) micrometastasis
External beam radiotherapy	60–70	40–47	20–23
Radioimmunotherapy	72–84	48–56	24–28

On the whole, the use of RIT seems warranted because of its different approach and complementarity relative to chemotherapy. For optimal results, RIT should be directed at the treatment of minimal residual disease, in which case its efficacy depends on various parameters (Table 75.1) which have not yet been clearly evaluated concerning their relative individual importance. This uncertainty accounts for the diversity of methodological conditions (choice of antibody, radionuclide, injection route, etc.) in the numerous phase I–II clinical trials carried out within the last 10 years. Although considerable caution should be exercised in comparing these different results, they provide the basis for a first analysis of the utility of RIT and for guiding future technological advances.

Table 75.3 B-cell malignancies

Reference	No. of patients	MAb (dose/cycle)	Radionuclide (activity)	Response rate	Complications		
					Haematological	HAMA	Others
10	28	Lym-1 (1 mg/ 5–10 mCi)	^{131}I fractionated low doses (30–60 mCi per injection). Total dose: 30–800 mCi	CR = 2/28 PR = 17/28	Thrombocytopenia: 10%	2/18	Fistula: 2/18
11	10	Lym-1 (1 mg/ 5–10 mCi)	^{131}I fractionated high doses (60–150 mCi per injection). Total dose: 60–400 mCi	CR = 2/6 PR = 1/6	Thrombocytopenia: 30%		
18,19	8†	Lym-1 (10–35 mg)	^{67}Cu (0.6–10.4 mCi)	PR = 3/8	0	0/5	0
12,13	17	B1 or F5 or MB1 or Anti-idiotype (58–1168 mg)	^{131}I single high dose with autologous bone marrow transplantation (232–700 mCi)	CR = 14/17 PR = 1/17	Myelosuppression: 14/16	0/10	Hypothyroidism: 2/10
Saletan SL, Norvitch ME, Rosen SJ et al‡	13	Lym-1 (30–67 mg)	^{131}I (50–267 mCi in one or two injections)	PR = 4/13	Myelosuppression	3/13	
14	10	MB1 (40 mg)	^{131}I (25–300 mCi in one or two injections)	CR = 1/9 PR = 1/9	Thrombopenia grade III–IV and/or neutropenia grade III–IV: 4/9	2/9	0
15	12	OKB7	^{131}I (90–160 mCi in three or four injections)	PR = 1/12	Neutropenia grade IV: $\frac{1}{12}$		Hypothyroidism: 2/12
17	7	LL2 (3.3–7.3 mg)	^{131}I (31–102 mCi in one or three injections)	PR = 2/5	Myelotoxicity grade III–IV: 5/7	1/7	0
16	5	Anti-idiotype (1000–2320 mg)	^{90}Y 10–20 mCi per cycle (1–4 cycles)	CR = 1/4	Mild haematological toxicity	0	0
Total	110			CR = 20% PR = 30%		13%	

† Pharmacokinetic studies
‡ A phase I/II escalating-dose safety, dosimetry and efficacy study of radiolabeled mono-clonal antibody Lym-1. American Cynamid Co, Medical Research Oncology Division, Clinical Research Oncology, Real River, NY

CURRENT RESULTS OF CLINICAL STUDIES

Systemic approach

Haematological malignancies

Among haematological malignancies, lymphomas are quite suitable for treatment with radiolabelled monoclonal antibodies since they are radiosensitive and involve immunosuppressed patients. Chemo- and radiotherapy have proved effective, but the prognosis with these techniques varies greatly according to histological grade with an overall failure rate which remains high, indicating the need for new treatment methods, including RIT.

The main data for RIT trials in B lymphomas are summarized in Table 75.3. The largest series reported by DeNardo et al[10,11] showed a 60% response rate in 38 patients treated with fractionated low doses (n = 28) or a maximal tolerated dose (n = 10) of ^{131}I-Lym-1 (Figs 75.2 and 75.3). Eary et al[12,13] obtained 81% complete response during 4–39 months using a single high injected dose of ^{131}I (with various monoclonal antibodies) and autologous bone marrow transplantation. Other series with ^{131}I reported partial response rates between 30 and 60%.[14–17] With radiometals, DeNardo et al[18,19] reported three partial responses in eight patients who received very low doses (22.2–385 MBq or 0.6–10.4 mCi) of copper-67 for pharmacokinetic studies, whereas Parker et al[16] observed three responses in five patients receiving 1–4 cycles of 370–740 MBq (10–20 mCi) each of yttrium-90. Out of a total of 110 patients treated to date with various activities of radionuclides and monoclonal antibodies, the overall response rate is about 50% (20% complete response, 30% partial response).

Injection of murine antibodies induces acute reactions in about 50% of cases and can lead to production of human monoclonal antibodies (HAMA). Acute reactions, including pruritus, rash, chills, fever, discomfort and hypotension, are usually mild and responsive to symptomatic treatments. No anaphylactic-related deaths have been reported. Development of HAMA has been noted in only 13% of patients. Interestingly, no HAMA response was noted by Parker et al[16] in five patients when an anti-idiotype monoclonal antibody was used.

Haematological toxicity of platelets and white blood cells, resulting from bone marrow radiosensitivity, previous chemotherapy or in some cases lymphomatous bone marrow involvement, is considered to be a major obstacle to increasing the radionuclide activity. Eary et al[12] investigated this problem in a phase I/II trial using escalated radionuclide doses in autologously transplanted patients with less than 20% bone marrow involvement. No toxic complications were observed in lung, liver or kidney despite injected doses of up to 25.9 GBq (700 mCi).

Other haematological malignancies treated with radiolabelled antibodies include Hodgkin's disease,[20,21] chronic lymphocytic leukaemia,[22,23] cutaneous T-cell lymphoma[24,25] and acute leukaemia[26–28] (Table 75.4). In treatment of Hodgkin's disease, Order et al[29] developed an original method using polyclonal anti-ferritin antibodies derived from various animal species immunized with ferritin from Hodgkin's splenic infiltrates. In a first study, 37 patients with refractory Hodgkin's disease treated with ^{131}I-labelled anti-ferritin had a 40% response rate;[21] haematological toxicity was a limiting factor. In a second study,[20] 35 patients received external beam irradiation (4.5 Gy × 2) in previously untreated areas of known disease larger than 5 × 5 cm, followed by infusion of ^{90}Y anti-ferritin and bone marrow transplantation when the ^{90}Y dose was greater than 740 MBq (20 mCi) (19/35). The response rate was 62%, but three patients died of aplasia despite bone marrow transplantation.

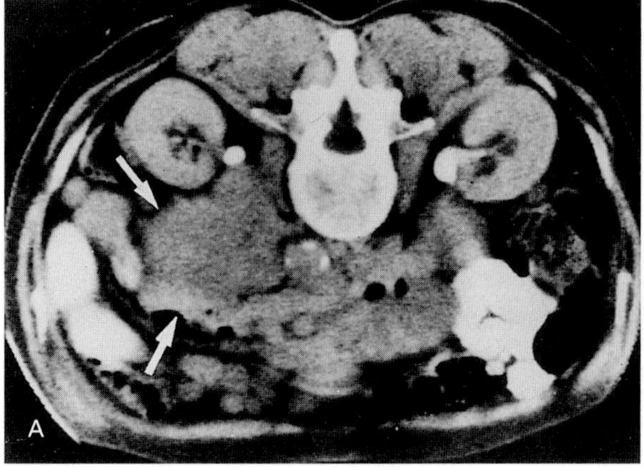

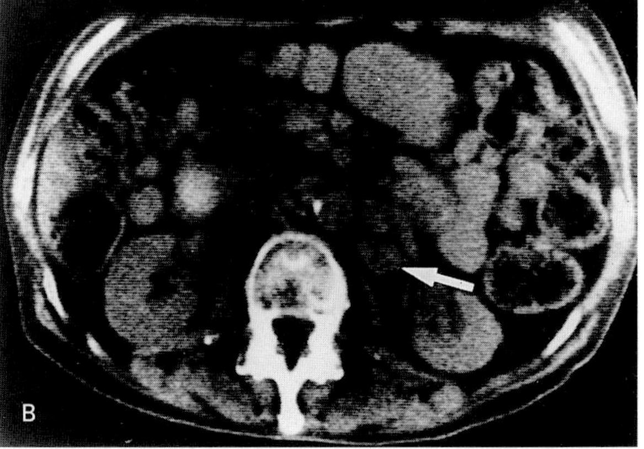

Fig. 75.2 Patients with Richter's syndrome, a malignant lymphomatous transformation of chronic lymphocyte leukaemia. Computed tomography of the abdomen at the level of the kidneys obtained before (A) and 14 months after (B) a series of injections of ^{131}I-Lym-1 (total activity 9.44 GBq or 255 mCi) revealed a dramatic decrease in the size of the abdominal mass (arrows). (Reproduced with permission from DeNardo et al.[23])

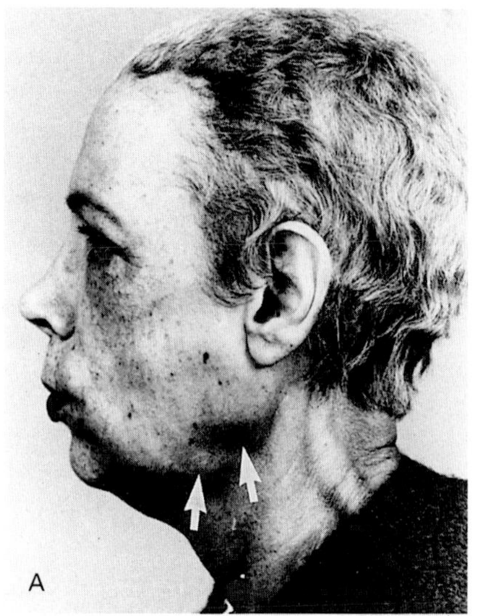

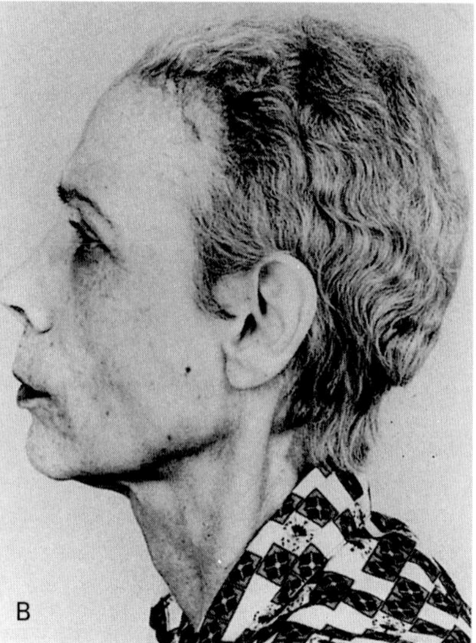

Fig. 75.3 Photographs of a patient with lymphoma before (A) and after (B) treatment with ^{131}I-Lym-1. (Reproduced with permission from DeNardo G L, DeNardo S J et al 1990 Radiation treatment of B-cell malignancies with immunoconjugates. In: Vaeth, Meyer (eds) The present and future role of MAbs in the management of cancer. Frontiers of radiation therapy and oncology, Vol 24. Karger, Basel, pp 194–201.)

Table 75.4 Other haematological malignancies

Reference	Disease	No. of patients	MAb (dose)	Radionuclide (dose)	Response rate*	Complications		
						Haematologic	HAMA	Others
22	CLL	4	T101 (5–10 mg)	^{131}I single injection (25–50 mCi)	0/4	0	0	0
23	CLL	2	Lym-1 (27–85 mg)	^{131}I fractionated low doses (160–324 mCi)	PR = 2/2	0	0	Ileovesical fistula: 1
25	CLL and CTCL	6	T101 (dose NR)	90Y (dose NR)	PR = 3/6	0	2	0
24	CTCL	5	T101 (10–17 mg)	^{131}I single injection (100–150 mCi)	PR = 2/5	Thrombocytopenia grade IV : 1	5	Dyspnoea : 2
26	ATL	6	IL-2 receptor (dose NR)	^{90}Y (5–10 mCi)	CR = 2/6 PR = 3/6	Granulocytopenia + thrombocytopenia : 1	NR	0
27	AML†	4	p-67 (4–9 mg)	^{131}I single injection (110–303 mCi)	CR = 4/4	–	1	0
28	AML	20	M-195 (3 mg/m^2)	^{131}I single dose escalation (50–210 mCi/m^2)	85% decrease in the absolute number of blasts mm^3 in bone marrow	Hypoplasia for doses > 160 mCi	40%	Bone pain : 2
21	Hodgkin's disease	37	Polyclonal antiferritin (3–10 mg)	^{131}I (50–100 mCi in one or two cycles)	CR = 1/37 PR = 14/37	Thrombocytopenia	0	0
20	Hodgkin's disease‡	35	Polyclonal antiferritin (1 mg/5–40 mCi)	^{90}Y fractionated injections (20–60 mCi) + bone marrow transplantation in 19/35	CR = 9/29 PR = 9/29	Death after prolonged bone marrow aplasia: 3	0	Pulmonary fibrosis : 1

* Only results in accordance with WHO critera are reported. Results are given for the number of evaluable patients.
† ^{131}I p-67 as part of a standard transplant regimen with cyclophosphamide and total-body irradiation.
‡ External beam irradiation prior to ^{90}Y anti-ferritin infusion.
CLL, chronic lymphocytic leukaemia; CTCL, cutaneous T-cell lymphoma; ATL, adult T leukaemia; AML, acute myeloid leukaemia; NR, not reported.

Treatment of refractory myeloid leukaemia with radiolabelled monoclonal antibodies significantly decreased blastic bone marrow involvement, indicating the feasibility of including a radiolabelled antimyeloid monoclonal antibody in a preparative bone marrow transplant regimen.[27,28]

Solid tumours

Hepatocarcinomas (Table 75.5) Order et al[29,30] pioneered the treatment of non-resectable hepatocarcinoma with radiolabelled polyclonal anti-ferritin antibodies derived from various species of animals. It was initially shown that high concentrations of ferritin exist around tumours and in stroma of malignancies clearly or apparently associated with a viral aetiology, such as hepatoma or Hodgkin's disease, and that this complex plays a physiological role in cellular immunity as well as in iron storage. It was then determined that ^{131}I anti-ferritin is selectively deposited in tumours and not in normal tissues. These deposits, related to an increase in vascular permeability directly correlated with vascular content, can be augmented by external irradiation.

In a first phase I–II trial,[29] 105 patients were treated with induction therapy [external beam irradiation (21 Gy in seven fractions) plus chemotherapy with 5-fluorouracil (5-FU)–doxorubicin on days 1, 3, 5 and 7 of irradiation] and one of the following protocols:

1. high-dose chemotherapy (5-FU–doxorubicin) followed by ^{131}I anti-ferritin (a single activity of 1.1–5.55 GBq or 30–150 mCi);
2. low-dose chemotherapy (5-FU–doxorubicin) associated with ^{131}I anti-ferritin (1.1 GBq plus 740 MBq or 30 mCi plus 20 mCi 5 days later in 1–4 cycles);
3. only ^{131}I anti-ferritin (1.1 GBq plus 740 MBq or 30 mCi plus 20 mCi 5 days later in 1–4 cycles).

Among 66 evaluable patients, 7% had complete and 46% partial response. Results were better in patients with

Table 75.5 Non-resectable hepatocarcinomas

Reference	No. of patients	MAb (dose)	Radionuclide (activity)	Results: Response rate	Results: Conversion to resectable status	Results: Overall survival	Results: Survival after surgical resection	Complications
35	11	Anti-AFP (dose NR)	^{131}I i.a.h. infusion (activity NR)	PR = 8/11 (73%)	NR	12 months: 36%	–	NR
34	20	IgG anti-ferritin (dose NR)	^{131}I i.a.h. or i.v. infusion (30–129 mCi)	PR = 13/20 (65%)	5/20 (25%)	NR	NR	Neutropenia+ thrombocytopenia 11/20 (55%)
33	25	IgG anti-ferritin (dose NR)	^{131}I i.a.h. infusion (10–139 mCi)	PR = 16/25 (64%)	7/25 (28%)	12 months : 52.5% 24 months : 28%	12 months : 83% 24 months : 75%	NR
29	105	IgG anti-ferritin (1 mg/8–10 mCi)	^{131}I* i.v. infusion 30 + 20 mCi/cycle (1– 4 cycle/s)	CR = 4/66† (7%) PR = 24/66 (36%)	5/66	24 months : 15%	–	Neutropenia grade III–IV: 12% Thrombocytopenia grade III–IV: 24% Persistent aplasia: one case
30	74	IgG anti-ferritin (1 mg/8–10 mCi)	^{131}I* i.v. infusion 30 + 20 mCi/cycle‡ (1– 4 cycle/s)	PR = 18/74† (24%) 11/48† (23%) after ^{131}I •7/26 (27%) after CT + ^{131}I	5/74 (7%)	NR	NR	Haematological toxicity grade III–IV: 28/48 (58%)
31	13	IgG anti-ferritin (1 mg/10–20 mCi)	^{90}Y i.v. infusion 20–37 mCi/cycle (1–2 cycle/s)	PR = 3/9†	1/9	NR	–	Neutropenia and/or thrombocytopenia grade III and IV when doses ⩾ 30 mCi
Total	248			CR + PR = 86/209 (41%)	23/194 (12%)			

* Induction therapy [external irradiation + chemotherapy (CT)] and ^{131}I anti-ferritin with or without CT.
† Evaluable patients
‡ Randomized trial.
NR, not reported; i.a.h., intra-arterial hepatic.

positive alphafetoprotein (AFP+, median survival 10.5 months) than in those who were AFP− (median survival 5 months).

After induction therapy, a randomized trial was designed to compare high-dose chemotherapy (5-FU–doxorubicin) every 3 weeks with low-dose chemotherapy (5-FU–doxorubicin) associated with ^{131}I anti-ferritin (1.1 GBq + 740 MBq or 30 mCi + 20 mCi 5 days later) every 8 weeks. In the event of tumour progression, cross-over therapy was carried out. It was concluded that there were no differences in survival between the two treatments: 7/26 patients achieved response with ^{131}I anti-ferritin after chemotherapy failure, and 7% of patients treated with ^{131}I anti-ferritin were converted from non-resectable to resectable status.[30]

Finally, in another phase I trial,[31] 13 patients treated with ^{90}Y anti-ferritin showed three partial responses, with haematological toxicity as a limiting factor in those receiving 1.1 GBq (30 mCi) or more of the radionuclide.

The overall results for patients treated with radiolabelled anti-ferritin indicate 11 conversions from non-resectable to resectable status, with survival beyond 3 years in 80% of these cases.[32]

Three Chinese trials[33–35] using either radiolabelled anti-AFP or anti-ferritin reported high response rates and high percentages of conversion to resectable status.

The response rate in 248 cases of non-resectable hepatoma was 41%, and conversion to resectable status 12%.

Cholangiocarcinomas Stillwagon et al[36,37] treated non-resectable cholangiocarcinomas using the same induction therapy as for hepatomas plus cyclic chemotherapy associated with ^{131}I anti-carcinoembryonic antigen (CEA) (1.1 GBq plus 740 MBq or 30 mCi plus 20 mCi 5 days later). The partial response rate was 33% in a first trial with 5-FU–doxorubicin[36] and 50% in a second trial with cisplatin added to 5-FU and doxorubicin.[37]

Other gastrointestinal malignancies Riva et al[38] reported good results in locally advanced or metastatic gastrointestinal (stomach, colon) cancers treated with cyclic intraperitoneal injections of ^{131}I anti-CEA. Other trials, most often using the intravenous route, failed to confirm these results.[39–41]

Neuroblastoma Despite progress in chemo- and radiotherapy, the prognosis for advanced stages of neuroblastoma remains poor. Cheung et al[42] in a phase I trial with murine IgG3 monoclonal antibody 3F8 specific for disialoganglioside GD2, studied 10 patients with metastatic neuroblastoma refractory to chemotherapy. Four patients received 122 MBq/kg (6 mCi/kg), three 296 MBq/kg (8 mCi/kg) and three 444 MBq/kg (12 mCi/kg) of ^{131}I-3F8. All developed grade IV pancytopenia. Eight received bone marrow transplantation, six showed stabilization and four partial response. In a phase I trial, Lashford et al[43] reported one partial response, one stabilization and two bone marrow aplasias in five refractory stage IV neuroblastomas treated with ^{131}I-UJ13A.

Gliomas (Table 75.6) As the blood–brain barrier is a major obstacle to intravenously injected drugs, some authors have used direct intratumoral administration or internal carotid artery injection of radiolabelled monoclonal antibody in cases of brain tumour. Brady et al[44] treated 14 high-grade astrocytomas with ^{125}I-labelled anti-epidermal growth factor (anti-EGF) after positive localization was determined with ^{111}In anti-EGF. Iodine-125, an Auger electron emitter, concentrates near the nucleus after internalization of anti-EGF. Results were encouraging,

Table 75.6 Brain tumours

Reference	Histological type	No. of patients	Injection route	MAb	Radionuclides (activity)	Response rate	Complications		
							Haematological	HAMA	Neurological
45	Gliomas	10	Intratumoral	BC2 anti-tenascine (0.8–5.8 mg per injection)	^{131}I (11–148 mCi in 1–3 injections)	CR = 1/10 (17 months) PR = 2/10 (11,12 months) S = 3/10 (5, 8, 9 months)	0	2/10	Headache: 4/10 Seizure: 1/10
	Recurrent astrocytomas grade III–IV	8	Internal carotid artery injection	Anti-EGF (1 mg/10 mCi per injection)	^{125}I (117–130 mCi in three injections)	PR = 4/8 S = 1/8	0	0	0
44	Astrocytomas* grade III–IV	6	Internal carotid artery injection	Anti-EGF (1 mg/10 mCi per injection)	^{125}I (117–130 mCi in three injections	CR = 2/6 PR = 1/6	0	0	0
46	Gliomas	6	Intratumoral	UJ13A+ Eric – 1	^{131}I (21–60 mCi in a single injection)	PR = 3/4	0	0	0

* External radiation therapy (60 Gy) + ^{125}I anti-EGF in non-pretreated patients.
S, Stabilization.

especially in non-pretreated patients who received external radiotherapy plus ^{125}I anti-EGF: 2/6 complete responses, 1/6 partial response. Riva et al[45] and Papanastassiou et al[46] reported responses in recurrent gliomas.

Melanoma Despite advances in characterization and production of monoclonal antibody to melanoma-associated antigens and in biodistribution of anti-melanoma monoclonal antibody, clinical results have been disappointing, probably because these tumours are most often radioresistant and highly variable in antigen expression.[47] However, Carasquillo et al[48] reported some transient objective responses in 15 patients using Fab fragments of an ^{131}I-labelled monoclonal antibody that recognizes the human melanoma-associated antigen P97.

Breast carcinoma DeNardo et al[49,50] used ^{131}I-cL6 (chimeric L6) to treat 11 locally advanced or metastatic breast cancers (740 MBq to 2.59 GBq/m^2 or 20–70 mCi/m^2, 1–4 cycles). Six of nine evaluable patients showed partial remission up to 5 months and three had grade IV haematological toxicity (Fig. 75.4).

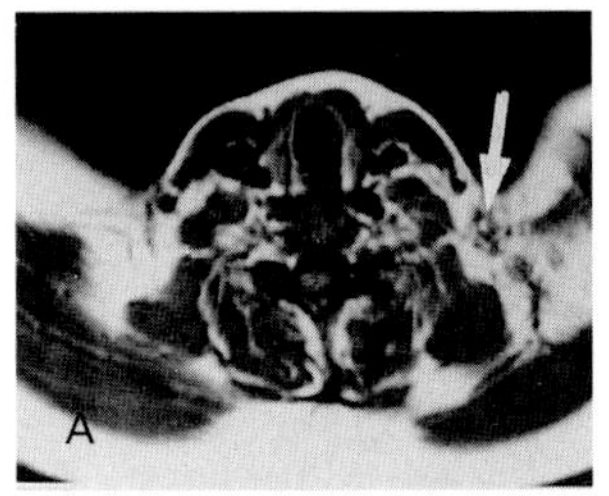

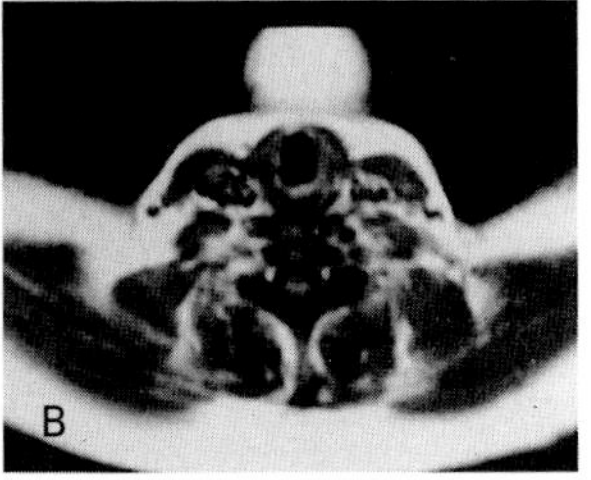

Fig. 75.4 Regression of tumour in cervical nodes in response to ^{131}I-cL6 therapy demonstrated by magnetic resonance imaging (MRI) before therapy (A) and 1 month after a second therapy dose (B). (Reproduced with permission from DeNardo et al.[49])

Intracavitary approach

Intraperitoneal route

In recent years, several phase I–II clinical trials of RIT have been carried out in Europe (UK, Italy) and the USA using various antibodies labelled with iodine-131 and yttrium-90.[51–62]

Iodine-131 was used to label seven different antibodies in five clinical studies comprising a total of 82 patients (Table 75.7). No response was observed in 26 patients with macroscopic tumour residues larger than 2 cm in diameter. In 30 patients with tumour residues smaller than 2 cm, only five cases of partial response were observed, in addition to one case of complete response in a patient with tumour residues smaller than 5 mm. A palliative effect, characterized by a transient disappearance of malignant ascites, was noted in three out of seven patients. In 15 patients with microscopic residual disease, seven cases of complete response were reported. Finally, in four patients with no evidence of disease (negative cytology on washings), no cases of relapse were noted.

In these 82 patients, toxicity was manifested mainly by 15 cases of myelosuppression when injected activities were

Table 75.7 Trial of intraperitoneal radioimmunotherapy with ^{131}I-labelled immunoconjugates

Antibody	Dose (mg)	Injected activity (mCi)	No. of patients	Residual disease prior to RIT		Response		Toxicity	References
HMFG 1 HMFG 2 AUA 1 H 17 E2		20–158	35	Macro > 2 cm Macro < 2 cm Micro NED	10 15 6 4	Macro > 2 cm Macro < 2 cm Micro	0 2 PR 3 CR	Catheter-related: 2 Myelosupression (> 100 mCi) : 6 (one irreversible)	53
HMFG 2	6–15	100–150	7	Macro < 2 cm Micro	6 1	No response		Reversible myelosuppression: 7	52
MOV 18	8–23	100	13	Macro < 5 mm Micro	5 8	Macro < 5 mm Micro	1 CR 4 CR	Reversible myelosuppression: 1	58
OC 125	10–60	20–120	20	Macro < 2 cm Macro > 2 cm	16 4	Macro > 2 cm Macro < 2 cm	0 3*	Reversible myelosuppression	57
2G3	5–50	15–150	7	Malignant ascites		Palliation	3	No myelosuppression	59
Total			82	Macro > 2 cm Macro < 2 cm Malignant ascites Micro NED	26 30 7 15 4	0 1 CR, 5 PR Palliation 7 CR Persistent NED	 3 4		

* Documented decrease in tumour burden of short duration.
NED, No evidence of disease.

above 3.7 GBq (100 mCi), including one case of irreversible myelosuppression. There were complications in only two cases due to insertion of the intraperitoneal catheter. The length of time that the catheter must remain in place constitutes one limitation of intraperitoneal chemotherapy as compared with intraperitoneal RIT, which requires only a single injection of radiolabelled antibody.

Yttrium-90 was used to label three different antibodies in three clinical studies comprising a total of 54 patients (Table 75.8). In 40 patients with a residual disease of variable size, only two partial responses and one transient response were noted. In 14 patients with no evidence of disease, only two cases of relapse were observed over a 20-month period. Toxicity was manifested by myelosuppression which varied in intensity according to the level of yttrium-90 activity injected. The in vivo stability of radiolabelling was not optimal with the DTPA used as chelating agent in these studies, and released yttrium-90 was taken up by bone and irradiated the bone marrow.

Human anti-mouse antibody (HAMA) production was a common factor in most patients injected with these two radionuclides.[63]

Taken together, these clinical studies with ^{131}I- or ^{90}Y-labelled antibodies (a total of 136 patients) confirm the results of experimental studies performed in vitro using multicell spheroid models. The only indication for potentially effective RIT is the clinical situation of minimal residual disease, especially microscopic, whether cytologically confirmed or not. Clinical studies concerning a large number of patients satisfying this indication are required to determine the role of intraperitoneal RIT as second-line treatment for ovarian carcinoma.

Intrathecal route

Another clinically studied intracavitary approach for RIT is the intrathecal route. In a study involving 15 patients (nine evaluable cases), Moseley et al[64,65] injected one of five different antibodies depending on the histopathological nature of the tumours. These antibodies were labelled with iodine-131 activities ranging from 407 MBq to 2.22 GBq (11–60 mCi). The results must be interpreted with caution because of the difficulty of assessing response to treatment (only cytological evaluation was performed). There were six responses among the nine evaluable cases. It is particularly noteworthy that two patients had a complete response, with no recurrence after 26 and 48 months. Toxicity was manifested in 7/15 cases by aseptic meningitis, in 3/8 by reversible bone marrow suppression (in patients receiving the highest activities: 2.04 and 2.22 GBq or 55 and 60 mCi) and in two cases by seizures.

Intravesical route

A third and promising intracavitary approach currently under investigation is the intravesical route for RIT of superficial tumours of the urinary bladder. As these tumours are only a few millimetres thick and the cells are directly exposed to the vesical cavity, they are presumably well suited to selective irradiation by beta-emitters with an appropriate range (a few millimetres). To date, experimental studies have been conducted in animal models,[66] and one clinical study has demonstrated the feasibility of this new approach by quantifying the uptake of ^{111}In-labelled antibody in tumour and normal tissues.[67]

Table 75.8 Trials of intraperitoneal radioimmunotherapy with ^{90}Y-labelled immunoconjugates

Antibody	Dose (mg)	Injected activity (mCi)	No. of patients	Residual disease prior to RIT		Response	Toxicity	Reference
OC 125	4–6	3–21	12	Macro > 2 cm	4	Transient CR: 1	Moderate thrombocytopenia: 3	62
				Macro < 2 cm	7	0		
				NED	1	Relapse after 13 months		
HMFG 1 AUA 1	15–35	5–25	14 evaluable	Macro < 2cm	6	Macro > 2 cm 0	Reversible myelosuppression all cases	60
				Macro < 2 cm	10	Macro < 2 cm 1 PR		
				Micro	1	Micro 0*		
HMFG 1	NI	5–25	28	Macro < 2 cm	8	0		61
				Macro < 2 cm	6	Macro < 2 cm 1 PR		
				Micro	1	0		
				NED	13	Persistent NED 12 (20 months)		
Total			54	Macro > 2 cm	15	1 Transient CR		
				Macro < 2 cm	23	2 PR		
				Micro	2	0		
				NED	14	Persistent NED 12		

* The patient was injected with only 6 mCi.
NI, not indicated; NED, no evidence of disease.

LIKELY PROSPECTS FOR THE COMING DECADE

Radioimmunotherapy, which has served a largely palliative function until now, should become curative within the next decade. To attain this objective, it will be necessary to deliver an adequate irradiation dose to the entire tumour target without causing significant damage to the more radiosensitive normal tissues, particularly bone marrow. Several methodological approaches, applicable in the short or longer term, are expected to raise the therapeutic index.

A first approach consists in increasing tumour uptake of radioantibody. An increase has been obtained in animal models by using interferon to enhance the antigenic expression of some tumour cells[68] or by managing accessibility to tumour cells from blood vessels (alteration of tumour blood flow, vascularity and vascular permeability) through the use of local irradiation, vasoactive drugs or lymphokines.[69] The use of these different methods in animal models has allowed tumour uptake to be increased by a factor of 2 or 3. The utility of this promising approach must be confirmed by clinical feasibility studies in patients within the next few years before RIT trials can be undertaken.

A second approach consists in reducing the concentration of radioactivity in normal tissues by applying a two-step pretargeting technique. This approach, which uses bifunctional antibodies[70] or the avidin–biotin system,[71] has already been studied in animal models and evaluated in clinical studies in patients. In patients who had undergone surgery for colorectal cancer, injection of a bifunctional anti-CEA/anti-DTPA indium antibody followed 3 or 4 days later by injection of a ^{111}In-labelled DTPA bivalent hapten gave tumour-to-normal tissue ratios 24 h after the second injection that were 4–5 times as high as those obtained 3 days after injection of $F(ab')_2$ fragments of the same anti-CEA antibody directly labelled with indium-111.[70] The increase in these ratios (particularly tumour to liver) resulted in a reduction in the activity of normal tissues, whereas tumour uptake was similar to or even slightly lower than that obtained with the directly labelled antibody. Clinical studies, initially performed for diagnostic purposes, will be extended in the next few years to therapeutic indications through the use of suitable beta-emitting radionuclides. It is hoped that the irradiation doses delivered to tumour targets, as compared with normal tissues, will be greater than those currently possible with directly labelled antibodies. This supposes (though it has not been demonstrated) that tumour uptake will not be relatively reduced by a saturation mechanism after injection of a large quantity of bifunctional antibody and radiolabelled hapten.

Other parameters, including radiosensitivity and tumour size, need to be considered in order to obtain optimal RIT efficiency. The most favourable situation concerns radiosensitive tumours (lymphoma, neuroblastoma, small-cell lung cancer) and micrometastases which all have cells directly accessible to radioantibody injected by an intracavitary route or by a systemic route in case the microtumours are still on the luminal surface of the vascular endothelium.[72] This situation in which micrometastases are directly and rapidly accessible to injected antibody is particularly suitable to alpha-emitting radionuclides, which have a more favourable linear energy transfer for tumoricidal irradiation than do beta-emitting radionuclides. The feasibility of this approach has recently been demonstrated in an animal model,[73] but many problems remain to be solved before clinical application can be undertaken in patients.

CONCLUSION

Immunospecific targeting with radiolabelled monoclonal antibodies, introduced clinically at the end of the 1970s, was initially used for immunoscintigraphic diagnostic applications. Ten years after the first clinical studies, immunoscintigraphy had demonstrated its usefulness for early diagnosis of recurrences of certain types of cancer. The first radioimmunotherapy studies were performed more recently in a context of rather general scepticism because of the low tumour uptake (less than 0.02% ID/g) of antibody injected by the systemic route. However, interesting and promising clinical results have now been obtained for specific indications in radiosensitive tumours (lymphomas) by systemic injection or in easily accessible small tumours by intracavitary injection.

Even though many problems still need to be solved, the future of RIT can now be viewed with some optimism. Provided that indications are limited to clinically favourable situations of microscopic tumours easily accessible by the bloodstream or endocavitary route, the technological and methodological approaches currently being developed will make it possible to deliver irradiation doses likely to be tumoricidal and thus curative in conditions of acceptable radiotoxicity controlled by haematopoietic growth factors. The immunogenicity of murine antibodies will continue to be a limiting factor until the clinical use of human or reshaped antibodies ultimately becomes feasible.

REFERENCES

1. Grossbard M L, Press O W, Appelbaum F R, Bernstein I D, Nadler L M 1992 Monoclonal antibody-based therapies of leukemia and lymphoma. Blood 80: 863–878
2. Ychou M, Ricard M, Lumbroso J et al 1993 Potential contribution of I-131-labelled monoclonal anti-CEA antibodies in the treatment of liver metastases from colorectal carcinomas: pretherapeutic study with dose recovery in resected tissues. Eur J Cancer 29A: 1105–1111

3. Vaughan A T M, Anderson P, Dykes P W, Chapman C E, Bradwel A R 1987 Limitations to the killing of tumours using radiolabelled antibodies. Br J Radiol 60: 567–578
4. Hoefnagel C A 1989 The clinical use of 131I-meta-iodobenzylguanidine (MIBG) for the diagnosis and treatment of neural crest tumors. Thesis, University of Amsterdam
5. Samaan N A, Schultz P N, Haynie T P, Ordonez N G 1985 Pulmonary metastasis of differentiated thyroïd carcinoma: Treatment results in 101 patients. J Clin Endocrinol Metab 65: 376–380
6. Schlumberger M, Arcangioli O, Piekarski J D, Tubiana M, Parmentier C 1988 Detection and treatment of lung metastases of differentiated thyroid carcinoma in patients with normal chest X-rays. J Nucl Med 29: 1790–1794
7. Chatal J F, Saccavini J C, Gestin J F et al 1989 Biodistribution of Indium-111-labeled OC125 monoclonal antibody intraperitoneally injected into patients operated on for ovarian carcinomas. Cancer Res 49: 3087–3094
8. Bardies M, Thedrez P, Gestin J F et al 1992 Use of multicell spheroids of ovarian carcinoma as an intraperitoneal radioimmunotherapy: uptake, retention kinetics and dosimetric evaluation. Int J Cancer 50: 984–991
9. Fowler J F 1990 Radiobiological aspects of low dose rates in radioimmunotherapy. Int J Radiat Oncol Biol Phys 18: 1261–1269
10. DeNardo G L, DeNardo S J, O'Grady L F, Levy N B, Adams G P, Mills S L 1990 Fractionated radioimmunotherapy of B-cell malignancies with 131I-Lym-1. Cancer Res 1990; 50 (suppl): 1014–1016
11. DeNardo G L, DeNardo S J, Mills S N, Lewis J P, O'Grady L F, Levy N B 1990 Treatment of B cell malignancies in patients using I-131-LYM-1 (abstract no 71). J Nucl Med 31: 723
12. Eary J F, Press O W, Badger C C et al 1990 Imaging and treatment of B-cell lymphoma. J Nucl Med 31: 1257–1268
13. Eary J F, Press O W, Appelbaum F R et al 1992 Update: radioimmunotherapy of B-cell lymphoma with I-131 anti-pan B cell antibodies (abstract no 162). J Nucl Med 33: 863
14. Kaminski M S, Fig L M, Zasadny K R et al 1992 Imaging, dosimetry and radioimmunotherapy with iodine 131-labeled anti-CD37 antibody in B-cell lymphoma. J Clin Oncol 10: 1696–1711
15. Czuczman M S, Straus D J, Divgi C R et al 1990 A phase I dose escalation trial of 131I-labeled monoclonal antibody OKB7 in patients with non-Hodgkin's lymphoma (abstract). Blood 76 (suppl): 345a
16. Parker B A, Halpern S E, Miller R A, Hupf H, Fricke J, Roston I 1991 Radioimmunotherapy of lymphoma with anti-idiotype monoclonal antibody. Antib Immunoconjug Radiopharm 4: 203
17. Goldenberg D M, Horowitz J A, Sharkey R M et al 1991 Targeting, dosimetry and radioimmunotherapy of B-cell lymphomas with iodine-131-labeled LL2 monoclonal antibody. J Clin Oncol 9: 548–564
18. DeNardo G L, DeNardo S J, Meares C F et al 1991 Pharmacokinetics of Copper-67 conjugated Lym-1, a potential therapeutic radioimmunoconjugate, in mice and in patients with lymphoma. Antib Immunconjug Radiopharm 4(4): 777–785
19. DeNardo G L, DeNardo S J, Meares C F 1991 Pharmacology of 67Cu-BAT-Lym-1 monoclonal antibody in patients with B cell lymphoma (abstract no 318). J Nucl Med 32: 984
20. Vriesendorp H M, Herpst J M, Germack M A et al 1991 Phase I-II studies of yttrium-labeled antiferritin treatment for end-stage Hodgkin's disease, including Radiation Therapy Oncology Group 87-91. J Clin Oncol 9: 918–928
21. Lenhard R E, Order S E, Spunberg J J, Asbell S O, Leibel S A 1985 Isotopic immunoglobulin: a new systemic therapy for advanced Hodgkin's disease. J Clin Oncol 3: 1296–1300
22. Zimmer A M, Kaplan E H, Kazikiewicz J M et al 1988 Pharmacokinetics of I-131 T101 monoclonal antibody in patients with chronic lymphocytic leukemia. Antib Immunoconjug Radiopharm 1: 291–303
23. DeNardo G L, DeNardo S J, O'Grady L F et al 1988 Pilot study of radioimmunotherapy of B-cell lymphoma and leukemia using I131 Lym-1 monoclonal antibody. Antib Immunoconjug Radiopharm 1: 17–33
24. Rosen S T, Zimmer A M, Goldman-Leikin R et al 1987 Radioimmunodetection and radioimmunotherapy of cutaneous T-cell lymphomas using an 131I-labeled monoclonal antibody: an Illinois Cancer Council study. J Clin Oncol 5: 562–573
25. Raubitschek A A 1990 Yttrium-90-labeled T101 in the treatment of hematologic malignancies. Fifth International Conference on Monoclonal Antibody Conjugates for Cancer, 1990, San Diego, CA.
26. Waldmann T A, Pastan I H, Gansow O A, Junghans R P 1992 The multichain interleukin-2 receptor: a target for immunotherapy. Ann Intern Med 116: 148
27. Appelbaum F R, Matthews D C, Eary J F et al 1992 The use of radiolabeled anti-CD33 antibody to augment marrow irradiation prior to marrow transplantation for acute myelogenous leukemia. Transplantation 54: 829–833
28. Schwartz M A, Lovett D R, Redner A et al 1991 Therapeutic trial of radiolabelled monoclonal antibody M195 in relapsed or refractory myeloid leukemias (abstract). Blood 78 (suppl 1): 54a
29. Order S, Pajak T, Leibel S et al 1991 A randomized prospective trial comparing full dose chemotherapy to 131I antiferritin: an RTOG study, Int J Radiot Oncol Biol Phys 20: 953–963
30. Order S E, Stillwagon G B, Klein J L et al 1985 I-131 antiferritin: a new treatment modality in hepatoma: an RTOG study. J Clin Oncol 3: 1573–1582
31. Order S E, Vriesendorp H M, Klein J L, Leichner P K 1988 A phase I study of 90 Yttrium antiferritin: dose escalation and tumor dose. Antibod Immunoconjugates Radiopharmaceut 2: 163–168
32. Sitzmann J V, Order S E, Klein J L, Leichner P K, Fishmann E K, Smith G W 1987 Conversion by new treatment modalities of nonresectable hepatocellular cancer. J Clin Oncol 5: 1566–1573
33. Tang Z Y, Liu K D, Bao Y M et al 1990 Radioimmunotherapy in the multimodality treatment of hepatocellular carcinoma with reference to second-look resection. Cancer 65: 211–215
34. Liu K D, Tang Z Y, Bao Y M, Lu J Z, Qian F, Yuan A N, Zhao H Y 1989 Radioimmunotherapy for hepatocellular carcinoma (HCC) using 131I-anti HCC isoferritin IgG: preliminary results of experimental and clinical studies. Int J Radiat Oncol Biol Phys 16: 319–323
35. Liu Y K, Yang K Z, Wu Y D, Gang Y Q, Zhu D N 1983 Treatment of advanced primary hepatocellular carcinoma by 131I-anti-AFP. Lancet 1: 531–532
36. Stillwagon G B, Order S E, Klein J L et al 1987 Multimodality treatment of primary nonresectable intrahepatic cholangiocarcinoma with 131I anti-CEA. A radiation therapy oncology group study. Int J Radiat Oncol Biol Phys 13: 687–695
37. Stillwagon G B, Order S E, Haulk T et al 1991 Variable low dose rate irradiation (131I-anti-CEA) and integrated low dose chemotherapy in the treatment of nonresectable primary intrahepatic cholangiocarcinoma. Int J Radiat Oncol Biol Phys 21: 1601–1605
38. Riva P, Tison V, Franceshi G, Riva N, Casi M, Moscatelli G 1992 Successful treatment of metastatic gastrointestinal cancer by means of radioimmunotherapy (abstract no 161). J Nucl Med 33: 863
39. Abdel-Nabi H, Spaulding M, Goldrosen M et al 1991 Phase I trial of IP administered Y-90 labeled CYT-103 MOAB for refractory colorectal carcinomas (abstract no 609). J Nucl Med 32: 1052
40. Divgi C R, Kemeny N, Cordon-Cardo C et al 1991 Phase I radioimmunotherapy trial with 131I-labeled monoclonal antibody (MAB) CC49 in patients with metastatic colorectal carcinoma. Proc Annu Meet Am Soc Clin Oncol 10: A699
41. Begent R H, Ledermann J A, Bagshawe K D et al 1990 Phase I/II study of chimeric B72.3 antibody in radioimmunotherapy of colorectal carcinoma. Br J Cancer 62: 487
42. Cheung N K V 1989 Phase I study of monoclonal antibody I-131 3F8 targeted radiation therapy of human neuroblastoma. Radiology 173: 420
43. Lashford L, Jones D, Pritchard J, Gordon I, Breatnach F, Kemshead J T 1987 Therapeutic application of radiolabeled monoclonal antibody UJ13A in children with disseminated neuroblastoma. Natl Cancer Inst Monogr 3: 53–57
44. Brady L, Woo D, Rackover M et al 1990 Radioimmunotherapy with 125I-EGF-425 in patients with brain tumors: preliminary results of a phase II clinical trial. Antib Immunoconj Radiopharm 3: 40

45. Riva P, Arista A, Sturiale C et al 1992 Treatment of intracranial human glioblastoma by direct intratumoral administration of 131I-labelled anti-tenascin monoclonal antibody BC-2. Int J Cancer 51: 7–13
46. Papanastassiou V, Tzanis S, Pizer B et al 1991 Targeted radiation therapy for malignant glioma. British Neuro-Oncology Group, Eleventh Annual Meeting, Glasgow, Scotland, UK, July 11–12, 1991
47. Larson S 1991 Biologic characterization of melanoma tumors by antigen-specific targeting of radiolabeled anti tumor antibodies. J Nucl Med 32: 287–291
48. Carrasquillo J A, Krohn K A, Beaumier P et al 1984 Diagnosis of and therapy for solid tumors with radiolabeled antibodies and immune fragments. Cancer Treat Rep 68: 317–328
49. DeNardo G L, DeNardo S J, O'Grady L F, Mills S L, Leuris J P, Macey D T 1991 Radioimmunotherapy with I-131 chimeric L-6 in advanced breast cancer. In: Ceriani R L (ed) Breast epithelial antigens. Plenum Press, New York, pp 227–232
50. DeNardo S J, O'Grady L F, Warhoe K A et al 1992 Radioimmunotherapy in patients with metastatic breast cancer (abstract no 160). J Nucl Med 33: 862
51. Stewart J S, Hird V, Snook D et al 1988 Intraperitoneal 131I and 90Y-labelled monoclonal antibodies for ovarian cancer: pharmacokinetics and normal tissue dosimetry. Int J Cancer 3: 71–76
52. Ward B, Mather S, Shepherd J et al 1988 The treatment of intraperitoneal malignant disease with monoclonal antibody guided 131I radiotherapy. Br J Cancer 58: 658–662
53. Stewart J S, Hird V, Snook D et al 1989 Intraperitoneal radioimmunotherapy for ovarian cancer: pharmacokinetics, toxicity and efficacy of I131 labeled monoclonal antibodies. Int J Radiation Oncol Biol Phys 16: 405–413
54. Muto M G, Finkler N J, Kassis A I et al 1992 Intraperitoneal radioimmunotherapy of refractory ovarian carcinoma utilizing iodine-131-labeled monoclonal antibody OC 125. Gynecol Oncol 45: 265–272
55. Epenetos A A, Munro A J, Stewart S et al 1987 Antibody-guided irradiation of advanced ovarian cancer with intraperitoneally administered radiolabelled monoclonal antibodies. J Clin Oncol 5: 1890–1899
56. Malamitsi J, Skarlos D, Fotiou S et al 1988 Intracavitary use of two radiolabeled tumor-associated monoclonal antibodies. J Nucl Med 29: 1910–1915
57. Finkler N J, Muto M G, Kassis A I, Weadock K, Tumeh S S, Zurawski V R, Knapp R C 1989 Intraperitoneal radiolabeled OC 125 in patients with advanced ovarian cancer. Gynecol Oncol 34: 339–344
58. Buraggi G L, Crippa F, Gasparini M, Seregni E, Bombardieri E, Mongioj V, Gavoni N 1993 Radioimmunotherapy of ovarian cancer with I-131 Mov 18: preliminary results. Communication in radioactive isotopes in clinical medicine and research. In: Crippa F (ed) Radioimmunotherapy of ovarian cancer. 20th Badgastein Symposium, 1992. Int J Biol Markers 8: 187–191
59. Buckman R, De Angelis C, Shaw P et al 1992 Intraperitoneal therapy of malignant ascites associated with carcinoma of ovary and breast using radioiodinated monoclonal antibody 2G3. Gynecol Oncol 47: 102–109
60. Stewart J S, Hird V, Snook D et al 1990 Intraperitoneal yttrium-90-labeled monoclonal antibody in ovarian cancer. J Clin Oncol 8: 1941–1950
61. Hird V, Stewart J S, Snook D et al 1990 Intraperitoneally administered 90Y-labelled monoclonal antibodies as a third line of treatment in ovarian cancer. A phase 1–2 trial: problems encountered and possible solutions. Br J Cancer 10: 48–51
62. Hnatowich D J, Mardirossian G, Rose P G et al 1991 Intraperitoneal therapy of ovarian cancer with Yttrium-90-labeled monoclonal antibodies: preliminary observations. Antib Immunoconjug Radiopharm 4: 359–371
63. Muto M G, Finkler N J, Kassis A I, Lepisto E M, Knapp R C 1990 Human anti-murine antibody responses in ovarian cancer patients undergoing radioimmunotherapy with the murine monoclonal antibody OC 125. Gynecol Oncol 38: 244–248
64. Moseley R P, Davies A G, Richardson R B et al 1990 Intrathecal administration of 131I radiolabelled monoclonal antibody as a treatment for neoplastic meningitis. Br J Cancer 62: 637–642
65. Moseley R P, Papanastassiou V, Zalutsky M R et al 1992 Immunoreactivity, pharmacokinetics and bone marrow dosimetry of intrathecal radioimmunoconjugates. Int J Cancer 52: 38–43
66. Russell P J, Ho Shon I, Boniface G R et al 1991 Growth and metastasis of human bladder cancer xenografts in the bladder of nude rats. Urol Res 19: 207–213
67. Bamias A, Keane P, Krausz T, Williams G, Epenetos A A 1991 Intravesical administration of radiolabeled antitumor monoclonal antibody in bladder carcinoma. Cancer Res 51: 724–728
68. Guadagni F, Schlom J, Johnston W W et al 1989 Selective interferon-induced enhancement of tumor associated antigens on a spectrum of freshly isolated human adenocarcinoma cells. J Natl Cancer Inst 81: 502–512
69. DeNardo G, DeNardo S, Kukis D, Diril H, Suey C, Meares C 1991 Strategies for enhancement of radioimmunotherapy. Nucl Med Biol 18: 633–640
70. Le Doussal J M, Barbet J, Delaage M 1992 Bispecific-antibody-mediated targeting of radiolabeled bivalent haptens: Theoretical, experimental and clinical results. Int J Cancer 7: 58–62
71. Paganelli G, Belloni C, Magnani P et al 1992 Two-step tumour targetting in ovarian cancer patients using biotinylated monoclonal antibodies and radioactive streptavidine. Eur J Nucl Med 19: 322–329
72. Zanzonico P 1992 Radioimmunotherapy of micrometastases: A continuing evolution. J Nucl Med 33: 2180–2183
73. Huneke R B, Greg Pippin C, Squire R A, Brechbiel M W, Gansow O A, Strand M 1992 Effective alpha-particle-mediated radioimmunotherapy in murine leukemia. Cancer Res 52: 5818–5820

76. Palliation of bone pain

A. J. McEwan

Painful bone metastases are a common cause of presentation or referral to family physicians, hospital specialists and clinical oncologists.[1–5] Symptoms associated with bone metastases are common and contribute to significant reduction in quality of life in the patient population affected. In addition to pain, these symptoms may also include those associated with hypercalcaemia, the sequelae of pathological fractures, neurological deficits, immobility and loss of independence.[6,7] These symptoms may also be compounded by overt depression and feelings of isolation, anxiety and fear.[8,9]

This group of patients is large and the symptoms are often difficult to control. Bonica[10] suggests that pain is a major symptom in up to 70% of patients with advanced cancer, with between 50% and 80% having inadequate pain relief through medical interventions. Twycross & Lack[11] have identified the factors which influence a patient's perception of pain (Fig. 76.1), demonstrating the complex nature of pain syndromes.

Clearly, management strategies which aim to provide pain palliation must not only include direct or indirect treatment of the cause of pain, but must also include an evaluation of the whole patient and the environment from which he or she may come.[12]

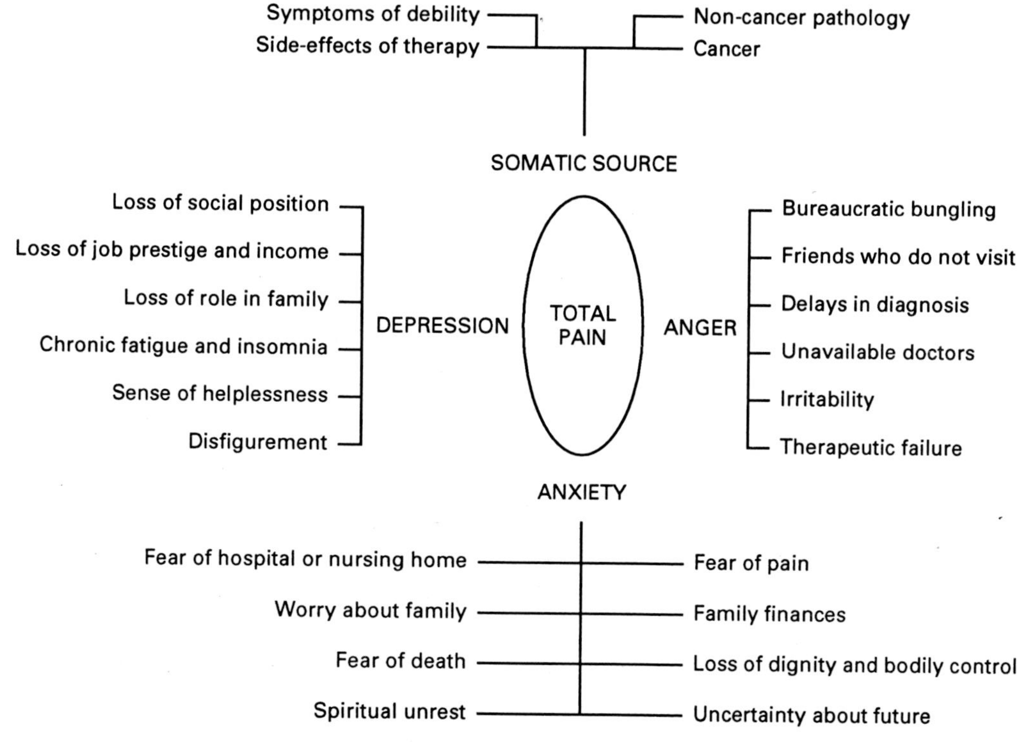

Fig. 76.1

Typically seven main strategies may be utilized to provide this direct or indirect therapy of painful bone metastases: (1) non-narcotic analgesics; (2) narcotic analgesics; (3) non-steroidal anti-inflammatory drugs; (4) hormone therapy; (5) chemotherapy; (6) local field external beam radiotherapy; (7) wide field external beam therapy.

An eighth treatment strategy should be added; the systemic administration of bone seeking radiopharmaceuticals. Although the use of these compounds was first reported almost 50 years ago, their role in the comprehensive management of cancer patients has not gained wide acceptance, despite the considerable use of phosphorus-32 in the 1960s and 1970s.[13–15]

The reasons for the lack of acceptance are complex, and include limited clinical trial data, narrow experience of their use within the clinical community, concerns about radiation safety and toxicity, cost and an imperfect understanding of optimum dosage schedules.

There is now, however, a wide body of literature on a number of current and potential radiopharmaceuticals which supports the use of these compounds as an effective – and cost effective – approach to pain palliation.[16]

PAINFUL BONE METASTASES

Bone metastases are most common in patients with primary carcinomas of the breast, prostate and lung, where autopsy evidence suggests up to 85% of patients have cancer metastatic to bone. Almost any cancer may metastasize to bone; cancers of the kidney, thyroid, cervix, bladder and gastrointestinal tract account for approximately 15–20% of the patient population presenting with bone metastases. Bone pain may be a significant symptom in up to 50% of the most common cancers and up to 5% in patients with gastrointestinal neoplasms.[6,17,18]

The development of bone metastases is a complex process whereby populations of cells with metastatic potential spread, usually haematogenously, to bone where a series of interrelated steps occur leading to arrest of the cells in the bone marrow, extravasation of tumour cells, invasion of bone and bone destruction and remodelling.[19] Direct invasion of bone may occur, particularly in pelvic and oropharyngeal cancers; cancers of the breast and lung may also invade the thoracic cage adjacent to the primary tumour.

Most metastases are associated with bones with a high proportion of red marrow; the most common sites are in the axial skeleton and include the vertebral bodies, pelvis and ribs, followed by the sternum, skull, femora, humeri and scapulae. Bone metastases are usually multiple; solitary lesions are most likely to be seen in patients with renal cell carcinoma or neuroblastoma.[12,20,21] At the time of presentation with pain it is likely that the patient will have multiple sites.

The radiographic appearance of bone metastases may be either lytic or blastic. This reflects, but does not exactly mirror, the local effects of bone metastases which may be those of bone destruction (osteolysis) or increased bone formation (osteosclerosis); both effects may occur simultaneously.[22–24] Most primary cancers produce a mixed pattern, although osteolysis is predominant. Osteolytic metastases are only seen in patients with myeloma, and prostate cancer usually produces sclerotic metastases.[20]

Bone destruction is mediated by osteoclasts stimulated by osteoclast stimulating factors produced in the tumour–bone environment.[23–25] The predominant factors are believed to be prostaglandins. The mechanisms of pain production in bone metastases include (1) stimulation of nerve endings by prostaglandins, kinins, substance P or histamine released by the osteolytic process; (2) periosteal stretching; (3) pathological fractures; and (4) local invasions.[12] Strategies to control pain must include each of these considerations.

BACKGROUND TO PAIN PALLIATION

Although the use of systemic radiotherapy to palliate pain was first reported in 1941, it was not until the 1980s that the exciting potential of this form of therapy was fully recognized and that well-constructed trials were instituted.

In addition to the radiopharmaceuticals reported before 1980, a number of new compounds have been described which have entered clinical trials. Two radiopharmaceuticals are now licensed in most countries, strontium-89 and phosphorus-32 orthophosphate, and two are in phase II and phase III trials – rhenium-186 HEDP and samarium-153 EDTMP.

These additions to the palliative armamentarium require major changes in the traditional ways in which most areas of nuclear medicine have been practised. Nuclear medicine practitioners utilizing these new radiopharmaceuticals must recognize that they are entering into a commitment to long-term patient care, to a collaborative relationship with referring physicians and to the long-term development of assessment and clinical trial methodology.

This chapter will address the problems of pain palliation in patients with cancer metastatic to bone, techniques available for pain palliation,[26] available radiopharmaceuticals and strategies for the clinical use of these compounds.

PALLIATIVE THERAPIES

The two main strategies of palliating this large group of patients remain radiotherapy and the graduated use of analgesics, both non-narcotic and narcotic. There are, in addition, a number of other treatments which have been utilized, with varying degrees of success (Table. 76.1).[12]

Table 76.1 Palliative treatment in patients with cancer metastatic to bone

Local field radiotherapy
Wide field radiotherapy
Non-narcotic analgesics
NSAIDS
Narcotic analgesics
Hormone therapy
Chemotherapy
Surgery
Interventional anaesthetic techniques
Unsealed source isotope therapy

Radiotherapy

Ionizing radiation was first reported as an effective palliative therapy within months of Roentgen's first description[27] and many reports of efficacy were available for review in 1933.[28] Subsequently, a very large body of literature has described remarkably consistent efficacy,[29] although there have been few prospective or placebo controlled trials.

Local radiotherapy has been shown to be effective in both retrospective and prospective trials,[29–40] with relief having been reported to have occurred in 80–100% of patients (Table 76.2). There is no consensus as to the most effective treatment regime;[41] the RTOG randomized trial comparing schedules of 800 cGy in one fraction; 2000 cGy in five fractions and 3000 cGy in 10 fractions gave equal response rates.[30] Reanalysis of the data[42] did suggest, however, that patients receiving the higher fractionated doses had better complete response rates. Local therapy is effective in patients with both solitary and multiple metastases and is also used as either primary or adjuvant therapy in the treatment of patients with (impending) pathological fractures[17,43,44] or spinal cord compression.[45–47]

In patients with multiple sites of pain, wide field radiotherapy has been advocated as an effective palliative treatment, either administered as upper or lower hemibody therapy, or as sequential hemibody therapy.[48–53] Typically 6–7 Gy are given as a single fraction to the upper half and 7–8 Gy to the lower half with a 2–4 week delay between the two treatments.[50,54] Partial relief of pain has been reported in 55–100% of patients; a lower percentage (5–50%) report complete palliative efficacy.

Toxicity in local field irradiation is minimal; in wide field radiation therapy toxicity may include thrombocytopenia, gastrointestinal symptoms and pneumonitis. These adverse effects have been reported in 2–32% of patients.[52]

Pain relief following external beam radiotherapy typically occurs within 48 h of treatment,[41,52] although it may, rarely, be delayed for up to 2 weeks. The duration of response is variable; most patients will have a meaningful response for at least 4 weeks and of these 39–48% still have effective relief at 24 weeks.[32] Figures for response rates in wide field radiotherapy are lower, although onset of relief is usual at 2 days. However, a good response may persist for up to 50% of the patient's remaining life.

Hormone therapy

Prostate and breast cancer are the two neoplasms with a propensity for metastatic spread to bone in which hormone manipulation has been shown to be effective as palliative therapy.[55,56] In metastatic breast cancer the therapeutic options include tamoxifen, aminoglutethimide and castration. Response is seen more commonly in oestrogen receptor positive patients, where about 50% of patients will show meaningful palliation.[17,57]

A wide range of therapeutic options is available for patients with prostate cancer, including castration, oestrogens, anti-androgens and total androgen blockage. Pain relief in this group of patients after initiation of therapy is often rapid and dramatic with responses commonly reported at 24 h.[55,57,58]

'Flare' responses may occur in up to 30% of patients. The duration of response after hormone therapy may be prolonged (median of 12 months)[57] but eventual relapse with recurrent pain is the rule. Once first line hormone therapy has failed, second line treatment is unlikely to give response rates above 30%.

Table 76.2 Reported frequency of pain relief after local radiotherapy for bone metastases – data from prospective studies

Author	Reference	Patients treated	Dose (Gy)	No. of fractions	Days	Overall + %	Complete + %
Tong	30	72	20	5	5	90	53
		74	40.5	15	19	92	61
		613	15–30	5–10	5–12	89	53
Madsen	31	27	20	2	8	48	–
		30	24	6	18	47	–
Price	32	140	8	1	1	85	27
		148	30	10	12	85	27
Price	33	21	4	1	1	43	5
Cole	34	16	8	1	1	100	–
		13	24	6	15	100	–

Data from Bates[41]

Chemotherapy

Effective palliation of pain to single or combination drug regimes is seen in most cancers metastatic to bone except prostate.[17,59,60] Response rates of 20–80% have been reported, with rates varying significantly between cancers.[12] Responses are usually seen within 2 weeks of commencing treatment and may be sustained for up to several months. Toxicity is related to the combination of chemotherapy agents used and most commonly include nausea and vomiting and myelosuppression.

Analgesics

Analgesic therapy is the mainstay of treatment for patients with painful bone metastases. The World Health Organization (WHO)[61] has developed a strategy which utilizes a graduated approach to the introduction of analgesics, starting with NSAIDS and then proceeding to 'weak' opioids and 'strong' opioids, in combination, if necessary, with NSAIDS and non-narcotic analgesics.[62]

Using this graduated approach most patients' symptoms can be controlled. The WHO recommends that a single opioid be titrated to give satisfactory pain relief and administered on a round-the-clock basis; 'break-through' medication may be administered on a pro rata basis. All treatment plans should be made with a clear understanding of the pharmacology of the opioid being used, particularly where continuous infusion techniques are required.[63] Using this regimen, either by using increasing doses or by changing medication, pain relief can be sustained in most patients. Side-effects are common and may include drowsiness, mood changes and constipation; careful attention to prescribing practice is required to minimize these effects.

RADIONUCLIDE THERAPY FOR PAINFUL BONE METASTASES

Background

Phosphorus-30 was the first radioactive isotope artificially produced in 1933.[64] Phosphorus-32 was described in 1932 and produced in significant quantities in 1934.[65,66] The bone seeking qualities of strontium were first described by Stoeltzner in 1874.[67] Strontium-89, a long lived radioactive isotope of strontium was first described in 1937.[68] Within 5 years of discovery of the radioactive isotopes of each of these compounds, they had both been used in clinical studies evaluating therapeutic efficacy as palliative treatments in metastatic cancer and as primary therapy in leukaemia and multiple myeloma.[68,69]

For the next 4 decades these were effectively the only compounds available for unsealed source therapy, being used intermittently over those years at a time when clinical trial methodology was imperfectly developed.

Subsequent to the 1970s, several new compounds have been postulated as alternative therapies (Table 76.3). All these compounds offer some theoretical advantages in the planning of palliative therapy. However, there are four important compounds which appear to have early indications of clinical relevance and which are in various stages of clinical development.[16,70]

Several authors have attempted to define the physical characteristics of the 'ideal' radiopharmaceutical for palliative therapy.[16,71,72] The basic principles underlying the use of any form of unsealed source treatment regime are that the absorbed dose to metastatic sites should offer a significant therapeutic advantage when compared with the absorbed dose to normal tissues. In addition, the treatment should be cost effective, easy to administer, should not pose an external radiation protection problem and should localize in all sites of skeletal metastatic disease (Table 76.4).

All the compounds currently in clinical trials fulfil these criteria with some degree of imperfection; this will be discussed in the following sections.

The absorbed dose to bone metastases is a function of the energy deposited within the tumour, which may be defined by parameters such as concentration of radiopharmaceutical at the tumour site, retention time and beta particle energy.[72–74] Parameters such as dose rate may also be important, but the radiobiology of very low dose

Table 76.3 Radiopharmaceuticals for palliative therapy

Radionuclide	Pharmaceutical	Half-life (days)	Max beta energy MeV	Mean beta energy MeV	Maximum range in tissue mm (max)	Maximum range in tissue mm (HV)	Gamma-photon keV (%)
Sr-89	Chloride	50.5	1.46	0.58	6.7	0.63	0
P-32	Orthophosphate	14.3	1.71	0.69	8.0	0.76	0
I-131	Diphosphonate	8.0	0.61	0.19	2.4	0.23	365 (81)
Re-186	Phosphonate	3.8	1.07	0.36	4.7	0.44	137 (9)
Re-188	Phosphonate	0.7	2.12	0.73	10.2	0.97	155 (10)
Sm-153	Chelate	1.95	0.8	0.23	3.4	0.32	103 (28)
Y-90	Citrate	2.7	2.27	0.93	11.0	1.04	0
Sn-117m	Chelate	13.6	IT				159 (86)

Table 76.4 Characteristics of an 'ideal' radiopharmaceutical for palliative therapy in patients with bone metastases

Selective retention in bone
Rapid soft tissue clearance
Selective uptake at metastatic sites relative to normal bone
Cost effective
Stable and easy to transport
Simple production process
$T_p > T_B$
E max > 0.8 MeV and < 2.0 MeV
Distribution should be predicted from bone images

rate (VLDR) radiation therapy is ill understood[75,76] and the importance of dose rate in palliative therapy at the ranges of VLDR therapy have not been tested clinically or in animal models. Current calculations of dose administered with any of the four radiopharmaceuticals are less than would be predicted to be effective using the high dose rate model of external beam radiotherapy. This anomaly reflects the limited understanding of VLDR radiobiology, the imprecision of dosimetry calculations and a less than clear understanding of optimum dosage schedules. It is still not apparent, for example, whether strontium-89 is best administered as a single, large dose or as smaller, fractionated dose over a 6–9 month period. In parallel with progress in developing clinical trial methodology for unsealed source therapy is a requirement to develop experimental in vitro techniques to understand VLDR radiobiology.

Several authors[13,70,77] have stressed the desirability of an imageable gamma-photon for these compounds, pointing to the value of imaging the biodistribution of the compound on a population by population and patient by patient basis and of the role of the imageable photon in assessing dosimetry. However, the gamma-ray does cause radiation protection problems, and may lead to requirements for admission.

It is our contention[13] that the imageable photon is not an essential requirement for these compounds. In all cases the distribution of the radiopharmaceutical is accurately predicted by ^{99m}Tc-MDP bone imaging, a simple routine procedure. By the time the radiopharmaceutical is available for use in phase III clinical trials or routine practice the biodistribution and whole body dosimetry studies will have been performed using tracer methodology (available for all isotopes but ^{32}P) and pharmacokinetic modelling. There will be, therefore, no requirement for the routine availability of imaging in the clinic. Tracer methodology is available for those centres wishing to develop tumour dosimetric techniques.

The most important factor in the development of these therapeutic agents is the conduct of well-designed, carefully controlled clinical trials that conform to standard cooperative group methodology such as that of the Radiation Therapy Oncology Group or Eastern Cooperative Oncology Group and which measure response by accepted testing methodologies.[65,78]

Phosphorus-32

Physical characteristics

Phosphorus-32 is a radioisotope of phosphorus which decays by beta emission, with a half-life of 14.3 days. For palliative therapy ^{32}P is now supplied as the orthophosphate, provided in a sterile non-pyrogenic solution with a concentration of 25 MBq per µl of NaH_2PO_4. Historically ^{32}P has not only been administered as orthophosphate but also polymetaphosphate, HEDP and pyrophosphate.[79–82]

Biodistribution and dosimetry

Phosphate is widely distributed in the body, contributing particularly to energy metabolism and to neuromuscular function, haematopoiesis and bone metabolism. The skeletal system is the largest phosphate pool in the body, comprising approximately 85% of the total pool. Within bone phosphorus is bound, as inorganic phosphate, to the hydroxyapatite matrix and turns over slowly. Within soft tissue and in the bone marrow phosphate distribution is predominantly intracellular, where it is found in the nucleus and cytoplasm. Excretion is predominantly by the renal route, although some faecal excretion does occur.[65,83–88]

Dosimetry estimates for ^{32}P therapy have been reported at intervals since 1950 (Table 76.5). The data have utilized physiological assumptions of ^{32}P skeletal distribution,[89–91] animal biodistribution studies,[92,93] and in vivo Bremsstrahlung imaging to calculate the uptake and retention data required for dosimetry modelling. In addition, Potsaid and coworkers[99] have assessed skeletal and bone marrow dosimetry of ^{32}P-HEDP in a series of five patients with metastatic prostate cancer. Using pharmacokinetic data obtained from these five patients and historical human and animal biodistribution data,[81,69–99] they presented data for bone to bone and bone to bone marrow doses as follows: cortical bone to bone 38 rad/mCi; trabecular bone to bone marrow 62 rad/mCi; bone marrow to bone marrow 19 rad/mCi.

Table 76.5 Skeletal dosimetry estimates for ^{32}P

Author	Date	Reference	Absorbed dose estimate (rads/mCi)	Notes
Friedell	1950	89	25	Assume 33% ^{32}P retained in bone
Low-Beer	1952	92	52	Whole body retention data
Seltzer	1964	90	30	Assume bone uptake; T_B 19 days
Mays	1973	94	15	T_E 14.1 days
Spiers	1976	93	63	Direct bone assay
Kereiakes	1980	95	63	
ICRP 52	1988	91	41	Assumes 30% bone uptake

The range of skeletal absorbed doses reported (25–63 rad/mCi) reflects the difficulty of calculation encountered. No direct measurement of uptake at metastatic sites has been reported, although animal and human biodistribution data suggest therapeutic ratios ranging from 1 to 10. Moreover, the target organ for toxicity – the bone marrow – appears to receive a relatively high dose in relationship to dose to metastases with contributions from both inorganic matrix uptake and uptake in the cellular compartment of the bone marrow space.[65,99,100]

In view of the difficulties of in vivo localization of ^{32}P, Wallace and Ross have described a technique for labelling radiophosphorus with technetium-99m which they have postulated as a possible in vivo tracer of ^{32}P metabolism. No dosimetric data were available from this study.[101]

Clinical use of phosphorus-32

Increased ^{32}P retention in myeloproliferative disorders was reported several times between 1939 and 1941,[102–106] and by 1945 there were 10 clinical reports of ^{32}P therapy, predominantly in haematological malignancies but also in patients with bone metastases. In 1946, Reinhard was able to publish a literature review which included the treatment results in 155 patients.[85] The potential of the compound for palliative therapy was recognized at this time; other than in the treatment of polycythaemia rubra vera, no efficacy in haematological malignancies was seen.

Friedell & Storaasli[89] first reported significant palliative efficacy in 10 patients with breast cancer metastatic to bone (83% response). The ^{32}P was administered at a dose of 2 mCi every 5 days – the average administered dose was 18.2 mCi over 40 days. In 1958, Maxfield reported a series of 158 patients treated with ^{32}P and testosterone with an overall 92% response rate.[107] The use of testosterone was based on data[108] suggesting that androgen stimulation increased uptake of phosphate by bone; this study demonstrated that testosterone administration increased the therapeutic ratio, with a 15–20 fold increase of ^{32}P uptake at sites of metastatic disease.

The extensive literature on the use of ^{32}P in the palliation of patients with cancer metastatic to bone has recently been reviewed by Silberstein et al[65] and by Montebello & Hartson-Eaton.[100] Table 76.6 is a synthesis of these and other data which summarizes the published literature on the efficacy of ^{32}P.[79,80,89,107,109–135]

Phosphorus-32 has been used as an individual agent in a variety of different dosage schedules. Typically between 8 and 20 mCi have been administered, in fractionated schedules over 7–40 days, although single doses of as low as 3 mCi have been used. In addition, adjunct treatment with testosterone and parathormone have been suggested as ways of potentiating therapeutic efficacy.

Based upon these initial results many reports appeared confirming efficacy of ^{32}P and testosterone; however, only one study[110] directly compared ^{32}P with ^{32}P and testosterone; in this study a difference in subjective response was seen – 50% for ^{32}P and 86% for ^{32}P and testosterone, although patient numbers were small. Androgen therapy, however, has a direct effect on hormone sensitive tumours and administration is not without potential adverse effects. Corwin reported increase in pain in the group treated with testosterone, whilst Fowler & Whitmore[109,110] noted subjective or objective adverse events in 87% of patients whom they treated; in 15% these adverse events were described as 'irreversible'. In addition, they reviewed 138 patients in the literature and found unfavourable responses in 93% with 7% showing serious morbidity.

In spite of the single report by Corwin, the literature does not support any additional clinical advantage to the concomitant administration of testosterone.[65,100]

Parathormone (PTH) has also been used as adjunct therapy to the administration of ^{32}P.[111] The rationale for the use of PTH is the mobilization of calcium and phosphate in bone associated with an increase in urinary excretion of phosphate. The combination of these two physiological effects is an increased absorption of ^{32}P in bone. Results of the use of these strategies is mixed and there is no convincing rationale for improved efficacy in patients treated with PTH.

This data review suggests that there is no meaningful difference in reported response rates between the three regimens. The response rates ranged from 20 to 100% with most series reporting response rates between 70% and 90%. Responses were reported as occurring between 5 and 14 days after injection and as being sustained for up to 6 months, although the average duration of response appears to have been between 2 and 4 months.

However, the series reviewed in Table 76.6 is notable for the absence of coherent clinical trial design. Virtually all studies used different dosing schedules for both the ^{32}P and the adjunct treatments; there are no consistent or quantitative evaluations of response and no consistent reporting format for either duration or quality of response. In addition, all reports have been based on retrospective reviews and no placebo controlled trials have been undertaken. Predominantly the trials reported treatments in patients with metastatic prostate and breast cancers; no meaningful differences in response rates between the two cancers were evident. Clinical improvement did not show any evidence of a dose–response effect.

Toxicity

Treatment toxicity is primarily reported as being related to myelosuppression; pancytopenia, thrombocytopenia and leukopenia were the most commonly reported toxicities. The nadir was usually reached by 5–6 weeks after injection with recovery being seen maximally at 2–3 months. Two deaths were reported in the series, both occurring at

Table 76.6 Reports of phosphorus-32 therapy in patients with cancer metastatic to bone

Author	Year	Reference	Patients treated	Patients responding	% responding	Adjunct therapy	Administered activity (mCi)
Friedell	1950	89	12	10	83	0	18.2 F
Kaplan	1960	79	8	7	87.5	0	20 F
Corwin	1970	110	8	4	50	0	16 F
Potsaid	1976	99	5	1	20	0	3–9 F
Werner	1980	80	8	7	87.5	0	10–12 S
Maxfield	1958	107	158	145	92	T	7–20 F
Vermooten	1959	113	27	20	75	T	7–20 F
Wildermuth	1960	114	5	4	80	T	8–20 F
Parson	1962	115	10	10	100	T	12.6 F po
Mandel	1962	116	14	11	79	T	9–14 F
Smart	1965	117	9	8	89	T	8.7 F
Walton	1965	118	53	39	73.5	T	9–15 F
Joshi	1965	119	13	13	100	T	12–15 F IV or po
Donati	1966	120	12	11	92	T	12.6 F IV or po
Morin	1967	121	6	6	100	T	5–7 S
Morales	1970	112	13	11	85	T	10.5 F
Corwin	1970	110	14	12	86	T	7–16 S or F
Hilts	1972	123	5	5	100	T	12 F
Edland	1974	124	42	36	86	T	9–10.5 F
Roberts	1979	125	46	34	74	T	10.5 F
Riva	1983	126	87	59	68	T	4–24 F
Ariel	1985	127	30	22	73	T	10 F
Aziz	1986	128	15	12	80	T	10–12 F
Burnet	1990	129	46	40	87	T	12 F
Tong	1967	111	8	6	75	P	5–20 F
Tong	1973	130	15	15	100	P	21 F
Pinck	1973	131	32	22	69	P	20 F
Merrin	1974	132	8	7	88	P	10 S
Johnson	1977	133	33	18	55	P	12 F
Cheung	1980	134	48	31	65	P, T	9–18 F
Glaser	1981	135	24	14	58	P, T	12 F
Sub total-0			41	29	71	0	
Sub total-T			605	498	82	T	
Sub total-P			168	113	67	P	
Total			814	640	79.2	0,P,T	

Notes: 0 = no adjunct therapy
T = testosterone
P = parathormone
F = fractionated dosing
S = single dosing

approximately the nadir,[134,136] and both as probably due to pancytopenia.

In addition, many series reported the occurrence of cord compression; however, this historical comparison, whilst incomplete, does not appear to suggest an incidence that is greater than would be predicted in this patient population.

Two studies[100,128] have compared the efficacy of ^{32}P therapy and hemibody radiotherapy. Both had comparable rates of efficacy. Toxicity was probably reduced in the ^{32}P group. These, however, are based on historical data; no direct comparison of the two modalities has been performed.

Summary

Most series reporting the efficacy of phosphorus-32 have used orthophosphate as carrier, although several other carriers have been evaluated. The main criticisms of the reports have been concisely stated by Silberstein et al,[65] who have stressed the absence of trial methodology.

However, response rates of the order of 70–80% appear to be valid and toxicity, although consistently reported and often severe, has rarely been life threatening. ^{32}P remains one of two compounds currently licensed.

Samarium-153 – ethylenediaminetetramethylene phosphonate (EDTMP)

Physical characteristics

Goeckeler et al first reported the synthesis of a series of ^{153}Sm complexes in 1987,[137] of which EDTMP was regarded as demonstrating the optimum combination of high bone uptake, rapid blood clearance and low soft tissue retention. This compound was subsequently developed as a potential therapeutic agent for assessment in animal and human studies.

Samarium-153 is a reactor produced radioisotope by neutron irradiation of samarium-152. Samarium-153 has a complex decay scheme, with a principal β_{max} energy of 0.81 MeV. It also emits a gamma-photon of 103 keV.[138,139] (Table 76.3)

When complexed with EDTMP it produces a stable complex with a labelling efficiency of greater than 90%.

Biodistribution and dosimetry

Biodistribution has been studied in rabbits, rats and dogs. Within 3 h most of the administered dose is localized in the skeleton, with less than 2% in soft tissue. Excretion is predominantly by the renal route. Distribution is comparable to that seen with ^{99m}Tc-MDP.[137]

Singh et al,[140] in a series of human biodistribution studies, have shown increased uptake at the site of metastatic lesions, with lesion to bone, bone to soft tissue and lesion to soft tissue being shown, respectively to be 4.04, 2.47 and 5.98.

Based on available biodistribution data, Logan et al, Heggie, and Eary et al[77,141,142] have calculated human dosimetry for this compound, confirming the marrow as the dose limiting organ (Table 76.7). Logan has estimated the whole body dose at 0.044 rad/mCi.

Clinical data

Initial reports of potential efficacy were reported in a dog population with spontaneous osteosarcoma. In two parallel studies, one was a dose escalation study of single and multiple doses of ^{153}Sm-EDTMP in normal dogs,[143] using haematological toxicity as an end point. Myelosuppression was seen in all dogs, with a dose response being evident. In the second study 40 dogs with spontaneous osteosarcoma were treated with either one single dose of 1 mCi or two doses administered one week apart.[144]

The results of this latter study showed seven dogs in complete remission, 25 with a partial remission and eight with no response. Small lesions were shown to respond better than large, an expected finding. Severe myelosuppression was noted with the fractionated treatment, although recovery, albeit incomplete, was usual.

Based partly on these preliminary data a series of phase I and II human trials have been undertaken (Table 76.8).

Phase I studies by Eary et al[145] and Turner et al[146] have used a dose schedule of up to 4.5 mCi/kg, giving total administered doses of up to 299 mCi. In both these series reversible myelosuppression was seen which was dose related. In phase II studies Turner & Claringbold[147,148] and Sandeman et al[149] both used marrow absorbed dose as the defining parameter by which administered dose was calculated, Turner & Claringbold giving up to 2 Gy and Sandeman et al up to 3 Gy.

Reversible myelosuppression was again reported, although Sandeman et al attribute two toxic deaths to thrombocytopenia.[150]

Responses typically were seen within 2 weeks of administration and were sustained for between 4 and 40 weeks, although Turner & Claringbold report 8 weeks as being the average. All authors report successful retreatment in selected patients.

Response rates of the order of 60–80% again seem predictable, similar to those reported in the ^{32}P trials, although a more coherent strategy of assessing response has been adopted. No placebo controlled trial of the efficacy of ^{153}Sm-EDTMP has been performed.

Table 76.7 Dosimetry estimates for ^{153}Sm EDTMP

		(Max) Absorbed dose (rads/mCi)			
Author	Reference	Bone	Marrow	Kidney	Bladder
Logan	77	11.28	3.82	0.4	4.55
Heggie	141	8.6	6.9		
Eary	142	25	5.7	0.65	3.6

Rhenium-186 etidronate (HEDP)

Physical characteristics

Etidronate is a diphosphonate which is presently in clinical trials as a palliative pharmaceutical in patients

Table 76.8 Review of ^{153}Sm EDTMP as palliative therapy for painful bone metastases

Author	Year	Reference	Patients treated	Patients responding	% Responding	Administered activity (mCi/Kg)
Turner	1989	148	19	15	79	
Turner	1989	146	34	22	65	0.28–0.48
Turner	1991	147	23	14	61	2 Gy MD
Sandeman	1992	149	14	7	50	1.5–3 Gy MD
Eary	1990	145	20	18	90	53–299 mCi

Note: MD = marrow dose

with cancer metastatic to bone, in addition to its possible clinical indication in the routine management of osteoporosis.

A discussion of the potential of ^{186}Re-HEDP as a possible therapeutic agent was published in 1979;[150] subsequently, descriptions of the chemical synthesis of the compound, and formulation of preparations for human use, were reported.[151–153] Technetium and rhenium are both Group VII metals.[139] Rhenium-186 decays with the emission of a beta particle, maximum energy 1.07 MeV; a low abundance (9.5%) gamma-ray is also produced in the decay (Table 76.3). ^{186}Re-HEDP and ^{99m}Tc-HEDP both show high in vitro stability and show high bone to soft tissue ratios and rapid blood clearance.

Biodistribution and dosimetry

Animal biodistribution studies have confirmed high uptake and retention in bone, with up to 14% of the injected dose remaining in the skeleton 96 h after injection. There is rapid urinary excretion with 43% of injected dose at 1 h and 70% at 6 h being found in the urine.[154]

Human biodistribution data confirms animal data. In patients with bone metastases, 21–38% of the injected dose is retained in the skeleton at 3 h after injection.[77] These data have been confirmed by de Klerk et al.[155]

Maxon et al have calculated dosimetry in patients with bone metastases (two breast, three prostate, one thyroid).[156] Mean doses to bone, marrow, tumour, kidney and bladder wall were, respectively, 3.2, 2.8, 41, 4.1 and 1.8 rad/mCi. An important component of these data has been the development of fixed and variable models of bone uptake and retention which this group are currently utilizing to build a microdosimetric model of bone therapy with systemic radionuclides. This approach to dosimetry calculations appears to offer a real opportunity to improve our ability to assess dose response and predictors of response.

Clinical trials

In 1991 Maxon published the results of a double blind cross-over placebo controlled trial of the efficacy of ^{186}Re-HEDP.[157] Thirteen evaluable patients with bone metastases were randomized to receive either ^{186}Re-HEDP or placebo (^{99m}Tc-MDP) and followed for 12 weeks; a cross-over injection at 4 weeks occurred if the patient failed to respond. This study confirmed the efficacy of the active compound when compared with placebo, and is one of only two appropriately controlled trials in the unsealed source literature.

The same group have also reported the efficacy of ^{186}Re-HEDP in a series of 20 patients administered as a single dose of 33 mCi.[158] Relief was reported in 80% of patients, usually occurring by 2 weeks and sustained for 7–8 weeks after injection. Doses to metastatic lesions were estimated at about 2600 rads.

Zonnenberg et al demonstrated comparable efficacy (90%) in a group of 10 patients with metastatic breast and prostate cancer, with a mean duration of response of 5 weeks (range 1–10 weeks).[159] Repeat treatments have also been shown to be safe and effective.[160]

Phase II and III trials are now underway in North America and in Europe to confirm the efficacy and define clinical utility of this compound. Radiation protection problems may be seen in some jurisdictions, but the lower doses administered when compared with ^{153}Sm-EDTMP suggest that these will be limited.

Strontium-89

Physical characteristics

Strontium-89 is a pure beta-emitting isotope of strontium with a max beta particle energy of 1.46 MeV, which was first used in clinical practice by Pecher,[68] who reported palliative efficacy in bone metastases (Table 76.3). Although strontium-89 does not decay with the emission of a gamma-photon, strontium-85 does decay with the emission of a 514 keV gamma-photon which has been used in tracer studies to assess biodistribution and dosimetry. Strontium-89 is administered as strontium chloride and is now licensed in most jurisdictions. It is delivered in vials containing 4 mCi ^{89}Sr. Excretion is mainly by the renal route, with physiological handling of ^{89}Sr mimicking that of calcium.[161] The strontium is incorporated into the inorganic matrix, with uptake being increased at sites of metastatic tumour.

Initial data on strontium kinetics and dosimetry in volunteers were published by the ICRP.[162] Subsequently, Blake and coworkers have completed a detailed series of biodistribution and dosimetry estimates in patients with prostate cancer metastatic to bone.[163–169] Whole-body retention of the radiopharmaceutical was shown to reflect metastatic burden; at 90 days post-injection the retention varied between 11% and 88% of injected dose depending upon the extent of metastatic disease. Normal bone turnover was more rapid, with a lesion to normal bone ratio of approximately 10:1.

Calculated dose to individual metastases varied between 380 and 2262 rad/mCi.[167] Marrow doses were typically one tenth of doses to metastatic sites. The same group have also assessed the effects of renal plasma clearance of strontium on retention and have shown a complex relationship between this parameter and metastatic burden in defining whole-body retention.

Breen et al have also performed dosimetric studies, showing broadly comparable doses to both normal bone and to metastatic sites.[170]

Clinical experience

Eighteen papers (Table 76.9)[171–188] have described clinical response rates in patients with cancer metastatic to bone. These have mostly described experience in patients with prostate and breast cancer, although several authors have shown, possibly impaired, efficacy in patients with other cancers.[173,175,176,179,187] Before the mid-1980s the data may be criticized for lack of coherent trial design, for ill-defined response criteria, and for inconsistent dosing schedules.

However, since the data of Robinson et al[184] and Laing et al[186] a standard dose of 4 mCi has been developed, with the ability to retreat after 3 months using the same activity. There has also been a significant improvement in trial design[161] and conformity to standard reporting practice, for example using RTOG criteria for response and toxicity.

Responses in patients with breast and prostate cancer have typically occurred within 2 weeks of injection and have been sustained for 3–6 months. About one-third of responders become pain free. Retreatment is safe[161] and likely to be effective if palliation was achieved with the first dose.

Toxicity is limited to myelosuppression, usually thrombocytopenia. This is usually mild, with less than 2% of the toxic events reported appearing to involve falls in platelet count below 50 000. Recovery is usual, although not necessary to baseline levels. McEwan et al[185] have demonstrated the safety of the technique in patients with a prior history of extensive irradiation.

No dose response has been observed, although the data of Laing suggest that doses of below 30 μCi/kg are ineffective.

One double blind cross-over placebo controlled trial has been reported[189] in which 32 patients were randomized to receive either strontium-89 spiked with strontium-85 or stable strontium spiked with strontium-85. Assessment and cross-over occurred at 6 weeks. Twenty-six patients were evaluable, demonstrating a significant advantage to strontium-89 therapy.

With the confirmation of palliative efficacy in this large reported series, several groups have attempted to define the clinical role of this radiopharmaceutical further. Porter[190,191] published the results of a series of 126 patients randomized to receive 10.8 mCi of strontium-89 or placebo at time of first radiotherapy requirements. Significant improvements in quality of life, pain scores, analgesic scores, time to new sites of pain, future radiotherapy requirements, and falls in PSA and alkaline phosphatase were shown in this group of advanced prostate cancer patients. The data appear to suggest the ability of strontium-89 to modify the progression of metastatic disease, which may lead to the development of strategies for the adjuvant use of strontium-89 earlier in the progress of the disease.

McEwan et al have performed a cost benefit study of a subset of these patients demonstrating that cost savings were accrued by the active group in terms of radiotherapy, drug costs and tertiary hospital stay costs.[192]

Dearnaly et al[187] have compared historical, matched data comparing the efficacy of ^{89}Sr with hemibody irradiation. Comparable response rates between the two groups were seen, implying the comparable efficacy of a systemically administered radiopharmaceutical to standard hemibody techniques. These data appear to be confirmed by the study of Kirk et al who showed ^{89}Sr to be as effective as hemibody radiotherapy and possibly more effective than local field radiotherapy.[193]

Table 76.9 Review of strontium-89 as palliative therapy for painful bone metastases

Author	Year	Reference	Patients treated	Patients responding	% Responding	Administered activity
*Schmidt	1974	171	10	8	80	10–20 μCi
*Firusian	1976	172	11	8	73	30 μCi/kg
Kutzner	1978	173	15	12	80	0.8–2.7 μCi
*Firusian	1978	174	43	33	77	15–30 μCi/kg
Hayek	1980	175	17	7	42	1–2 mCi
Correns	1979	176	12	8	67	1–2 mCi
Kimmig	1983	177	12	11	90	3 mCi
Buchali	1983	178	70	60	86	1 mCi
Silberstein	1985	179	45	23	51	1–4.5 mCi
†Reddy	1986	180	47	43	91	30–40 μCi/kg
Kloiber	1987	181	10	5	50	10–60 μCi/kg
†Robinson	1987	182	109	81	74	30–40 μCi/kg
Tennvall	1988	183	11	5	45	3–6 mCi F
Buchali	1988	184	21	14	67	3 × 2 mCi F
McEwan	1990	185	26	20	77	40 μCi/kg
Laing	1991	186	83	62	75	30–60 μCi/kg
Fossa	1992	187	23	11	48	4 mCi
Dearnaly	1992	188	24	23	96	30–60 μCi/kg
Total			589	434	70.5	

Note: * and † series include common patients.

Now that clinical efficacy has been established it is evident that the clinical community must develop effective strategies to ensure that this cost effective therapy is used in the most effective and appropriate settings.[194] Mertens[195] and Ackery & Yardley[196] have suggested possible strategies to enhance the effectiveness of strontium-89 by the use of radiosensitizers, chemotherapy agents, biological response modifiers, and simple physiological strategies.

Other radiopharmaceuticals

One other compound with potential therapeutic application has recently been described. Sn-117m(4+) DTPA (Table 76.3) is a bone seeking chelate which has been shown in animal[197,198] and human[199] studies to have high concentration in the body and rapid blood and soft tissue clearance. This isotope has a 13.6 day half-life and decays with emission of low energy conversion electrons with a short path length, possibly reducing potential marrow toxicity.

Preliminary clinical studies have indicated a bone dose of 200–300 rad/mCi and a marrow dose of 4–7 rad/mCi, suggesting a significant therapeutic ratio. The lesion to normal tissue ratio varied from 1 to 15. The authors advocate an administered dose of approximately 9 mCi. No efficacy or toxicity data are available, and future clinical trials are awaited with interest.

RADIATION SAFETY

Most jurisdictions require admission of patients administered with the doses of gamma-emitting isotopes discussed in this chapter, although for ^{153}Sm-EDTMP and ^{186}Re-HEDP this is unlikely to require more than an overnight stay. As beta-emitters, ^{32}P and ^{89}Sr do not require hospitalization.

All these radiopharmaceuticals are excreted in the urine and patients should be advised on appropriate hygiene and care. No additional special precautions are required. The beta-emitters are not a radiation hazard to hospital staff, family members or crematorium staff.[196]

OVERVIEW

Pain palliation is effectively provided by all forms of radiation therapy. It is interesting to note that all techniques give comparable response rates, with all series suggesting that between 70% and 90+% of patients will respond. Complete responses are typically seen in about 30% of responders.

External beam techniques have the advantage of a more rapid response time, whilst the unsealed source therapy agents, particularly strontium-89, may offer a more sustained response, particularly when compared with hemibody radiotherapy. In addition there is the opportunity for retreatment with the systemic therapy agents. The opportunity to treat, safely, multiple painful sites – and multiple silent sites – is a clear advantage to these latter agents.

Of the four compounds, strontium-89 has the most coherent database and the best developed clinical trial methodology to support clinical use. Responses for this compound appear to develop a little slower, but to be consistently more sustained than for the other three compounds. However, the data provided by the current phase II and III trials for ^{153}Sm-EDTMP and ^{186}Re-HEDP will give a clearer indication of their future clinical role. It might be that there will be an advantage in their relatively higher dose rate in less blastic metastases, whilst the long half-life and retention of strontium-89 will have advantages in the more blastic metastatic disease.

ROUTINE CLINICAL USE OF UNSEALED SOURCE THERAPY IN PAIN PALLIATION

The role of palliative therapy for advanced metastatic cancer is to improve the quality of remaining life and to help the patient and his or her family through the terminal stages of the disease. Prolongation of survival is an unlikely benefit; indeed, as the results of the Trans Canada study[190,191] show, increased survival is improbable in this population of patients.

With this palliative intent in mind, it is imperative that the physician involved in palliative unsealed source therapy be involved as early as possible in this phase of the patient's management, and that he or she be involved in the follow-up and further evaluation of the patient. The nuclear medicine physician must be aware of and be familiar with the clinical use of the other palliative modalities discussed earlier in this chapter. If there is to be appropriate use of the palliative radiopharmaceuticals, then that use must be in the widest possible context of the management of that patient. The role of external beam radiotherapy and opiate analgesics must be clearly understood, and isotope therapy instituted within the parameters of a well-defined treatment plan.

The greatest clinical experience is presently with strontium-89 and so the following comments will be related specifically to this radiopharmaceutical, although the general principles will apply to any of the four radiopharmaceuticals discussed in this chapter. Table 76.10 outlines relative contraindications for administration of strontium-89.

When a patient is referred for therapy, the initial clinical examination should assess painful sites, level of pain, analgesic requirements and quality of life. If clinical examination reveals the presence of an impending cord compression or pathological fracture, then strontium-89 is absolutely contraindicated; the patient should be referred for urgent radiotherapy opinion.

Table 76.10 Contraindications for the use of palliative unsealed source therapy

Impending pathological fracture
Impending cord compression
Solitary very painful metastatic site
Platelet count < 80 000
White cell count < 2.0
Concomitant chemotherapy
Projected survival of less than 2 months

A solitary, very painful, metastatic site is only a relative contraindication to strontium-89 therapy. This is an appropriate indication for single field external beam radiotherapy where pain relief will be more certain and will occur more rapidly. Based on the data of Porter et al[190] and Kirk et al[193] however, there may be an indication for the use of strontium-89 in an adjunct setting. The external beam irradiation may unmask other sites of pain, possibly in the short term, probably in the long term. These will eventually require additional radiotherapy and will certainly require increasing analgesic use. The evidence from these two studies suggests that time to new pain is increased and so it may well be appropriate under these circumstances to treat the patient with strontium-89 at the same time as radiation therapy is administered.

All forms of unsealed source therapy may cause myelosuppression, particularly in patients with compromised bone marrow. Patients with depressed platelets may develop symptomatic thrombocytopenia and should be treated only with extreme caution. The count nadir occurs at about 4–6 weeks, so close patient follow-up is crucial. For this reason it is not recommended that unsealed source therapy be given at the same time as, or immediately before, myelotoxic chemotherapy.

The patient most likely to benefit from strontium-89 therapy may be defined as a patient with prostate or breast cancer with several bone metastases and multiple flitting pains, particularly if poorly controlled by non-narcotic analgesics or NSAIDS. Survival should be projected to be at least 3 months. Outside these parameters there are no well-defined indicators as to which patient or patient associated symptoms are most likely to respond.

Studies with all four radiopharmaceuticals have shown efficacy with repeat administrations, particularly if the patient has responded to the first treatment. Treatment should be initiated as soon as significant pain recurrence is noted – toxicity can be predicted with a modest degree of certainty by the toxicity and recovery noted after the first treatment.[164] Robinson et al[194] have suggested offering repeat therapies every 3 months, almost on a prophylactic basis, to prevent recurrence of pain. Anecdotal evidence suggests that those patients with less osteoblastic metastases than those of prostate and breast cancer may require treating at intervals of less than 3 months.

Patients in whom unsealed source therapy is felt to be appropriate should have the same care and attention given to the development of their treatment plan as any patient attending for radiotherapy or analgesic therapy. When the patient attends for consultation a treatment goal should be clearly articulated and discussed; the aspirations and possible morbidity of the therapy should be enumerated and, if appropriate, the risk–benefit ratio described; the treatment goal should be clearly outlined to the patient and the patient's family; confirm that metastatic disease is the cause of the patient's bone pain; consider the patient's condition – terminally ill patients will not respond to strontium-89 treatment.[200] Robinson et al[194] have outlined a treatment plan for strontium-89 therapy including requirements for follow-up, patient information and management of pain medication.

Unsealed source therapy for bone metastases is a simple, cost effective, repeatable and very effective form of palliative therapy which has been shown to be good clinical practice in the patient with advanced cancer. Despite the paucity of hard data before the mid-1980s, there is now convincing evidence of its effectiveness. The nuclear medicine community is best placed to offer this to patients in need. However, in the past there has been reluctance to make the necessary changes in practice to ensure that the community is fully involved in this area of unsealed source therapy.[123] The required changes in practice have been clearly enumerated;[201] we owe it to our patients to ensure that they are completely instituted.

REFERENCES

1. Stjernswärd J 1985 Cancer pain relief: an important global health issue. Clin J Pain 1: 95–97
2. Saunders G M 1985 The management of terminal illness. Edward Arnold, London
3. Daut R L, Cleeland C S 1982 The prevalence and severity of pain in cancer. Cancer 50: 1913–1918
4. Twycross R G, Fairfield S 1982 Pain in far advanced cancer. Pain 14: 303–310
5. Foley K M, Arbit E 1989 The management of cancer pain. In: DeVita V T, Hellman S, Rosenberg S A, eds. Cancer: principles and practice of oncology. 3rd ed. Lippincott, Philadelphia. pp 2064–2087
6. Paterson A H G 1987 Bone metastases in breast cancer, prostate cancer and myeloma. Bone 8 (Suppl 1): 17–22
7. Stoll B A 1983 Natural history, prognosis, and staging of bone metastases. In: Stoll B A, Parbhoos S, eds. Bone metastases: monitoring and treatment. Raven Press, New York. pp 1–20
8. Cleeland C S 1984 The impact of pain on patients with cancer. Cancer 54: 26, 35–41
9. Bond M R 1979 Psychologic and emotional aspects of cancer pain. In: Bonica J J, Ventafridda V, eds. Advances in pain research and therapy, Vol 2. Raven Press, New York. pp 81–88
10. Bonica J J 1985 Treatment of cancer pain: current status and

future needs. In: Fields H L et al, eds. Advances in pain research and therapy, Vol 9. Raven Press, New York. pp 589–616
11. Twycross R G, Lack S A 1983 Symptom control in far advanced cancer: pain relief. Pitman Books, London
12. Nielsen O S, Munro A J, Tannock I F 1991 Bone metastases: pathophysiology and management policy. J Clin Oncol 9 (3): 509–524
13. McEwan A J B 1993 Editorial. Pain palliation and nuclear medicine. Eur J Nucl Med 20: 1–3
14. Kim S I, Chen D C P, Muggia F M 1988 A new look at radionuclides therapy in metastatic disease of bone (review and prospects). Anticancer Res 8: 681–684
15. Hoskin P J 1991 Editorial. Palliaton of bone metastases. Eur J Cancer 27 (8): 950–951
16. Hosain F, Spencer R P 1992 Radiopharmaceuticals for palliation of metastatic osseous lesions: biologic and physical background. Semin Nucl Med 22 (1): 11–16
17. Lote K, Walloe A, Bjersand A 1986 Bone metastasis. Prognosis, diagnosis and treatment. Acta Radiol Oncol 25: 227–232
18. Patanaphan V, Salazar O M, Risco R 1988 Breast cancer: metastatic patterns and their prognosis. South Med J 81: 1109–1112
19. Fidler I J, Radinsky R 1990 Genetic control of cancer metastasis. J Natl Cancer Inst 82: 166–168
20. Jacobs S C 1983 Spread of prostatic cancer to bone. Urology 21: 337–344
21. Berrettoni B A, Carter J R 1986 Mechanisms of cancer metastasis to bone. J Bone Joint Surg 68A: 308–312
22. Carter R L 1985 Patterns and mechanisms of bone metastases. J Royal Soc Med 78 (Suppl 9): 2–6
23. Carter R L 1985 Patterns and mechanisms of localized bone invasion by tumours: studies with squamous carcinomas of the head and neck. Critical Rev Clin Lab Sci 22: 275–315
24. Galasko C S B 1982 Mechanisms of lytic and blastic metastatic disease of bone. Clin Orthop 169: 20–27
25. Garrett I R 1993 Bone destruction in cancer. Semin Oncol 20 (Suppl 2): 4–9
26. Foley K 1987 Pain syndromes in patients with cancer. Med Clin North Am 71 (2): 169–184
27. Kuttig H 1984 Radiotherapy of cancer pain. In: Zimmerman M, Drings S, Wagner S (eds) Pain in the cancer patient. Recent Results in Cancer Research 89: 190–194
28. Leddy E T 1930 Roentgen treatment of metastasis to the vertebrae and bones of the pelvis from carcinoma of the breast. Am J Roent Radiat Therapy 24: 657–672
29. Hoskin P J 1988 Scientific and clinical aspects of radiotherapy in the relief of bone. Cancer Survey 7: 69–86
30. Tong D, Gillick L, Hendrickson F R 1982 The palliation of symptomatic osseous metastases. Final results of the Radiation Therapy Oncology Group. Cancer 50: 893–899
31. Madsen E L 1983 Painful bone metastasis: efficacy of radiotherapy assessed by the patients: a randomised trial comparing 4 Gy X 6 versus 10 Gy X 2. Int J Radiat Oncol Biol Phys 9: 1775–1779
32. Price P, Hoskin P J, Easton D, Austin A, Palmer S G, Yarnold J R 1986 Prospective randomised trial of single and multifraction radiotherapy schedules in the treatment of painful bony metastases. Radiother Oncol 6: 247–255
33. Price P, Hoskin P J, Easton D, Austin A, Palmer S G, Yarnold J R 1988 Low dose single fraction radiotherapy in the treatment of metastatic bone pain: a pilot study. Radiother Oncol 12: 297–300
34. Cole D J 1989 A randomised trial of a single treatment versus conventional fractionation in the palliative radiotherapy of painful bone metastases. Clin Oncol 1: 59–62
35. LeBourgeois J P, Casset J M 1976 Irradiation concentrée des metastases osseuses. Journal de Radiologie Medicale 58: 737–739
36. Hendrickson F, Shehata W, Kirchner A 1976 Radiation therapy for osseous metastasis. Int J Radiat Oncol Biol Phys 1: 275–278
37. Gilbert H, Kagan A, Nussbaum H et al 1977 Evaluation of radiation therapy for bone metastases: pain relief and quality of life. Am J Roent 129: 1095–1096
38. Ambrad A J 1978 Single dose and short, high dose fractionation radiation therapy for osseous metastases. Int J Radiat Oncol Biol Phys 4: 207–208
39. Martin W M C 1983 Multiple daily fractions of radiation in the palliation of pain from bone metastases. Clin Rad 34: 245–249
40. Trodella L, Ansili-Cefaro G, Turrisiani A. Marmiroli L, Cellini N, Nardone L 1984 Pain in osseous metastases: results of radiotherapy. Pain 18: 387–396
41. Bates T 1992 A review of local radiotherapy in the treatment of bone metastases and cord compression. Int J Radiat Oncol Biol Phys 23: 217–221
42. Blitzer P H 1985 Reanalysis of the RTOG study of the palliation of symptomatic osseous metastases. Cancer 55: 1468–1472
43. Malawer M M, Delaney T F 1989 Treatment of metastatic cancer to bone. In: De Vita Jr V T, Hellman S, Rosenberg S A, eds. Cancer, principles and practice of oncology. Lippincott, Philadelphia. pp 2298–2317
44. Cheng D S, Seitz C B, Eyre H J 1980 Nonoperative management of femoral, numeral and acetabular metastases in patients with breast carcinoma. Cancer 45: 1533–1537
45. Findlay G F G 1984 Adverse effects of the management of malignant spinal cord compression. J Neurol Neurosurg Psychiatr 47: 761–766
46. Kagan A R 1988 Radiation therapy for metastases and myeloma. Spine 2: 343–349
47. Rate W R, Solin L H, Turrisi A T 1988 Palliative radiotherapy for metastatic malignant melanoma: brain metastases, bone metastases, and spinal cord compression. Int J Radiat Oncol Biol Phys 15: 859–864
48. Salazar O M, Rubin P, Keller B et al 1978 Systemic (half-body) radiation therapy: response and toxicity. Int J Radiat Oncol Biol Phys 4: 937–941
49. Salazar O M, Rubin P, Hendrickson F R et al 1981 Single-dose half-body irradiation for the palliation of multiple bone metastases from solid tumors: a preliminary report. Int J Radiat Oncol Biol Phys 7: 773–781
50. Salazar O M, Rubin P, Hendrickson F R et al 1986 Single-dose half-body irradiation for palliation of multiple bone metastases from solid tumors: final Radiation Therapy Oncology Group report. Cancer 58: 29–36
51. Qasim M M 1977 Single dose palliative irradiation for bony metastasis. Strahlentherapie 153: 531–532
52. Qasim M M 1981 Half body irradiation in metastatic carcinomas. Clin Radiol 32: 214–219
53. Fitzpatrick P J, Rider W D 1976 Half body radiotherapy. Int J Radiat Oncol Biol Phys 1: 197–207
54. Rubin P, Salazar O, Zagars G et al 1985 Systemic hemibody irradiation for overt and occult metastases. Cancer 55: 2210–2221
55. Chisholm G D 1990 Carcinoma of the prostate: reasons for endocrine treatment prior to symptomatic metastases. In: Schroder F H, ed. Treatment of prostatic cancer: facts and controversies. Progress in clinical and biological research, Vol 359. Wiley-Liss, New York. pp 1–6
56. Lippman M E, Lichter A S, Danforth D N 1988 Diagnosis and management of breast cancer. Saunders, Philadelphia
57. Stoll B A 1983 Hormonal therapy – pain relief and recalcification. In: Stoll B A, Parbhoo S, eds. Bone metastases: monitoring and treatment. Raven Press, New York. pp 321–342
58. Smith J A 1987 New methods of endocrine management of prostate cancer. J Urol 137: 1–10
59. Marsoni S, Hurson S, Eisenberger M 1985 Chemotherapy of bone metastases. In: Garrattini S, ed. Bone resorption, metastasis and diphosphonates. Raven Press, New York. pp 181–195
60. Tannock I 1985 Is there evidence that chemotherapy is of benefit to patients with carcinoma of the prostate? J Clin Oncol 3: 1013–1021
61. World Health Organization 1986 Cancer pain relief. World Health Organization, Geneva
62. Ferrer-Brechner T, Ganz P 1984 Combination therapy with ibuprofen and methadone for chronic cancer pain. Am J Med 77 (Suppl): 78–83

63. Campa J A, Payne R 1992 The management of intractable bone pain: a clinician's perspective. Semin Nucl Med 22 (1): 3–10
64. Joliot F, Curie I 1934 Artificial production of a new kind of radioelement. Nature 133: 201–202
65. Silberstein E B, Elgazzar A H, Kapilivsky A 1992 Phosphorus-32 radiopharmaceuticals for the treatment of painful osseous metastases. Semin Nucl Med 22: 17–27
66. Lawrence E O, Cooksey D 1936 On the apparatus for the multiple acceleration of light ions to high speeds. Phys Rev 50: 1131–1136
67. Treadwell A deG, Low-Beer B V A, Friedell H L, Lawrence J H 1942 Metabolic studies on neoplasm of bone with the aid of radioactive strontium. Am J Med Sci 204: 521–530
68. Pecher C 1942 Biological investigations with radioactive calcium and strontium: preliminary report on the use of radioactive strontium in the treatment of metastatic bone cancer. University of California Publications in Pharmacology, Vol. 2. pp 117–149
69. Lawrence J H, Wasserman L R 1950 Multiple myeloma: a study of 24 patients treated with radioactive isotopes (P^{32} and Sr^{89}). Ann Intern Med 33: 41–55
70. Holmes R A 1993 Radiopharmaceuticals in clinical trials. Semin Oncol 20 (Suppl): 22–26
71. Troutner D E 1987 Chemical and physical properties of radionuclides. Nucl Med Biol 14: 171–176
72. Wegst A V 1987 Methods of calculating radiation absorbed dose. Nucl Med Biol 14: 269–271
73. Logan K W 1987 Quantitative SPECT imaging for diagnosis and dosimetry in radionuclide therapy. Nucl Med Biol 14: 205–209
74. Volkert W A, Goeckler W F, Ehrhardt G J et al 1991 Therapeutic radionuclides: production and decay property consideration. J Nucl Med 32: 174–175
75. Held K D 1987 Radiobiology: biologic effects of ionizing radiations. In: Harbert J C (ed) Nuclear medicine therapy. Thieme, New York. pp 257–284
76. Maxon H R, Thomas S R, Hertzberg V S et al 1992 Rhenium-186 hydroxyethylidene diphosphonate for the treatment of painful osseous metastases. Semin Nucl Med 22: 33–40
77. Logan K W, Volkert W A, Holmes R A 1987 Radiation dose calculations in persons receiving injection of Samarium-153 EDTMP. J Nucl Med 28: 505–509
78. Porzsolt F, Tannock I 1993 Goals of palliative cancer therapy. J Clin Oncol 11: 378–381
79. Kaplan E, Fels I G, Kotlowski B R 1960 Therapy of carcinoma of the prostate metastatic to bone with P-32 labeled condensed phosphate. J Nucl Med 1: 1–13
80. Werner B, Isacson C, Lundell G et al 1980 ^{32}P-pyrophosphate in the treatment of persistent metastatic bone pain. Acta Radiol Oncol 19: 327–329
81. Tofe A J, Francis M D, Slough C L et al 1976 P-33 EHDP and P-32 (EHDP, PPi, and Pi) tissue distributions in consideration of palliative treatment for osseous neoplasms. J Nucl Med 17: 548 (Abstract)
82. Marshak A 1940 Uptake of radioactive phosphorus by nuclei of liver and tumors. Science 92: 460–461
83. Stoff J S 1982 Phosphate homeostasis and hypophosphatemia. Am J Med 72: 489–495
84. Kaufman C E, Felsenfield A J, Vabatta J B 1984 Maintenance of body fluid potassium, calcium, magnesium and phosphorus. In: Frohlich E D, ed. Pathophysiology. 3rd edn. Lippincott, Philadelphia. p 265
85. Reinhard E H, Moore C V, Bierbaum O S et al 1946 Radioactive phosphorus as a therapeutic agent. A review of the literature and analysis of the results of treatment of 155 patients with various blood diseases, lymphomas and other malignant neoplastic disease. J Lab Clin Med 31: 107–195
86. Harrison H E, Harrison H C 1979 Disorders of calcium and phosphate metabolism in childhood and adolescence. Saunders, Philadelphia. pp 15–46
87. Wilkinson R 1976 Absorption of calcium, phosphorus and magnesium. In: Nordin B E C, ed. Calcium, phosphate and magnesium metabolism. Churchill-Livingstone, New York. pp 36–113
88. Cabrejas M L, Mendez Falcon M A, Mran M Z 1979 The intestinal absorption of phosphate in normal human subjects. Int J Nucl Med Biol 6: 45–48
89. Friedell H L, Storaasli J P 1950 The use of radioactive phosphorus in the treatment of carcinoma of the breast with widespread metastases to the bone. Am J Roent Rad Ther 64: 559–575
90. Seltzer R A, Kereiakes J G, Saenger E L 1964 Radiation exposure from radioisotopes in pediatrics. New Engl J Med 271: 84–90
91. International Commission on Radiological Protection Publication 53 1988 Radiation dose to patients from radiopharmaceuticals. Pergamon, Oxford. p 84
92. Low-Beer B V A, Blais R S, Scofield N E 1952 Estimation of dosage for intravenously administered P-32. Am J Roentgenol 67: 28–41
93. Spiers F W, Beddoe A H, King S D et al 1976 The absorbed dose of bone marrow in the treatment of polycythemia by ^{32}P. Br J Radiol 49: 133–140
94. Mays C W 1973 Cancer induction in man from internal radioactivity. Health Phys 25: 585–592
95. Kereiakes J G, Rosenstein M 1980 Handbook of radiation doses in nuclear medicine and diagnostic x-ray. CRCP, Boca Raton. p. 161
96. Francis M D, Slough C L, Tofe A J 1976 Distribution and effect of P-32 HEDP in normal and bone tumor bearing dogs. J Nucl Med 17: 538 (Abstract)
97. Bigler R E, Rosen G, Tofe A J et al 1976 Comparative distribution of P-32 and Tc-99m diphosphonates in patients with osteogenic sarcoma. J Nucl Med 17: 548 (Abstract)
98. Hall J N, Tokars R P, O'Mara R E 1975 P-32 diphosphonate: a potential therapeutic agent. J Nucl Med 16: 532 (Abstract)
99. Potsaid M S, Irwin Jr R J, Castronov F P et al 1978 [^{32}P] Diphosphonate dose determination in patients with bone metastases from prostatic carcinoma. J Nucl Med 19: 98–104
100. Montebello J F, Hartson-Eaton M 1989 The palliation of osseous metastasis with ^{32}P or ^{89}Sr compared with external beam and hemibody irradiation: a historical perspective. Cancer Invest 7: 139–160
101. Wallace J C, Ross I T H 1977 Method to quantify uptake of radiophosphorus in therapy of metastatic bone disease using ^{99}Tc^{m} radiophosphate. Br J Rad 50: 664–666
102. Chievitz O, Heversy G 1935 Radioactive indicators in the study of phosphorus metabolism in rats. Nature 163: 754–755
103. Lawrence J H, Scott K G 1939 Comparative metabolism of phosphorus in normal and lymphomatous animals. Proc Soc Exp Biol Med 40: 694–696
104. Lawrence J H, Tuttle L W, Scott K G et al 1940 Studies on neoplasms with the aid of radioactive phosphorus. I. The total phosphorus metabolism of normal and leukemic mice. J Clin Invest 19: 267–271
105. Kenny J M, Marinelli L D, Woodard H Q 1941 Tracer studies with radioactive phosphorus in malignant neoplastic disease. Radiology 37: 683–687
106. Erf L A 1941 Retention of radiophosphorus in whole and aliquot portion of tissues of patients dead of leukemia. Proc Soc Exp Biol NY 47: 287–289
107. Maxfield J R, Maxfield J G S, Maxfield W S 1958 The use of radioactive phosphorus and testosterone in metastatic bone lesions from breast and prostate. South Med J 51: 320–328
108. Hertz S 1950 Modifying effect of steroid hormone therapy of human neoplastic disease as judged by radioactive phosphorus (P-32) studies. J Clin Invest 29: 821 (Abstract)
109. Fowler J E, Whitmore W F 1982 Considerations for the use of testosterone with systemic chemotherapy in prostatic cancer. Cancer 49: 1373–1377
110. Corwin S H, Malament M, Small M et al 1970 Experiences with P-32 in advanced carcinoma of the prostate. J Urol 104: 745–748
111. Tong E C K, Rubenfeld S 1967 The treatment of bone metastases with parathormone followed by radiophosphorus. Am J Radiol 99: 422–434
112. Potsaid M, Irwin R, Castronova F et al 1976 Phosphorus-32 EHDP clinical study of patients with prostate carcinoma bone metastases. J Nucl Med 17: 548–549 (Abstract)
113. Vermooten V, Maxfield J R, Maxfield J G S 1959 The use of

radioactive phosphorus in the management of advanced carcinoma of the prostate. West J Surg Obstet Gynecol 67: 245–249
114. Wildermuth O, Parker D, Archambeau J L et al 1960 Management of diffuse metastasis from carcinoma of the prostate. JAMA 172: 1607–1611
115. Parsons R L, Campbell J L, Thormley M W 1962 Experience with P-32 in the treatment of metastatic carcinoma of the prostate: a follow-up report. J Urol 88: 812–813
116. Mandel P R, Chiat H 1962 Radioactive phosphorus for carcinoma of the breast with diffuse metastatic bone disease. NY State J Med 62: 1970–1976
117. Smart J G 1965 The use of P-32 in the treatment of severe pain from bone metastases of carcinoma of the prostate. Br J Urol 37: 139–147
118. Walton R J 1965 Palliative treatment of osseous metastases from carcinoma of the breast and carcinoma of the prostate with radioactive phosphorus and testosterone. J Can Assoc Radiol 16: 213–216
119. Joshi D P, Seery W H, Golberg L G 1965 Evaluation of phosphorus-32 for intractable pain secondary to prostatic carcinoma metastases. JAMA 193: 621–623
120. Donati R M, Ellis H, Gallagher N I 1966 Testosterone potentiated P-32 therapy in prostatic carcinoma. Cancer 19: 1088–1090
121. Morin L J, Stevens J C 1967 Radioactive phosphorus in the treatment of metastasis to bone from carcinoma of the prostate. J Urol 97: 130–132
122. Morales A, Connolly J G, Burr R C 1970 The use of radioactive phosphorus to treat pain in metastatic carcinoma of the prostate. Can Med Assoc J 103: 372–373
123. Hilts S V 1972 Nuclear medicine in the management of metastatic bone cancer. Ariz Med 29: 329–333
124. Edland R W 1974 Testosterone potentiated radiophosphorus therapy of osseous metastases in prostatic cancer. Am J Radiol 120: 678–683
125. Roberts D J 1979 ^{32}P-Sodium phosphate treatment of metastatic malignant disease. Clin Nucl Med 4: 92–93
126. Riva P 1983 Radiometabolic therapy with ^{32}P in bony metastases: experience on 127 patients. J Nucl Med All Sci 27: 183–187
127. Ariel I M, Hassouna H 1985 Carcinoma of the prostate. The treatment of bone metastases by radioactive phosphorus (^{32}P). Int Surg 70: 63–66
128. Aziz H, Choi K, Sohn C et al 1986 Comparison of ^{32}P therapy and sequential hemibody irradiation (HBI) for bony metastases as methods of whole body irradiation. Am J Clin Oncol 9: 264–268
129. Burnet N G, Williams G, Howard N 1990 Phosphorus-32 for intractable bony pain from carcinoma of the prostate. Clin Oncol 2: 220–223
130. Tong E C K, Finkelstein P 1973 The treatment of prostatic bone metastases with parathormone and radioactive phosphorus. J Urol 109: 71–75
131. Pinck B D, Alexander S 1973 Parathormone potentiated radiophosphorus therapy in prostatic carcinoma. Urology 1: 201–204
132. Merrin C, Bakshi S 1974 Treatment of metastatic carcinoma of the prostate to bone with parathormone and radioactive phosphorus. J Surg Oncol 6: 67–72
133. Johnson D E, Haynie T P 1977 Phosphorus-32 for intractable pain in carcinoma of prostate. Urology 9: 137–139
134. Cheung A, Driedger A A 1980 Evaluation of radiophosphorus in the palliation of metastatic bone lesions from carcinoma of the breast and prostate. Radiology 134: 209–212
135. Glaser M G, Howard N, Waterfall N 1981 Carcinoma of the prostate: the treatment of bone metastases by radiophosphorus. Clin Radiol 32: 695–697
136. Storaasli J P, King R L, Krieger H et al 1961 Palliation of osseous metastases from breast carcinoma with radioactive phosphorus alone and in combination with adrenalectomy. Radiology 76: 422–429
137. Goeckeler W F, Edwards B, Volkert W A, Holmes R A, Simon J, Wilson D 1987 Skeletal localization of Samarium-153 chelates: potential therapeutic bone agents. J Nucl Med 28: 495–504
138. Holmes R A 1992 [^{153}Sm] EDTMP: a potential therapy for bone cancer pain. Semin Nucl Med 22: 41–45
139. Ketring A R 1987 ^{153}Sm-EDTMP and ^{186}Re-HEDP as bone therapeutic radiopharmaceuticals. Nucl Med Biol 14: 223–232
140. Singh A, Holmes R A, Farhangi M 1989 Human pharmacokinetics of Samarium-153 EDTMP in metastatic cancer. J Nucl Med 30: 1814–1818
141. Heggie J C P 1991 Radiation absorbed dose calculations for Samarium-153-EDTMP localized in bone. J Nucl Med 32: 840–844
142. Eary J F, Collins C, Stabin M et al 1993 Samarium-153-EDTMP biodistribution and dosimetry estimation. J Nucl Med 34: 1031–1036
143. Lattimer J C, Corwin Jr L A, Stapleton J et al 1990 Clinical and clinicopathologic effects of Samarium-153-EDTMP administered intravenously to normal beagle dogs. J Nucl Med 31: 586–593
144. Lattimer J C, Corwin Jr L A, Stapleton J et al 1990 Clinical and clinicopathologic response of canine bone tumor patients to treatment with Samarium-153-EDTMP. J Nucl Med 31: 1316–1325
145. Eary J F, Collins C, Appelbaum F R 1990 Sm-153-EDTMP treatment of hormone refractory prostate carcinoma. J Nucl Med 31: 755 (Abstract)
146. Turner J H, Claringbold P G, Hetherington E L, Sorby P, Martindale A A 1989 A phase I study of Samarium-153 ethylenediaminetetramethylene phosphonate therapy for disseminated skeletal metastases. J Clin Oncol 7: 1926–1931
147. Turner J H, Claringbold P G 1991 A phase II study of treatment of painful multifocal skeletal metastases with single and repeated dose Samarium-153 ethylenediaminetetramethylene phosphonate. Eur J Cancer 27: 1084–1086
148. Turner J H, Martindale A A, Sorby P 1989 Samarium-153-EDTMP therapy of disseminated skeletal metastases. Eur J Nucl Med 15: 784–795
149. Sandeman T F, Budd R S, Martin J J 1992 Samarium-153-labelled EDTMP for bone metastases from cancer of the prostate. Clin Oncol 4: 160–164
150. Mathieu L, Chevalier P, Galy G et al 1979 Preparation of 186-Rhenium labelled HEDP and its possible use in the treatment of osseous neoplasms. Int J Appl Radiat Isot 30: 725–727
151. Eary J F, Durack L, Williams D, Vanderheyden J-L 1990 Considerations for imaging Re-188 and Re-186 isotopes. Clin Nucl Med 15: 911–916
152. Deutsch E, Libson K, Vanderheyden J L et al 1986 The chemistry of rhenium and technetium as related to the use of isotopes of these elements in therapeutic and diagnostic nuclear medicine. Int J Nucl Med Biol 13: 465–477
153. Vanderheyden J L, Heeg M J, Deutsch E 1985 Comparison of the chemical and biological properties of trans-[Tc $(DMPE)_2Cl_2]^+$ and trans-Re $(DMPE)_2Cl_2]^+$, when DMPE = 1,2-Bis (dimethylphosphine) ethane: single-crystal structural analysis of trans-[Re $(DMPE)_2Cl_2]PF_6$. Inorg Chem 24: 1666–1673
154. Pipes D W, Deutsch E 1993 Rhenium Re-186 etidronate injection. Drugs of the future. In press
155. de Klerk J M H, van Dijk A, van het Schip A D, Zonnenberg B A, van Rijk P P 1992 Pharmacokinetics of Rhenium-186 after administration of Rhenium-186-HEDP to patients with bone metastases. J Nucl Med 33: 646–651
156. Maxon H R, Deutsch E A, Thomas S R 1988 Re-186 (Sn)HEDP for treatment of multiple metastatic foci in bone: human biodistribution and dosimetric studies. Radiology 166: 501–507
157. Maxon H R, Schroder L E, Hertzberg V S et al 1991 Rhenium-186(Sn)HEDP for treatment of painful osseous metastases: results of a double-blind crossover comparison with placebo. J Nucl Med 32: 1877–1881
158. Maxon H R, Schroder L E, Thomas S R et al 1990 Re-186 (Sn)HEDP for treatment of painful osseous metastases: initial clinical experience in 20 patients with hormone-resistant prostate cancer. Radiology 176: 155–159
159. Zonnenberg B A, de Klerk J M H, van Rijk P P 1991 Re-186-HEDP for treatment of painful bone metastases in patients with metastatic prostate or breast cancer. Preliminary results. J Nucl Med 32: 1082 (Abstract)

160. Englaro E E, Schroder L E, Thomas S R, Williams C C, Maxon H R 1992 Clin Nucl Med 17: 41–44
161. Porter A, Mertens W 1991 Strontium 89 in the treatment of metastatic prostate cancer. Can J Oncol 1: 11–18
162. International Commission on Radiological Protection Publication 30 1979 Metabolic data for strontium: limits for intakes of radionuclides by workers, Part 1. Pergamon, Oxford: pp 77–78
163. Blake G M, Zivanovic M A, McEwan A J, Ackery D M 1986 Sr-89 therapy: strontium kinetics in disseminated carcinoma of the prostate. Eur J Nucl Med 12: 447–454
164. Blake G M, Zivanovic M A, McEwan A J, Condon B R, Ackery D M 1987 Strontium-89 therapy: strontium kinetics and dosimetry in two patients treated for metastasising osteosarcoma. Br J Rad 60: 253–259
165. Blake G M, Zivanovic M A, McEwan A J, Batty V B, Ackery D M 1987 ^{89}Sr radionuclide therapy: dosimetry and haematological toxicity in two patients with metastasising prostatic carcinoma. Eur J Nucl Med 13: 41–46
166. Blake G M, Gray J M, Zivanovic M A, McEwan A J, Fleming J S, Ackery D M 1987 Strontium-89 radionuclide therapy: a dosimetric study using impulse response function analysis. Br J Rad 60: 685–692
167. Blake G M, Zivanovic M A, Blaquiere R M, Fine D R, McEwan A J, Ackery D M 1988 Strontium-89 therapy: measurement of absorbed dose to skeletal metastases. J Nucl Med 29: 549–557
168. Blake G M, Wood J F, Wood P J, Zivanovic M A, Lewington V J 1989 ^{89}Sr therapy: strontium plasma clearance in disseminated prostatic carcinoma. Eur J Nucl Med 15: 49–54
169. Blake G M, Zivanovic M A, Lewington V J 1989 Measurements of the strontium plasma clearance rate in patients receiving ^{89}Sr radionuclide therapy. Eur J Nucl Med 15: 780–783
170. Breen S L, Powe J E, Porter A T 1992 Dose estimation of strontium-89 radiotherapy of metastatic prostatic carcinoma. J Nucl Med 33: 1316–1323
171. Schmidt C G, Firusian 1974 89-Sr for the treatment of incurable pain in patient with neoplastic osseous infiltrations. Int J Clin Pharmacol 9: 199–205
172. Firusian N, Mellin P, Schmidt C G 1976 Results of ^{89}Strontium therapy in patients with carcinoma of the prostate and incurable pain from bone metastases: a preliminary report. J Urol 116: 764–768
173. Kutzner J, Grimm W, Hahn K 1978 Palliative strahlentherapie mit Strontium-89 bei ausgedehnter skelettmetastasierung. Strahlentherapie 154: 317–322
174. Firusian N 1978 Endoossale isotopen-therapie maligner skeleterkrankungen. Z. Krebsforsch 91: 143–156
175. Hayek D, Ritschard J, Zwahlen A, Courvoisier B, Donath A 1980 Emploi du strontium-89 dans le traitement antalgique des métastases osseuses. Schweiz med Wschr 110: 1154–1159
176. Correns H-J, Mebel M, Buchali K, Schnorr D, Seidel C, Mitterlaechner E. Strontium 89 therapy of bone metastases of carcinoma of the prostate gland. Eur J Nucl Med 4: 33–35
177. Kimmig B, Hermann H J, Kober B 1983 Nuklearmedizinishe therapie von knochen-metastasen. Rötgenblätter 36: 216–219
178. Buchali K, Correns H J, Schnorr D, Schürer M, Sydow K, Lips H 1984 89-Strontium – therapy of skeletal metastases of prostatic carcinoma. Proceedings of the 1984 Bad Gastein International Radiopharmaceutical Conference pp 151–156
179. Silberstein E B, Williams C 1985 Strontium-89 therapy for the pain of osseous metastases. J Nucl Med 26: 345–348
180. Reddy E K, Robinson R G, Mansfield C M 1986 Strontium 89 for palliation of bone metastases. J Nat Med Assoc 78: 27–32
181. Kloiber R, Molnar C P, Barnes M 1987 Sr-89 therapy for metastatic bone disease: scintigraphic and radiographic follow-up. Radiology 163: 719–723
182. Robinson R G, Spicer J A, Preston D F, Wegst A V, Martin N L 1987 Treatment of metastatic bone pain with Strontium-89. Nucl Med Biol 14: 219–222
183. Tennvall J, Darte L, Lundgren R, Mohamed El Hassan A 1988 Palliation of multiple bone metastases from prostatic carcinoma with Strontium-89. Acta Oncol 27: 365–369
184. Buchali K, Correns H-J, Schuerer M, Schnorr D, Lips H, Sydow K 1988 Results of a double blind study of 89-Strontium therapy of skeletal metastases of prostatic carcinoma. Eur J Nucl Med 14: 349–351
185. McEwan A J B, Porter A T, Venner P M, Amyotte G 1990 An evaluation of the safety and efficacy of treatment with Strontium-89 in patients who have previously received wide field radiotherapy. Antibody, Immunoconjugates, and Radiopharmaceuticals 3: 91–97
186. Laing A H, Ackery D M, Bayly R J et al 1991 Strontium-89 chloride for pain palliation in prostatic skeletal malignancy. Br J Rad 64: 816–822
187. Dearnaly D P, Bayly R J, A'Hern R P, Gadd J, Zivanovic M M, Lewington V J 1992 Palliation of bone metastases in prostate cancer. Hemibody irradiation or Strontium-89. Clin Oncol 4: 101–107
188. Fosså S D, Paus E, Lochoff M, Melbye Backe S, Aas M 1992 ^{89}Strontium in bone metastases from hormone resistant prostate cancer: palliation effect and biochemical changes. Br J Cancer 66: 177–180
189. Lewington V J, McEwan A J, Ackery D M et al 1991 A prospective, randomised double-blind crossover study to examine the efficacy of Strontium-89 in pain palliation in patients with advanced prostate cancer metastatic to bone. Eur J Cancer 27: 954–958
190. Porter A T, McEwan A J B, Powe J E et al 1993 Results of a randomized phase-III trial to evaluate the efficacy of Strontium-89 adjuvant to local field external beam irradiation in the management of endocrine resistant metastatic prostate cancer. Int J Radiat Oncol Biol Phys 25: 805–813
191. Porter A T, McEwan A J B 1993 Strontium-89 as an adjuvant to external beam radiation improves pain relief and delays disease progression in advanced prostate cancer: results of a randomized controlled trial. Semin Oncol 20 (Suppl 2): 38–43
192. McEwan A J B, Amyotte G A, McGowan D G, MacGillivray J A, Porter A T 1994 Retrospective analysis of the cost effectiveness of treatment with Metastron (Strontium-89 chloride) in patients with prostate cancer metastatic to bone. Nucl Med Commun: In press
193. Kirk D, Quilty P M, Russell J M et al 1991 A comparison of the clinical and economic effectiveness of Metastron (strontium 89) and conventional radiotherapy in metastatic prostate cancer. Presented at the 22nd Congress Société International D'Urologie, Sevilla, Spain
194. Robinson R G, Preston D F, Spicer J A, Baxter K G 1992 Radionuclide therapy of intractable bone pain: emphasis on Strontium-89. Semin Nucl Med 22: 28–32
195. Mertens W C 1993 Radionuclide therapy of bone metastases: prospects for enhancement of therapeutic efficacy. Semin Oncol 20 (Suppl 2): 49–55
196. Ackery D, Yardley J 1993 Radionuclide-targeted therapy for the management of metastatic bone pain. Semin Oncol 20 (Suppl 2): 27–31
197. Srivastava S C, Meinken G E, Richards P et al 1985 The development and in-vivo behavior of tin containing radiopharmaceuticals. I. Chemistry, preparation and biodistribution in small animals. Int J Nucl Med Biol 12: 167–174
198. Oster Z H, Som P, Srivastava S C et al 1985 The development and in-vivo behaviour of tin containing radiopharmaceuticals. II. Autoradiographic and scintigraphic studies in normal animals and in animal models of bone disease. Int J Nucl Med Biol 12: 175–184
199. Atkins H L, Mausner L F, Srivastava S C et al 1993 Biodistribution of Sn-117m(4+) DTPA for palliative therapy of painful osseous metastases. Radiology 186: 279–283
200. Kagan A R 1992 Radiation therapy in palliative cancer management. In: Perez C A, Brady L W, eds. Principles and practice of radiation oncology. 2nd edn. Lippincott, Philadelphia. pp 1495–1507
201. Henkin R E 1993 Therapy in nuclear medicine – a bone of contention. J Nucl Med 34: 1037–1038 (Editorial)

77. Alternative approaches to targeting therapy

M. Fischer

The aims of selective targeting of therapy are to increase the effectiveness of treatment while limiting radiation or chemotoxicity to normal tissue. This can be achieved by increasing local concentrations of radiopharmaceutical agents with low systemic exposure. Locoregional radionuclide therapy should create an advantageous concentration gradient between tumour or cavity fluid and radiation burden to surrounding tissue. Alternative radionuclide therapy includes different techniques for targeting radiopharmaceuticals to tumours via direct intravascular (intra-arterial, intralymphatic), intracavitary (pericardial, pleural, peritoneal space) or intralesional and also intra-articular injection in inflammatory diseases.

DIRECT INTRALESIONAL INJECTION

During the early 1950s several centres reported direct intralesional injection of radionuclides (^{32}P chromic phosphate colloid) into inoperable tumours.[1] This procedure was later superseded by brachyradiotherapy using implanted seeds.

DIRECT INTRACYSTIC INJECTION

Craniopharyngiomas and some other intracerebral tumours are characterized by a cystic component that may lead to raised intracranial pressure or local pressure effects. Neurosurgery of these lesions may be hazardous. Morbidity and mortality of neurosurgical removal of craniopharyngiomas remain high. Fluid aspiration is often followed by rapid reaccumulation of fluid. Sclerosant or cytotoxic drugs may be injected or instilled into the cyst by direct stereotactic puncture. The use of beta-emitting radiolabelled colloids avoids systemic resorption and is therefore a more attractive option. The technique can be used to target higher absorbed radiation doses to tumour than can be achieved using conventional external beam radiotherapy. The use of ^{90}Y, ^{186}Re or ^{32}P colloids has been shown to ablate the epithelial lining of the cyst, effectively preventing fluid reaccumulation. Dose-dependent decrease in size or even collapse of the cyst may be observed. Several groups have reported significant long-term benefits in patients with craniopharyngiomas, cystic gliomas, cystic grade IV astrocytomas and other cystic lesions.[2–4] Because of the short range of beta-emitters in tissue, intracystic radionuclide therapy is influenced by the dose administered to the cyst wall, thickness of the wall and location of the cyst. No beneficial effect on solid portions of a tumour or thick or calcified cyst walls can be expected. Solid tumours, mixed tumours with small cysts and predominantly intrasellar tumours are, therefore, unlikely to respond to this approach.[5,6] Administered activity depends on the volume of the cyst; a formula for calculation was given by Taasan *et al.*[4] Activities ranged from 18 MBq to 56 MBq (0.5–1.5 mCi) in a volume of 0.1–0.5 ml in craniopharyngiomas, the calculated doses to the cyst lining being from 100 to 400 Gy, assuming a non-uniform dispersal of the radioisotope in the cyst fluid but adherence to the cyst wall[7] and 4–92.5 MBq (0.1–2.5 mCi) in cystic astrocytomas (Fig. 77.1).

Treatment should be followed by imaging either using bremsstrahlung (^{90}Y, ^{32}P) or gamma emission (^{186}Re) to

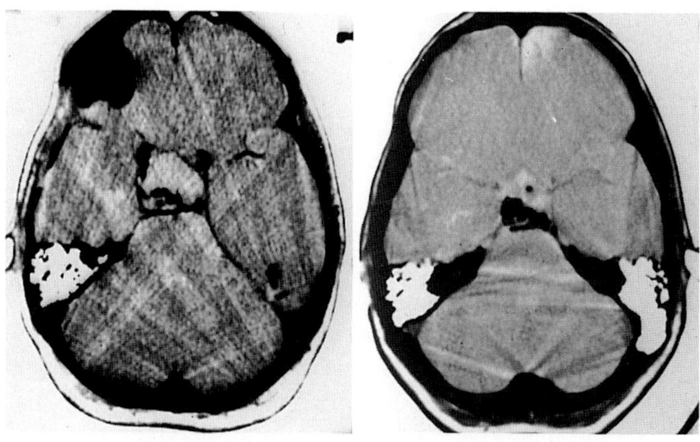

Fig. 77.1 Computed tomography of a craniopharyngioma treated with 200 Gy of ^{32}P colloid. Time between the first (left) and second (right) Cts is 11 months (September 1988 to August 1989). (Courtesy of Dr Taren & Dr Shapiro, University of Michigan, Ann Arbor, MI, USA.)

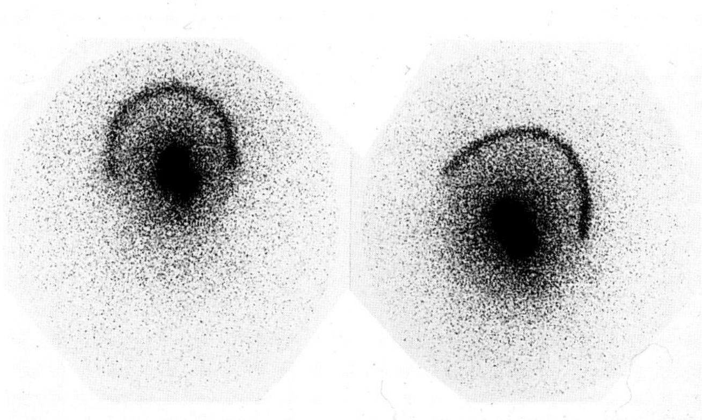

Fig. 77.2 Bremsstrahl scan of a large suprasellar cystic craniopharyngioma after administration of ^{32}P colloid in anterior (left) and left lateral (right) projection (with a marker over scalp). (Courtesy of Dr Taren & Dr Shapiro, University of Michigan, Ann Arbor, MI, USA.)

confirm the localization of the radionuclides in the cyst (Fig. 77.2). The advantages of this procedure are minimal risk, delivery of larger tumoricidal doses to the area of the tumour, reducing the rate of cystic fluid reaccumulation, reducing the cyst size and low radiation burden to normal brain tissue.

INTRAVASCULAR INJECTION

Intra-arterial

Direct intra-arterial injection of pharmaceutical agents results in a high delivery to the vascular bed fed by the perfusing arteries. This is true if the drug undergoes extensive deposition in the tumour vascular bed. Radiopharmaceutical delivery can be enhanced by selective permanent or temporary occlusion of the intratumoral precapillary arterioles to enhance tumor-to-normal tissue ratio, by semiselective vasoactive agents or by radiosensitizers. As the radiopharmaceutical is confined to the extracellular space, this approach can deliver a high radiation dose to the tumour surface, but intracellular fluid diffusion is limited. Intra-arterial therapy is, therefore, only applicable to small tumours.

The hepatic arterial therapy by infusion is based on the fact that vascular supply of hepatic tumours derives almost exclusively from the hepatic arteries (about 95%), in comparison with normal liver, which is supplied predominantly by the portal venous system (about 70%). Direct hepatic arterial injection of radiopharmaceutical agents can therefore be used for targeted therapy. Systemic toxicity is minimized by using drugs which have a high affinity for tumours (greater than 80% extraction). This intra-arterial approach is reserved for inoperable tumours, which may become resectable following treatment. Endoarterial embolizing tumour therapy with radionuclides has the maximum selectivity with highest radiation doses to the tumour and negligible exposure of normal tissue.

The observation that oil contrast media are retained in hepatic arteries generated interest in the use of intra-arterial ^{131}I-labelled lipiodol or ethiodol to treat liver tumours. This approach is of value for small tumours (<4.5 cm) in the absence of portal–systemic shunting. Treating more than 100 patients with ^{131}I-labelled lipiodol or ethiodol, the authors concluded that the smaller the tumour the better was the therapeutic effect.[8] Larger tumours respond better to combination therapy comprising ^{131}I lipiodol, intra-arterial chemotherapy, hepatic artery embolization and hyperthermia.

Injection of 74 MBq to 4.4 GBq (2–120 mCi) of ^{131}I lipiodol resulted in tumour shrinkage and palliation.[9] In the majority of patients with hepatocellular carcinoma, tumour shrinkage of > 50% but no complete remission was observed. Mean absorbed doses were calculated with 62.4 ± 50 Gy to the tumour, 5.5 ± 8.7 Gy to the normal liver and 2.9 ± 2.2 Gy to the lung.[10]

The substitution of radiolabelled ceramic or resin microspheres for lipiodol significantly reduced lung deposition. Injecting these microspheres labelled with ^{32}P or ^{90}Y, doses of 100–200 Gy were delivered with response rates of 39–68% and some preliminary evidence of prolongation of survival. A disadvantage of these resin or ceramic particles is leaching of free yttrium, which results in high bone marrow uptake and myelosuppression.[11] The incorporation of ^{90}Y or ^{32}P into the matrix of glass microspheres eliminated this problem, but, because of greater density of glass particles compared with blood, the distribution of glass microspheres may be less uniform than plastic, activated microspheres. Nevertheless, it was possible to deliver 15 times more microspheres to 2-mm-diameter liver tumours or nodules than nearby normal liver tissue.[11] High radiation doses can be tolerated by the human liver when delivered as a series of beta-emitting point sources.[12] This high radiation exposure does not influence normal liver function. Careful positioning of the intra-arterial catheter is essential to prevent embolization of gastrointestinal vessels. Side-effects, observed after application of radiolabelled particles are the same as after ^{131}I lipiodol: fever, elevation of liver enzymes and gastrointestinal symptoms.[13,14] The same authors reported palliation and, in most patients, stabilization of disease using ^{90}Y glass microspheres.

Intralymphatic

A small number of studies have used ^{32}P-tri-*n*-octylphosphate (80 MBq) (2 mCi) mixed with ^{131}I lipiodol (20 MBq) (0.5 mCi) for intralymphatic infusion in patients with suspicion of micrometastases of malignant melanoma of the lower limb. These radiopharmaceuticals are stored only in normal lymph nodes but not in tumour tissue.

Therefore, larger tumours or lymph node metastases (> 8 mm) cannot be treated effectively. Intralymphatic radionuclide therapy is contraindicated in the presence of lymphatic obstruction or large tumours. Radiopharmaceutical extravasation may lead to local radiation necrosis, and lung fibrosis may result from high pulmonary uptake.

INJECTION INTO SEROUS CAVITIES

The aim of direct injection of pharmaceuticals into serous cavities in patients with malignant effusions is to control the effusion and to 'kill' single malignant cells or clusters of cells. The ideal drugs for this approach are those with slow egress from the cavity and a rapid systemic clearance. Local tissue concentrations can be increased by incorporating drugs into particles or mixture with microspheres.[15]

This form of therapy, using either cytostatics or radionuclides, is likely to be most effective in treating small tumour volumes because the drugs are distributed outside the tumour cells and are limited by the depth of diffusion or maximum range of radioactive emission. The mechanism of intracavitary chemotherapy differs from radionuclide therapy because drugs may enter the peripheral cells and be transported via the capillaries of the tumour.[16]

Various radionuclides have been recommended for intracavitary therapy: ^{32}P, ^{90}Y and more recently Auger-electron emitting halogens ^{123}I and ^{80m}Br halodeoxyuridines (XUdR).[17] The high-energy gamma emission of ^{198}Au necessitated inpatient isolation and the radionuclide is no longer available in most countries.

Intrapericardial therapy

Following pericardiocentesis in patients with pericardial effusions, 185–1100 MBq (5–30 mCi) of ^{32}P colloid is instilled. A success rate between 40 and 91% in stopping the reaccumulation of the effusions has been reported.[18,19] No severe side-effects occurred, but constrictive pericarditis following repeated intrapericardial injections of the tracer was observed.

Intrapleural therapy

Instillation of cytostatics or radionuclides into the pleural space should be regarded as palliative therapy in patients with malignant effusions, although this approach may be more effective in mesothelioma. Very few series of patients with malignant pleural effusion treated with instillation of cytostatics have been reported. Mitoxantrone is suitable because of its low lipophilicity and low pleural clearance. In 67–93% complete or partial remission was observed without any side-effects. The results seem to be dose dependent.[20,21] Similar results have been reported for radionuclide therapy, instilling 220–370 MBq (6–10 mCi) of ^{32}P or 2.5–4.0 GBq (68–110 mCi) of ^{90}Y per pleural cavity, directly into the effusion or after mixing with sodium chloride. Before instillation, an injection of diagnostic radiocolloid is recommended to avoid focal accumulation of the therapeutic dose by non-uniform tracer distribution. During the first 6–8 h after instillation the patient should change position to guarantee a homogeneous tracer distribution and fixation to the parietal and visceral pleura. Effectiveness was observed in 50–74%,[22,23] but had no significant influence on the survival rate of metastatic carcinomas. In constrast to ^{198}Au, which caused myelosuppression in rare cases, no side-effects were reported for ^{32}P and ^{90}Y.

Intraperitoneal therapy

Intraperitoneal instillation may be performed as adjuvant therapy in patients with ovarian carcinoma following first surgical procedure or after second-look laparotomy in stage I (FIGO classification) to prevent tumour expansion from single cells.[24] Patients with malignant ovarian cancer benefit from chemotherapy followed by radionuclide therapy. Even bulky metastases may be cured by adjuvant radionuclide therapy following systemic chemotherapy. This procedure, however, has to be considered as palliative therapy of malignant effusions.

370 MBq to 4.0 GBq (10–110 mCi) of ^{32}P colloid or 2.5–4.0 GBq (68–110 mCi) of ^{90}Y in a volume of >100 ml sodium chloride should be infused. Prior scintigraphy with ^{99m}Tc-labelled colloid is recommended to show uniform distribution of the tracer over the serosal surface. Frequent turning of the patient ensures uniform distribution of the administered radionuclide. The estimated dose to the peritoneum is about 30 Gy per 370 MBq (10 mCi) of ^{32}P. The therapeutic effect is dose dependent. Using high doses of ^{198}Au (>7.4 GBq) (>200 mCi) the 5-year survival rate increased to 47.5% from 31.4% with <7.4 GBq (<200 mCi). Further improvement may be observed by combining radionuclide therapy with external beam irradiation and/or chemotherapy.[24]

In 29 patients with minimal residual disease (<2 cm) 4-year survival rates for ^{32}P therapy combined with chemotherapy were 50%, for chemotherapy alone 22%.[23] The effectivity in patients with malignant effusion is about 85%. In rare cases only (5%) severe side-effects (mostly ileus) were observed after ^{198}Au therapy. ^{32}P and ^{90}Y cause fewer side-effects. Complications were described after combining external beam irradiation prior to intraperitoneal ^{32}P, perhaps as a result of focal accumulation of the radiotracer.

INTRA-ARTICULAR THERAPY

For local treatment of rheumatoid synovitis several approaches exist. Intra-articular injection of corticosteroids or cytostatics result in only temporary improvement in most patients. Patients with persistent synovial effusions due to rheumatoid arthritis and other inflammatory joint diseases, pigmented villonodular synovitis and haemophilic joint diseases which do not respond to conservative treatment within 6 months should be managed with radionuclide synoviorthesis or surgical synovectomy. This form of radionuclide therapy is discussed in Chapter 88.

REFERENCES

1. Shapiro B, Fig L M, Carpi A 1992 General principles and perspectives of cancer therapy with radiopharmaceuticals. In: Carpi A, Sagripanti A, Mittermayer C (eds) Progress in clinical oncology. Sympomed, Munich, pp 68–111
2. Shapiro B, Fig L M, Carey J, Kallus M, Taren J, Hood T 1990 Intracavitary therapy of cystic brain tumors with P-32 chromic phosphate colloid. In: Schmidt H A E, Chambron J (eds) Nuclear medicine. Quantitative analysis in imaging and function. Schattauer, Stuttgart, pp 574–576
3. Askienazy S, Turak B, Piketty M L et al 1990 Colloidal 186Re in the endocavitary irradiation of cystic craniopharyngiomas. J Nucl Med 31: S143
4. Taasan V, Shapiro B, Taren J A et al 1985 Phosphorus-32 therapy of cystic Grade IV astrocytomas: technique and preliminary application. J Nucl Med 26: 1335–1338
5. Bernstein M, Gutin P H 1985 Interstitial irradiation of skull base tumors. Can J Neurol Sci 12: 366–370
6. Kobayashi T, Kageyama N, Ohara K 1981 Internal irradiation for cystic craniopharyngiomas. J Neurosurg 55: 896–903
7. Kallus M A, Fig L M, Arcamano M, Hood T, Taren J A, Shapiro B 1989 Treatment of cystic brain tumor: distribution of 32-P-chromic phosphate colloid (32-P-CPC) in cyst fluid. J Nucl Med 30: 833
8. Rentsch M, Triller J, Rosler H, Geiger L, Noelpp U, Baer H U 1990 Ein Tumor-retentionsregister für Microsphären als Grundlage für die selektive Radionuklidembolisierungstherapie von Tumoren mit 90-yttrium Microspharen. In: Höfer R, Bergmann H, Sinzinger H (eds) Radioaktive Isotope in Klinik und Forschung. Badgastein, pp 12–13
9. Park C H, Yoo H S, Suh J H 1990 Critical evaluation of I-131-lipiodol therapy for hepatocellular carcinoma. Eur J Nucl Med 16: S143
10. Le Jeune J J, Bourget P, Victor G, Therain F, Lemaire B, Collet H 1990 I-131 lipiodol in the treatment of hepatocellular carcinoma: results of a multicenter phase II study of fifty patients. Eur J Nucl Med 16: S143
11. Roberson P L, Ten Haken R K, McShan D L, McKeever P E, Ensminger W D 1992 Three-dimensional tumor dosimetry for hepatic yttrium-90-microsphere therapy. J Nucl Med 33: 735–738
12. Gray B N, Burton M A, Kelleher D, Matz L 1990 Tolerance of the liver to the effects of yttrium-90 radiation. Int J Radiat Oncol Biol Phys 18: 619–623
13. Herba M J, Illescas F F, Thirwell M P et al 1988 Hepatic malignancies: improved treatment with intraarterial Y-90. Radiology 169: 311–314
14. Houle S, Yip K, Shepperd F A, Rotstein L E, Paul K, Sniderman K W 1990 Intraarterial yttrium-90 glass microspheres for internal radiation therapy of hepatocellular carcinoma. Eur J Nucl Med 16: S142
15. Levin B 1987 Locoregional therapy: what are we learning about its limitations and future applications? In: Seeber S, Aigner K R, Enghofer E (eds) Die lokoregionale Tumortherapie. De Gruyter, Berlin, pp 5–11
16. Loffler T 1987 Intraperitoneale Chemotherapie: Grundlagen, pharmakologische Aspekte, Kathetertechnik und Behandlungsindikationen. In: Seeber S, Aigner K R, Enghofer E (eds) Die lokoregionale Tumortherapie. De Gruyter, Berlin, 51–60
17. Gatley S J, Harper P V, Stark V, Pan M-L, DeSombre E R 1989 On the suitability of I-123 and Br-80m Halodeoxyuridines (XUdR) for Auger electron radiotherapy of intraperitoneal cancer. J Nucl Med 30: 833
18. Firusian N 1980 32-P-therapy for malignant pericardial effusion. Onkologie 3: 12–17
19. Hermann H J 1982 Nuklearmedizin. Urban & Schwarzenberg, Munich.
20. Hoffman W, Hansmann E, Weidmann B, Osieka R, Seeber S 1987 Experimentelle und klinische Erfahrungen zur intrakavitaren Tumortherapie mit Mitoxantron (Novantron). In: Seeber S, Aigner K R, Enghofer E (eds) Die lokoregionale Tumortherapie. De Gruyter, Berlin, pp 95–102
21. Musch E, Mackes K G, Bode U, Werner A, Merkle E, Peiss J 1987 Intrapleurale Applikation von Mitoxantron. In: Seeber S, Aigner K R, Enghofer E (eds) Die lokoregionale Tumortherapie. De Gruyter, Berlin, pp 71–80
22. Biersack H J 1979 Die Behandlung der Pleuritis carcinomatosa mit Radionukliden. Der Nuklearmediziner 2: 268–275
23. Hoefnagel C A 1991 Radionuclide therapy revisited. Eur J Nucl Med 18: 408–431
24. Vahrson H 1979 Radiogold/-yttrium-Behandlung der Peritonitis carcinomatosa. De Nuklearmediziner 2: 276–283

78. Functional analysis of cancer therapy effects in other organs

R. A. Valdés Olmos

In clinical oncology, nuclear medicine functional studies are performed for monitoring of organ function and detection of injury related to cancer therapy.[1] In two of the major modalities of cancer therapy, radiotherapy and chemotherapy, there is an increasing tendency to intensify the anti-tumour effect with a curative intent which may be associated with a higher risk of injury to normal organs and tissues, and possible deterioration of the quality of life of the patient. Moreover, to overcome toxicity of normal organs, new cancer therapy regimens have, over the last decade, incorporated a wide spectrum of alternatives varying from new anti-cancer drugs, protective agents, antiemetics, and biological response modifiers to bone marrow transplantation and use of various haematopoietic growth factors.[2,3] All this makes it necessary in clinical nuclear medicine to recognize not only the toxic effects of conventional cancer therapy but also the modified organ response associated with complementary treatment.

CARDIAC INJURY

The most frequently observed condition of iatrogenic cardiac damage in oncology is the cardiotoxicity by chemotherapy containing anthracyclines. Rarely, administration of chemotherapy, such as that containing vinca alkaloids, cisplatin, cyclophosphamide or 5-fluouracil, can lead to myocardial ischaemia and infarct.[4] A less documented entity is the radiation-induced cardiac injury; in contrast to cardiotoxicity by anthracyclines, in which histological myocyte damage correlates with the cumulative dose,[5] the radiation effect is mainly focused on the myocardial capillaries and less frequently the coronary macrovasculature.[6]

Anthracycline-associated cardiotoxicity

The principal anthracycline cardiotoxicity is a dose-dependent chronic condition characterized by progressive, mostly irreversible, left ventricular dysfunction which can lead to overt heart failure and cardiomyopathy. The prevalence of congestive heart failure increases from <2% at a total cumulative dose up to 400 mg/m^2 to more than 20% at 700 mg/m^2 or over.[7] Serial monitoring of the systolic heart function by determination of the left ventricular ejection fraction (LVEF) at rest remains the parameter most used to detect early cardiotoxicity. Since congestive heart failure is preceded by a progressive drop in LVEF, discontinuation of anthracycline therapy is recommended after an absolute decrease in LVEF by 10 EF units or more from baseline or when LVEF declines below 50% (or 30% in cases with abnormal baseline). This does reduce the incidence and the severity of congestive heart failure considerably.[8] LVEF decrease must be interpreted with caution, however, as variations may be caused by differences in the angulation of the camera, data processing and radiopharmaceuticals used.[9] The sympathetic tone fluctuations and emotional stress may also induce significant variations in the LVEF. To distinguish the chronic dose-dependent cardiac dysfunction from transient positive inotropic effects observed during or shortly after anthracycline administration[10] or occasional acute reversible cardiodepressive effects mostly associated with ECG abnormalities,[11] LVEF studies must be performed at least 3 weeks after a previous chemotherapeutic course. Diagnosis of cardiotoxicity may be improved by the detection of wall motion abnormalities, especially in the anteroseptal ventricular areas,[12,13] or early changes in the peak filling rate (PFR) of the left ventricle[14,15] which may precede LVEF decline. The contribution of exercise LVEF to the detection of cardiotoxicity remains controversial[16] and is frequently impractical, for example in many patients with advanced cancer, an optimal performance of exercise may be difficult.

Adverse anthracycline effects on the heart pump function may be reduced when the drug is administered by continous infusion rather than by bolus injection[17] or when cardioprotective agents such as the iron-chelating bispiperazinedione ICRF-187 is added to the chemotherapeutic scheme.[18]

In spite of well-established LVEF criteria to overcome

anthracycline-associated cardiotoxicity, the overall probability of developing congestive heart failure is still considerable (Fig. 78.1) and the high incidence of late cardiac sequelae recently reported in long-term survivors who had received chemotherapy containing anthracyclines for leukaemia and osteosarcoma[19–21] implies that long-lasting subclinical injury is not uncommon and may possess a high risk when retreatment with anthracyclines is required. The current trend of treatment intensification and increasing chances of prolonged survival for a significant number of patients calls for more sensitive, reliable and non-invasive methods to assess cardiac injury, replacing invasive procedures such as endomyocardial biopsy, which until now has been the only technique able to correlate abnormal cellular changes with the cumulative anthracycline dose. The introduction of ^{111}In-labelled anti-myosin antibody (Fab) in cardiotoxicity has facilitated the direct visualization of heart muscle cell injury since the tracer

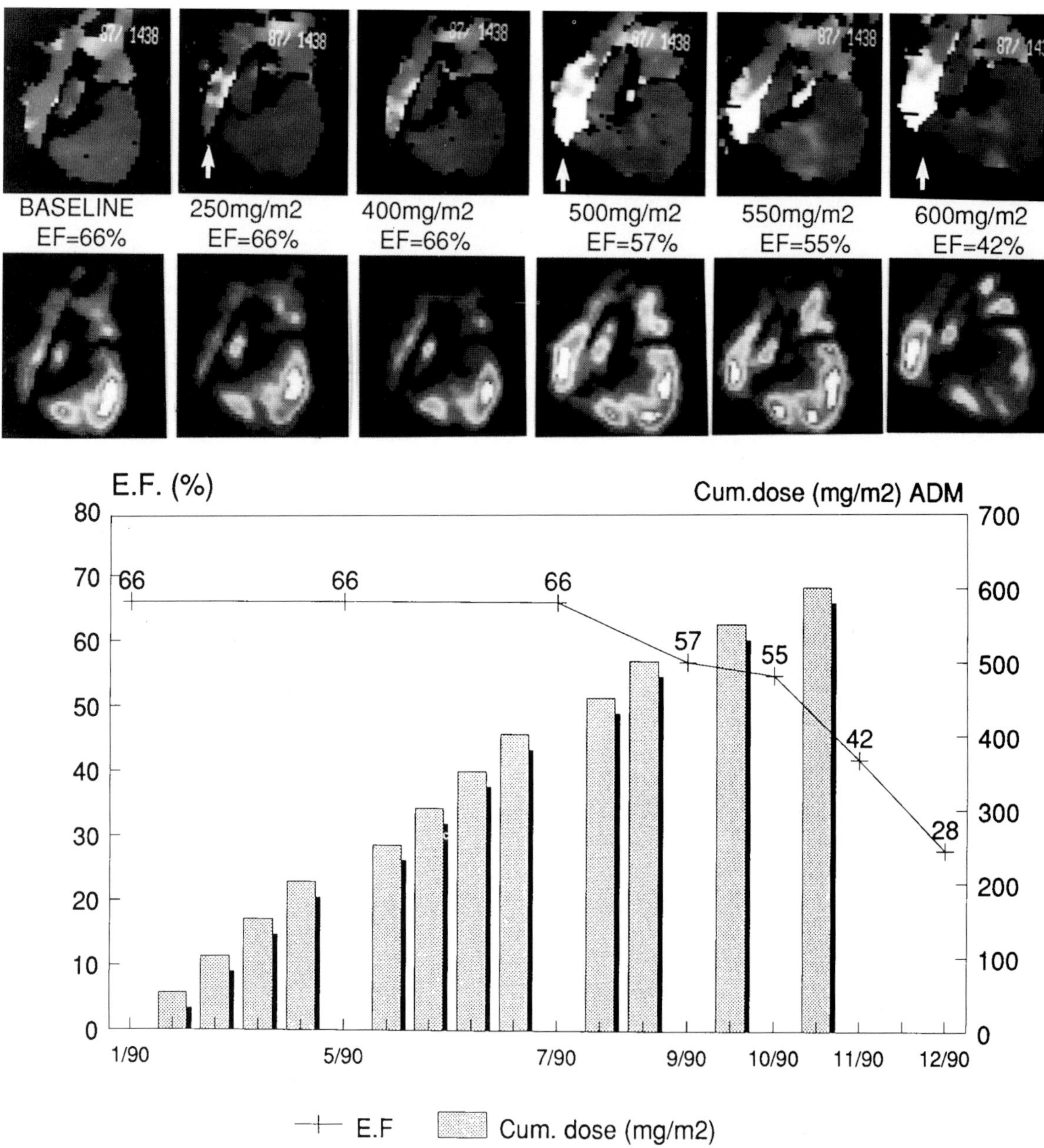

Fig. 78.1 Anthracycline-related cardiotoxicity. Serial measurements of LVEF in a 36-year-old patient treated with doxorubicin for advanced breast carcinoma; in spite of the discontinuation of therapy after initial decline of LVEF to 42% at 600 mg/m^2, a more pronounced LVEF decrease indicates irreversible damage leading to overt congestive heart failure. Sequential LAO Fourier phase–amplitude images show progressive abnormal phase changes (arrows) and subsequent dilation of the right atrium accompanied by increasing ventricular amplitude deterioration and dilation, principally of the left ventricle. Note that focal changes precede deterioration of global LVEF.

binds to myosin when the myocyte has been irreversibly damaged by doxorubicin administration.[22] The degree of anti-myosin myocardial uptake, measured by 48 h heart-to-lung ratios on planar anterior images, correlates with the cumulative dose of anthracycline,[23] and intensive uptake, with ratios higher than 1.9, may predict onset of congestive heart failure before LVEF deterioration.[24] Complementary planar LAO and SPECT images may be useful to demonstrate anti-myosin uptake by the myocardium, which may persist for a few months after cessation of chemotherapy,[25] and to study its distribution pattern, which is mostly diffuse (Fig. 78.2). Damage of the cardiac neurones by anthracyclines has been reported to occur prior to myocyte impairment: the myocardial accumulation of ^{125}I-MIBG at 4 h reflects the adrenergic neuronal intravesicular concentration, and a doxorubicin dose-dependent decrease in this parameter may indicate neurone injury.[26] The myocardial adrenergic derangement appears to correlate with the severity of LVEF decrease in cardiotoxicity[1,27] with an increase in the 4-h ^{123}I-MIBG washout values (Fig. 78.3).

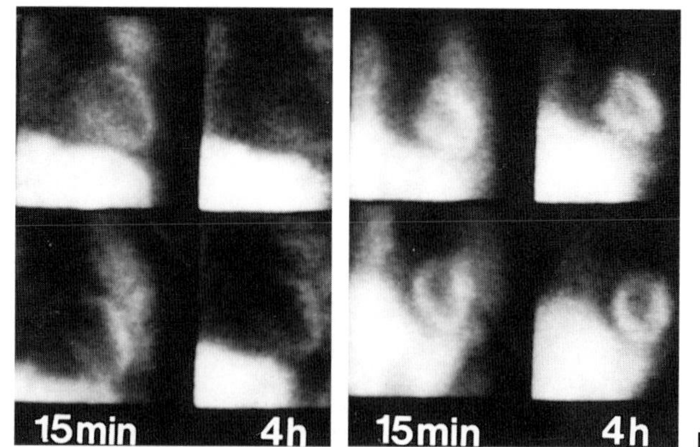

Fig. 78.3 Planar ^{123}I-MIBG heart scintigraphy (anterior and LAO views) showing reduced uptake and decreased 4 h myocardial retention, indicating myocardial adrenergic derangement, in a 37-year-old patient who had developed severe cardiotoxicity (A); in contrast (B), in another patient with normal LVEF at 300 mg/m^2, uptake and myocardial retention are not abnormal. (Reproduced with permission from Valdés Olmos et al.[1])

Radiation-induced cardiac damage

The incidence of radiation pericarditis and other clinical events after radiotherapy of the thorax has diminished significantly since the improvement in irradiation techniques. However, the risk of subclinical injury remains, since modern methods of mantle field planning in Hodgkin's disease may include more than 50% of the heart, and the proportion tends to increase when extensive mediastinal disease must be irradiated. In breast cancer, irradiation of the internal mammary nodes may involve 20–30% of the heart within the high-dose region, particularly when the left chain is irradiated. A cardiodepressive effect may be observed shortly after irradiation, and LVEF tends to decrease with recovery of the function only 2 months later.[28]

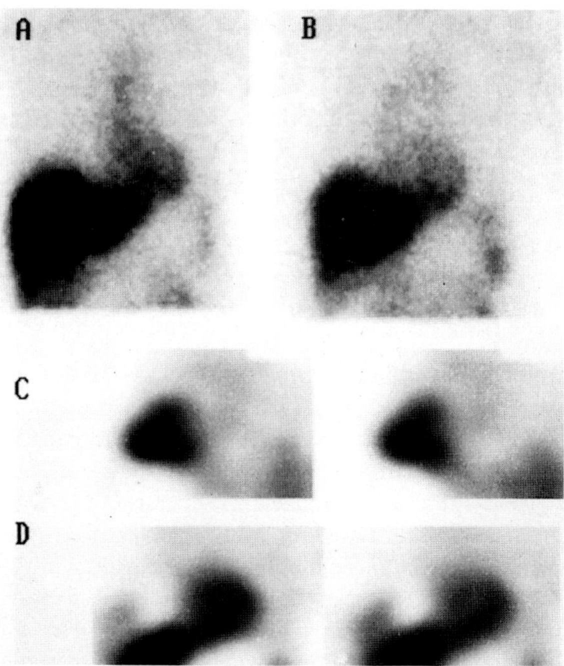

Fig. 78.2 Anterior (A), LAO (B) and SPECT (C and D) images showing intensive uptake of ^{111}In anti-myosin in the left ventricle in a 58-year-old patient who had developed moderate cardiotoxicity during doxorubicin treatment. Note, on SPECT slices, that myocardial damage is diffuse.

Damage to the myocardial capillaries by radiation is a slowly developing process over several years, leading to progressive myocardial fibrosis and late cardiac dysfunction with abnormal LVEF at rest, impaired LVEF response at exercise, contractility abnormalities and PFR reduction.[29,30] In patients with radiation-induced small-vessel disease, reversible perfusion defects on ^{201}Tl SPECT, anatomically not correlated with the epicardial coronary vessels, may be observed, whereas in cases of persistent defects myocardial fibrosis must be considered.[31]

KIDNEY TOXICITY

Cisplatin and ifosfamide are the chemotherapeutic drugs most likely to cause renal damage, especially in children. Radiotherapy of abdominal malignancies involving the kidneys frequently leads to radiation nephropathy.

Chemotherapy-induced tubular injury

Cisplatin, essential in the therapy of germ cell tumours, and ifosfamide, effective against solid tumours, especially in children, are both nephrotoxic in a dose-dependent manner.[32] In the case of cisplatin, proximal tubular

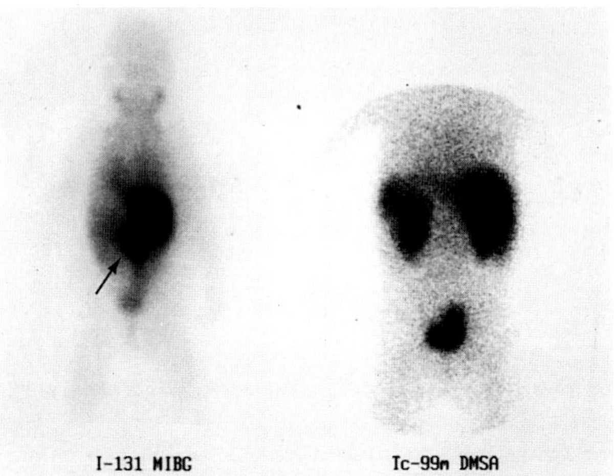

Fig. 78.4 Severe ifosfamide-induced nephrotoxicity in a 4-year-old patient who had been treated for inoperable neuroblastoma (indicated by an arrow on the ^{131}I-MIBG posterior image). On the ^{99m}Tc-DMSA posterior image, reduced kidney uptake and increased liver/spleen activity are observed. Kidney retention is also decreased with abnormal increased bladder accumulation.

impairment precedes alterations in glomerular filtration rate and effective plasma renal flow, and its early detection by laboratory measurements has been advocated, together with the induction of diuresis by infusion of mannitol and saline or frusemide, and the use of the new platinum derivatives such as carboplatin, as a strategy to overcome nephrotoxic effects.[33] The use of ifosfamide has been associated with the development of Fanconi's syndrome, a generalized disorder of the proximal tubule of the kidney (Fig. 78.4).[34] Progressive diminishment of ^{99m}Tc-DMSA absolute kidney uptake may be observed when the cumulative ifosfamide dose increases, showing a better correlation than other indicators of tubular function such as serial measurements of urine levels of beta-2-microglobulin.[35] Decline of ^{99m}Tc-DMSA uptake at low cumulative ifosfamide doses may be transient and function tends to recover after drug discontinuation, but when treatment is restarted a more pronounced and pesistent decrease indicates irreversible tubular damage (Fig. 78.5).

Radiation nephropathy

Radiation-induced kidney damage may involve the endothelial cells of the glomeruli, the parenchymal cells or the renal tubules. The nephropathy often progresses slowly, in a number of cases leading to complete atrophy of the irradiated renal tissue, and its clinical course may be complicated by anaemia, hypertension or renal failure. Divided renal function by renography may be useful to document unilateral nephropathy, but when both kidneys are irradiated, absolute ^{99m}Tc-DMSA kidney uptake can assess the extent of renal injury better.[36] In patients with non-Hodgkin's lymphoma of the stomach whose left kidney is irradiated with doses higher than 40 Gy, a decline of the renal function is observed from approximately 6 months after irradiation onwards, decreasing to about 30% of pretreatment ^{99m}Tc-DMSA uptake values by 30–54 months.[37] In patients irradiated for vertebral or rib malignancies, kidney areas included in the radiation fields may show transient increased uptake on bone scintigraphy.[38] Progressive kidney dysfunction in unilateral radiation nephropathy, frequently accompanied by compensatory increased function of the contralateral kidney, can lead to irreversible total loss of function of the affected kidney (Fig. 78.6) and eventually to hypertension.[39]

LUNG DAMAGE

Bleomycin is the chemotherapeutic agent most commonly associated with lung toxicity. Other agents which may cause pulmonary toxicity are nitrosoureas, cyclophosphamide, busulphan and methotrexate. In radiotherapy, lung injury may be associated with any treatment involving the thoracic region.

Chemotherapy-associated pulmonary toxicity

The lung toxicity of bleomycin and nitrosoureas, which is characterized by alveolar epithelial disruption, intra-alveolar fluid and protein leakage, and focal necrosis of type I pneumocytes in the early phase, is related to the cumulative dose and may lead to pulmonary fibrosis in the late period.

In the early period of the disease, accumulation of ^{67}Ga is frequently found and scintigraphy may be used to assess the extent and severity of toxicity by bleomycin,[40] nitrosureas[41] and other agents such as cyclophosphamide.[42] Increased permeability in injured lung areas may be observed on ^{99m}Tc-DTPA aerosol studies.[43,44]

Adverse lung effects of thoracic irradiation

In radiotherapy of chest malignancies, radiation pneumonitis may appear 2–6 months after irradiation and lung fibrosis may occur after 6 months. Besides causing injury of the type II pneumocytes and the capillary endothelial cells, irradiation also induces the persistent release of fibroblast stimulant cytokines from alveolar macrophages, which may enhance the late pulmonary interstitial fibrosis.[45] ^{67}Ga, in contrast to chest radiographs, is almost invariably abnormal in cases of clinical radiation pneumonitis, and in 20% of the asymptomatic irradiated patients. In the latter category, scans return to normal within 5 months, and in symptomatic patients ^{67}Ga follow-up may be useful to assess the response to steroid therapy.[46] In our experience at the Netherlands Cancer Institute increased uptake of

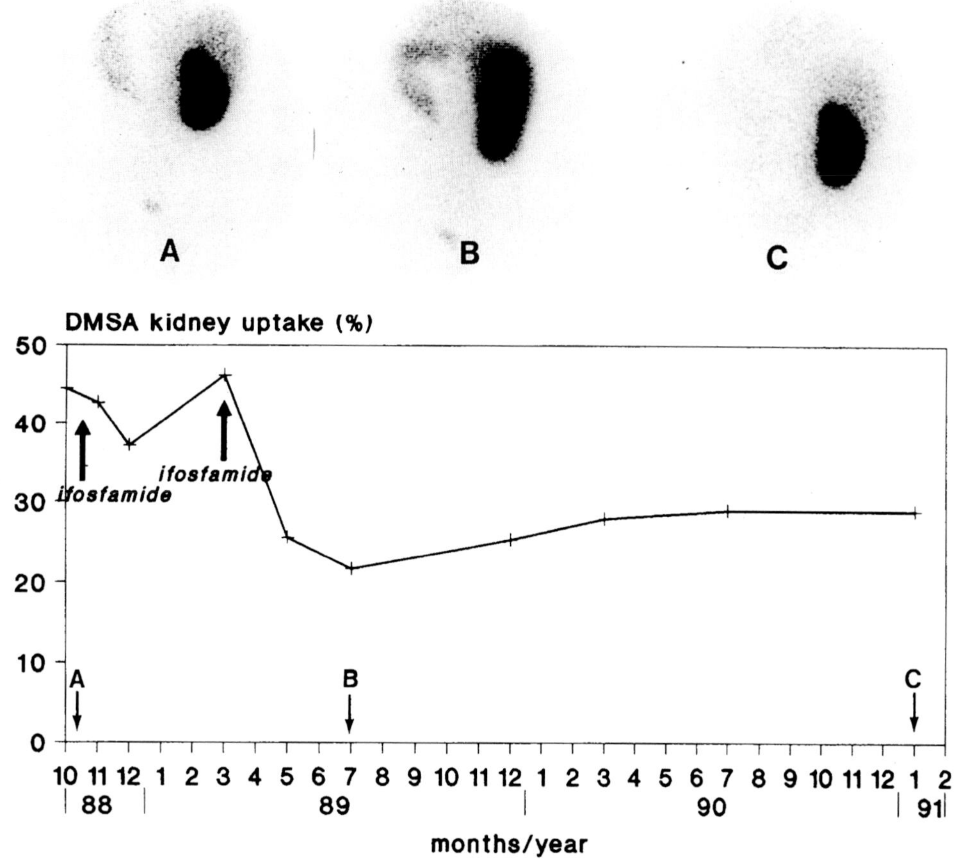

Fig. 78.5 Ifosfamide-induced tubular injury. Serial ^{99m}Tc-DMSA absolute kidney uptake in a 5-year-old patient showing transient decline and recovery of uptake to normal values after initial courses of chemotherapy; after restarting the treatment, a more pronounced decrease of the function without complete recovery after 2 years indicates irreversible tubular damage. Note the diminished uptake of the right kidney on sequential posterior scintigrams initially accompanied by increased liver activity. Left kidney has been resected because of a nephroblastoma.

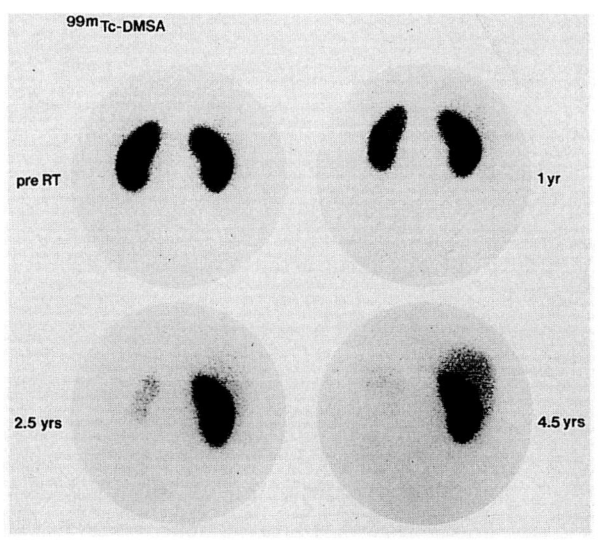

Fig. 78.6 The 'vanishing kidney' in a radiation nephropathy. Scintigraphic 5 year follow-up of kidney function with ^{99m}Tc-DMSA in an adult patient treated for a malignant lymphoma of the stomach, showing progressive loss of function of the left kidney, which had received a high irradiation dose (40 Gy). The right kidney, irradiated with 13 Gy, remains normal and even shows compensatory hypertrophy. (Reproduced with permission from Valdés Olmos et al.[1])

^{111}In-octreotide in normal lung tissues may also be observed shortly after radiotherapy of thoracic malignancies. After mantle field irradiation for Hodgkin's disease, loss of lung perfusion in irradiated areas is usually more pronounced than ventilation changes,[47] and may be accompanied in cases of radiation pneumonitis by altered permeability.[48]

DIGESTIVE TRACT

The most frequent acute gastrointestinal toxicities from cancer therapy are chemotherapy-induced nausea and vomiting. Less frequent is acute ulceration and diarrhoea, which can occur with both radiotherapy and chemotherapy. Nuclear medicine procedures are most often ordered by clinicians for recognizing the late radiation-induced small bowel injuries, and, less frequently, for the assessment of injuries to the liver, oesophagus and large bowel.

Small bowel radiation damage

Generally, the early effects of bowel irradiation reflect

epithelial stem cell injury, whereas the late effects are predominantly the results of slowly evolving vascular injury. The latent period between completion of the course of radiotherapy and the subsequent development of late bowel damage is usually 6–24 months.[49] In damage of the small bowel, diarrhoea is the most frequent symptom, which is principally caused by bile acid malabsorption as a result of terminal ileitis or ileal resection; however, in a number of patients diarrhoea may be caused by intraluminal bacterial overgrowth by stasis due to strictures, fistulas or resection. In patients with bile acid malabsorption ^{75}Se-HCAT retention is abnormally reduced, and when this test is combined with a test sensitive for colonization (e.g. one of the breath tests or the Schilling test) cases with bacterial overgrowth may be differentiated. This may facilitate how to treat the diarrhoea: by cholestyramine and/or antibiotics.[50–53] The ^{75}Se-HCAT test may also be helpful to evaluate the effect of alternative anti-diarrhoea agents such as loperamide which, by prolonging the intestinal transit, may improve the bile acid absorption in the remnant distal ileum of patients without extensive ileal injury and thereby the clinical condition.[54]

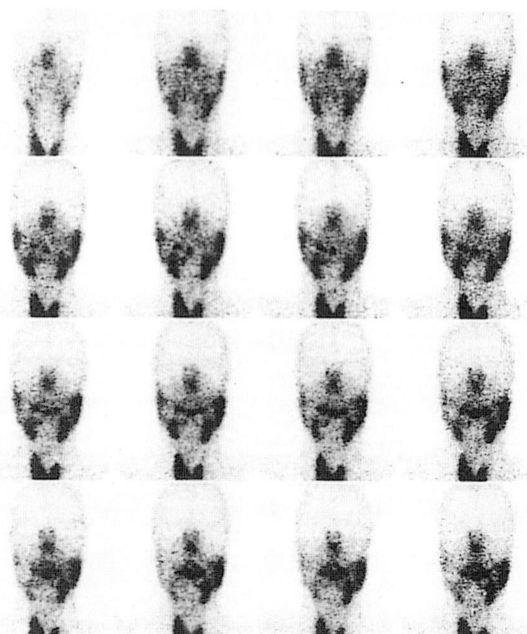

Fig. 78.7 Sequential ^{99m}Tc salivary scintigraphy of an adult patient showing a normal excretion response of the salivary glands of the non-irradiated right side after carbachol stimulation. By contrast, the salivary glands of the left side, which had been irradiated with a dose of 40 Gy, show impaired excretion response.

SALIVARY GLANDS

Post-irradiation xerostomia is an important side-effect of radiotherapy of head and neck cancer, leading to chronic oral disease with subjective distress, and a pronounced decrease in quality of life. The condition may be aggravated by poor oral hygiene, soft-tissue ulcerations, dental caries and tooth decay, may lead to osteoradionecrosis of the mandible and may predispose to oesophageal injury as a result of decreased acid clearance from the oesophagus. The principal radiation-induced damage occurs in the acinar and ductal systems.[55] The salivary glands possess an iodide-trapping mechanism which is radioresistant up to about 30 Gy, and since ^{99m}Tc pertechnetate, like radioiodine, is concentrated in the intralobular ductule cells, sequential ^{99m}Tc scintigraphy is particularly useful to study the effects of radiation (Fig. 78.7). The uptake of ^{99m}Tc by the major salivary glands decreases progressively after radiation doses higher than 50 Gy,[56] and the excretion response to the parasympathetic stimulant carbachol, not impaired below 25 Gy, is often reduced at higher radiation levels and becomes almost invariably abnormal above 45 Gy.[1] Salivary dysfunction may also occur after therapy of thyroid carcinoma with more than 5.55 GBq of ^{131}I,[57] and is almost always present after treatment with cumulative doses over 37 GBq.[58] In radiation-induced sialadenitis, an acute disorder after radiotherapy, increased ^{67}Ga uptake, frequently found in the affected gland, usually decreases after 6 months.[59]

SKELETON AND BONE MARROW

Bone marrow toxicity is one of the major adverse effects of cancer therapy. Bone marrow regeneration after radiotherapy, as studied by ^{111}In chloride scintigraphy, appears to depend on age and is significantly greater in patients under 18 years.[60] When large volumes are irradiated, bone marrow ablation may occur in the radiation fields, but non-irradiated bone marrow may become more active, for instance in femora and humeri.[3] In irradiated areas (Fig. 78.8), bone or bone marrow scintigraphy usually shows diffusely reduced uptake[61,62] which coincides with MRI findings.[63] Bone uptake of non-irradiated areas tends to decrease too, although this can only be perceived by quantitative measurements,[64] and may be influenced by bed rest.[65] In children and adolescents, irradiation may affect the growing skeleton, contributing to a decrease in final height.[66]

In chemotherapy, the flare response of bone metastases with increased uptake in bone lesions, considered to be an expression of a favourable osteoblastic response to treatment, is the most frequent short-term induced effect.[67] When chemotherapy is combined with haematopoietic growth factors to reduce myelotoxicity, diffuse increased bone uptake, probably to be explained by bone marrow changes, may be observed in addition to the flare response.[68]

An additional serious cause of morbidity in patients with potentially curative benefit from chemotherapy,

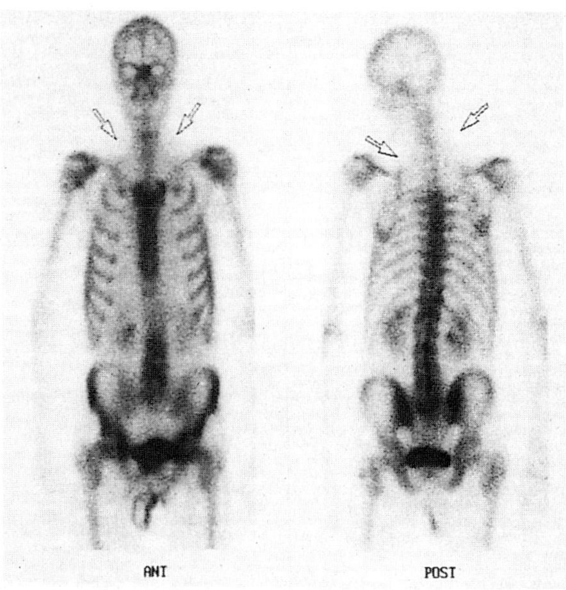

Fig. 78.8 Characteristic decreased bone uptake in irradiated skeleton areas (arrows) of an adult patient who had received radiotherapy for advanced breast carcinoma 1 year previously.

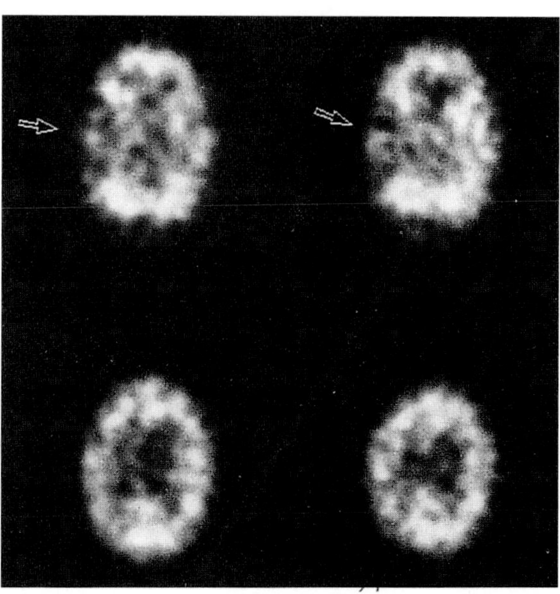

Fig. 78.9 Transaxial ^{99m}Tc-HMPAO SPECT slices showing reduced brain perfusion (arrows) due to necrosis in a patient who had received external beam irradiation for an astrocytoma 19 months previously.

radiotherapy or high-dose corticosteroids, such as used in the treatment of Hodgkin's lymphoma, is the onset of osteonecrosis, which mostly affects the femoral heads, and less frequently the humeral head, mandible and knees. Very early in the development of this condition, bone scintigraphy may show either a photon deficiency at the necrosis site or the 'doughnut sign' with increased activity surrounding the necrotic centre.[69]

ADVERSE BRAIN EFFECTS

Radiation necrosis, which may be progressive and lethal, is the major dose-limiting complication of brain irradiation. Combined radiotherapy and chemotherapy may lead to leucoencephalopathy. In contrast to transient adverse effects occurring shortly after radiation, late radiation injury is mostly progressive and irreversible and may be fatal.[70] Most radiation injuries reflect events occurring in the vasculoconnective tissue stroma and not in functioning mature nerve cells, whereas chemotherapy, sparing the vasculature, is cytoxic by acting directly on the glial cells and may produce diffuse white matter necrosis.[3] A particular sequel of brain irradiation is the expression of adverse neurocognitive effects, with decline of IQ scores, in children treated for brain tumours.[71] On PET scintigraphy, and also on SPECT (Fig. 78.9), late radiation necrosis is accompanied by reduced metabolism and perfusion in areas in which the blood–brain barrier is defective.[72] In patients with clinical deterioration the scintigraphic demonstration of diminished metabolism in irradiated tumour sites is an essential aid to distinguish areas of necrosis from tumour recurrence, which is usually associated with increased metabolism; CT and/or MRI, after treatment, are usually non-conclusive in this respect.[73,74]

Administration of cytokine biological response modifiers, such as interleukin 2, may be associated with the development of parkinsonian rigidity, depression or dementia which is mostly accompanied by changes in the

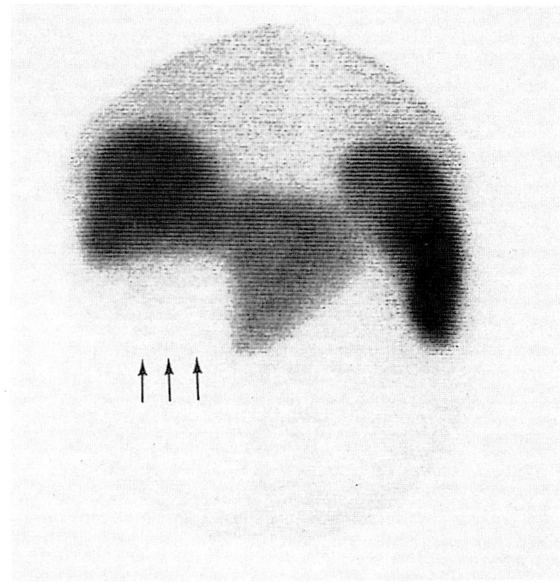

Fig. 78.10 Radiation injury to the liver in an adult patient who had received 60 Gy for a gall bladder carcinoma 4 months before the radiocolloid scan, seen as a large filling defect in the inferior area of the right lobe (arrows) which had been included in the radiation fields. Ultrasonography and CT had been unable to demonstrate abnormalities. (Reproduced with permission from Valdés Olmos et al.[1])

distribution of ^{99m}Tc-HMPAO in frontal, parietal and basal ganglia areas.[75]

MISCELLANEOUS

The steadily increasing number of patients considered cured of cancer makes continuous surveillance and characterization of adverse cancer therapy effects imperative. In long-term survivors of childhood cancer, estimated to be 1 in 900 young adults by the year 2000, a great variety of impairments, affecting practically every organ system, has gradually been identified.[76,77] In addition to the injuries described above, adverse effects of irradiation on thyroid function may be expected in patients receiving more than 26 Gy to the thorax and neck[66] and scintigraphy with ^{99m}Tc or ^{123}I may be helpful to identify radiation lesions to the thyroid or induced hypothyroidism, whereas ^{67}Ga may enable the localization of inflammatory areas. In liver injury, ^{99m}Tc colloid may show the loss of function of the part of the liver involved in the radiation field (Fig. 78.10), which frequently leads to late atrophy of the entire lobe.[1] The most common chemotherapy-associated long-term liver injury may be observed following treatment with methotrexate and 6-mercaptopurine.[78] In cases of severe toxicity accompanied by hepatocellular necrosis and bile stasis, evaluation using hepatobiliary agents such as ^{99m}Tc-IDA derivatives may be useful, whereas in cases of chemotherapy-associated hepatic veno-occlusive disease,[4] liver scintigraphy using ^{99m}Tc colloid is helpful. In radiation-induced enterocolitis, areas of increased inflammatory activity in small bowel and colon may be localized using labelled leucocytes,[79] and in post-irradiation oesophagitis coating of ^{99m}Tc sucralphate may help to document ulcerations.[1]

REFERENCES

1. Valdés Olmos R A, Hoefnagel C A, Van der Schoot J B 1993 Nuclear medicine in monitoring of organ function and detection of injury related to cancer therapy. Eur J Nucl Med 20: 515–546
2. Powis G P 1991 Toxicity of anticancer drugs to humans: a unique opportunity to study human toxicology. In : Powis M, Hacker M P (eds) The toxicity of anticancer drugs. Pergamon Press, New York, pp 1–8
3. Rubin P, Constine L S, Nelson D F 1992 Late effects of cancer treatment: radiation and drug toxicity. In: Perez C A, Brady L W (eds) Principles and practice of radiation oncology. Lippincot, Philadelphia, pp 124–161
4. Doll D C, Yarbro J W 1992 Vascular toxicity associated with antineoplastic agents. Semin Oncol 19: 580–596
5. Billingham M E, Mason J W, Bristow M R, Daniels J R 1978 Anthracycline cardiomyopathy monitored by morphologic changes. Cancer Treat Rep 62: 865–872
6. Awad H K 1991 Late reacting tissues: radiation-induced heart disease. In: Awad H K (ed) Radiation oncology. Kluwer, Dordrecht, pp 449–456
7. Legha S S, Benjamin R S, Mackay B et al 1982 Reduction of doxorubicin-induced congestive heart failure. Ann Intern Med 96: 133–139
8. Schwartz R G, McKenzie W B, Alexander J et al 1987 Congestive heart failure and left ventricular dysfunction complicating doxorubicin therapy. Seven-year experience using serial radionuclide angiocardiography. Am J Med 82: 1109–1118
9. Dey H M, Kassamali H 1988 Radionuclide evaluation of doxorubicin cardiotoxicity: the need for cautious interpretation. Clin Nucl Med 13: 565–568
10. Pauwels E K J, Horning S J, Goris M L 1983 Sequential equilibrium gated radionuclide angiocardiography for the detection of doxorubicin cardiotoxicity. Radiother Oncol 1: 83–87
11. Strashun A 1992 Adriamycin, congestive cardiomyopathy, and metaiodobenzylguanidine. J Nucl Med 2: 215–220
12. Alcan K E, Robeson W, Graham M C, Palestro C, Oliver F H, Benua R S 1985 Early detection of anthracycline-induced cardiotoxicity by stress radionuclide cineangiography in conjunction with Fourier amplitude and phase analysis. Clin Nucl Med 10: 160–166
13. Barendswaard E C, Prpic H, van der Wall E E, Camps J A J, Keyzer H J, Pauwels E K J 1991 Right ventricle wall motion abnormalities in patients treated with chemotherapy. Clin Nucl Med 16: 513–516
14. Lee B H, Goodenday L S, Muswick G J, Yasnoff W A, Leighton R F, Skeel R T 1987 Alterations in left ventricular diastolic function with doxorubicin therapy. J Am Coll Cardiol 9: 184–188
15. Massing J L, Caillot D, Casasnovas R O et al 1992 Early detection of anthracycline cardiotoxicity: interest of radionuclide angiography analysis of left ventricular (L V) filling parameter (abstract). Eur J Nucl Med 19: 667
16. Knesewitsch P, Göldel N H, Fritsch S, Moser E 1987 Equilibrium radionuclide ventriculography in the evaluation of adriamycin cardiotoxicity. II. Results under exercise. Nuklearmedizin 26: 212–219
17. Workman P 1992 Infusional anthracyclines; is slower better? If so, why? Ann Oncol 3: 591–594
18. Speyer J L, Green M D, Kramer E et al 1988 Protective effect of the bispiperazinedione ICRF-187 against doxorubicin-induced cardiac toxicity in women with advanced breast cancer. New Engl J Med 319: 745–752
19. Stinherz L J, Steinherz P G, Tan C T C, Heller G, Murphy 1991 Cardiac toxicity 4 to 20 years after completing anthracycline therapy. JAMA 266: 1672–1677
20. Lipshultz S E, Colan S D, Gelber R D, Perez-Atayde A R, Sallan S E, Sanders S P 1991 Late cardiac effects of doxorubicin therapy for acute lymphoblastic leukemia in childhood. N Engl J Med 324: 808–815
21. Geidel S, Garn M, Grävinghoff L et al 1991 Kardiomyopathie nach osteosarkombehandlung: ein beitrag zur kardiotoxizität von adriamycin. Klin Pädiatr 203: 257–261
22. Hiroe M, Ohta Y, Fujita N et al 1992 Myocardial uptake of ^{111}In monoclonal antimyosin Fab in detecting doxorubicin cardiotoxicity in rats. Morphological and hemodynamic findings. Circulation 86: 1965–1972
23. Carrió I, Estorch M, Berná L et al 1991 Assessment of anthracycline-induced myocardial damage by quantitative indium 111 myosin-specific monoclonal antibody studies. Eur J Nucl Med 18: 806–812
24. Carrió I, Estorch M, Berná L, Duncker D, Torres G 1992 Early detection of patients at risk of congestive heart failure during adriamycin therapy by means of In-111 antimyosin studies (abstract) J Nucl Med 33: 895
25. Estorch M, Carrió I, Berná L et al 1990 Indium-111-antimyosin scintigraphy after doxorubicin therapy in patients with advanced breast cancer. J Nucl Med 31: 1965–1969
26. Wakasugi S, Wada A, Hasegawa Y, Nakano N, Shibata N 1992 Detection of abnormal cardiac adrenergic neuron activity in adriamycin-induced cardiomyopathy with iodine-125-metaiodobenzylguanidine. J Nucl Med 33: 208–214
27. Valdés Olmos R A, ten Bokkel Huinink W W, Greve J C, Hoefnagel C A 1992 I-123 MIBG and serial radionuclide angiocardiography in doxorubicin related cardiotoxicity. Clin Nucl Med 17: 163–167

28. Lagrange J L, Darcourt J, Benoliel J, Bensadoun R J, Migneco O 1992 Acute cardiac effects of mediastinal irradiation: assessment by radionuclide angiography. Int J Radiat Oncol Biol Phys 22: 897–903
29. Burns R J, Bar-Shlomo B Z, Druck M N et al 1983 Detection of radiation cardiomyopathy by gated radionuclide angiography. Am J Med 74: 297–302
30. Savage D E, Constine L S, Scwartza R D, Rubin P 1990 Radiation effects on left ventricular function and myocardial perfusion in long term survivors of Hodgkin's disease. Int J Radiat Oncol Biol Phys 19: 721–727
31. Maunory C, Pierga J Y, Valette H, Tchernia G, Cosset J M, Desgrez A 1992 Myocardial perfusion damage after mediastinal irradiation for Hodgkin's disease: a thallium-201 single photon emission tomography study. Eur J Nucl Med 19: 871–873
32. Skinner R, Pearson A D J, Coulthard M C et al 1991 Assessment of chemotherapy-associated nephrotoxicity in children with cancer. Cancer Chemother Pharmacol 28: 81–92
33. Daugaard G, Abildgaard U 1989 Cisplatin nephrotoxicity. Cancer Chemother Pharmacol 25: 1–9
34. Pratt C B, Meyer W H, Jenkins J J et al 1991 Ifosfamide, Fanconi's syndrome, and rickets. J Clin Oncol 9: 1495–1499
35. Anninga J K, De Kraker J, Hoefnagel C A, Voûte P A 1990 Ifosfamide induced nephrotoxicity evaluated by ^{99m}Tc-DMSA renal scintigraphy (abstract). Med Pediatr Oncol 18: 406
36. Anninga J K, Hoefnagel C A, Dewit L 1990 The role of quantitative 99mTc-DTPA renography and 99mTc-DMSA scintigraphy in detection and follow up of radiation nephropathy. In: Schmidt H A E, Chambron J (eds) Nuclear medicine. Quantitative analysis in imaging and function. Schattauer, Stuttgart, pp 417–419
37. Dewit L, Anninga J K, Hoefnagel C A, Nooijen W J 1990 Radiation injury in the human kidney: a prospective analysis using specific scintigraphic and biochemical end points. Int J Rad Oncol Biol Phys 19: 977–983
38. Palestro C, Fineman D, Goldsmith S J 1988 Acute radiation nephritis. Its evolution on sequential bone imaging. Clin Nucl Med 13: 789–791
39. Verheij M, Dewit L, Valdés Olmos R A, Hoefnagel C A 1992 Captopril 99m-Tc-DTPA renography in patients with radiation-induced renovascular hypertension. In: Schmidt H A E, Höfer R (eds) Nuclear medicine in research and practice. Schattauer, Stuttgart, pp 545–548
40. Richman S D, Levenson S M, Bunn P A, Flinn G S, Johnston G S, DeVita V T 1975 67Ga accumulation in pulmonary lesions associated with bleomycin toxicity. Cancer 36: 1966–1972
41. Sostman H D, Putman C E, Gamsu G 1981 Diagnosis of chemotherapy lung. AJR 136: 33–40
42. MacMahon H, Bekerman C 1978 The diagnostic significance of gallium lung uptake in patients with normal chest radiographs. Radiology 127: 189–193
43. O'Doherty M J, Van de Pette J E, Page C J, Bateman N T, Singh A K, Croft D N 1986 Pulmonary permeability in hematologic malignancies. Effects of the disease and cytotoxic agents. Cancer 58: 1286–1288
44. Ugur Ó, Caner B, Balbay M D et al 1993 Bleomycine lung toxicity detected by technetium-99m diethylene triamine penta-acetic acid aerosol scintigraphy. Eur J Nucl Med 20: 114–118
45. Rubin P, Finkelstein J, Shapiro D 1992 Molecular biology mechanisms in the radiation induction of pulmonary injury syndromes: interrelationship between the alveolar macrophage and the septal fibroblast. Int J Radiat Oncol Biol Phys 24: 93–101
46. Kataoka M, Kawamura M, Itoh H, Hamamoto K 1992 Ga-67 citrate scintigraphy for the early detection of radiation pneumonitis. Clin Nucl Med 17: 27–31
47. Boersma L J, Damen E M F, de Boer RW et al 1992 Three-dimensional superimposition of SPECT and CT data to quantify radiation-induced ventilation and perfusion changes of the lung, as a function of the locally delivered dose. In: Schmidt H A E, Höfer R (eds) Nuclear medicine in research and practice. Stuttgart, Schattauer, pp 44–47
48. Suga K, Ariyoshi I, Nishigauchi et al 1992 Altered regional clearance of 99mTc-DTPA in radiation pneumonitis. Nucl Med Commun 13: 357–364
49. Galland R B, Spencer J 1990 The natural history of clinically established radiation enteritis. In: Galland R B, Spencer J (eds) Radiation enteritis. Edward Arnold, London, pp 136–146
50. Ludgate S M, Merrick M V 1985 The pathogenesis of post-irradiation chronic diarrhoea: measurement of SeHCAT and B12 absorption for differential diagnosis determines treatment. Clin Radiol 36: 275–278
51. Miholic J, Vogelsang H, Schlappack O, Kletter K, Szepesi T, Moeschl P 1989 Small bowel function after surgery for chronic radiation enteritis. Digestion 42: 30–38
52. Valdés Olmos R A, den Hartog Jager F C A, Hoefnagel C A, Taal B G 1991 Imaging and retention measurements of selenium 75 homocholic acid conjugated with taurine, combined with carbon 14 glycochol breath test to document ileal dysfunction due to late radiation damage. Eur J Nucl Med 18: 124–128
53. Danielsson A, Nyhlin H, Persson H, Stendahl U, Stenling R, Suhr O 1991 Chronic diarrhoea after radiotherapy for gynaecological cancer: occurrence and aetiology. Gut 32: 1180–1187
54. Valdés Olmos R A, den Hartog Jager F C A, Hoefnagel C A, Taal B G 1991 Effect of loperamide and delay of bowel motility on bile acid malabsorption caused by late radiation damage and ileal resection. Eur J Nucl Med 18: 346–350
55. Awad H K 1991 Early reacting tissues: the digestive tract. In: Awad H K (ed) Radiation oncology. Kluwer, Dordrecht, pp 291–322
56. Tsujii H 1985 Quantitative dose–response analysis of salivary function following radiotherapy using sequential RI-sialography. Int J Rad Oncol Biol Phys 11: 1603–1612
57. Delprat C C, Hoefnagel C A, Marcuse H R 1983 The influence of ^{131}I therapy in thyroid cancer on the function of salivary glands. Acta Endocrinol 252 (suppl): 73–74
58. Albrecht H H, Creutzig H 1976 Functional scintigraphy of the salivary gland after high dose radio-iodine therapy. Fortschr Röntgenstr 125: 546–551
59. Beckerman C, Hoffer P B 1976 Salivary gland uptake of 67Ga-citrate following radiation therapy. J Nucl Med 17: 685–687
60. Sacks E L, Goris M L, Glatstein E, Gilbert E, Kaplan H S 1978 Bone marrow regeneration following large field radiation. Influence of volume, age, dose, and time. Cancer 42: 1057–1065
61. Cox P H 1974 Abnormalities in skeletal uptake of ^{99m}Tc polyphosphate complexes in areas of bone associated with tissues which have been subjected to radiation therapy. Br J Radiol 47: 851–856
62. Reske S N, Karstens J H, Gloekner W et al 1989 Radioimmunoimaging for diagnosis of bone marrow involvement in breast cancer and malignant lymphoma. Lancet 2: 299–301
63. Yankelevitz D F, Henschke C I, Knapp P H, Nisce L, Fi Y, Cahill P 1991 Effect of irradiation therapy on thoracic and lumbar bone marrow: evaluation with M R imaging. AJR 157: 87–92
64. Israel O, Gorenberg M, Frenkel A et al 1992 Local and systemic effects of radiation on bone metabolism measured by quantitative SPECT. J Nucl Med 33: 1774–1782
65. Charkes N D, Silverman C 1992 Does radiotherapy affect regional bone formation? J Nucl Med 33: 1780–1782
66. Hubbard S M, Longo D L 1991 Treatment-related morbidity in patients with lymphoma. Curr Opin Oncol 3: 852–862
67. Coleman R E, Mashiter G, Whitaker K B, Moss D W, Rubens R D, Fogelman I 1988 Bone scan flare predicts successful systemic therapy for bone metastases. J Nucl Med 29: 1354–1359
68. Stokkel M P M, Valdés Olmos R A, Hoefnagel C A, Richel D J 1993 Tumor and therapy associated abnormal changes in bone scintigraphy: old and new phenomena. Clin Nucl Med 18: 821–828
69. Mankin H J 1992 Nontraumatic necrosis of bone (osteonecrosis). N Eng J Med 326: 1473–1478
70. Sheline G E, Wara W M, Smith V 1980 Therapeutic irradiation and brain injury. Int J Radiat Oncol Biol Phys 6: 1215–1228
71. Silber J H, Radcliffe J, Peckham V et al 1992 Whole-brain irradiation and decline in intelligence: the influence of dose and age on IQ score. J Clin Oncol 10: 1390–1396
72. Valk P E, Dillon W P 1991 Radiation injury of the brain. AJR 156: 689–706
73. O'Tuama L A, Janicek M J, Barnes P D et al 1991 ^{201}Tl/^{99m}Tc-HMPAO SPECT imaging of treated childhood brain tumors. Pediatr Neurol 7: 249–257

74. Coleman R E, Hoffman J M, Hanson M W, Sostman H D, Schold S C 1991 Clinical application of PET for the evaluation of brain tumors. J Nucl Med 32: 616–622
75. Podoloff D A, Kim E E, Haynie T P 1992 SPECT in the evaluation of cancer patients: not quo vadis; rather, ibi fere summus. Radiology 183: 305–317
76. Hammond G D 1992 Late adverse effects of treatment among patients cured of cancer during childhood. CA-Cancer J Clin 42: 261–262
77. DeLatt C A, Lampkin B C 1992 Long-term survivors of childhood cancer: evaluation and identification of sequelae of treatment. CA Cancer J Clin 42: 263–282
78. Perry M C 1982 Hepatoxicity of chemotherapeutic agents. Semin Oncol 9: 65–74
79. Levi S, Hodgson H J 1990 The medical management of radiation enteritis. In: Galland R B, Spencer J (eds) Radiation enteritis. Edward Arnold, London, 176–198

SECTION 6

Nuclear medicine in disorders of bones and joints

79. Bone scintigraphy: the procedure and interpretation

I. P. C. Murray

With a revolutionary impact similar to that of radioiodine on the investigation of thyroid disease in the 1950s, skeletal scintigraphy has become indispensable to the investigation of disorders affecting bone. Reflecting the exquisite sensitivity with which alterations in physiology can be displayed, skeletal scintigraphy cannot be considered as merely an investigation supplementary to radiology. The two modalities exist in a symbiosis which is critical to the evaluation of many skeletal problems, radiography demonstrating the anatomical alterations often resulting from changes in bone mineral content; skeletal scintigraphy indicating the aberrant metabolic status produced by modifications of bone vascularity and osteoblastic activity. In many instances, the radionuclide study will reveal an abnormality long before radiological alteration; in some it may indicate which area should most appropriately undergo radiological examination, while in others it may be of value by demonstrating a pattern of abnormal changes which will reinforce a radiological opinion. It may also indicate whether the radiologically demonstrable lesion is of clinical significance. Awareness of the indications for skeletal scintigraphy and the alterations which most characteristically will be encountered is therefore mandatory in the investigation of skeletal disease whether neoplastic, inflammatory or traumatic.

THE PROCEDURE

Radiopharmaceuticals

The propensity for certain radionuclides to concentrate in bone was first recognized in the early 1920s with the observation of the effects of ingested salts by painters of luminous watch dials and the subsequent demonstration that the uptake was in bone. Actual metabolic studies with radionuclides were commenced in 1935 by Chievitz & Hevesy[1] with ^{32}P orthophosphate and extended in the early 1940s with the use of fluorine-18 (^{18}F), calcium-45 (^{45}Ca) and strontium-89 (^{89}Sr). A wide variety of radionuclides were evaluated in the succeeding years for their bone-seeking properties. Successful bone imaging, however, was not achieved until 1961 with the use of strontium-85 (^{85}Sr) by Fleming et al.[2] Subsequent reports of intensive clinical studies indicated that the procedure was capable of detecting lesions well before radiological change. The radionuclide was, however, far from ideal because of a large radiation dose and the necessity to wait for at least 24–48 h to allow excretion of unbound radioactivity before the scanning could be undertaken. Improvement resulted from the introduction of ^{87m}Sr by Charkes[3] with its shorter half-life, but a troublesome and persistent background from the soft tissues still negated satisfactory images. The alternative, ^{18}F, advocated first by Blau et al,[4] was much more satisfactory, particularly with a faster blood clearance and improved skeletal visualization. Its main disadvantage, however, was not merely cost, being cyclotron produced, but its very short half-life of 1.83 h, which limited availability.

Nevertheless, the experience with ^{18}F made it clear that skeletal scintigraphy offered as much as other nuclear medicine procedures which had rapidly become routine. Much of their value lay in the use of technetium-99m (^{99m}Tc) radiopharmaceuticals, reflecting the ideal properties of this radionuclide for clinical use. The search for a technetium-labelled bone-seeking agent was based on the phosphate complexes in view of the effect of phosphonates in the treatment of bone disorders. The first practical agent, however, was the technetium polyphosphate described by Subramanian & McAfee.[5] Subsequent studies concentrated on optimizing the chain lengths of the polyphosphates, with varying success, but excellent images were provided by a triphosphate used by Murray et al.[6] The quality of this agent was not surprising since subsequently it was shown that, as a result of terminal autoclaving, the radiopharmaceutical was dominantly pyrophosphate, an agent later shown to be highly efficient in routine skeletal scintigraphy.[7] Soon, however, a variety of labelled diphosphonates, notably hydroxyethylidene diphosphonate (HEDP), were introduced and, following extensive clinical trials, such as that by Pendergrass et al,[8] subsequently became the bone-scanning agents of choice. Many agents have undergone extensive evaluation and comparison, but methylene diphosphonate (medronate. MDP), developed by Subramanian et al,[9] remains the most widely used agent. This radiopharmaceutical gained popularity because of more rapid blood clearance and higher skeletal affinity than those formerly in use. These virtues also led to the advocacy of the use of hydroxyethylidene diphosphonate (HEDP) and later of hydroxymethylene diphosphonate (HMDP). However, the results of a multicentric comparison of HMDP and MDP reported by Delaloye et al[10] failed to identify a significant clinical difference. Superior skeletal visualization has been demonstrated using dicarboxypropane diphosphonate (DPD), but several clinical trials, including that by Pauwels et al,[11] also failed to show any clinical difference even although DPD had a higher blood-to-soft tissue ratio (B/ST). Fogelman[12] has emphasized that visualization of a focal lesion depends on the contrast between the lesion and the surrounding bone, the lesion-to-bone ratio (L/B). The contrast between bone and soft tissue (B/ST) merely leads to an improved bone scan and not necessarily improved visualization of lesions. This concept is supported by the clinical experience of Rosenthall et al[13] and Smith et al[14] using dimethylamino diphosphonate (DMAD), with which lesions were identified that would not be visualized with MDP. Confirming this experience, Fogelman[12] pointed out that DMAD has an extremely low uptake by normal bone but an extremely high L/B ratio. He postulated that, although not acceptable for routine use, this radiopharmaceutical could well have a valuable role to play in selected cases, for example when an equivocal lesion was noted with MDP or when a patient with a known primary tumour complains of bone pain and yet no abnormality is seen on the MDP scintigraphic study.

The bone-seeking properties of the phosphonates have also been utilized to achieve preferential uptake of the complexes labelled with other radionuclides in skeletal lesions. As discussed in Chapter 76, the major clinical role has been to target metastatic deposits and provide localized radiation sufficient to provide significant palliation of pain.

The sensitivity with which skeletal scintigraphy demonstrates lesions in bone is offset by the lack of specificity, the mechanisms of uptake being induced by many pathological disorders. The aim of considerable research in nuclear medicine throughout the world is, therefore, to harness the potential of specific lesion identification by the use of labelled monoclonal antibodies against tumour antigens (Ch. 68). Research into bone tumours has predominantly been related to osteogenic sarcoma. A range of monoclonal antibodies which react with osteosarcoma cells have been developed. One of these, designated 791T/36, was found to localize in human osteosarcoma xenografts maintained in immuno-deprived mice. Labelling of the antibody with ^{131}I enabled detection of the uptake at the xenograft site.[15] Following the report by Farrands et al[16] of the successful in vivo localization of this antibody in a patient with osteogenic sarcoma, it was employed by Perkins et al[17] in a further 14 patients with various skeletal lesions. Positive localization was seen in seven of nine patients with primary bone tumours, four of which were osteosarcomas. However, uptake was noted in two patients with osteomyelitis. It was suggested that the antibody might be more appropriate for targeting therapeutic agents, for example being conjugated to cytotoxic drugs. More recently, Sakahara et al[18] have reported their experience with another monoclonal antibody, OST7, which was shown to have a high degree of specificity to human osteogenic sarcoma and selectively localized in the osteogenic sarcoma xenografts of nude mice. The different pharmacokinetics noted by them, using whole antibody or antibody fragments and with different radiolabels, ^{131}I or ^{111}In, does however highlight the problems which must be overcome before such agents can be used in routine clinical immunoscintigraphy.

Other radionuclides may be utilized in studies to complement the technetium phosphate skeletal imaging, although none has such ideal physical properties. The mechanisms producing their selective localization often provide supplementary information solving particular problems. Gallium citrate (^{67}Ga), with a physical half-life of 78 h, is known to localize in tumours by mechanisms which have been deeply researched although not fully elucidated. Certainly they do involve binding to transferrin and reaction with transferrin receptors on tumour cell membranes. As discussed in Chapter 62, ^{67}Ga has been found to have its most useful role in the diagnosis and staging of lymphomas. Variable results have been encountered in attempts to differentiate benign from malignant lesions, but some workers have found it useful in the assessment of primary bone tumours, especially in the delineation of tumour size and in the evaluation of therapy. However, for these purposes, it now seems that thallium-201 (^{201}Tl) is more reliable. Accumulation of ^{67}Ga also occurs within inflammatory lesions. The concentration in leucocytes also probably involves transferrin, with the intracellular binding site being lactoferrin. While more specific than the technetium bone-seeking agents in its propensity for sites of neoplasm or infection, some gallium is normally deposited in the skeleton and there will also be mild preferential accumulation reflecting vascularity in areas of body repair such as healing fractures. Interpretation of combined radionuclide studies does therefore require comparison of the distribution patterns obtained, evaluating dissimilarity of the avidity of the lesion for technetium agents and radiogallium. Localization of infection can also be achieved with the use of leucocytes labelled with indium (^{111}In), with a physical half-life of 2.8 days, but false positives reflecting uptake in fractures and tumours have been reported. A variety of methods for labelling leucocytes with ^{99m}Tc have been advocated and, more recently, increasing attention has been paid to ^{99m}Tc polyclonal immunoglobulins and anti-granulocyte monoclonal antibodies. Marrow imaging can be undertaken with a variety of colloids of varying particle size, labelled with technetium, or by utilizing acidic ^{111}In chloride.

Instrumentation

At the time of the initial availability of the technetium phosphate complexes, most departments used a rectilinear scanner or a standard gamma-camera with a 250 mm field of view. The potential of the new technique was immediately obvious, but the procedure was time-consuming, many views being required to complete a skeletal survey. The introduction of dual headed rectilinear scanners provided an improvement by allowing whole-body images to be obtained even although the resolution and quality was such that 'spot views' were required of areas considered to be suspicious. The advent of cameras with 400 mm fields of view further facilitated the quality of imaging, particularly when scanning beds became available and permitted whole-body images. However, the resolution was still less than that of the same instrument used in the static mode. Difficulties were also encountered since the size of most instruments required a double sweep over the body, which frequently produced a 'zipper' at the overlap, often coinciding with the spine. The growing popularity of bone scintigraphy, allied with the advantages of whole-body surveys, which not only save time but avoid moving patients in pain, played a large part in the introduction of the maxi-camera with a field of view of 500 mm.

Further improvement has accompanied the current generation of gamma-cameras, with digital imaging providing even higher quality and the capacity to 'zoom' and thus magnify areas of interest for detailed study. In particular, the capacity to rotate the camera head and hence perform single photon emission computed tomography (SPECT) has had a major impact on the diagnostic accuracy of skeletal scintigraphy. This technique has, of course, a critical role in many procedures investigating various systems, but experience has shown that it is indispensable in identifying various clinical problems affecting the skeleton. Markedly improved visualization of an abnormality can often arise from the ability of SPECT to remove the activity from overlying/underlying tissues which otherwise would obscure the image at the depth of interest. This is perhaps typified by the removal of the hyperaemia often lying over the avascular head of femur and the contribution of the activity below, arising from the acetabulum. More importantly, this ability to achieve an accurate image of a body section at a prescribed depth is critical in being able to separate bony structures which are overlapping in planar images. Such overlap is inevitable in viewing a vertebra in which the body is superimposed on the posterior elements where a variety of small lesions can occur in different sites. As a consequence, lesional contrast is improved, permitting not only improved detection but also, by displaying the slices in transaxial, coronal and sagittal projections, a perception of three-dimensional anatomy which improves localization and more exact delineation of the size of the lesion. Interpretation usually requires review of this spatial information in all three planes, but in some instances that provided in one plane may be of particular value. Thus, in SPECT examinations of the knee, the greatest information may well be obtained from the transaxial images since this plane, is, of course, at right angles to the anteroposterior projection of the planar images and only achievable by SPECT. The improved diagnostic accuracy in several clinical situations has been such that SPECT is almost mandatory when investigating these patients. In view of the longer time of the examination, this can indeed provide difficulties in maintaining patient throughput since many of the indications for SPECT are associated with common problems, such as low back pain. However, multiheaded cameras, either dual or triple, do provide a solution because of the shorter time required for a SPECT study. Further, there is evidence that the use of such instruments can, because of the greater sensitivity providing higher resolution, achieve a significant increase in diagnostic sensitivity over that achieved by single headed SPECT.[19]

Technique

The dose of ^{99m}Tc medronate utilized varies according to departmental policy, usually being 800 MBq. The dose for children is calculated using the usual formula related to weight with a minimum of 80 MBq considered necessary. After reconstitution of the lyophilized reagent with the required activity of ^{99m}Tc pertechnetate, the agent should be allowed to incubate for 15 min and the dose drawn immediately prior to injection. The reconstituted vial should be utilized within 8 h.

In many patients, when there is a localized problem, evaluation of the regional vascularity is valuable. This 'three-phase' study comprises a flow phase, a blood pool image and standard static views. Further static images 24 h later have been advocated as a 'four-phase study'. The dynamic flow requires rapid sequential images every 3 s for 30 s. A further image is obtained at 1 min. Although usually referred to as 'blood pool', it probably more correctly reflects the alterations in the bone extracellular fluid resulting from changes in capillary permeability.

The timing of the static images following injection is a matter of opinion, influenced by convenience to the patient and the workload. Bone uptake is maximum at 2 h, by which time a significant proportion of unbound radiopharmaceutical will have been excreted by the kidneys, but some workers still believe that it is worthwhile waiting for 4 h to ensure minimal soft-tissue retention. To reduce the latter and minimize bladder radiation, the patient should be encouraged during the interval to drink fluids and void prior to the commencement of the scan. On occasions the patient may be unable to void, thus rendering views of the pelvis non-diagnostic because of the activity in the urinary bladder. It may therefore be necessary to perform static imaging of the pelvis at 24 h.

Unless the clinical problem is clearly local, a whole-body image is desirable. Techniques vary. A preferred method is to acquire a desired count density (e.g. 900 K) over the anterior chest and obtain all other views for the same time. A high-quality whole-body survey can now be achieved in approximately 7–8 min for each of the anterior and posterior views. A high-resolution collimator is preferred to maximize detail both in the sweeps and in the spot views, which are undertaken as indicated to study any particular area. It does appear to offer the best compromise between resolution and imaging time. Supplementary images are often necessary. Some of these may be obtained with particular positioning of the patient for optimal visualization of an area. Difficulties encountered in viewing osseous structures in the pelvis because of radioactive urine in the bladder can often be overcome by imaging from a subpubic projection (Fig. 79.1). Superior images of the lumbar spine are, for example, achieved with the patient sitting and the back flexed (Fig. 79.2). Oblique views will frequently permit improved identification of the site of an osseous abnormality, but several projections may be required to delineate lesions in the feet and ankles precisely. This often is simplified with the use of the pinhole collimator, as shown for example by Mandell et al[20] in improving the identification of tarsal coalitions. This collimator has a much more common role in routine scintigraphy of the skeleton than in other systems. The magnified images achievable, with fine detail, are often critical in providing optimal information, as demonstrated for example by Bahk et al.[21] Many consider that its use is essential in the assessment of hip disorders, particularly in children in whom scintigraphy should be undertaken in both external (frog-leg) and maximal internal rotation.

The decision whether to undertake SPECT and obtain more precise location in any area will reflect the clinical problem and the information already obtained from the planar images. It may be apparent that SPECT is the appropriate procedure to ensure adequate assessment of a patient's symptoms. In others, it may be considered to be a necessary supplement to the planar studies in order to localize abnormalities more precisely or to attempt to demonstrate abnormalities at symptomatic sites when planar images are normal. There are a number of different acquisition protocols and processing techniques which can be used for bone SPECT. Each department should establish its own preferred protocol regarding collimators, acquisition times and angular sampling as well as post-acquisition filtering techniques.

The method employed to interpret a SPECT study is essentially a matter of personal preference. In general, review at the computer terminal is undertaken with manipulation of the display. Initially 16-image displays of all three planes are studied but, in order to maximize appreciation of the three-dimensional anatomy, the use of a program for review of interrelated files permits simultaneous assessment of lesion localization in all three sets (Fig. 79.3). Any abnormality visualized on one set of

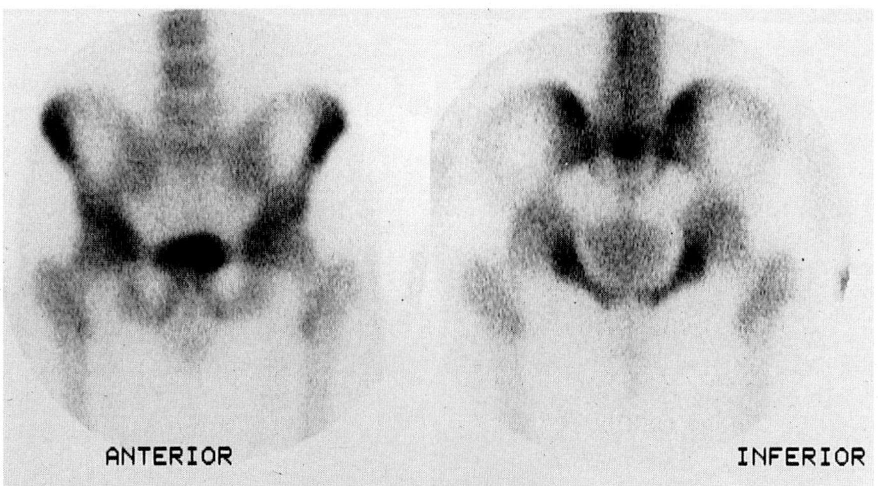

Fig. 79.1 In standard and anterior views of the pelvis, radioactive urine may obscure osseous structures, particularly the pubic symphysis. Caudal views from a subpubic projection overcome the problem.

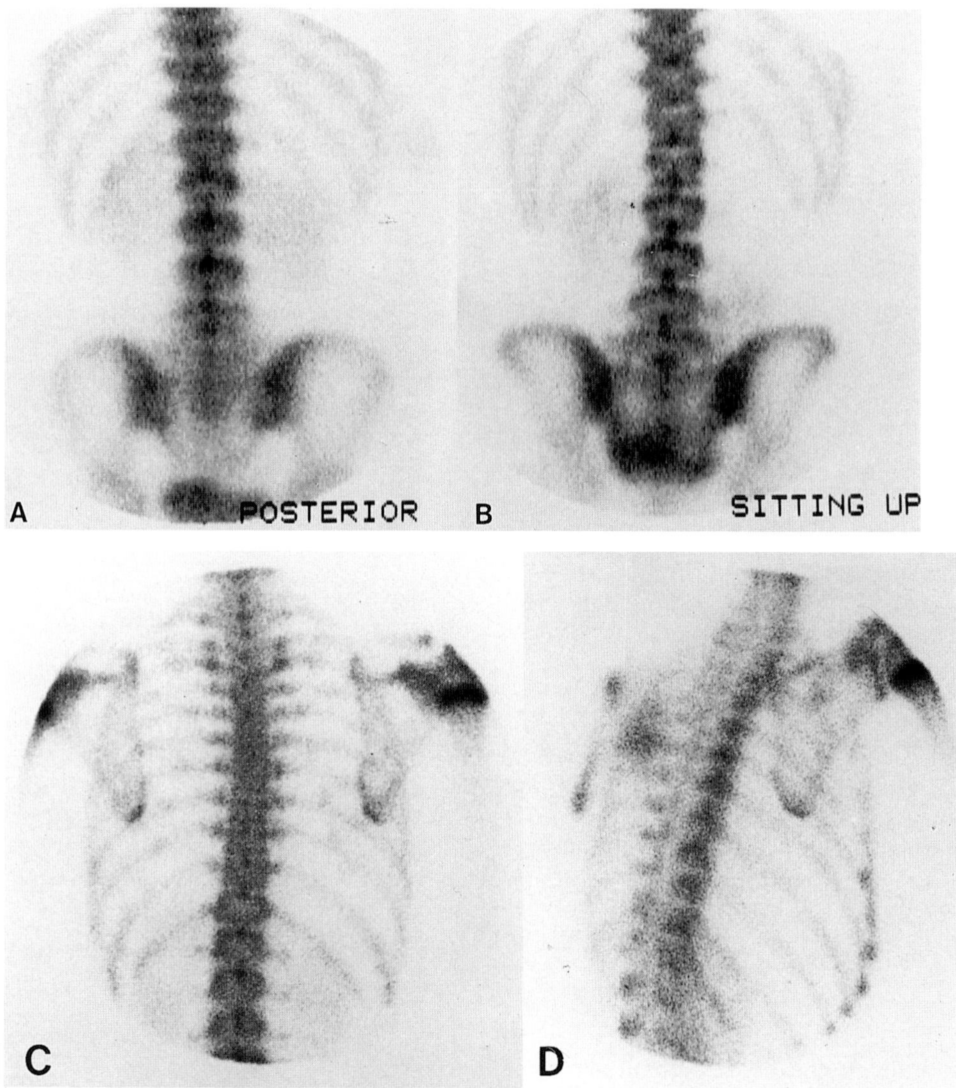

Fig. 79.2 The effect of positioning involved in improving scan quality. Superior delineation of the vertebrae is achieved with the patient sitting and back flexed (B) compared with lying prone (A). In addition to the conventional posterior projection (C), oblique views (D) permit assessment of the vertebral body and the spinous processes separately.

sectional images should be identified on the other two. In order to avoid misinterpretation of statistical fluctuations being abnormal, any alteration should be demonstrable in at least two adjacent slices. Three-dimensional surface displays, while providing interesting images, have generally been unhelpful in the evaluation of skeletal disorders, although Shih et al[22] suggested the technique was useful by demonstrating the relationships of bone to other structures.

A variety of methods to quantitate alterations in the fate of the ^{99m}Tc phosphate complexes have been advocated, but few have found any routine application despite enthusiasm by the protagonists. Most have arisen from attempts to optimize the diagnostic information when the alterations in the images are slight or equivocal. The simplest approach has been to generate an uptake ratio comparing the activity in a region of interest over an area of bone suspected to be abnormal with that over an area of normal bone, either adjacent or on the contralateral side, or in soft tissue. This approach has been used in studying avascular necrosis of the hip, but probably most frequently applied in attempts to achieve an improved diagnosis of ankylosing spondylitis. The characteristic increased MDP uptake in the sacroiliac joints can only be reliably observed at a stage when radiographic changes have also developed. In order to identify the disorder earlier, many attempts have been made to use a sacroiliac joint–S1 ratio but have usually been frustrated by the wide normal range resulting from variations with age and sex. These problems have also beset the use of a count profile drawn across the

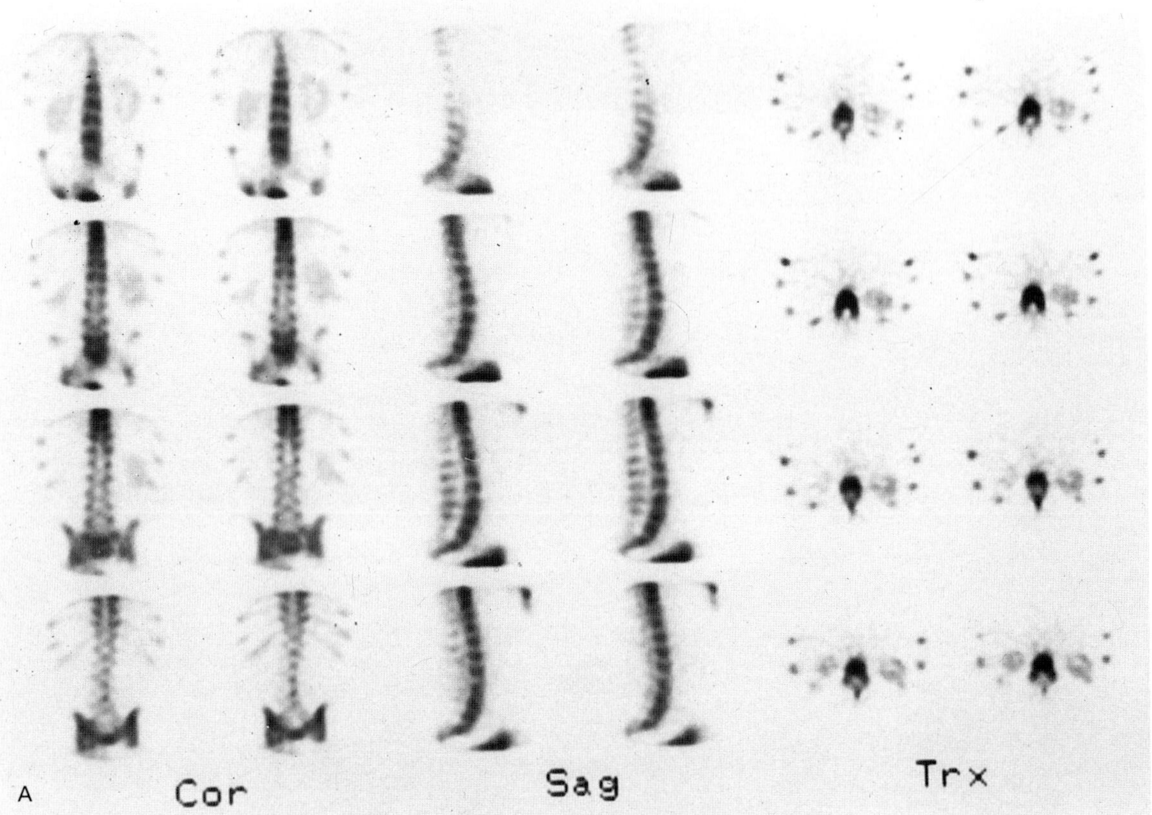

Fig. 79.3 (A) Normal SPECT of the spine. Selected images from serial sections in the three projections (Cor; coronal; Sag, sagittal; Trx, transaxial). These permit visualization of the individual vertebral bodies, spinal cord, pedicles and spinous processes.

sacroiliac region. The difficulties are less important when using lesion–bone or lesion–soft tissue ratios in the same individual in serial studies monitoring response to treatment. This can also be achieved with studies of whole-body retention of the bone radiopharmaceuticals as described by Fogelman et al.[23] This method, however, while capable of demonstrating accelerated bone turnover, does require a shadow-shield whole-body monitor. The alternative, assessing the retention of ^{99m}Tc diphosphonates by measuring the urinary output over 24 h, is negated by the difficulties inherent in achieving complete collection. Quantitative SPECT has been shown by Front et al[24] to be capable of documenting changes in bone metabolism and useful in monitoring response to treatment in patients with endocrine abnormalities.[25]

MECHANISMS

Clinical experience and numerous experimental studies have combined to provide an understanding of the mechanisms involved in the uptake of the technetium phosphate complexes into the skeleton and the manner in which abnormalities are demonstrated. It has become clear that several factors are involved, but many aspects remain to be clarified.

Closely related to the rate of concentration in bone are alterations in blood flow and in extraction efficiency. Decreased delivery, as in avascular disorders such as Perthes' disease, is, not surprisingly, associated with reduced accumulation. Increased vascularity, as in Paget's disease, is characteristically associated with increased radiopharmaceutical concentration in the extracellular fluid by passive diffusion and which, operating with other mechanisms, permits intense bone uptake. However, paradoxically, a diffuse increase in uptake also results from inhibition of sympathetic control[26] and there is a lack of a linear relationship between increases in blood flow and accumulation of the phosphate complexes.[27] Moreover, experimental studies have shown that, whatever role vascular alterations may have, they cannot explain the high preferential uptake at sites such as the epiphyseal plates, metabolic bone tumours and fractures, situations in which changes in the extraction ratio are markedly enhanced.[28] Thus, although altered blood flow will affect the delivery of the radioactivity, the key factor influencing the concentration of the radiopharmaceutical in the bone extracellular

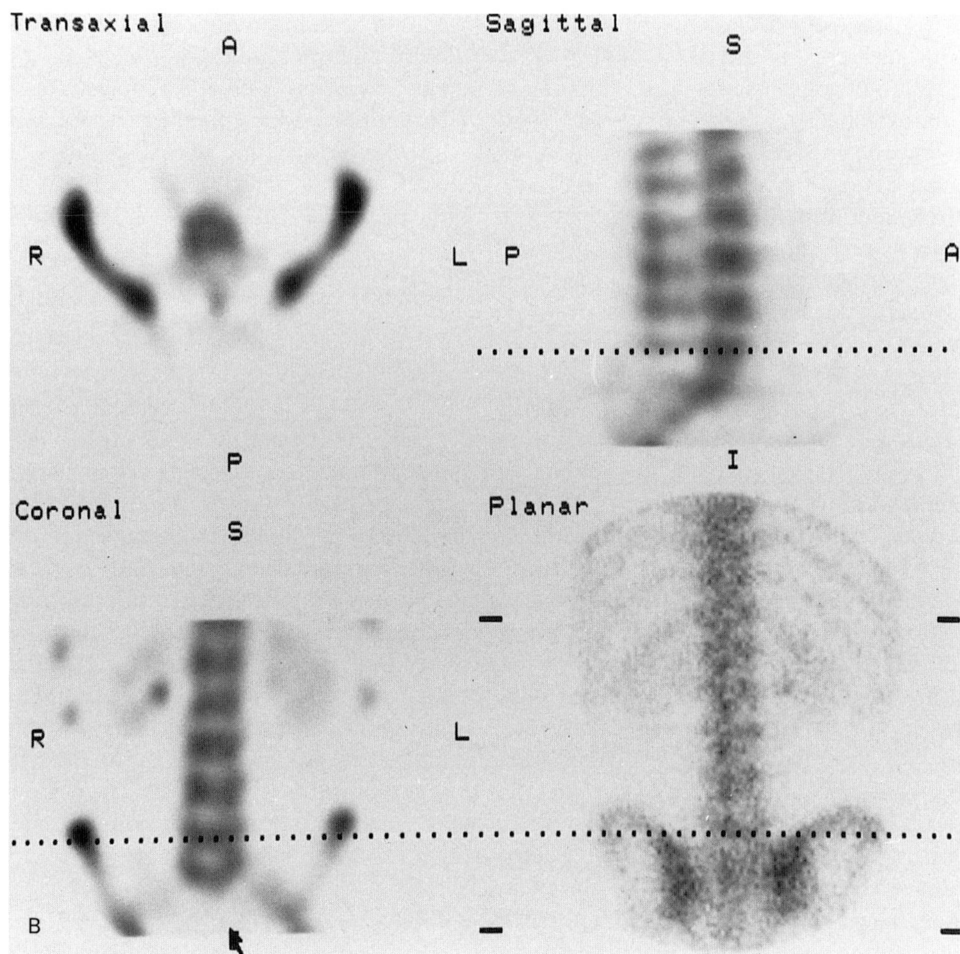

Fig. 79.3 **(B)** By selection of the appropriate sections from each plane, those which demonstrate the abnormality most clearly can be placed adjacent to each other and allow precise assessment of size and site of the change. Top left, transaxial; top right, sagittal; bottom left, coronal; bottom right, planar view. The dotted line indicates the level relevant to the appropriate plane displayed.

fluid is, almost certainly, the opening of microvasculature pathways which are normally closed. Not only does this permit higher concentrations in the extracellular fluid, but access to areas of reactive new bone formation is achieved. The relationship of such changes in the vasculature and fluid compartments to the increase in uptake associated with osteoneogenesis was shown in animals by Lavender et al,[27] who demonstrated an approximately 100% increase in flow at an osteotomy site but an 800% increase in MDP uptake. It is also compatible with clinical observations of the skeletal uptake in various circulatory disorders and the demonstration that lesions which do not induce an osteoblastic reaction, for example myeloma, are associated with only minimal or even no discernible focal accumulation. Alterations in the extraction efficiency from blood into bone are also in keeping with the generalized increased avidity noted in metabolic bone diseases.

Experimental studies have shown that there is selective localization of radioactivity below the laminar osteoid and on the actively bone-forming mineralizing layer, implying a reaction at the hydroxyapatite crystal surface.[29] Compatible with such autoradiographic experiments has been the demonstration that the absorption of the diphosphonate complexes onto immature calcium phosphate with a low Ca–P molar ratio, as is present at the calcifying front, is significantly greater than onto mature crystalline hydroxyapatite.[30]

There is evidence that there may be supplementary binding sites in addition to the mineral component. In particular, based on studies comparing bone which had either been demineralized or in which collagen had been altered, there does appear to be a role of preferential binding with the collagen moiety.[31] This may well be of greater relative importance in metabolic bone disease in which there is a significant correlation between the bone-to-soft tissue ratio for pyrophosphate uptake and the urinary hydroxyproline–creatinine ratio, evidence of the presence of immature collagen.[32] Investigations continue in order to elucidate the actual nature of the complex which reacts with bone and the precise mechanism of the reaction on the bone surface.

Numerous examples of extraosseous accumulation of the technetium phosphate complexes have also had relevance in studying the mechanisms of localization. In some instances, this deposition appears to be the same reaction with hydroxyapatite as in bone, simply related to neogenesis in lesions such as osteosarcoma, although changes in capillary permeability at the tumour borders may contribute. It has, however, been of interest to note that the bone-seeking agents are not always concentrated in metastatic visceral calcification even when this is radiologically evident, for example that associated with chronic renal failure. The discrepancy may well reflect the nature of the calcium phosphate deposit which, in uraemia, is similar to magnesium whitlockite, high in magnesium with 30% as pyrophosphate, which may prevent the transformation to apatite.[33] In contrast, the deposit in hypercalcaemic patients is brushite, later transformed to apatite, so that when the solubility product for calcium and phosphate is exceeded, there is hydroxyapatite crystal precipitation in the tissues. A variety of other mechanisms have been postulated to explain extraosseous deposits in other pathological states, for example reaction with immature collagen in healing scars, or binding to receptor sites on tissue enzymes, such as acid or alkaline phosphatase in lesions such as breast cancer.[34] More complex mechanisms, however, are certainly involved in the development of technetium phosphate complex deposition in necrotic muscle, as in myocardial infarct or rhabdomyolysis. Alterations in cell membrane viability and integrity result in abnormal intracellular flux of ionic calcium and precipitation of calcium salts.[35] The subsequent deposition of the technetium phosphate complexes appears to involve factors such as binding onto amorphous calcium phosphate, crystalline hydroxyapatite and also calcium complexes within myofibrils.[36]

INTERPRETATION

The sensitivity with which lesions are demonstrated with scintigraphy usually reflects the observation of a relatively obvious area of focally increased uptake. In most instances this results from the osteoblastic response of bone to the local insult whatever the actual aetiology. In general, it indicates the reparative process, visualized radiologically as sclerotic lesions. However, even bone destruction with osteoclastic activity, such as occurs with metastatic invasion, is usually associated with reactive attempts at bone repair, and the resultant change in bone metabolism will be seen as radiopharmaceutical uptake even at the site of radiologically lytic lesions. Indeed, this physiological mechanism is often associated with an avidity that produces an abnormality exaggerating the actual size of the lesion. However, some of the alterations may be subtle, particularly those caused by reduced osteoblastic activity or diminished vascularity. Interpretation of a skeletal scintigraphic study therefore requires not only images of high quality, with appropriate supplementary views, but careful scrutiny, bearing in mind the normal variants and the non-osseous artefacts which may occur, and also evaluation in light of the particular clinical problem and the radiological findings.

Normal variants

In the majority of patients, a whole-body study is desirable. This will permit assessment of the overall distribution of the radiopharmaceutical, noting factors such as an unexpected increase or decrease in the overall uptake throughout the skeleton, alterations in the pattern of accumulation, undue retention in the tissues or areas where more detailed spot views are desirable. It is logical that both anterior and posterior views are obtained and reviewed in parallel, comparing any alterations, and remembering, for example, that, because of normal lordosis, the lower lumbar vertebrae are often best evaluated in the anterior view. In particular, however, study of the symmetry about the midline is critical, and even in a limited study, scintigraphs of the corresponding contralateral side must be reviewed. The evaluation of symmetry is of such importance that initially the possibility of any

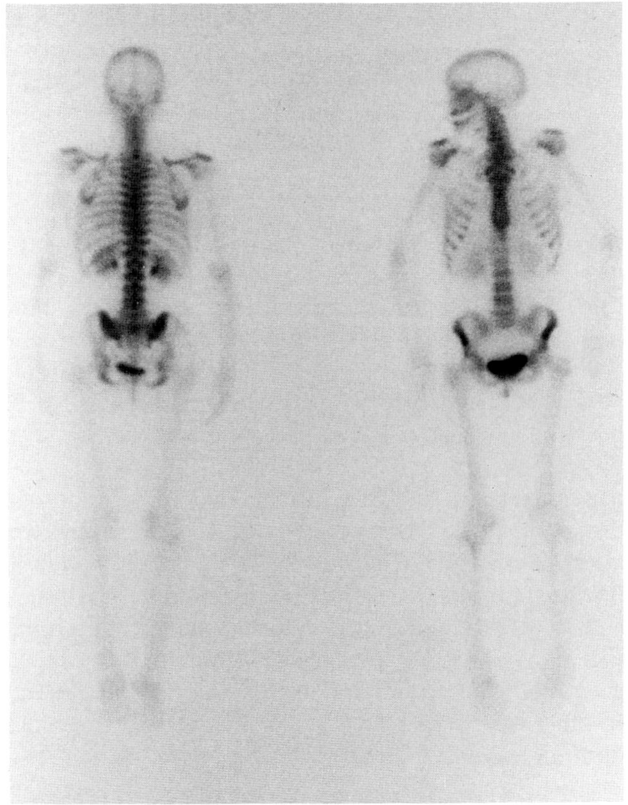

Fig. 79.4 Normal whole-body survey demonstrating varying uptake at different sites and the right–left symmetry about the midline.

rotation of the patient must be excluded. In the normal whole-body sweep (Fig. 79.4), there will be some variation in the avidity of uptake, being lower in the arms and legs and greater in areas associated with higher bone turnover. The greater accumulation in the sacroiliac areas, for example, reflects weight bearing. This, in some patients, may be a factor causing asymmetry in uptake. Thus, for example, even the altered gait resulting from the pain of a stress fracture is frequently associated with diffuse increased accumulation in the asymptomatic foot. The effect of normal muscle stress may result in areas of relatively high uptake, e.g. the scapular tips, which are usually sufficiently prominent that further views of the arms in different positions may be required to elucidate whether there is a lesion in underlying ribs. Similarly, increased accumulation may be noted in muscle insertions such as the deltoid tuberosity or in the posterior ribs at the insertions of the ileocostalis thoracis portion of the erector spinae muscles. A similar appearance of 'stippling' of the ribs may also be observed in the child because of 'shine-through' from the increased uptake in the costochondral junctions occurring normally at these growth sites (Fig. 79.5). In studies undertaken following pregnancy, aberration from the normal distribution will result from the effects of pelvic diastasis, especially in the symphysis pubis (Fig. 79.6).

It is, of course, particularly important to remember that in the child, intense uptake is to be expected in the metaphyseal–epiphyseal areas of the long bones. This uptake diminishes with increasing age until epiphyseal fusion is complete. In the child, particular attention must be paid to the metaphyseal–epiphyseal areas of the long bones. This, in part, reflects the predilection for the

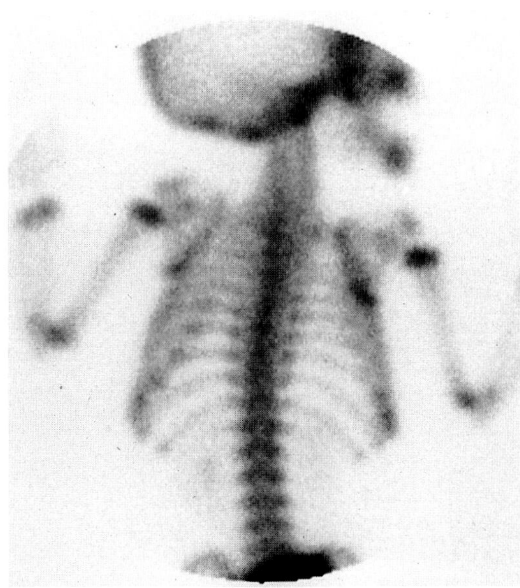

Fig. 79.5 Normal costochondral uptake in the child may be sufficiently intense to be visualized as 'rib stippling' in the posterior view.

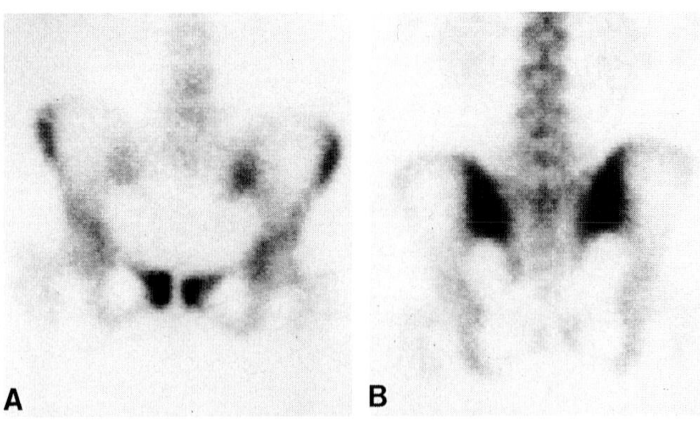

Fig. 79.6 Pelvic diastasis associated with pregnancy induces increased accumulation in the sacroiliac joints with the pubic symphysis demonstrable post partum (A, anterior; B, posterior).

metaphysis in the child for disorders such as osteomyelitis or metastasis. The changes in the vascular supply to these areas with growth from the neonate through childhood must be remembered since they will influence the likely site of the development of focal disease in haematogenous infection. Being associated with high levels of physiological activity, intense uptake in the growth centres is to be expected. The growth plate is divided into three cartilaginous zones: resting, proliferative and hypertrophic. Within the last lies the zone of provisional calcification in which osteoblasts deposit seams of osteoid, which Christensen & Krogsgoord[37] showed to be the site of uptake of bone-seeking radiopharmaceuticals. In preambulatory children the meta-epiphyseal complex demonstrates intensely increased accumulation as compared with the diaphysis and it is difficult to distinguish between the epiphysis and the epiphyseal growth plate. Thus, in these infants, the growth complexes are usually of a globular shape (Fig. 79.7). However, as a child begins to walk the epiphyseal plate becomes more identifiable as a linear band of preferential uptake. This uptake becomes even more marked as fusion approaches. The activity of the meta-

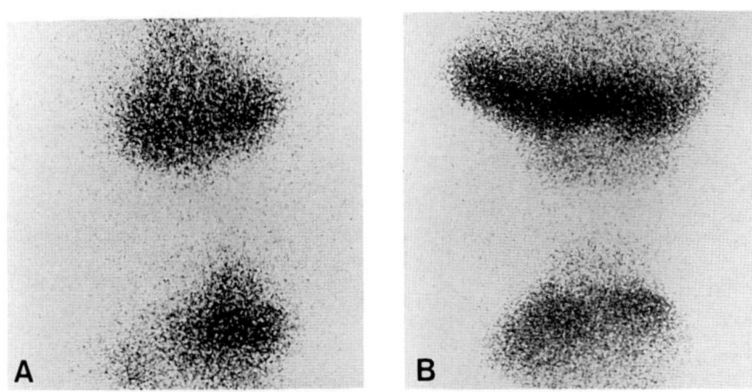

Fig. 79.7 The infantile growth complex is visualized (A), even with magnification views with the pinhole collimator, as a globular appearance, whereas, at later ages, the components of the growth complex can be identified, as in a 15-month-old boy (B) in whom flattening of the elliptical growth plate is commencing.

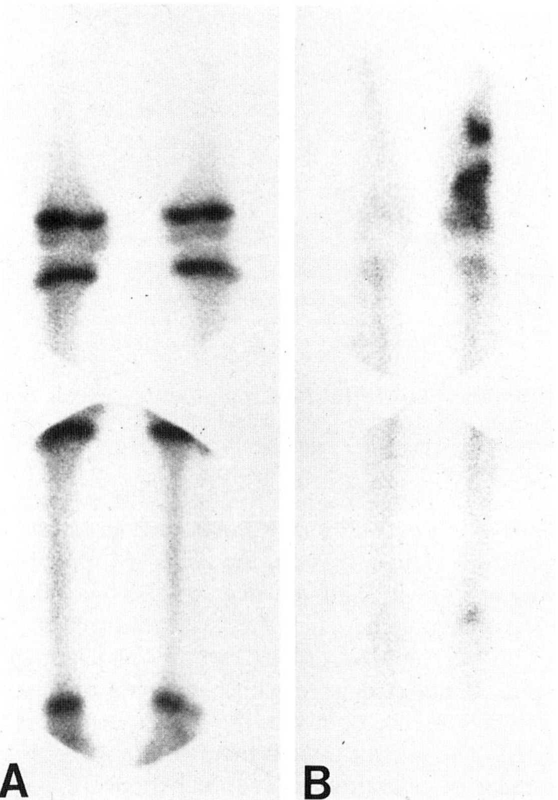

Fig. 79.8 The normal growth complex uptake with preferential and linear accumulation in the growth plate of an 8-year-old boy (A) can be compared with the absence of this normal pattern in an 8-year-old girl receiving long-term steroid therapy for leukaemia which has involved bone (B). The abnormal distribution in the femur reflects leukaemic infiltration.

physis adjacent to the plate is approximately equal to the epiphyseal activity and, while there is a gradient between the plate and diaphysis through the zones of provisional calcification, the edge of the plate should be well demarcated (Fig. 79.8). Any blurring of the edge should arouse suspicion. Alterations in the expected appearance of the growth plate may identify abnormal growth and development. Profound metabolic dysfunction resulting from disorders such as chronic renal failure, or produced by long-term steroid therapy, can be associated with reduction in uptake in the growth plate or even delayed appearance of accumulation in ossific centres. Asymmetrical reduction in activity may result from radiotherapy. The effect of trauma is variable. In some instances, there will be a reactive increase in uptake in the growth plate, but if there is a transepiphyseal fracture the cessation of physiological activity will be obvious because of the diminished accumulation of radioactivity. Such changes may be readily visible, but Harcke[38] has pointed out that simple inspection may not identify growth plate pathology involving only a portion of the physis. He recommended growth plate quantification whereby a count profile of a slice across the plane is computer generated, with comparison with the contralateral physis or studied in four segments. This technique was recommended in particular to evaluate the efficacy of epiphysidesis.

Other areas in which preferential uptake may be noted in the normal child include the base of the skull in infants, while in older children there may well be persistent active uptake in the suture between the sphenoid and the basiocciput (Fig. 79.9). Study of the accumulation in the cranial

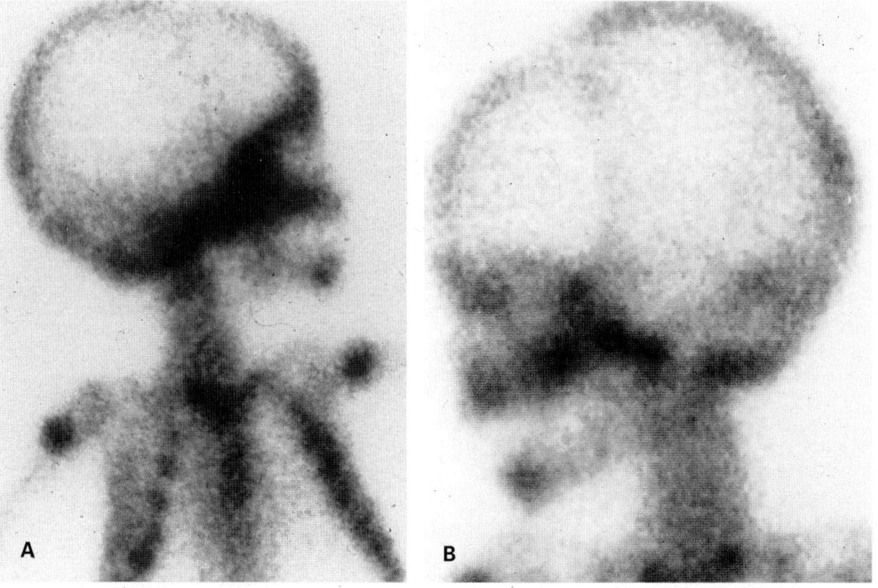

Fig. 79.9 Skull appearances in children. (A) The characteristic increased accumulation in the base of the skull noted normally in a 3-month-old child. (B) Normal scintigraphic appearances of the skull in a 6-year-old child: persistence of uptake in the sutures and in the base of the skull, with activity particularly evident in the suture between the sphenoid and basiocciput.

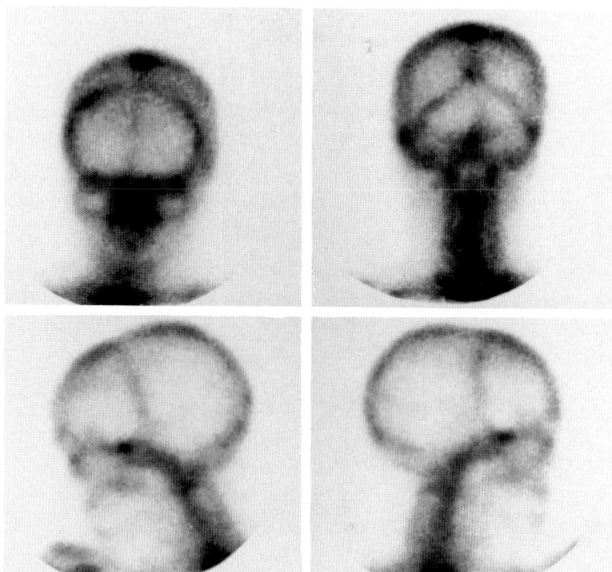

Fig. 79.10 Renal osteodystrophy. Views of the skull in various projections, demonstrating undue prominence of accumulation in the sutures.

sutures may be critical in the identification of craniosynostosis. Gates & Dore[39] described the pattern in this disorder, whereby the initial finding was focal osteoblastic activity identified on the study as increased radionuclide accumulation in a portion of the involved suture. As the abnormal fusion process extended along the suture like the closing of a zipper, there was a corresponding spread of the radioactivity. With complete fusion, uptake diminished. Persistent visualization of the sutures of the skull in later life may be normal, but such accumulation, if marked, is commonly associated with disorders of metabolism such as renal osteodystrophy (Fig. 79.10). However, as noted by Harbert & Desai,[40] persistent uptake in the line of the sutures may be observed as small foci which are totally innocent but cause concern if metastases are suspected. In contrast, diffuse uptake in the calvarium and the frontal region is evidence of hyperostosis frontalis interna. Diffusely increased accumulation over the entire calvarium may merely reflect ageing, although frequently associated with intense chemotherapy. When intense, often associated with alterations throughout the skeleton, such accumulation may be the result of metabolic disorders.[41] Ageing is usually accompanied by reduced overall skeletal uptake and frequently by symmetrical periarticular accumulation, mainly indicative of degenerative arthritic change. Such asymptomatic joint alteration in older subjects occurs mainly in the large joints but not infrequently is most obvious in the sternoclavicular and acromioclavicular joints. Calcified costal cartilages are often demonstrable, and uptake in the thyroid and hyoid cartilages can occur. Similarly, calcification in the femoral arteries can be noted. In the female, mild diffuse uptake in the breast is not usual. In initial dynamic flow studies involving views of the pelvis, the vascularity of the menstruating uterus may be very apparent (Fig. 79.11).

The resolution obtainable with modern instrumentation has resulted in marked improvement in image quality. This is particularly obvious in the spine where, particularly in the lower thoracic and lumbar vertebrae, the disc spaces, pedicles and spinous processes are readily identified. Delineation of cervical and thoracic vertebrae is less clear-cut. However, the spinous processes are usually well seen, in particular that of C7, and the costotransverse joints may be prominent. Persistence of the vertebral transverse process epiphysis may be noted as an area of focally increased uptake.[42] Such visualization, as in other

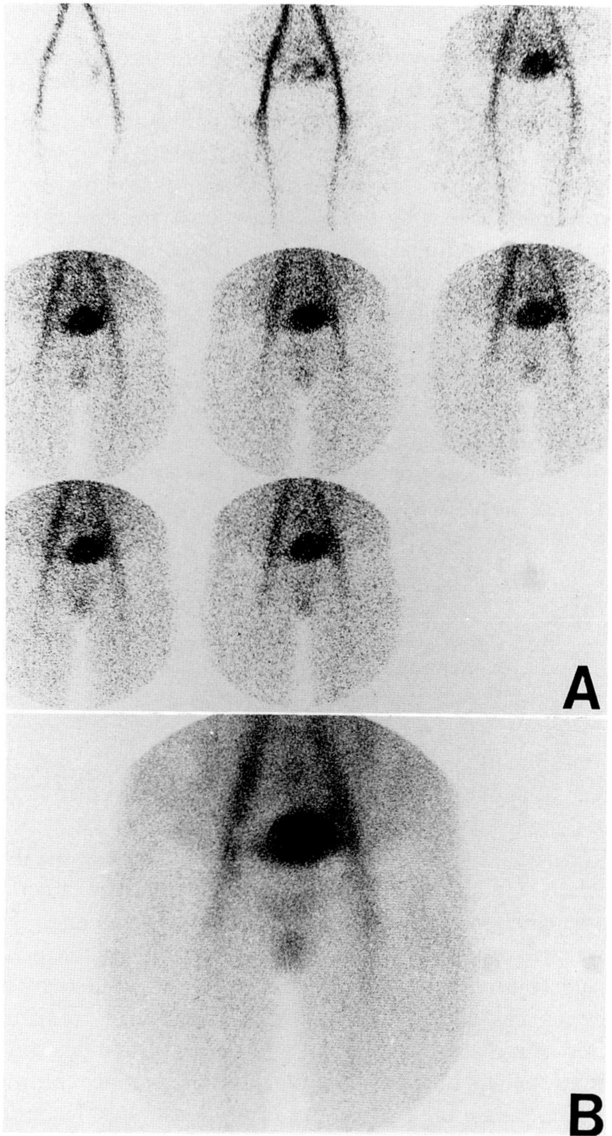

Fig. 79.11 Uterus in menstruation. A routine dynamic flow study (A) and blood pool phase (B) in standard views of the pelvis identifies increased vascularity.

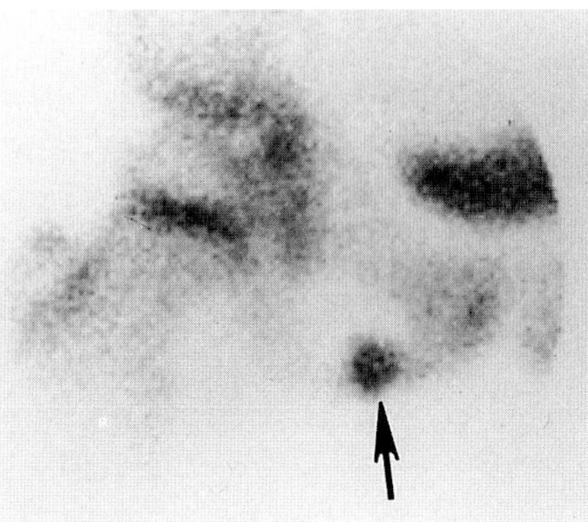

Fig. 79.12 Ischiopubic synchondrosis. Views with a pinhole collimator permit clear identification of a typical focus of mild discrete accumulation.

sites such as the ischio-pubic synchondrosis,[43] may occur normally as growth plates become intensely active at the initiation of fusion, but is of more significance in symptomatic individuals with a history of trauma (Fig. 79.12). Uptake in other normal radiographic variants in the extremities, particularly those of which the presence of congenital synchondroses may predispose to injury, such as an accessory navicular, and ossicles in which there may be premature degenerative change, for example the os styloideum, is abnormal and crucial in evaluating the symptomatic patient.[44] Fink-Bennett & Shapiro[45] drew attention to the importance of recognizing that focal uptake occurs frequently as a normal variant at the fibrocartilaginous junction of the sternum and manubrium, the angle of Louis, and should not be confused with an osseous abnormality.

Artefacts

It might seem superfluous to emphasize that correct function of the equipment is essential for satisfactory scintigraphy, but the effect of an improperly set photopeak in producing a false-positive bone scan, with multiple areas of apparently focal osseous uptake, has been shown by Tondeus & Ham.[46]

The quality control of current radiopharmaceuticals is such that it is now uncommon to encounter the effects of poor labelling associated with free pertechnetate. The latter will result in the specific trapping of the radionuclide by the thyroid, stomach and salivary gland. Uptake by the thyroid alone has been reported in hyperthyroidism,[47] whereas it is unusual in metastatic visceral calcification in which specific uptake in the stomach is the most common feature.[48] The biodistribution of the radiopharmaceutical can be altered by in vivo reaction, particularly those exchange reactions in which the radionuclide detaches from the pharmaceutical and adheres to another com-

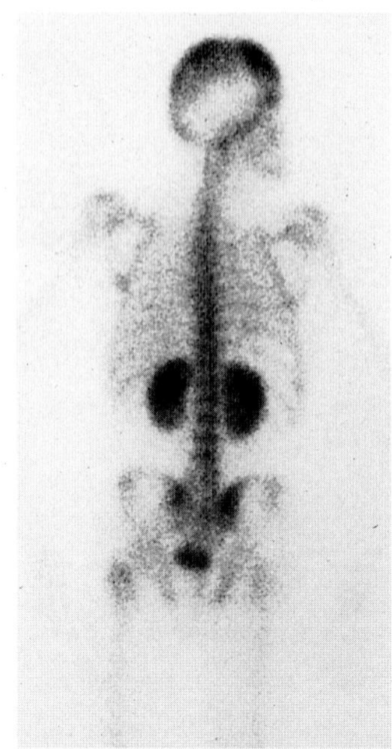

Fig. 79.13 Thalassaemia. The 'hot kidneys' associated with chronic iron overload induced by repeated blood transfusions.

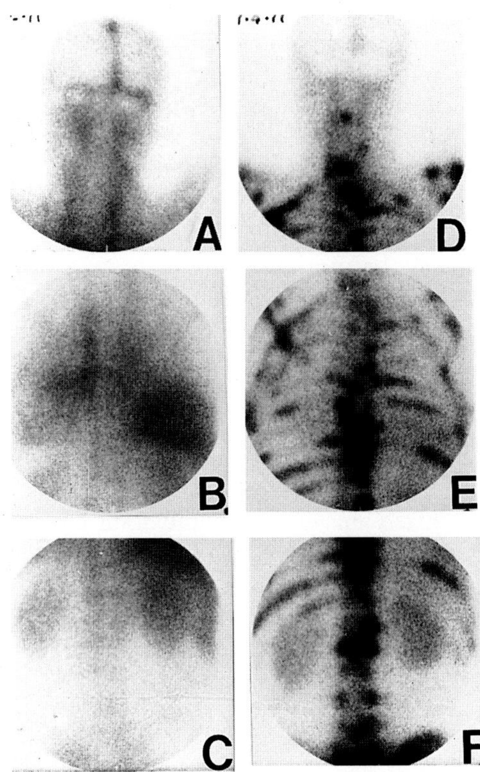

Fig. 79.14 The effect of iron on the biodistribution of ^{99m}Tc pyrophosphate. Routine scintigraphy in a 64-year-old man with prostatic carcinoma undertaken 24 h after an intravenous Imferon infusion showed, in views of the cervical (A), thoracic (B) and lumbar (C) spine, marked blood pool activity with gross reduction of bone uptake. Studies of the same patient obtained two weeks later (D–F) show extensive skeletal metastases with negligible blood pool activity. (Reproduced with permission from Choy et al.[49])

pound which may have different organ specificity or biological fate. Typical of these is the decreased bone uptake and intense renal accumulation which may occur in patients with chronic iron overload,[49] such as those with haemochromatosis or those receiving frequent blood transfusions (Fig. 79.13). It is possible that the renal uptake may be due to the displacement of ^{99m}Tc in a form preferentially excreted or to the creation of a new complex which has kidney-seeking properties. An acute effect in which there appears to be a direct complex seen between intravenous iron dextran and the technetium bone-seeking agents results in marked blood pool labelling and gross reduction in bone uptake[50] (Fig. 79.14), while localized accumulation is frequently observed at sites where intramuscular iron dextran has been administered[15] (Fig. 79.15). Similar mechanisms are postulated as being responsible for the considerable splenic MDP accumulation, noted by Spencer et al[52] in the spleen of a patient with autoimmune haemolytic anaemia, in light of the marked increase in splenic haemosiderin. Augmented renal uptake is noted shortly after administration of chemotherapeutic drugs[53] (Fig. 79.16). 'Hot' kidneys were noted by Bernard et al[54] in 6 of 600 patients. Two had received mitoxantrone, one had had a single injection of calcitonin, one was hypocalcaemic and one had undergone radiotherapy. No aetiological factor was identified in the other patient. A variety of disorders were present in the 13 patients with 'hot kidneys' in the 2056 studies reviewed by Koizumi et al,[55] including cirrhosis and diabetic mellitus. The findings also occurred after amphotericin B therapy, in nephrocalcinosis and with myoglobulinuria.

A similar mechanism of competition is almost certainly responsible for the phenomenon whereby markedly reduced uptake in bone of ^{99m}Tc-MDP is encountered in patients receiving therapy with etidronate disodium (EHDP).[56] This effect of EHDP on the biodistribution of MDP was initially demonstrated by Watt & Hill[57] in the rat, there being a typical carrier effect with a dose-related interference in skeletal MDP uptake. The duration of this effect is unknown but is important in view of the increasing use of this form of therapy in many bone disorders, including Paget's disease, hypercalcaemia and osteoporosis. Because of the 20–30 day biological half-life of EHDP in the skeleton there is concern that the effect may last for months. However, although undertaken in a patient who had received only a single dose of EHDP, serial studies undertaken by Sandler et al[58] did show normal biodistribution of MDP had returned at 15 days. Orzel et al[59] encountered no difficulty in using serial bone scans at 5–6 month intervals to assess the therapeutic response of oral diphosphonates for myositis ossificans.

Perhaps the most common iatrogenic alteration in bone uptake is the induction of areas of reduced uptake by radiotherapy (Fig. 79.17). Such defects, rare in regions receiving less than 20 Gy, usually occur between 4 and 6 months following radiotherapy and can persist for 18 months.[60] As shown by Ferris & Ziessman,[61] the acute

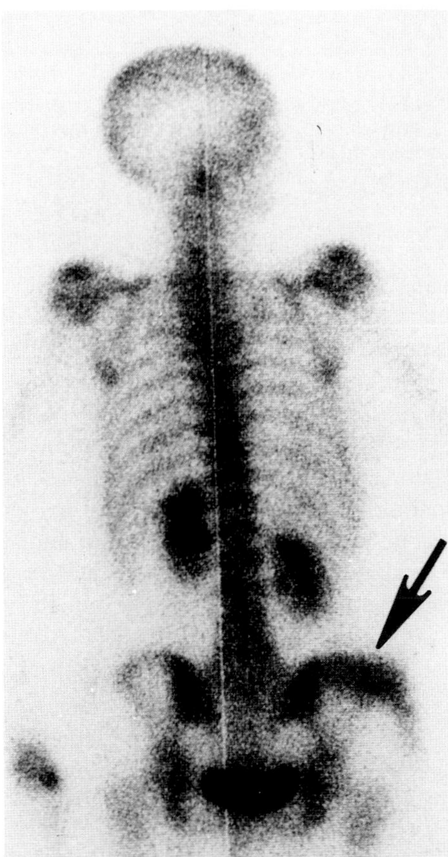

Fig. 79.15 Intramuscular iron injections. Extraosseous accumulation in right buttock.

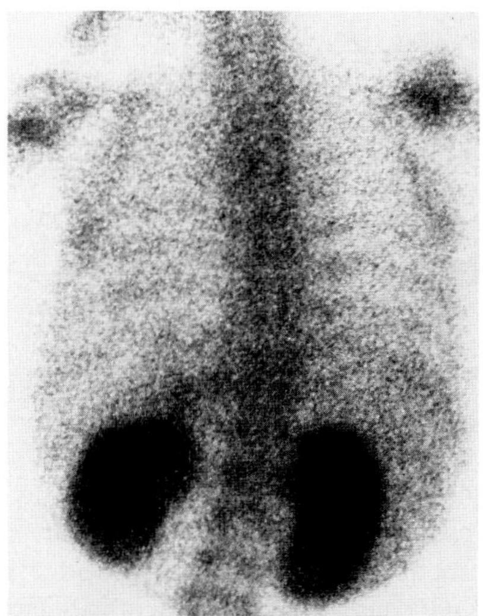

Fig. 79.16 Effect of chemotherapy. Preferential accumulation in the kidneys following treatment of a child with neuroblastoma.

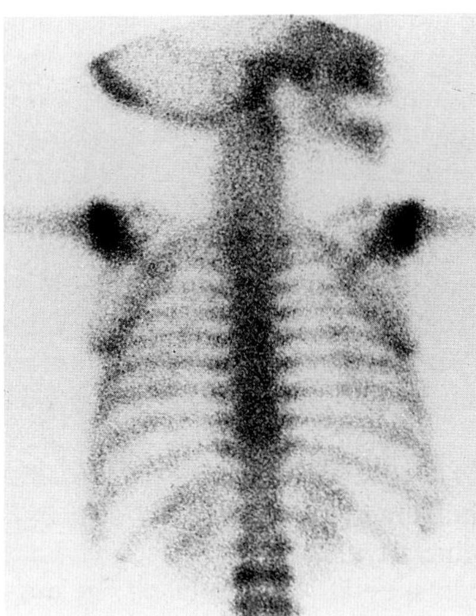

Fig. 79.17 Radiation-induced photopenia identified as reduced accumulation in several vertebral bodies, the area of the radiation port for the treatment of para-aortic nodes in a child with orchidoblastoma.

inflammatory soft-tissue phase of radiation injury is accompanied by evidence of hyperaemia in the blood flow and blood pool phases of the bone scan. Israel et al,[62] using SPECT to quantitate MDP uptake as an indicator of bone metabolism, did find an early period of increased metabolism after irradiation. However, in all 28 patients studied, there was a significant reduction in uptake compared with bone metabolism prior to irradiation. The surprising observation was that, while the decrease was more pronounced in bone which had received irradiation than in the non-irradiated bone, there was still a significant decrease in the non-irradiated bone. They postulated that this might have been induced by a systemic factor released into circulation from the irradiated tissue. Commenting on these findings, Charkes & Silverman[63] suggested that the reduction in uptake might be the result of associated bed rest, which so rapidly causes changes in bone metabolism: reduced bone formation and increased bone resorption.

The renal excretion of radiopharmaceutical unbound to bone can lead to considerable difficulty in interpretation but can also provide unexpected diagnostic information. The kidneys are usually readily visualized, but alterations in the normal uptake, shape or site may well be of significance, as has been shown in many series, in most of which the prevalence has been approximately 15%. Some workers, for example Chayes & Strashun,[64] have suggested special modifications of the procedure to enhance the opportunity of obtaining additional diagnostic information by identifying renal abnormalities. Generally, however, the effort is not considered worthwhile, provided it is remembered that such changes can be present incidentally and the renal images routinely examined. Reduced kidney uptake, particularly if asymmetrical, may indicate the presence of renal disease, as may a difference in size. A persistent high tissue background will be produced by the retention of the radiopharmaceutical resulting from impaired renal function, often masking the skeletal uptake to a degree that the study is uninterpretable. More often, poor visualization of the kidneys will be the result of the alterations in biodistribution resulting from skeletal disease with enhanced uptake of radiopharmaceutical by normal bone. This 'faint kidney' sign is therefore usually associated with the 'superscan' typical of generalized metabolic disorders or resulting from gross metastatic involvement (Fig. 79.18). Reviewing 215 patients with abnormal renal images, Adams et al[65] observed this sign in 34, none of whom had renal disease. Kajubi & Chayes[66] identified the 'superscan' by the unusual avid early uptake into the vertebrae. Asymmetry in size may be obvious with the demonstration of a small or non-functioning kidney indicating the need for additional investigation. Low-lying kidneys can cause difficulties in studying the pelvis, but displacement of normally sited kidneys by adrenal and retroperitoneal tumours may be obvious. Extraosseous uptake by such neoplasms can

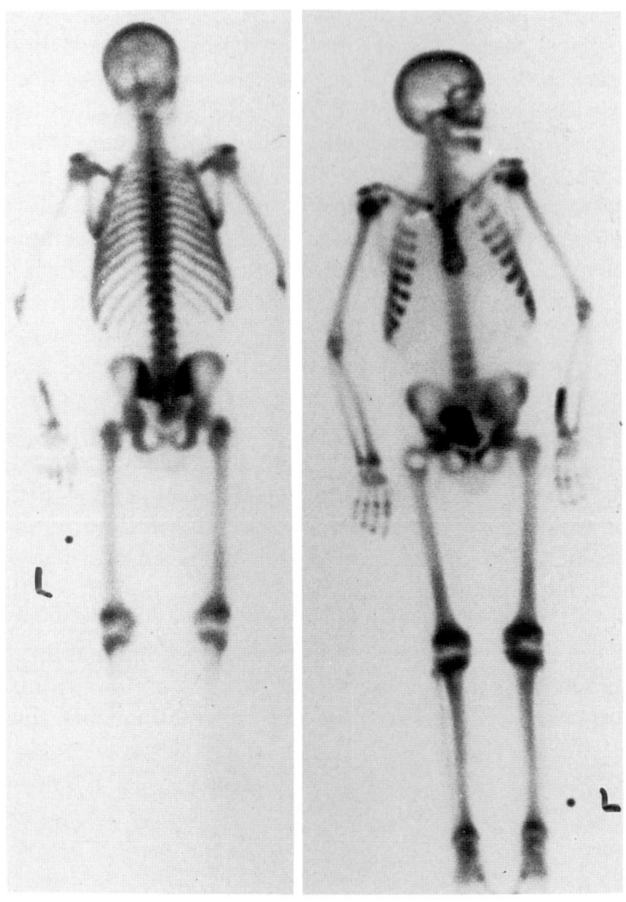

Fig. 79.18 Advanced renal osteodystrophy. The generalized increase in accumulation throughout the skeleton results in images of excellent quality, the 'superscan'.

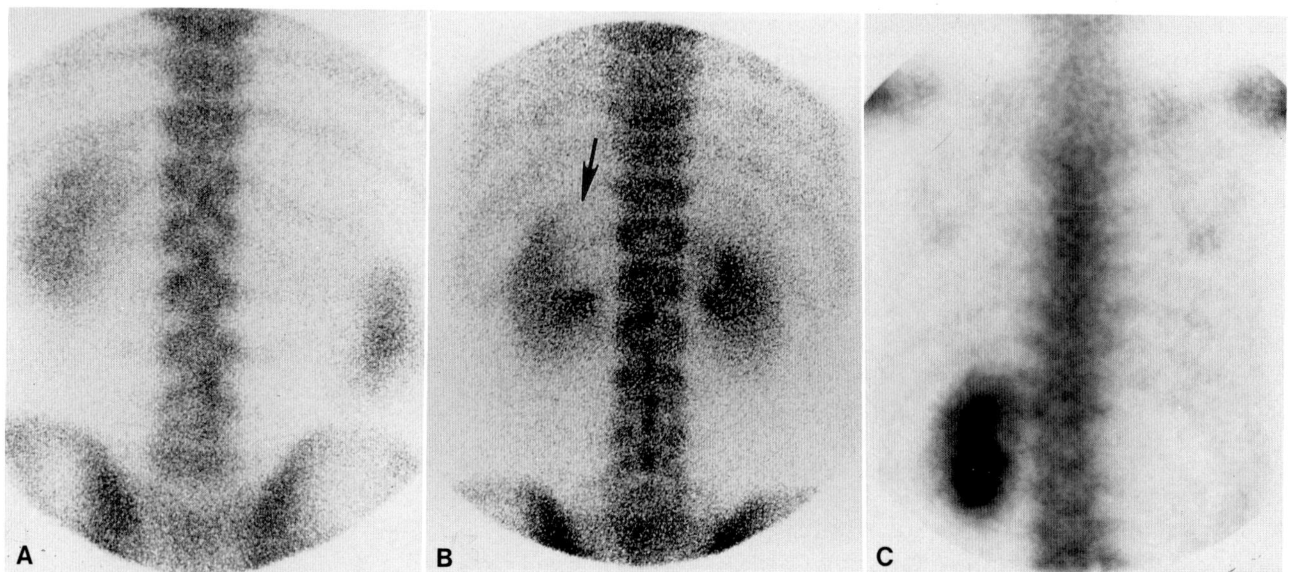

Fig. 79.19 Renal pathology noted in routine bone scintigraphy. (A) Hypernephroma: displacement and reduction of the normal renal accumulation in the right kidney by a large tumour. (B) Hypernephroma: distortion of the contour of the upper pole of the left kidney by a lesion subsequently shown to be due to this neoplasm. (C) Wilms' tumour: total absence of accumulation in the right kidney in an 8-year-old girl presenting with a loin mass, subsequently demonstrated to be a Wilms' tumour.

occur, and often they will cause distortion of the renal outline. This also may be the manifestation of a kidney tumour or other intrarenal space-occupying lesions, for example cysts, which will frequently be identified by the non-uniformity of the distribution of the radiopharmaceutical or even, on occasion, by the non-visualization of the entire kidney (Fig. 79.19). Retention of radioactive urine in the pelvicalyceal system may be very obvious (Fig. 79.20). The reported prevalence of this abnormality has varied greatly in various series, in some exceeding 20%. Adams et al,[65] however, stressed that the finding of such retention of radioactive urine was of little significance if the study had been performed in the supine position. This was confirmed by Haden et al,[67] who in a series of 531 patients found that, of 44 who had renal retention in the supine position, 33 (75%) drained in the upright position. Only 11 patients (2.1%) were shown to have obstructive uropathy. The frusemide washout study was not helpful in identifying these patients. Focal renal uptake, often in a linear pattern, which could be mistaken for urine retention, adrenal accumulation or a rib abnormality, can occur

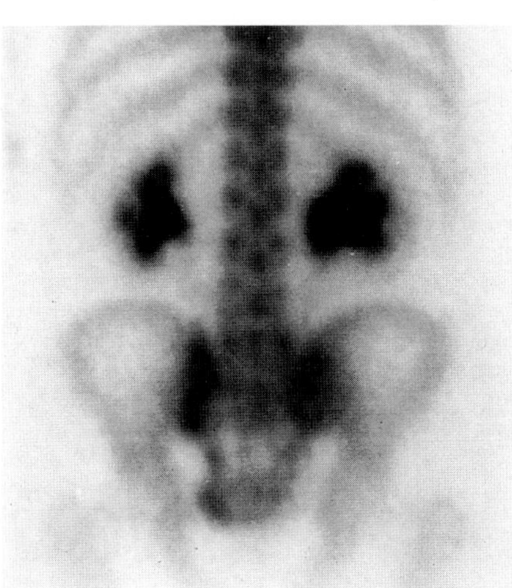

Fig. 79.20 Retention of radioactive urine in dilated pelvicalyceal systems and in the ureter, resulting from obstruction to urinary outflow.

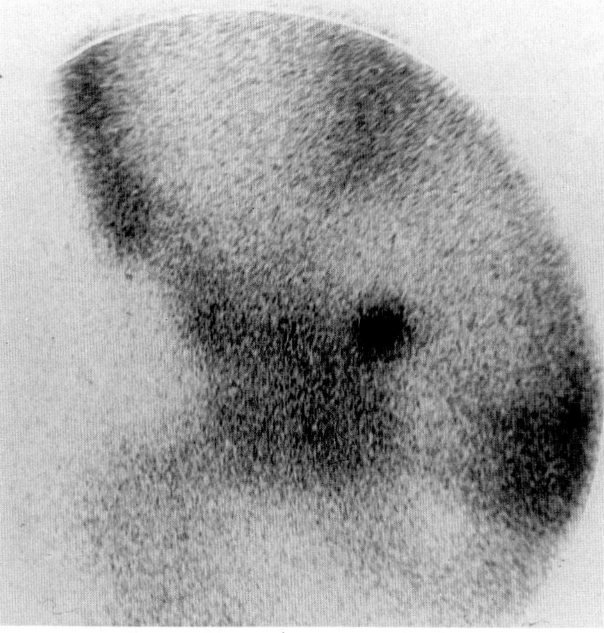

Fig. 79.21 Diverticulum of bladder. Focus of accumulation resulting from residual radioactive urine.

in acute radiation nephritis, corresponding to the stage of interstitial haemorrhage and necrotizing vasculitis. In four of such patients reported by Palestro et al,[68] this extraosseous accumulation had resolved in further studies 11–13 months later. Marked retention of radioactive urine in the ureters may indicate obstruction to outflow by intrapelvic neoplasia. Small pools of radioactive urine can, however, cause considerable difficulty in differentiation from foci in bones, especially if lying in the renal pelvis underlying ribs, in the ureters or in bladder diverticulae (Fig. 79.21). Further views after patient movement and repositioning or using different projections may be of value. While it is imperative to attempt complete bladder emptying immediately prior to scintigraphy, residual bladder activity frequently negates optimal studies, particularly of the pubis and ischia. Supplementary images, including using decubitis positions and particularly of the pelvic inlet with caudal projections, achieved by sitting on the camera, may be rewarding (Fig. 79.22). Additional imaging 24 h later may be required. Similar delayed studies may also be necessary to visualize bone in patients who have undergone urinary diversion surgery, particularly if there is the demonstration of large colonic collections of radioactive urine. Attempts must be made to move ileal urine reservoir bags away from osseous structures. On occasion, bizarre images may reveal unsuspected abnormalities such as vesicocolonic fistulae. Observation of shape and position of the bladder may unmask intrapelvic pathology. It is essential to remember the possibility of spots of contamination by radioactive urine simulating foci of osteoblastic activity, particularly if they overlie bone. Although such contamination is frequently suspected because of the marked intensity of the radioactivity, differentiation may require removal of clothing or washing of skin (Fig. 79.23). Somewhat similarly, failure to remove a tampon with absorbed radioactivity could lead to a mistaken diagnosis of osteitis pubis (Fig. 79.24).

Radioactive urine in the bladder is responsible for frequently encountered artefacts in SPECT studies of the pelvis. Because the amount of activity is varying during acquisition, 'streaking' occurs in the reconstructed images and can overlap bony structures of interest. Further, the intense bladder activity may be such as to cause pixel overload, resulting in adjacent 'cold' areas, which may lie in the region of the femoral heads, usually the main sites of diagnostic interest. A number of techniques have been advocated, to prevent these artefacts, but none has gained universal acceptance. The post-acquisition computer processing method described by Bunker et al[69] has been favoured, and in a comparative study by O'Connor & Kelly[70] was superior. However, while they found that the image quality was significantly improved, they suggested caution in interpretation, particularly the medial aspects of the hips.

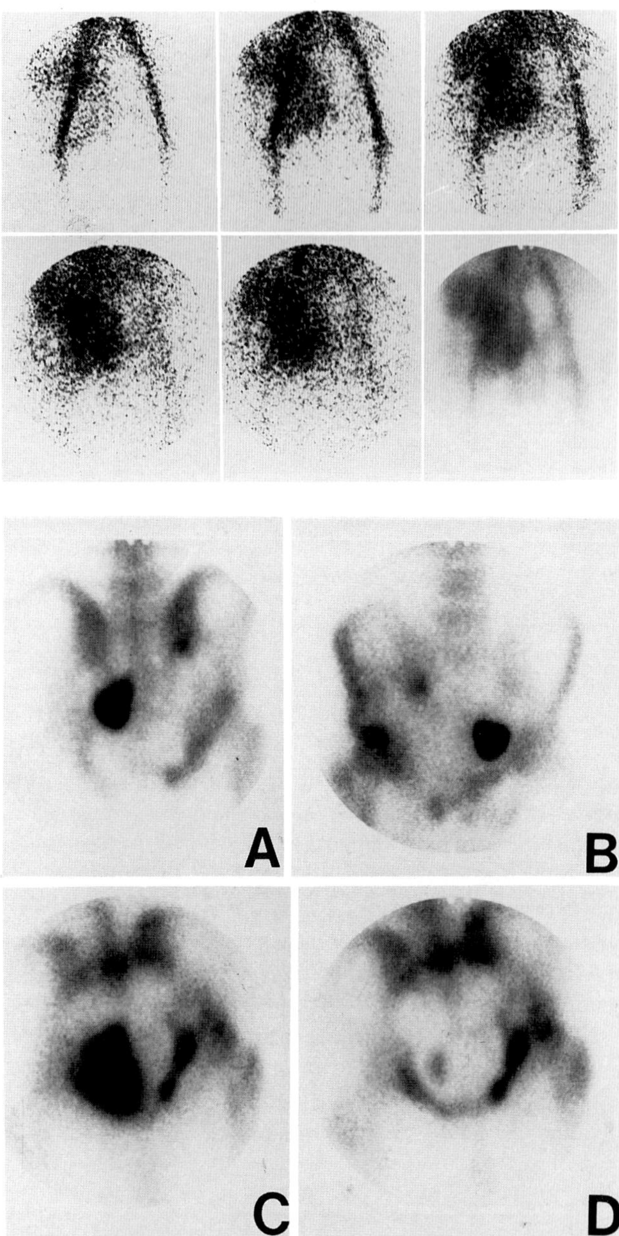

Fig. 79.22 (Top) Dynamic flow study and blood pool phase of the pelvis in a 31-year-old man complaining of persistent right hip pain following an injury 12 months previously. A large hypervascular area was demonstrable with persistent hyperaemia in the blood pool image (bottom right). (Bottom) In both the anterior (A) and posterior (B) views of the pelvis, there is increased accumulation throughout the right ischium and also the right sacroiliac joint. This abnormal ischial uptake is most clearly demonstrated in the subpubic views of the pelvic inlet. In these views, in particular, displacement of the bladder activity to the left is noted both before (C) and after (D) voiding. This vascular intrapelvic mass, arising from the right ischium, was established histologically to be an aggressive giant cell tumour.

Alterations in skeletal uptake can occur in a variety of systemic disorders, not infrequently being visualized in a pattern typical of the particular disorder. Local pathology, however, may affect the uptake of the radiopharmaceu-

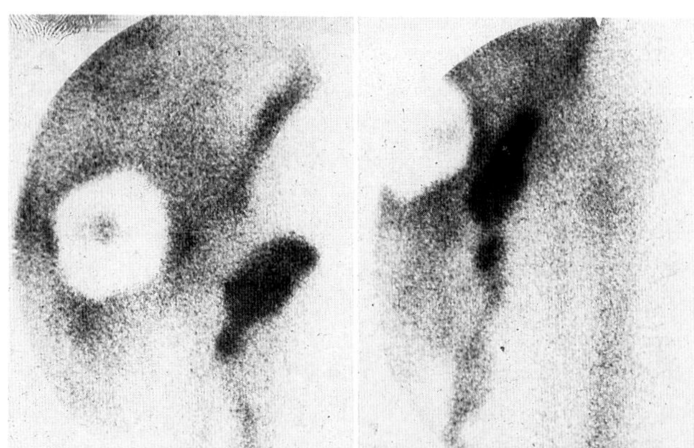

Fig. 79.23 Artefact caused by radioactive urine contamination noted as a focus of accumulation (left), which was suspected as the cause in view of the intensity in comparison with normal bone, although lying approximately in the bony outline, and which was confirmed by movement of the clothing (right).

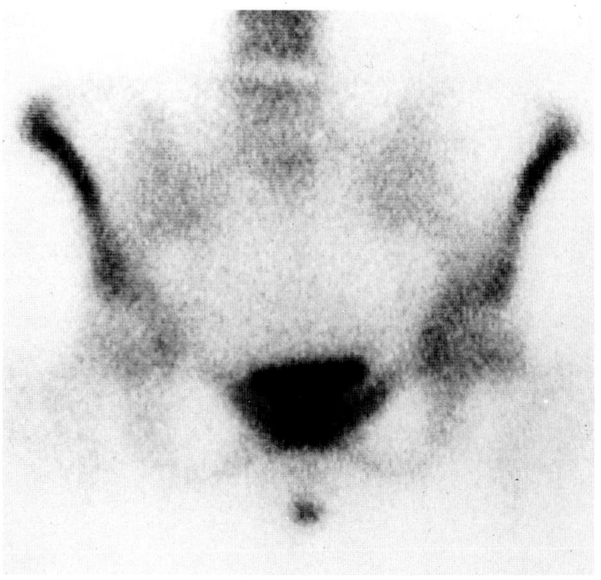

Fig. 79.24 Abnormal pubic symphysis uptake was compatible with stress injury induced by horse riding but was the result of radioactivity absorbed onto a tampon. Removal of the tampon resulted in normal images.

tical. Increased accumulation throughout an entire bone can be associated with various vascular disturbances. Such extended uptake throughout the femur was reported by Glasier et al[71] as the result of thrombosis in the right femoral vein. Chronic venous insufficiency is recognized as a cause of periosteal bone formation. Gensburg et al[72] reported this as being associated with marked uptake on scintigraphy in two patients. They expressed surprise that this scan abnormality had been so rarely noted in view of the frequency of the condition. They suggested that the long-standing nature of the periosteal process, presumably resulting from impaired periosteal blood supply, may not be sufficiently active to induce increased radionuclide uptake despite the common radiographic change of thick undulating periosteal reaction. Resnick & Niwayama,[73] pointing out that periostitis may be detected in 10–60% of patients with chronic venous stasis, also commented that arterial insufficiency has been associated with periosteal bone proliferation. Preferential radionuclide uptake, localized to bone 2–3 weeks after the acute ischaemic insult, was reported by Simpson[74] in two patients in whom arterial embolism had occurred. Similar increased bone uptake was found by Glasier et al[71] in another patient in whom septic embolism had occurred. A widely recognized cause of increased osseous accumulation in the axial skeleton is that occurring in paralysed limbs. Prakash et al[75] identified this phenomenon in all three hemiparetic patients studied and in five of nine paraplegic patients. Normal localization in the affected limbs was identified in three hemiparetic patients and in the remaining four paraplegic patients. In the latter, however, the paraplegia had existed for longer than 9 years. They pointed out that in the first several years of disuse, although there is a gross increase in bone absorption, bone formation is increased up to twice normal. Further, radiographic studies by Dequeker[76] have shown increased periosteal new bone formation occurring in disuse osteoporosis. However, patients with a long-standing paralysis have decreased osteogenesis as well as bone absorption in paralysed limbs, postulated by Prakash et al[75] as being the probable cause for the lack of increased localization in patients with a long-standing paralysis.

Extravasation of the radiopharmaceutical at the injection site is usually very obvious but the consequent occurrence of uptake in an axillary lymph node, although rare, can cause difficulty and require care to differentiate from a rib lesion. Marked accumulation of ^{99m}Tc-MDP at the site of extravasation of the radiographic contrast medium, iodothalamate meglumide, has been described by Aquino & Villaneuva-Meyer.[77]

Failure to remove metallic and other objects, such as coins, necklaces, belts and breast prostheses, will cause the attenuation of ^{99m}Tc, as will pacemakers. These areas of absent uptake are usually readily identified by the non-anatomical site and shape. Similarly, there is usually little difficulty recognizing the rounded photopenia resulting from the gastric air bubble, especially in children.

Extraosseous uptake

Non-skeletal accumulation of the technetium phosphate complexes is not uncommon, and a myriad of case reports have appeared, leading to numerous lists and tables. Even the most extensive, such as that by McAfee & Silberstein,[78] have become outdated as additional examples are recorded. The range is such that, while a number of mechanisms have been postulated,[79] it is considered that no single one can be responsible and that often there may be an interaction of two or more. The occurrence of this phenomenon varies from common disorders, in which it may play a key diagnostic role, to those in which the observation assists in the evaluation of the clinical problem or perhaps unveils a totally unsuspected and unrelated disease, to those which are rare, bizarre and of little clinical significance. Recognition of the abnormality may just arouse curiosity (Fig. 79.25), but it may be of critical clinical relevance, and cannot be ignored.

Factors affecting the normal distribution of the radiopharmaceutical will produce readily identifiable abnormalities. Retention in soft tissue generally will occur in severe renal dysfunction, but will also be obvious in the affected limb in lymphoedema. Rodman et al[80] reported the findings in inferior vena cava obstruction: soft-tissue accumulation below the mid-thorax with normal radiopharmaceutical clearance above this level. Retention of radioactivity within the soft tissue has occasionally been noted in association with deep venous thrombosis, and Zuckier et al[81] observed uptake localized in the thrombi. Chronic venous thrombosis may also result in diffuse soft-tissue accumulation[72] and can also induce subcutaneous ossification, which Truit et al[82] suggested was best delin-

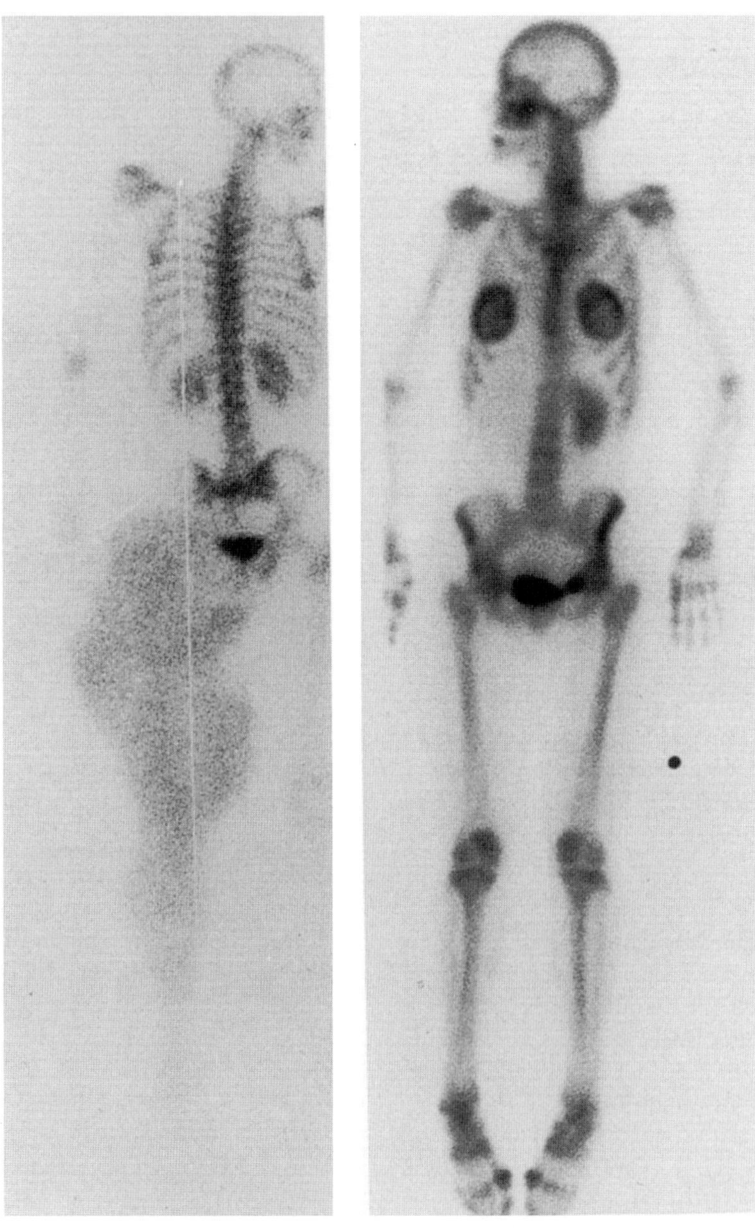

Fig. 79.25 Extraosseous uptake. (A) Massive neurofibromatosis: diffuse uptake throughout left leg. (B) Silicone injections: selective uptake in sites of breast augmentation 15 years before.

eated by SPECT. The scintigraphic changes of periostitis may also be demonstrable. These changes also are associated with arterial occlusion and ischaemia, in which more focal and intense uptake resulting from muscle infarction can be obvious.[74]

The site of the extraosseous localization may be obvious, such as in a pleural effusion or ascitic collection (Fig. 79.26). With a few exceptions, uptake in such collections has been associated with malignancy, Siegel et al[83] showing that 90% of the activity occurring in a pleural effusion is in the non-cellular fluid phase. However, in reporting such accumulation in a patient with sympathetic pleural effusion and reviewing the literature, Cole et al[84] suggested that tumour involvement with the pleural space or involvement of the pleura is not a prerequisite for MDP accumulation, which may be the result of disruption of pleural permeability by mechanisms which remain obscure. Increased pulmonary uptake of MDP can occur following radiotherapy or in radiation pneumonitis. It has also been noted by Vaquer et al[85] in *Pneumocystis carinii* pneumonia with reversal of uptake following specific therapy, which paralleled that of ^{67}Ga. Diffuse uptake in other organs is less common than the focal accumulation resulting from numerous pathological processes. However, splenic accumulation in a pattern differing from that associated with more discrete uptake in infarction, tumour deposits and splenic haematoma can occur in a wide range of haematological disorders, including leukaemia, lymphoma, glucose 6-phosphate deficiency, thalassaemia and sickle cell disease. Many of the patients in whom it has been reported were transfusion dependent, and the localization probably reflects the resulting haemosiderosis with transchelation of ^{99m}Tc. In a study of 38 patients with sickle cell diseases, Silberstein et al[86] found that all those whose spleens were visualized with bone scintigraphy had functional asplenia, identified as lack of uptake of ^{99m}Tc sulphur colloid. In contrast, only half of those whose spleens did not accumulate the bone-seeking radiopharmaceutical had functional asplenia.

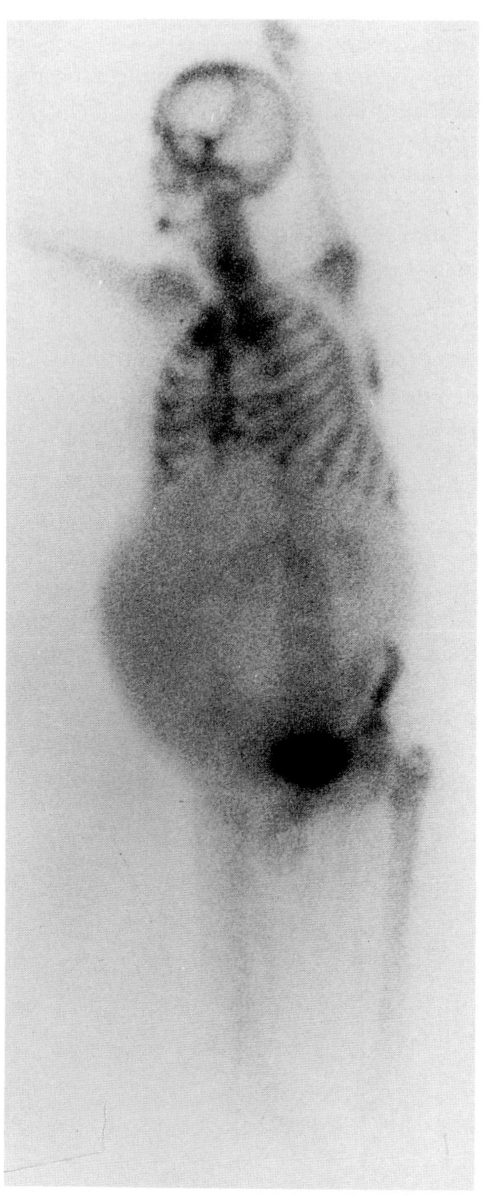

Fig. 79.26 Gross ascites causing abnormal accumulation.

The mechanisms whereby ^{99m}Tc bone-seeking radiopharmaceuticals localize in ischaemic or dying cells has been the basis of considerable interest[83,84] in view of the frequency and significance of the findings. Abnormal ionic calcium flux following altered cell membrane integrity is a major factor and results in changes in the intracellular solubility of calcium and phosphate and precipitation of calcium salts[87]. Binding of the ^{99m}Tc phosphate agents to calcium either as amorphous calcium phosphate or complexed to myofibrils and other macromolecules in the myoplasm may well explain the preferential uptake, although transchelation of technetium may also be involved[88]. Uptake in myocardial infarction was initially an incidental observation,[89] but it was realized that it occurred with such frequency that 'hotspot' imaging using the bone-seeking radiopharmaceuticals for detecting avid focal accumulation in the myocardium became a routine and sensitive means of detecting acute myocardial necrosis (Ch. 99). The alteration is, however, non-specific, and similar uptake can occur in unstable angina, myocardial contusion, pericarditis and ventricular aneurysm. With views in appropriate projections it should be possible to differentiate readily the localized uptake reflecting areas of tissue necrosis induced by cardioversion (Fig. 79.27). Diffuse myocardial accumulation has been reported in hypercalcaemia, amyloidosis, alcoholic cardiomyopathy and adriamycin-induced cardiotoxicity. Care is required to ensure that the uptake readily visualized as associated with cerebral infarction is not an osseous lesion (Fig. 79.28). Intense accumulation may also be encountered in infarcts of the spleen, particularly related to the sickle cell crisis; in the liver, resulting

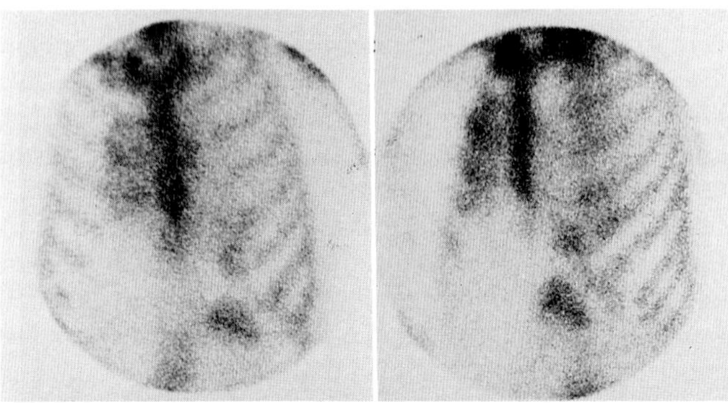

Fig. 79.27 Soft-tissue injuries induced by cardioversion. Numerous foci of extraosseous accumulation.

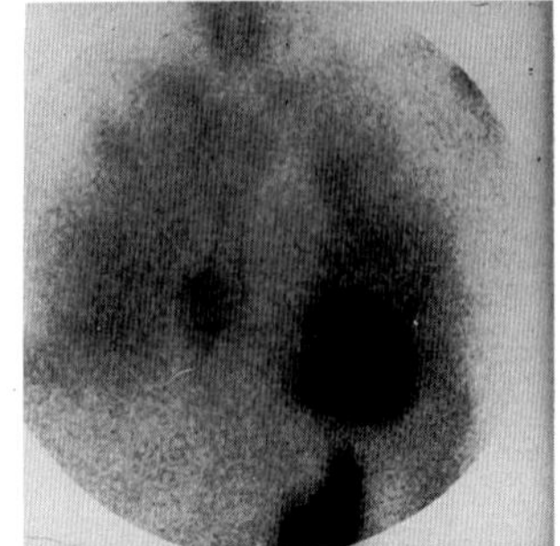
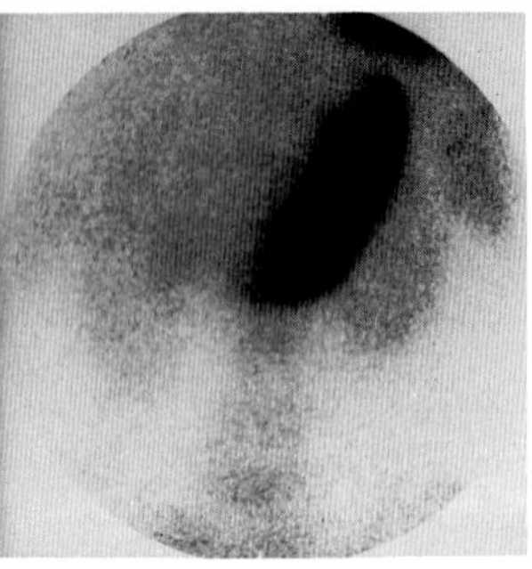

Fig. 79.29 Metastatic visceral calcification demonstrated in a patient with hypercalcaemia associated with gross metastatic disease from carcinoma of the breast; moderately abnormal accumulation is obvious in the lungs and thyroid while the myocardial and gastric uptake is intense.

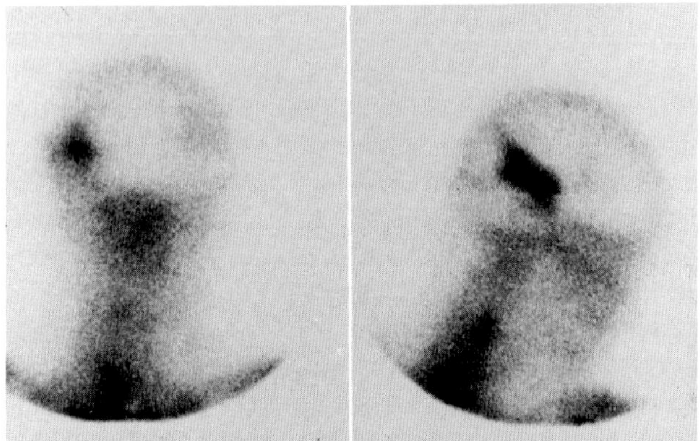

Fig. 79.28 Right hemispheric cerebral infarction. Extraosseous accumulation observed as intense uptake.

from ischaemic hepatopathy; and in centrilobular necrosis, from necrotizing enterocolitis of the newborn.

Diffuse uptake in multiple organs is most likely to be the result of metastatic visceral calcification. The hypercalcaemia usually associated may be induced by hyperparathyroidism, the secondary disorder often producing more striking abnormalities than the primary, or be evidence of malignancy. Varied carcinomas, lymphoma and multiple myeloma have all been noted as the primary pathology. While the uptake in the stomach is the most common site, Choy & Murray[49] emphasized that it can occur in the myocardium, lungs, kidneys and thyroid (Fig. 79.29), and noted the variation in the speed with which the alterations in the different organs is reversed following therapy. Uptake in liver and spleen has also been reported. They also drew attention to the relative rarity with which abnormal MDP uptake has been noted in uraemic patients despite an autopsy rate of pulmonary calcification of 60%. Radiological change is also not common. Only 3 of 30 patients reported by De Graaf et al[90] had radiological change, but only one had scintigraphic demonstration of increased pulmonary uptake. The discrepancy appears to arise from the different chemical nature of the deposits. De Jonge et al[91] suggest that such differences may also explain the relatively rare finding of gastric uptake from bone-seeking radiopharmaceuticals in uraemic patients, despite gastric calcification occurring in approximately 60%.

Mild superficial uptake, usually in a linear pattern and identifiable as lying in body folds, can result from hyperhidrosis, most often demonstrable in the very obese subject. Diffuse uptake may be observed in the breast. This can occur in the entirely normal breast, although perhaps more commonly visualized in the gynaecomastia induced by hormonal therapy for prostatic cancer. The accumulation may be somewhat more focal when associated with either benign or malignant pathology but is nonspecific (Fig. 79.30). However, Holmes et al[92] noted that 95% of benign lesions were associated with bilateral uptake compared with only 25% of malignant lesions. They suggested that further investigation was only warranted when unilateral breast uptake was observed. In 75% of patients studied by Bledin et al,[93] non-mammary uptake of no pathological significance was noted in the ribs on the mastectomy side.

Intense focal accumulation in muscle may identify rhabdomyolysis with a mechanism similar to that causing uptake in myocardium. It occurs most frequently following muscle injury, particularly unusual or excessive

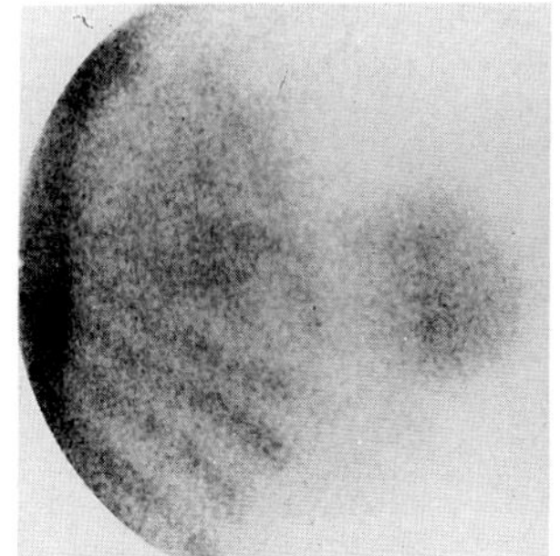
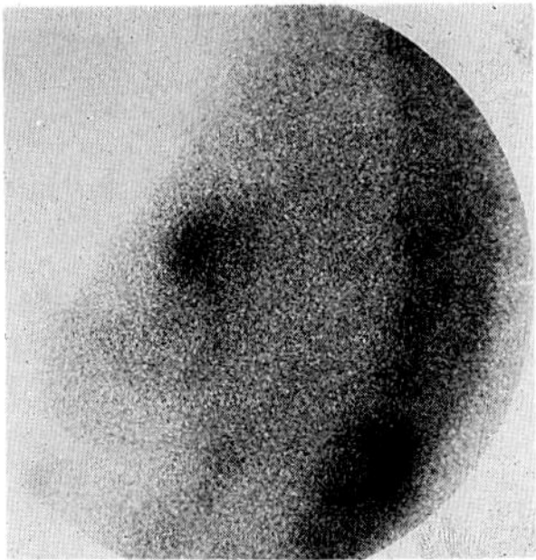

Fig. 79.30 Extraosseous accumulation. Right: Normal breast, diffuse uptake. Left: Carcinoma of breast, focal activity.

exertion, a variety of sporting activities having been reported as responsible. Scintigraphy was advocated by Delpassand et al[94] as a valuable method of assessing the degree of muscle damage following electrical burns. Non-traumatic causes in which muscle uptake of MDP has been reported include alcohol and cocaine intoxication. Less intense but diffuse accumulation in muscle can be observed in a variety of muscle disorders, such as polymyositis, muscular dystrophy, carcinomatous myopathy, paraneoplastic syndromes, scleroderma and dermatomyositis. It may be induced by exercise in the McArdle syndrome.[95] The resolution of the scan changes following therapy can be of clinical value, as for example in patients with polymyositis.[96] However, abnormal muscle uptake of the bone-seeking radiopharmaceuticals is most frequently the result of heterotopic bone formation or myositis ossificans. This disorder is characterized by an initial inflammatory lesion in muscle with subsequent ossification, probably resulting from transformation of primitive mesenchyme-derived cells into bone-forming cells. It can occur in a rare regressive congenital disorder, myositis ossificans progressiva, in which there is widespread calcification of muscle readily demonstrable as extraosseous accumulation of ^{99m}Tc-MDP.[97] However, myositis ossificans is most commonly seen after direct muscle trauma (Fig. 79.31), as a complication of paralysis (Fig. 79.32) or complicating hip arthroplasty, in which it occurs in over 50% of cases. The valuable role of achieving early diagnosis using skeletal scintigraphy was shown by Orzel et al[59] in 50 patients, in 43 of whom myositis

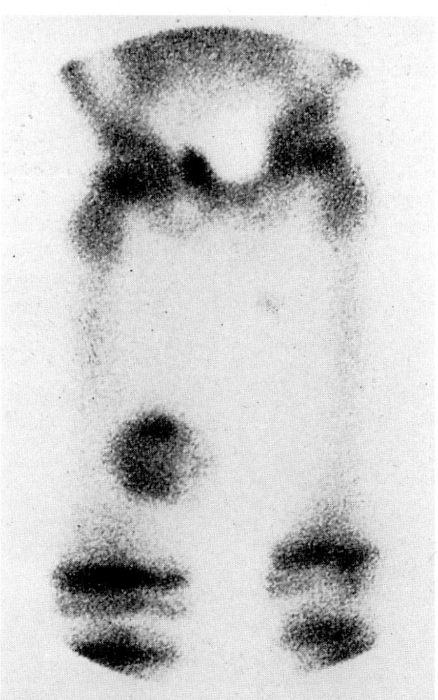

Fig. 79.31 Myositis ossificans. Intense extraosseous accumulation in the lower thigh.

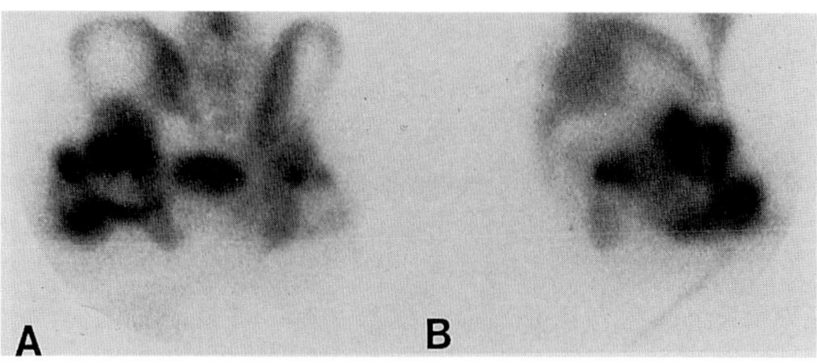

Fig. 79.32 Heterotopic calcification. Prolonged immobilization (A) Anterior and (B) right lateral projections of the pelvis, showing the gross extraosseous accumulation reflecting heterotopic calcification.

ossificans was confirmed and correctly excluded in the remaining seven. They emphasized the importance of undertaking a three-phase study since the flow and blood pool phases were more impressive in 15/43 than the soft-tissue uptake. In three, only these early images were initially abnormal, although the diagnostic muscle uptake was identified by a further study 1 week later. Radiographic documentation followed the radionuclide investigation by an average of 15 days. In 14 patients treated with oral etidrone disodium, a response characterized by resolution of the scintigraphic changes was demonstrated in seven. These had all been started on therapy prior to a radiological change. No scintigraphic response was observed in four patients in whom treatment was started after extensive soft-tissue calcification had been documented by radiography. Mulheim et al[98] also advocated serial studies, particularly in order to identify maturation and thus permit assessment of the optimal time for surgical resection since this condition may recur if the metabolic activity has not been stabilized. Serial studies will also determine the efficacy of treating tumoral calcinosis[99] in which the intense extraosseous uptake and site is so typical (Fig. 79.33). Extraosseous localization in unusual sites and often of bizarre shape can be associated with many benign

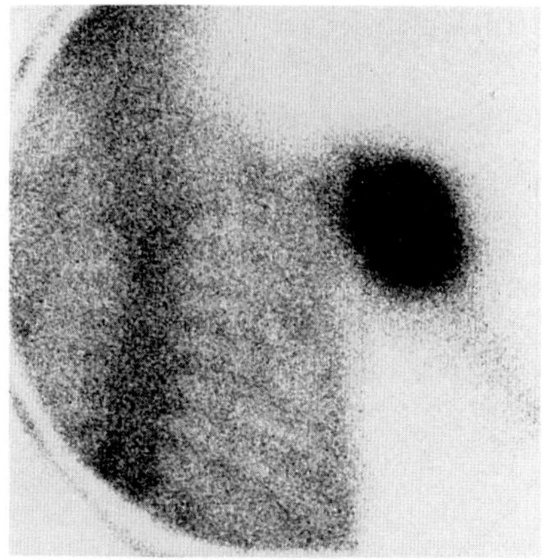

Fig. 79.33 Tumoral calcinosis. Intense accumulation in ectopic calcification in a 3-year-old girl.

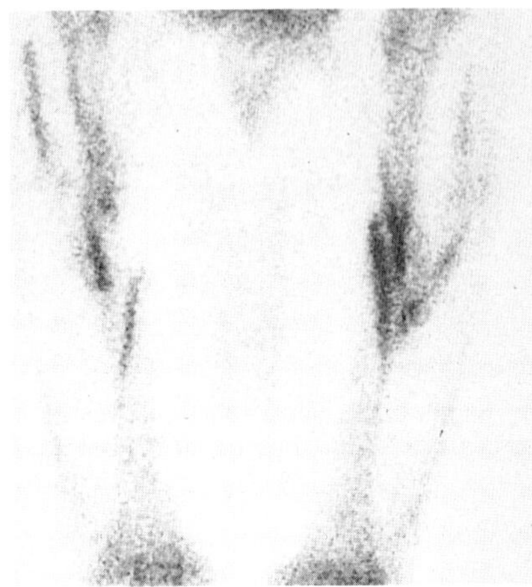

Fig. 79.34 Extraosseous uptake visualized as streaks of accumulation in the numerous sites of pethidine injections.

abnormalities, including calcifying haematomas and scars, or in sites of drug administration (Fig. 79.34).

Perhaps the most avid accumulation of ^{99m}Tc-MDP in soft tissues is that occurring in amyloid deposits. On occasions, these may be so extensive that uptake in bone is reduced. Commenting that many reports in the literature had doubtful diagnostic proof, Janssen et al[100] undertook a detailed study of 18 patients with five different forms of the disease. Their results showed that, with regard to the involvement of the thyroid, tongue, salivary glands, nervous system, intestines, liver, spleen and kidneys, bone scintigraphy can play a very important role in the evaluation of amyloidosis associated with inflammatory conditions (AA amyloidosis) or that associated with plasma cell dyscrasia (AL amyloidosis). They found MDP to be preferable to pyrophosphate, contradicting the earlier suggestion by Lee et al.[101] A surprising finding was the visualization of the kidneys in anuric amyloidotic patients, in contrast to the lack of any uptake in anuric controls. The role of skeletal scintigraphy in identifying myocardial

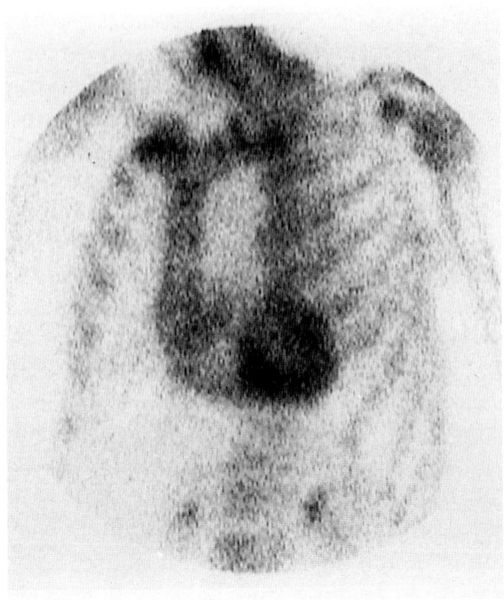

Fig. 79.35 Cardiac amyloidosis associated with marked uptake in the myocardium.

involvement remains controversial. Very avid accumulation of ^{99m}Tc-MDP can occur (Fig. 79.35). However, Janssen et al[100] observed no cardiac uptake in 6/9 patients with apparent clinical and echocardiographic involvement of the heart, whereas accumulation was found in three patients with normal echocardiography. Considerable attention has been paid to the use of these bone-scanning agents in identifying cardiac amyloidosis in view of the associated major morbidity and mortality. Wizenberg et al,[102] for example, found intense diffuse myocardial uptake in all of 10 consecutive patients with tissue-proven amyloidosis. Falk et al,[103] finding similar intense uptake in 9/11 patients with an ECG suggestive of amyloidosis, compared with only 2/9 with normal electrocardiograms, concluded that it was a sensitive and specific test. Gertz et al[104] agreed that the intense diffuse myocardial accumu-

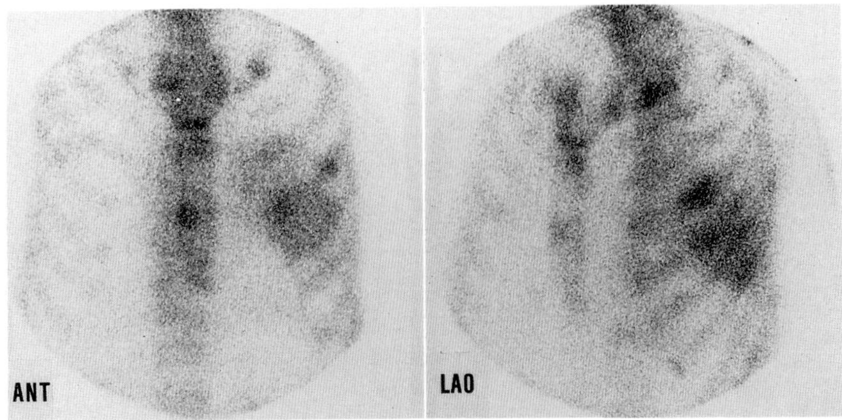

Fig. 79.36 Carcinoma of the lung. Extraosseous accumulation in the primary tumour is observed in the anterior and left anterior oblique view, with metastatic lesions in bone.

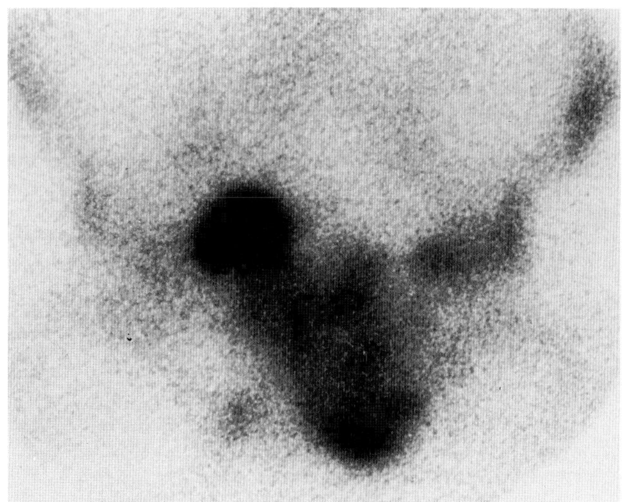

Fig. 79.37 Metastases from prostatic carcinoma. Extraosseous uptake with gross accumulation in nodal metastases, differentiated from urinary contamination by repeated studies following washing.

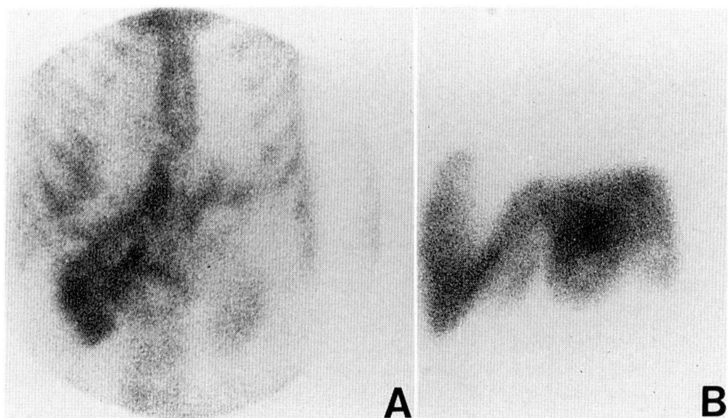

Fig. 79.38 Hepatic metastases from carcinoma of the lung. Intense extraosseous accumulation with bizarre outline, observed in an anterior view with skeletal scintigraphy (A), is confirmed as extraosseous uptake of the radiopharmaceutical, by comparison with the area of absent accumulation identified with standard liver scintigraphy with ^{99m}Tc sulphur colloid (B).

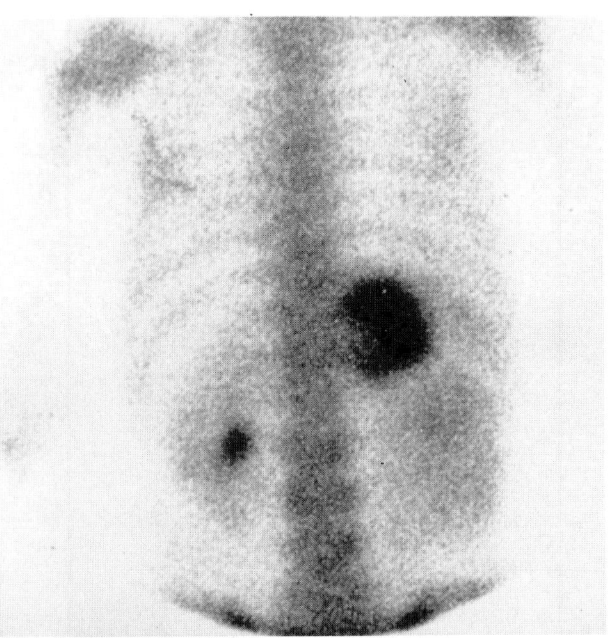

Fig. 79.39 Neuroblastoma. Intense extraosseous accumulation occurring, as frequently observed, in the primary site.

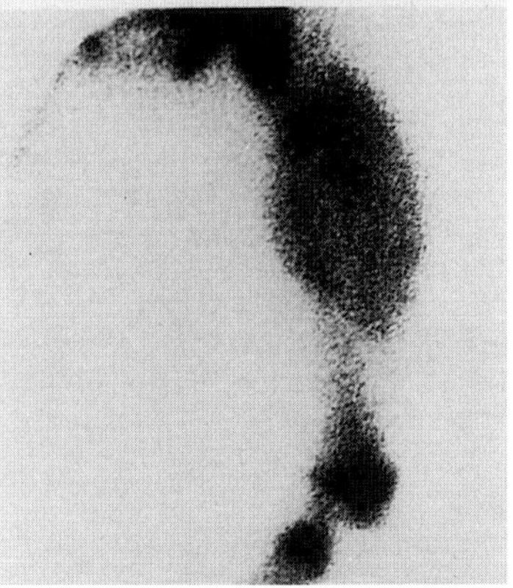

Fig. 79.40 Fibrosarcoma. Extraosseous accumulation in the thigh in a 4-year-old boy.

lation is specific for amyloid cardiomyopathy but pointed out that they could only identify it in 3/20 patients with the disorder. Lesser uptake was found in another 14 but of an intensity present in 15/20 control subjects.

There are few malignant tumours in which the uptake of the bone-seeking radiopharmaceuticals have not been described as an incidental finding on routine skeletal scintigraphy (Fig. 79.36). Although the observation of extra-osseous accumulation should never be ignored and an explanation sought, frequently such a finding has little clinical significance, other than providing confirmation of known diagnostic information. On occasion, however, it may be of importance in identifying non-osseous metastatic deposits which have been unsuspected, for example in lymph nodes (Fig. 79.37) or, more commonly, within the liver (Fig. 79.38). Certainly the uptake which may be found in metastases of osteogenic sarcoma, especially in lung, warrants routine serial studies in the management and follow-up of these children. The frequency with which these can be identified is somewhat controversial, but the increased sensitivity may well result from the use of SPECT. As marked accumulation in the primary lesion is demonstrable in the majority of cases of neuroblastoma (Fig. 79.39), visualization of such uptake when this neoplasm is suspected provides important diagnostic support. Nearly all malignant soft-tissue tumours accumulate the bone agents (Fig. 79.40), as do approximately 50% of the benign tumours. Chew et al[105] suggests that the major role of skeletal scintigraphy in these patients is to assist in the planning of surgical treatment by evaluation of the relationship of the primary tumour to adjacent bone and identifying whether direct involvement of bone has occurred.

REFERENCES

1. Chievitz O, Hevesy G 1935 Radioactive indicators in the study of phosphorus metabolism in rats. Nature 136: 754–755
2. Fleming W H, McIlraith J D, King E R 1961 Photoscanning of bone lesions utilising strontium-85. Radiology 77: 635–636
3. Charkes N B 1969 Some differences between bone scans made with 87mSr and 85Sr. J Nucl Med 10: 491–494
4. Blau M, Nagler W, Bender M A 1962 Fluorine-18: a new isotope for bone scanning. J Nucl Med 3: 332–334
5. Subramanian G, McAfee J G 1971 A new complex for 99m-Tc for skeletal imaging. Radiology 99: 192–196
6. Murray I P C, McKay W J, Robson J, Sorby P, Boyd R E 1972 Skeltec, a thermo-stable 99mTc agent for skeletal scintigraphy. J Nucl Med 13: 445
7. Huberty J P, Hattner R S, Powell M R 1974 A 99m-Tc-pyrophosphate kit: a convenient, economical and high quality skeletal-imaging agent. J Nucl Med 15: 124–126
8. Pendergrass H P, Potsaid M S, Castronovo F P 1973 The clinical use of 99m-Tc-diphosphonate (HEDSPA). Radiology 107: 557–562
9. Subramanian G, McAfee J G, Blair R J, Kallfelz F A, Thomas F D 1975 Technetium-99m-methylene diphosphonate – a superior agent for skeletal imaging: comparison with other technetium complexes. J Nucl Med 16: 744–755
10. Delaloye B, Delaloye-Bischof A, Dudczak R et al 1985 Clinical comparison of 99mTc-HMDP and 99mTc-MDP. A multi-centric study. Eur J Nucl Med 11: 182–185
11. Pauwels E K J, Blom J, Camps J A J, Hermans J, Rijke A M 1983 A comparison between the diagnostic efficacy of 99mTc-MDP, 99mTc-DPD and 99mTc-HDP for the detection of bone metastases. Eur J Nucl Med 25: 166–169
12. Fogelman I 1987 99mTc diphosphonate bone-scanning agents. In: Fogelman I (ed) Bone scanning in clinical practice. Springer, London, p 3
13. Rosenthall L, Stern J, Arzoumanian A 1982 A clinical comparison of MDP and DMAD. Clin Nucl Med 7: 403–406
14. Smith M L, Martin W, McKillop J H, Fogelman I 1984 Improved lesion detection with dimethyl-amino-diphosphonate: a report of two cases. Eur J Nucl Med 9: 519–520
15. Pimm M V, Embleton M J, Perkins A C, Price M R, Robins R A, Robinson G E, Baldwin R W 1982 In vivo localization of anti-osteogenic sarcoma 791T monoclonal antibody in osteogenic sarcoma xenografts. Int J Cancer 30: 75–85
16. Farrands P A, Perkins A, Sully L et al 1983 Localisation of human osteosarcoma by antitumour monoclonal antibody. J Bone Joint Surg 65B: 638–640
17. Perkins A C, Armitage N C, Hardy J G, Wastie M L, Pimm M V, Hardcastle J D 1985 The immunoscintigraphy of bone tumours using an 131I-labelled anti-osteosarcoma monoclonal antibody. In: Donato L, Britton K (eds) Immunoscintigraphy. Gordon & Breach, New York
18. Sakahara H, Endo K, Nakashima T et al 1987 Localization of human osteogenic sarcoma xenografts in nude mice by a monoclonal antibody labelled with radioiodine and indium-111. J Nucl Med 28: 342–348
19. Lee M H, Moon D H, Na H W et al 1992 Diagnosis of femoral head avascular necrosis by triple head high resolution. J Nucl Med 33: 936
20. Mandell G A, Harcke H T, Hugh J, Kumar S J, Maas K W 1990 Detection of talocalcaneal coalitions by magnification bone scintigraphy. J Nucl Med 31: 1797–1801
21. Bahk Y W, Kim O K, Chung S K 1987 Pinhole collimator scintigraphy in differential diagnosis of metastasis, fracture, and infections of the spine. J Nucl Med 28: 447–451
22. Shih W J, Magoun S, Stipp V et al 1991 Volume three-dimensional display of Tc-99m HMDP skull, cervical vertebral, thoracic vertebral, lumbar vertebral, and/or pelvic SPECT images by triple head camera. J Nucl Med 32: 913–914
23. Fogelman I, Bessant R G, Turner J G, Citrin D L, Boyle I T, Greig W R 1978 The use of whole-body retention of Tc-99m diphosphonate in the diagnosis of metabolic bone disease. J Nucl Med 19: 270–275
24. Front D, Israel O, Jerushalmi J et al 1989 Quantitative bone scintigraphy using SPECT. J Nucl Med 30: 240–245
25. Israel O, Front D, Hardoff R, Ish-Shalom S, Jerushalmi J, Kolodny G M 1991 In vivo SPECT quantitation of bone metabolism in hyperparathyroidism and thyroxicosis. J Nucl Med 32: 1157–1161
26. Sagar V V, Piccone J M, Charkes N D 1979 Studies of skeletal tracer kinetics. III. Tc-99m (Sr) methylenediphosphonate uptake in the canine tibia as a function of blood flow. J Nucl Med 20: 1257–1261
27. Lavender J P, Khan R A A, Hughes S P F 1979 Blood flow and tracer uptake in normal and abnormal canine bone: comparison with Sr-85 microspheres, Kr-81m, and Tc-99m MDP. J Nucl Med 20: 413–418
28. Charkes N D, Makler Jr P T, Phillips C 1978 Studies of skeletal tracer kinetics. 1. Digital computer solution of a five-compartmental model of (18F) fluoride kinetics in humans. J Nucl Med 19: 1301–1309
29. Tilden R L, Jackson J, Enneking W F 1973 99m-Tc-polyphosphate: histological localisation in human femurs by autoradiography. J Nucl Med 14: 576–578
30. Francis M D, Ferguson D L, Tofe A J, Bevan J A, Michaels S E 1980 Comparative evaluation of three diphosphonates: in-vivo absorption (C-14 labelled) and in-vivo osteogenic uptake (Tc-99m complexed). J Nucl Med 21: 1185–1189
31. Kaye M, Silverton S, Rosenthall L 1975 Technetium-99m-pyrophosphate studies in-vivo and in-vitro. J Nucl Med 16: 40–45
32. Wiegmann T, Kirsch J, Rosenthall L, Kaye M 1976 Relationship between bone uptake of 99m-Tc-pyrophosphate and hydroxyproline in blood and urine. J Nucl Med 17: 711–714
33. Alfrey A C, Solomones C C, Ciricilla J, Miller N L 1976 Extraosseous calcification. Evidence for abnormal pyrophosphate metabolism in uremia. J Clin Invest 57: 692–699
34. Zimmer A M, Isitman A T, Holmes R A 1975 Enzymatic inhibition of diphosphonate: a proposed mechanism of tissue uptake. J Nucl Med 16: 353–356
35. Wahner H W, Dewanjee M K 1981 Drug induced modulation of Tc-99m-pyrophosphate tissue distribution: what is involved? J Nucl Med 22: 555–559
36. Siegel B A, Engel W K, Derrer E C 1977 Localization of technetium-99m diphosphonate in acutely injured muscle. Neurology 27: 230–238
37. Christensen S B, Krogsgoord O W 1981 Localization of Tc-99m MDP in epiphyseal growth plates of rats. J Nucl Med 22: 237–245
38. Harcke H T 1986 Quantitative scintigraphy of bone growth, bone ischaemia, and the sacroiliac joint. In: Grainger R G, Allison D J (eds) Diagnostic radiology: an Anglo-American textbook of imaging. Churchill Livingstone, Edinburgh, pp 520–534
39. Gates G F, Dore E K 1975 Detection of craniosynostosis by bone scanning. Radiology 115: 665–671
40. Harbert J, Desai R 1985 Small calvarial bone scan foci – normal variations. J Nucl Med 26: 1144–1148
41. Senda K, Itoh S 1987 Evaluation of diffusely high uptake by the calvaria in bone scintigraphy. Ann Nucl Med 1: 23–26
42. Mandell G A, Harcke H T 1987 Scintigraphy of persistent vertebral transverse process epiphysis. Clin Nucl Med 12: 359–362
43. Cawley K A, Dvorak A D, Wilmot M D 1983 Normal anatomic variant: scintigraphy of the ischiopubic synchondrosis. J Nucl Med 24: 14–16
44. Lawson J P 1985 Symptomatic radiographic variants in extremities. Radiology 157: 625–631
45. Fink-Bennett D M, Shapiro E E 1984 The angle of Louis. A potential pitfall ('Louie's hot spot') in bone scan interpretation. J Clin Nucl Med 6: 352–354
46. Tondeus M, Ham H R 1989 A case of false-positive bone imaging. Clin Nucl Med 14: 547
47. Peterdy A E 1985 The diagnosis of thyroid disease on bone scans. Clin Nucl Med 10: 177–179
48. Choy D, Murray I P C 1980 Metastatic visceral calcification identified by bone scanning. Skeletal Radiol 5: 151–159

49. Choy D, Murray I P C, Hoschl R 1981 The effect of iron on the biodistribution of bone scanning agents in humans. Radiology 140: 197–202
50. Hiltz A H, Iles S E 1990 Abnormal distribution of Tc-99m Iminodiphosphonate due to iron dextran therapy. Clin Nucl Med 15: 818–819
51. Van Antwerp J D, Hall J N, O'Mara, R E, Schuyler E H 1975 Bone scan abnormality produced by interaction of Tc-99m diphosphonate with iron dextran (Imferon). J Nucl Med 16: 577
52. Spencer R, Sziklas J J, Rosenberg R J et al 1990 Splenic uptake of Tc-99m MDP: possible relationship to hemosiderin. Clin Nucl Med 15: 582
53. Lutrin C L, McDougall I R, Goris M L 1978 Intense concentration of technetium 99m PYP in kidneys of children treated with chemotherapeutic drugs for malignant disease. Radiology 128: 165–167
54. Bernard M S, Hayward M, Hayward C et al 1990 Evaluation of intense renal parenchymal activity ('Hot Kidneys'). Clin Nucl Med 15: 254–256
55. Koizumi K, Tonami N, Hisada K 1981 Diffusely increased Tc-99m MDP uptake in both kidneys. Clin Nucl Med 6: 362–365
56. Krasnow A Z, Collier B D, Isitman A T et al 1988 False-negative bone imaging due to Etidronate therapy. Clin Nucl Med 13: 264–267
57. Watt I, Hill P 1981 Effects of acute administration of ethane hydroxydiphosphonate (EHDP) on skeletal scinitgraphy with technetium-99m-methylene disphosphonic acid (Tc-MDP) in the rat. Br J Radiol 54: 592–596
58. Sandler E D, Parisi M T, Hattner R S 1991 Duration of Etidronate effect demonstrated by serial bone scintigraphy. J Nucl Med 32: 1782–1784
59. Orzel J A, Rudd T G, Nelp W B 1984 Heterotopic bone formation (myositis ossificans) and lower extremity swelling mimicking deep venous thrombosis. J Nucl Med 25: 1105–1107
60. Hattner R S, Hartmeyer J, Wara W M 1982 Characterization of radiation-induced photopenic abnormalities on bone scans. Radiology 145: 161–163
61. Ferris J V, Ziessman H A 1988 Technetium-99m MDP imaging of acute radiation-induced inflammation. Clin Nucl Med 13: 430–432
62. Israel O, Gorenberg M, Frenkel A et al 1992 Local and systemic effects of radiation on bone metabolism measured by quantitative SPECT. J Nucl Med 33: 1774–1782
63. Charkes N D, Silverman C 1992 Does radiotherapy affect bone formation? J Nucl Med 33: 1780–1782
64. Chayes Z W, Strashun A M 1980 Improved renal screening on bone scans. Clin Nucl Med 5: 94–97
65. Adams K J, Shuler S E, Witherspoon I R et al 1980 A retrospective analysis of renal abnormalities detected in bone scans. Clin Nucl Med 5: 1–7
66. Kajubi S K, Chayes Z W 1985 Superscan prediction – another benefit for early renal views in bone scans. J Nucl Med 26: 428–429
67. Haden H T, Katz P G, Konerding K F 1988 Detection of obstructive uropathy by bone scintigraphy. J Nucl Med 29: 1781–1785
68. Palestro C, Fineman D, Goldsmith S T 1988 Acute radiation nephritis: Its evaluation on sequential bone imaging. Clin Nucl Med 13: 787–791
69. Bunker S R, Handmaker H, Torre D M et al 1990 Pixel overflow artifacts in SPECT evaluation of the skeleton. Radiology 174: 229–232
70. O'Connor M K, Kelly B T 1990 Evaluation of techniques for the elimination of 'hot' bladder artifacts in SPECT of the pelvis. J Nucl Med 31: 1872–1875
71. Glasier C M, Seibert M D, Williamson M D 1987 The gamut of increased whole bone activity in bone scintigraphy in children. Clin Nucl Med 12: 192–197
72. Gensburg R S, Kawashima A, Sandler C M 1988 Scintigraphic demonstration of lower extremity periostitis secondary to venous insufficiency. J Nucl Med 29: 1279–1282
73. Resnick D, Niwayama G 1981 Diagnosis of bone and joint disorders. W B Saunders, Philadelphia, p 2996
74. Simpson A J 1977 Localization of 99mTc-pyrophosphate in an ischaemic leg. Clin Nucl Med 2: 400–403
75. Prakash V, Kamel N J, Lin M S et al 1978 Increased skeletal localisation of 99m-Tc-diphosphonate in paralysed limbs. Clin Nucl Med 48–50
76. Dequeker J 1971 Periosteal and endosteal surface remodelling in pathologic conditions. Invest Radiol 6: 260–265
77. Aquino S, Villaneuva-Meyer J 1992 Uptake of Tc-99m MDP in soft tissues related to radiographic contrast media extravasation. Clin Nucl Med 17: p 974
78. McAfee J G, Silberstein E B 1984 Non-osseous uptake. In Differential diagnosis in nuclear medicine. Silberstein E B, McAfee J G (eds) McGraw Hill, New York, pp 300–318
79. Brill D R 1981 Radionuclide imaging of nonneoplastic soft tissue disorders. Semin Nucl Med 11: 177–288
80. Rodman D J, Atkinson L K, Maxwell D D et al 1990 Bone scan in inferior vena cava obstruction. Clin Nucl Med 15: 740–743
81. Zuckier L S, Patel K A, Wexler J P et al 1990 The hot clot sign: a new finding in deep venous thrombosis on bone scintigraphy. Clin Nucl Med 15: 790–793
82. Truit C L, Hartshorne M F, Peters V J 1988 Subcutaneous ossification of the legs examined with SPECT. Clin Nucl Med 13: 423–425
83. Siegel M E, Walker Jr W J, Campbell J L 1975 Accumulation of Tc-99m-diphosphonate in malignant pleural effusions: detection and verification. J Nucl Med 16: 883–885
84. Cole T J, Balseiro J, Lippman H R 1991 Technetium-99m-Methylene-Diphosphonate (MDP) uptake in sympathetic effusion: an index of malignancy and a review of the literature. J Nucl Med 32: 325–327
85. Vaquer R A, Dunn E K, Subrahmanya B et al 1989 Reversible pulmonary uptake and hypertrophic pulmonary osteoarthropathic distribution of technetium-99m-methylene diphosphonate in a case of *Pneumocystis carinii* pneumonia. J Nucl Med 30: 1563–1567
86. Silberstein E B, Delong S, Cline J 1984 Tc-99m diphosphonate and sulphur colloid uptake by the spleen in sickle disease: interrelationship and clinical correlates: concise communication. J Nucl Med 25: 1300–1303
87. Dewanjee M K, Kahn P C 1976 Mechanism of localization of 99m Tc-labelled pyrophosphate and tetracycline in infarcted myocardium. J Nucl Med 17: 639–646
88. Buja L M, Tofe A J, Kulkarni P V et al 1977 Sites and mechanisms of localization of technetium-99m phosphorus radiopharmaceuticals in acute myocardial infarct and other tissues. J Clin Invest 60: 724–740
89. Bonte F J, Parkey R W, Graham K D, Moore J, Stokely E M 1974 A new method for radionuclide imaging of myocardial infarct. Radiology 110: 473–474
90. de Graaf P, Schicht I M, Pauwels E K J, te Velde J, de Graaf J 1978 Bone scintigraphy in renal osteodystrophy. J Nucl Med 19: 1289–1296
91. de Jonge F A A, Pauwels E K J, Hamby N A T 1991 Scintigraphy in the clinical evaluation of disorders of minimal and skeletal metabolism in renal failure. Eur J Nucl Med 18: 839–855
92. Holmes R A, Manoli R S, Isitman A T 1975 Tc-99m labelled phosphates as an indicator of breast pathology. J Nucl Med 16: p. 536
93. Bledin A G, Kim E E, Haynie T P 1982 Bone scintigraphic findings related to unilateral mastectomy. Eur J Nucl Med 7: 500–501
94. Delpassand E S, Dhekne R D, Barron B J et al 1991 Evaluation of soft tissue injury by Tc-99m bone agent scintigraphy. Clin Nucl Med 16: 309–314
95. Swift T R, Brown M 1978 99m-Tc pyrophosphate muscle labelling in McArdle syndrome. J Nucl Med 19: 295–297
96. Otsuka N, Fukunaga M, Ono S et al 1988 Visualization of soft tissue by Technetium-99m MDP in polymyositis. Clin Nucl Med 13: 291–293
97. Guze B H, Schelbert H 1989 The nuclear medicine bone image and myositis ossificans progressiva. Clin Nucl Med 14: 161–162
98. Muheim G, Donath A, Rossier A B 1973 Serial scintigrams in the course of ectopic bone formation in paraplegic patients. AJR 118: 865–869
99. Leicht E, Berberich R, Lauffenburger T, Haas H G 1979 Tumoral calcinosis: accumulation of bone seeking tracers in the calcium deposits. Eur J Nucl Med 4: 419

100. Janssen S, Piers D A, Rijswijk M H et al 1990 Soft-tissue uptake of 99m Tc-diphosphonate and 99m Tc-pyrophosphate in amyloidosis. Eur J Nucl Med 16: 663–670
101. Lee V W, Caldarone A G, Falk R H et al 1983 Amyloidosis of heart and liver: comparison of Tc-99m pyrophosphate and Tc-99m methylene diphosphonate for detection. Radiology 148: 239–242
102. Wizenberg T A, Muz J, Sohn Y H et al 1982 Value of positive myocardial technetium-99m-pyrophosphate scintigraphy in the non-invasive diagnosis of cardiac amyloidosis. Am Heart J 103: 468–473
103. Falk R H, Lee V W, Rubinow A et al 1983 Sensitivity of technetium-99m-pryophosphate scintigraphy in diagnosing cardiac amyloidosis. Am J Cardiol 51: 826–830
104. Gertz M A, Brown M L, Hauser M F et al 1987 Utility of technetium Tc 99m pyrophosphate bone scanning in cardiac amyloidosis. Arch Int Med 147: 1039–1044
105. Chew F S, Hudson T M, Enneking W F 1981 Radionuclide imaging of soft tissue neoplasms. Semin Nucl Med 11: 277–288

80. The evaluation of malignancy: primary bone tumours

I. P. C. Murray

For a considerable period after the introduction of the technetium phosphate complexes, skeletal scintigraphy had a limited role in the diagnosis of primary bone tumours. Subsequent therapeutic advances have been such that early diagnosis and staging is even more critical and requires maximum use of all diagnostic modalities, including skeletal scintigraphy. There has been growing awareness that fairly characteristic scintigraphic patterns can be identified and that radionuclide studies, often using the technetium agents and other radionuclides in combination, offer complementary information in the evaluation of the primary lesion, assessment of the tumour size and in monitoring therapy.

EVALUATION OF THE PRIMARY LESION

The lesser metabolic activity of a benign tumour should be expected to be associated with a less intense accumulation of the radiopharmaceutical. While generally true, it cannot be totally relied upon. Nevertheless, a negative scintigraphic study can be of diagnostic assistance, particularly when radiological interpretation is difficult. Thus, for example, no scintigraphic alteration is to be expected in a simple bone cyst, unless traumatized, whereas fibrous dysplasia is characterized by a well-delineated intense uptake. Similarly, no alteration is associated with the radiological abnormality of the fibrous cortical defect.[1] While unusual, varying degrees of accumulation may occur in non-ossifying fibromas.[2] In contrast, intense circumscribed uptake can be demonstrated in ossifying fibromas (Fig. 80.1), although quite non-specific, being identical, for example, with those

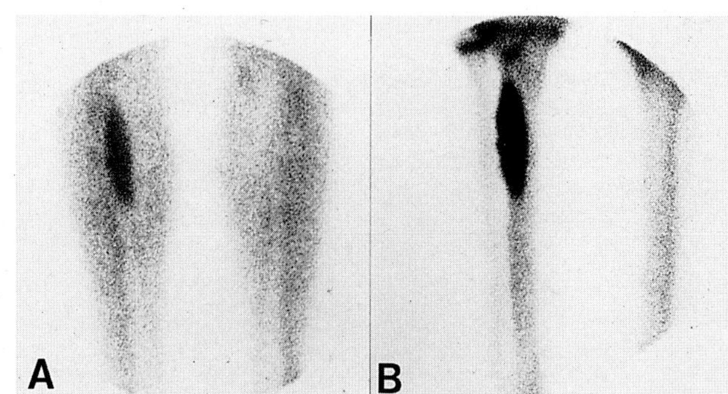

Fig. 80.2 Adamantinoma in upper tibia, demonstrated by discrete vascularity in the blood pool phase (A), and a well-delineated and intense area of uptake in the delayed images (B).

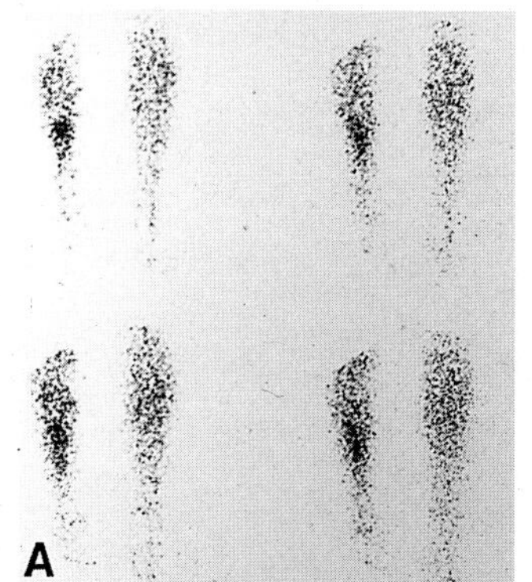

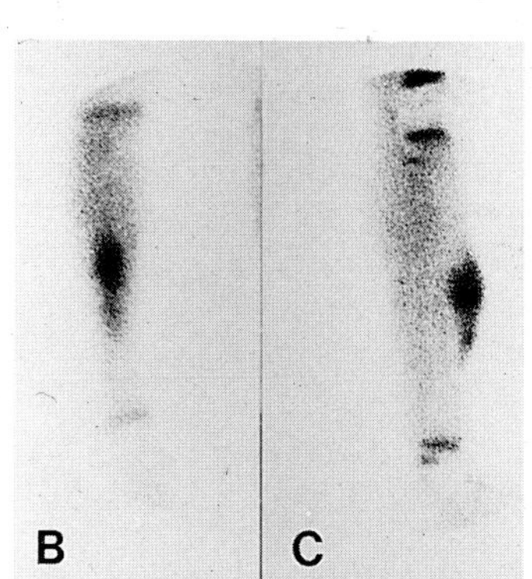

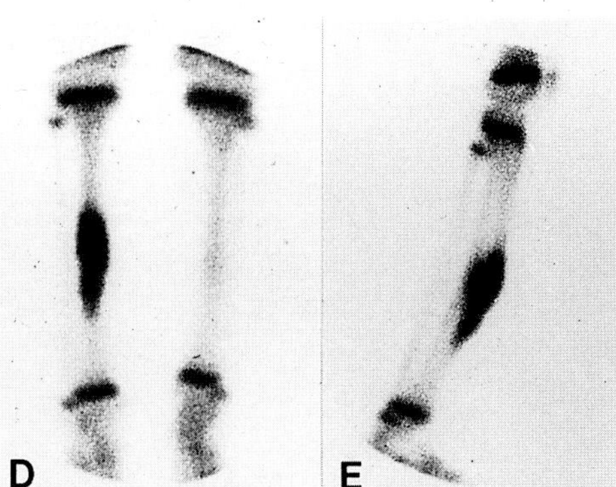

Fig. 80.1 Osteofibrous dysplasia (ossifying fibroma). In the dynamic phase (A) an intense focal area of vascularity is noted. (B and C) A well-localized area of hyperaemia becomes evident in the blood pool in both the anterior and medial projections (D and E). In the delayed image, accumulation is intense and well delineated. In the later projection it is identified as lying in the anterior aspect of the tibial shaft.

occurring in fibrous dysplasia and in adamantinoma (Fig. 80.2). The degree of vascularity noted in the latter in the initial stage may be less marked. In benign tumours, the lesion margin is typically clearly delineated. Bone islands are not usually visualized scintigraphically but mild focal uptake may be seen, merely reflecting the normal mild metabolic activity of the bone island and only demonstrable because of the size of the particular lesion.[3] Visualization of osteochondroma will also depend on the status of ossification (Fig. 80.3), waning with the fusion of the adjacent epiphysis, so that radionuclide uptake after skeletal maturation must cause concern, particularly in patients with multiple exostoses.[4] The malignant change which can occur in patients with multiple enchondromas (Fig. 80.4) can be difficult to ascertain scintigraphically. Although Pearlman and Steiner[5] suggested that it was not possible to determine whether such cartilaginous tumours were benign or malignant by evaluation of the intensity and uniformity of uptake, a lesion which is not only significantly larger but displays marked avidity, particularly in the pattern of that encountered in chondrosarcoma (Fig. 80.5), heightens suspicion. Serial studies are of value in indicating the need for biopsy. Chondroblastoma, however, is normally characterized by uniform distribution and only minimal uptake (Fig. 80.6) although Humphrey et al[6] reported three cases which were hyperaemic and displayed marked avidity.

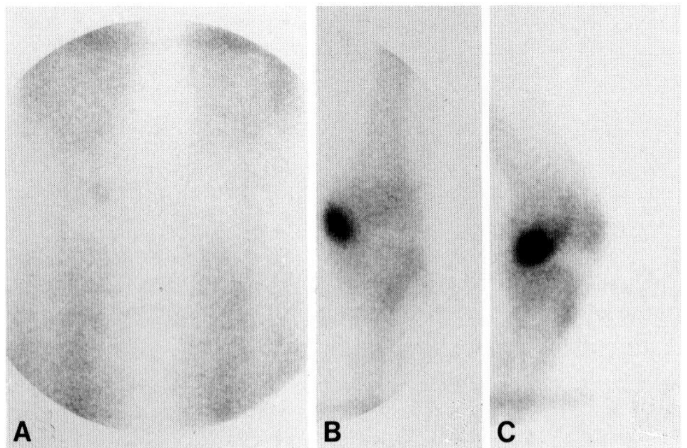

Fig. 80.3 Osteochondroma on medial aspect of left proximal tibia. Significant vascularity is absent in the initial blood pool phase (A), but the lesion becomes demonstrable in the standard static views (B and C).

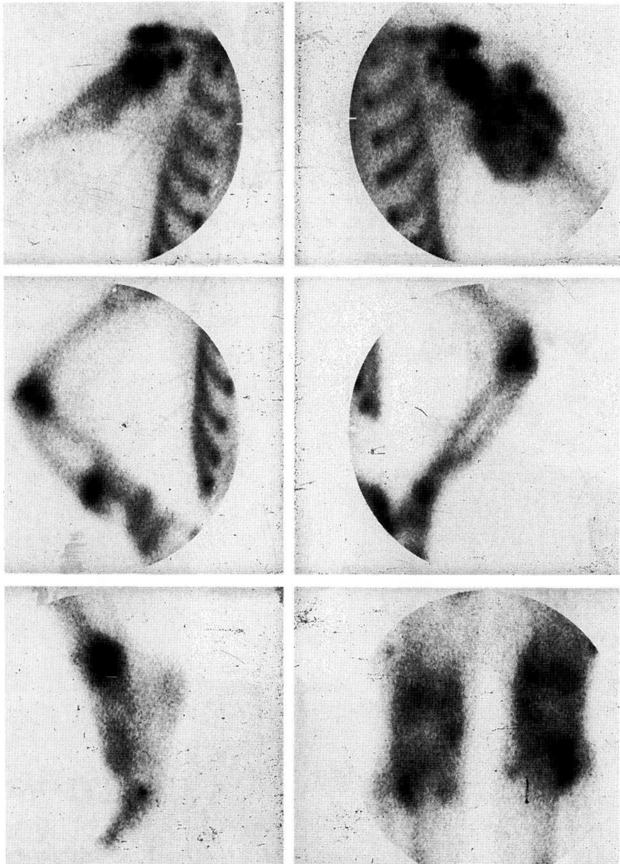

Fig. 80.4 Diaphyseal aclasis. Multiple foci of increased accumulation, of varying size and intensity, and associated bone distortion demonstrate continuing activity of osteochondromas.

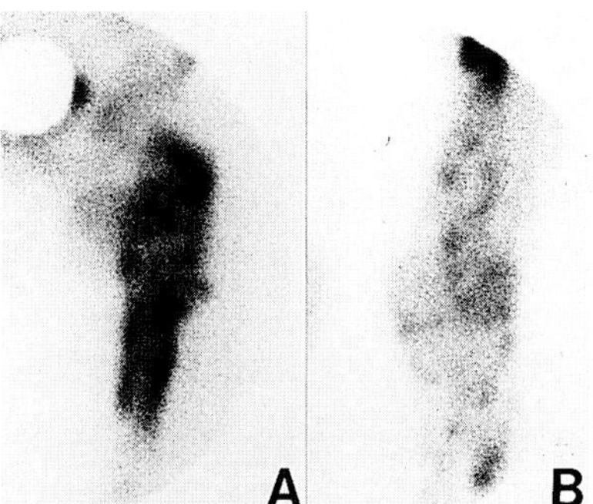

Fig. 80.5 Chondrosarcoma complicating Ollier's disease. Increased accumulation is present in the femur (A), with patchy distribution and focal areas of increased uptake. This accumulation contrasts with the small and less intense foci noted in benign lesions in the lower femur and upper tibia (B).

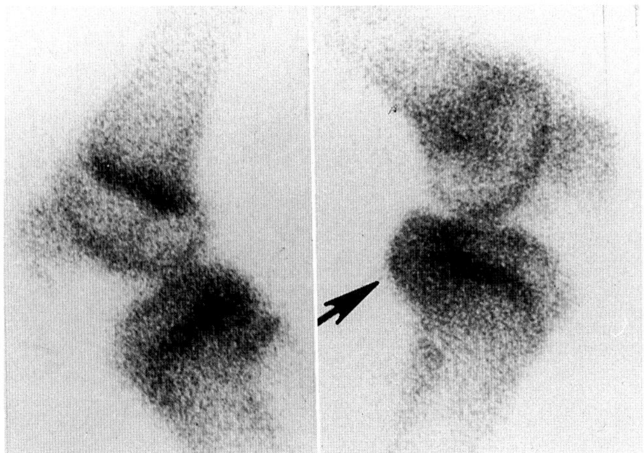

Fig. 80.6 Chondroblastoma in a 15-year-old presenting with a mildly painful swelling of the posterior aspect of the left upper tibia, associated with only minor and totally uniform accumulation.

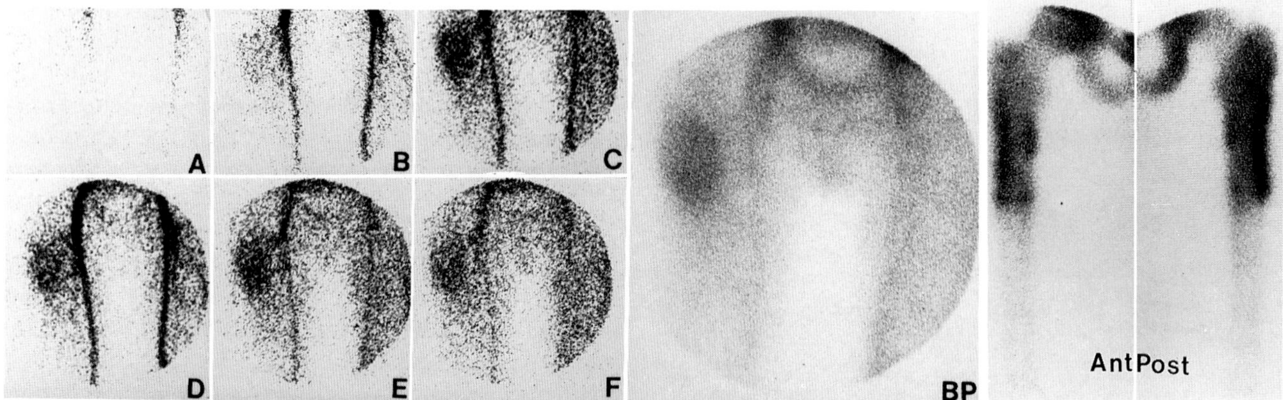

Fig. 80.7 Three-phase scintigraphy identifying an extraosseous sarcoma. The dynamic (A – F) and blood pool (BP) images of the right femur reveal an area of hypervascularity of the lateral aspect of the upper femur. Anterior (Ant) and posterior (Post) views show cortical accumulation of the radiopharmaceutical, more marked on the lateral aspect, indicating the osseous reaction to the extraosseous tumour.

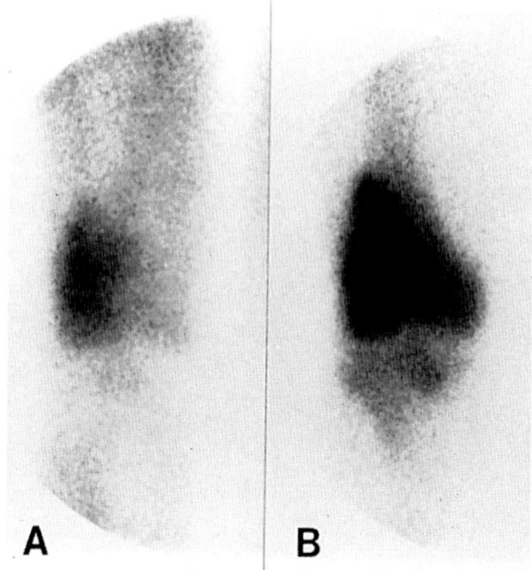

Fig. 80.8 Osteogenic sarcoma. The blood pool image (A) demonstrates the vascularity of the tumour, but in the delayed views (B) the accumulation of radionuclide has extended considerably into surrounding bone.

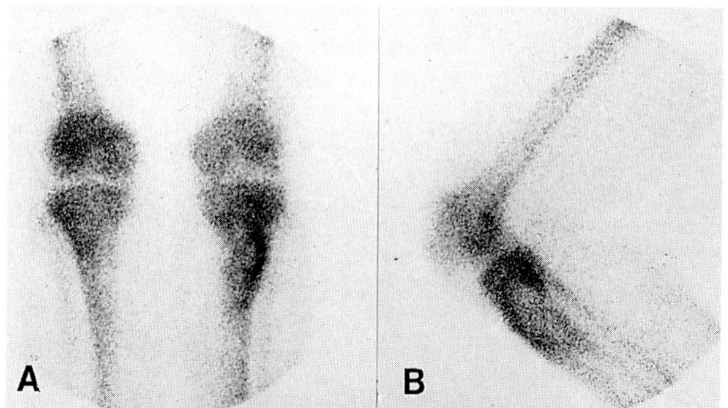

Fig. 80.9 Aneurysmal bone cyst. In delayed images (A, anterior; B, medial), an aneurysmal bone cyst in the upper tibia is visualized as a 'doughnut', a rim of increased uptake surrounding a photopenic area which, in the initial phases, has been the site of well-delineated localized and intense vascularity.

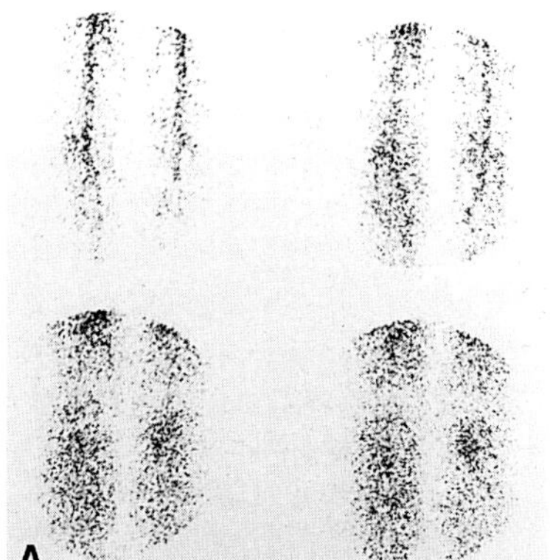

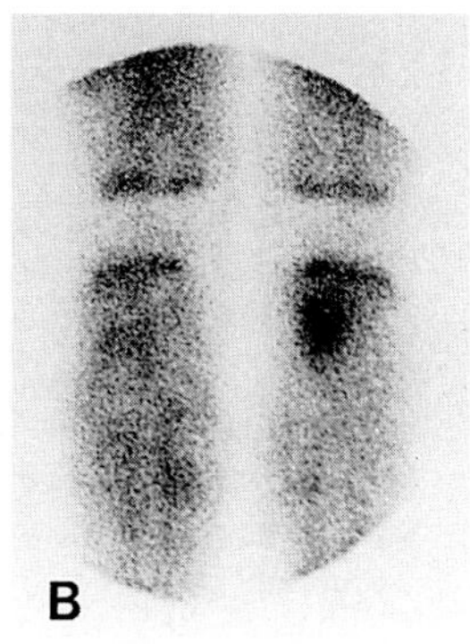

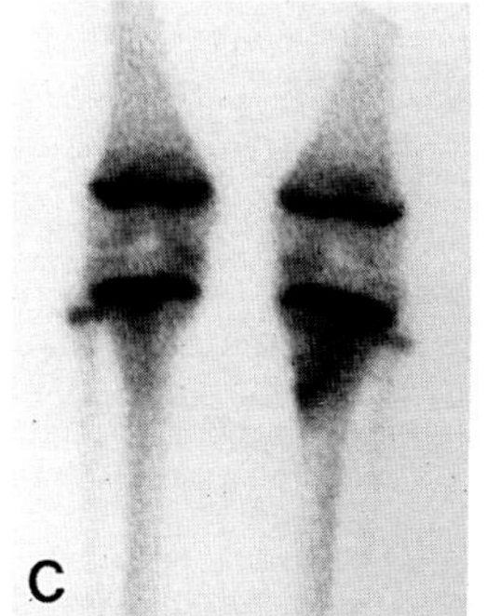

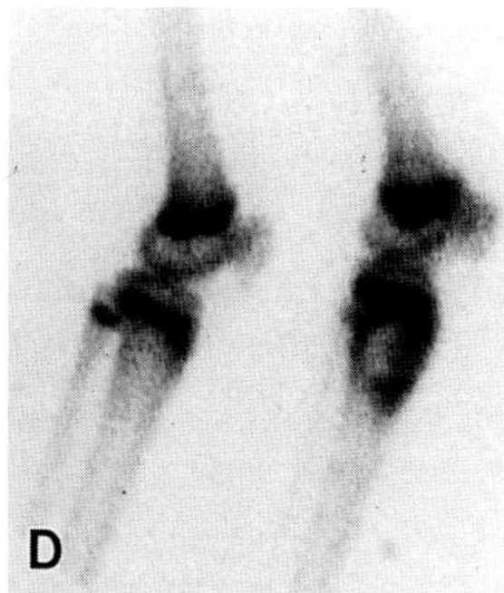

Fig. 80.10 Chondromyxoid fibroma. In the dynamic phase (A), the scintigraphic pattern shows a mild restricted area of increased vascularity, which is observed as a focal area of hyperaemia in the blood pool phase (B), and which corresponds to the photopenic centre of the tumour visualized in the subsequent delayed views (C and D) particularly in the medial projection.

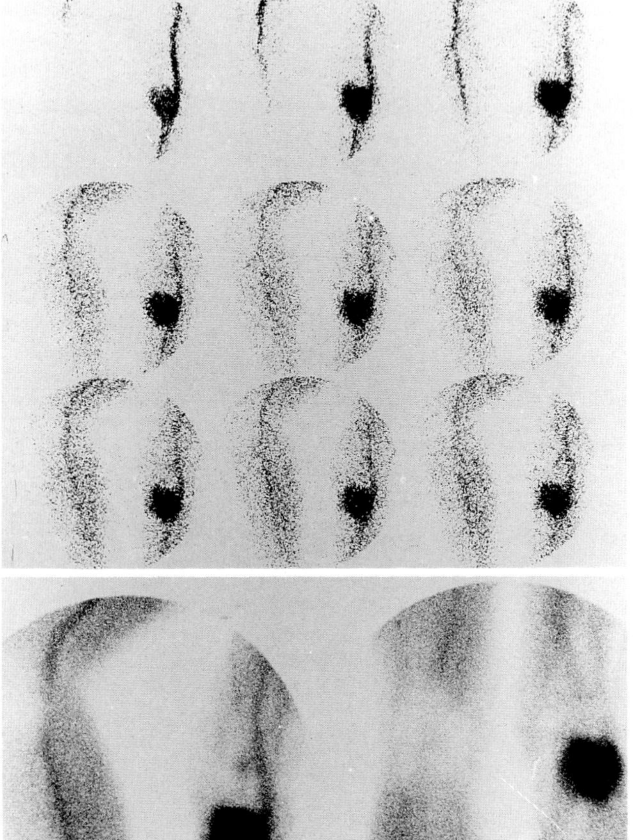

Fig. 80.11 Giant cell tumour. Intense vascularity is demonstrated in both the dynamic and blood pool phases in the large lesion in the distal femur.

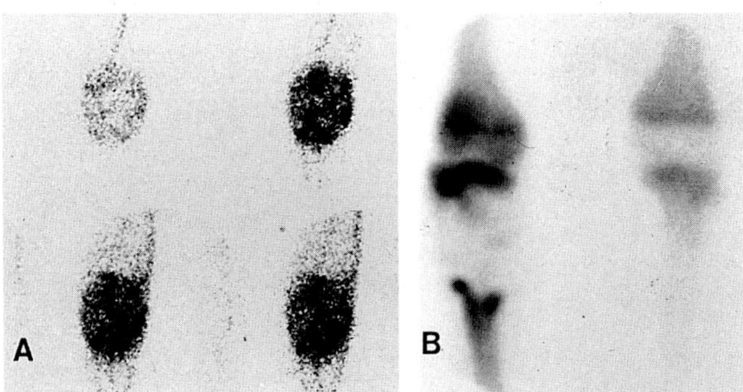

Fig. 80.12 Malignant fibrous histiocytoma. A very large and extremely vascular abnormality is observed in the dynamic phase (A) in the site of this tumour in a 12-year-old boy. In the delayed views (B), the tumour totally replaces bone, there being no radiopharmaceutical accumulation and only moderate osteoblastic response in adjacent aspects of the tibia.

Three-phase scintigraphy is usually rewarding. Malignant tumours are usually highly vascular. Evidence of local hyperaemia may also be helpful in identifying a soft-tissue mass which may not show uptake of the radiopharmaceutical in the subsequent images, although these can be valuable in defining bony reaction or invasion by extraosseous tumours (Fig. 80.7).[7] A local flush may be noted in some benign lesions, for example being common in osteoid osteoma[8] and osteoblastoma.[9] When compared with the later delayed images, the vascular studies may be of value in delineating tumour size (Fig. 80.8). A particular pattern may be observed. In aneurysmal bone cyst, for example, the lesion is usually visualized as a ring of increased uptake surrounding an area of diminished uptake, present in 16 of 25 patients reported by Hudson.[10] In the initial dynamic and blood pool phases, an intense hyperaemic focus can often be demonstrated in this photopenic centre (Fig. 80.9). A similar appearance has been noted in chondromyxoid fibroma (Fig. 80.10), but in giant cell tumour, in which a 'doughnut' is also a common finding in the delayed images, the initial vascularity is characteristically more marked and generalized (Fig. 80.11). The unusual association of evidence of gross vascularity and a major photopenic lesion, reflecting the bone destruction,

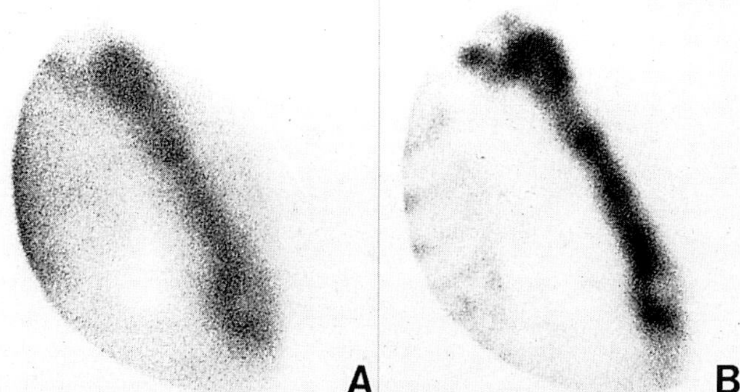

Fig. 80.13 Haemangiosarcoma of the humerus. Blood pool phase (A) demonstrates intense vascularity, the subsequent static views (B) showing marked increased uptake in a patchy fashion.

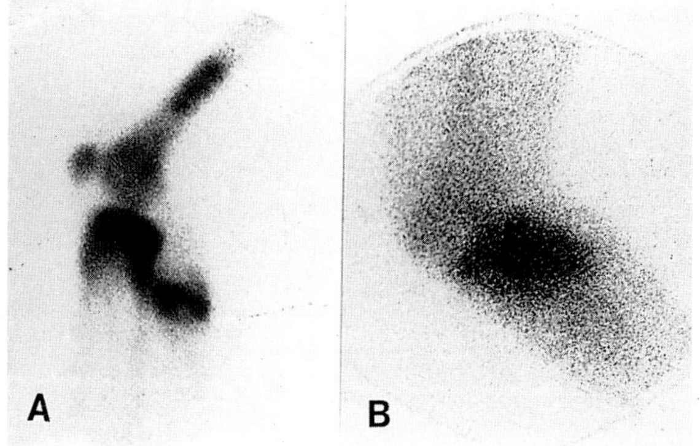

Fig. 80.14 Role of ^{67}Ga scanning. (A) Abnormal ^{99m}Tc-MDP uptake was demonstrable in an osteogenic sarcoma arising in the upper fibula with extraosseous extension and in a second site in the lower femoral shaft. (B) The intense ^{67}Ga uptake which occurred in the osteogenic sarcoma demonstrated the tumour size more accurately. However, no ^{67}Ga accumulated in the femoral lesion, subsequently shown to be a benign enchondroma.

may be observed in malignant fibrous histiocytoma (Fig. 80.12). The dramatic vascularity observed with three-phase scintigraphy in the multiple lesions of skeletal angiomatosis is strikingly discordant with the delayed images in which a 'doughnut' is seen. Toxey and Achong[11] noted that the areas of early vascularity were photopenic and surrounded by a rim of only slightly increased activity. Intense vascularity and marked uptake of the radiopharmaceutical in a patchy pattern associated with bone distortion, unlike the changes of Paget's disease, occurs in haemangiosarcoma (Fig. 80.13).

In an attempt to improve the specificity of scintigraphy in differentiating malignant from benign lesions, Simon and Kirchner[12] compared imaging with ^{99m}Tc phosphonate and ^{67}Ga in 57 patients. With the former agent they noted that the degree of intensity was greater in almost all the malignant lesions and emphasized that, if diffusely increased activity in contiguous bone was present, the lesion was likely to be malignant. However, they suggested that ^{67}Ga studies may well provide better identification of malignant tumours. They observed marked preferential uptake in all malignant tumours, except chondrosarcoma, whereas if a tumour showed no increased activity, as in 6 of 38 lesions, it was always benign (Fig. 80.14). It was also noted that contiguous bone accumulation of ^{67}Ga was not present in either malignant or benign bone tumours. A close relationship between the degree of increased medronate accumulation and ^{67}Ga uptake in osteogenic sarcoma was noted by Yeh et al,[13] using a semiquantitative method to evaluate tumour avidity. High or moderate ^{67}Ga uptake seemed to be associated with hypervascular tumours and was most often noted in predominantly osteoblastic tumours. Preferential ^{67}Ga accumulation in Ewing's sarcoma has also been demonstrated.[14] Increased uptake was observed by Estes et al[15] in all 28 patients with this tumour, being very avid in 24. However, because of the variability with which bone tumour margins are defined with ^{67}Ga, increasing attention has been paid to the use of ^{201}Tl as a tumour-seeking agent (Ch. 63). Tumour localization of this radionuclide is influenced by blood flow and tumour mass but is predominantly dependent on several metabolic processes, particularly Na^+K^+-ATPase activity. Consequently, preferential uptake reflects cellular activity and accumulation is related to cellular viability. This is upheld by the observation by Ramanna et al[16] of the 'doughnut' appearance of high-grade sarcomas in which a highly intense zone of uptake surrounds a relatively low level of activity at the site of tumour necrosis typical of these rapidly growing neoplasms. In their series and others, all malignant tumours concentrated ^{201}Tl (Fig. 80.15). This was also found by Van der Wall et al,[17] but they emphasized that ^{201}Tl uptake was not detectable in 16 of 17 bone abnormalities proved to be benign, thus providing a predictive value of a negative study of 90%. ^{99m}Tc-methoxyisobutylisonitrile (MIBI) has also been used to improve the detection of bone tumours. Caner et al[18] noted uptake of this radiopharmaceutical in 36/42 malignant tumours. However, five of the six not visualized were Ewing's sarcoma. There was a significant overlap between the lesion–normal bone ratios for benign and malignant lesions.

Skeletal scintigraphy is indispensable in the diagnosis of osteoid osteoma in view of the sensitivity with which it can be detected. Lisbona and Rosenthall,[19] for example, identified the lesion in 20 symptomatic patients in whom radiography was positive in 11. Of the 13 who also had conventional tomography, only 11 were positive. Making up 12% of benign tumours, it should be suspected if there is the typical history of bone pain occurring at rest and relieved by prostaglandin inhibitors such as aspirin. Such a history is not always elicited and a bone scan is warranted in a child or young adult with persistent pain, especially when this pain is in areas associated with radiological difficulty: the spine, neck of femur and small bones of the

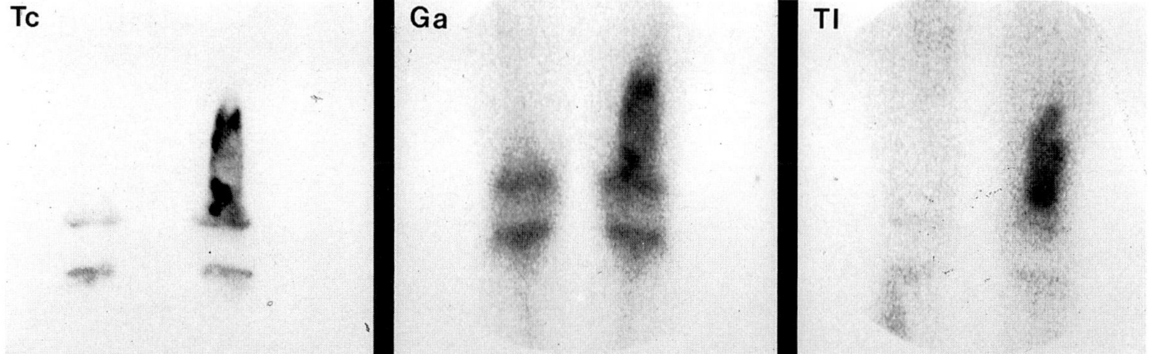

Fig. 80.15 Tumour scintigraphy with different radiopharmaceuticals. The site of an osteogenic sarcoma in the lower femur is readily identified with ^{99m}Tc-MDP (Tc), the uptake being most intense on the periphery of the tumour. The probability of the lesion being malignant is upheld by the preferential accumulation of ^{67}Ga, the distribution being similar to that of MDP. Scintigraphy with ^{201}Tl is also abnormal, providing further clear evidence of possible malignancy, but the accumulation differs and is most intense in the tumour centre, where the osteoblastic change was less evident.

hands and feet. A negative study virtually excludes the diagnosis. The identification of the nidus as a typical intense focus of uptake within the area of abnormal osteoblastic activity is important, not merely in the diagnosis but also in therapy, on occasion the demonstration of a persistent abnormality explaining the continuous symptomatology (Fig. 80.16). Precise siting is often critical to surgery in limiting the amount of bone required to be removed, particularly when the tumour arises in the posterior elements of a vertebra, the site of 10% of osteoid osteomas. This localization is readily achieved with the use of SPECT (Fig. 80.17). A variety of methods using the technetium phosphate agents have been employed to permit the intra-operative localization. These have included marking the site using scintigraphy immediately prior to surgery, intraoperative imaging and exact localization with a small probe during the operation, and monitoring the activity of removed bone fragments and of the site to ensure complete excision.[20] Reviewing experience with these different methods, Harcke et al[21] favoured the probe technique. Similar scintigraphic findings are encountered in osteoblastoma, which is considered by many to be differentiated from an osteoid osteoma by exceeding a diameter of 1.5–2 cm.

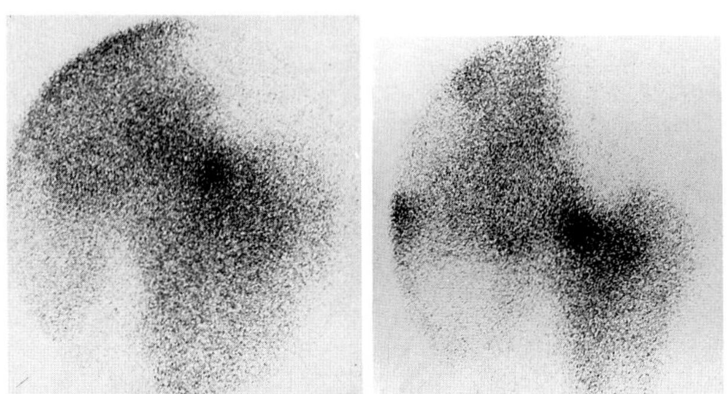

Fig. 80.16 Osteoid osteoma. Pinhole images identify the focal activity of the nidus in the left femoral neck (left). A repeat study (right), 9 months after surgery, explains continuing pain to be due to the persistence of the nidus. Observe some surrounding bone reaction.

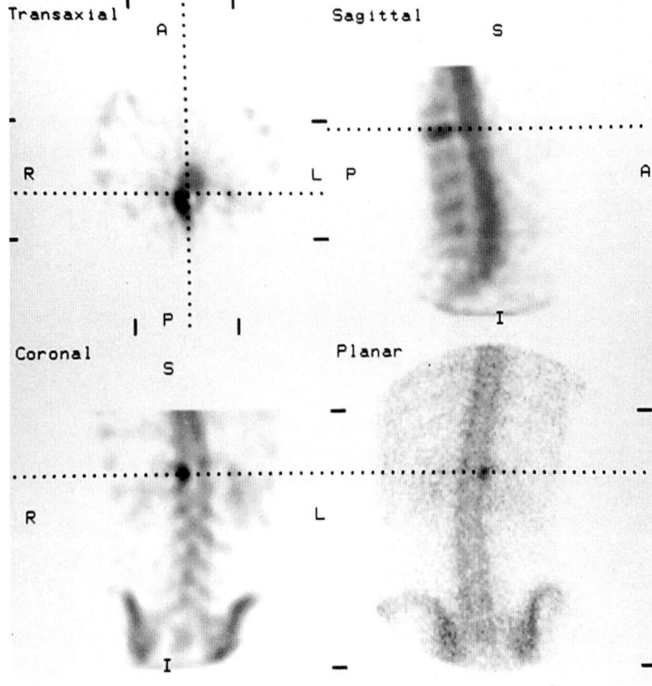

Fig. 80.17 Osteoid osteoma. Planar views readily identified the small intense uptake in the lower thoracic spine. With SPECT the lesion was clearly delineated and localized exactly in the posterior lamina on the right.

As reported by Goodgold et al,[22] giant cell tumours characteristically are visualized as a rim of moderately intense accumulation surrounding a photopenic centre (Fig. 80.18). These changes were also noted by Peimer et al[23] and Levine et al,[24] although in both series several patients did demonstrate uniformly increased uptake throughout the tumour. While this may reflect scintigraphic techniques, the variability in the distribution within the tumour can be observed in different lesions when presenting in multicentric sites (Fig. 80.19). It was evident in the study of 23 patients with giant cell tumour by Van Nostrand et al,[25] who noted differing degrees of activity in the tumours, the 'doughnut' only being present in 52%. More particularly, they concluded that scintigraphy could not differentiate benign from malignant giant cell tumours.

Increasing experience with skeletal scintigraphy has suggested that some different types of tumours tend to demonstrate particular recurring combinations of alterations. This concept was examined by McLean and Murray,[26] who studied 51 patients, comprising 22 with osteogenic sarcoma, 16 with Ewing's sarcoma and 14 with chondrosarcoma. They assessed the scintigraphic studies for the overall intensity of accumulation, the pattern of distribution, the degree of distortion of the bony outline and the scintigraphic margin of the lesion. Although no feature was unique to a particular tumour and the

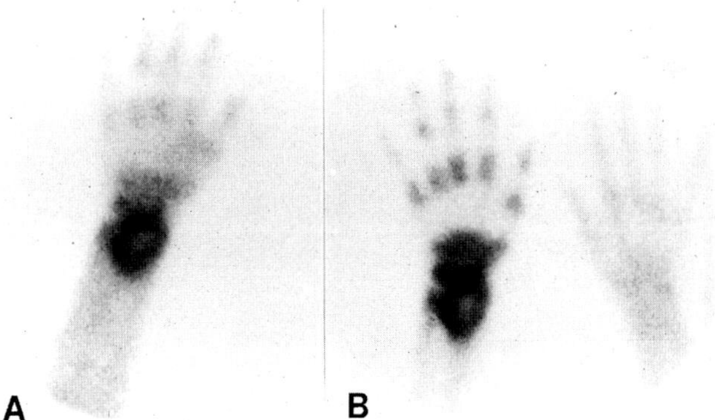

Fig. 80.18 Giant cell tumour of the radius, characteristically subarticular. Blood pool phase (A) and later static views (B) show significant vascularity and a typical 'doughnut' appearance.

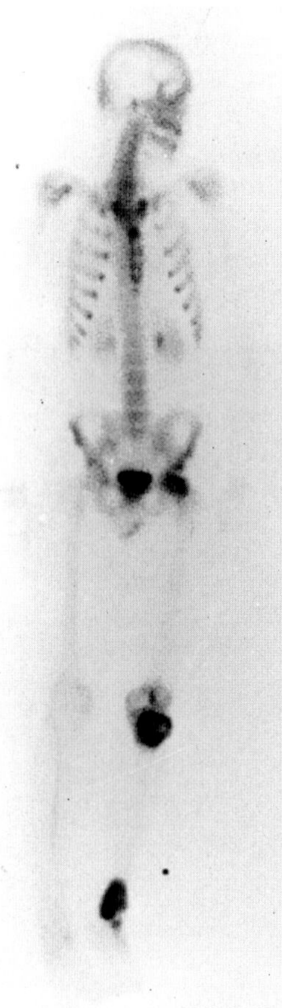

Fig. 80.19 Multicentric giant cell tumours in left leg identified in a whole body survey (left). The dominant lesion in the proximal end of the left tibia presents a typical 'doughnut' appearance.

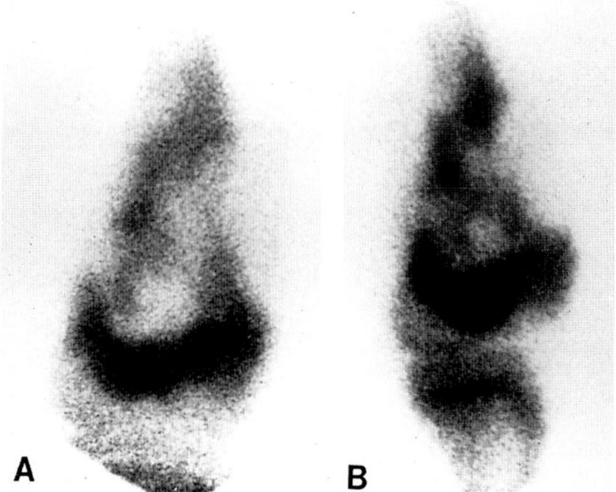

Fig. 80.20 Osteosarcoma in the distal femoral metaphysis. A typical pattern of accumulation is demonstrated in the anterior (A) and lateral (B) views, with the distortion of the bony outline and growth plate and the patchy but intense uptake which is observed so frequently in this malignant neoplasm.

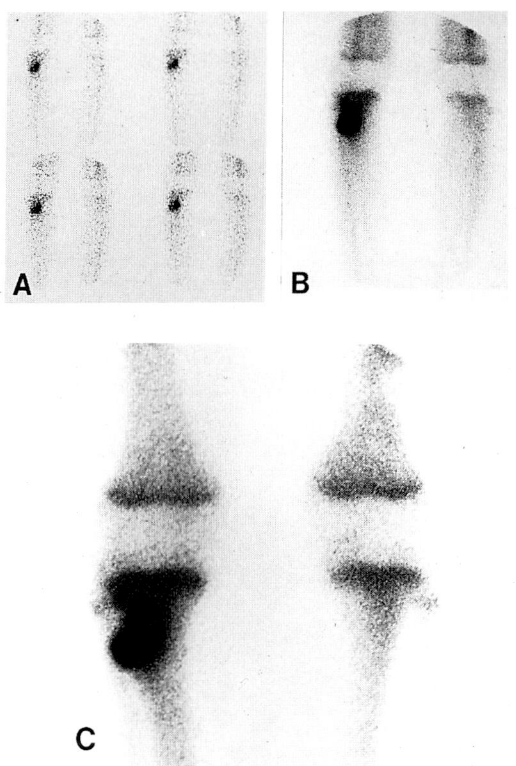

Fig. 80.21 Osteogenic sarcoma. Intense vascularity is demonstrated in a small, well-delineated area in both the dynamic (A) and blood pool (B) phases. In the delayed images (C), accumulation is demarcated clearly but is very intense and causes considerable bony distortion.

spectrum of grading of each feature for any one tumour overlapped with another, a certain combination of features occurred more frequently for each, allowing suggestion of a specific neoplasm as the most likely diagnosis. Thus, in osteogenic sarcoma, accumulation was almost always markedly increased, but the distribution characteristically demonstrated a patchiness of areas of decreased accumulation within the overall high uptake. The bony outline usually showed marked distortion and the margin of the lesion was very ill-defined (Fig. 80.20). However, in some patients there was a more circumscribed abnormality in which the accumulation was uniform but markedly increased and associated with greatly increased vascularity (Fig. 80.21). SPECT may be very useful in localizing precisely the different siting of paraosteal and periosteal osteosarcoma (Figs 80.22 and 80.23) and their less aggressive nature will be reflected by considerably lesser degrees of avidity for the radiopharmaceutical. In Ewing's sarcoma, intense accumulation is also common, but the distribution of uptake tends to be much more homogeneous than in osteosarcoma, the distortion less marked and less irregular (Fig. 80.24). The margin of the tumour is usually poorly delineated. In chondrosarcoma, the avidity of radiopharmaceutical uptake varies but the typical pattern of distribution is moderately increased uptake throughout the tumour with scattered focal areas

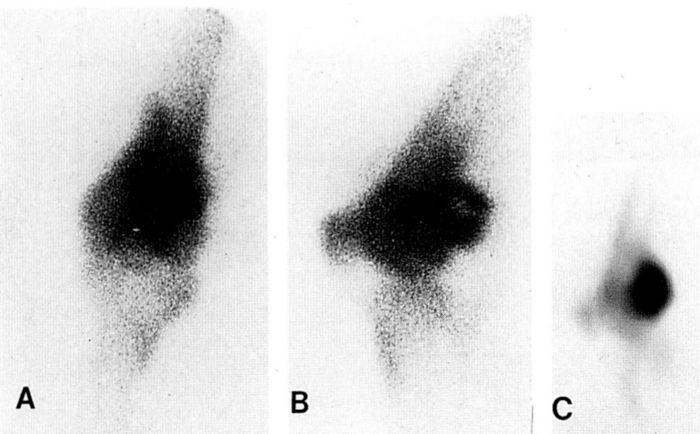

Fig. 80.22 Paraosteal osteogenic sarcoma. In the anterior view of the knee (A), abnormal accumulation in an irregular distribution can be observed in the distal end of the femur. In the lateral projection (B), the focal nature of the parosteal lesion can only just be differentiated from the reactive hyperaemia in the femur. However, the tumour is clearly delineated and localized with SPECT (C).

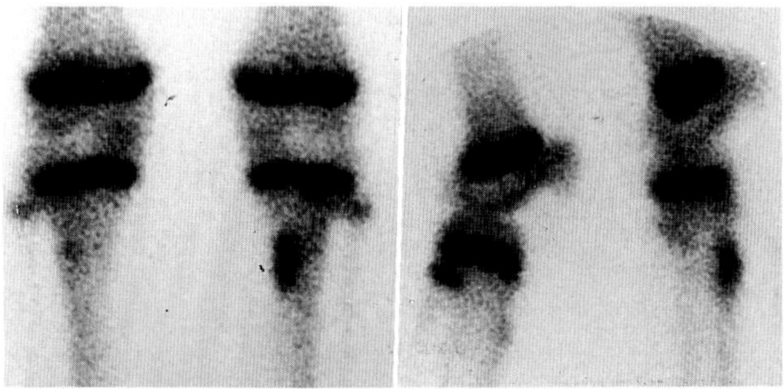

Fig. 80.23 Periosteal sarcoma. The less aggressive nature of this form of sarcoma is reflected by the degree of radionuclide avidity localized to the tibial cortex in this lesion.

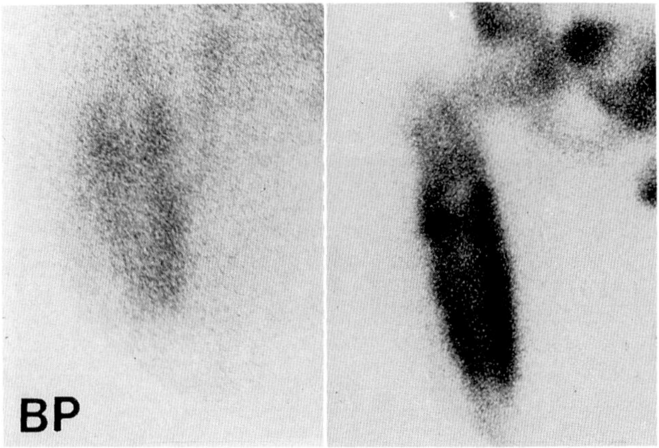

Fig. 80.24 Ewing's sarcoma. Characteristic pattern in the upper right femur; considerable hyperaemia in the blood pool phase and intense accumulation with a reasonably homogeneous distribution, mild and uniform bone distortion and poorly delineated scintigraphic margins in the later image.

of more intense accumulation (Fig. 80.25). The bony outline is usually only mildly distorted and the tumour margin well defined. The pattern was similar to that previously described in several patients by Hudson et al.[27] These authors were not, however, able to correlate the scintigraphic appearances and the histological grading of chondrosarcoma, as Perlman and Steiner[5] had also failed to do.

Despite the tendency for typical appearances to be observed in each tumour, there is no unique pattern for any, and scintigraphy cannot be used as the sole investigation. Indeed, photopenia has been reported to be associated with osteogenic sarcoma[28] (Fig. 80.26) and with Ewing's sarcoma.[29] Nevertheless, the association of scinti-

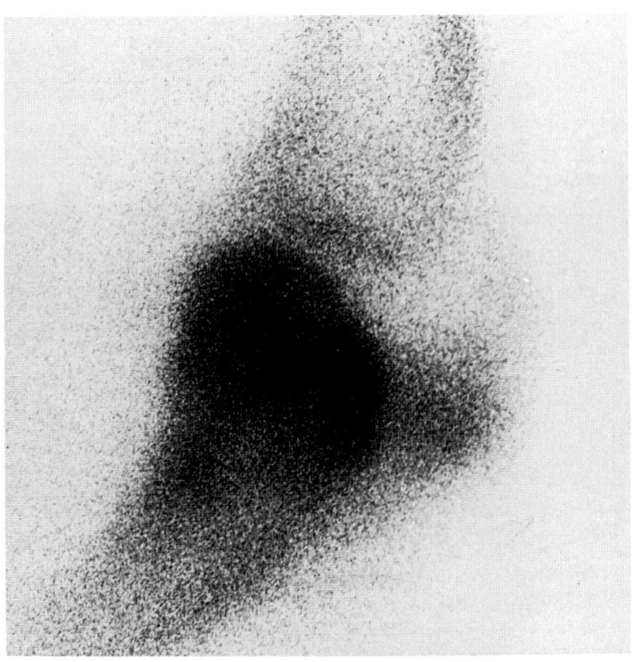

Fig. 80.25 Chondrosarcoma. Characteristic scintigraphic pattern in the distal femur with accumulation being moderately well circumscribed, with minimal bony distortion and a pattern of distribution identifying foci of increased uptake throughout the lesion.

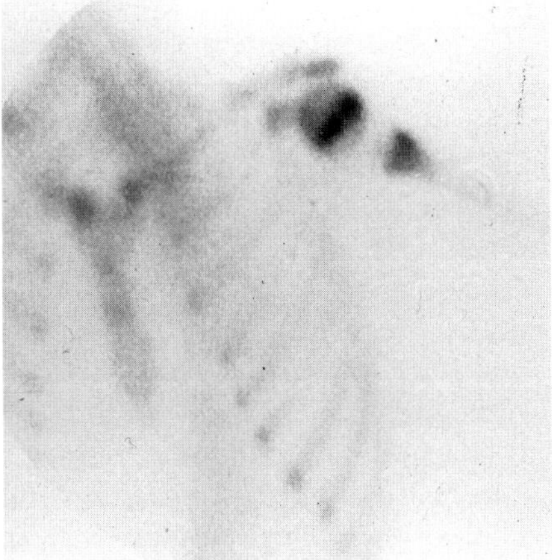

Fig. 80.26 Osteogenic sarcoma. In the upper humeral metaphysis there is a clear area of absent accumulation at the site of an osteogenic sarcoma, with only mild reduction in osteoblastic reaction on the proximal and distal aspects.

graphic changes should engender suspicion of a particular type. This suspicion will be heightened by the degree of preferential localization of ^{67}Ga or ^{201}Tl.

SIZE OF LESION

The precise delineation of the limits of the primary tumour is essential for the appropriate planning of remedial surgery or radiotherapy. Controversy continues as to the reliability of the bone scan in defining the size of the primary bone tumours. Thrall et al[30] drew attention to the abnormal radionuclide deposition adjacent to a number of focal skeletal lesions, and Goldman and Braunstein[31] noted that 10 of 13 patients exhibited a relative increase in radioactivity at the ends of the long bones of the affected extremity which might be mistaken for haematogenous metastases. However, Papanincolaou et al,[32] in 20 patients with osteogenic sarcoma, found an excellent correlation between pathology and scintigraphy and, in 46 of 48 patients with this tumour investigated by McKillop et al,[33] there was good agreement between the scintigraphic images, radiographs and pathological findings in defining the limit of the tumour. These reports, however, conflict with the experience of others. Chew and Hudson[34] reported overestimation of the size of the tumour by scintigraphy in 11 of 18 patients with osteogenic sarcoma, resulting from marrow hyperaemia, medullary reactive bone or periosteal new bone as well as disuse osteoporosis. In their study of 23 patients with giant cell tumour, Van Nostrand et al[25] observed extended patterns of activity in 19, yet in none was there true tumour extension. Increased uptake beyond the true tumour margin does appear to be less common in medullary chondrosarcomas. Hudson and Chew[27] noted that the uptake corresponded accurately to the anatomical extent in 15 of 18 tumours.

Since the area of abnormal radionuclide uptake with the ^{99m}Tc diphosphonate complexes may overestimate the actual tumour size, affecting surgical decisions such as the optimal level for amputation, Simon and Kirchner[12] suggested that ^{67}Ga scintigraphy might be more useful in determining the tumour limits since contiguous activity is not demonstrable. While it can provide improved delineation of a tumour, emission tomography (SPECT) has not proved capable of overcoming the main consequence of extended uptake observed in standard planar scintigraphy, masking the presence of 'skip' metastases within the medullary canal (Fig. 80.27). This occurred in two of four patients with such lesions in a series of 18 patients studied by Chew and Hudson.[34] Intramedullary extension can be detected accurately by emission tomography, although there can be difficulties in the evaluation of long bone osteosarcoma.[35] Hudson et al[36] pointed out that magnetic resonance imaging can define tumour spread within marrow but may also demonstrate reactive abnormality beyond the true tumour margin. Bone marrow scintigraphy has been used successfully in osteogenic sarcoma by Miller and Ettinger[37] for the assessment of both proximal and distal extent of tumour and in the detection of metastases to the bone marrow. Marrow scintigraphy was found to be particularly of value in Ewing's sarcoma in revealing unsuspected focal marrow involvement.[38]

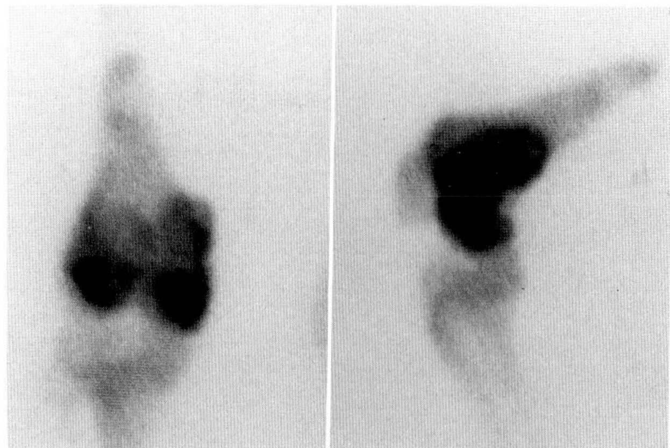

Fig. 80.27 'Skip' metastases from an osteogenic sarcoma. Appropriate exposure permits their identification within the reactive uptake extending proximally from the site of the primary tumour in an 18-year-old youth.

A whole-body survey is imperative at the time of diagnosis of a primary bone malignancy since demonstration of distant disease will radically alter therapeutic decision. However, metastases at presentation were only encountered in osteogenic sarcoma in 1/56 (2%) of the series reported by Goldstein et al,[39] 1/48 (2%) by McKillop et al[33] and 4/62 (6%) by Murray and Elison.[40] Metastatic disease at the time of diagnosis is, however, considerably more common in Ewing's sarcoma, skeletal metastases being identified by scintigraphy in 3/28 (11%) of a series studied by Goldstein et al[41] and 2/38 (5%) by Murray and Elison,[40] but in 25 (35%) of 72 patients reported by Nair.[42] It is important to be aware that focal uptake in the contralateral leg may be caused by stress fractures induced by the changes of weight bearing.[43]

EVALUATION OF THERAPY

The range of therapeutic options now available and the consequent marked improvement in survival demands even closer attention to choosing the appropriate protocols for primary bone tumours than formerly. Evaluation of the efficacy of chemotherapy in each individual is critical, there being a significantly higher disease-free survival rate in patients who respond well than in non-responders. Identification of preoperative response identifies a regimen appropriate for post-operative therapy and by inducing regression of the tumour facilitates limb-salvaging approaches. Response is primarily assessed by clinical observa-

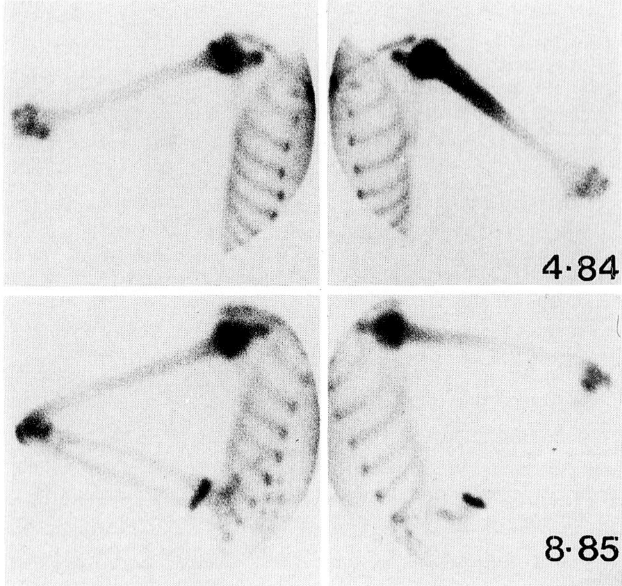

Fig. 80.28 Ewing's sarcoma. The response to chemotherapy is evident by comparing the original scintigraphs with the characteristic changes of this tumour in the left upper humerus (4.84) with a normal appearance 16 months later, following treatment.

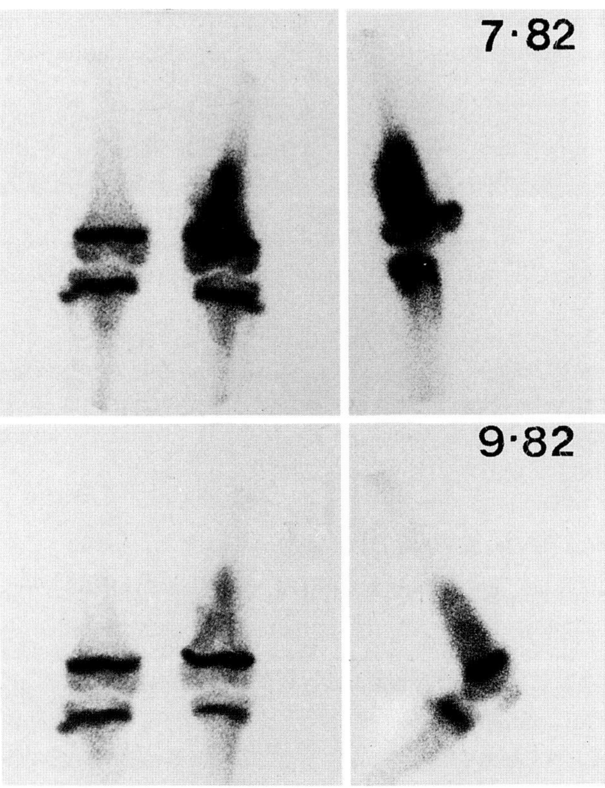

Fig. 80.29 Osteogenic sarcoma. Use of preoperative chemotherapy. Comparison of the original scintigraphs (7.82) in anterior and medial projections, with those 6 weeks later (9.82), showing the marked reduction in avidity, diminution in tumour size and clearer delineation of the upper margin of the tumour.

tion and by clinical evaluation of the tumour after resection but scintigraphy offers a further useful parameter.

Bone scanning with ^{99m}Tc diphosphonates can demonstrate reduction in the avidity of the tumour, often most dramatically seen in Ewing's sarcoma (Fig. 80.28). Tumour shrinkage may also be demonstrable, especially in osteogenic sarcoma (Fig. 80.29). In serial investigations of 13 patients, Knop et al[44] undertook serial studies in 30 patients to evaluate the effect of preoperative chemotherapy. Changes in the blood pool images and in MDP plasma clearance provided accuracies in presurgical prediction of tumour regression of 88% and 96% respectively. Even at the halfway stage of chemotherapy they found that a poor response could be reliably predicted. Three-phase skeletal scintigraphy combined with determination of plasma clearance of the radiopharmaceutical was utilized by Sommer et al,[45] who suggested that a reduction in clearance predicted response with an accuracy of up to 100%.

The reliability of bone scanning in monitoring therapy has been questioned. Erlemann et al[46] found an accuracy with bone scanning in the assessment of response of 80% for osteogenic sarcoma and only 50% for Ewing's sarcoma. The overall accuracy of 73.7% compared unfavourably with 85.7% obtained with dynamic MRI imaging with gadolinium-DTPA enhancement. Alternative procedures have been advocated; Yeh et al[13] used a semiquantitative measurement of tumour/non-tumour

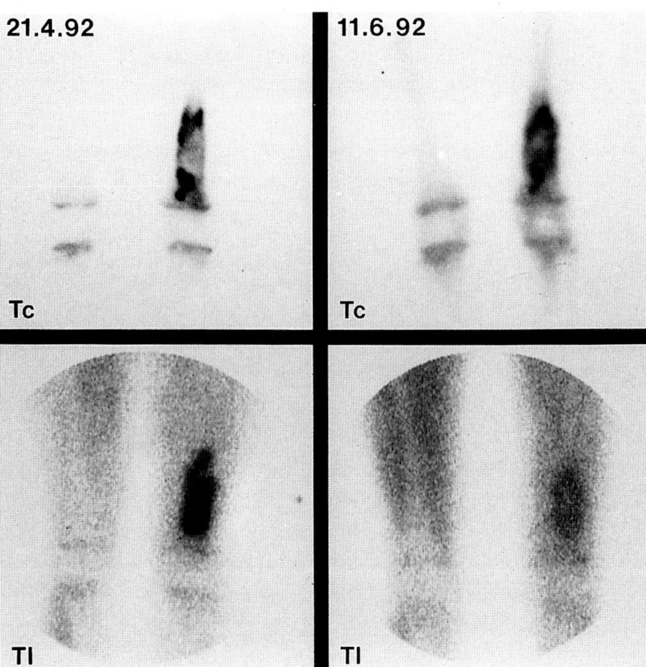

Fig. 80.30 Evaluation of chemotherapeutic response. In a comparison of studies before (21.4.92) and after 2 weeks of chemotherapy (11.6.92), the ^{99m}Tc-MDP images showed evidence of increased osteoblastic activity and no significant change in tumour size, whereas the avidity and size of ^{201}Tl images were markedly reduced, in keeping with the considerable tumour regression which was obvious clinically.

avidity of ^{67}Ga as a method to assess response in osteogenic sarcoma, finding that decreased ^{67}Ga uptake, associated with such response, occurred earlier and more consistently than changes in the accumulation of the technetium phosphate complexes. The experience by Estes et al[15] was similar in a study of 30 patients with Ewing's sarcoma. Decreased intensity of ^{67}Ga following therapy was noted in all patients, while MDP uptake diminished in 23 of 28 studies. However, the degree of uptake of ^{67}Ga following therapy was markedly less and relapses later occurred in only four patients in whom the uptake remained equal to normal bone. While there was subsequent relapse in 7/11 patients in whom MDP uptake remained obvious, it was suggested that the residual uptake was more related to other factors such as bone remodelling. This was also blamed by Ramanna et al[16] for the inaccurate correlation of bone scanning with response.

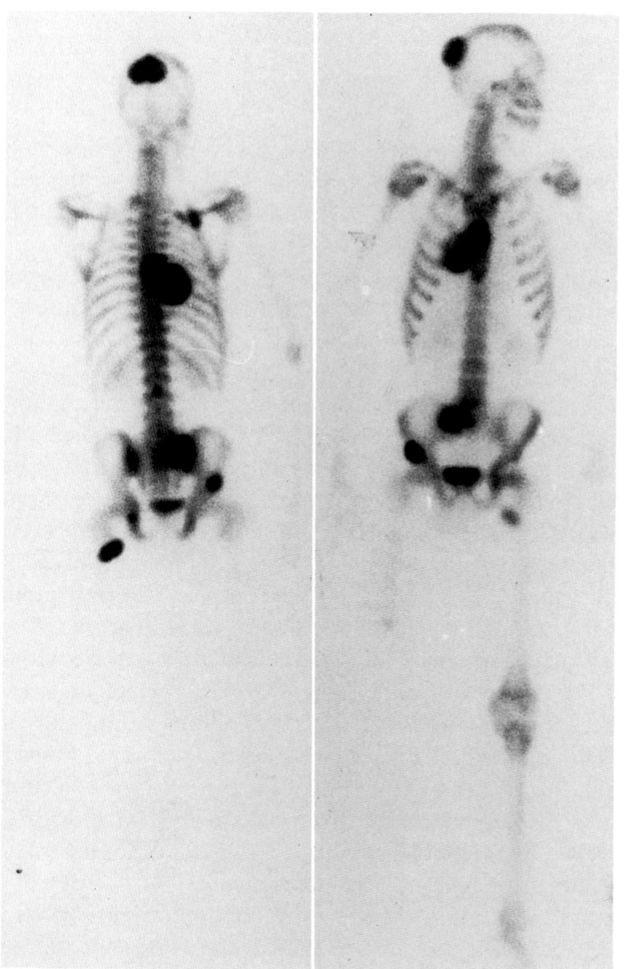

Fig. 80.31 Osteogenic sarcoma. Whole-body skeletal surveys in a boy who had previously undergone amputation of the right leg, providing demonstration of accumulation of the radiopharmaceutical in distant metastases. These include osseous metastases in the occipitoparietal region, right scapula, right sacroiliac joint and ilium as well as extraosseous deposits, not merely in the common site in the lungs, but also in the soft tissue in the buttocks.

They found that ^{201}Tl was superior to ^{67}Ga, identifying 7/8 patients in whom there was histological demonstration of >95% tumour necrosis, whereas in only four of these was there reduction in ^{67}Ga uptake (Fig. 80.30).

The improved efficiency of therapy for primary malignant bone tumours is such that the survival rates are markedly altered. Routine serial bone scintigraphy has therefore established an important role in the evaluation of progress. Attention must be paid to the site of the primary tumour to ascertain if there has been local recurrence. Increased uptake in the stump usually diminishes by 6 months. In their 48 patients with osteogenic sarcoma, McKillop et al[33] noted that there was intense focal uptake at the stump in five patients either persisting beyond 6 months or developing later. Three of these subsequently demonstrated local recurrent tumour. The major role of sequential studies is, however, the detection of metastases (Fig. 80.31). The changing indications for these serial studies, related to improved therapy, were initially demonstrated by Goldstein et al,[39] who observed the appearance of bone metastases in 21 (37%) of 56 patients with osteogenic sarcoma. Actuarial analysis of the data of McNeil and Hanley,[47] indicated that patients with osteosarcoma show an almost linear increase in the recurrence of bone metastases between 5 and 29 months after diagnosis, the rate being approximately 1% per month. Confirmation was provided by the studies by McKillop

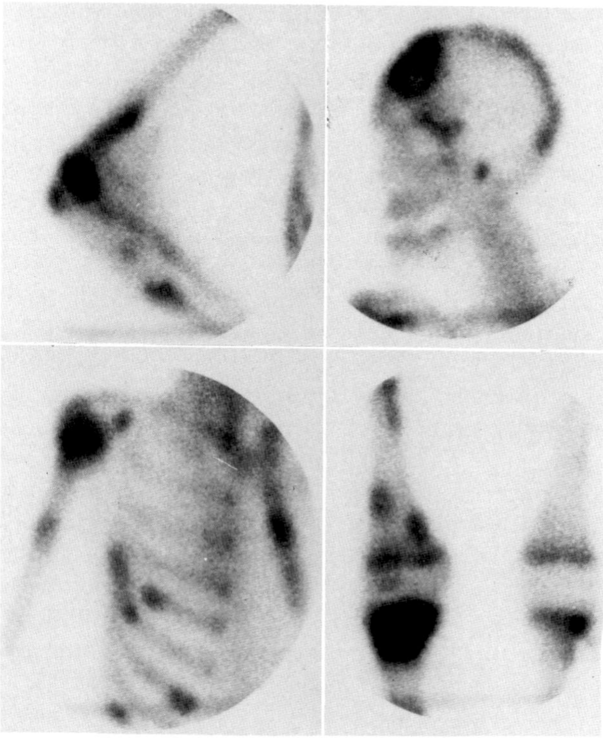

Fig. 80.32 Ewing's sarcoma. Disseminated metastases indicated by multiple areas of focal increased uptake in numerous sites throughout the skeleton.

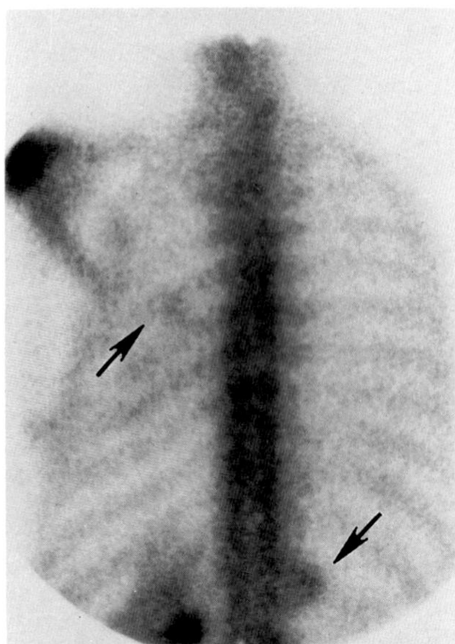
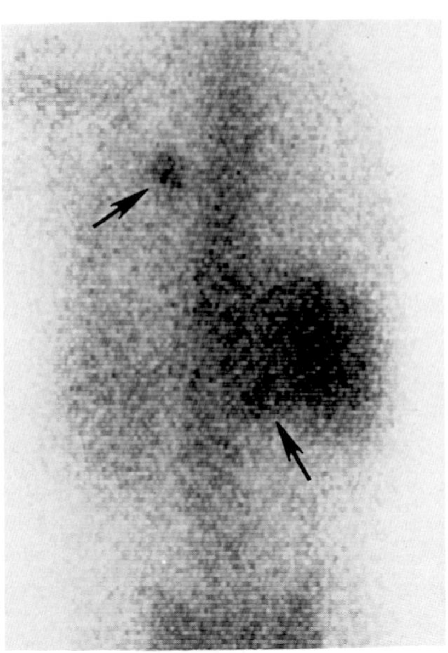

Fig. 80.33 Osteogenic sarcoma. Extraosseous accumulation in non-skeletal metastases demonstrated during skeletal scintigraphy (A) in the left lung and right renal bed, confirmed subsequently with gallium scintigraphy in identical sites (B).

et al,[33] who demonstrated bone metastases in 20 (43%) of 47 patients, and by Murray and Elison,[40] who noted that skeletal metastases developed in 11 (23%) of 48 patients initially free of metastatic disease. Pulmonary metastases remain more common, developing in 29/56 (52%) of the series described by Goldstein et al,[39] 28/47 (60%) by McKillop et al[33] and 27/48 (56%) by Murray and Elison.[40] The role of bone scanning in the long-term management of patients with osteosarcoma was clearly shown by the sequence in which the metastases developed in the patients in these series. Bone metastases developed prior to or simultaneously with lung metastases in 5/31 (16%), 7/33 (21%) and 7/37 (19%) respectively. Awareness that scintigraphic interpretation requires asymmetrical uptake, especially in the pelvis and the sacroiliac joints, may reflect stress related to altered weight bearing. Goldstein et al[39] noted such asymmetry in 26 of 36 patients who had undergone amputation, in 65% this being in the site opposite to the amputation. The asymmetry was on the involved side, however, in three of five patients with a surgically implanted prosthesis.

Regular scintigraphy is also indicated in Ewing's sarcoma. Goldstein et al[41] reviewed 28 patients with Ewing's sarcoma; of 22 patients free from metastases at presentation, 10 (45%) subsequently developed bone metastases. The experience of Murray and Elison[40] is similar; 10 (33%) of 30 patients free of disease at diagnosis later developing distant bone metastases (Fig. 80.32). The skeletal metastases were demonstrated prior to or simultaneously with lung metastases in 9/32 (41%) of the series reported by Goldstein et al[41] and in 10/17 (59%) in that of Murray and Elison.[40]

The extraosseous accumulation of the bone-seeking radiopharmaceuticals, associated with a large variety of cancers, may be obvious in metastases from osteogenic sarcoma, particularly those within the lungs. There is, however, divergence of opinion regarding the frequency of the phenomenon. Hoefnagel et al[48] noted diphosphonate uptake in 11 of 12 patients with pulmonary metastases, two being noted by scintigraphy prior to X-ray tomography. On the other hand, Goldstein et al[39] observed uptake in metastases in only 5/29 patients and McKillop et al[33] in 4/28 patients' lung metastases. The unreliability of the use of skeletal scintigraphy in the identification of extraosseous metastatic disease was clearly demonstrated by Vanel et al[49] even using SPECT, which has been advocated by Kirk and Schulz.[50] Gallium scintigraphy has been utilized to demonstrate such pulmonary lesions (Fig. 80.33), and Ohta et al[51] reported clear-cut accumulation in lung metastases from osteosarcoma using ^{99m}Tc-labelled dimercaptosuccinic acid (DMSA V) and emission tomography. The incidental occurrence of accumulation of the technetium bone-seeking radiopharmaceuticals in extraosseous metastatic deposits from osteogenic sarcoma in a variety of other sites has been reported, but uptake in non-skeletal metastases from Ewing's sarcoma is rare.

REFERENCES

1. Conway J J, Gooneratne N, Simon G 1975 Radionuclide evaluation of distal femoral metaphyseal irregularities which simulate neoplasm. J Nucl Med 16: 521
2. Brenner R J, Hattner R, Lilien D L 1979 Scintigraphic features of nonosteogenic fibroma. Radiology 131: 727–730
3. Hall F M, Goldberg R P, Davies J A K, Fainsinger M H 1980 Scintigraphic assessment of bone island. Radiology 135: 737–742
4. Epstein D A, Levin E J 1978 Bone scintigraphy in hereditary multiple exostoses. AJR 130: 311–333
5. Perlman R J, Steiner C E 1978 Chondrosarcoma – correlative study of nuclear imaging and histology. Bull Hosp Jt Dis Orthop Inst 39: 153–164
6. Humphry A, Gilday D L, Brown R G 1980 Bone scintigraphy in chondroblastoma. Radiology 137: 497–499
7. Enneking W F, Chew F S, Springfield D S, Hudson T M, Spanier S S 1981 The role of radionuclide bone-scanning in determining the resectibility of soft-tissue sarcomas. J Bone Joint Surg 63A: 249–257
8. Smith F W, Gilday D L 1980 Scintigraphic appearances of osteoid osteoma. Radiology 137: 191–195
9. Martin N L, Preston D F, Robinson R G 1976 Osteoblastoma of the axial skeleton shown by skeletal scanning. J Nucl Med 17: 187–189
10. Hudson T M 1984 Scintigraphy of aneurysmal bone cysts. AJR 142: 761–765
11. Toxey J, Achong D M 1991 Skeletal angiomatosis limited to the hand: radiographic and scintigraphic correlation. J Nucl Med 18: 1912–1914
12. Simon M A, Kirchner P T 1980 Scintigraphic evaluation of primary bone tumours: comparison of technetium-99m phosphonate and gallium citrate imaging. J Bone Joint Surg 62A: 758–764
13. Yeh S D J, Rosen G, Caparros B, Benua R S 1984 Semi-quantitative gallium scintigraphy in patients with osteogenic sarcoma. Clin Nucl Med 9: 175–183
14. Frankel R S, Jones A E, Cohen J A, Johnson K W, Johnston G S, Pomeroy T C 1974 Clinical correlations of ^{67}Ga and skeletal whole-body radionuclide studies with radiography in Ewing's sarcoma. Radiology 110: 597–603
15. Estes D N, Magill H L, Thompson E I, Hayes E A 1990 Primary Ewing's sarcoma: Follow-up with Ga-67 scintigraphy. Radiology 177: 449–453
16. Ramanna L, Waxman A, Binney G, Waxman S, Mirra J, Rosen G 1990 Thallium-201 scintigraphy in bone sarcoma: comparison with gallium-67 and technetium MDP in the evaluation of chemotherapeutic response. J Nucl Med 31: 567–572
17. Van der Wall H, Murray I P C, Huckstep R L, Philips R L 1993 The role of thallium scintigraphy in excluding malignancy in bone. Clin Nucl Med 18: 551–557
18. Caner B, Kitapcl M, Unlu M et al 1992 Technetium-99m-MIBI uptake in benign and malignant bone lesions: a comparative study with technetium-99m-MDP. J Nucl Med 33: 319–324
19. Lisbona R, Rosenthall L 1979 Role of radionuclide imaging in osteoid osteoma. AJR 132: 77–80
20. Ghelman B, Thompson F M, Arnold W D 1981 Intra-operative localisation of an osteoid osteoma. J Bone Joint Surg 63A: 826–827
21. Harcke H T, Conway J J, Tachdjian M O et al 1985 Scintigraphic localisation of bone lesions during surgery. Skeletal Radiol 13: 211–216
22. Goodgold H M, Chen D P, Majd M, Nolan N G, Malawer M 1984 Scintigraphic features of giant cell tumour. Clin Nucl Med 9: 526–530
23. Peimer C A, Schiller A L, Mankin H J, Smith R J 1980 Multicentric giant cell tumour of bone. J Bone Joint Surg 62A: 652–656
24. Levine E, De Smet A A, Neff J R, Martin N L 1984 Scintigraphic evaluation of giant cell tumor of bone. AJR 143: 343–348
25. Van Nostrand D V, Madewell J E, McNiesh L M, Kyle R W, Sweet D 1986 Radionuclide bone scanning in giant cell tumor. J Nucl Med 27: 329–338
26. McLean R G, Murray I P C 1984 Scintigraphic patterns in certain primary malignant bone tumours. Clin Radiol 35: 379–383
27. Hudson T M, Chew F S, Manaster B J 1982 Radionuclide bone scanning in medullary chondrosarcoma. AJR 139: 1071–1076
28. Siddiqui A R, Ellis J H 1982 'Cold spot' on bone scan at the site of primary osteosarcoma. Eur J Nucl Med 7: 480–481
29. Bushnell D, Shirazi P, Kitedar N, Blank J 1991 Ewing's sarcoma seen as a "cold" lesion on bone scans. Clin Nucl Med 8: 173–174
30. Thrall J H, Geslien G E, Corcoran R J, Johnson N C 1975 Abnormal radionuclide deposition patterns adjacent to focal skeletal lesions. Radiology 115: 659–663
31. Goldman A B, Braunstein P 1975 Augmented radioactivity on bone scans of limbs bearing osteosarcomas. J Nucl Med 16: 423–424
32. Papanicolaou N, Kózakewich H, Treves S, Goorin A, Emans J 1982 Comparison of the extent of osteosarcoma between surgical pathology and skeletal scintigraphy. J Nucl Med 23: 7–209
33. McKillop J H, Etcubanas E, Goris M L 1981 The indications for, and the limitations of bone scintigraphy in osteogenic sarcoma. Cancer 48: 1133–1138
34. Chew F S, Hudson T M 1982 Radionuclide bone scanning of osteosarcoma: falsely extended uptake patterns. AJR 139: 49–54
35. Coffre C, Vanel D, Contesso G et al 1985 Problems and pitfalls in the use of computed tomography for the local evaluation of long bone osteosarcoma. Skeletal Radiol 13: 147–153
36. Hudson T M, Hamlin D J, Enneking W F, Pettersson H 1985 Magnetic resonance imaging of bone and soft tissue tumours: early experience in 31 patients compared with computer tomography. Skeletal Radiol 13: 134–136
37. Miller J H, Ettinger L J 1985 Osteosarcoma. In: Miller J H, White L (eds) Imaging in paediatric oncology. Williams & Williams, Baltimore, pp 378–388
38. Miller J H, Ettinger L J 1985 Ewing and other osseous origin sarcomas. In: Miller J H, White L (eds) Imaging in paediatric oncology. Williams & Williams, Baltimore, pp 389–403
39. Goldstein H, McNeil B J, Zufall E, Jaffe N, Treves S 1980 Changing indications for bone scintigraphy in patients with osteosarcoma. Radiology 135: 177–180
40. Murray I P C, Elison B S 1986 Radionuclide bone imaging for primary bone malignancy. Clin Oncol 5: 141–158
41. Goldstein H, McNeil B J, Zufall E, Treves S 1980 Is there still a place for bone scanning in Ewing's sarcoma? J Nucl Med 21: 10–12
42. Nair N 1985 Bone scanning in Ewing's sarcoma. J Nucl Med 26: 349–352
43. Gorenberg M, Groshar D, Israel O, Ben-Arwsh M, Kolodwy G M, Front D 1992 Stress fractures associated with osteosarcoma of the lower limbs. J Nucl Med 33: 1699–1700
44. Knop J, Delling G, Heise U, Winkler K 1990 Scintigraphic evaluation of tumor regression during preoperative chemotherapy of osteosarcoma: Correlation of ^{99m}Tc-methylene diphosphonate parametric imaging with surgical histopathology. Skeletal Radiol 19: 165–172
45. Sommer H J, Knop J, Heise U, Winkler K, Delling G 1987 Histomorphometric changes of osteosarcoma after chemotherapy: correlation with 99m-Tc methylene diphosphonate functional imaging. Cancer 59: 252–258
46. Erlemann R F, Sciuk J, Bosse A 1990 Response of osteosarcoma and Ewing's sarcoma to preoperative chemotherapy: assessment with dynamic and static MR imaging and skeletal scintigraphy. Radiology 175: 791–796
47. McNeil B J, Hanley J 1980 Analysis of serial radionuclide bone images in osteosarcoma and breast carcinoma. Radiology 135: 171–176
48. Hoefnagel C A, Bruning P F, Cotten P, Marcuse H R, Van der Schoot J B 1981 Detection of lung metastases from osteosarcoma by scintigraphy using 99m-Tc-methylene-diphosphonate. Diagn Imaging 50: 277–284
49. Vanel D, Henry-Amar M, Lumbroso J et al 1984 Pulmonary evaluation of patients with osteosarcoma: roles of standard radiography, tomography, CT, scintigraphy and tomoscintigraphy. AJR 143: 519–523
50. Kirk G A, Schulz E E 1987 Usefulness of SPECT in evaluating osteosarcoma metastases to the lung. Clin Nucl Med 12: 356–358
51. Ohta H, Ishii M, Yoshizumi M 1985 Is ECT imaging with Tc(V)-99m dimercaptosuccinic acid useful to detect lung metastases of osteosarcoma? Clin Nucl Med 10: 13–15

81. The evaluation of malignancy: metastatic bone disease

Hans Van der Wall

The potential for skeletal scintigraphy was evident using the early bone-seeking agents since, despite the suboptimal quality of the images, they revealed tumour deposits in bone prior to radiological change. Initial interest with the introduction of the technetium phosphates was in the evaluation of their accuracy in detecting metastatic lesions in bone. In four series comparing scintigraphy with radiography in 1403 patients, 28% more abnormalities were demonstrated by scintigraphy. Only 1.5% of radiographic abnormalities were not detected by scintigraphy. Subsequent experience has fulfilled this early promise. The sensitivity of the radionuclide technique is based on the physiological basis for preferential uptake, which identifies as little as 5–15% alteration in local bone turnover. Delineation of a lytic lesion by conventional radiology requires a minimum size of 1 cm and a focal loss of at least 50% of bone mineral,[1] while at least a 30% increase in bone mineral content is necessary to appreciate sclerotic lesions.

ANATOMICAL CONSIDERATIONS

The spread of metastatic deposits to various organs, and especially the bones, is dependent upon the mechanical distribution of tumour cells by either direct, lymphatic or haematogenous routes. This is necessary but not sufficient for the establishment of metastases as the interplay of more complex mechanisms will determine if the tumour cells survive and multiply at these distant sites. It is well established that metastatic deposits have a proclivity to localize in the axial skeleton, which is difficult to explain given that most tumours embolize through the venous circulation and therefore should be trapped in the lungs via the caval or pulmonary venous system or in the liver via the portal venous system. In 1940, Batson[2] described a plexus of vertebral veins that formed rich anastomotic connections with veins of the brain, skull, neck, ribs, shoulder girdle, viscera and vertebral column. These were valveless structures that allowed retrograde blood flow when either thoracic or intra-abdominal pressures were raised. He suggested that this system permitted the haematogenous spread of the two most common malignancies (breast and prostatic carcinoma) to the axial skeleton. A wealth of observations have supported this premise.

More rarely, arterial dissemination may be implicated in the spread of bony metastases, as evidenced by purely cortical metastases. Characteristically, these occur in the appendicular skeleton and are thought to be transported to the cortex by the anastomotic branches between the nutrient and periosteal arteries. Such lesions have been reported as uniformly osteolytic and associated with a soft-tissue mass in approximately 50% of cases.[3] The diaphyseal and metadiaphyseal location of the majority of such lesions may be explained by the proximity to a nutrient artery.

Within the confines of the skeleton lies one of the largest organs in the body, the bone marrow. It contributes approximately 3.0 kg in males and 2.6 kg in females,[4] forming a large reservoir in dynamic continuum with the vascular compartment. The osseous component that provides architectural and metabolic support to marrow is cancellous bone, the interface at which osteoclasts, osteoblasts and osteocytes are active. Bone marrow has a rich arterial blood supply from the nutrient arteries that anastomose with transosteal vessels before forming an extensive and complex sinusoidal system. Red marrow is the vascular active form, while yellow marrow is the quiescent element. With ageing, red marrow is progressively concentrated in the axial skeleton. It is therefore not surprising that over 90% of metastases will lodge in the bone marrow prior to extension into the osseous structures. The ready availability of a high-volume, low-pressure venous delivery system and the presence of abundant substrate make it a fertile ground for metastatic disease.

PATHOLOGICAL CONSIDERATIONS

The organ-selective properties of metastases have been

known for over 100 years and were first explored by Stephen Paget in 1889;[5] this came to be known as the 'seed and soil' hypothesis. A considerable body of literature has accumulated that supports the concept of selective colonization of tissues by metastases. A recent review of this literature[6] details the importance of vascular endothelial receptors, adhesion molecules, mitogens, growth factors, cellular growth inhibitors and angiogenic factors. For example, it has been demonstrated that stromal cells produce a growth factor in the bone marrow that promotes the growth of prostatic adenocarcinoma cells at a rate faster than in the gland itself.

SCINTIGRAPHIC FINDINGS

Typical appearance

The osteoblastic response to almost all metastatic deposits will, because of the mechanisms of uptake in response to the insult of invasion of bone, result in a focus of preferential accumulation or a 'hot spot'. Most typically, multiple lesions of varying size, shape and intensity will be observed in an irregular distribution throughout the axial skeleton, with at least 10% occurring in the skull and appendicular skeleton. The latter can indeed be the site of solitary distant lesions sufficiently often to make their inclusion in a survey mandatory. The pattern of distribution of such abnormalities by site is illustrated in Fig. 81.1. On occasion, the dissemination of disease may be so extensive that the study may resemble the 'superscan' typical of metabolic bone disease and characterized by intense uptake throughout the skeleton and faint renal accumulation (Fig. 81.2). Careful assessment will usually identify the cause by indicating some patchiness of accumulation, particularly in the ribs and in the limbs, which often demonstrate less uptake than the rest of the skeleton.

Rarely, the appearance of a metastasis may take the form of a 'sunburst reaction' due to tumour extending subperiosteally and stimulating new bone formation. This appearance has classically been associated with primary bone tumours and may erroneously suggest this diagnosis. In a review of 70 such cases[7] due to metastatic disease, prostatic adenocarcinoma was found to be most frequent (29%), followed by carcinoma of the bronchus (10%) and neuroblastoma (10%). The scan appearance is of intense increase in accumulation extending outside the cortical outline with more patchy areas of intense uptake in the subperiosteal region.

In view of the pathogenesis of metastatic disease, it is possible that in the early phases, when disease is confined to the bone marrow, the bone scan should be normal. This was confirmed in patients with disseminated breast cancer, up to 25% of whom had evidence of bone marrow disease on scanning with an antibody to leucocytes, but no alteration in uptake on the polyphosphate bone scan.[8]

Atypical appearances

When a deposit is not associated with a typical osteoblastic response, the bone scan may be entirely normal. This false-negative study can reflect the relatively indolent nature of the lesion, but the absence of a reparative response may also indicate the aggressive nature of the tumour, implying an ominous prognosis. Such deposits more often appear as entirely 'cold' or photopenic spots with absent accumulation. In association with significant bone lysis, these photopenic abnormalities can be surrounded by a rim of significantly increased accumulation, indicating a periph-

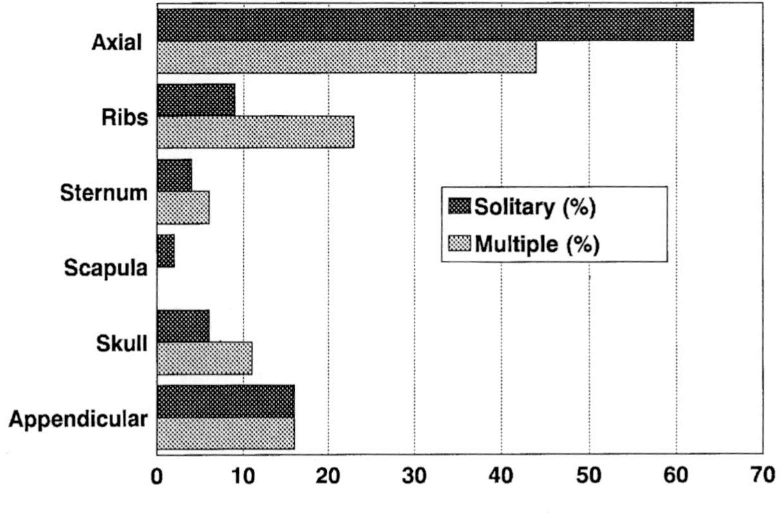

Fig. 81.1 Sites of skeletal metastases.

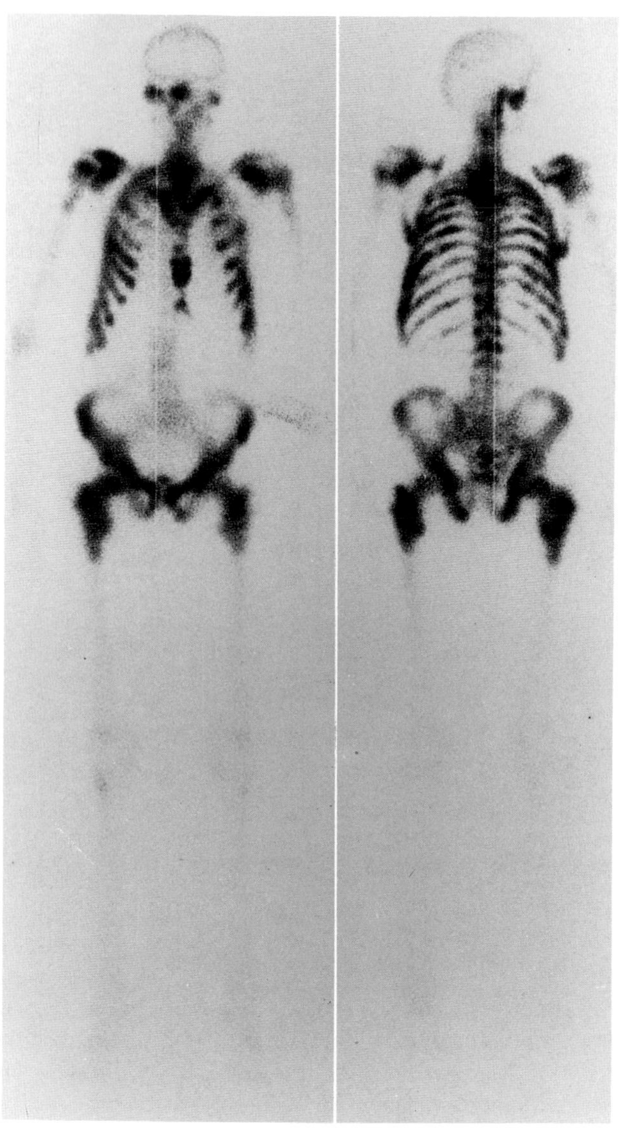

Fig. 81.2 Disseminated metastatic involvement from prostatic carcinoma presenting as increased accumulation with a patchy distribution throughout the axial skeleton, the limbs and skull being relatively spared and the renal accumulation markedly diminished, since, because of the marked skeletal accumulation, less radiopharmaceutical is available for excretion.

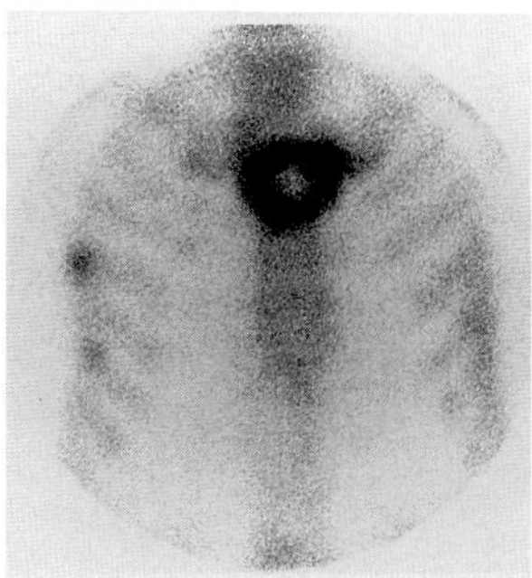

Fig. 81.3 Metastatic disease from breast carcinoma in a man, producing intense accumulation occupying the manubrium sternum with a 'doughnut' appearance resulting from the central photopenia, and also focal rib lesions.

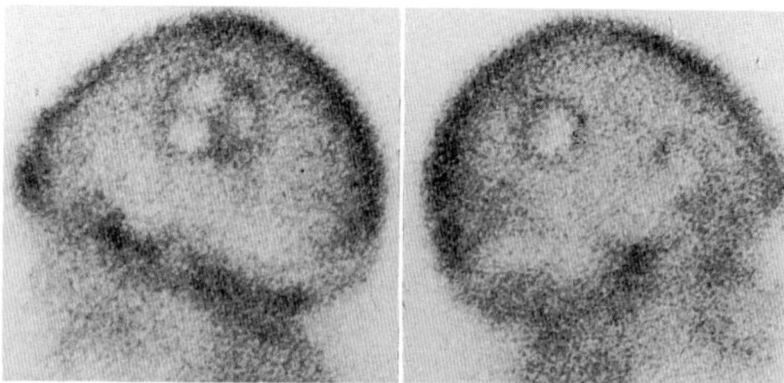

Fig. 81.4 Follicular thyroid cancer. Multiple metastases involving the skull, observed as discrete photopenic areas with only minimal osteoblastic reaction as a surrounding 'rim'.

eral reparative response (Fig. 81.3) This appearance may occur both in very aggressive tumours or, conversely, with neoplasms which characteristically are slow-growing, e.g. thyroid carcinoma (Fig. 81.4). In the latter, of course, the survey with ^{131}I is likely to be more rewarding, as may be the use of thallium-201 (^{201}Tl).

The solitary lesion

The visualization of a 'hotspot', even in an individual with a known carcinoma, is not specific for metastatic disease, although obviously the probability is very high when multiple widespread lesions are noted. The distribution of multiple lesions can be critical in interpretation of the study, e.g. the linear and curved pattern typical of several fractured ribs (Fig. 81.5) The greatest difficulty occurs with solitary lesions, which can result from many aetiologies (Fig. 81.6). The shape of the abnormality may be valuable since, for example, a metastatic deposit, invading along the rib, becomes elongated, while a rib fracture tends to be significantly more focal. There are, however, recorded exceptions to even this observation.[9] The significance of solitary lesions has been studied by several groups, summarized by McNeil.[10] Overall, 55% of solitary scan abnormalities were caused by neoplastic disease and 25% by trauma. Among patients with a known primary tumour, 70% of rib lesions were malignant and 80% of vertebral lesions were malignant. Tumeh et al,[11] however, in a review of 2851 patients with cancer, noted solitary rib lesions in only 1.4%, 90.2% being the result of a benign factor. Such difficulties in interpretation are of course influenced by the nature of the primary neoplasm and the distribution of secondary deposits, thoracic spine and rib lesions, for example, being the more frequent site of deposits in both breast and lung cancer. However, although 23 (18%) of 125 patients with carcinoma of the lung studied by Matsumato et al[12] had abnormal uptake

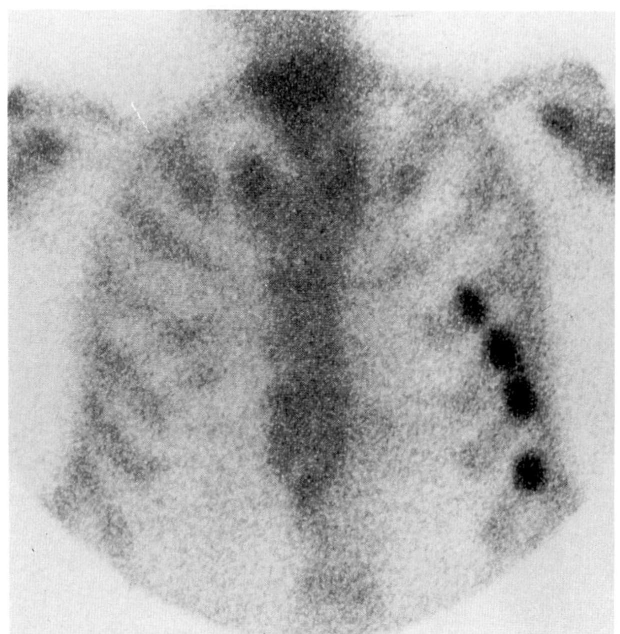

Fig. 81.5 Rib fractures. Characteristic foci visualized in a curved linear pattern.

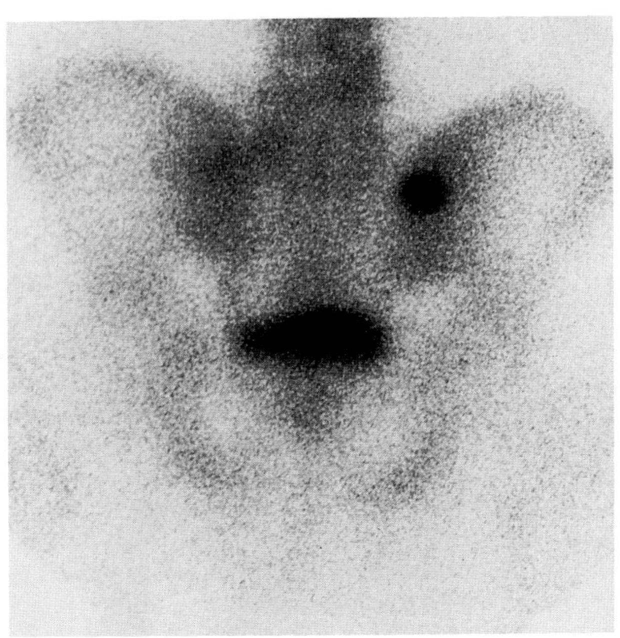

Fig. 81.6 Prostatic carcinoma. Discrete solitary lesion in the right sacroiliac joint, the only evidence of metastatic spread.

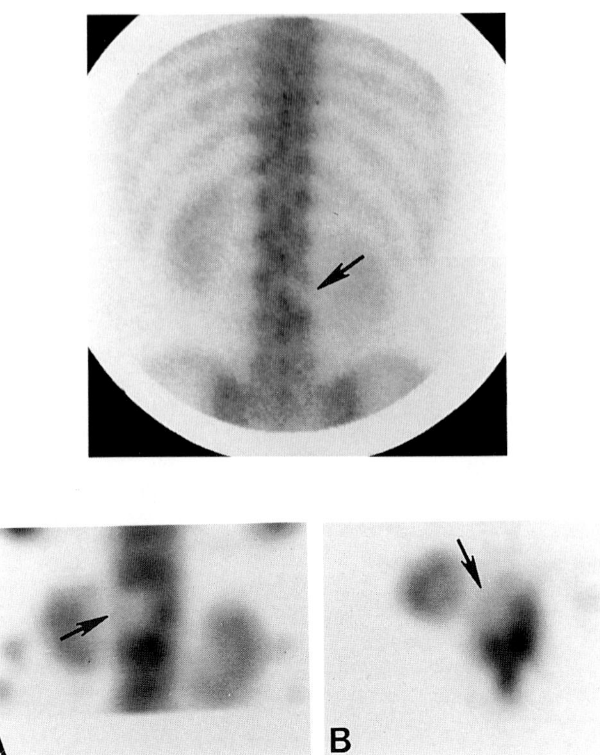

Fig. 81.7 (*Top*) The use of emission tomography. The only lesion with standard planar views in a patient with carninoma of the lung is an ill-defined reduction of activity in L3. (*Bottom*) SPECT demonstrates the metastasis as a clearly delineated photopenic area in both the coronal (A) and transaxial (B) sections.

only in the ribs, in 14 of these (61%) the lesion was benign. In contrast, 76% of isolated sternal abnormalities, which occurred in 3.1% of 1104 patients with breast cancer reviewed by Kwai et al,[13] were malignant. Emission tomography (SPECT) certainly offers assistance by more precise localization and assessment of size of a solitary abnormality, especially when present in a vertebra (Fig. 81.7). In particular, this will permit distinguishing a lesion in the body from one sited more laterally and reflecting arthritic change. The latter is frequently noted in the cervical spine, identified by its lateral position and intensity, which is usually significantly less than a metastasis (Fig. 81.8). Delbeke et al[14] compared MRI and bone scintigraphy in the evaluation of osseous spine metastases. They concluded that the modalities were complementary, the radionuclide study remaining the best screening procedure to show the location of abnormalities in the spine as well as identifying lesions elsewhere in the skeleton. MRI proved useful in differentiating metastases from other lesions in bone and demonstrating epidural masses and paravertebral extension of the tumour.

^{201}Tl scanning does offer an accurate alternative modality for the assessment of solitary lesions of bone. Uptake of the agent reflects a complex interplay of cellularity, metabolic status and blood flow, which are altered in tumours. Van der Wall et al[15] studied 25 lesions in 22 patients (including three coexistent benign abnormalities), 21 of which were in the appendicular skeleton. ^{201}Tl scanning for the identification of malignancy was found to have a sensitivity of 88% and a specificity of 94%. The

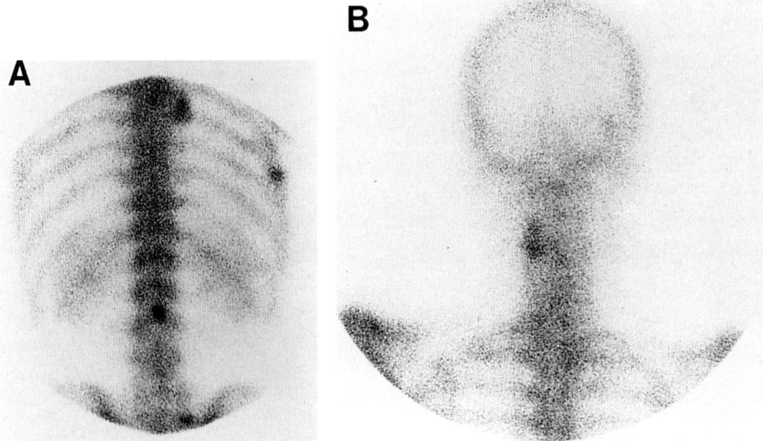

Fig. 81.8 Vertebral lesions. (A) Suspicion that an apparently solitary lesion in a spinous process is a metastasis, because of siting and intensity, is confirmed by observation of further foci, particularly in the ribs. (B) Arthritic change in the cervical spine differentiated from a metastasis by the siting and intensity.

predictive value of a positive scan, demonstrating preferential accumulation of ^{201}Tl, was 88%, while the negative predictive value of the study was 94%. Lesions that demonstrated no preferential ^{201}Tl accumulation included enchondromas, a haemangioma of bone, fibrous dysplasia, recent fractures and an osteochondroma. Abnormalities demonstrating intense ^{201}Tl accumulation included metastatic Ewing's sarcoma, colonic carcinoma, clear cell carcinoma of the kidney, lymphoma and adenocarcinoma of the breast and prostate.

INDICATIONS

The major indications for skeletal scintigraphy in patients with a known malignancy are for staging, assessment of bone pain, extent of bony disease and prior to or for charting response to therapy.

Staging

In view of the dramatic manner with which skeletal metastases are shown and the sensitivity of the technique, it could be argued that skeletal scintigraphy should be mandatory in the staging of many neoplasias, even when there are known metastases, since frequently the scan will demonstrate more extensive disease than previously suspected. However, it is obvious that it is difficult to establish that such a policy confers significant health benefit in terms of reduced cost and patient inconvenience or has beneficial consequences for patient management and outcome. Nevertheless, there is abundant proof of a major routine role in several cancers, notably breast and prostate, the evidence having been reviewed in detail by McKillop.[16] The importance of the staging examination will be analysed in detail under consideration of these specific malignancies.

Skeletal pain

One of the most difficult clinical problems that the patient with a known malignancy poses is the evaluation of skeletal pain. Palmer et al[17] studied 195 consecutive patients with either breast (131) or prostatic malignancy (64) by scintigraphy. The prevalence of skeletal malignancy was high, being 40% in patients with breast carcinoma and 63% in patients with prostatic carcinoma. There was a statistically significant correlation between bone pain and the presence of metastases. In patients with breast cancer reporting the presence of skeletal pain, 57% had metastases and 36% had none, the remainder being uncertain by scan criteria. In those who were asymptomatic, 19% had evidence of metastases. Among prostate cancer patients, metastases were present in 82% with skeletal pain and 34% with no pain. The lumbar spine represented the most painful site of metastases in both groups, almost half the patients with the abnormality complaining of site-specific pain. Apart from this site, pain was an unreliable indicator of the anatomical location of metastasis.

The clinical background is naturally of major significance in the consideration of such patients. In 138 patients with back pain and a previous history of malignancy, studied by Schutte & Park,[18] nearly 40% had an abnormality later proven to be a metastatic deposit. Bone pain, particularly without radiological abnormality, is therefore frequently an indication for skeletal scintigraphy, not merely when there is concern regarding a malignant aetiology, but in many other contexts, e.g. possible sports injuries, suspected infection, etc. The findings may be such as to answer the clinical problem, but in other instances will indicate the optimal site for a bone biopsy. The experience of Collins et al[19] is typical. Using percutaneous needle biopsy in 130 patients with lesions identified in bone scans, in 58 the abnormality being solitary, positive biopsy was achieved in 111, 45% revealing malignancy. In patients presenting with a pathological fracture, radionuclide surveys will not only reveal whether there is disseminated disease but also identify the most accessible biopsy site.

Evaluation of therapy

The atraumatic nature of skeletal scintigraphy permits ready utilization of sequential studies. This may be employed to observe alterations in lesions which have caused difficulty in evaluation or in the assessment of response to appropriate therapy. Changes in the scintigraphic findings may well accompany the treatment of metastatic lesions but can provide unexpected difficulties in interpretation. This arises from the 'flare phenomenon', in which healing of lesions is initially associated with an osteoblastic response and possibly an increase in blood flow due to an inflammatory response to the tumour destruction, manifested as increased activity.[20] There is subsequent regression of uptake. As Rossleigh et al[21] emphasized, small previously undetected lesions may become demonstrable, apparently as new sites, and cause concern that there has actually been further dissemination of disease. Such alterations are now well recognized as common in metastases from carcinoma of the breast,[22] but the frequency with which the phenomenon occurs in those from carcinoma of the prostate has been more controversial.[23] A more recent report from Johns et al[24] described the appearance in approximately 20% of a group of 26 patients treated with the hormonal agent leuprolide. The process has also been reported following the treatment of metastatic small-cell carcinoma of the lung.[25]

Difficulties may also arise because of a varying response to therapy, resulting in some lesions becoming better and some worse, although both will show increased activity.[26] Continued sequential scanning may be essential since, as healing progresses, the intensity of the lesion uptake diminishes and, by 6 months, it should be feasible to differentiate between response and progression. Thus, on occasion, it is gratifying to use such serial imaging to demonstrate complete regression.

BREAST CARCINOMA

Post-mortem studies indicate that 50–80% of females dying of breast cancer will have bone metastases. The predilection of metastases for bone marrow and bone has been well documented, and several studies have confirmed that bony metastases herald a poor prognosis, median survival being 24 months.[27] Several factors are predictive of the tendency of tumours to metastasize. Histologically, the presence of dense angiogenesis in the primary tumour (microvessel count > 100 per 200× field) is associated with metastases in almost 100% of patients.[28] Primary tumour size and clinical staging are also important predictors of the presence and progression of metastases. A similar prognostic role for a circulating tumour marker CA15-3 has also been shown to predict both soft-tissue and skeletal metastases. Prior to the introduction of the technetium phosphate agents, there was considerable divergence of opinion on the incidence of metastases in women presenting with breast cancer, the frequency of an abnormal bone scan with the earlier agents varying from 4 to 38%.

Staging

Numerous reports of experience with the technetium agents have appeared and, not surprisingly, the incidence of abnormal studies varies considerably, reflecting the staging of the lesion. The lack of consensus regarding the utility of the bone scan as a routine staging investigation was clearly reflected in an overview from a workshop on breast carcinoma held in 1988.[29] As the test has a low yield in Stage I or II disease, it was suggested that routine staging examinations should be confined to patients with only stage III or IV disease. However, a good case was made for a baseline bone scan in all patients to allow discrimination of new from long-standing findings in subsequent studies. In their extensive review of the role of scintigraphy in breast cancer, Fogelman & Coleman[30] summarized the results of 20 series from the literature. The detection rate of metastases in 1243 patients with stage I disease was 3%, in 1983 with stage II was 5% and in 801 with stage III was 18%. The results of baseline scans from a single centre were reviewed by Coleman et al[31] and may be more valid, given the uniformity of staging procedures. Scans were obtained in 1267 consecutive patients presenting with breast cancer. By staging of primary tumour size (T), 0.3% of patients with T1, 3% with T2, 8% with T3 and 13% with T4 had bone metastases. By clinical staging, none with stage I, 3% with stage II, 7% with stage III and 47% with stage IV had bone metastases. Importantly, 23% had bone scan abnormalities radiologically confirmed as benign disease. The false-positive rate for scintigraphy was confirmed at 1.6% after median follow-up of 3.5 years in 20 patients. The conclusion from this study was that in patients with a primary tumour less than 2 cm in diameter or clinical stage I routine staging bone scintigraphy is unjustified. Similarly, results from two recent studies[32,33] also found a lack of utility of routine bone scans in limited primary disease and clinical stage I and II patients.

Approximately 5% of patients will initially present with stage IV disease. Sherry et al[34] have identified a subset of patients with stage IV disease who have only skeletal metastases and significantly prolonged survival in comparison to those with both skeletal and extraskeletal disease. In this group, median survival was 33 months compared with 9 months in patients with extraskeletal disease. The bone scan is clearly of prognostic importance in this group.

Follow-up studies

In seven studies which reported the follow-up of 1520 women presenting with clinically early breast cancer and normal studies, 145 (9.5%) developed abnormal studies over follow-up periods between 1 and 5 years, the prevalence of abnormal scans ranging from 7 to 26% (Fig. 81.9). The mean time after presentation to development of bone scan abnormalities was about 2 years. The prevalence is obviously related to the stage of disease at presentation. Fogelman & Coleman[30] suggested that the policy for serial studies should be based on consideration of various prognostic factors in each patient, including tumour size, axillary lymph node involvement, histological grading and receptor status. Such statistics become increasingly important in light of the evidence of the increase in 2 year mortality in patients with abnormal scans, approximating 65% in patients with abnormal scans compared with 10% in those with normal scans.

The utility of routine yearly follow-up studies has also become questionable in light of several recent studies. Pedrazzini et al[35] followed 1601 patients with axillary lymph node-positive breast carcinoma for 4 years with yearly bone scintigraphy. While 8.5% had a first recurrence of disease in bone at a median of 48 months, only 2.4% had recurrence in the first 12 months. A total of 6900 bone scans were performed to yield this result, requiring an average of 50 scans for each abnormal study. The cost-effectiveness is therefore highly questionable. It is particularly important to consider this information in light of the results from the Eastern Cooperative Oncology Group study,[36] in which 65% of patients with skeletal metastases were identified by symptoms and 18% by scan criteria alone. Taken together these two studies indicate that, because of the low yield in early-stage disease, it may be prudent to scan only the symptomatic patients. The results of the scan will undoubtedly influence prognosis, and may change therapeutic strategies. While there is no evidence that earlier treatment of metastases improves survival, it has the clear advantage of directing attention to sites of potential pathological fracture so that further radiological evaluation and prophylactic treatment can reduce ensuing complications.

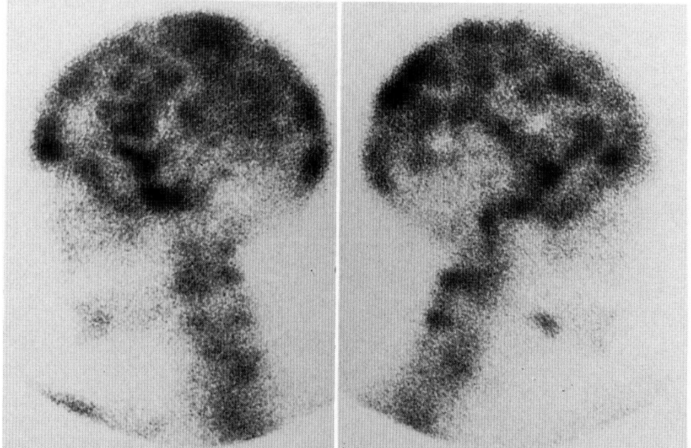

Fig. 81.9 Disseminated metastatic disease from carcinoma of the breast observed in the serial scan in a woman in whom a standard scan 1 year before had been entirely normal. Multiple foci of abnormal accumulation are demonstrated throughout the calvarium and cervical spine.

Difficulty in interpretation may be encountered following mastectomy. A variety of scintigraphic alterations may be induced, as reported by Bledin et al,[37] the commonest, in 38 of 51 patients, being apparently increased accumulation in the anterior upper ribs on the affected side, resulting from reduction in tissue attenuation.

PROSTATIC CARCINOMA

Prostate carcinoma is a major cause of mortality and morbidity in men over the age of 50 years. Approximately 50% of patients with metastatic disease die within 30 months and 80% within 5 years. Skeletal metastases occur in about 85% of patients dying of prostate cancer. The prognostic role of skeletal scintigraphy in prostatic carcinoma is similar to that in breast carcinoma. Lund et al[38] showed that patients with an abnormal scan on presentation have a mortality rate of approximately 45% at 2 years compared with 20% for those with a normal initial scan.

The natural history of prostatic carcinoma is variable. This was evaluated by George[39] in a study of 120 patients with initially localized disease and no bone scan evidence of skeletal disease, followed over 7 years. Endoscopic prostatic resection for relief of obstructive symptoms was the only therapy. While local tumour increased in size in 84%, only 13 patients developed skeletal metastases at a mean of 35.8 months. This strongly suggested a malignancy of limited biological potential. It supports the concept of latent versus progressive disease in younger patients, as this group was older and presented with obstructive symptoms in 90% of cases.

Staging

Bone is the only site of metastasis in 65% of patients presenting with metastatic tumour, and the frequency of abnormal bone scans at presentation is high. In six series, studying 956 patients, abnormal bone scans at presentation were present in 36.2%, the prevalence varying from 30 to 51%[16]. The frequency is related to the clinical staging, 5% in stage I, increasing to 10% in stage II, while for stage III it is 20%.[40]

The histological grade of the tumour is also predictive of the occurrence of metastases, as has been shown by Shih et al.[41] They found that patients with high Gleason histological grade tumours had a higher incidence of metastases (15 of 33 patients) than those with a low score (none of 16 patients). In particular, all patients with a 'superscan' appearance of widespread metastases demonstrated high histological grades.

Follow-up studies

The value of routine serial studies remains uncertain. Pollen et al[42] noted that patients with initially negative radionuclide studies but in whom scintigraphy showed progression of disease had a 41% chance of survival at 6 months and 7% at 12 months. For those in whom progression was not demonstrated, these probabilities were 88% and 60% respectively. Both Lund et al[38] and Huben & Schellhammer[43] found that approximately 20% developed abnormal scans in a follow-up period of 3 years. The latter, however, concluded that routine follow-up scintigraphy was not justifiable since all patients manifested progression by either bone pain or elevated serum enzymes.

A definite role for serial bone scanning in patients with established skeletal disease is in the assessment of therapy, particularly in the setting of trials for new or established agents (Fig. 81.10). Few patients with skeletal metastases have clinically measurable disease, and up to 30% may have normal serum acid phosphatase levels. The addition of prostate-specific antigen (PSA) may change such assessments. Terris et al[44] found that when post-operative levels of PSA were undetectable, follow-up bone scans were normal in 75.4% of 118 patients with initially localized disease. A rising PSA level was more predictive of the onset of skeletal metastases in 8.5%.

Soloway et al[45] described a simple scale for quantitation of the extent of disease (EOD) involving the skeleton by the number and size of lesions on a bone scan. They demonstrated a 2 year survival of 94% for grade 1 EOD (< 6 metastases, being < 50% of the size of a vertebral body) compared with 40% for grade 4 EOD ('superscan' or involvement of 75% of the ribs, vertebrae and pelvic bones). It is a simple system that has a good correlation with survival and may prove useful in assessing response to therapy.

LUNG CARCINOMA

Since so many patients with lung cancer present with disseminated metastatic disease, it is not surprising that a high prevalence of skeletal involvement is recorded, particularly in those with small-cell or anaplastic cancer. The role of skeletal scintigraphy lies, therefore, in the evalua-

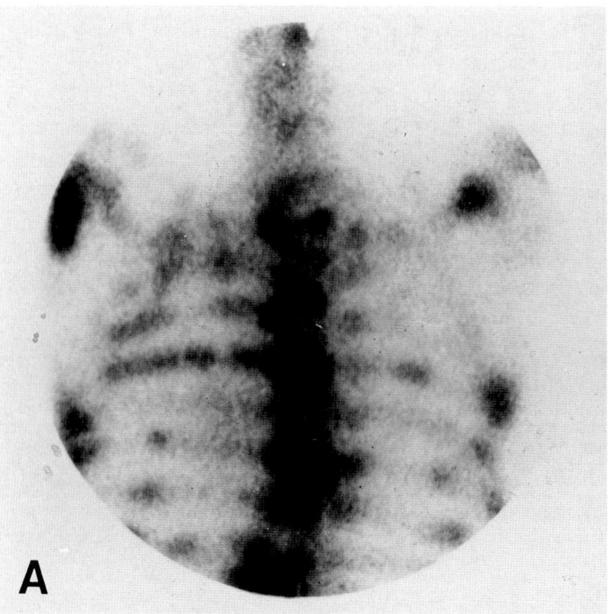

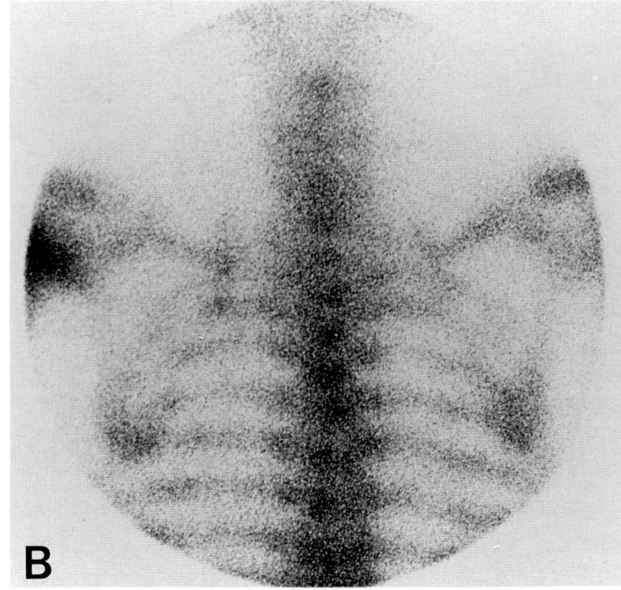

Fig. 81.10 Disseminated prostatic carcinoma. (a) Pretherapy scintigram, showing typical multiple foci of irregular size and intensity. (B) Sequential scan 1 year following hormonal therapy, with regression of metastatic lesions (evaluation of therapy).

tion of those in whom the primary lesion appears amenable to surgery, since 87% of 40 patients with abnormal scans studied by Gravenstein et al[46] had died within 6 months and another 10% by 12 months. Even in those with operable tumours, the study is probably only of clinical significance in symptomatic patients. Metastases were demonstrable in only 19% of patients without pain studied by Kies et al[47] and in 4% of those studied by Hooper et al,[48] compared with prevalences of 78% and 36% respectively in those with symptoms.

OTHER MALIGNANCIES

A philosophy based on clinical staging and potential cure also appears rational in the use of bone scanning in several other neoplasia, for example cervical, bladder and renal cancers, but in view of the incidence of skeletal metastases from these tumours, the procedure probably has its main role in assessment of those patients in whom there is a clinical suspicion of bone involvement. As Kim et al[49] emphasized, the frequency of 'cold lesions' associated with kidney tumours is relatively high. Variable scan appearances are associated with metastases from melanoma, and scintigraphy is probably only justified in advanced disease or in symptomatic patients.

Non-metastatic manifestations

In the initial study, particularly in patients with cancer of the lung, a frequent incidental observation will be the demonstration of changes associated with hypertrophic pulmonary osteoarthropathy. Widespread abnormalities throughout the skeleton are often visualized. In the 48 patients reviewed by Ali et al,[50] the extremities were invariably involved, although with asymmetry in 17%. With the exception of the humerus, the proximal and distal portions of each long bone were involved with equal frequency. Changes were also commonly demonstrable in the skull, scapulae, patellae and clavicles. The characteristic alteration in the long bones is intense pericortical uptake, the 'tramline sign' (Fig. 81.11). Changes in the hands may be obvious in the absence of clinical evidence of clubbing (Fig. 81.12). After treatment of the associated disease, there is usually rapid regression of the scintigraphic changes, and return of the scan to normal within 1 month of successful therapy has been reported.[51]

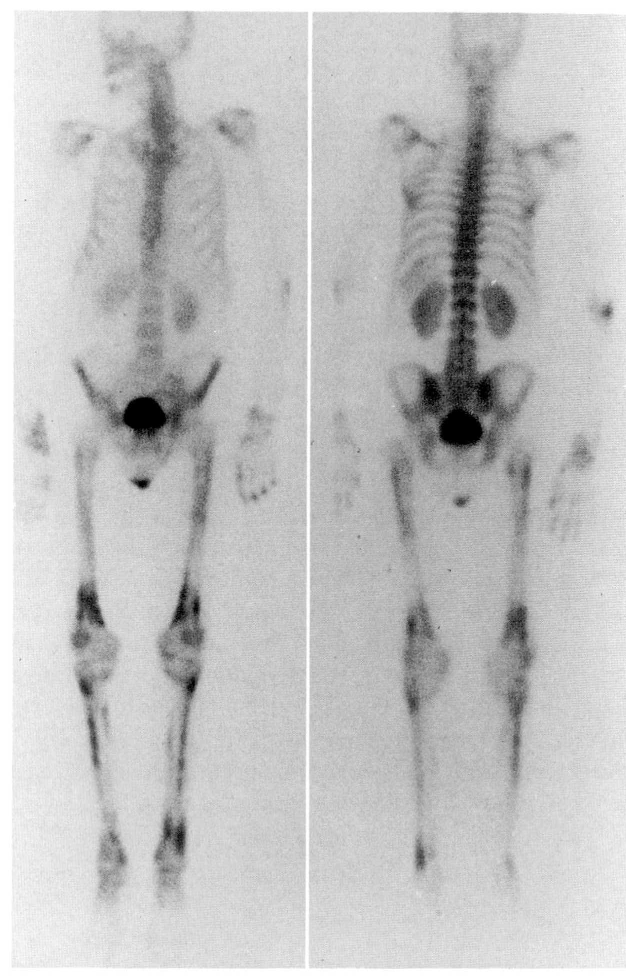

Fig. 81.11 Hypertrophic pulmonary osteoarthropathy. Characteristic pericortical uptake. The cortical 'stripes' of activity ('tramline sign') are evident as an irregular pattern in the long bones of the lower limbs, but are virtually absent in those of the upper limbs.

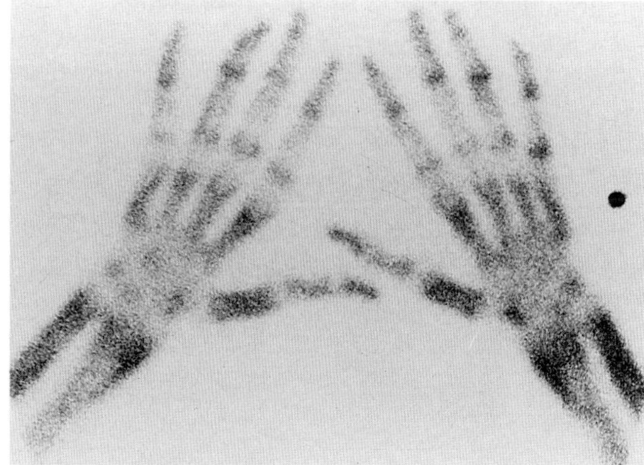

Fig. 81.12 Hypertrophic pulmonary osteoarthropathy. Characteristic appearances of the hands.

INFILTRATIVE DISORDERS

Proliferative changes in most of the bone marrow elements and its architectural milieu can produce changes in the bone scan appearance as a result of a reactive process or direct involvement. This is most commonly associated with abnormalities in the white blood cell elements.

Multiple myeloma

Despite some disparity in reported experience, it is now generally agreed that radiography is more reliable than bone scintigraphy in assessing the extent of multiple myeloma. This reflects the relative absence of reactive osteoneogenesis, possibly because of the production of an osteoblast-inhibitory factor in this disorder. Thus, while areas of increased uptake may be noted, there is often no abnormality and it is well recognized that the lesion may be 'cold' or photopenic (Fig. 81.13). Thus, the radionuclide image failed to show evidence of disease or underestimated the size at 27% of 562 sites in 51 patients reported by Woolfenden et al.[52] Uptake was increased in 95% of the 174 abnormal sites, but discrete areas of decreased uptake were present in 5%. Frank et al[53] studied 20 patients, finding 'hot lesions' in 11, 'cold' in five and 'mixed' in 2, and concluded that images that showed areas of increased uptake were almost always associated with fracture. In the series of Woolfenden et al,[52] however, fractures accounted for only 36% of radiographically abnormal sites with increased uptake on the radionuclide image. Accordingly, scintigraphy does appear to be worthwhile as a complementary investigation, especially in patients with bone pain. It allows the early identification of fractures, often preceding radiographic changes.

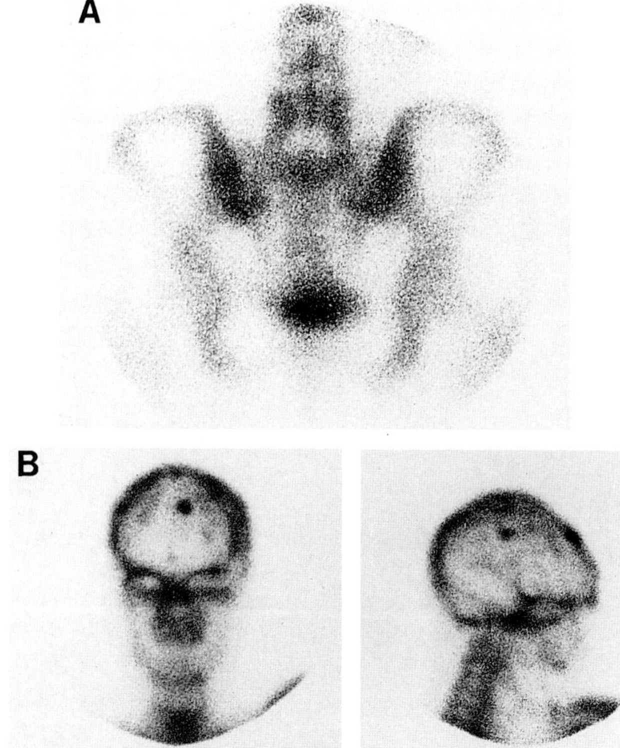

Fig. 81.13 (A) Plasmacytoma. Solitary, discrete, photopenic area with minimal osteoblastic response in L5. (B) Multiple myeloma. Patchy areas of increased activity scattered throughout the skull.

Leukaemia

Skeletal abnormalities may take a mixed form on bone scanning in leukaemia, with the changes in bone being most marked in the acute leukaemias of childhood. In one series, bone scanning revealed abnormal accumulation in 80% of cases at presentation, being most prevalent around the knees.[54] More rarely the accumulation may be reduced and the abnormalities present as 'cold' spots. The reduced accumulation may be on the basis of bone necrosis due to pressure effects from the leukaemic infiltration, direct osseous toxicity or secondary to therapy with either methotrexate or external beam irradiation.[55] The possibility of osteomyelitis must always be foremost in any interpretation of such changes, given the profound nature of the immune suppression from both the primary disease and the therapy.

Histiocytosis

As emphasized by Antonmattei et al,[56] a similar spectrum of scintigraphic findings occurs in the group of disorders classed as 'histiocytosis X'. Thus, although Gilday & Ash[57] observed only one false negative in 10 children, other authors have experienced a higher prevalence, only 35% of the individual lesions demonstrated on radiographs by Parker et al[58] being seen with the radionuclide examination. Crone-Munzebrock & Brassow[59] reported that in 70 patients, 53 bone lesions were detected by radiology, but only 32 were identified by scintigraphy, six being 'cold'. They commented that not infrequently there was a peripheral rim of activity surrounding the margins of the osteolysis (Fig. 81.14). They suggested, however, that recurrences were identified more readily by scintigraphy. The areas of increased uptake vary in intensity, but in the lower limbs tend to be more elongated and diffuse than other metastatic deposits in bone (Fig. 81.15). Westra

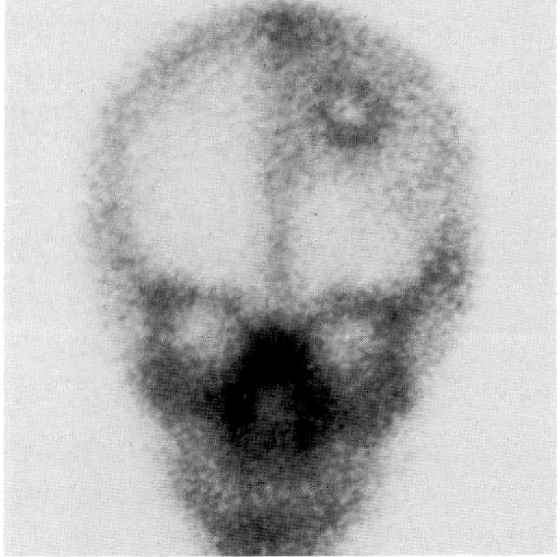

Fig. 81.14 Histiocytosis in a 5-year-old boy: skull lesion showing osteopenic area with a rim of reparative activity.

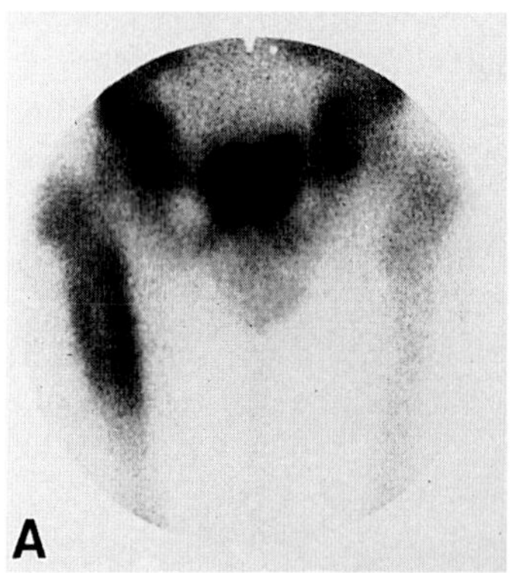

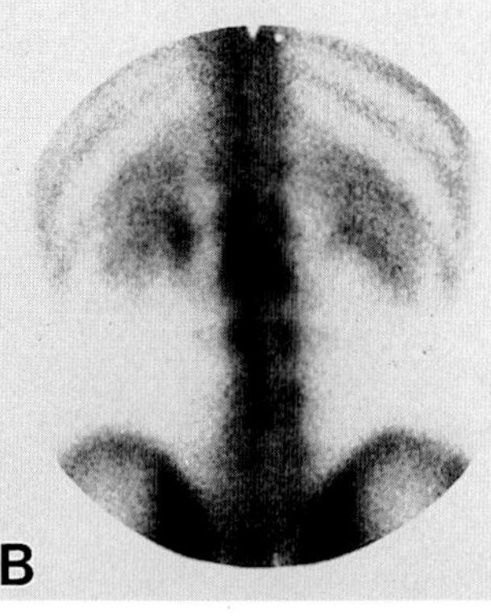

Fig. 81.15 Eosinophilic granulomas. (A) Infiltration of the right upper femur is identified as a diffuse area of increased accumulation with indistinct borders and little bony distortion. (B) A further deposit was demonstrated in L2.

et al[60] found the type of the disorder to be important, the radionuclide study being reliable in unifocal eosinophil granuloma but not in multifocal disease. Negative scans were observed at radiograpically demonstrable sites. More focal, extensive and intense abnormalities occur in 'malignant histiocytosis', lymphohistiocytic reticulosis, as might be expected in view of its more aggressive nature. Gallium scintigraphy is of value in staging this disorder, and Howman-Giles & Uren[61] have found this radionuclide to be of value in both the initial assessment and serial follow-up of patients with histiocytosis X.

Lymphoma

Although skeletal involvement is rare as a primary phenomenon, it occurs in up to one-third of patients with disseminated Hodgkin's disease. While it can be identified with technetium-phosphate scintigraphy, experience of the sensitivity of the investigation varies considerably. Eggenstein et al,[62] for example, concluded that bone scintigraphy is more reliable than radiography in Hodgkin's disease but less useful in non-Hodgkin's lymphoma, whereas Martin & Ash[63] reported that scintigraphy shows more extensive disease than radiography in non-Hodgkin's lymphoma. The appearances are variable, reflecting the osseous reaction, and while focal deposits may be demonstrable there is often a diffuse pattern of increased accumulation with poorly defined margins, which if symmetrical and widespread can cause difficulty in identification (Fig. 81.16). Overall, the investigation is probably best utilized in patients with bone pain, and alternative procedures, including gallium scintigraphy, are generally more likely to be rewarding. These combined radionuclide studies may be of value in the investigation of primary lymphoma of bone and primary reticulum cell sarcoma.

Myelofibrosis

Myelofibrosis fits into the spectrum of myeloproliferative disorders and most commonly follows an indolent course. The scan appearance may be normal or more rarely demonstrate a generalized increase in long bone accumulation due to bony reaction to marrow expansion. In its acute form, the disease is characterized by severe systemic features, culminating in a rapid and fatal outcome, and is thought to be a variant of acute leukaemia, possibly of the megakaryocyte lineage. Skeletal scintigraphy demonstrates multiple sites of increased accumulation due to either bony infiltration or necrosis.[64]

Systemic mastocytosis

This is a condition characterized by dense mast cell infiltration of a number of tissues, including bone marrow. Patients complain of bone pain, flushing, abdominal pain, diarrhoea and syncope, secondary to the secretion of mast cell-derived mediators such as histamine, prostaglandins and heparin. The skeleton is one of the most frequently involved organs of the body, with radiographs demonstrating diffuse or focal sclerotic, lytic and mixed lesions. Skeletal scintigraphy is more sensitive than radiographs and reveals more extensive abnormalities. Again, these may be detected as diffuse or focal increase in accumulation, with the extent of the abnormalities paralleling urinary and serum histamine levels.[65]

PAEDIATRIC TUMOURS

Introduction

The assessment of metastatic disease in childhood requires special care and attention to technique as well as a sound knowledge of the normal scan pattern. Immobilization of the patient is crucial and may be achieved by either physical restraint or chemical sedation. Acquisition of a three-phase study and whole-body images

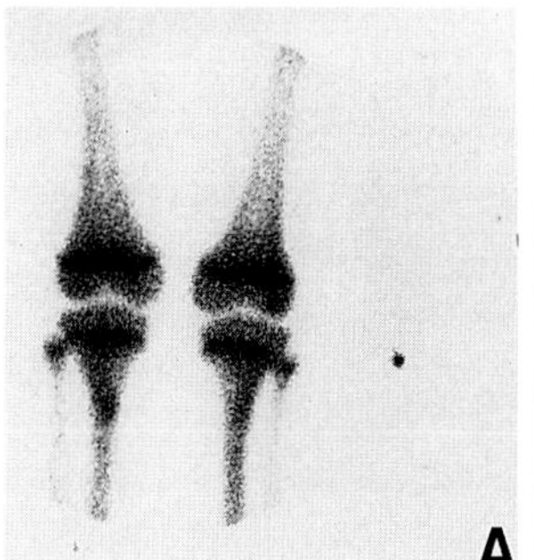

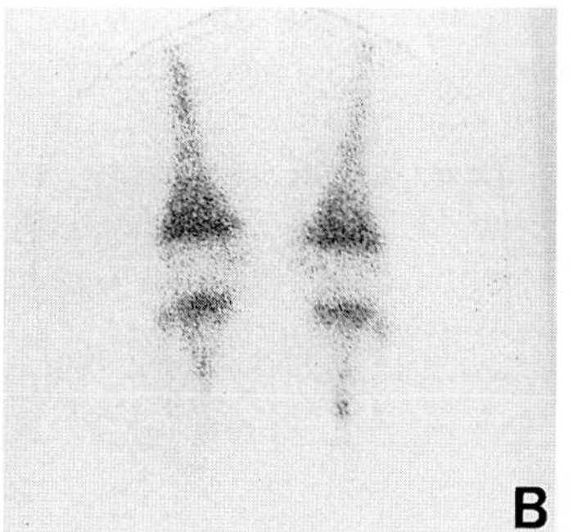

Fig. 81.16 Lymphoma. Although symmetrical, infiltration is manifest by metaphyseal accumulations (A), which are obscured by the growth plates. (B) Lymphomatous infiltration is confirmed by gallium scintigraphy.

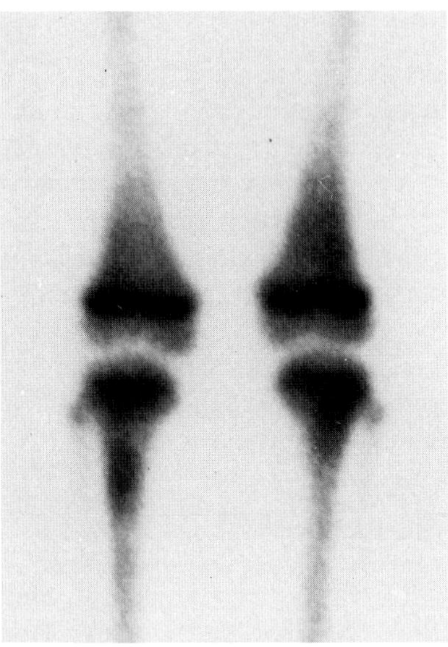

Fig. 81.17 Patient positioning. The growth plates in the femora and tibiae are presented perpendicular to the camera face, with no obliquity that can mask the metastatic neuroblastoma present in all metaphyses.

should be mandatory. Positioning is important as activity in the growth plates may blur or mask a focus of malignancy in the adjacent metaphysis if the camera face is not perpendicular to the physis, allowing better edge definition (Fig. 81.17). In small children, appropriate magnification is necessary to achieve spatial resolution, and this may be accomplished with pin-hole collimation or the acquisition of magnified images. Single photon emission computed studies (SPECT) may be invaluable in elucidation of alterations in sites such as the vertebral column and cranium. Appropriate care should be taken to avoid contamination of the patient by radioactive urine and the degradation of images of the pelvis by activity in the urinary bladder.

Neuroblastoma

Neuroblastoma is one of the most common extracranial solid tumours of childhood. It typically metastasizes to the skeleton, and bone scintigraphy holds a critical place in the staging process and in the management of these children. The sensitivity with which metastases are detected has been repeatedly shown, for example, by Howman-Giles et al,[66] who identified skeletal lesions in 29 of 49 children, and by Sty et al[67] in 7 of 13 cases. Podrasky et al[68] reviewed 42 studies in 35 children, finding metastases in 21. These and other authors have all found scintigraphy much more reliable than radiography, although Kaufman et al[69] did, in contrast, find that in 6 of 12 children a total of 18 lesions were present, 14 of which were only detected radiographically. They ascribed this to small lesion size and a lytic radiological appearance. Photopenic scintigraphic abnormalities with this tumour are well recognized.[70] The osseous metastases may be totally disseminated, the calvarium frequently being involved. Typically, however, they are metaphyseal in location, most frequently in the proximal humeri, distal femora and proximal tibiae (Fig. 81.18). If the blood supply is compromised or the tumour extends into the growth plate, the growth plate will show diminished accumulation. Asymmetry is common, being present in 24 of the 29 children recorded by Howman-Giles et al.[66] The abnormalities may be those usually associated with metastatic deposits, focal and intense. Not infrequently, however, the involvement may be visualized as diffuse increased juxta-articular deposition. In particular, the sharp linear edge of the growth plate becomes blurred.

Howman-Giles et al[66] drew attention to the frequency with which uptake was noted within the primary lesion, 17 of the 49 cases in their series. This phenomenon is now recognized as common in neuroblastoma and other neural crest tumours (Fig. 81.18). Podrasky et al[68] observed this uptake in 20 of 27 patients. It is of interest that it occurred in one of three with uncalcified tumour, whereas five of seven primary lesions with no uptake were calcified. Incidental uptake in extraosseous metastases is also not

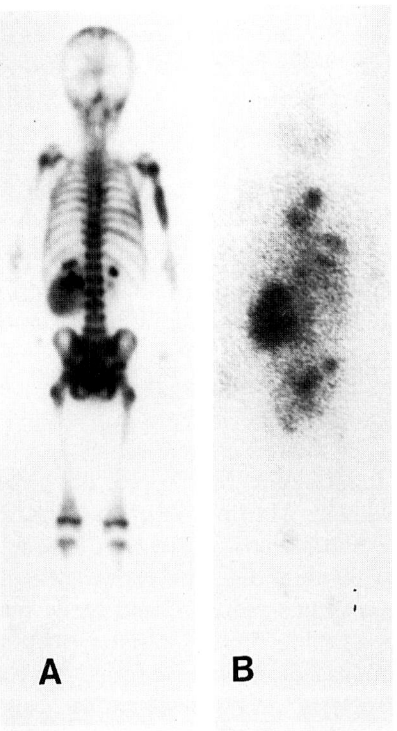

Fig. 81.18 Neuroblastoma. Posterior whole-body bone study (A) and corresponding ^{131}I-MIBG (B) study in the same projection. There is increased uptake of ^{99m}Tc-MDP in the primary lesion in the left adrenal gland, displacing the kidney, and numerous areas of increased accumulation, especially in the humeri and around the knees, pelvis and several ribs. All these abnormalities demonstrate ^{131}I-MIBG uptake. Additional foci of ^{131}I-MIBG uptake are present in lymph nodes in the right supraclavicular fossa and superior mediastinum.

infrequently observed. Mandell & Heyman[71] noted such lesions in numerous sites, commenting that calcification was uncommon and that vanillylmandelic (VMA) levels were only elevated in 63%. Alterations in renal outline or site or obstruction to urine outflow are often obvious.

The value of sequential studies has been emphasized by the review by Baker et al[72] of 40 children. Metastases were demonstrable in 11 at presentation, but in another 17, new or recurrent lesions were identified when previous studies had been normal. These authors also suggested that bone marrow scans can be valuable. It is now established that the use of metaiodobenzylguanidine (MIBG) labelled with either ^{123}I or ^{131}I is more rewarding (Ch. 67). The affinity of this radiopharmaceutical for the neurosecretory storage granules of chromaffin cells is particularly obvious in neuroblastoma (Fig. 81.18) identifying both the primary and metastatic lesions readily, as exemplified by the report of Hoefnagel et al[73] who, in 47 patients, found a sensitivity of 95%. Other neural crest tumours may concentrate MIBG but less consistently. Serial MIBG scintigraphy is valuable in assessing response to therapy, the demonstration of a negative study being particularly useful in assessing the suitability for marrow transplantation. The therapeutic use of the radiopharmaceutical has shown efficacy in some children (Ch. 74).

Caution should, however, be exercised concerning the potential for either ^{123}I or ^{131}I-MIBG to detect all sites of skeletal metastatic disease. Garty et al[74] reported that 29% of metastases were not detected by ^{131}I-MIBG, and Gordon et al[75] documented a false-negative rate of 21% for ^{123}I-MIBG. In contrast, Shulkin et al[76] found the two scintigraphic studies to be complementary, none of the 85 patients having a discordant result, although the ^{131}I-MIBG studies confirmed more extensive skeletal involvement.

Other tumours

Other childhood solid tumours frequently metastasize to bone, including rhabdomyosarcoma, retinoblastoma and hepatoblastoma. Scintigraphy with the bone-seeking agents frequently shows uptake in the primary lesions. It is invaluable, especially in association with radiogallium studies, in the search for metastatic bone disease, usually being superior to radiography. However, Sty et al[77] have shown that disseminated Wilms' tumour was a notable exception.

REFERENCES

1. Edelstyn G A, Gillespie P J, Grebell F S 1967 The radiological demonstration of osseous metastases: experimental observation. Clin Radiol 18: 158–162
2. Batson O V 1940 The function of the vertebral veins and their role in the spread of metastases. Ann Surg 112: 138–149
3. Hendrix R W, Rogers L F, Davis T M 1991 Cortical bone metastases. Radiology 181: 409–413
4. Vogler J B, Murphy W A 1988 Bone marrow imaging. Radiology 168: 679–693
5. Paget S 1889 The distribution of secondary growths in cancer of the breast. Lancet 1: 571–573
6. Zetter B R 1990 The cellular basis of site-specific tumour metastasis. N Engl J Med 322: 605–612
7. Bloom R A, Libson E, Husband J E, Stoker D J 1987 The periosteal sunburst reaction to bone metastases. A literature review and report of 20 additional cases. Skeletal Radiol 16: 629–634
8. Duncker C M, Carrio I, Berna L et al 1990 Radioimmune imaging of bone marrow in patients with suspected bone metastases from primary breast cancer. J Nucl Med 31: 1450–1455
9. Morgan K, Winer-Muran H, Massie D 1986 Complex rib fracture presenting as a solitary linear focus of increased uptake on bone scan imaging. Clin Nucl Med 11: 797
10. McNeil B J 1984 The value of bone scanning in neoplastic disease. Semin Nucl Med 14: 277–286
11. Tumeh S S, Beadle G, Kaplan W D 1985 Clinical significance of solitary rib lesions in patients with excess skeletal malignancy. J Nucl Med 26: 1140–1143
12. Matsumoto S, Shibuya H, Umehara I, Suzuki S 1987 Scintigraphic diagnosis of rib lesions in patients with lung carcinoma. Clin Nucl Med 12: 960–963
13. Kwai A H, Stomper P C, Kaplan W D 1988 Clinical significance of isolated scintigraphic sternal lesions in patients with breast cancer. J Nucl Med 29: 324–328
14. Delbeke D, Powers T A, Partain C L, Sandler M P 1988 Comparison of MRI and bone scintigraphy in the evaluation of osseous spine metastases. J Nucl Med 29: 763–767
15. Van der Wall H, Murray I P C, Huckstep R L, Philips R L 1993 The role of thallium scintigraphy in excluding malignancy in bone. Clin Nucl Med 18: 551–557
16. McKillop J H 1987 Bone scanning in metastatic disease. In: Fogelman I (ed) Bone scanning in clinical practice. Springer, London, pp 41–60
17. Palmer E, Henrikson K, McKusick K, Strauss H W, Hochberg F 1988 Pain as an indicator of bone metastasis. Acta Radiol 29: 445–449
18. Schutte H E, Park W M 1983 The diagnostic value of bone scintigraphy in patients with a low back pain. Skeletal Radiol 10: 1–4
19. Collins J D, Bassett L, Main G D, Kagan C 1979 Percutaneous biopsy following positive bone scans. Radiology 132: 439–442
20. Alexander J L, Gillespie P J, Edelstyn G A 1976 Serial bone scanning using technetium 99m diphosphonate in patients undergoing cyclical combination chemotherapy for advanced breast cancer. Clin Nucl Med 1: 13–16
21. Rossleigh M A, Lovegrove F T A, Reynolds P M, Byrne N J 1982 Serial bone scans in assessment of response to therapy in advanced breast carcinoma. Clin Nucl Med 7: 397–402
22. Rossleigh M A, Lovegrove F T A, Reynolds P M, Byrne N J, Whitney B P 1984 The assessment of response to therapy of bone metastases in breast cancer. Aust NZ J Med 14: 19–22
23. Pollen J J, Witztum K S, Ashburn W L 1984 The flare phenomenon on radionuclide bone scan in metastatic prostate cancer. AJR 142: 773–776
24. Johns W D, Garnick M B, Kaplan W D 1990 Leuprolide therapy for prostate cancer. An association with scintigraphic 'flare' on bone scan. Clin Nucl Med 15: 485–487
25. Cosolo W, Morstyn G, Arkles B, Zimet A S, Zalcberg J R 1988 Flare response in small cell carcinoma of the lung. Clin Nucl Med 13: 13–16
26. Condon B R, Buchannan R, Garvie N W et al 1980 The assessment of progression or secondary bone lesions following cancer of the breast or prostate using serial radionuclide imaging. Br J Radiol 54: 18–23
27. Coleman R E, Reubens R D 1987 The clinical course of bone metastases. Br J Cancer 55: 61–66
28. Weidner N, Semple J P, Welch W R, Folkman J 1991 Tumour

angiogenesis and metastasis. Correlation in invasive breast carcinoma. N Engl J Med 324: 1–8
29. Colman M, Mattheiem W 1988 Imaging techniques in breast cancer: Workshop report. Eur J Cancer Clin Oncol 24: 69–71
30. Fogelman I, Coleman R 1988 The bone scan and breast cancer. In: Freeman L M, Weissman H S (eds) Nuclear medicine annual. Raven Press, New York, pp 1–38
31. Coleman R E, Rubens R D, Fogelman I 1988 Reappraisal of the baseline bone scan in breast cancer. J Nucl Med 29: 1045–1049
32. Harinder S B, Sisley J F, Johnson R H 1993 Value of preoperative bone and liver scans and alkaline phosphatase in the evaluation of breast cancer patients. Am J Surg 165: 221–223
33. Cox M R, Gilliland R, Odling-Smee G W, Spence R A J 1992 An evaluation of radionuclide bone scanning and liver ultrasonography for staging breast cancer. Aust NZ J Surg 62: 550–555
34. Sherry M M, Greco F A, Johnson D H, Hainsworth J D 1986 Breast cancer with skeletal metastases at initial diagnosis. Cancer 58: 178–182
35. Pedrazinni A, Gelber R, Isley M, Castiglione M, Goldhirsch A 1986 First repeated bone scan in the observation of patients with operable breast cancer. J Clin Oncol 4: 389–394
36. Pandya K J, McFadden E T, Kalish L A, Tormey D C, Taylor 4th S G, Falkson G 1985 A retrospective study of the earliest indicators of recurrence in patients on Eastern Cooperative Oncology Group adjuvant chemotherapy trials for breast cancer. Cancer 55: 202–205
37. Bledin A G, Kim M P E, Haynie T P 1982 Bone scintigraphic findings related to unilateral mastectomy. Eur J Nucl Med 7: 500–501
38. Lund F, Smith P H, Suciu S 1984 Do bone scans predict the prognosis in prostatic cancer? A report of the EORTC protocol 30762. Br J Urol 26: 58–63
39. George N J R 1988 Natural history of localised prostatic cancer managed by conservative therapy alone. Lancet 1: 494–497
40. McNeil B J, Polak J F 1981 An update on the rationale for the use of bone scans in selected metastatic and primary bone tumours. In: Pauwels E K J, Schutte H E, Taconis W K (eds) Bone scintigraphy. University Press, Lieden pp 187–208
41. Shih W-J, Mitchell B, Wierzbinski B, Magocum S, Ryo U Y 1991 Prediction of radionuclide bone imaging findings by Gleason histologic grading of prostate carcinoma. Clin Nucl Med 16: 763–766
42. Pollen J J, Gerber K, Ashburn W L, Schmidt J D 1981 Nuclear bone imaging in metastatic cancer of the prostate. Cancer 47: 2585–2594
43. Huben R P, Schellhammer P F 1982 The role of routine follow-up bone scan after definitive therapy of localised prostatic cancer. J Urol 128: 510–512
44. Terris M K, Klonecke A S, McDougall I R, Stamey T A 1991 Utilisation of bone scans in conjunction with prostate-specific antigen levels in the surveillance for recurrence of adenocarcinoma after radical prostatectomy. J Nucl Med 32: 1713–1717
45. Soloway M S, Hardeman S W, Hickey D, Raymond J, Todd B, Soloway S, Moinuddin M 1988 Stratification of patients with metastatic disease on initial bone scan. Cancer 61: 195–202
46. Gravenstein S, Paltz M A, Pories W 1979 How ominous is an abnormal scan in bronchogenic carcinoma? JAMA 241: 2523–2524
47. Kies M S, Baker A W, Kennedy P S 1978 Radionuclide scans in the staging of carcinoma of the lung. Surg Gynecol Obstet 147: 175–176
48. Hooper R G, Beechler C R, Jonson M C 1978 Radioisotope scanning in the initial staging of bronchogenic carcinoma. Am Rev Resp Dis 108: 279–286
49. Kim E E, Bledin A G, Gutierrez C, Haynie T P 1983 Comparison of radionuclide images and radiographs with skeletal metastases from renal cell carcinoma. Oncology 48: 284–286
50. Ali A, Tetalman M R, Fordham E W, Turner D A, Chiles J T, Patel S L, Schmidt K D 1980 Distribution of hypertrophic pulmonary osteoarthropathy. AJR 134: 771–780
51. Freeman N H, Tonkin A K 1976 Manifestations of hypertrophic pulmonary osteoarthropathy in patients with carcinoma of the lung. Radiology 120: 363–365
52. Woolfenden J M, Pitt M J, Durie B G M, Moon T E 1980 Comparison of bone scintigraphy and radiography in multiple myeloma. Radiology 134: 723–728
53. Frank J W, LeBesque S, Buchanan R B 1982 The value of bone imaging in multiple myeloma. Eur J Nucl Med 7: 502–505
54. Clausen N, Gotze H, Pederson A, Riis-Petersen J, Tjalve E 1983 Skeletal scintigraphy and radiography at onset of acute lymphocytic leukemia in children. Med Pediatr Oncol 11: 291–296
55. Morrison S C, Adler L P 1991 Photopaenic areas on bone scanning associated with childhood leukemia. Clin Nucl Med 16: 24–26
56. Antonmattei S, Tetalman M R, Lloyd T V 1979 The multi-scan appearance of eosinophilic granuloma. Clin Nucl Med 4: 53–55
57. Gilday D L, Ash J M 1976 Benign bone tumours. Semin Nucl Med 6: 33–46
58. Parker B R, Pinckney L, Etcubanas E 1980 Relative efficacy of radiographic and radionuclide bone studies in the detection of the skeletal lesions of histiocytosis X. Radiology 134: 377–380
59. Crone-Munzebrock W, Brassow F 1983 A comparison of radiographic and bone scan findings in histiocytosis X. Skeletal Radiol 9: 170–173
60. Westra S J, van Woerden H, Postma A, Elema J D, Piers D A 1983 Radionuclide bone scintigraphy in patients with histiocytosis X. Eur J Nucl Med 8: 303–306
61. Howman-Giles R, Uren R 1988 The use of gallium 67 in histiocytosis X. Aust NZ J Med 18: 499
62. Eggenstein G, Drochmans A, De Roo M, Wildiers J, Devos P, Van der Schueren G 1978 Bone scintigraphy as detection method for bone and bone marrow involvement in malignant lymphoma with regard to other exploration techniques. J Belge Radiol 61: 471–474
63. Martin D J, Ash J M 1977 Diagnostic radiology in non-Hodgkin's lymphoma. Semin Oncol 4: 297–309
64. Marino G G, Robinson W L 1989 Acute myelofibrosis: correlation of radiographic, bone scan, and biopsy findings. J Nucl Med 30: 251–254
65. Rosenbaum R C, Frieri M, Metcalfe D D 1984 Patterns of skeletal scintigraphy and their relationship to plasma and urinary histamine levels in systemic mastocytosis. J Nucl Med 25: 859–864
66. Howman-Giles R, Gilday D L, Ash J M 1979 Radionuclide skeletal survey in neuroblastoma. Radiology 131: 497–502
67. Sty J R, Babbitt D P, Casper J T, Boedecker R A 1979 99m-Tc methylene diphosphonate imaging in neural crest tumours. Clin Nucl Med 4: 12–17
68. Podrasky A E R, Stark D D, Hattner R S, Gooding G A, Moss A A 1983 Radionuclide bone scanning in neuroblastoma: skeletal metastases and primary tumour localisation of 99m-Tc MDP. AJR 141: 469–472
69. Kaufman R A, Thrall J H, Keyes J W, Brown M L, Zaken J F 1978 False negative bone scans in neuroblastoma metastatic to the ends of long bones. AJR 130: 131–135
70. Fawcett H D, McDougall I R 1980 Bone scan in extra-skeletal neuroblastoma with hot primary and cold skeletal metastases. Clin Nucl Med 5(2): 49–50
71. Mandell G A, Heyman S 1986 Extra-osseous uptake of technetium-99m MDP in secondary deposits of neuroblastoma. Clin Nucl Med 11: 337–340
72. Baker M, Siddiqui A R, Provisor A, Cohen M D 1983 Radiographic and scintigraphic skeletal imaging in patients with neuroblastoma: concise communication. J Nucl Med 24: 467–469
73 Hoefnagel C A, Voute P A, deKraker J, Marcuse H R 1987 Radionuclide diagnosis and therapy of neural crest tumours using iodine-131 metaiodobenzylguanidine. J Nucl Med 28: 308–314
74. Garty I, Friedman A, Sandler M P, Kedar A 1989 Neuroblastoma: Imaging evaluation by sequential Tc-99m MDP, I-131 MIBG and Ga-67 citrate studies. Clin Nucl Med 14: 515–522
75. Gordon I, Peters A M, Gutman A, Morony S, Dicks-Mireaux C, Pritchard J 1990 Skeletal assessment in neuroblastoma – the pitfalls of Iodine-123-MIBG scans. J Nucl Med 31: 129–134
76. Shulkin B L, Shapiro B, Hutchinson R J 1992 Iodine-131-metaiodobenzylguanidine and bone scintigraphy for the detection of neuroblastoma. J Nucl Med 33: 1735–1740
77. Sty J R, Hernandez R J, Starshak R J 1984 Bone imaging in paediatrics. Grune & Stratton, Orlando, pp 85–92

82. Assessment of infection

Hans Van der Wall

While antibiotic therapy has revolutionized the treatment of most bacterial disease, the impact on osteomyelitis has been less marked. The incidence of acute haematogenous osteomyelitis in childhood has decreased, but the incidence of subacute infection has shown a persistent increase.[1] Early diagnosis remains the key to successful therapy. Improvements in radionuclide imaging, antibiotics and surgical techniques have made a considerable impact in reducing the morbidity of the condition over the past two decades.[2]

The term osteomyelitis embodies infection of both bone and marrow. It is a term of convenience, as the progression of infection may be from bone marrow with secondary spread to cortical bone or via the periosteal or soft tissues into cortical bone, with or without involvement of the marrow element. Manifestations of the infection can be varied, depending on the age of the patient, site of involvement, immunological status, nature of the infecting organism and portal of entry. Such infection may be acute and resolve with no sequelae or progress to chronic osteomyelitis if unrecognized or inadequately treated, as still happens in approximately 4% of cases.[1] Trauma, prosthetic devices and immunological or haematological disease may also predispose to the development of chronic infection.

Septic arthritis implies infection of the joint itself, which may be as a primary event or secondary to a focus of adjacent osteomyelitis.

MECHANISMS

Bone and joint structures may be contaminated by three primary routes.

1. Haematogenous spread. Dissemination of infection through the vascular route.
2. Contiguous sources. Infection may spread from adjacent soft tissue into bone or joint structures. This is exemplified by osteomyelitis of the facial bones secondary to dental or sinus infections.
3. Implantation. Infection may be implanted by penetrating injury or during or following surgery of bone or joint structures.

Of the three mechanisms, haematogenous spread is the most common source of osteomyelitis, tending to occur in long bones in children and in vertebrae in the adult.[3]

ANATOMICAL CONSIDERATIONS

Vascular anatomy

The vascular supply of tubular bones is derived from one or two nutrient arteries that arise from the diaphyseal vessels, penetrate the cortex and divide into variable and complicated sinusoidal networks. At the ends of the bone these arteries ramify with terminal branches of the metaphyseal and epiphyseal vessels. Within the bone marrow, the cortical branches divide and connect with capillaries of the Haversian system. At the surface of cortical bone the capillaries form connections with the periosteal plexuses. This ensures that superficial cortical bone derives a variable blood supply from both the periosteal and medullary arterial circulations. The effluent blood flow is initially into a venous sinus, which then unites with veins that follow the nutrient arteries, eventually draining into large venous channels.

The pattern of blood supply at the ends of the long bones is dependent upon age, and the important contribution of the variation in anatomy upon the pathology has been well described by Trueta.[4] In the infant (0–1 year), diaphyseal and metaphyseal vessels may perforate the open growth plate to reach and supply the epiphysis. With increasing growth during the childhood years (1–16 years) there is progressive involution of these vessels till eventually none penetrates the open growth plate. As the growth plate gradually closes, anastomotic channels are then established from the metaphysis into the epiphysis.

The blood supply of the hip is more complex and, given the propensity for complications following infection, requires detailed elucidation. Trueta[5] provided an elaborate description of the changes in blood supply with increasing age. From birth to 4 months the femoral head is supplied by the metaphyseal vessels and inconstantly by the artery in the round ligament. This pattern continues to a variable degree until the growth plate is fully established. As the growth plate becomes a barrier, the metaphyseal vessels contribute negligible supply to the head and virtually all nourishment arises from the lateral epiphyseal vessels. A second supply is progressively established through the ligamentum teres between the ages of 4 and 9 or 10 years. In adolescence, as the barrier of the growth plate begins to break down, vascular anastomoses are reformed from the metaphyseal circulation and the adult pattern is established.

Joints derive their blood supply from vessels that penetrate the capsule, forming a plexus in the deepest layer of the synovial membrane. These vessels terminate at the articular margins as the circulus articularis vasculosus. Articular cartilage is thought to derive a proportion of its nutrition from these anastomotic loops, but mostly from the synovial fluid.

Periosteal anatomy

In childhood, the periosteum is thicker and more loosely applied to the underlying cortical bone than in the adult. It may be easily lifted away from the cortical surface, leading to disruption of blood flow to the superficial cortex.

PATHOLOGICAL CONSIDERATIONS

The metaphyses of the long bones are the most common site of lodgement of organisms in haematogenous osteomyelitis. Blood flow is at its slowest in the capillaries of the metaphyseal marrow, in the region adjacent to the growth plate. One salient exception to the localization of infection in the metaphysis is in children affected by sickle cell disease. The shaft of long bones is more commonly affected than the metaphysis, near the site of entry of the nutrient arteries into the bone.[6] Rarely, primary infection of the epiphysis may occur via the large encircling artery (Hunter's circle) that supplies multiple branches to the peripheral metaphysis and entire epiphysis in older children.

The pathological processes that occur in osteomyelitis have been well characterized.[7] Once the infectious inoculum is lodged, an inflammatory reaction occurs (myelitis), leading to oedema and increasing exudative pressure within the marrow cavity that may compromise the local blood flow, causing significant tissue damage. If the infectious exudate penetrates the endosteum, it may then enter the Haversian and lacunar systems of the cortical bone (osteitis) and eventually spread to the periosteum (periostitis). At this level, especially in childhood, the periosteum may be lifted away, allowing the development of a significant infective collection (subperiosteal abscess) and stimulating the formation of new bone (involucrum). The abscess may spread along the shaft, but is constrained by the strong periosteal attachment at the epiphysis. As there is containment of these processes by the rigidity of the bony structures and the fibrous periosteum, the rising tissue pressures can lead to ischaemic injury and the formation of a sequestrum of devitalized cortical bone. Sequestra may provide tissue sanctuaries for the establishment of chronic infection. A similar situation can occur with smouldering subperiosteal infection stimulating osteoblastic reaction and new bone formation (involucrum), which together with a similar reaction at the medullary interface can envelop the inflammatory reaction. If this reaction becomes prolonged and exuberant it leads to the variant known as Garré's sclerosing osteomyelitis.[7]

Not all chronic infections take this destructive path, and occasionally the initial infection may be rapidly localized and walled off to create a bony abscess (Brodie's abscess) or undergo spontaneous sterilization.[7]

Histologically, the reaction of chronic infection differs from the acute process in several seminal areas. The cellular infiltrate is less marked and the predominant cells are lymphocytes and plasma cells, not the polmorphonuclear series. Thus suppuration and ischaemic destruction of bone go hand in hand with fibrous and bony repair. Sinus tracts may form within the cortex or result from penetration through the periosteum to the skin.

Any joint may be affected by septic arthritis, but those most commonly involved are the hip, knee, ankle, shoulder, sternoclavicular joint, elbow and wrist. Haematogenous seeding is the most common path of infection, with an inflammatory exudate originating in the synovium adding to the volume of synovial fluid. The increased volume of fluid may then raise the pressure within the constraining joint capsule and lead to tamponade of blood vessels, as happens in the hip, predisposing to ischaemic injury to the bone. The inflammatory reaction also leads to damage to the articular surface. Mediators involved in the process are thought to be plasminogen, bacterial toxins and proteases released by leucocytes.

THE SCINTIGRAPHIC EVALUATION OF INFECTION

Infection in bone leads to profound and early alterations in vascularity, often associated with a less intense response in surrounding but uninfected structures, secondary to neurohumoral changes.[8] A rapid osteoblastic response is also associated with such infection. In view of the local hypervascularity and the rapid reaction of bone to the insult of focal infection, it is not surprising that the mechanisms controlling the localization of bone-seeking agents operate to produce a typical intense accumulation. Such areas of uptake will occur at any site of infection related to bone and, particularly when unsuspected, this aetiology must be considered in the differential diagnosis of any abnormal study. The changes can be expected to occur rapidly in the course of any infection of the bones and joints. Skeletal scintigraphy is, therefore, of paramount importance in the early diagnosis, especially as the radiological alterations of bone destruction and periosteal new bone formation cannot be expected for 10–14 days or more after the onset.[9] It is recognized that such investigations of acute bone and joint infection may indicate the need for supplementary scintigraphy with other radionuclides. However, these are more likely to be essential in the elucidation of chronic infection or infection complicating pre-existing sites of bone disease, as the persistence of the reparative processes results in such marked abnormalities that the differentiation of continued infection in bone is extremely difficult. There is still controversy as to which of the alternative radionuclides is most appropriate in these varied chronic problems.

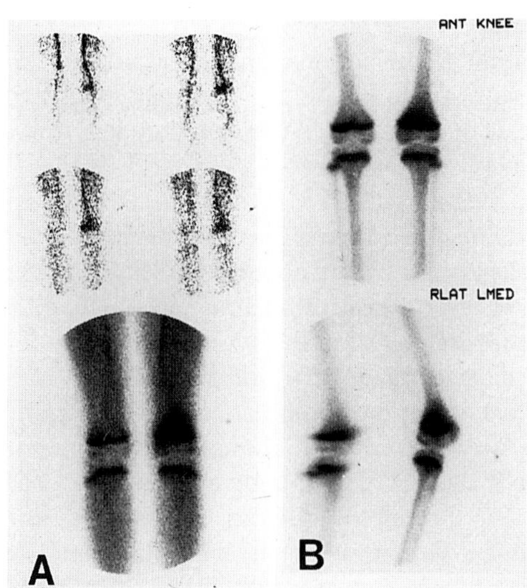

Fig. 82.1 Acute osteomyelitis in a child. The angiographic and blood pool phases (A) of the ^{99m}Tc-MDP study demonstrate intense hyperaemia in the distal metaphysis of the left femur, adjacent to the growth plate. Delayed images (B) reveal intense accumulation at this site, extending diffusely into the metadiaphyseal region.

Acute infection

Technetium phosphate scanning

Since the initiation of early treatment of acute haematogenous osteomyelitis will prevent irreversible changes, the obvious abnormalities noted with skeletal scintigraphy after the introduction of the technetium phosphate agents ensured that the procedure became commonplace. A large number of series followed, showing the extremely valuable role in diagnosis, almost all authors reporting sensitivities well in excess of 90%.[10–13] The high sensitivity of the technique has, however, been questioned by several authors,[14,15] particularly in the neonatal group.

Characteristically a 'three-phase' bone scan will demonstrate hyperaemia in both the early angiographic and 'blood pool' phase of the study and intense focal uptake in the 'delayed phase' within 48–72 h of the onset (Fig. 82.1). A pattern of 'extended' uptake has also been described by Glasier et al[16] in the setting of childhood osteomyelitis and by Taylor & Lawson[17] in the setting of adult osteomyelitis. Diffuse uptake along the shaft of long bones was demonstrated in the presence of infective periostitis, severe soft-tissue sepsis adjacent to bone and with hyperaemia secondary to focal osseous sepsis in 8 of 12 patients in these two studies. Hyperaemia leading to a diffuse increase in uptake has also been reported by Thrall et al.[18]

As the frequency of use of bone scans is increasing, it is gradually being recognized that not all abnormalities, and in particular infection, appear as 'hotspots'. Many authors have reported the occurrence of 'cold' lesions at the site of proven osteomyelitis.[19,20] This can best be understood in terms of the pathophysiology of osteomyelitis. Rising tissue pressure secondary to the inflammatory response to infection can lead to significant ischaemic injury to bone, and reduce the delivery of the radiopharmaceutical to the local area of devitalized bone. Furthermore, if the infective exudate lifts the periosteum away under pressure, then cortical blood flow may be interrupted, again reducing the delivery of the radiopharmaceutical to superficial cortical structures. A mixed scan appearance may then result, with a 'cold' lesion as well as regions of increased blood flow and delayed uptake in surrounding bone. Several authors have identified this pattern as being the result of subperiosteal abscess formation.[21–23] The pattern is an indication for urgent surgical decompression to prevent irreversible ischaemic injury and the development of a sequestrum.

Jones & Cady[21] have indicated that osteomyelitis is not the only cause of 'cold' lesions. Bone infarcts, sickle cell crises, aseptic necrosis, Perthes' disease and metastatic malignant disease can also cause a similar appearance. The observation further reinforces the importance of clinical data in scan interpretation.

It may be difficult to differentiate osteomyelitis from other inflammatory disorders such as cellulitis, septic arthritis and lesions associated with intense focal uptake such as the healing phase of a bone infarct in patients with sickle cell anaemia, particularly in view of the susceptibility of the last to salmonella osteomyelitis.[6] For this reason, Gilday et al[10] strongly recommended the routine combined use of the 'blood pool' study and delayed bone imaging. The procedure was later extended to the 'three-phase' study, by inclusion of the radionuclide angiogram portion by Maurer et al.[24] More recently, Alazraki et al[25] recommended the 'four-phase bone scan' with a 24 h image, finding this procedure of value in assessing osteomyelitis in patients with peripheral vascular disease. While some have found blood pool images to be non-contributory, most workers have found that the three-phase study is valuable, particularly at an early stage, by demonstrating the intense focal hyperaemia even if the later uptake is only mildly abnormal. Cellulitis (Fig. 82.2) will demonstrate a diffuse hyperaemic phase, but in the later studies progressive decrease of activity results in either a normal image or a diffuse non-focal accumulation.[11] Thus, using the combination of a blood pool phase with standard delayed view, Howie et al[12] correctly distinguished all cases of cellulitis or soft-tissue abscess from osteomyelitis. It is of interest that, in their series, 7 of the 55 children with proven osteomyelitis were initially considered to have false-negative studies, but it transpired that an abnormality in six had been misinterpreted as representing alternative pathology.

Children account for approximately 80% of all patients with osteomyelitis. Neonates contribute 7–10%, but the incidence in this subgroup appears to be increasing.[26] Various adult subgroups contribute to the remainder. The major studies indicate that there are two peaks in the incidence of osteomyelitis in childhood. Nade et al[26] found a peak in children under 1 year of age, while Trueta[27] and Blockey & Watson[28] found a second peak between the ages of 9 and 11 years.

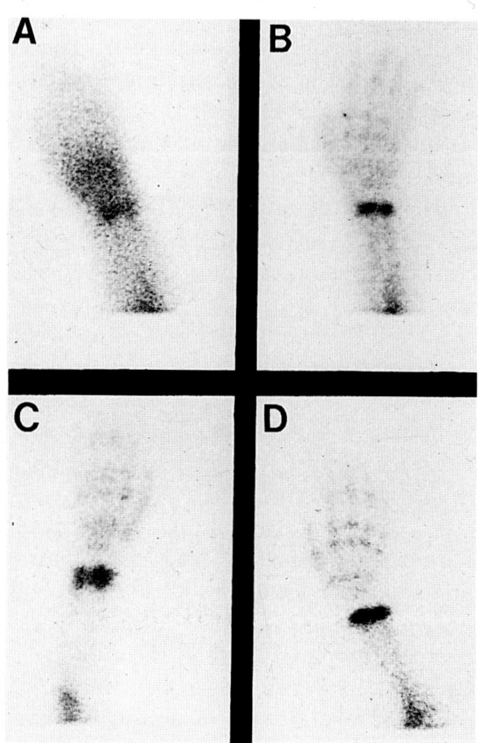

Fig. 82.2 Cellulitis in a 9-month-old girl. The blood pool study of the left hand (A) demonstrates diffuse increase in accumulation compared with the normal right hand (B), but the asymmetry does not persist in the subsequent delayed scans (C and D).

The primacy of paediatric cases creates a unique clinical problem as neonates and young children are less able to localize the site of infection and may present with refusal to move a limb or fever.[29] A diagnosis cannot be established in approximately 10% of limping children even after careful history, examination, appropriate radiology and blood tests.[30] Amongst 50 consecutive patients falling into this category, 24 were subsequently shown to have a focus of bone, joint or soft-tissue sepsis. Aronson et al[30] concluded that bone scanning was sensitive, specific, accurate and cost-effective in arriving at a definitive diagnosis.

The high incidence of osteomyelitis in childhood also creates a number of technical problems for scintigraphic imaging. Immobilization of the patient is crucial and may be achieved by either physical restraint or chemical sedation. Acquisition of a three-phase study and whole-body images should be mandatory. Positioning is important as activity in the growth plates may blur or mask a focus of infection in the adjacent metaphysis if the camera face is not perpendicular to the physis, allowing better edge definition. In small children, appropriate magnification is necessary to achieve spatial resolution, and this may be accomplished with pinhole collimation or the acquisition of magnified images. Single photon emission computerized studies (SPECT) may be invaluable in elucidation of alterations in sites such as the vertebral column (Fig. 82.3) and cranium. The procedure can, for example, readily delineate the changes induced by mastoiditis in the child, in whom the diagnosis can be less obvious prior to the development of the mastoid air cells. In the adult, SPECT can readily demonstrate the extension of infection into the base of the skull.

Appropriate care should be taken to avoid contamination of the patient by radioactive urine and the degradation of images of the pelvis by activity in the urinary bladder.

Reporting of such studies in children requires knowledge of the temporal changes in anatomy in the various age groups and careful comparison of the affected limb or joint with the contralateral side. Ideally, the images should be acquired in the same projections for a fixed time rather than for counts. The importance of considering relevant clinical data in reporting scans cannot be overstated. This was amply illustrated by Sundberg et al[31] in a study of the detection of suspected septic arthritis in 106 children. If scans were reported blindly, with no knowledge of clinical information, the test had a sensitivity of 13%. If the relevant clinical data were considered during reporting, the sensitivity increased to 70%. Howie et al[12] correctly reported 56 of 62 sites of osteomyelitis while blinded to the clinical details. A further five cases were correctly reported when the clinical data were taken into considera-

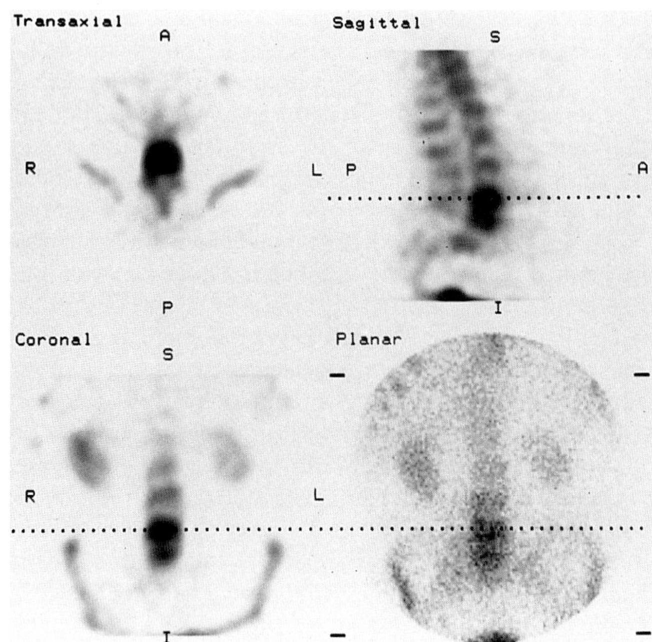

Fig. 82.3 Vertebral osteomyelitis in an 8-year-old boy. SPECT study demonstrating intense uptake in the body of the fourth lumbar vertebra, extending into the posterior aspect of the body on the right side. The extent and precise anatomical siting is clearly seen in all three projections.

tion. Further support for the importance of clinical data in scan reporting has been provided by McCoy et al.[32]

While major surgical intervention at a site of sepsis can lead to major changes in accumulation that confound the scan diagnosis, needle aspiration of areas of suspected bone and joint sepsis does not. Canale et al[33] and McCoy et al[32] showed that needle aspiration does not affect bone scans performed within the following 48 h.

In uncomplicated cases of osteomyelitis, when pre-existing bone disease is not present and the radiograph is normal, the overall sensitivity of three-phase bone scanning is 94% and the specificity 95%. Schauwecker[34] included six major series in his review of osteomyelitis. The scan was positive in 182 of 194 cases and correctly excluded the disease in 360 of 380 cases. He found a sharp contrast in the grouped results from 14 series if any cause of bone remodelling was present, complicating the diagnosis of infection. While the sensitivity remained high at 95% (250 of 262 cases) the specificity was markedly reduced at 33% (110 of 330 cases). It is a clear reflection of the exquisite sensitivity of bone scanning in the detection of any alteration in bone turnover.

Neonatal osteomyelitis The biology and natural history of neonatal osteomyelitis differs significantly from childhood osteomyelitis in a number of aspects. Premature infants' survival rates are much higher as technological methods of life support have improved. Unfortunately, the high dependency of these infants makes invasive monitoring and prolonged intravenous access essential and, coupled with an immature immune system, results in a high risk of a variety of infections. Complications during pregnancy or delivery and venous or umbilical artery catheterization for prolonged periods carry a high risk of osteomyelitis.[35] Rarely, fetal scalp monitoring has led to cranial infection and repeated heel punctures for blood sampling have led to calcaneal infection.[2] Similarly, suprapubic bladder puncture in the neonate may be complicated by osteomyelitis of the pubic bones.

Up to 20% of low-risk and 75% of high-risk cases of neonatal osteomyelitis may be multifocal with up to 50% having transphyseal spread of infection[36] (Fig. 82.4). An adjacent joint effusion may be present in 60–70% of cases. The diffuse nature of the disease, the propensity for complications and the paucity of associated signs[2] highlights the importance of an investigation that offers a whole-body image and additional information about the vascular supply of the epiphysis.

A major controversy persists with regard to the sensitivity of technetium phosphate scintigraphy in neonatal osteomyelitis. Ash & Gilday[15] considered it to be futile in light of their experience in 10 infants with 20 sites of osteomyelitis, only six being demonstrable as abnormal. They suggested that this might reflect the differences in the disorder between the infant and the older child, including the different anatomy, with many vessels penetrating the epiphyseal plate. Others have experienced similar difficulty, noting varying patterns including the non-visualization of the entire normal growth complex. In total contrast, however, Bressler et al[38] demonstrated abnormal radionuclide localization in all of 25 sites of proven osteomyelitis in 15 infants aged less than 6 weeks.

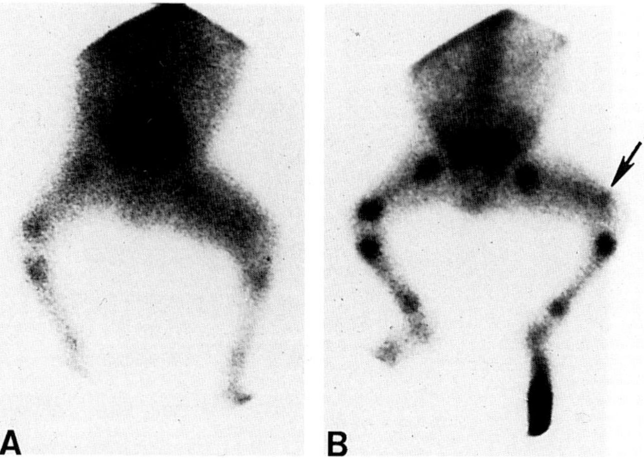

Fig. 82.4 Osteomyelitis. Studies in a neonate of 34 weeks' gestation, presenting with cellulitis of the left thigh. The blood pool phase (A) demonstrates diffuse accumulation in this thigh, which becomes less marked in the delayed scan (B). However, in the latter study, total absence of radionuclide uptake in the left distal femoral epiphysis was consistent with osteomyelitis, which was confirmed subsequently (Reproduced with permission from Murray.[37])

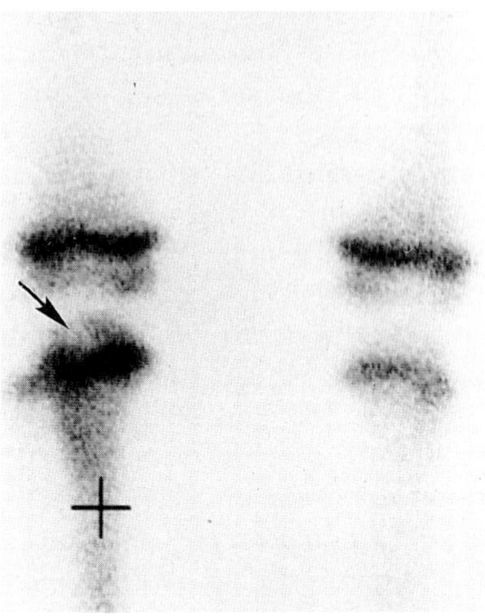

Fig. 82.5 Epiphyseal osteomyelitis.^{99m}Tc-MDP study from a 6-year-old male with staphylococcal osteomyelitis and septic arthritis. A 'cold' area (arrow) is clearly seen in the lateral aspect of the right upper tibial epiphysis. Diffusely increased periarticular and growth plate accumulation is also present in the right knee.

No difference in the scintigraphic appearances were noted in comparison with older children. The difference in experience might, in part, reflect improved instrumentation and the ability to separate abnormal foci from the intense globular growth plate of the neonate, particularly utilizing a pinhole collimator. They emphasized the incidence of diffuse multifocal osteomyelitis in the neonate, their studies demonstrating 10 additional unsuspected foci of infection. Such multifocal disease can create problems since symmetrical metaphyseal involvement can be difficult to recognize and total-body surveys are mandatory.

Childhood osteomyelitis As discussed earlier, few metaphyseal vessels penetrate the epiphysis in the childhood years. The physis forms a natural barrier to spread of infection from the metaphysis to the epiphysis, although rarely subacute infection of the epiphysis may occur as a primary event.[39] Purely epiphyseal lesions are uncommon, and are usually associated with a Brodie's abscess adjacent to the growth plate, with subsequent penetration across the growth plate into the epiphysis. These abnormalities may show either increased or decreased uptake (Fig. 82.5) depending upon the site and degree of vascular compromise resulting from increased tissue pressure.

In general, the epiphysis and joint are relatively protected from the ischaemic process resulting from infection of metaphyseal bone. While involvement of all bones has been reported, the most commonly involved are the femur and tibia[40] (Fig. 82.6). However, involvement of unusual sites of infection can lead to major difficulties in diagnosis. Haematogenous osteomyelitis of the pelvis in childhood is a good example (Fig. 82.7). The clinical manifestation may be quite diverse, presenting as disturbance of gait, pain on hip abduction or even abdominal pain as the sole symptom. It reinforces the necessity of obtaining a whole-body image capable of revealing unsuspected sites of pathology.

The usefulness and high sensitivity of the bone ^{99m}Tc phosphate bone scan in childhood osteomyelitis has been established in numerous studies. More recently the sensitivity for diagnosis has been reported at 96%[13] in a series of 116 cases of acute osteomyelitis. This included 23 patients with involvement of the pelvic bones. Just as importantly, another large series reported the negative predictive value at 93% and the positive predictive value at 90%.[12] Of the 280 patients in this series, bone scanning

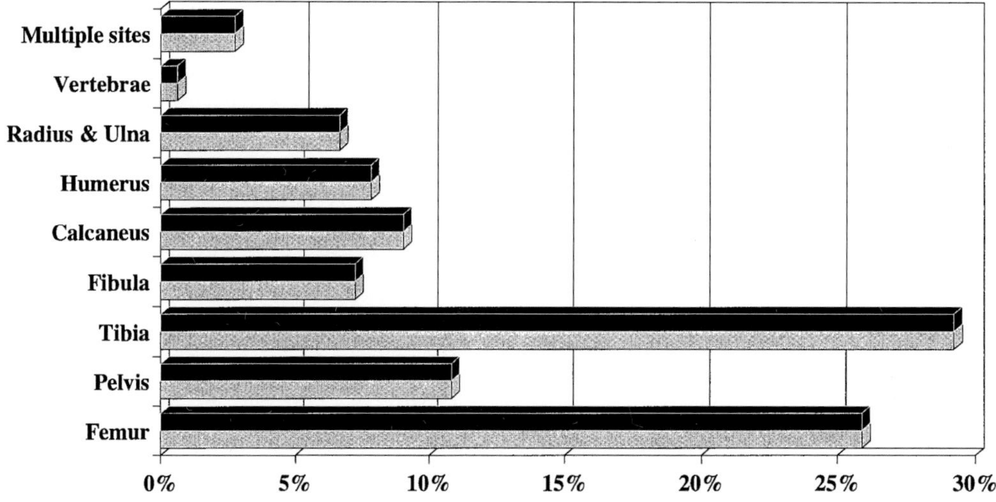

Fig. 82.6 Major sites of childhood osteomyelitis. (Data based on 391 patients from Craigen et al[1] and Scott et al.[13])

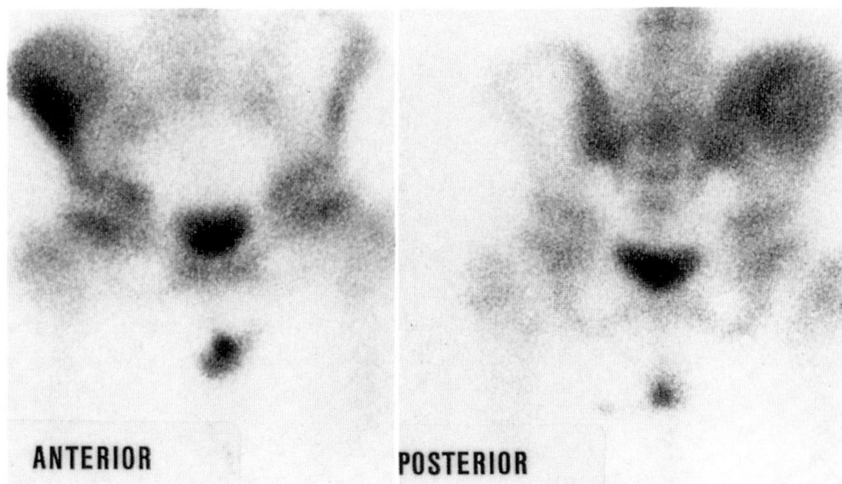

Fig. 82.7 Osteomyelitis of the ilium in an 11-year-old boy, characterized by diffuse increase in accumulation with a central area of relatively diminished uptake.

correctly identified 11 of 12 patients with osteomyelitis of the pelvic bones. It again highlights the value of bone scanning in the clinical differentiation of osteomyelitis from others disorders.

Multifocal osteomyelitis Multifocal osteomyelitis has largely been a problem in patients with predisposing conditions such as immunodeficiency, intravenous drug abusers, those receiving prolonged intravenous therapy and in neonates, particularly if premature.[2] Howman-Giles & Uren[41] reviewed their experience in a series of 136 infants and children with osteomyelitis and no predisposing conditions. 27 patients (19%) were found to have multifocal disease on bone scan. They found two peaks of disease, one in neonates (38% of cases) and the other in children aged 9–12 years (46% of cases). Even in the older age group, a high proportion of patients had non-specific complaints or presented with an acute septicaemic illness. Osteomyelitis was unsuspected on the basis of clinical information. These data suggest a surprisingly high proportion of cases of multifocal disease in comparison with the findings of the series of Scott et al[13] and Craigen et al,[1] who reported less than 5% of cases as being multifocal.

McCoy et al[32] also reported a group of patients with staphylococcal sepsis and multiple sites of increased uptake on bone scan that failed to progress after the institution of appropriate antibiotic therapy. Nade[3] has theorized that these were probably areas of aborted infection. The bone scan findings of multiple sites of clinically occult infection should be used as a guide for biopsying the most accessible lesion. Biopsy is essential in establishing the correct diagnosis as multifocal sites of increased accumulation on bone scan may also be due to metastatic malignant disease. It reflects the proclivity of metastases to lodge in the metaphyseal region, in common with haematogenous osteomyelitis.

Discitis of childhood. This is a clinical syndrome that occurs in childhood at a mean age of 6 years, presenting with back pain, refusal to walk, low-grade fever and a raised sedimentation rate. While clinically indistinguishable from pyogenic vertebral osteomyelitis, cultures are negative and the clinical course benign.[2] Scintigraphy reveals localization of activity in the involved disc space as well as in the adjacent vertebral end plates[43] (Fig. 82.8).

Adult haematogenous osteomyelitis While haematogenous osteomyelitis is relatively uncommon in the adult, there are various subgroups that are more susceptible to infection. Intravenous drug abusers have a high incidence of both haematogenous and traumatically implanted osteomyelitis. Haematogenous disease tends to localize in the vertebral column and pelvis,[2] while the directly implanted disease tends to be peripheral.[17] Osteomyelitis may also occur in severely immunosuppressed patients or complicate prolonged intravenous therapy or parenteral nutrition.[2] Hughes et al[43] has recently drawn attention to the poor recognition of bone and joint sepsis in 34 patients infected by the human immunodeficiency virus.

The more complex entities of osteomyelitis in the vertebral column and in the setting of neuropathic bone disease are considered in relation to the use of other scintigraphic agents for the detection of infection.

Other scintigraphic agents

As experience with the technetium phosphate complexes has continued to accumulate, it has become recognized that false-negative results can occur. This was highlighted by Sullivan et al,[14] leading to the acceptance that negative studies with the technetium phosphate complexes in patients with a high clinical suspicion of osteomyelitis

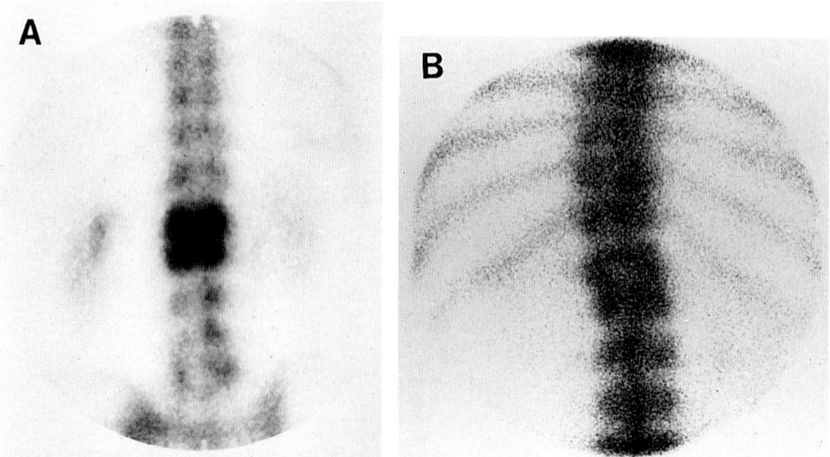

Fig. 82.8 Acute discitis. (A) Scan of the spine in a 10-year-old boy who presented with pain in the buttocks, identified as referred pain caused by discitis, characterized by intense accumulation in the neighbouring vertebrae. (Reproduced with permission from Murray.[37]) (B) Loss of joint space and anatomical deformity but uniform accumulation of the radiopharmaceutical indicative of healed discitis.

should undergo alternative scintigraphic investigations. The grouped results for all scintigraphic modalities are shown in Table 82.1.

^{67}Gallium Greatest attention has been paid to the use of gallium (^{67}Ga) in view of its known capacity to localize in areas of pus, supported by experimental evidence in animals. One of its unfortunate characteristics is the weak bone-scanning properties for which it was initially proposed as a primary bone-scanning agent. Although there has been some variability in the results and even some evidence that uptake can in part result from sterile reparative bone processes, most have concluded that ^{67}Ga is more sensitive in detecting osteomyelitis than technetium phosphates,[44] and that specific uptake occurs earlier.[45] This is in accord with many clinical observations. Direct comparative studies have been undertaken. Handmaker & Giammona[46] showed that both technetium and ^{67}Ga studies were positive at the same time in 8 of 17 children with acute osteomyelitis, while positive ^{67}Ga studies were identified in five in whom the technetium study was negative, although three later became positive. Lewin et al[47] showed that combined scintigraphy raised the sensitivity for detecting osteomyelitis from 0.65 with technetium phosphate alone to 1.00 with both procedures, although positive scans due to lesions other than osteomyelitis occurred. While it has been suggested that both agents be injected simultaneously in a routine fashion in suspected osteomyelitis, it is generally conceded that, because of greater cost and radiation burden, limited availability, as well as the extension of time before the study can be completed, ^{67}Ga should be reserved for those in whom there is a high clinical suspicion of disease not clearly defined by the standard bone scan.

Table 82.1 Comparison of various scintigraphic methods for the detection of osteomyelitis. (From Schauwecker[34].)

Method	Sensitivity (%)	Specificity (%)	No. of studies
^{99m}Tc phosphate			
Uncomplicated	94	95	6
Complicated	95	33	14
^{67}Ga	81	69	15
^{111}In chloride	92	81	2
^{111}In leucocytes	88	85	16
^{99m}Tc-HMPAO leucocytes	87	81	6
^{111}In polyclonal IgG	98	86	3

These supplementary investigations with alternative radionuclides may be of particular value in elucidating infection in various situations in which the standard skeletal scintigraphy may be equivocal, for example disc space infection in children which, although infrequent, usually presents considerable diagnostic difficulty. Gates[42] suggested that the appearances reported by him in four children may be unique to the disorder: marked narrowing of the intervertebral disc spaces with abnormal increased radionuclide uptake in the adjacent vertebral bodies in which accumulation is predominantly the location of the primary ossification centres in the pedicles. The changes may be vividly demonstrated with SPECT. However, while there have been reports in which SPECT was positive despite normal planar scans, the use of the pinhole views does identify the typical 'wafer' uptake in adjacent vertebral end plates, providing differentiation from vertebral osteomyelitis (Fig. 82.9). Atkinson et al[48] studied 19 children with suspected pathology involving

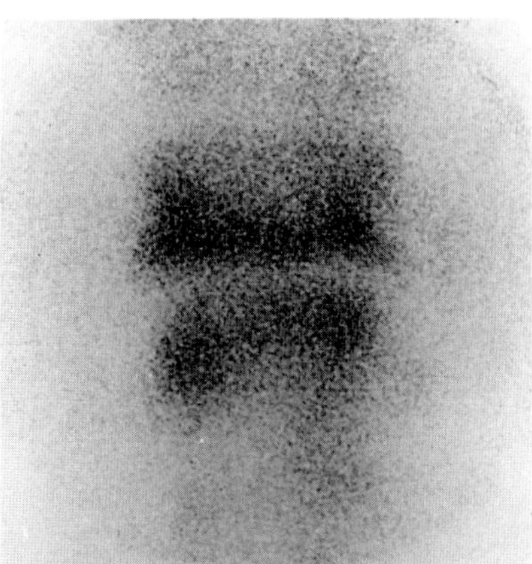

Fig. 82.9 Discitis. Characteristic 'wafer' accumulation in the borders of verebral bodies.

the vertebral column and found the radionuclide study to be abnormal in all 11 cases of discitis, osteomyelitis and two tumours. However, Wenger et al[49] pointed out that the changes can be equivocal and ^{67}Ga was indicated. Bruschwein et al[50] reviewed their experience in 100 patients in whom disc space infection was suspected. In 19 in whom infection was present, the ^{67}Ga scan was positive in 17, in three being the only localizing investigation. In five patients with pyogenic vertebral osteomyelitis reported by Haase et al,[51] all had positive phosphate and ^{67}Ga studies, but they comment, in particular, on the paravertebral uptake of ^{67}Ga, suggestive of soft-tissue abscess, giving the appearance of a 'butterfly', which they believe unique.

Considerable difficulty may be experienced using phosphate scintigraphy in assessing the presence of acute osteomyelitis in the diabetic foot in view of the not infrequent reparative changes of previous infection, concurrent cellulitis or degenerative arthritic change. Park et al[52] suggested that the three-phase study could be valuable if particular care was paid to the discrepancy between the vascular phases in terms of the degree and extent of hyperaemia and the persistence of focal uptake in the later static images. Thus, they identified 20 of 21 patients with acute osteomyelitis but did emphasize the difficulties related to the alternative disease. Alazraki et al,[25] assessing osteomyelitis in patients with diabetes and peripheral vascular disease, advocated the addition of the 24 h image, the 'four-phase study', and suggested that this permitted the correct diagnosis to be achieved in four more of the 21 studies, resulting in an accuracy of 85% as compared with 80% for three-phase scintigraphy. Nevertheless, it was of interest that, of six patients in whom ^{67}Ga scintigraphy was undertaken, this correctly identified infection in all patients, whereas phosphate scintigraphy was correct in only five. There is general support for the use of ^{67}Ga in unravelling the diagnostic problems with the diabetic foot. The differentiation of sepsis in soft tissue from that in bone and of recurrence of acute infection in bone which shows persistent phosphate abnormalities from diabetic osteoarthropathy poses a major challenge. The bone scan alterations resulting from the latter, to an extent reflecting sympathetic denervation, can be marked, showing increased concentration in all phases, although Park et al[52] suggested that initial hyperaemia was less common. Eymontt et al[53] noted that there was usually a combination of diffuse and focal uptake, reflecting hyperaemia and new bone formation. The latter is probably responsible for the slight increase in ^{67}Ga accumulation which may be seen. The assessment of the ^{67}Ga study can be difficult and involves comparison of both the distribution and intensity of uptake of this radionuclide with that of the preceding technetium phosphate. Lack of anatomical congruence as well as of avidity is important: the more intense and focal ^{67}Ga concentration, the more likely is bone infection (Fig. 82.10). Views in multiple projections are usually essential to achieve this comparison. As the discrepancies in the studies may be subtle, it is particularly important to undertake the investigations prior to the introduction of antibiotic therapy, which may rapidly ameliorate the degree of ^{67}Ga accumulation. Nevertheless, it may be virtually impossible to differentiate infection from neurogenic arthropathy, in which there may be not only marked technetium uptake but also intense accumulation of ^{67}Ga. Sayle et al[54] recommended the use of ^{111}In chloride as a means to overcome the difficulties which may be encountered in differentiating cellulitis from osteomyelitis because of the tendency for bone scintigraphy to overestimate the extent of the disease.

Differentiation of osteomyelitis from bone infarction depends considerably on the timing of the study. In the early stages of fulminant infection there may be a large photopenic area. Typically, however, the hyperaemia and focal uptake will be demonstrated within 2 days. In contrast, after bone infarction, the 2 day scan will usually either be normal or permit delineation of a photopenic

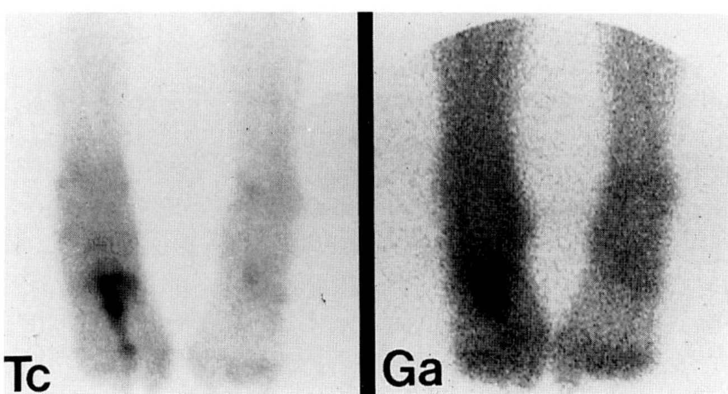

Fig. 82.10 Osteomyelitis. Study from a patient with diabetic neuropathy in the lower limbs and an ulcer in the sole of the right foot. ^{99m}Tc-MDP scan shows intense accumulation in the middle toe of the right foot. The corresponding ^{67}Ga study demonstrates intense accumulation at the same site and extension into the adjacent soft tissues.

area. Lutzker & Alavi[55] found such areas in 9 of 12 patients with sickle cell anaemia studied within 12 days of the onset of symptoms. However, Gelfand & Harcke[56] found focal increase in 10 of 34 sites of infarction in 30 patients, indistinguishable from osteomyelitis. Later, during the revascularization phase, 'pinhole' views may permit visualization of the pattern of peripheral 'stripes' characterizing revascularization from the periosteum. This clinical problem was thoroughly investigated by Amundsen et al[57] with combined technetium and ^{67}Ga scintigraphy in 18 patients. They concluded that neither investigation by itself could reliably differentiate osteomyelitis from infarction but that the combined studies correctly identified focal infection in all four instances.

Schauwecker's[34] review of the 15 major series considering ^{67}Ga and/or the ^{99m}Tc phosphate bone scan for the detection of osteomyelitis found an overall sensitivity of 81% (209 of 257 cases) and a specificity of 69% (188 of 272 cases). Bone remodelling from any other cause clearly appeared to affect the specificity, particularly in the case of neuropathic change.

^{111}In chloride. ^{111}In chloride falls within the same group of the periodic table as ^{67}Ga and possesses similar biological behaviour. It binds to transferrin and localizes at sites of infection by the same mechanisms as ^{67}Ga, with the exception of its weak bone-scanning properties. Few reports have been published in regard to its usefulness in acute osteomyelitis. It has been evaluated in prosthetic joint infection and chronic osteomyelitis.[54]

Labelled leucocytes. The major current controversy relates to the possible advantages of labelled leucocytes over ^{67}Ga, particularly in acute osteomyelitis. Experimental studies in rabbits have indicated earlier positive accumulation at sites of infection using ^{111}In oxine-labelled white cells than ^{99m}Tc-MDP.[58] Clinical experience has tended to uphold this view, but many authors, for example Ehrlich et al,[59] have experienced a significant incidence of false positives.

The superiority of labelled leucocytes resides in the ability to detect infection at sites of bone remodelling. Studies in the setting of infection at sites of bony non-union complicating fracture illustrate this advantage. Seabold et al[60] and Esterhai et al[61] utilizing ^{111}In-labelled leucocytes demonstrated a sensitivity of 84% and 100% and a specificity of 97% and 100% respectively. Maurer et al[62] also reported high sensitivity and specificity in a small group of patients with neuropathic joint disease, but experienced difficulty separating bone and soft-tissue infection. Schauwecker et al[63] were able to demonstrate good delineation of bone from soft-tissue infection by addition of the ^{99m}Tc phosphate bone scan to the leucocyte study, achieving an accuracy of 89% (Fig. 82.11).

Vertebral osteomyelitis poses problems when imaged with ^{111}In-labelled leucocytes. Several authors (e.g. Rüther et al[64]) have reported low sensitivities for the diagnosis. A 'cold' defect has been reported in up to 40% of cases.[65] The reason for reduced accumulation at sites of vertebral infection may be related to chronicity or prior antibiotic therapy. Palestro et al[66] found that the addition of a ^{99m}Tc sulphur colloid bone marrow scan to the leucocyte study led to good improvements in sensitivity and accuracy in 22 of 73 patients with skeletal infection.

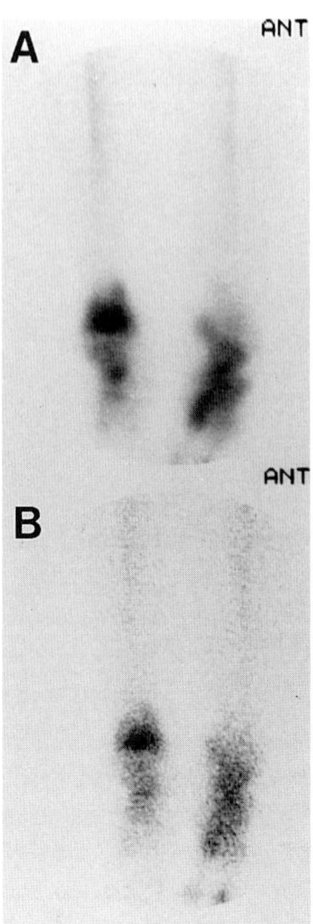

Fig. 82.11 Osteomyelitis. Study in a patient with diabetic osteoarthropathy and suspected osteomyelitis of the right lower tibia. The ^{99m}Tc-MDP study illustrates intense uptake at the distal end of the right tibia as well as other sites of intense accumulation in both feet. The corresponding ^{111}In leucocyte study demonstrates intense preferential uptake in the distal end of the right tibia only, subsequently proven to be the result of osteomyelitis. Only minimal increase in uptake is seen at the other sites of increased accumulation present in the bone scan.

Disadvantages of ^{111}In leucocyte labelling have been listed by a number of workers. The radionuclide is cyclotron produced and costly, and the procedure of cell labelling may take up to 2.5 h if predominantly pure granulocytes are labelled. Unfavourable dosimetry precludes its safe use in children in view of prolonged retention in the spleen and bone marrow. Furthermore, false-positive studies for infection have been found in the setting of recent fractures and metastatic carcinoma.[67] The degree of uptake may, however, be significantly less than in the setting of infection.[34]

Because of the limitations associated with ^{111}In use, several methods of labelling leucocytes with ^{99m}Tc have been attempted. Most experience amongst the alternative agents has been with ^{99m}Tc hexamethylpropyleneamine oxime (HMPAO). The major advantages are the widespread availability in kit form, ability to administer a larger dose with a reduced radiation burden and performance of SPECT imaging. These clear-cut advantages should lead to greater sensitivity of the technique. Schauwecker[34] found the sensitivity to be 87% and the specificity 81% in six published trials. Lantto et al[68] showed the agent to be more accurate at localization of lesions than ^{99m}Tc phosphate scanning, and more specific in detecting infection at sites of pre-existing disease.

The efficacy of ^{99m}Tc tin colloid labelling of leucocytes by phagocytic engulfment remains to be established. It has the promise of ease and speed of labelling and the convenience of production in a kit form.

Immunoglobulins. ^{111}In-labelled immunoglobulins have been studied in various clinical settings and are thought to be accumulated in inflammatory tissue by binding of the Fc portion of the IgG molecule.[69] Polyclonal IgG is labelled with ^{111}In and injected intravenously followed by imaging at 24–48 h. The labelling process takes approximately 10 min and yields a high labelling efficiency (> 97%). Oyen et al[70] have shown equal sensitivity compared with ^{111}In-labelled leucocytes, but higher degrees of lesional uptake, in 16 patients with low-grade osteomyelitis. This may be related to more rapid blood clearance and favourable biodistribution, allowing four times as much activity to be injected. Sites of fracture and prosthetic joint loosening displayed no preferential accumulation. The same group found a sensitivity of 86% and a specificity of 84% for the detection of osteomyelitis in 16 diabetic patients investigated for osteomyelitis complicating neuropathic foot disease.[71]

Labelled antibodies. Technically, the antibodies are directed against antigens present on granulocytes and therefore should have similar sensitivities to labelled leucocytes. However, as these are mouse antibodies, the human anti-mouse antibody (HAMA) response remains a distinct limitation to repeated use. Labelling with either ^{99m}Tc or ^{123}I takes approximately 10–20 min and yields over 95% labelling efficiency. Patients are studied at 4–6 h after injection. Hotze et al[72] studied 30 patients with suspected peripheral or vertebral osteomyelitis. In this unselected patient population, the sensitivity for peripheral osteomyelitis was found to be 89% and the specificity 63%. In vertebral osteomyelitis, the sensitivity was 57% and the specificity 75%. While the agent was shown to be useful in peripheral osteomyelitis, Sciuk et al[73] described eight patients with vertebral osteomyelitis in whom the abnormality was 'cold'. This was thought to be nonspecific for infection.

Seybold et al[74] studied two antibodies labelled with either ^{123}I or ^{99m}Tc in 70 patients with acute or chronic osteomyelitis. Sensitivity was reported at 97%, specificity at 92% and accuracy 95% with a positive predictive value of 95%. This group, however, performed SPECT imaging wherever appropriate. Unfortunately, the number of cases of axial infection was not reported.

The mixed nature of these two reports clearly indicates the need for further study, especially in unselected groups of patients with both axial and appendicular infection. Seybold et al[74] conclude that despite the advantages of the agents, the method should be restricted to situations in which other modalities have failed.

^{99m}Tc-labelled nanocolloid. This agent is formed by the attachment of ^{99m}Tc to a 30-nm-diameter particle of human serum albumin and is thought to diffuse into areas of increased capillary permeability. Rapid blood clearance allows good contrast and permits imaging within 4 h. It has been shown to be superior to ^{67}Ga in 39 patients with suspected bone and joint infections[75] and as sensitive as labelled leucocytes for the detection of peripheral osteomyelitis.[76] However, in a limited series, it too lacked sensitivity for the detection of vertebral osteomyelitis.[64]

Other modalities

Although the bone changes associated with osteomyelitis may take 10–14 days to become apparent on plain radiography,[9] the soft-tissue abnormalities may imply the diagnosis earlier.[77] Plain radiography of the suspected site is therefore clearly mandatory as it may indicate precise siting and demonstrate suspected or coexistent abnormalities.

Computerized tomography (CT) has been used for cortical imaging in the past but has largely been replaced by magnetic resonance imaging (MRI). Schauwecker[34] reviewed 11 series and found an overall sensitivity of 95% and specificity of 88%. The problem remains specificity, as any cause of marrow disease may masquerade as osteomyelitis, even when due to trauma or tumour.[78] In a study of ^{99m}Tc phosphate imaging, both MRI and CT were shown to have similar sensitivities for the detection of osteomyelitis, with MRI being the most specific. It provided precise spatial resolution and indicated the extent of soft-tissue involvement more accurately in 22 patients.[79]

Ultrasound has also shown some potential in the diagnosis of early osteomyelitis. It relies on the presence of subperiosteal fluid adjacent to bone as the bone itself remains impenetrable. Abiri et al[80] studied 48 patients prospectively and demonstrated osteomyelitis in 10 of 12 patients subsequently proven to have osteomyelitis. A role for ultrasound has yet to be established in larger series as the problems of local skin disease and pain may preclude adequate imaging.

Septic arthritis

In children, in particular, the painful hip is a common problem in which skeletal scintigraphy has a major role to

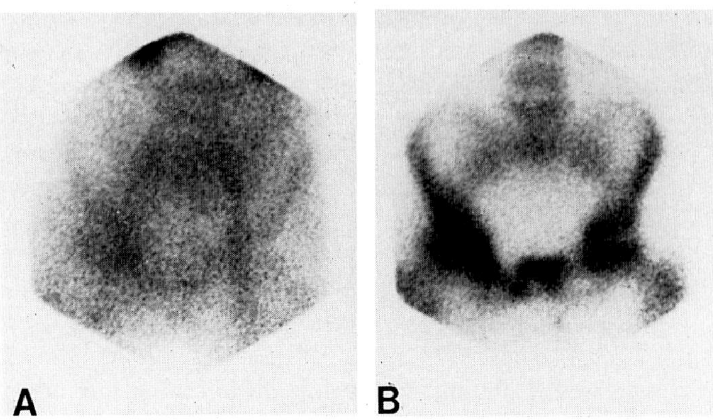

Fig. 82.12 Septic arthritis in the right hip of a 13-year-old boy. The blood pool study (A) shows diffuse hyperaemia in the right hip joint. In the delayed views (B), the accumulation is even more intense, but remains diffuse. (Reproduced with permission from Murray.[31])

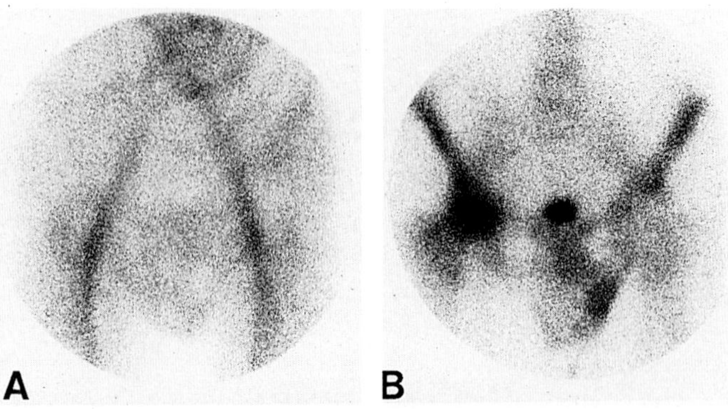

Fig. 82.13 Synovitis of the right hip demonstrated as asymmetrical and localized accumulation in the standard delayed images (B) without significant hyperaemia in the preceding blood pool study (A).

play. The consequences of septic arthritis are such that the diagnosis must be reached urgently in order to permit early intervention. Characteristic changes may be encountered: marked hyperaemia and local concentration in the dynamic and 'blood pool' phases and increased juxta-articular accumulation in the delayed images (Fig. 82.12). Comparison with the contralateral asymptomatic joint is essential, either by visualization of both in the spot views or by performing the study on each side with the same preset time rather than preset counts. Depending on the patient's size, pinhole views may be extremely valuable, by improving delineation, especially of the hip joint, and can be rewarding. Many investigators have found that it has a particular role in the evaluation of the painful hip. While the study can be entirely normal in transient synovitis, increased uptake can occur in the static images albeit less intense than in septic arthritis[81] (Figs 82.13 and 82.14). However, there is rarely similar hyperaemia in the initial phases.

Some investigators have indicated that the bone scan is a relatively insensitive and non-specific investigation in the diagnosis of septic arthritis[46] requiring the use of ^{67}Ga to increase sensitivity to above 50%. This, however, discounts two important prognostic variables that may be gleaned from the bone scan, especially in the hip, where the consequences of infection can be devastating. The early and delayed phases sometimes demonstrate photopenia corresponding to the femoral head, indicating tamponade of the retinacular vessels by a tense joint effusion and requiring urgent decompression to prevent avascular necrosis (Fig. 82.15). The importance of identifying joint effusions has been emphasized by Kloiber et al,[82] who noted an area of diminished delivery in the blood pool images in 10 of 38 children with hip pain of recent onset, eight of whom had joint aspirations confirming the presence of an effusion. In the later images, nine had reduced uptake involving the entire proximal femoral ossification centre. Such findings confirm the critical importance of the early diagnosis of septic arthritis since, of the three in whom the complete absence of femoral head activity resulted from septic arthritis, follow-up studies showed no

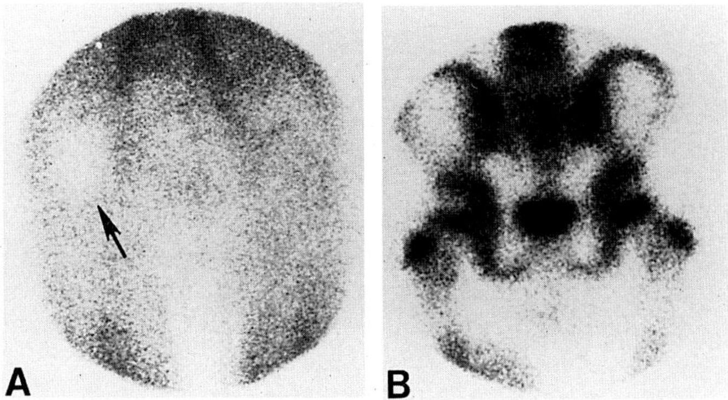

Fig. 82.14 Joint effusions. (A) Evidence of an intra-articular effusion in the right hip is provided by an area of absent accumulation in the blood pool phase, although, owing to transient synovitis, no asymmetry of accumulation is evident in the later statis views (B).

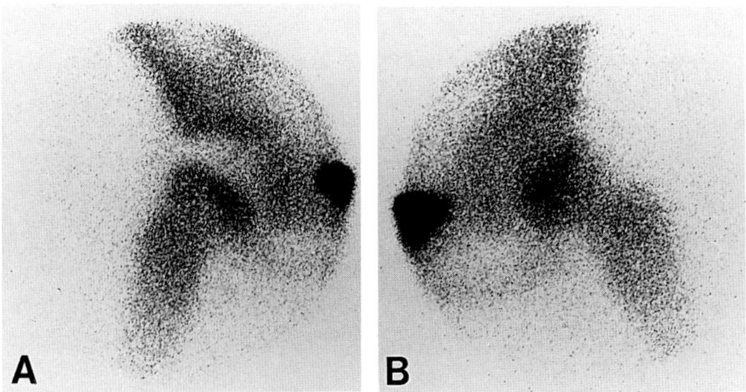

Fig. 82.15 Leukaemia. Delayed views, with pinhole collimation, of the hips in a 10-year-old boy show diminished accumulation in the right hip (A), the result of a sterile joint effusion compared to the normal left hip (B).

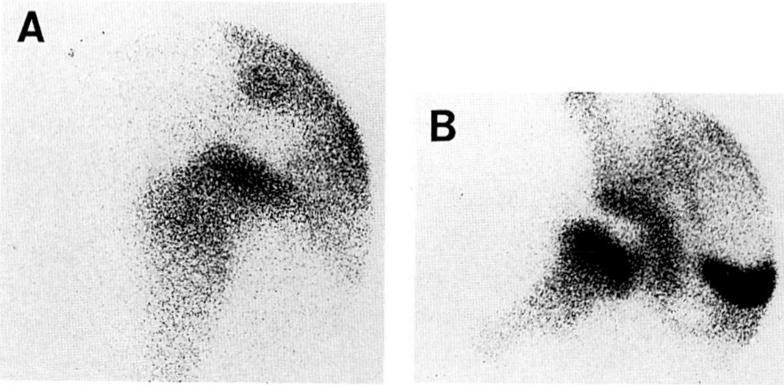

Fig. 82.16 Septic arthritis. Views of the hip in a 1½-year-old boy who had been receiving antibiotic therapy for a *Haemophilus* infection for 3 weeks, demonstrating total absence of uptake throughout the right femoral head due to secondary ischaemia (A). A further study 1 year later (B) demonstrates continuing absence of revascularization of the proximal femoral epiphysis with distortion of the bony outline and the epiphyseal plate. (Reproduced with permission from Murray.[37])

improvement in one child, infarction later being proved (Fig. 82.16). Even with early surgery these patients have a worse prognosis as demonstrated in long-term follow-up.[83] It was found that 22% of 55 children with a 'cold hip' had septic arthritis confirmed at surgery. Six of the 55 children in this group had detrimental effects in the involved hip at 3 months after the infection.

The mechanism and consequences of such findings may be understood in terms of the special anatomy of the hip joint, as discussed. Animal studies have confirmed that maintenance of intra-articular pressure at 50 mmHg for 12 h can lead to infarction of the femoral head.[84] While arthrocentesis has no effect on the scan finding in septic arthritis,[85] arthrography with volumes of contrast agent under 6 ml can lead to transient femoral head ischaemia with no long-term sequelae.[86] This was reflected by a reduction in uptake of ^{99m}Tc phosphate in the femoral head, with later return of activity to normal.

The presence of coexistent osteomyelitis in the neck of the femur has been shown to be a poor prognostic variable. Bennett & Namnyak[87] described eight cases amongst 43 patients with septic arthritis, of whom seven demonstrated long-term morbidity. Howie et al,[12] for example, identified the presence of focal osteomyelitis in the femoral neck in four of eight patients with septic arthritis of the hip, but did not include details of long-term follow-up.

Septic sacroiliitis can cause particular difficulty in diagnosis. Experience with bone scintigraphy has varied but, as emphasized by Kumar & Balachandran,[88] unilateral disease is best appreciated in the anterior pelvic view. Skeletal scintigraphy was the most contributory in five patients reported by Horgan et al,[89] who found the blood pool images to be of particular value although noting the ^{67}Ga scans were also useful (Fig. 82.17).

Such observations indicate that the major role of skeletal scintigraphy in suspected septic arthritis is not merely to provide confirmation by showing a characteristic pattern, but to identify vascular compromise and associated osteomyelitis and the need to aspirate bone as well as the joint. The urgency is such that, if the clinical suspicion is sufficiently high despite a negative study, aspiration is preferable to waiting for a ^{67}Ga study. There is no doubt that supplementary ^{67}Ga scintigraphy improves the overall diagnostic accuracy. Rosenthall et al[90] have shown that a combined study does raise the sensitivity for the detection of septic arthritis from 54% with ^{99m}Tc-MDP alone to 84%. While both studies are often indicated when the clinical problem is less acute and the suspicion less high, the complementary investigations may be of more practical value in the adult, particularly when infection is suspected in a joint with pre-existing disease, e.g. rheumatoid arthritis, in which abnormal bone images would be expected.

Chronic infection

Chronic osteomyelitis is a rare phenomenon as a complication of cases of acute infection where no predisposing cause is apparent. Most recent series have found a progression rate of approximately 4% of cases to chronic osteomyelitis.[1] The reasons for this low prevalence are many, the advances in antibiotics and early surgical intervention being the most

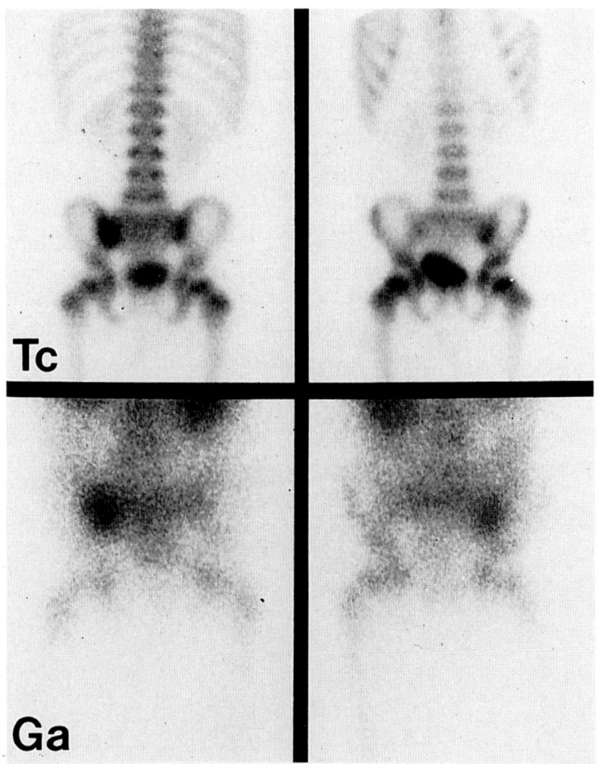

Fig. 82.17 Septic sacroiliitis. ^{99m}Tc-MDP study illustrates increased accumulation in the left sacroiliac joint. The corresponding ^{67}Ga study also shows intense uptake in the septic left sacroiliac joint.

important. Chronic sepsis of bone is a more common problem in the setting of immunosuppression, systemic illness, compound trauma, post-operatively or as a complication of chronic sepsis in an adjacent non-osseous structure. It may also prove to be a devastating complication in association with the insertion of orthopaedic devices such as prosthetic joints, a specialized area of imaging which is addressed in the next chapter.

Chronic osteomyelitis is not a single entity but encompasses a spectrum of disease that is defined in terms of the immunological status of the host, pre-existing bone disease and the nature of the infecting organism (e.g. bacterial *vs.* fungal). The nature of these interactions will determine the sites of involvement and will clearly dictate the path of scintigraphic imaging. A number of chronic infective and non-infective disease processes have been described which display features that make them readily identifiable or may lead to diagnostic confusion.

Technetium phosphate scanning

Chronic recurrent multifocal osteomyelitis. This is a rare form of osteomyelitis of unknown aetiology that occurs between the ages of 19 months and 27 years (Fig. 82.18). No infective organism has been identified. Lesions are usually present in the metaphyses, with a proclivity for the tibia and femur, and may be symmetrical, leading to diagnostic confusion with metastatic disease. Other sites that may be involved are the clavicle, fibula, short bones and the axial skeleton. Biopsy demonstrates the features of non-specific osteomyelitis. Treatment with antibiotics does not alter the course, although approximately 25% of patients will have an elevated anti-streptolysin O titre. A further association with pustulosis palmoplantaris has been noted in 25% of cases.

Malignant external otitis. This is a potentially fatal infection that spreads from soft tissues into the cranial structures in diabetic and immunosuppressed patients. The common causative organisms are *Pseudomonas aeruginosa* and more rarely, *Proteus*, *Klebsiella* and *Staphylococcus* species. Bone scanning is sensitive and careful imaging, especially with SPECT, can reveal the true extent of disease and demonstrate spread to the apex of the petrous temporal bone and base of skull (Fig. 82.19). If scintigraphy is utilized to assess therapy, then the power of bone scanning is diminished by ongoing accumulation at the site of repair and ^{67}Ga or an alternative agent such as nanocolloid[91] will need to be considered. Imaging with ^{67}Ga may also be a problem because of physiological uptake in the parotid gland, a potential source of confusion owing to its proximity to the mastoid bone.

Granulomatous osteomyelitis. Tuberculosis is the most common cause of granulomatous osteomyelitis, particularly because of the increasing prevalence of the disease in patients infected by the human immunodeficiency virus. Other causes are brucellosis,[92] coccidiomycosis and blastomycosis, in all of which bone scintigraphy has proven valuable. A common feature in this group of infections is the presence of multiple sites of involvement, varying from 30% to 50%. The vertebrae are a common site of involvement, and diagnostic confusion with malignant disease may arise when multifocal involvement is present (Fig. 82.20). In the recent past, the incidence of skeletal tuberculosis has been affected by the proportion of African and Asian migrants in the community. Skeletal involvement has been reported in 3% of patients with tuberculosis in the USA.[93] The most frequent and severe form of osseous involvement is tuberculous spondylitis,[94] with sacroiliac involvement being reported in 10% of cases.[93] The bone scan may demonstrate focal non-specific increase in accumulation at the site of infection or, more rarely, diffuse increase in accumulation which is indistinguishable from metastatic disease.[95]

El-Desouki[92] reported a series of 214 patients with brucellosis and musculoskeletal symptoms. Bone scanning revealed abnormal uptake at 319 sites in 196 patients, 47.7% having multifocal involvement. Plain radiography identified abnormalities in 52 of 214 patients. The lumbar spine and sacroiliac joint were the two most commonly affected areas.

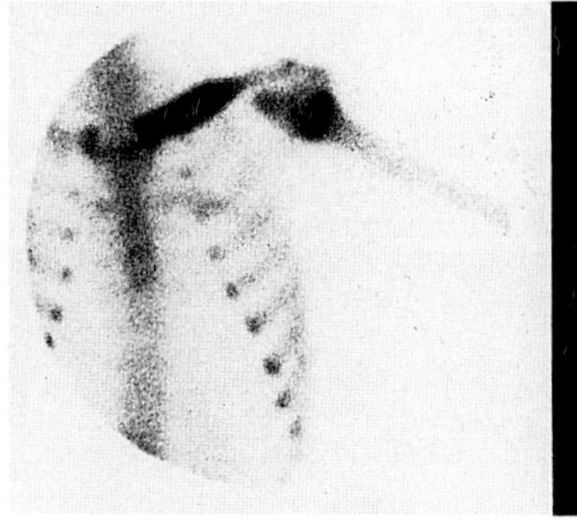
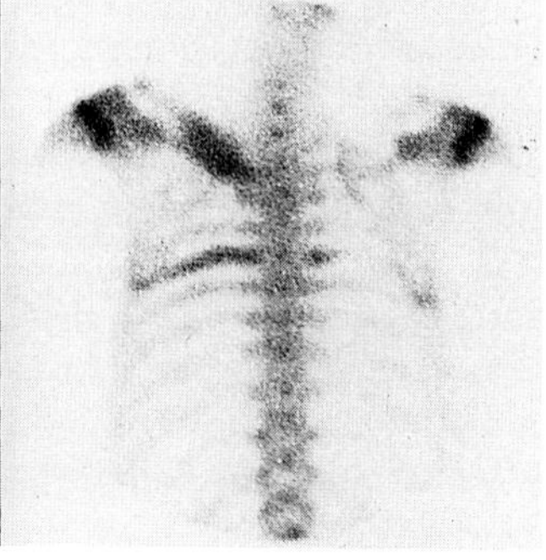

Fig. 82.18 Chronic recurrent multifocal osteomyelitis. ^{99m}Tc-MDP study demonstrating typical intense avidity in the affected clavicle and ribs.

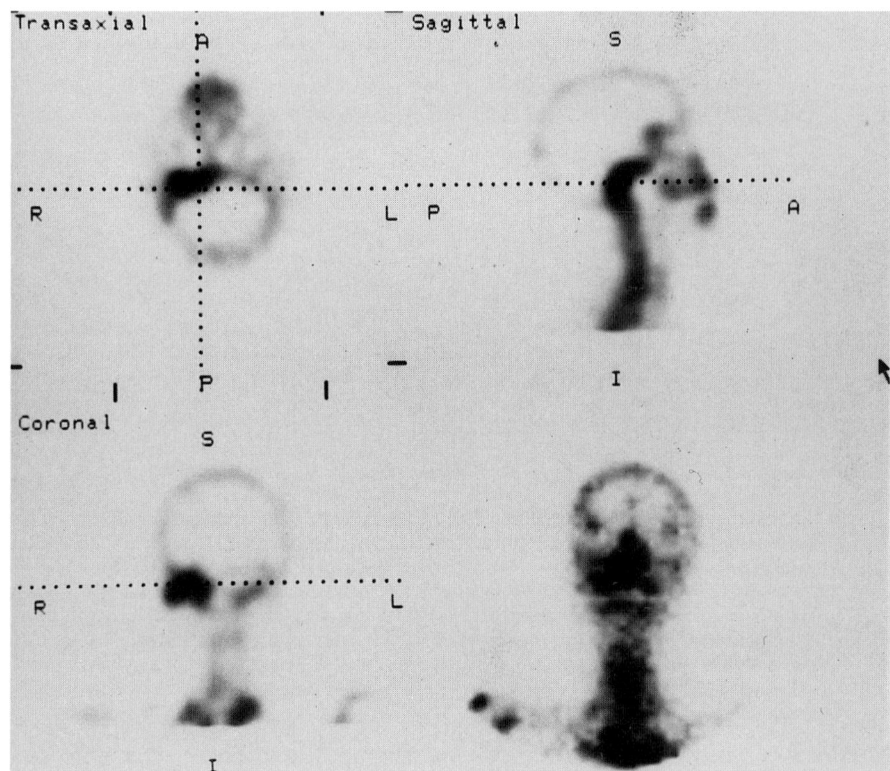

Fig. 82.19 Malignant external otitis. ^{99m}Tc-MDP SPECT study demonstrating intense accumulation extending from the right mastoid region to the apex of the petrous temporal bone. The patient had poorly controlled insulin-dependent diabetes mellitus. Biopsy revealed *Pseudomonas aeruginosa* infection.

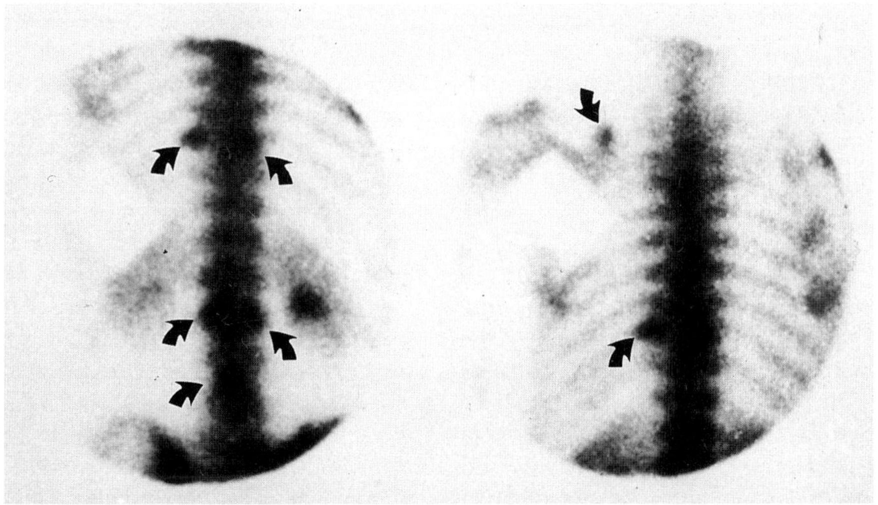

Fig. 82.20 Coccidiomycosis. Numerous small but intense foci reveal the disseminated nature of the infection.

Fungal osteomyelitis Infection with *Candida, Aspergillus* and *Rhizopus* species is also becoming more common in severe primary immunosuppressive states or following therapy of malignant disease or organ transplantation. These abnormalities may also be multifocal and do not possess any specific features. Biopsy is necessary for the diagnosis and the bone scan may be crucial in determining the most accessible site.

The problems that beset ^{99m}Tc phosphate scintigraphy relate to its specificity, as the sensitivity of the technique

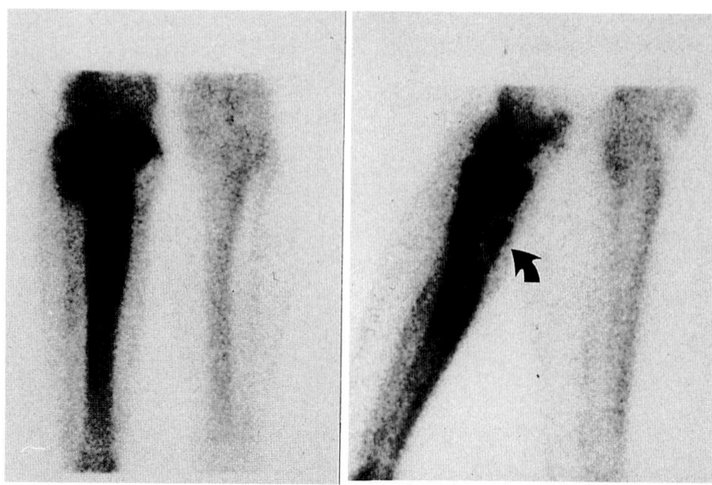

Fig. 82.21 Chronic osteomyelitis. ^{99m}Tc-MDP study in a patient who suffered a compound fracture of the right tibia requiring multiple operative procedures and instrumentation which precluded the use of CT or MRI. The scan demonstrates intense accumulation in a distorted and thickened right tibia with a 'cold' defect in its anterior surface with faintly increased accumulation in the central aspect. At surgery, this proved to be chronic sclerosing osteomyelitis with a sequestrum at the site of the 'cold' defect.

approaches 100%. It reflects the mechanism of accumulation, with preferential localization at sites of osteoblastic activity, making the separation of infection from the reparative process difficult. The vascular integrity of tissue can be easily conveyed, and instrumentation which can interfere with radiological and magnetic resonance imaging poses no major problems (Fig. 82.21). Suspicion of infection may be heightened by incongruent hyperaemia in the angiographic and blood pool phases, relative to the stage of the healing process. Its utility is in confirming a pathological process in bone as opposed to soft tissue, and therefore in its high negative predictive value.

Other scintigraphic techniques

^{67}Ga. While ^{67}Ga localizes at sites of infection by a number of mechanisms, it also possesses weak bone-scanning properties. Problems of specificity that affect the ^{99m}Tc phosphate agents will therefore also apply in cases of chronic infection. This problem has been addressed by comparison of the intensity of ^{67}Ga accumulation with that of the ^{99m}Tc phosphate agents. A high sensitivity and specificity may be obtained when the intensity of ^{67}Ga accumulation exceeds that in the bone scan. Al-Sheikh et al[96] reported a sensitivity of 80% and a specificity of 83% in 21 patients. In sharp contrast, Seabold et al[60] found a sensitivity of 22% and a specificity of 100% in 49 patients with suspected infection at sites of fracture non-union. They found a significant number of false-negative studies in patients in whom the intensity of accumulation was equal in the two studies, a criterion that Tumeh et al[97] had earlier reported as being associated with a low prevalence of disease. The major technical difference between the two studies was that the latter group undertook the ^{67}Ga study at 24 h following injection, rather than 48 h. The marked difference between such results in many ways highlights the overall problems that plague ^{67}Ga scanning from both a technical standpoint and in the subjective nature of the reporting process.

^{111}In chloride. There is a limited body of literature that considers the role of ^{111}In chloride in the detection of chronic osteomyelitis. In contrast to ^{67}Ga, it has no bone-scanning properties and in the main contribution from Sayle et al[54] did not demonstrate accumulation at sites of non-healing fractures of 3–8 months' duration. Images obtained at 48–72 h detected 54 true positives, seven true negatives, four false positives and three false negatives for an overall sensitivity of 95% and specificity of 64%. The low specificity may well have been due to the small number of 'normals' studied. In comparison, the results of the bone scan in 46 patients led to a specificity of 20%.

Labelled leucocytes. The main cellular infiltrate at the site of chronic osseous sepsis is composed of lymphocytes and mononuclear cells, with a paucity of polymorphonuclear cells. Nevertheless, many series attest to the success of labelled leucocyte scintigraphy in the diagnosis of chronic infection. Part of the explanation may be that the labelling process also non-specifically labels lymphocytes. Early experience reported that infection of greater than 6 weeks' duration did not demonstrate significant ^{111}In leucocyte accumulation, whereas labelled lymphocytes were positive. Several groups have since found better results, reporting a sensitivity of approximately 86% and a specificity of approximately 84% for ^{111}In-labelled leucocytes. Rüther et al[64] demonstrated a sensitivity of approximately 90% and a specificity of 57% utilizing ^{99m}Tc-HMPAO-labelled leucocytes. The low specificity was due to accumulation at the sites of fracture or surgery. Experience with the detection of chronic vertebral infection has been problematic in all series, as with the acute situation, with sensitivities of approximately 50–60%. Few data are currently available about the role of ^{99m}Tc tin colloid-labelled leucocytes in the detection of chronic infection.

Other agents. Small numbers of patients with chronic osteomyelitis have been studied with a variety of other scintigraphic agents. None of these series has been large enough to influence the major role of bone, ^{67}Ga and labelled leucocyte scintigraphy. Sciuk et al[73] compared ^{99m}Tc-labelled human immunoglobulin with ^{99m}Tc-labelled anti-granulocyte antibodies in 25 patients with chronic osteomyelitis. For peripheral disease the sensitivity of the techniques was 83% and 100% respectively, while specificity was 100% for both. Axial infection was problematic, with none of the sites being detected by the monoclonal antibody and a sensitivity of only 63% for human immunoglobulin. This is in agreement with Rüther et al,[64] who found a sensitivity of 95% for the same antibody at peripheral sites, with poor axial sensitivity. Their group also studied the efficacy of ^{99m}Tc-labelled nanocolloid, finding a high sensitivity (95%) for peripheral disease, and again, poor sensitivity at axial sites. Other antibodies have also been successfully used in chronic infection,[74] but the small patient numbers and the expense of the technique have prevented widespread acceptance.

The addition of ^{99m}Tc sulphur colloid imaging can significantly enhance the utility of labelled leucocyte scanning. Palestro et al[65] demonstrated in 73 patients that incongruity of distribution of the two agents accurately reflects the presence of infection in more complicated cases. Sites of infection stimulate uptake of labelled leucocytes, and by the same mechanism will displace or infarct normal marrow elements, leading to reduced accumulation of the marrow scanning agent. The addition of marrow scanning led to improvement in the sensitivity of labelled leucocyte scanning from 86% to 100% and specificity from 12% to 94%.

CONCLUSION

In spite of the complex array of scintigraphic techniques that are available for the detection of infection, the bone scan remains the first line of investigation after plain radiography. It is only when infection is superimposed at sites of pre-existing bone disease or the question of recurrent or persistent infection arises that other scintigraphic techniques or modalities should be considered. This decision should be based on considerations of radiation exposure, cost, availability and utility. The current body of evidence suggests that ^{67}Ga imaging should be supplanted by labelled leucocytes as the second scintigraphic technique after bone scanning. Preferably, the radionuclide used for labelling should be ^{99m}Tc rather than ^{111}In because of the radiation burden and cost involved. Bone scanning remains necessary for spatial localization and its high negative predictive value, which can render other forms of imaging unnecessary. There may well be a limited role for other scintigraphic techniques under special circumstances which require more rigorous definition.

REFERENCES

1. Craigen M A C, Watters J, Hackett J S 1992 The changing epidemiology of osteomyelitis in children. J Bone Joint Surg 74-B: 541–545
2. Waldvogel F A, Vasey H 1980 Osteomyelitis: the past decade. N Engl J Med 303: 360–370
3. Nade S 1983. Acute haematogenous osteomyelitis in infancy and childhood. J Bone Joint Surg 65B: 109–119
4. Trueta J 1959 The three types of acute haematogenous osteomyelitis. J Bone Joint Surg 41B: 671–680
5. Trueta J 1957 The normal vascular anatomy of the human femoral head during growth. J Bone Joint Surg 39B: 358–394
6. Adeyokunnu A A, Hendrickse R G 1980 Salmonella osteomyelitis in childhood: a report of 63 cases seen in Nigerian children of whom 57 had sickle cell anaemia. Arch Dis Childh 55: 953–957
7. Cotran R S, Kumar V, Robbins S L 1989 The musculoskeletal system. In: Cotran R S, Kumar V, Robbins S (eds) Robbins pathologic basis of disease, 4th edn. W B Saunders, Philadelphia, pp 1315–1371
8. Shim S S 1968 Physiology of blood circulation of bone. J Bone Joint Surg 50A: 812–817
9. Handmaker H, Leonards R 1976 The bone scan in inflammatory osseous disease. Semin Nucl Med 6: 95–105
10. Gilday D L, Paul D J, Paterson J 1975 Diagnosis of osteomyelitis in children by combined blood pool and bone imaging. Radiology 117: 331–335
11. Majd M, Frankel R S 1976 Radionuclide imaging in skeletal inflammatory and ischaemic disease in children. AJR 126: 832–841
12. Howie D W, Savage J P, Wilson T G, Paterson D 1983 The technetium phosphate bone scan in the diagnosis of osteomyelitis in childhood. J Bone Joint Surg 65A: 431–437
13. Scott R J, Christofersen M R, Robertson W W, Davidson R S, Rankin L, Drummond D S 1990 Acute osteomyelitis in children. J Pediatr Orthop 10: 649–652
14. Sullivan D C, Rosenfield N S, Ogden J, Gottschalk A 1980 Problems in the scintigraphic detection of osteomyelitis in children. Radiology 135: 731–736
15. Ash J M, Gilday D L 1980 The futility of bone scanning in neonatal osteomyelitis: concise communication. J Nucl Med 21: 417–420
16. Glasier C M, Seibert J J, Williamson S L 1987 The gamut of increased whole bone activity in bone scintigraphy in children. Clin Nucl Med 12: 192–197
17. Taylor C R, Lawson J P 1986 Periostitis and osteomyelitis in chronic drug addicts. Skeletal Radiol 15: 209–212
18. Thrall J H, Geslien G E, Corcoron R J, Johnson M C 1975 Abnormal radionuclide deposition patterns adjacent to focal skeletal lesions. Radiology 115: 659–663
19. Russin L D, Staab E V 1976 Unusual bone scan findings in acute osteomyelitis. J Nucl Med 17: 617–619
20. Barron B J, Dhekne R D 1984 Cold osteomyelitis radionuclide bone scan findings. Clin Nucl Med 9: 392–393

21. Jones D C, Cady R B 1981 'Cold' bone scans in acute osteomyelitis. J Bone Joint Surg 63B: 376–378
22. Murray I P C 1982 Photopenia in skeletal scintigraphy of suspected bone and joint infection. Clin Nucl Med 7: 13–20
23. Allwright S J, Miller J H, Gilsanz V 1991 Subperiosteal abscess in children: scintigraphic appearances. Radiology 179: 725–729
24. Maurer A H, Chen D C P, Camargo E E, Wong D F, Wagner Jr H, Alderson P O 1981 Utility of three phase scintigraphy in suspected osteomyelitis. J Nucl Med 22: 941–949
25. Alazraki N, Dries D, Datz F, Lawrence P, Greenberg E, Taylor Jr A 1985 Value of a 24-hour image (four phase bone scan) in assessing osteomyelitis in patients with peripheral vascular disease. J Nucl Med 26: 711–717
26. Nade S, Robertson F W, Taylor T K F 1974 Antibiotics in the treatment of acute osteomyelitis and acute septic arthritis in children. Med J Aust 2: 703–705
27. Trueta J 1968 Studies of the development and decay of the human frame. Heinemann, London
28. Blockey N J, Watson J T 1970 Acute osteomyelitis in children. J Bone Joint Surg 52B: 77–87
29. Cole W G, Dalziel R E, Leitl S 1982 Treatment of acute osteomyelitis in childhood. J Bone Joint Surg 64B: 218–223
30. Aronson J, Garvin K, Seibert J, Glasier C, Tursky E A 1992 Efficiency of the bone scan for occult limping toddlers. J Pediatr Orthop 12: 38–44
31. Sundberg S B, Savage J P, Foster B K 1989 Technetium phosphate bone scan in the diagnosis of septic arthritis in childhood. J Pediatr Orthop 9 (5): 579–585
32. McCoy J R, Morrisey R T, Seibert J 1981 Clinical experience with the technetium-99m scan in children. Clin Orthop 154: 175–180
33. Canale S T, Harkness R M, Thomas P A, Massie J D 1985 Does aspiration of bones and joints affect results of later bone scanning? J Pediatr Orthop 5: 23–26
34. Schauwecker D S 1992 The scintigraphic diagnosis of osteomyelitis. AJR 158: 9–18
35. Lim M O, Gresham E L, Franken Jr E A, Leala R D 1977 Osteomyelitis as a complication of umbilical artery catheterisation. Am J Dis Child 131: 142–144
36. Mok P M, Reilly B J, Ash J M 1982 Osteomyelitis in the neonate. Radiology 145: 677–682
37. Murray I P C 1980 Bone scanning in the child and young adult II. Skeletal Radiol 5: 65–76
38. Bressler E L, Conway J J, Weiss S C 1984 Neonatal osteomyelitis examined by bone scintigraphy. Radiology 152: 685–688
39. Green N E, Beauchamp R D, Griffin P P 1981 Primary subacute epiphyseal osteomyelitis. J Bone Joint Surg 63A: 107–114
40. Jaffe H L 1972 Metabolic, degenerative and inflammatory diseases of bones and joints. Lea & Febiger, Philadelphia
41. Howman-Giles R, Uren R 1991 Multifocal osteomyelitis in childhood. Review by bone scan. Clin Nucl Med 17: 274–278
42. Gates G F 1977 Scintigraphy of discitis. Clin Nucl Med 2: 20–25
43. Hughes R A, Rowe I F, Shanson D, Keat A C S 1992 Septic bone, joint and muscle lesions associated with human immunodeficiency virus infection. Br J Rheumatol 31: 381–388
44. Norris S H, Watt I 1981 A radionuclide uptake in the evolution of experimental osteomyelitis. Br J Radiol 54: 207–211
45. Graham G D, Lundy N M, Fredrick R J, Hartshorne M F, Bereger D E 1983 Scintigraphic detection of osteomyelitis with 99m-Tc-MDP and 67 Ga-Citrate. J Nucl Med 24: 1019–1022
46. Handmaker H, Giammona S T 1984 Improved early diagnosis of acute inflammatory skeletal-articular disease in children: a two-way radiopharmaceutical approach. Pediatrics 73: 661–669
47. Lewin J S, Rosenfield N S, Hoffer P B, Downing D 1986 Acute osteomyelitis in children: combined Tc-99m and Ga-67 imaging. Radiology 158: 795–804
48. Atkinson R N, Patterson D C, Morris L L, Savage J P 1978 Bone scintigraphy in discitis and related disorders in children. Aus NZ J Surg 48: 374–377
49. Wenger D R, Bobechkow P, Gilday D L 1978 The spectrum of inter-vertebral disc-space infection in children. J Bone Joint Surg 60A: 100–108
50. Bruschwein D A, Brown M L, McLeod R A 1980 Gallium scintigraphy in the evaluation of disk-space infections: concise communication. J Nucl Med 21: 925–927
51. Haase D, Martin R, Marrie T 1980 Radionuclide imaging in pyogenic vertebral osteomyelitis. Clin Nucl Med 5: 533–537
52. Park H, Wheat L J, Siddiqui A R et al 1982 Scintigraphic evaluation of diabetic osteomyelitis: concise communication. J Nucl Med 23: 569–573
53. Eymontt M J, Alavi A, Dalinka M K, Kyle G C 1981 Bone scintigraphy in diabetic osteoarthropathy. Radiology 140: 475–477
54. Sayle B A, Fawcett H D, Wilkey D J, Cierny III G, Mader J T 1985 Indium-111 chloride imaging in chronic osteomyelitis. J Nucl Med 26: 225–229
55. Lutzker L G, Alavi A 1976 Bone and marrow imaging in sickle-cell disease: diagnosis of infarction. Semin Nucl Med 6: 83–91
56. Gelfand M J, Harke H T 1978 Skeletal imaging in sickle cell disease. J Nucl Med 19: 698
57. Amundsen R R, Siegal M J, Siegel B A 1984 Osteomyelitis and infarction in sickle-cell hemoglobinopathies: differentiation by combined technetium and gallium scintigraphy. Radiology 153: 807–812
58. Raptopoulos V, Doherty P W, Goss T P, King M A, Johnson K, Gantz N M 1982 Acute osteomyelitis: advantage of white cells in early detection. AJR 139: 1077–1082
59 Ehrlich L, Martin R H, Saliken J C 1984 Indium-111 WBC scintigraphy in adult osteomyelitis. J Nucl Med 25: 42
60. Seabold J E, Nepola J V, Conrad G R, Marsh J L, Montgomery W J, Bricker J A, Kirchner P T 1989 Detection of osteomyelitis at fracture nonunion sites: comparison of two scintigraphic methods. AJR 152: 1021–1027
61. Esterhai J L, Goll S R, McCarthy K E, Velchik M, Alavi A, Brighton C T, Heppenstall R B 1987 Indium-111 leucocyte scintigraphic detection of subclinical osteomyelitis complicating delayed and nonunion of long bone fractures: a prospective study. J Orthop Res 5: 1–6
62. Maurer A H, Millmond S H, Knight L C et al 1986 Infection in diabetic osteoarthropathy: use of indium labelled leucocytes for diagnosis. Radiology 61: 221–225
63. Schauwecker D S, Park H M, Burt R W, Mock B H, Wellman H N 1988 Combined bone scintigraphy and indium-111 leucocytes in neuropathic foot disease. J Nucl Med 29: 1651–1655
64. Rüther W S, Hotze A, Möller F, Bockisch A, Heitzmann P, Biersack H J 1990 Diagnosis of bone and joint infection by leucocyte scintigraphy: a comparative study with 99mTc-HMPAO leucocytes, 99mTc-labeled antigranulocyte antibodies and 99mTc-labeled nanocolloid. Arch Orthop Trauma Surg 110: 26–32
65. Eisenberg B, Powe J E, Alavi A 1991 Cold defects in In-111 labeled leucocyte imaging of osteomyelitis in the axial skeleton. Clin Nucl Med 16: 103–106
66. Palestro C J, Roumanas P, Swyer A J, Kim C K, Goldsmith S J 1992 Diagnosis of musculoskeletal infection using combined In-111 leucocyte and Tc-99m sulfur colloid marrow imaging. Clin Nucl Med 17: 269–273
67. Abreu S H 1989 Skeletal uptake of indium-111 labeled white blood cells. Semin Nucl Med 19: 152–155
68. Lantto T, Kaukonen J P, Kokkola A, Laitinen R 1992 Tc-99m HMPAO labeled leucocytes superior to bone scan in the detection of osteomyelitis in children. Clin Nucl Med 17: 7–10
69. Rubin R H, Fischman A J, Callahan R J et al 1989 111-In labeled nonspecific immunoglobulin scanning in the detection of focal infection. N Engl J Med 321: 935–940
70. Oyen W J G, Claessens R A M J, van Horn J R, van der Meer J W M, Corstens F H M 1990 Scintigraphic detection of bone and joint infections with Indium-111 labeled nonspecific polyclonal immunoglobulin G. J Nucl Med 31: 403–412
71. Oyen W J G, Netten P M, Lemmens A M et al 1992 Evaluation of infectious diabetic foot complications with Indium-111-labeled human nonspecific immunoglobulin G. J Nucl Med 33: 1330–1336
72. Hotze A L, Briele B, Overbeck B et al 1992 Technetium-99m-labeled anti-granulocyte antibodies in suspected bone infections. J Nucl Med 33: 526–531
73. Sciuk J, Brandau W, Vollet B et al 1991 Comparison of technetium 99m polyclonal human immunoglobulin and technetium 99m

monoclonal antibodies for imaging chronic osteomyelitis. Eur J Nucl Med 18: 401–407
74. Seybold K, Frey L D, Locher J 1992 Immunoscintigraphy of infections using 123-I and 99m-Tc-labeled monoclonal antibodies. Advanced experiences in 230 patients. Angiology 43: 85–90
75. Abramovici J, Rubinstein M 1988 Tc-99m nanocolloids: an alternative approach to the diagnosis inflammatory lesions of bone and joints. Eur J Nucl Med 14: 244
76. Streule K, de Schrijver M, Fridrich R 1988 Tc-99m labelled HSA nanocolloids vs In-111 oxine labelled granulocytes in detecting skeletal septic processes. Nucl Med Commun 9: 59–67
77. Ferguson A B 1975 Orthopaedic surgery in infancy and childhood, 4th edn. Williams & Wilkins, Baltimore
78. Schlesinger A E, Hernandez R J 1992 Diseases of the musculoskeletal system in children: Imaging with CT, sonography and MR. AJR 158: 729–741
79. Beltran J, Noto A M, McGhee R B, Freedy R M, McCalla M S 1987 Infections of the musculoskeletal system: high field strength MR imaging. Radiology 164: 449–454
80. Abiri M M, Kirpekar M, Ablow R C 1989 Osteomyelitis: detection with US. Radiology 172: 509–511
81. Heyman S, Goldstein H A, Crowley W, Treves S 1980 The scintigraphic evaluation of hip pain in children. Clin Nucl Med 5: 109–115
82. Kloiber R, Pavlosky W, Portner O, Gartke K 1983 Bone scintigraphy of hip joint effusions in children. AJR 140: 995–999
83. Uren R F, Howman-Giles R 1991 The 'cold hip' sign on bone scan. A retrospective review. Clin Nucl Med 16: 553–556
84. Woodhouse C G 1964 Dynamic influences of vascular occlusion affecting the femoral head. Clin Orthop 32: 119–129
85. Traughber P D, Manaster B J, Murphy K, Alazraki N P 1986 Negative bone scans of joints after aspiration or arthrography: Experimental studies. AJR 146: 87–91
86. Mandell G A, Harcke H T, Bowen J R, Sharkey C A 1989 Transient photopenia of the femoral head following arthrography. Clin Nucl Med 14: 397–404
87. Bennett O M, Namnyak S S 1992 Acute septic arthritis of the hip joint in infancy and childhood. Clin Orthop Related Res 281: 123–132
88. Kumar R, Balachandran S 1983 Unilateral septic sacro-iliitis. Importance of the anterior view of the bone scan. Clin Nucl Med 413–415
89. Horgan J G, Walker M, Newman J H, Watt I 1983 Scintigraphy in the diagnosis and management of septic sacroiliitis. Clin Radiol 34: 87–91
90. Rosenthall L, Kloiber R, Damteu B, Al-Majid H 1982 Sequential use of radiophosphate and radiogallium imaging in the differential diagnosis of bone, joint, and soft tissue infection: quantitative analysis. Diagn Imaging 51: 249–258
91. Malamitsi J, Maragoudakis P, Papafragou K et al 1993 Preliminary results on scintigraphic evaluation of malignant external otitis. Eur J Nucl Med 20: 511–514
92. El-Desouki, M 1991 Skeletal brucellosis: assessment with bone scintigraphy. Radiology 181: 415–418
93. Salomon C G, Ali A, Fordham E W 1986 Bone scintigraphy in tuberculous sacroiliitis. Clin Nucl Med 11: 407–408
94. Pritchard D J 1975 Granulomatous infections of bones and joints. Orthop Clin N Am 6: 1029–1047
95. Nocera R M, Sayle B, Rogers C, Wilkey D 1983 Tc-99m MDP and Indium-111 chloride scintigraphy in skeletal scintigraphy. Clin Nucl Med 8: 418–420
96. Al-Sheikh W, Sfakianakis G N, Mnaymneh W et al 1985 Subacute and chronic bone infections: diagnosis using In-111, Ga-67 and Tc-99m MDP bone scintigraphy, and radiology. Radiology 155: 501–506
97. Tumeh S S, Aliabadi P, Weissman B N, McNeil B J 1986 Chronic osteomyelitis: bone and gallium scan patterns associated with active disease. Radiology 158: 685–688

83. Chronic infection: radionuclide diagnosis of the infected joint replacement

Christopher J. Palestro

While synthetic replacements are available for a multitude of joints in the human body, the two joints most often artificially reconstructed and about which the most data are available, are the hip and the knee. Total hip and total knee replacements are each performed approximately 120 000 times annually in the United States. For the most part the results of these procedures, in terms of relief of pain and restoration of function, have been very satisfactory. Complications do arise, however, and include heterotopic ossification, loosening, dislocation, fracture, and infection. Infection of a joint replacement is a particularly serious problem inasmuch as failure to diagnose and adequately treat this complication virtually assures that any revision arthroplasty performed will be doomed to failure.

Diagnosing the infected joint replacement, even with the myriad of sophisticated techniques currently available, is a difficult task. Clinical history, physical examination, erythrocyte sedimentation rate, peripheral leucocyte count, plain radiography, and joint aspiration and culture, suffer from insensitivity, non-specificity, or both, and are of limited value. Radionuclide techniques used to diagnose the infected joint replacement include ^{99m}Tc-MDP bone scintigraphy, ^{67}Ga citrate, and ^{111}In-labelled leucocyte scintigraphy, alone and in various combinations.

BONE SCINTIGRAPHY

Over the past 15 years the role of bone scintigraphy in the diagnosis of postoperative complications of joint arthroplasty has been evaluated by numerous investigators. Gelman et al[1] reviewed the results of bone scintigraphy performed on 21 painful joint replacements, including 17 hip and four knee prostheses. They reported an overall accuracy of 85% in the hips and 100% in the knees for this technique. Weiss et al,[2] using focally increased uptake at the tip of the femoral component or in the region of the acetabular component as the criteria for an abnormal study, reported that bone scintigraphy was 100% sensitive and 77% specific for diagnosing infection or loosening of the total hip replacement. As promising as these early results were, it must be borne in mind that they reflected the ability of bone imaging to detect complications of joint replacement generally, not infection specifically. Williamson et al[3] were among the first investigators to suggest that patterns of periprosthetic uptake around hip

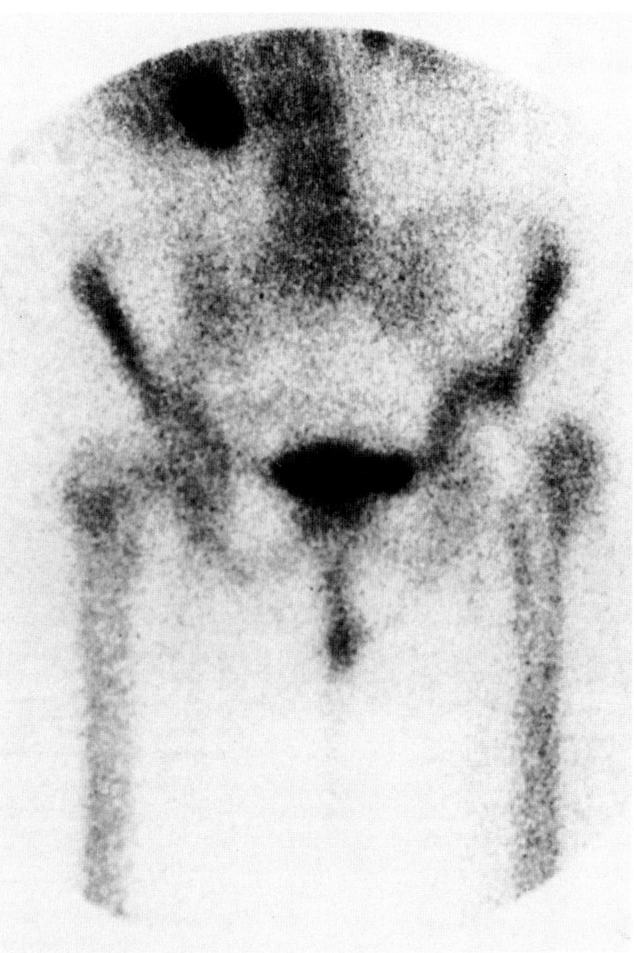

Fig. 83.1A Normal appearance of a left total hip replacement on bone scintigraphy: periprosthetic activity is indistinguishable from that in the adjacent non-articular bone.

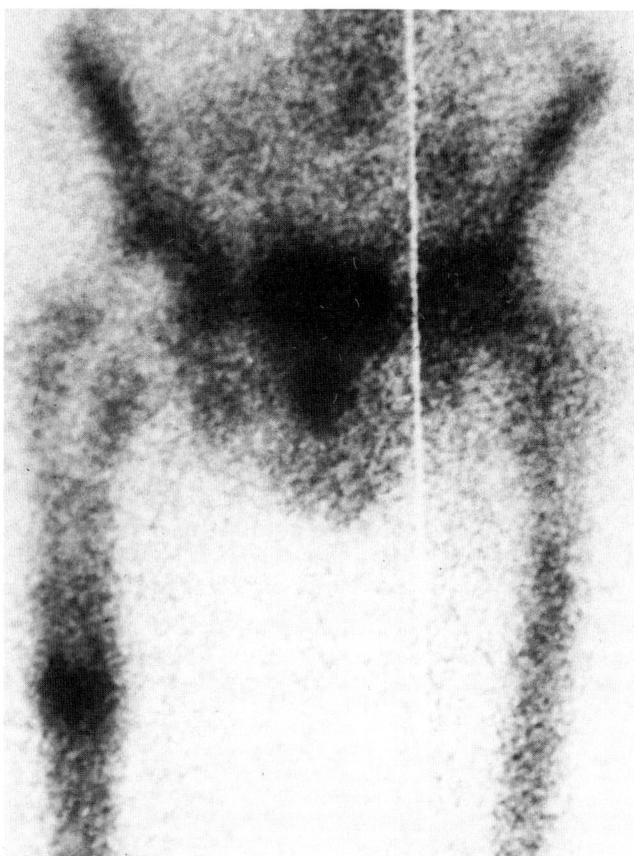

Fig. 83.1B Bone scan shows intense focal uptake at the tip of the femoral component of a right total hip replacement, a pattern which is generally associated with loosening without infection.

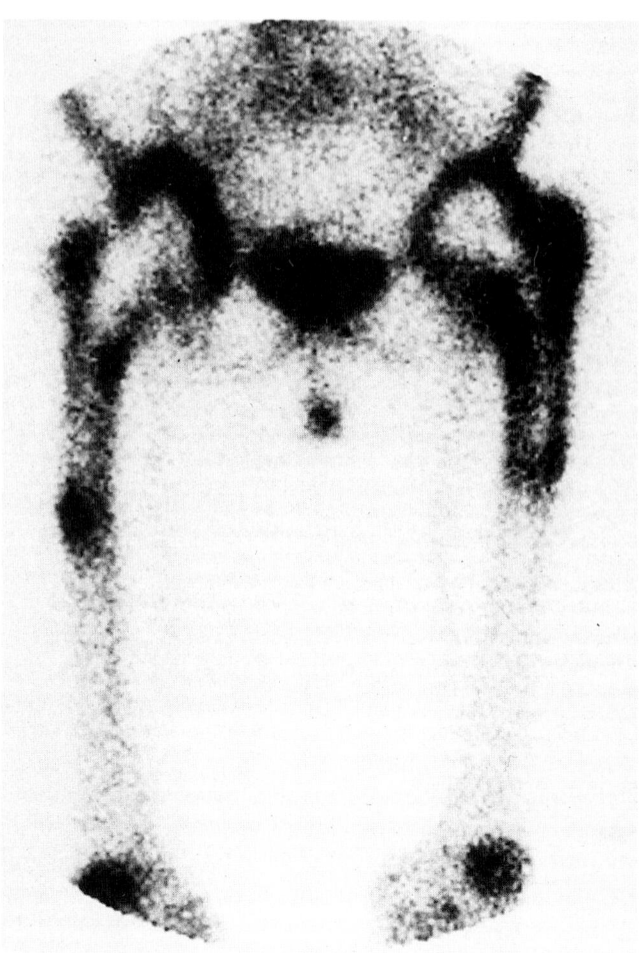

Fig. 83.1C There is diffuse periprosthetic activity around the femoral component of a left total hip replacement, which is generally associated with infection. Note also the intense uptake around the acetabular component as well as the tip of the femoral component of the right total hip replacement. A loose but uninfected right hip replacement was surgically removed; the left hip replacement was asymptomatic and received no additional work-up.

prostheses were useful to differentiate between loosening and infection. They found that while focal periprosthetic uptake was associated with loosening, diffuse uptake around both the femoral and acetabular components was associated with infection (Fig. 83.1). Other investigators, however, have reported conflicting results. Williams et al[4] reviewed 38 total hip replacements, of which 14 were subsequently found to be infected. While all 14 demonstrated the diffuse pattern of periprosthetic uptake, this pattern was also present in 13 uninfected prostheses, and these authors concluded that it was not possible to distinguish infected from uninfected hip replacements based solely on patterns of periprosthetic uptake of ^{99m}Tc-MDP. Mountford et al[5] found that, although the diffuse pattern of periprosthetic uptake was associated primarily with infection, this pattern was present in only five out of 11 (45%) infected joint replacements these investigators studied. Aliabadi et al[6] reported that bone scintigraphy was 75% sensitive and 96% specific for diagnosing loosening with or without infection, but they found that this procedure did not permit the separation of those patients with, from those patients without, infected prostheses. They also noted that while an abnormal study indicated a prosthetic abnormality, a negative study did not exclude one. We[7] recently reviewed the role of bone scintigraphy for diagnosing infected total knee replacements and found that the study was neither sensitive (76%) nor specific (50%) for this purpose. Moreover, the limited data that is available suggests that in contrast to osteomyelitis in general, three-phase bone scintigraphy does little to improve the accuracy of routine bone scanning for diagnosing joint replacement infection.[7–9]

Perhaps the single most important limitation to bone scintigraphy is the non-specificity of the procedure. Increased activity present on the images reflects increased bone mineral turnover, which can result from any of a number of conditions, in addition to infection. This problem is further complicated by the numerous patterns of periprosthetic uptake associated with asymptomatic hip and knee replacements. During the first year following implantation of a total hip replacement, periprosthetic

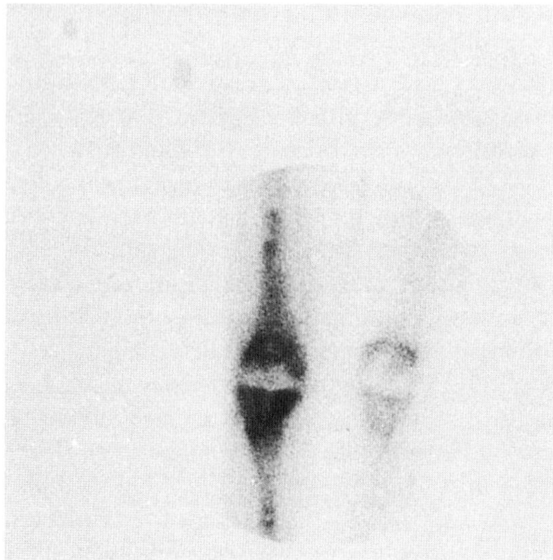

Fig. 83.2A Bilateral total knee replacements implanted 4 years prior to imaging. The right was loose, the left asymptomatic.

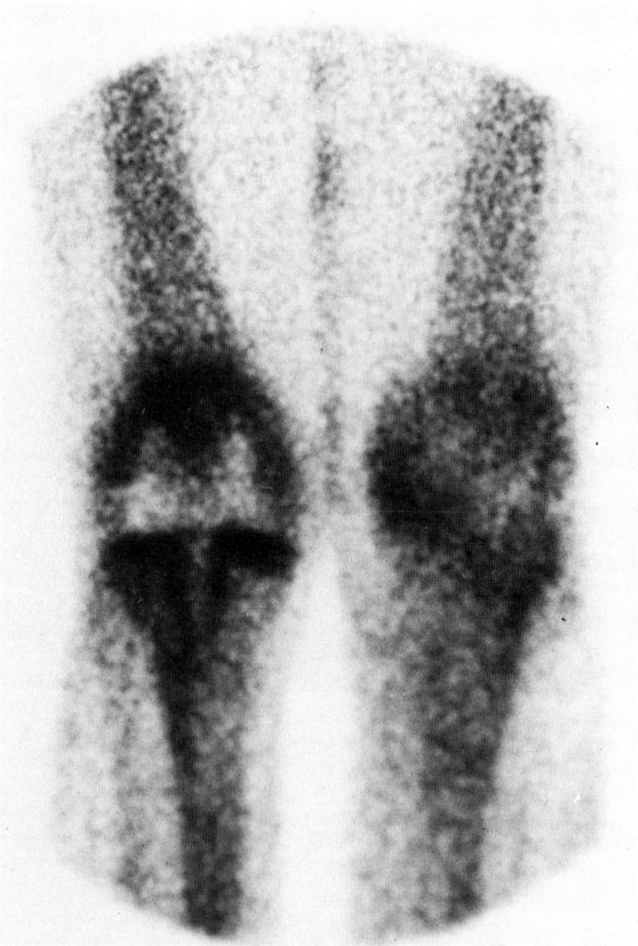

Fig. 83.2B Increased activity around both femoral and tibial components in a patient with a 5-year-old asymptomatic right total knee replacement. The pattern of uptake around this asymptomatic prosthesis is virtually indistinguishable from the pattern of uptake around the loosened right knee replacement in Fig. 83.2A.

uptake patterns are very variable; beyond 1 year, in the case of the cemented hip replacement, most asymptomatic patients will have a normal scan. Ten per cent of patients will, however, have definite persistent uptake beyond this time, even in the absence of any complications.[10] In the case of the cementless or porous coated hip replacement, persistent uptake beyond 1 year is even more prevalent.[11,12] Assessment of the total knee replacement with bone scintigraphy is even more problematic than that of hip replacements, with 63% of femoral components and 89% of tibial components demonstrating persistent periprosthetic activity more than 12 months after implantation[13] (Fig. 83.2B). It has been suggested that if the utility of bone scintigraphy is to be maximized it may be necessary to perform serial imaging, including baseline studies. While this undoubtedly would be helpful, this is a luxury not usually available in the normal clinical setting.

Recognizing the limitations inherent in bone scintigraphy, other radionuclide techniques in addition to, or instead of, bone imaging having been used to diagnose the infected joint replacement.

BONE–GALLIUM SCINTIGRAPHY

Though its mechanisms of uptake are not well understood, the propensity of gallium to accumulate in infection was first recognized during the early 1970s, and numerous investigators have studied the role of this radionuclide in the diagnosis of joint arthroplasty infection. Reing et al[14] evaluated 79 patients with both bone and gallium scintigraphy. Twenty of the 79 patients were subsequently found to have infected joint replacements. Although bone scintigraphy (criteria not specified) was abnormal in 20 (100%) of 20 infected prostheses, confirming the sensitivity of the procedure, the study was also abnormal in 50 (85%) of 59 uninfected prostheses, rendering it very nonspecific (specificity: 15%). In contrast, 19 out of 20 infected prostheses were abnormal on gallium scintigraphy while none of the 50 uninfected prostheses were abnormal on gallium imaging indicating that the technique was not only sensitive (95%) but specific (100%) as well. Ten additional patients in this series with negative bone scans who did not undergo gallium imaging were subsequently confirmed to be infection-free. These authors concluded that while a negative bone scan is strong evidence against an infected joint replacement, an abnormal study is nonspecific, and the addition of gallium imaging under these conditions greatly enhances the accuracy of the radionuclide diagnosis of the infected joint replacement. Rushton et al[15] reviewed bone and gallium imaging in 51 patients with painful hip arthroplasties, as well as 34 control patients, and came to the same conclusions.

Rosenthall et al[16] evaluated bone–gallium imaging in 46 patients with a variety of orthopaedic hardware and made

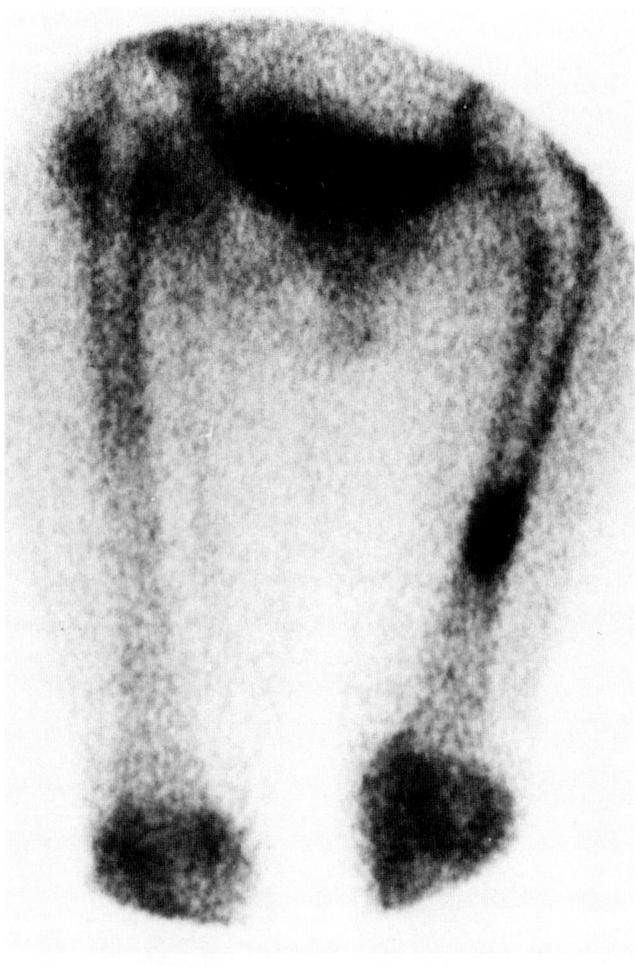

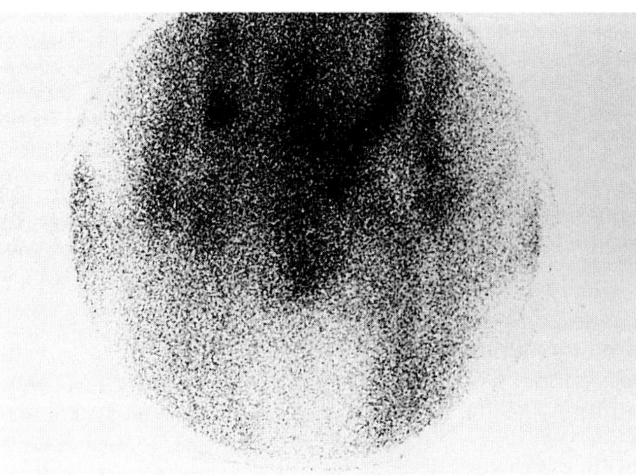

Fig. 83.3 Sequential bone–gallium imaging of a left total hip replacement. Mild diffuse periprosthetic uptake with superimposed focal uptake at the tip of the femoral component is noted on the bone image (A). No abnormal periprosthetic uptake is present on the gallium image (B). The combined study is negative for infection.

several important observations about the significance of different patterns of periprosthetic uptake of these two radiotracers. They found that a negative gallium study excluded infection with a high degree of certainty (12/12), regardless of the results of the bone study. Of 16 patients in their series with a similar distribution of both radiotracers (spatially congruent images), none had infection, and one had an aseptic bursitis. In 18 patients the distribution of the two radiotracers was different (spatially incongruent images) and 16 of these 18 had infection; the remaining two patients had aseptic synovitis. Based on their observations, these investigators concluded that when bone and gallium images are spatially congruent or when the gallium image is negative, regardless of the results of bone scintigraphy, infection is very unlikely (unless the uptake of gallium is intense) while spatially incongruent images are highly suggestive of infection (Figs 83.3 and 83.4). Williams et al[4] identified abnormal gallium uptake in 13 (93%) out of 14 infected joint replacements, and in only two (8%) out of 24 uninfected joint replacements. When they evaluated combined bone–gallium scintigraphy, however, they found that only seven (50%) of the 14 infected joint replacements demonstrated spatially incongruent bone–gallium images; in the other seven infected joint replacements, the images were spatially congruent. Merkel et al[17] prospectively evaluated sequential bone–gallium imaging in a canine model. The combined studies were classified as positive for infection if the distribution of the two tracers was spatially incongruent or, when the distribution was spatially congruent, if the intensity of uptake of gallium exceeded the intensity of uptake of MDP. Studies were classified as negative for infection if the images were spatially congruent and the intensity of gallium uptake was less than that of MDP. Studies in which both the spatial distribution and intensity of uptake of the two radiotracers were congruent, were classified as equivocal (Fig. 83.5). In this series the sensitivity, specificity, and accuracy of bone–gallium images for diagnosing the infected joint replacement were 61%, 71%, and 67%, respectively. In a larger retrospective review of 130 patients with painful orthopaedic prostheses, using the same interpretative criteria, these investigators reported very similar results.[18] Gomez-Luzuriaga et al[19] evaluated 40 patients with painful total hip replacements, who subsequently underwent surgery. Twenty of the 40 hip replacements studied were infected. Classifying sequential bone–gallium images as positive for infection when the images were spatially incongruent or when gallium uptake was more intense than that of MDP, they reported a sensitivity, specificity, and accuracy of 70%, 90% and 80% respectively.

Sequential bone–gallium imaging has proven most accurate when the gallium images are negative, or when the distribution of the two radiotracers is spatially incongruent. Unfortunately, these patterns are encountered in a minority of the patients studied, and consequently this combined technique offers only a modest improvement over bone scintigraphy alone.

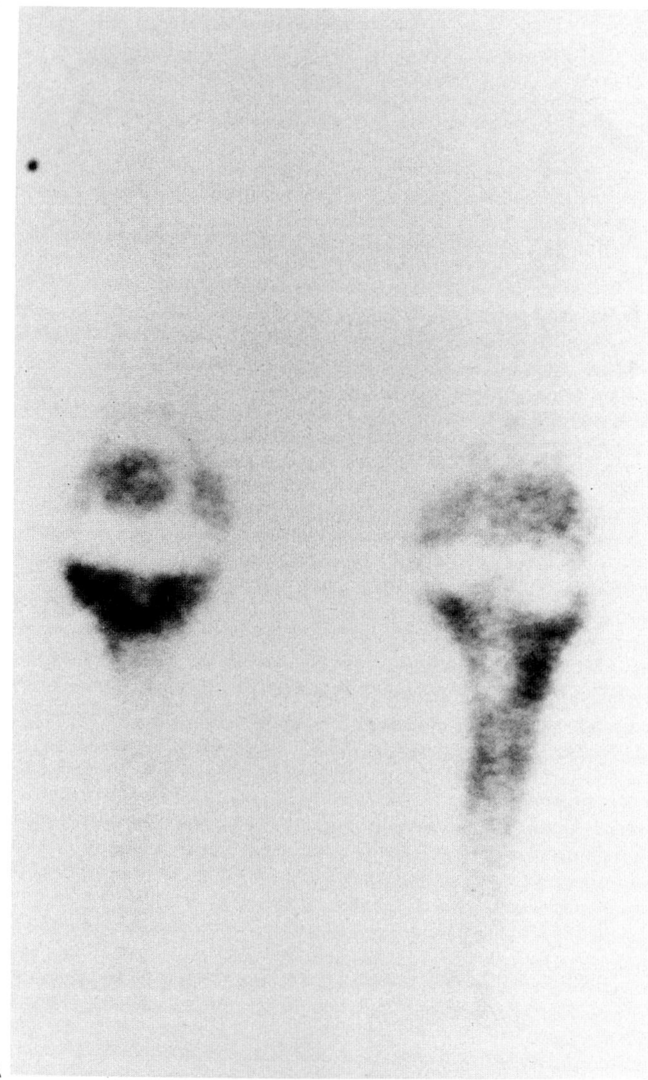

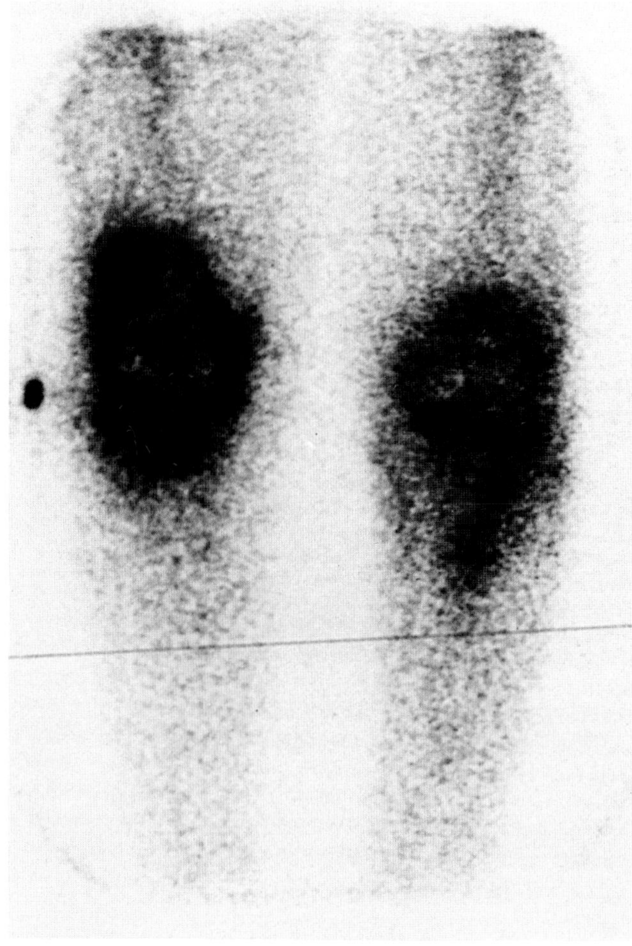

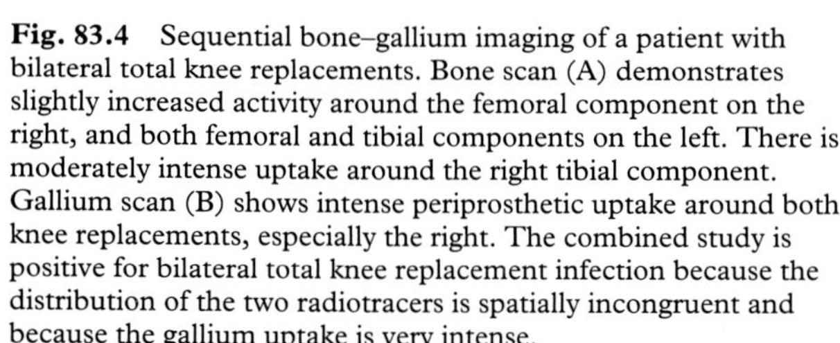

Fig. 83.4 Sequential bone–gallium imaging of a patient with bilateral total knee replacements. Bone scan (A) demonstrates slightly increased activity around the femoral component on the right, and both femoral and tibial components on the left. There is moderately intense uptake around the right tibial component. Gallium scan (B) shows intense periprosthetic uptake around both knee replacements, especially the right. The combined study is positive for bilateral total knee replacement infection because the distribution of the two radiotracers is spatially incongruent and because the gallium uptake is very intense.

Labelled leucocyte imaging

Labelled leucocyte imaging is, at least theoretically, the ideal technique for diagnosing the infected joint replacement because, in general, white cells do not accumulate at sites of increased bone mineral turnover in the absence of infection. In one of the early investigations of the role of labelled leucocyte imaging in orthopaedics, Propst-Proctor et al[20] found the technique to be extremely sensitive for detecting acute musculoskeletal infection, including infected joint replacements. Equally important, these investigators noted that non-infectious conditions such as heterotopic ossification, metastatic disease, and degenerative arthritis did not demonstrate white cell accumulation, suggesting that the technique was not only sensitive, but specific as well. Although these initial findings were encouraging, subsequent investigations yielded conflicting results regarding the utility of white cell imaging in musculoskeletal infection. McKillop et al[21] compared ^{67}Ga and labelled leucocyte imaging in 15 painful prostheses, six of which were infected. Without specifying their interpretative criteria, they reported sensitivities and specificities of 50% and 100% respectively for leucocyte imaging, and 86% and 82% respectively for gallium. They concluded that the low sensitivity of leucocyte imaging in their series was the result of the chronic, low-grade inflammation present in their patients. In contrast, Pring et al[22] using labelled granulocytes to evaluate 60 prosthetic joints, including 11 that were infected, reported a sensitivity of 100% and a specificity of 89.5% for this technique. In their series, studies in which periprosthetic white cell activity was at least as intense as normal marrow activity were classified as positive for infection. Magnuson et al[8], using similar criteria, reported a sensitivity and specificity of 88% and 73% respectively,

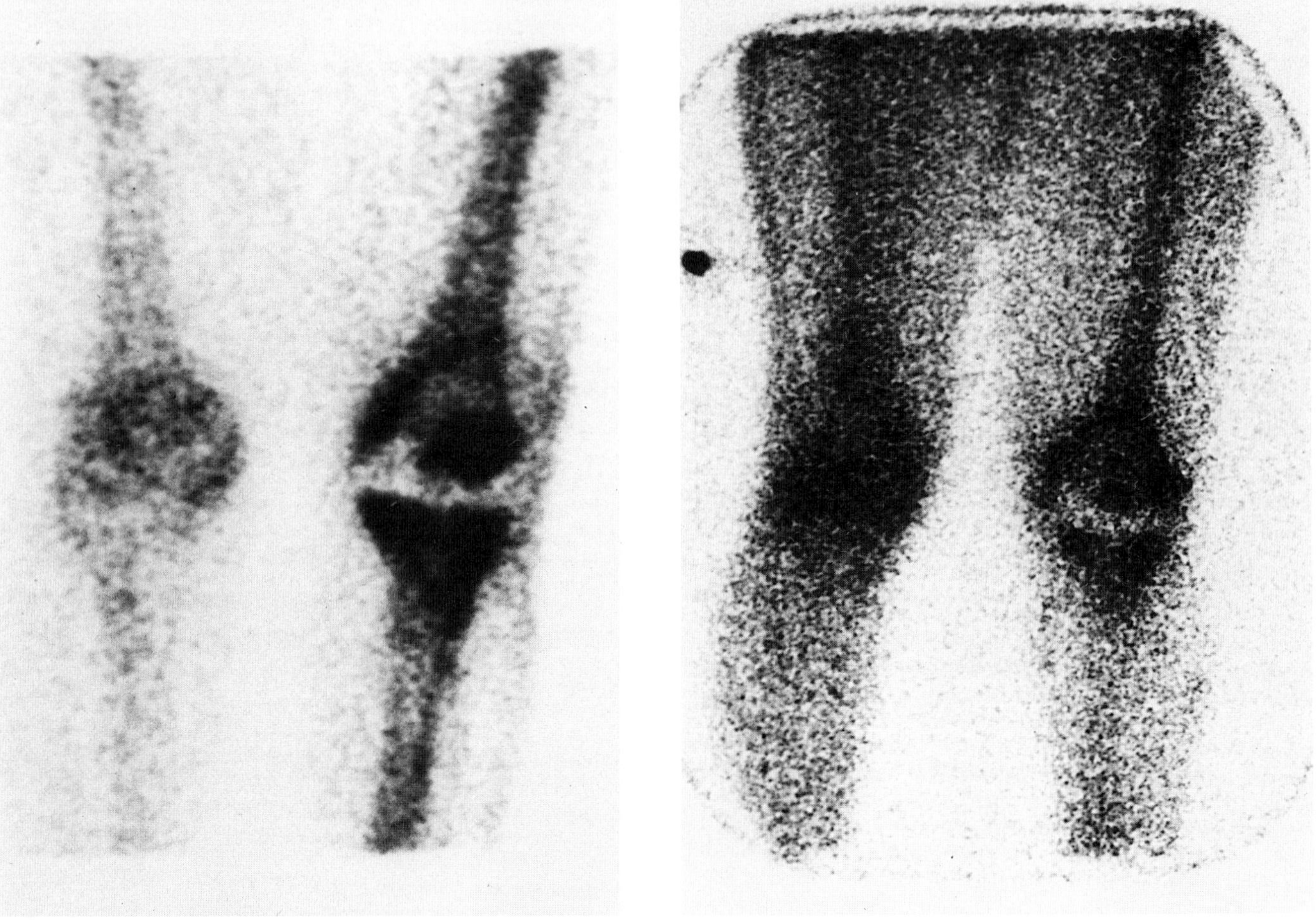

Fig. 83.5 Bone (A) and gallium (B) images of a left total knee replacement are congruent both spatially and in terms of intensity of uptake, and therefore the study is equivocal for infection.

for diagnosing infected orthopaedic hardware using labelled leucocyte imaging. Wukich et al[23] evaluated 24 total joint replacements. They classified images as positive for infection when focally increased activity, compared to adjacent bone, was identified. Using this criterion, they reported that labelled leucocyte imaging was 100% sensitive, but only 45% specific for joint replacement infection. Johnson et al[24] evaluated hip replacements and also reported a high sensitivity (100%) but a low specificity (50%) for this technique. We evaluated total knee and total hip replacements.[7,25] Using any periprosthetic activity at all as the criterion for infection we reported a sensitivity of 89% and a specificity of 50% for total knee prosthesis infection. Using only periprosthetic activity more intense than the contralateral knee activity as the criterion for a positive study, the sensitivity was unchanged at 89%, while the specificity rose to 75%. Using these same two criteria for total hip replacements, the specificity of the study improved from 23% when any periprosthetic uptake was considered positive for infection, to 61%, when only activity more intense than the contralateral side was considered positive for infection. Unlike the knee prostheses, however, the sensitivity of the technique decreased from 100% to 65%, when activity greater than the contralateral side was the criterion for a positive study.

With its theoretical superiority to both bone and sequential bone–gallium scintigraphy, the surprisingly inconsistent, and for the most part disappointing, results that have been reported for the labelled leucocyte diagnosis of the infected orthopaedic implant require some analysis.

Several investigators have suggested that, while labelled leucocyte imaging is very useful for diagnosing acute musculoskeletal infection, it is less satisfactory for the chronic, indolent, low grade infection, usually associated with infected orthopaedic hardware. Al-Sheikh et al[26] found virtually no difference between labelled leucocyte and gallium imaging in patients with suspected musculoskeletal infection who had been symptomatic for at least 1 month. Thirteen of the 21 patients they studied had orthopaedic hardware in place. These investigators considered leucocyte activity to be abnormal when the intensity of activity in the region of interest was greater than the contralateral side. Using this criterion for a positive study, they found leucocyte imaging to be 80% sensitive for diagnosing chronic bone infection. They also noted that even when this hyperactivity was present, it was not always easy to detect. Prchal et al[27] compared the results of leucocyte imaging in musculoskeletal infection in patients who had been symptomatic for less than 6 weeks to those who had been symptomatic for more than 6 weeks. They classified studies as positive for acute infection when the intensity of white cell uptake exceeded the intensity of liver and spleen uptake while uptake more intense than marrow, but less intense than liver and spleen was felt to be consistent with chronic infection. The sensitivity of the technique for acute infection was 100%, but only 50% for chronic infection. Schauwecker et al[28] reported that the sensitivity of leucocyte imaging for diagnosing acute osteomyelitis was 100%, but for chronic osteomyelitis the sensitivity fell to 60%. These authors did not, however, indicate whether or not duration of symptoms was used to classify patients as having an acute or chronic process. Finally we have observed a relationship between the appearance of vertebral osteomyelitis on leucocyte imaging, and the duration of patient symptoms.[29] We found that patients with vertebral osteomyelitis who were symptomatic for 2 weeks or less all had increased activity (compared to adjacent normal activity) on white cell studies; beyond this 2 week period some patients had increased uptake of white cells, and two patients even had 'normal' activity. The majority, however, had decreased or absent labelled white cell activity at the site of infection.

That the intensity of labelled leucocyte uptake decreases with time is not surprising when one considers the fundamentals of the technique. Generally speaking a mixed population of leucocytes is labelled which, in the majority of patients, is composed primarily of neutrophils. It stands to reason, therefore, that the procedure will be most useful for detecting those conditions, such as an acute bacterial infection, that incite a neutrophilic response. The procedure will be less useful in conditions that incite other than a neutrophilic response, or in conditions where the neutrophilic response has waned as a result of treatment with antibiotics or steroids, or has simply subsided over time.

If chronicity of infection were the sole, or even the principal explanation for the unsatisfactory labelled leucocyte results that have been reported, then the reported results should consistently reflect low sensitivity. Some investigators however, studying similar patient populations, have reported just the opposite: high sensitivity, but low specificity for the technique.[23,24] Moreover, as already noted in patients with hip prostheses, we were able to dramatically alter the sensitivity (and specificity) of the technique merely by changing the criteria for a positive study.[25]

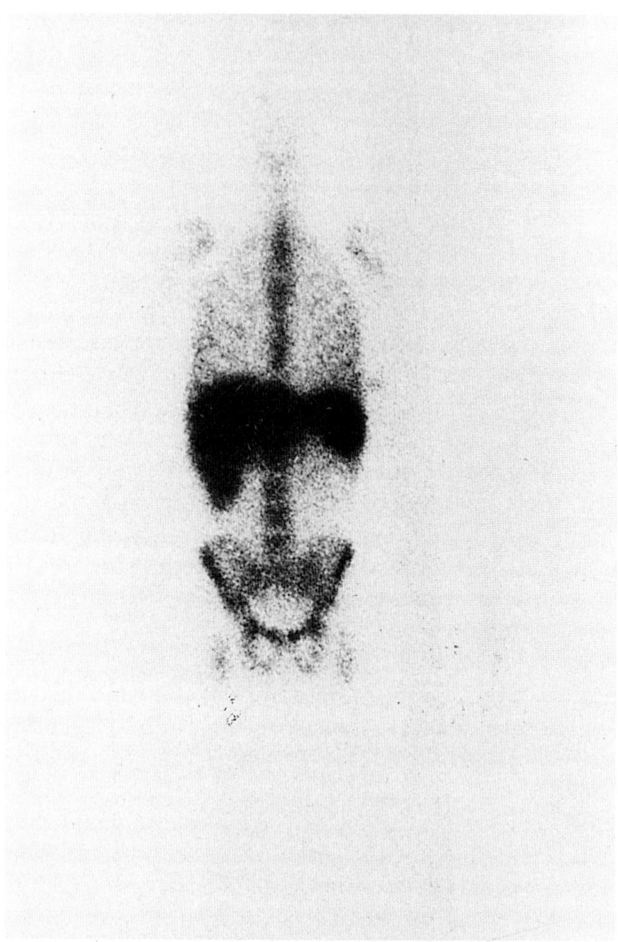

Fig. 83.6 Anterior ^{111}In labelled leucocyte image of a 40-year-old man demonstrates normal physiologic distribution of marrow activity.

The explanation of the often contradictory results reported for labelled leucocyte imaging, even in similar patient populations, lies not so much with the acute or chronic nature of the infection per se, but rather with an inability to arrive at a satisfactory method for interpretation of these studies. Typically, labelled white cell images, like most other radionuclide procedures, are interpreted by comparing the intensity of uptake in the region of interest to the intensity of uptake in some, presumably normal, reference point. When the study is performed for the evaluation of orthopaedic infection, the reference point usually selected is the bone marrow. In the normal adult up to approximately 70 years of age, the normal distribution of haematopoietically active marrow is limited to the axial skeleton, and proximal third of the humeri and femurs (Fig. 83.6). Those studies in which uptake of labelled leucocytes in the region of interest, exceeds the uptake in the preselected normal reference point, are classified as abnormal or positive for infection. A prerequisite for the success of the procedure, therefore, is that the degree of uptake in the abnormal zone exceeds the degree of uptake in the normal zone, a situation which does not always occur, as borne out by the previous discussion.

There is a second, even more fundamental, problem with labelled leucocyte imaging, that needs to be addressed. While the normal distribution of haematopoietically active marrow is confined to the axial skeleton and proximal humeri and femurs, there is considerable individual to individual variation. Conditions such as tumour, previous radiation therapy, sickle cell disease, and Paget's disease, can result in unusual and even bizarre distributions of 'normal' marrow. It is likely, moreover, that the placement of orthopaedic hardware such as prostheses, rods, plates, etc., stimulates the conversion of fatty into haematopoietically active marrow, further complicating the 'normal' distribution of functioning marrow. Under these circumstances, it may be virtually impossible to separate functioning marrow, atypical in location, from infection (Fig. 83.7).

Efforts to improve the accuracy of labelled leucocyte imaging have focused on the use of one of two combined modalities: leucocyte–bone and leucocyte–marrow imaging. Several investigators have reported that combined leucocyte–bone imaging is superior to conventional leucocyte imaging for diagnosing complicating osteomyelitis in general, and infected orthopaedic hardware in particular. Al-Shiekh et al[26] reported that the sensitivity of labelled leucocyte imaging for diagnosing subacute and chronic bone infection in 21 orthopaedic patients was 80%, while the specificity was only 50%. When they interpreted the white cell images together with bone scans, using criteria similar to that used for interpreting sequential bone–gallium images, the specificity of the study rose to 75%, while the sensitivity remained at 80%. In the series of Wukich et al,[23] the specificity for diagnosing joint replacement infection rose from 45% for white cell imaging alone to 85% for leucocyte–bone imaging, although the sensitivity dropped from 100% to 85%. Johnson et al[24] reported similar results in the assessment of total hip arthroplasties, noting that the combined technique offered a higher specificity (95% *vs.* 50%) at the expense of a somewhat lower sensitivity (88% *vs.* 100%).

In contrast to the foregoing results, obtained primarily in hip replacements, our results in total knee replacements were far less satisfactory. We obtained a sensitivity of 67% and a specificity of 78% for the combined technique, *vs.* a sensitivity and specificity of 89% and 75%, respectively, for leucocyte imaging alone.[7] Recent work by Oswald et al[11] also suggests that the combined leucocyte bone technique has serious limitations. They found that in 15% of asymptomatic patients with porous coated hip arthroplasties, leucocyte–bone images were incongruent, and they concluded that, at least in patients with the porous coated variety of hip replacement, incongruence of leuco-

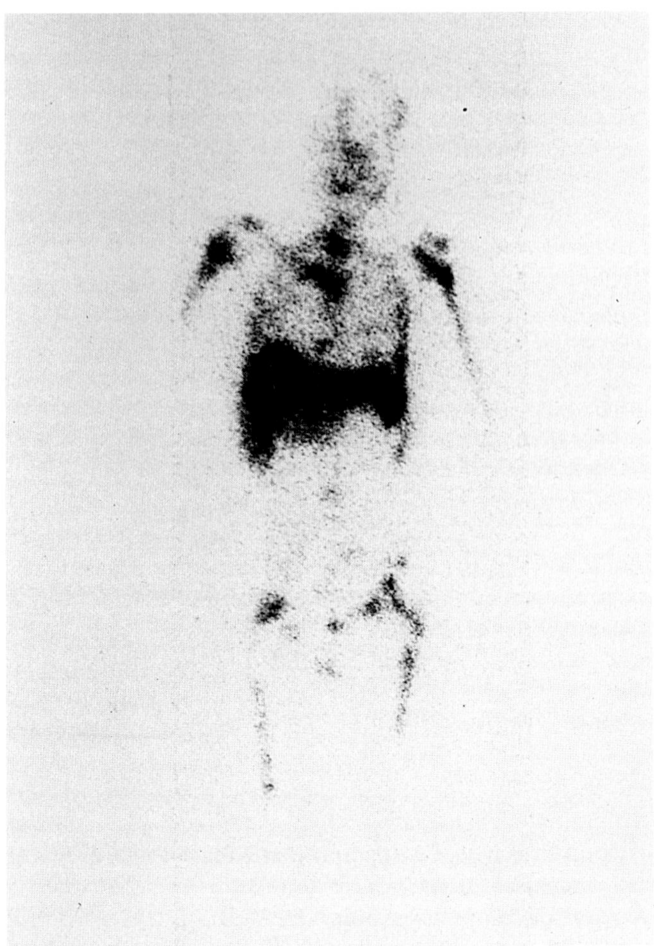

Fig. 83.7 Anterior ^{111}In labelled leucocyte image of a 43-year-old woman with disseminated breast carcinoma metastases. Note not only the presence of marrow expansion into the distal humeri and femurs, but also the irregular nature of the distribution and the varying intensities of tracer uptake by the marrow. In this patient, the selection of a normal marrow reference point is difficult, to say the least, making it virtually impossible to confirm the presence or absence of osteomyelitis. (This patient had no bony infection.) Areas of apparently increased marrow activity, which could be incorrectly interpreted as sites of infection (or even tumour) merely represent sites of residual functioning marrow, surrounded by photopenic tumour deposits (which do not concentrate the radiotracer).

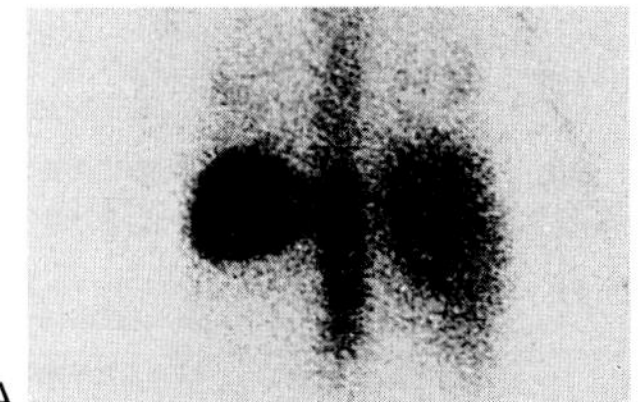

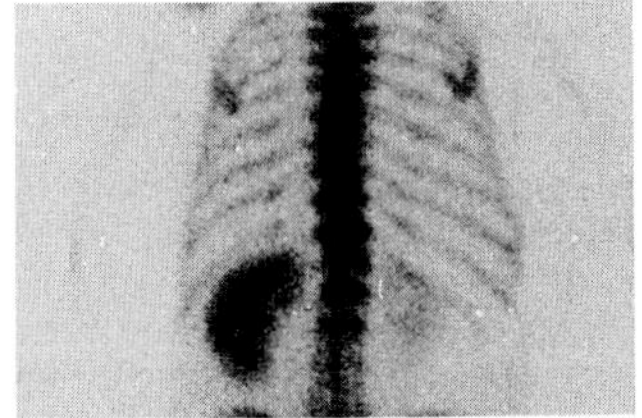

Fig. 83.8 ^{111}In labelled leucocyte (**A**) and ^{99m}Tc-MDP (**B**) images of the lower thoracic and lumbar spines performed on a patient undergoing radiation therapy at the time of imaging. Note the intense hyperactivity on the leucocyte images compared to the bone images. According to criteria used for interpretation of leucocyte–bone imaging, this study would be classified as positive for osteomyelitis. In point of fact these images illustrate the different (acute) effects that radiation therapy exerts on cortical bone and marrow.

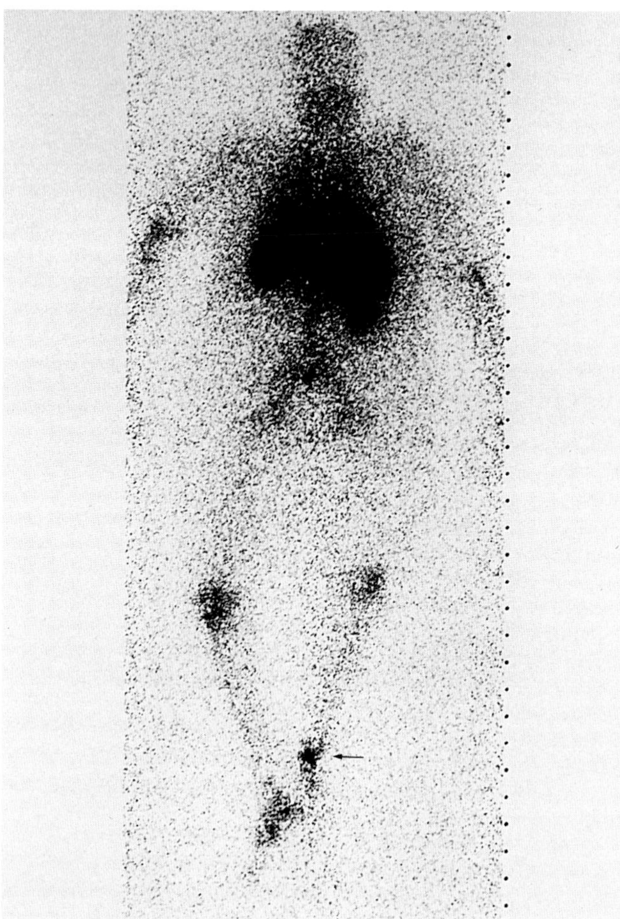

Fig. 83.9A Posterior whole-body labelled leucocyte image performed on a young woman with S-C haemoglobinopathy. The marrow activity is generally diminished, except for a focal area in the right ankle (arrow).

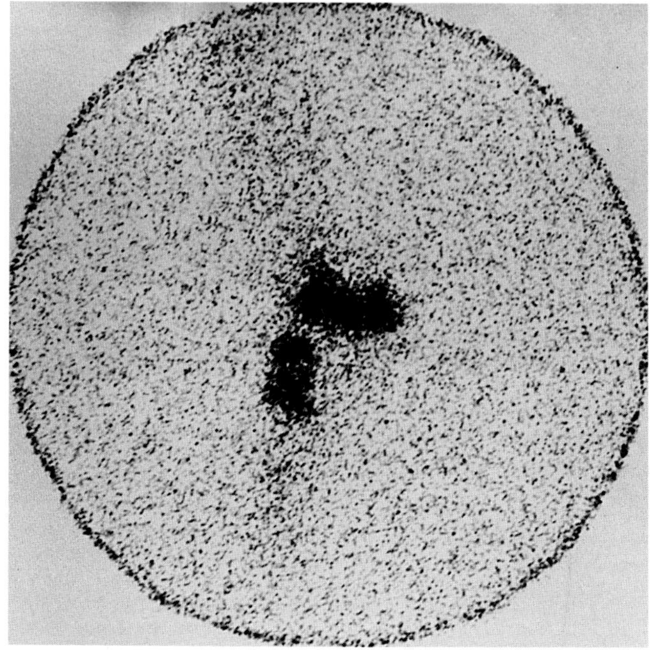

Fig. 83.9B Lateral view of the right ankle demonstrating intense leuocyte uptake in the talus, calcaneus, and distal tarsal bones.

cyte-MDP activity at the prosthetic tip is of little clinical utility. Part of the problem with the combined leucocyte bone technique is that, while ^{99m}Tc-MDP accumulates in bone, labelled leucocytes accumulate in marrow. Conditions that affect marrow may or may not affect bone and vice versa. Even when a particular entity affects both bone and marrow, the effects may be dramatically different, as we have reported in patients undergoing radiation therapy[30] (Fig. 83.8).

LEUKOCYTE–MARROW IMAGING

While some investigators have combined labelled leucocyte imaging with bone scintigraphy in an effort to improve the accuracy of the technique for diagnosing the infected joint replacement, we, and others, have studied combined leucocyte–marrow imaging for this same purpose. Both labelled leucocyte and sulphur colloid images reflect radiotracer accumulation in the reticuloendothelial cells, or fixed macrophages, of the marrow. We have previously demonstrated that the distribution of marrow activity is similar on leucocyte and sulphur colloid images,

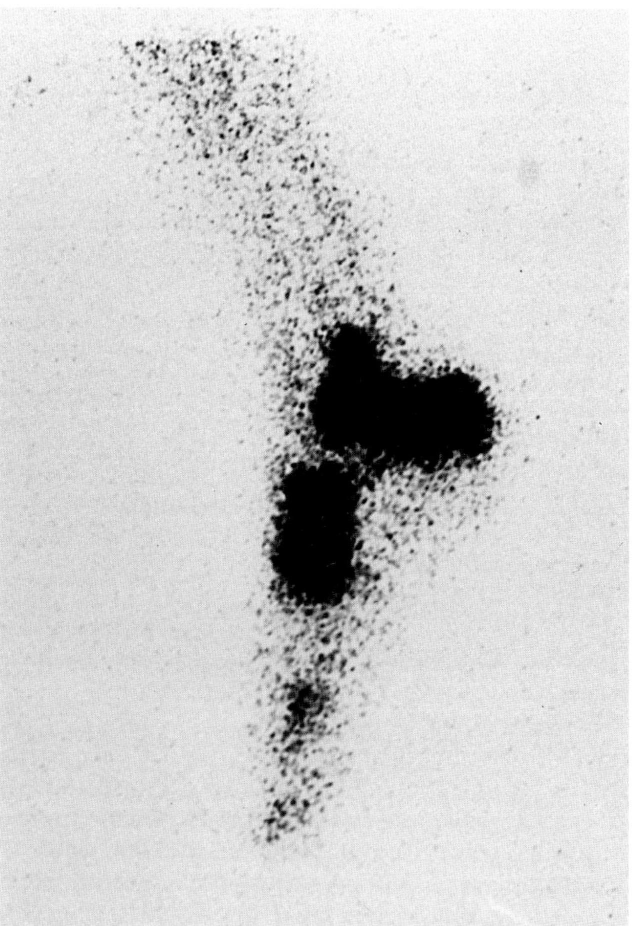

Fig. 83.9C Lateral view obtained after injection of sulphur colloid, confirms that this is functioning marrow, not infection.

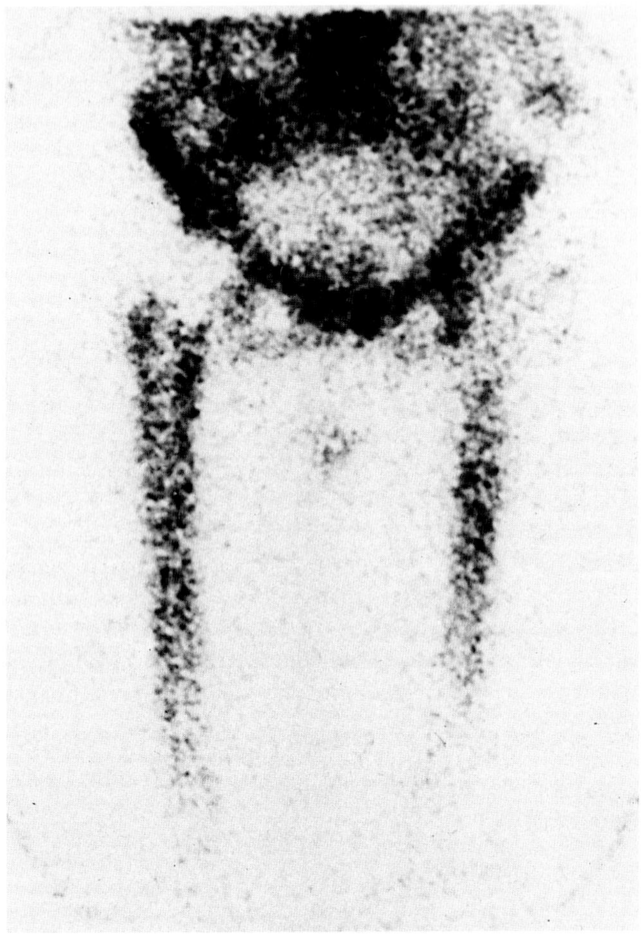

Fig. 83.10A Anterior labelled leucocyte image demonstrates diffuse periprosthetic uptake around the femoral component of a right total hip replacement. This uptake is more intense than the contralateral side.

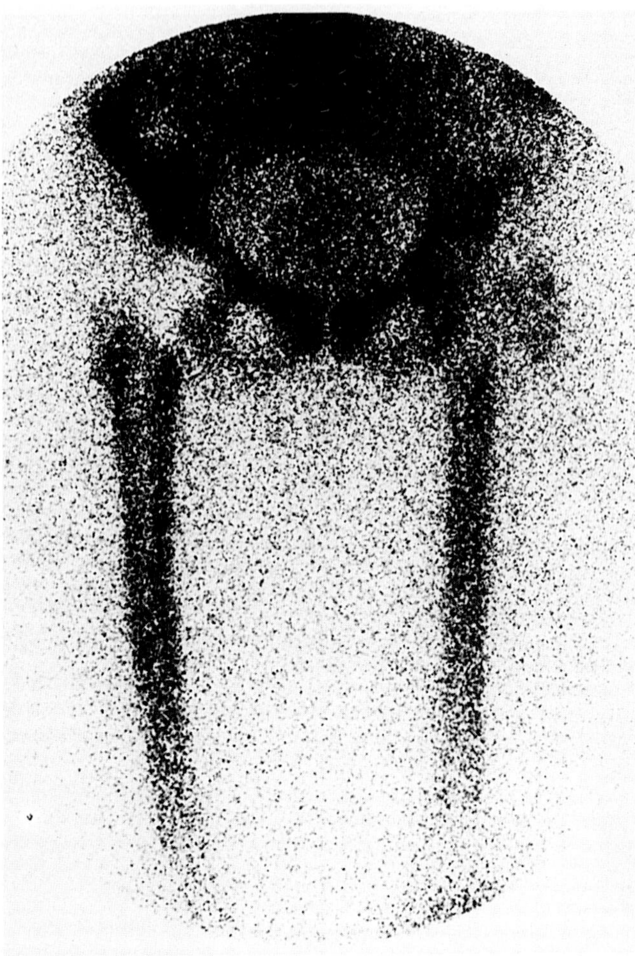

Fig. 83.10B The distribution of periprosthetic activity on the sulphur colloid marrow image is identical to that noted on the labelled leucocyte study. These images are congruent, and the combined leucocyte marrow images are therefore negative for infection.

both in normal individuals as well as in individuals with underlying marrow abnormalities[31] (Fig. 83.9). These images are, in other words, spatially congruent. The one exception to this congruent pattern is infection, i.e. osteomyelitis, which exerts opposite effects on labelled leucocytes and sulphur colloid. While stimulating uptake of white cells, osteomyelitis suppresses uptake of sulphur colloid. In osteomyelitis, therefore, in contrast to other conditions that affect the marrow, leucocyte and marrow images are dissimilar, or spatially incongruent.

In what was one of the earliest descriptions of the leucocyte–marrow imaging technique, Mulamba et al[32] reported a sensitivity of 92% and a specificity of 100% for diagnosing infected hip replacements with combined leucocyte marrow imaging. (They did not, however, provide the results of labelled leucocyte images interpreted in isolation.) We reviewed the results of labelled leucocyte imaging performed on 92 total hip replacements, including 50 which were also studied with sulphur colloid marrow imaging[24] (Fig. 83.10). The results of leucocyte imaging, interpreted in isolation, varied with the criterion selected for a positive study. When any periprosthetic activity was considered positive for infection, the sensitivity of the technique was 100%, yet the specificity was only 23%. When only periprosthetic activity more intense than the contralateral side was considered positive for infection, the sensitivity fell to 65%, while the specificity rose to 61%. In contrast, when the leucocyte and marrow images were interpreted together, and the criterion for a positive study was the presence of periprosthetic labelled leucocyte activity without corresponding activity on the sulphur colloid image (incongruent images) the sensitivity of the study was 100%, and the specificity 97%. We subsequently obtained equally satisfactory results using this technique to evaluate painful knee prostheses, and found leucocyte–marrow imaging to be superior to bone scintigraphy (including three-phase) alone, leucocyte imaging alone, and combined leucocyte–bone imaging in this population[7] (Figs 83.11 and 83.12). These very satisfactory results have been reported by other investigators as well, with the overall accuracy of the technique ranging between 89% and 98%.[33,34] The reason why leucocyte–marrow imaging has proved so valuable is that this procedure eliminates the fundamental problem inherent in labelled leucocyte imaging of musculoskeletal infection: the inability of the technique, based upon patterns of distribution or intensity of uptake, to separate marrow from infection.

Fig. 83.11 Images performed on woman with a painful 2-year-old left total knee replacement. In addition to bilateral femoral shaft activity, the labelled leucocyte image (A) demonstrates activity around both the femoral and (especially) the tibial components. Sulphur colloid image

Being confronted by numerous techniques, how then does one approach the radionuclide diagnosis of the infected joint replacement, or orthopaedic hardware in general? While there are as many answers to this question as there are procedures available, my recommendations are as follows. The first procedure that should be performed is labelled leucocyte imaging. If there is no periprosthetic activity present on the images, the study is negative for infection, and the radionuclide work-up is complete. The addition of sulphur colloid imaging adds nothing to the diagnosis under these circumstances, and need not be performed. More often, however, it is the case that there is at least some periprosthetic activity. In this situation, upon completion of the white cell study, marrow imaging should be performed. If the distribution of the two radiotracers is spatially congruent (regardless of intensity), the study is negative. If the images are spatially incongruent, and the incongruence results from leucocyte image activity without corresponding marrow image activity (*not* vice versa) the prosthesis is infected. For those situations in which, for whatever reason, labelled leucocyte imaging cannot be performed, then sequential bone–gallium imaging should be the radionuclide procedure used.

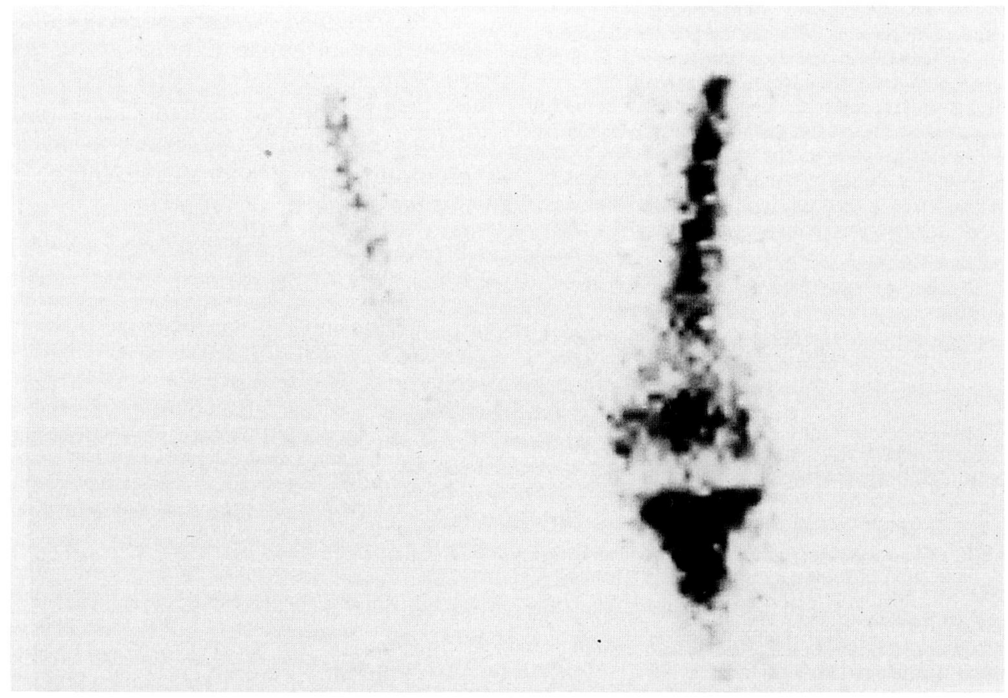

Fig. 83.11 (B) demonstrates a nearly identical distribution of radiotracer. The leucocyte marrow images are congruent, indicating that there is no infection. A loose, but uninfected prosthesis was surgically confirmed. (Reproduced with permission from Palestro et al[7].)

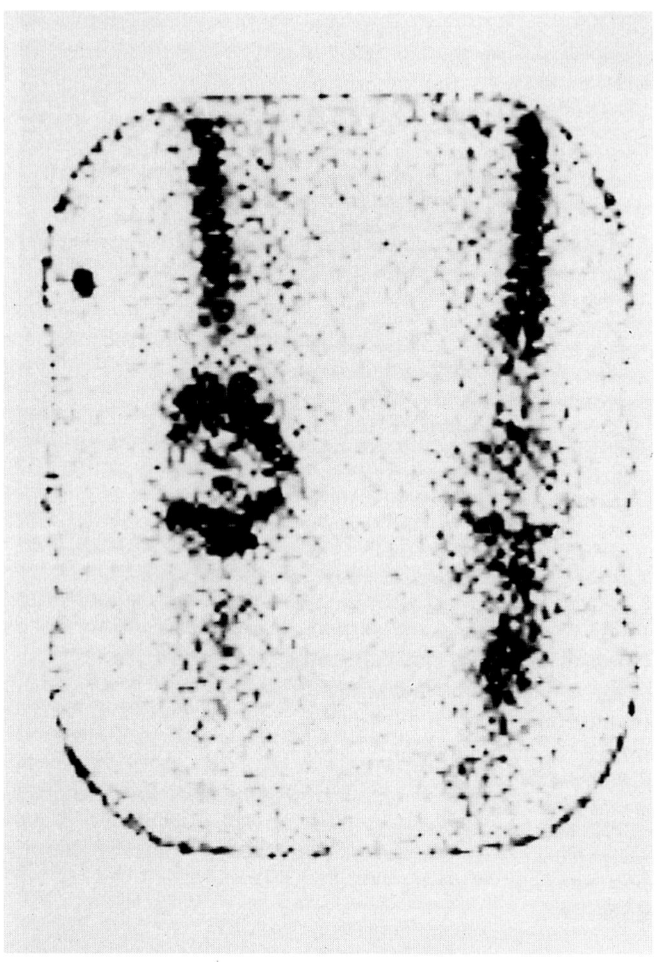

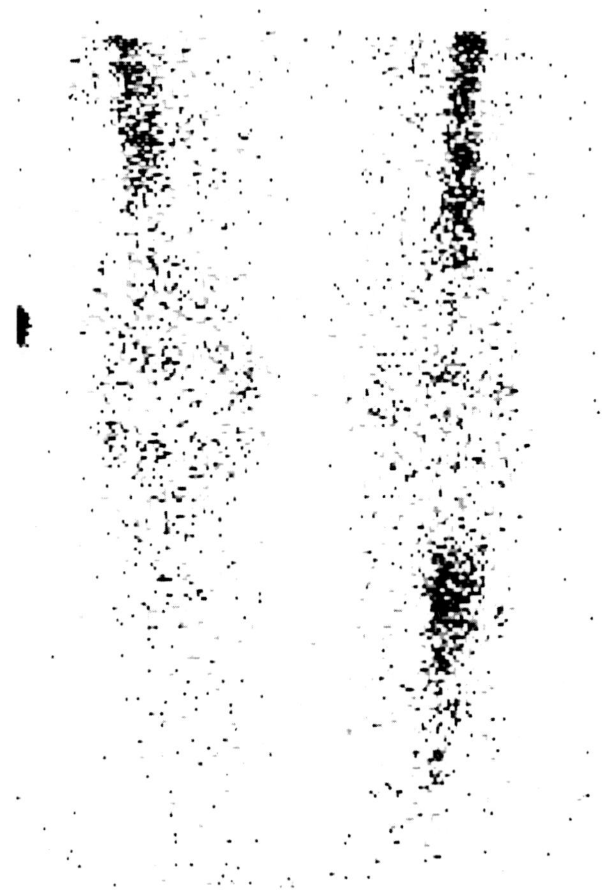

Fig. 83.12 An 85-year-old man with 4-year-old bilateral knee replacements was studied for possible infection. Labelled leucocyte image (A) demonstrates bilateral femoral shaft activity as well as intense periprosthetic uptake around both components of the right knee replacement and the proximal aspect of the tibial component of the left knee replacement. Activity on the sulphur colloid image (B) is limited to the femoral shafts and distal left tibia. The leucocyte marrow images of both knees are incongruent and consistent with bilateral infected knee replacements, which was subsequently confirmed at surgery. (Reproduced with permission from Palestro et al[7].)

The radionuclide diagnosis of the infected joint replacement (and orthopaedic hardware in general) has a long and complicated history, and each new development has resulted in improved patient care. Though it is my belief that at the present time leucocyte–marrow imaging is the procedure of choice for this diagnostic dilemma, it is also my hope that in the near future, simpler single isotope studies that yield superior results will be available.

REFERENCES

1. Gelman M I, Coleman R E, Stevens P M, Davey B W 1978 Radiography, radionuclide imaging, and arthrography in the evaluation of total hip and knee replacement. Radiology 128: 677–682
2. Weiss P E, Mall J C, Hoffer P B, Murray W R, Rodrigo J J, Genant H K 1979 ^{99m}Tc-methylenediphosphonate bone imaging in the evaluation of total hip prostheses. Radiology 133: 727–729
3. Williamson B R J, McLaughlin R E, Wang G J, Miller C W, Teates C D, Bray S T 1979 Radionuclide bone imaging as a means of differentiating loosening and infection in patients with a painful total hip prosthesis. Radiology 133: 723–726
4. Williams F, McCall I W, Park W M, O'Connor B T, Morris V 1981 Gallium-67 scanning in the painful total hip replacement. Clin Rad 32: 431–439
5. Mountford P J, Hall F M, Wells C P, Coakley A J 1986 ^{99}Tc^{m}-MDP, ^{67}Ga-citrate and ^{111}In-leucocytes for detecting prosthetic hip infection. Nucl Med Comm 7: 113–120
6. Aliabadi P, Tumeh S S, Weissman B N, McNeil B J 1989 Cemented total hip prosthesis: radiographic and scintigraphic evaluation. Radiology 173: 203–206
7. Palestro C J, Swyer A J, Kim C K, Goldsmith S J 1991 Infected knee prosthesis: diagnosis with In-111 leukocyte, Tc-99m sulfur colloid, and Tc-99m MDP imaging. Radiology 179: 645–648
8. Magnuson J E, Brown M L, Hauser M F, Berquist T H, Fitzgerald R H Jr, Klee G G 1988 In-111-labeled leukocyte scintigraphy in suspected orthopedic prosthesis infection: comparison with other imaging modalities. Radiology 168: 235–239
9. Sciuk J, Puskas C, Greitemann B, Schober O 1992 White blood cell scintigraphy with monoclonal antibodies in the study of the infected endoprosthesis. Eur J Nucl Med 19: 497–502

10. Utz J A, Lull R J, Galvin E G 1986 Asymptomatic total hip prosthesis: natural history determined using Tc-99m MDP bone scans. Radiology 161: 509–512
11. Oswald S G, Van Nostrand D, Savory C G, Callaghan J J 1989 Three-phase bone scan and indium white blood cell scintigraphy following porous coated hip arthroplasty: a prospective study of the prosthetic tip. J Nucl Med 30: 1321–1331
12. Oswald S G, Van Nostrand D, Savory C G, Anderson J H, Callaghan J J 1990 The acetabulum: a prospective study of three-phase bone and indium white blood cell scintigraphy following porous-coated hip arthroplasty. J Nucl Med 31: 274–280
13. Rosenthall L, Lepanto L, Raymond F 1987 Radiophosphate uptake in asymptomatic knee arthroplasty. J Nucl Med 28: 1546–1549
14. Reing C M, Richin P F, Kenmore P I 1979 Differential bone-scanning in the evaluation of a painful total joint replacement. J Bone Joint Surg 61-A: 933–936
15. Rushton N, Coakley A J, Tudor J, Wraight E P 1982 The value of technetium and gallium scanning in assessing pain after total hip replacement. J Bone Joint Surg 64-B: 313–318
16. Rosenthall L, Lisbona R, Hernandez M, Hadjipavlou A 1979 ^{99m}Tc-PP and ^{67}Ga imaging following insertion of orthopedic devices. Radiology 133: 717–721
17. Merkel K D, Fitzgerald R H Jr, Brown M L 1984 Scintigraphic examination of total hip arthroplasty: comparison of indium with technetium-gallium in the loose and infected canine arthroplasty. In: Welch R B, ed. The hip. Proceedings of the Twelfth Open Scientific Meeting of the Hip Society, Atlanta. pp 163–192
18. Merkel K D, Brown M L, Fitzgerald R H Jr 1986 Sequential technetium-99m HMDP-gallium-67 citrate imaging for the evaluation of infection in the painful prosthesis. J Nucl Med 27: 1413–1417
19. Gomez-Luzuriaga M A, Galan V, Villar J M 1988 Scintigraphy with Tc, Ga and In in painful total hip prostheses. Int Orthop 12: 163–167
20. Propst-Proctor S L, Dillingham M F, McDougall I R, Goodwin D 1982 The white blood cell scan in orthopedics. Clin Ortho Rel Res 168: 157–165
21. McKillop J H, McKay I, Cuthbert G F, Fogelman I, Gray H W, Sturrock R D 1984 Scintigraphic evaluation of the painful prosthetic joint: a comparison of gallium-67 citrate and indium-111 labelled leukocyte imaging. Clin Rad 35: 239–241
22. Pring D J, Henderson R G, Keshavarzian A et al 1986 Indium-granulocyte scanning in the painful prosthetic joint. AJR 146: 167–172
23. Wukich D K, Abreu S H, Callaghan J J et al 1987 Diagnosis of infection by preoperative scintigraphy with indium-labeled white blood cells. J Bone Joint Surg 69-A: 1353–1360
24. Johnson J A, Christie M J, Sandler M P, Parks P F, Homra L, Kaye J J 1988 Detection of occult infection following total joint arthroplasty using sequential technetium-99m HDP bone scintigraphy and indium-111 WBC imaging. J Nucl Med 29: 1347–1353
25. Palestro C J, Kim C K, Swyer A J, Capozzi J D, Solomon R W, Goldsmith S J 1990 Total-hip arthroplasty: periprosthetic indium-111-labeled leukocyte activity and complementary technetium-99m-sulfur colloid imaging in suspected infection. J Nucl Med 31: 1950–1955
26. Al-Sheikh W, Sfakianakis G N, Mnaymneh W et al 1985 Subacute and chronic bone infections: diagnosis using In-111, Ga-67 and Tc-99m MDP bone scintigraphy, and radiography. Radiology 155: 501–506
27. Prchal C L, Kahen H L, Blend M J, Barmada R 1987 Detection of musculoskeletal infection with the indium-111 leukocyte scan. Orthopedics 10: 1253–1257
28. Schauwecker D S, Park H M, Mock B H et al 1984 Evaluation of complicating osteomyelitis with Tc-99m MDP, In-111 granulocytes, and Ga-67 citrate. J Nucl Med 25: 849–853
29. Palestro C J, Kim C K, Swyer A J, Vallabhajosula S, Goldsmith S J 1991 Radionuclide diagnosis of vertebral osteomyelitis: indium-111-leukocyte and technetium-99m-methylene disphosphonate bone scintigraphy. J Nucl Med 32: 1861–1865
30. Palestro C J, Kim C K, Vega A, Goldsmith S J 1989 Acute effects of radiation therapy on indium-111-labeled leukocyte uptake in bone marrow. J Nucl Med 30: 1989–1991
31. Palestro C J, Charallel J, Vallabhajosula S, Greenberg M, Goldsmith S J 1987 In-WBC as a bone marrow imaging agent. J Nucl Med 27: 574 (Abstract)
32. Mulamba L'A H, Ferrant A, Leners N, deNayer P, Rombouts J J, Vincent A 1983 Indium-111 leucocyte scanning in the evaluation of painful hip arthroplasty. Acta Orthop Scand 54: 695–697
33. King A D, Peters A M, Stuttle A W J, Lavender J P 1990 Imaging of bone infection with labelled white blood cells: role of contemporaneous bone marrow imaging. Eur J Nucl Med 17: 148–151
34. Seabold J E, Nepola J V, Marsh J L et al 1991 Postoperative bone marrow alterations: potential pitfalls in the diagnosis of osteomyelitis with In-111-labeled leukocyte scintigraphy. Radiology 180: 741–747 scintigraphy.

84. Vascular manifestations

I. P. C. Murray

Since changes in blood flow are a significant factor affecting the extraction ratio of the bone-seeking radiopharmaceuticals, it is not surprising that major scintigraphic abnormalities are demonstrable in those skeletal disorders in which altered vascular delivery occurs. These are usually evident in the initial components of the three-phase study to an extent that the dramatic abnormalities in the later static images are totally explicable. Indeed, the effect of altered delivery on the skeletal uptake is such that not only is scintigraphy critical in the assessment of the extent of the disorder but sequential studies are invaluable in assessing progress or monitoring therapy. The vascular insult may be major, such as occurs in trauma, acute or repetitive, but may result from disturbance of the capillary microcirculation. Thus, Sy et al[1] postulated that a useful application of skeletal scintigraphy was imaging of the hands in assessing the vascular status in obliterative vascular disorders, for example scleroderma, in which characteristic accumulation may occur in the distal phalanges (Fig. 84.1). Similar alterations are associated with occupational acro-osteolysis, in which the capillary alterations and sluggish blood flow induced by PVC exposure are aggravated by trauma.[2] Sequential studies show regression following change in occupation (Fig. 84.2). In a variety of disorders in which vascular disruption is not a major aetiological factor, the incidental vascular consequences may permit the bone scan to play a major role in their identification.

PAGET'S DISEASE

Although the initial change in Paget's disease is an intense osteoclastic resorption of bone, this is followed by intense osteoblastic activity accompanied by intense vascularity, replacement of normal lamellar bone with connective tissue with a significant immature collagen content and, ultimately, subperiosteal new bone formation resulting in the characteristic cortical thickening. All of these are fundamental to the mechanisms by which the technetium phosphate complexes localize in bone, and it is not surprising that the changes visualized with skeletal scintigraphy are probably more marked in this disorder than in any other. This is of considerable importance in view of its

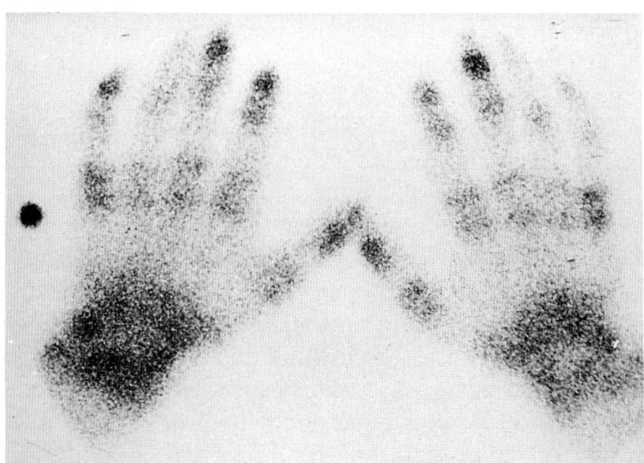

Fig. 84.1 Scleroderma. Foci of accumulation confined to the terminal phalanges.

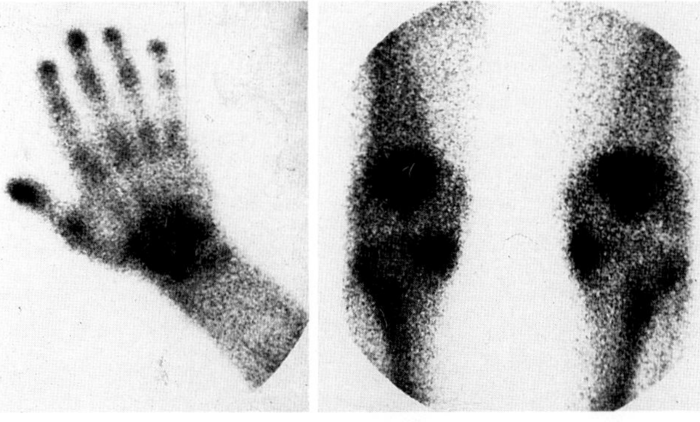

Fig. 84.2 Occupational acro-osteolysis. Scintigraphy in a PVC worker, showing areas of increased uptake, particularly in the terminal digits, both patellae and tibial condyles – all sites of occupational or weight-bearing stress. Similar abnormalities were evident in the left hand and in both feet. Following immediate change of occupation, scintigraphic activity regressed almost completely during the next 3 years.

prevalence, approximately 4–5% in elderly individuals, this probably being an underestimate in view of the frequency with which unsuspected disease is noted totally incidentally in patients undergoing bone scanning for unrelated conditions. While environmental and hereditary factors have been considered important in the aetiology, current evidence favours the disease being due to a slow viral infection of the osteoclast. However, while there are similarities in the distribution of the disease compared with haematogenous osteomyelitis, the haemodynamic changes are such as to warrant consideration of this disease in relation to vascular disorders. Certainly, the initial phases of a routine scintigraphic study are characterized by the intense increase in vascular delivery. This may be sufficiently great that, for example, if the skull is being examined, the radionuclide angiogram of the flow phase may show the preferential diversion through the external carotid arteries and identify the 'steal' from the intracerebral circulation which may result in symptoms of cerebral vascular insufficiency.

The experience of skeletal scintigraphy has had a major impact on many concepts regarding Paget's disease, since the characteristic, yet asymptomatic, lesions are encountered incidentally but regularly in the course of the investigation of some other suspected skeletal disorders. Accordingly, it rapidly became clear that in any patient with Paget's disease, total body surveys are mandatory. While monostotic disease (Fig. 84.3) is relatively common, accounting for approximately 10–25% in various series, such surveys will frequently identify multiple sites of involvement with varying degrees of activity (Fig. 84.4). Many areas of Pagetoid change will not be detected by radiography, confirmed by a number of series, for example 20% in that by Mazieres et al,[3] 16% in that by Vellenga et al[4] and 26% in that by Fogelman & Carr.[5] Fogelman & Carr[5] drew attention to the fact that, while 33 of 127 sites of disease in 23 patients were not visualized on radiographs, one-third of these were in areas difficult to evaluate with standard views, for example scapulae, ribs and sternum. Of course, further lesions can only become visible on radiography when more than 30–50% of the bone has been resorbed. The discrepancy between the modalities is also

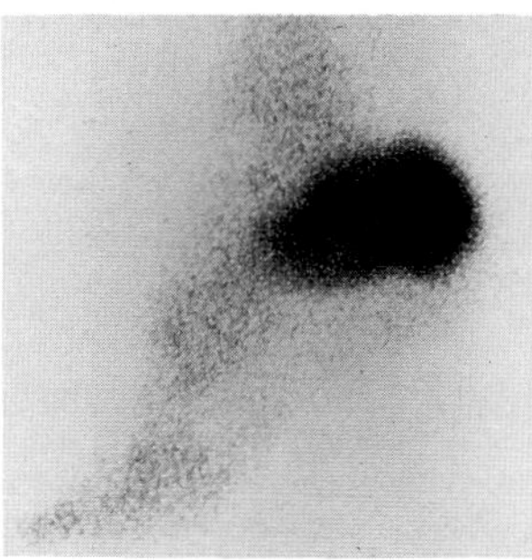

Fig. 84.3 Monostotic Paget's disease involving the calcaneus.

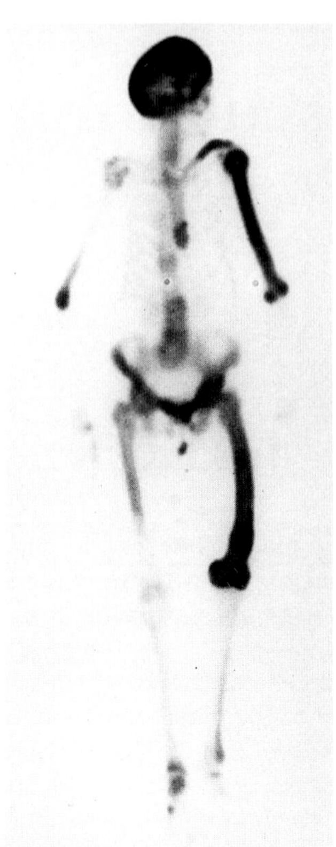

Fig. 84.4 Paget's disease. Characteristic scintigraphy showing polyostotic involvement with diffuse accumulation but varying avidity in different sites.

closely related to the activity of the disease, especially as lesions clearly abnormal on scintigraphy but radiologically normal are generally asymptomatic and therefore probably at early stages of the disorder. Even although a minority of Pagetoid lesions are symptomatic, the most metabolically active are those with the highest uptake and those most likely to be symptomatic. Nevertheless, as shown by Fogelman & Carr,[5] the weight-bearing bones with scintigraphic changes are more likely to be associated with symptoms. It is therefore of particular interest that these authors found headache to be rare in patients with skull involvement even although such involvement is usually manifest as grossly avid accumulation (Fig. 84.5).

The distribution of lesions seen with scintigraphy differs little from that identified radiologically, the pelvis, spine (particularly the lumbar), femur, tibia and skull being most commonly involved. Typically the scintigram shows intense accumulation of the radiopharmaceutical throughout the affected bone with a uniform distribution. Preservation of the normal anatomical configuration is characteristic and assists in the differentiation of Paget's disease from other scan abnormalities. The avidity at the different sites throughout the body may vary considerably. In general, the lesion appears at the articular end, progressing along the shaft, often producing an appearance with the advancing edge having a sharp V-shaped outline, paralleling the 'flame-shape' resorption seen radiologically (Fig. 84.6). In the purely lytic stage, the uptake may be low grade with relatively greater accumulation at the advancing edge. This phenomenon is most commonly observed in the skull, presenting as osteoporosis circumscripta (Fig. 84.7). The major factor affecting the radionuclide uptake does appear to be the cellular activity, reflecting the metabolic status of the disorder, although mild uptake may persist in the 'burnout' or treated lesions, probably the consequence of continuing bone remodelling. However, 'burnout' lesions without metabolic activity and therefore not visible on the bone scan will be detected radiologically with sclerotic changes.

While the pattern of activity is usually uniform, conforming to the bony outline, it may occasionally be somewhat patchy (Fig. 84.8). This causes problems of interpretation, particularly in the pelvis, when alternative pathologies such as metastatic disease pose a clinical problem. Since both can occur simultaneously, each lesion must then be assessed individually. On occasion, metastatic lesions can be identified as being photopenic. Even a fracture with reactive change may be extremely difficult to identify since focal increased uptake is superimposed on the generalized high uptake. The major concern lies in the identification of a complicating osteogenic sarcoma even although it occurs in less than 1% of patients with Paget's disease. This must be suspected when there is local and significant distortion of the bony outline. Shirazi et al[6] pointed out the difficulties in differentiating Paget's

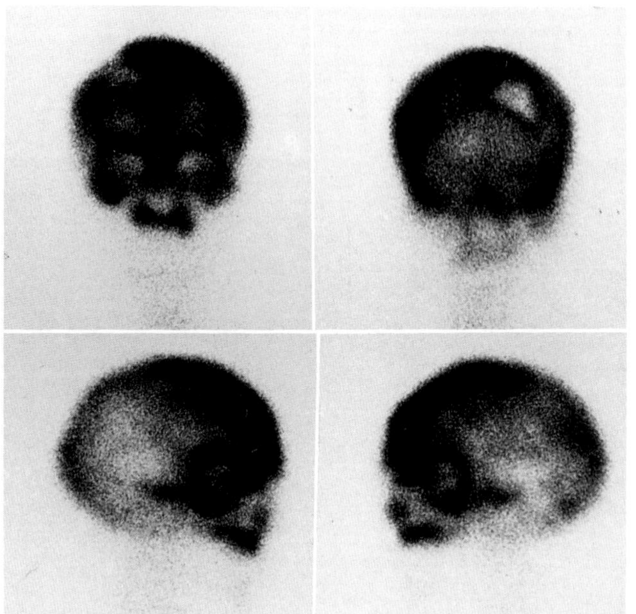

Fig. 84.5 Paget's disease. Characteristic alterations involving the skull.

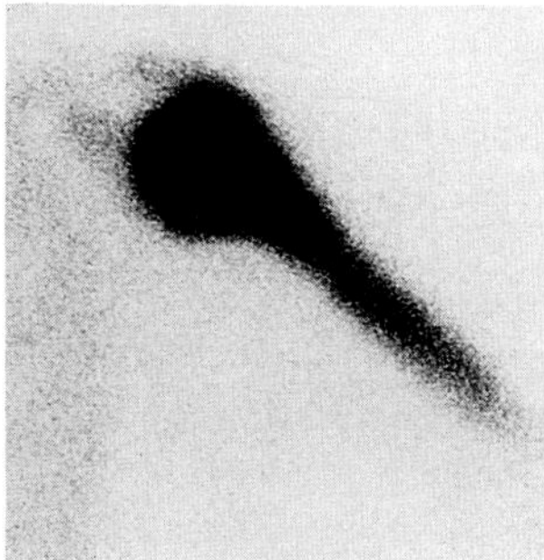

Fig. 84.6 Paget's disease. Intense accumulation in the upper humerus in a characteristic pattern.

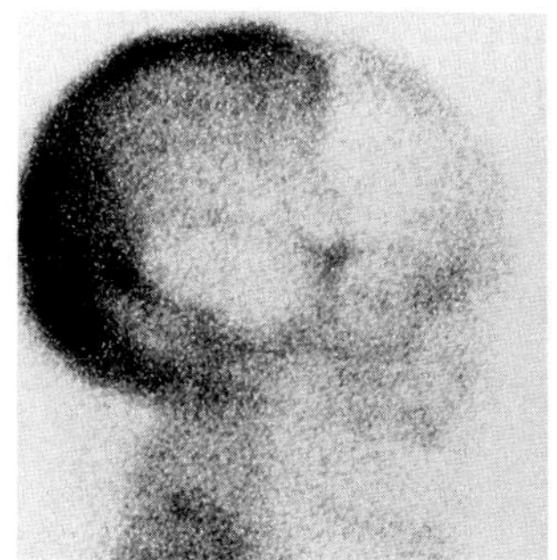

Fig. 84.7 Paget's disease. Typical scintigraphic alterations in osteoporosis circumscripta.

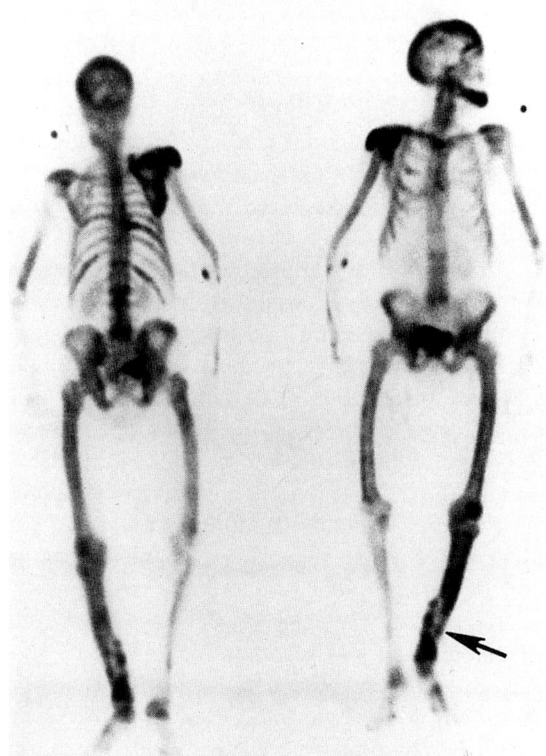

Fig. 84.8 Paget's disease. The difficulties in interpretation arising from the variability of the scintigraphic appearances of Paget's disease is demonstrated by the whole body survey in a 77-year-old male. The distribution is patchy and irregular, particularly in the vertebral column and ribs, raising suspicion of metastatic disease especially as there is evidence of an osteosarcoma in the left tibia (Fig. 84.9). Pulmonary metastases were identified later, but none in bone.

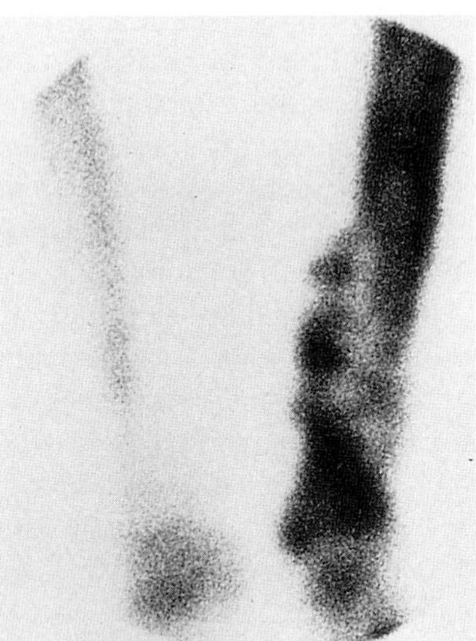

Fig. 84.9 Malignant change in Paget's disease. Osteosarcoma visualized as a clearly defined area, with patchy areas of uptake, within intense accumulation in the left tibia. Metastases developed later in the lungs, but none in bone (cf. Fig. 84.8).

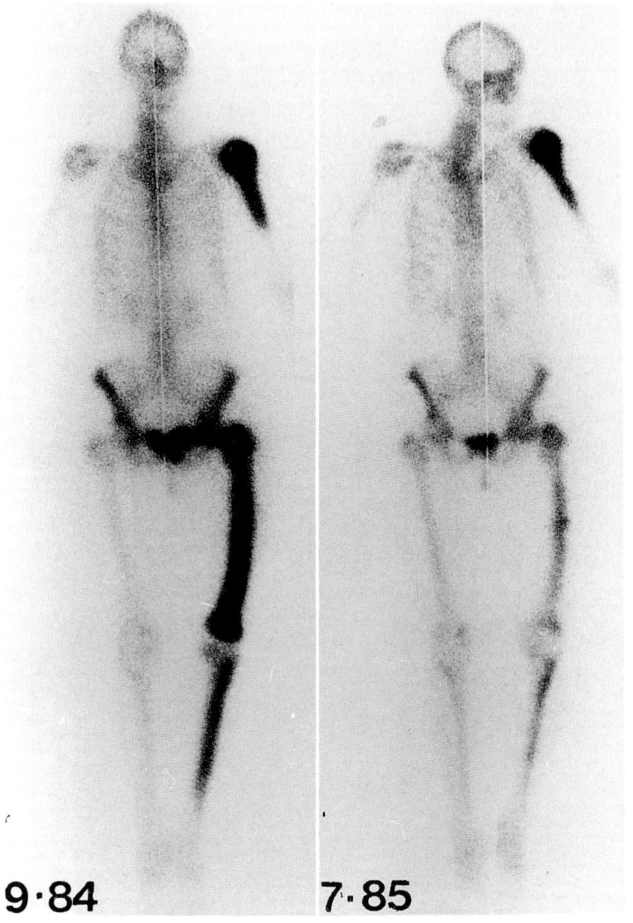

Fig. 84.10 Paget's disease. Evaluation of therapy with calcitonin, comparing the characteristic scintigraphic appearances, particularly in the left femur and tibia and left humerus, with the appearances following 9 months' therapy.

disease from this complication because of the intense uptake occurring in both, although they emphasized that the typical finding associated with osteosarcoma was the extraskeletal extension of activity beyond the margins of bones. However, it has been recognized that reduced uptake in sarcoma is much more common (Fig. 84.9), 13 of the 17 patients reported by Smith et al[7] having decreased accumulation of ^{99m}Tc-MDP, although less apparently reduced in the remaining four. Yeh et al[8] recommended the use of supplementary ^{67}Ga scintigraphy, reporting that preferential gallium uptake at the site of sarcoma could be identified.

The introduction of appropriate therapy is usually followed by satisfactory reduction of symptoms accompanied by significant regression of the scintigraphic abnormalities (Fig. 84.10). Attempts have been made to evaluate the overall activity of the disease in various ways in order to permit monitoring of such response to therapy. The vascularity so typical of the disease and obvious in the diagnostic study can also be of value in assessing therapy. The changes in perfusion were studied by Boudreau et al,[9] who considered them to be more reliable in the bone scan as an indicator of disease activity, correctly anticipating the eventual rise or fall in alkaline phosphatase. However, the clinical usefulness of this technique is limited by the fact that only one disease area can be assessed within the gamma-camera field of view. Further, not all lesions will respond to therapy equally. Vellenga et al[10] introduced a qualitative grading of the intensity and extent of the scan changes in every site, deriving an overall scintigraphic index. Subsequently these authors[10] found that computer quantitation of changes in radioactivity, comparing involved bone with areas of normal bone, was comparable, but overall more sensitive in detecting alterations induced by therapy. In 27 patients in whom the scintigraphy was performed after diphosphonate therapy, significant alterations were detected by quantitation alone in 40%. Other approaches have been recommended by various authors, but have not gained widespread acceptance. Smith et al,[11] for example, did show that a 24 h whole-body retention of ^{99m}Tc phosphonate measurement did accurately reflect disease activity. Alternative imaging radiopharmaceuticals have also not found a significant clinical role. Waxman et al[12] suggested that ^{67}Ga accumulation reflected biochemical changes more accurately than diphosphonate. The role of ^{201}Tl remains uncertain since experience differs in various series as to the frequency of the uptake of this radionuclide in Paget's disease. Dunn et al[13] noted the absence of accumulation of ^{111}In leucocytes in sites of Paget's disease associated with positive uptake of MDP and ^{67}Ga. Although Palestro et al[14] demonstrated a correlation between the extent of photopenia occurring with ^{111}In leucocyte imaging with the disease stage, the procedure has no role in monitoring treatment as it indicates the loss of marrow through displacement by abnormal proliferating or sclerotic osteoid tissue.

While observation of deterioration of the appearances in a bone scan will provide a sensitive means of anticipating the recurrence of the disease during clinical remission, there is little predictive value in obtaining a study which is unchanged, and the general consensus is that there is little justification in obtaining serial bone scans on the chance that an alteration might be noted and thus anticipate the relapse. However, the continued introduction of new and increasingly effective drugs for the treatment of Paget's disease has emphasized that there is a role for the bone scan in the assessment of the efficacy of such treatment. Difficulties arise from the natural history of the disease, which results in a variation in intensity of radiopharmaceutical uptake in lesions, reflecting the changes in bone resorption and bone formation. This was demonstrated by Patel et al[15] in untreated patients. In comparison, after treatment, they observed an overall improvement but, although the changes in the lesions were usually of a greater degree than is normal, there was no uniform pattern. Indeed, while uptake was normalized in 20 lesions, new abnormal sites developed in five patients. In contrast, Vellenga et al found that a uniform decrease in all Pagetoid sites followed the use of both combined calcitonin and EHDP[16] and of pamidronate.[17] A variable response followed pamidronate therapy in the study by Ryan et al,[18] who emphasized that the scan appearances may change from predominantly uniform to predominantly focal, risking the possibility of causing confusion with metastatic deposits. While normalization was not required for relief of symptoms, they concluded that the bone scan appearances did assist in the assessment of need for further treatment.

FIBROUS DYSPLASIA

Since fibrous dysplasia is characterized by fibrous replacement of portions of the medullary cavities of bone or bones, the scintigraphic appearances have similarities to those in Paget's disease. Similar intense hyperaemia and marked radiopharmaceutical accumulation are to be expected. While the margins are usually well delineated, lack of preservation of the bony outline provides differentiation (Fig. 84.11). Rarely, there may be multiple small discrete focal areas of increased accumulation causing suspicion of metastatic bone disease. Machida et al,[19] reviewing 26 patients found that 4 of 40 cystic lesions and 2 of 30 radiologically 'ground glass' lesions did not show the typical increased uptake. Hardoff & Gips[20] identified a lesion in the skull only with the use of SPECT, which they also found to be useful to define accurately the site and extent of lesions. The mandibular lesions of cherubism can usually be readily identified.[21] The extent of craniofacial fibrous dysplasia is usually obvious, but as up to 25%

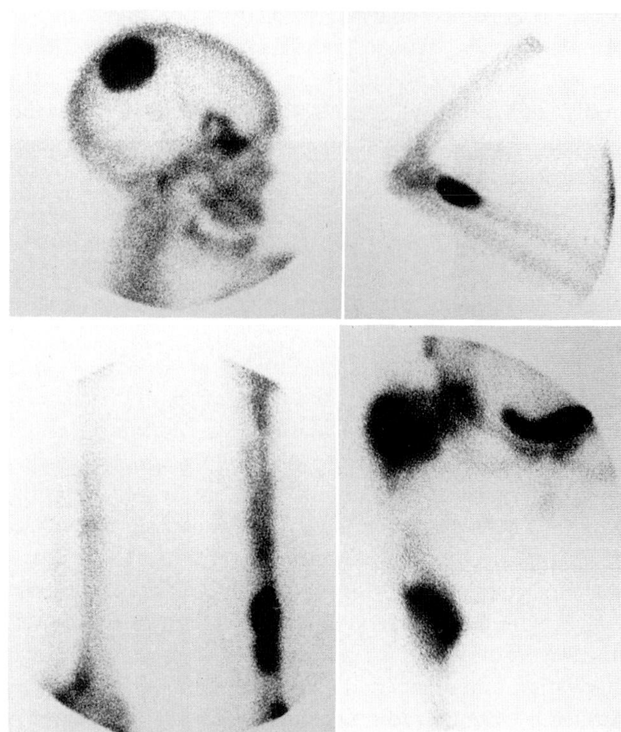

Fig. 84.11 Polyostotic fibrous dysplasia. Multiple areas of well-delineated and intense accumulation in numerous sites.

of these children have at least one other site of involvement elsewhere in the skeleton a whole-body study is warranted. Identification of such polyostotic involvement is one of the main indications for the skeletal scintigraphy, since many of the lesions will be asymptomatic. The scintigraphic changes in the McCune–Albright syndrome, in which polyostotic fibrous dysplasia is a characteristic component have been studied by Pfeffer et al.[22] They found that the distribution of the lesions varied somewhat from those occurring in idiopathic fibrous dysplasia,[23] although the skull, facial bones and legs were similarly the most commonly involved. In view of the pathological changes it is not surprising that there is intense gallium accumulation in the sites of fibrous dysplasia and decreased uptake of indium-labelled leucocytes in these sites.

OSTEONECROSIS

A variety of pathological events may be responsible for the disruption of blood supply causing necrosis of bone. They include mechanical interruption of the arterial flow, occlusion by thombosis or embolism, sludging within the vessel or damage to vessel wall and obstruction to the venous return. One alone may be sufficient to produce crucial oxygen deprivation or there may be an interaction of several, culminating in the catastrophe.[24] Despite intensive study, the exact cause of the vascular insufficiency in several conditions characterized by bone necrosis, for example Perthes' disease, remains uncertain. Common to all, however, is the death of the osteocytes, which occurs rapidly, experimental studies showing that 12 h may be sufficient. Surrounding bone responds with hyperaemia and fibrous deposition, providing a zone from which revascularization commences in a few weeks. Blood vessels, 'cutting cones', invade the dead bone, removing the necrotic tissue by osteoclastic resorption and introducing osteoblasts for the synthesis of new bones by 'creeping substitution'. It is only at this stage that radiological features become apparent, whereas bone scintigraphy readily identifies the formative events. The chronological appearances of the scan alterations reflect the sequential pathological processes. In animal studies, the initial marrow death may be identified by scanning with ^{99m}Tc antimony colloid.[25] The sensitivity of the ^{99m}Tc diphosphonates to demonstrate the absence of uptake in viable osteocytes by 72 h was shown by Ruland et al,[26] who also observed that no alterations in MRI images were apparent for 6 weeks. Subsequently the revascularization and associated exuberant osteoblastic repair is revealed by intense radiopharmaceutical accumulation. As these observations have been fully upheld with routine clinical experience, skeletal scintigraphy has a major role in the diagnosis and management of the various conditions characterized by ischaemic necrosis of bone.

Bone infarction may occur at a single site or be disseminated. If the latter, the infarcts often are the result of a systemic disorder in which the disease is characterized by occlusion of small vessels. Typical of these is sickle cell disease, in the course of which sickle cell crises are associated with multiple infarcts, some of which are asymptomatic (Fig. 84.12). All areas will, however, be demonstrable within 2 days as regions of photopenia. It is of importance to note the extraosseous uptake in splenic infarcts which may occur. Revascularization results from collateral channels, predominantly the periosteal supply, where it is observed as peripheral stripes of increased uptake which extend as the healing process proceeds.[27] The exception to this sequence, as Greyson & Kassel[28] emphasize, may occur at the epiphyseal location if the epiphyseal collaterals are adequate (Fig. 84.13). In these circumstances, no true infarct would occur, but with ischaemia sufficient to stimulate osteoblastic response increased uptake would be noted without an initial 'cold' area. Such an occurrence would enhance the difficulty in differentiating such infarction from osteomyelitis. This may be frequently suspected in sickling crises. Gallium scintigraphy may be required, Armas & Goldsmith[29] showing that the uptake will be decreased or absent in acute infarction and normal in healing infarcts which show increased uptake on the bone scan. It may be invaluable in differentiating septic infarction from fulminating infection with photopenia.

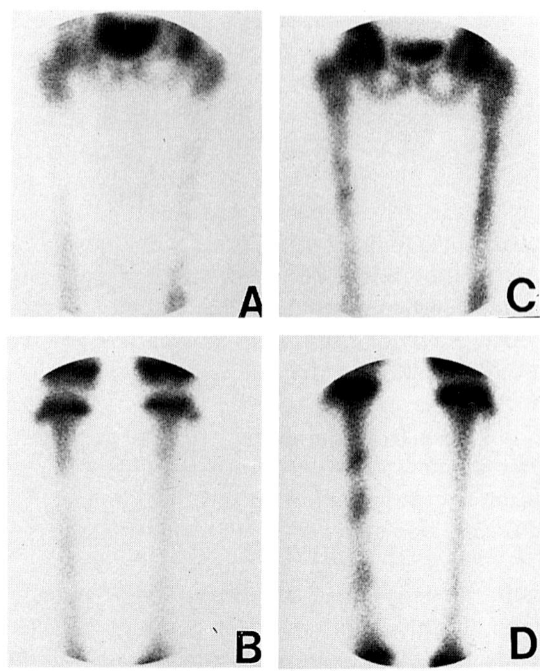

Fig. 84.12 Sickle cell disease. Views of the legs of an 8-year-old child presenting with bone pain, demonstrating multiple areas of decreased accumulation indicative of sites of bone infarction (A and B). A further study (C and D) 4 weeks later demonstrates increased uptake in these areas, the result of revascularization.

Similar mechanisms operate in Gaucher's disease, in which the intramedullary circulation is reduced by the accumulation of cerebroglycosides. The scan changes of the resulting bone ischaemia were reviewed by Israel et al,[30] finding the expected reduction in uptake initially and subsequently the increased accumulation. They did identify increased uptake at an early stage in one patient as the result of a fracture and in another caused by osteomyelitis, confirmed by preferential ^{67}Ga localization. Bilchik & Hayman[31] emphasized the similarity between the clinical features of 'pseudo-osteomyelitis' in the bone crises of this disorder and those of bone infection and the value of observing the photopenia in the first few days. Radiation osteonecrosis, although dose-related, probably results from alterations in the microvasculature rather than direct radiation damage to the bone cells. The similar changes, characterized by absent uptake, which result from frostbite,[32] are probably the result of alterations in the vessel walls leading to erythrocyte sludging.

Post-traumatic necrosis

The diversity of experience regarding the incidence of avascular necrosis of the femoral head following a subcapital fracture of the femoral neck parallels the differences in opinion regarding the indications for endoprosthetic replacement, even although the results of the use of this as a primary procedure in unselected patients have been

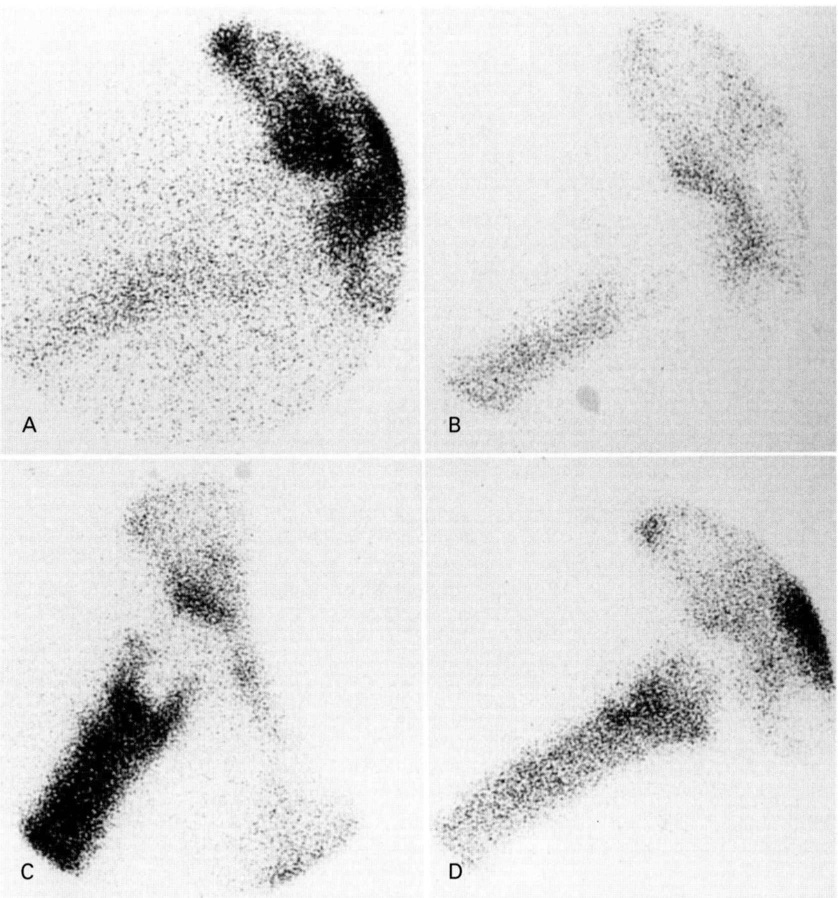

Fig. 84.13 Septic infarction of femur. Serial studies in a 14-month-old girl presenting with fever and marked swelling of the right thigh. (A) Pinhole view of right hip on admission, with markedly reduced uptake in femoral head, neck and upper shaft, more extensive than expected from even fulminant osteomyelitis. A gallium study was identical. (B) Study performed 1 week later with similar changes. (C) Study after a further 2 weeks, demonstrating intense accumulation in the femoral shaft with peripheral 'stripes' of periosteal revascularization of the septic infarction in the upper femur. (D) Further pinhole view obtained 9 weeks after admission, showing further revascularization of the infarcted femur.

satisfactory. The preoperative identification of those at high risk is obviously desirable. While there is significant correlation between the degree of displacement of the femoral head and ischaemia, radiology is not sufficiently reliable and has led to numerous studies attempting to evaluate the role of skeletal scintigraphy in the early demonstration of the effect of the disruption of the blood supply. The scan appearances will depend on the time since injury since they closely parallel pathological changes in the femoral head, confirmed by the close correlation between MDP scintigraphy and simultaneous tetracycline labelling. Thus, initially it may be possible to identify a 'cold' area in the head indicating the avascularity and reduced delivery of the radiopharmaceutical (Fig. 84.14). There may be a 'doughnut', the image of this photopenic centre surrounded by the region of hyperaemia and reactive change. Subsequently the photopenic area diminishes as there is ingrowth of osteoblasts upwards into the head so that ultimately, as healing progresses, there is uniform intense radioactivity throughout. Many investigators have found observation of these changes to be reliable in ascertaining the viability of the femoral head. Lucie et al,[33] studying 53 patients with femoral neck fracture, noted entirely normal images in 17/19 femoral heads shown to be viable but abnormalities in 31/34 in whom avascular necrosis was confirmed. Despite their accuracy of prediction of 92.5%, controversy still surrounds the value of the procedure and various alternatives to standard planar scintigraphy have been suggested. Stromqvist et al,[34] for example, obtained ratios comparing the fractured with the intact side and concluded that MDP imaging performed within 3 weeks reveals reduced capital activity in about 50% of fractures and that imaging can predict their healing course. Many of the problems reflect the difficulties in actually visualizing the femoral head itself. Initially the bone abnormality may be masked by soft-

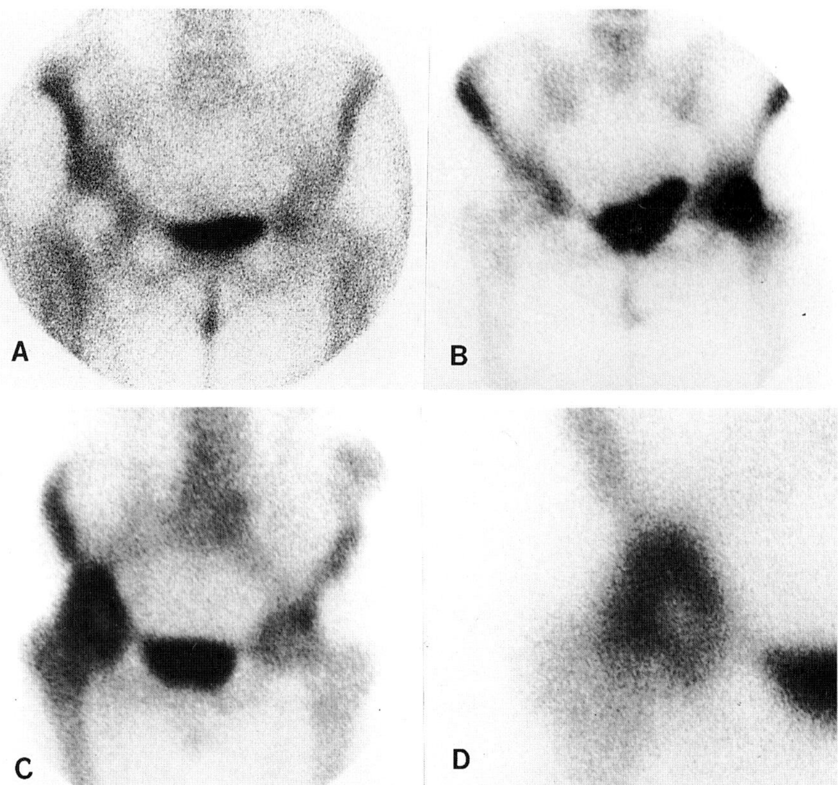

Fig. 84.14 Avascular necrosis of the femoral head. (A) Femoral head ischaemia is demonstrated as total lack of accumulation soon after the injury, prior to evidence of uptake at the fracture site. (B) Total revascularization is visualized with intense increased uptake throughout a femoral head. (C) Advanced revascularization is evident in the femoral head but a small ill-defined area of diminished accumulation can just be visualized within the avid accumulation. (D) A magnification view obtained by 'zoom' delineated the 'cold' area poorly demonstrated in (C), surrounded by activity resulting from bone healing and secondary osteoarthritis in the acetabulum.

tissue hyperaemia, and in the reparative phase by the ring of activity due to bony healing and secondary hip joint osteoarthritis. These problems can be overcome by the use of emission tomography (SPECT) (Fig. 84.15). Thus, Collier et al[35] were able to identify the photopenic defect of avascular necrosis in 17 of 20 involved hips, whereas with planar imaging only 11 were detected. They suggested that a major role for the procedure was in the identification within the revascularizing femoral head of the persistent photopenic defect resulting from incomplete femoral head revascularization. They commented that there was no instance in which pinhole views demonstrated a defect unidentified by SPECT. Geuen et al[36] found that in adults, SPECT revealed eight patients with alterations in the femoral head indicative of avascular necrosis, whereas only five of these abnormalities were seen on pinhole images. The difficulties experienced with SPECT due to the 'bladder artefact' to a certain extent reflects the change in radioactivity in the bladder due to the increasing accumulation of urine throughout the study. Improved studies are possible with a shorter acquisition time using multiheaded cameras. Lee et al[37] using triple headed SPECT, found that the sensitivity in detecting femoral head avascular necrosis was 97% compared with 82% with planar studies, higher than previously reported using single headed SPECT.

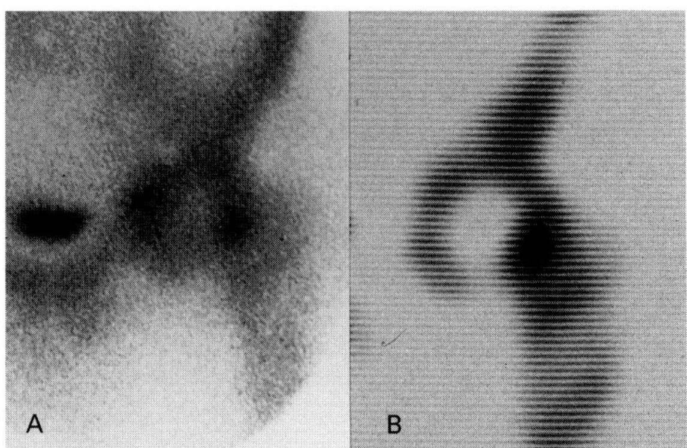

Fig. 84.15 SPECT in the identification of avascular necrosis. In a patient with a fractured neck of femur there is again a 'doughnut' appearance in the planar view (A). SPECT (B) permits clear identification of the linear uptake at the fracture site and the total absence of accumulation in the femoral head indicating avascular necrosis which had been marked by the superficial hyperaemia.

In view of the fact that death of the myeloid elements precedes osteocytic death, radiocolloid imaging has been

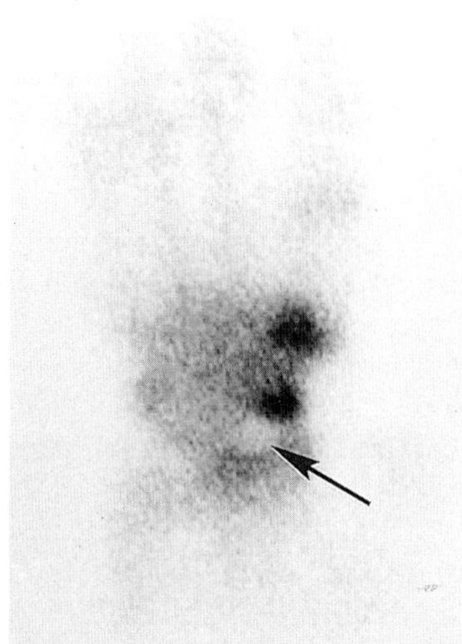

Fig. 84.16 Avascular necrosis of the scaphoid. Whereas the distal pole of a fractured scaphoid shows focal increased uptake there is a void in the proximal pole indicative of avascular necrosis. Reaction to the trauma is also noted with accumulation in the metacarpophalangeal joint.

claimed to be superior to the technetium phosphate agents in determining the viability of the femoral head within the first 24 h. Employing ^{99m}Tc sulphur colloid, Myers et al[38] believed that it was possible to predict avascular necrosis with 95% accuracy. Phillips et al[39] identified 24/28 femoral heads shown to be avascular by tetracycline labelling, although there were four false positives in 30 patients. Williams et al,[40] however, found entirely normal hip uptake of colloid in only 27% of 28 normal patients, the others having variable degrees of diminished accumulation. Turner[25] preferred ^{99m}Tc antimony colloid, which is associated with significantly greater marrow uptake, and found that 11 of 12 patients with diminished accumulation subsequently developed osteonecrosis. However, inactive bone marrow in two patients prevented interpretation. Similarly, Spencer et al[41] were unable to identify colloid uptake in the femoral head in the majority of patients. Because of this difficulty, reflecting the paucity of marrow activity in the femoral head, particularly in the elderly, colloid scintigraphy has not gained popularity.

The possibility of avascular necrosis of the scaphoid is often of concern. It is possible to identify the small necrotic fragment, usually proximal, as photopenic[42] (Fig. 84.16), while the demonstration of the focal area of hyperaemia and increased uptake does provide reassurance in indicating ongoing revascularization. Reinus et al[43] found that bone scans were more sensitive than MRI although less specific. Shafq et al[44] found scintigraphy of value in the identification and follow-up of aseptic necrosis of the talus following injury.

Steroid-induced osteonecrosis

It is difficult to predict which patients receiving steroid therapy will develop osteonecrosis. Estimates of the frequency range from 2–4% to over 25%. While the risk increases with the dose and duration, there is no clear correlation with either factor. This variability probably reflects the variety of mechanics postulated as being responsible for osteonecrosis in patients receiving exogenous steroids. The relative role of the different pathological changes remains controversial,[24] although a major factor is now considered to be the impedance of blood flow, arterial and venous, caused by an increase in the size of marrow fat cells. The differing changes which can be observed with scintigraphy suggest that the aetiology can indeed be multifactorial. On occasion, a large photopenic area, similar to those resulting from major vascular disruption, may be noted, for example in a humeral or femoral head. It is more likely that such areas will be associated with intense hyperconcentration of the radiopharmaceutical indicative of revascularization, since this will usually have commenced prior to the onset of symptoms. Such evidence of major osteonecrosis is less common than the demonstration of patchy increased accumulation, sometimes with a pattern of numerous areas of linear increased uptake (Fig. 84.17). Such findings are totally compatible with the hypothesis that steroid-induced

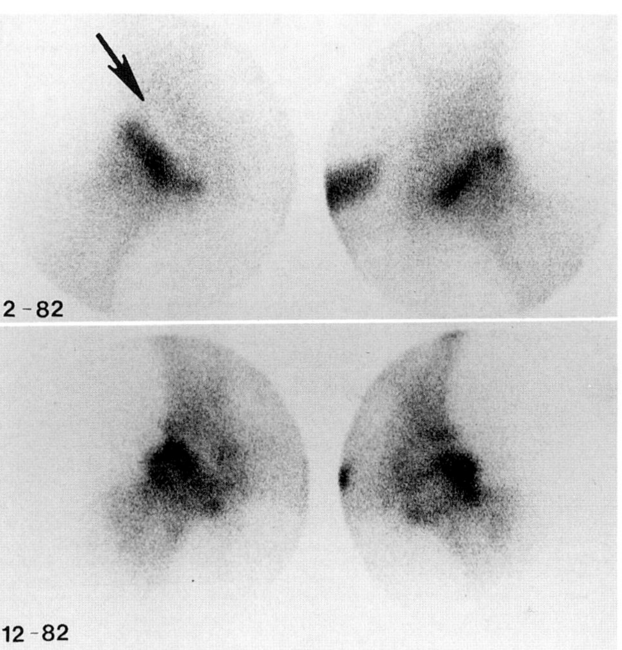

Fig. 84.17 Steroid-induced osteonecrosis. Serial changes in the hips in an asthmatic patient on long-term steroid therapy: initial study (February 1982) shows bilateral flattening of the femoral heads, with ischaemia changes on the right (arrow), associated with linear areas of increased accumulation indicative of insufficiency fractures. Ten months later (December 1982) increased accumulation is associated with revascularization, but further areas of patchy increased accumulation are indicative of continuing microfractures.

osteonecrosis is related to the retardation of repair of fatigue microfractures, which become more obvious, ultimately resulting in sufficient weakening of the bone structure to produce collapse. In other instances, the uptake in multiple small irregular areas is compatible with the alterations in microcirculation due to postulated changes such as intravenous fat emboli, erythrocyte sludging, etc. Nevertheless, the sensitivity with which all these various changes can be demonstrated, usually many months prior to radiography, have established a useful role for skeletal scintigraphy in elucidating the aetiology of pain in patients susceptible to this complication of steroid therapy. Conklin et al[45] undertook a detailed study of 36 patients with systemic lupus erythematosus being treated with prednisone, comparing skeletal scintigraphy and radiography with measurement of bone marrow pressure. Ischaemic necrosis was detected by the radionuclide study with a sensitivity of 89% compared with 41% achieved radiologically. Increased accumulation was demonstrated in 27 joints, whereas a photopenic area was noted in seven hips.

Caisson disease

Although the concept of vascular occlusion in this disorder resulting from bubbles related to decompression has been questioned and alternative mechanisms similar to those in steroid-induced osteonecrosis have been postulated, the pattern of the scintigraphic changes commonly seen are usually large, commonly juxta-articular, and thus compatible with major vessel occlusion. It has been suggested by MacLeod et al[46] that the major role of scintigraphy is in the prediction of which lesions will develop necrosis and thus forecast the risk of later articular structural deformity.

Spontaneous necrosis

The aetiology of focal necrosis occurring spontaneously, presenting as pain in the knees in the elderly without antecedent history of trauma or medication, remains obscure. The diagnosis may not be considered because of normal radiographs and pre-existing degenerative arthritis. It should perhaps be suspected because of the sudden onset of pain, 29/34 of the patients reported by Al-Rowaith et al[47] recalling the exact moment. Confirmation is readily provided by a bone scan with focal increased blood flow, hyperaemia and intense localized and well-delineated uptake in the delayed images (Fig. 84.18). While it may occur in the medial tibial plateau,[48] typically the femoral condyles are affected, most commonly the medial. This was involved in 37 knees in the study by Al-Rowaith et al,[47] the lateral being the site in only three, and in all the 40 knees investigated in detail by Greyson et al.[49] They identified different phases. In the acute phase, the characteristic scan changes were obvious. While there could be reversion to normal within 6 months, most progressed to the subacute phase in which the delayed images showed little change but the early vascular changes steadily diminished. With progression of healing, the bone scan of the late stage showed reversion of the original abnormality to normal in some patients. In others, if an articular defect had developed, shown radiologically, focal uptake was present at the point of altered weight bearing on the deformed articular surface.

THE OSTEOCHONDROSES

This term has been considered historical and inexact, 'post-traumatic necrosis of individual bone' being preferred as indicating the role of chronic stress superimposed onto the other postulated aetiological factors. It does, however, encompass the avascular disorders of various bone, most having acquired eponyms, in which skeletal scintigraphy has become recognized as highly sensitive in establishing the early diagnosis.

The scintigraphic patterns are those typical of vascular

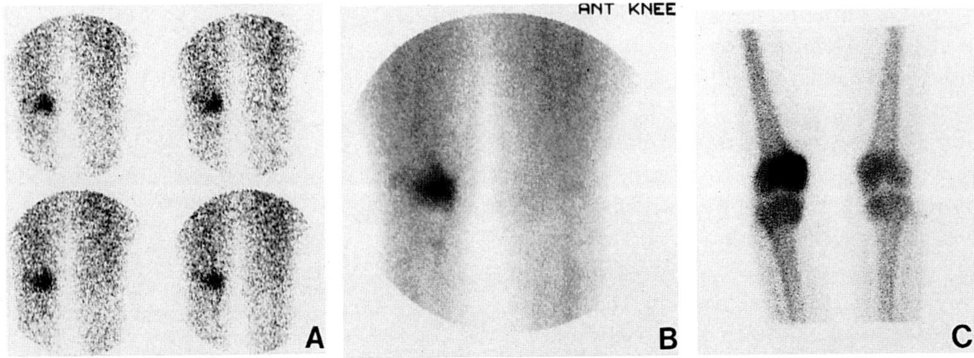

Fig. 84.18 Spontaneous osteonecrosis. Typical pattern of localized increased vascularity in the vascular phases (A and B) and intense accumulation in the medial femoral condyle in the delayed image (C).

abnormalities, with the appearance depending on the time of investigation in relation to the onset and progress of the disorder. Thus, the study may show the discrete photopenic area indicative of osteocyte death followed by an edge of advancing revascularization, climaxing with the entire area demonstrating hyperconcentration of the radiopharmaceutical, ultimately subsiding towards normal as healing progresses. Radiological alterations lag far behind and, indeed, may never be demonstrated.[50]

Legg–Calve–Perthe's disease

Because of its frequency and the dire consequences of delayed diagnosis, the greatest attention in attempting to elucidate the aetiology of these conditions has been directed to Legg–Calve–Perthe's disease (LCPD). While this disorder occurs between the ages of 3 and 12 years, the peak incidence is at 5–7 years, which also is the transition period in which the blood supply of the femoral head in the child is particularly susceptible to ischaemic insult. Trueta[51] showed that at these ages metaphyseal blood supply to the epiphysis is virtually negligible, while the round ligament has not yet provided vessels penetrating the epiphysis. The only source of blood supply to the epiphysis is provided by the lateral epiphyseal vessels, which group tightly around the lateral aspect of head. However, LCPD cannot simply be characterized as a local ischaemic disorder in the otherwise normal child. Mechanical obstruction of the extraosseous vessels in the hip has never been demonstrated, discounting the possibility of acute transient synovitis leading to tamponade of the retinacular vessels, nor has there been any evidence of a significant frequency of the occurrence of LCPD developing in later years in children in whom transient synovitis has occurred. Burwell[52] has summarized a vast body of literature that implicates delayed bone age, abnormal stature and low growth velocity, disproportionate skeletal growth, hormonal abnormalities and congenital anomalies and defects. The unifying theory remains localized disharmony between the growth of cartilage and bone. It is probable that an ischaemic event of unknown aetiology renders the femoral epiphysis avascular and thus vulnerable to trauma, even that of normal childhood activities. Sequential microfractures with partial healing and disruption of the normal ossification pathway perpetuate the ischaemia, culminating in avascular necrosis of part or all of the femoral head. As a consequence, absence of delivery and accumulation of the bone-seeking radiopharmaceuticals is so readily demonstrated that scintigraphy has a critical role in differentiating this disorder from other causes of the 'irritable hip' causing a limp in children; 48 of 131 children in the series studied by Sutherland et al,[53] 58 of 133 in that by Cavailloles et al[54] and 38 of 164 in that of Carty et al.[55] The changes, described by Danigelis et al,[56] confirmed by these and other authors, do depend on the stage of disease, but the photopenic void in the proximal femoral epiphyses is absolutely characteristic (Fig. 84.19). This abnormality is so readily shown by pinhole imaging, particularly with the hip in maximum medial rotation, that SPECT is unlikely to be required. Similarly, quantitation of the changes in blood flow or of accumulation in the femoral head has not proved advantageous, particularly because the changing configuration of the head causes difficulty in placing the regions of interest. Using conventional planar imaging, Sutherland et al[53] found a sensitivity of 0.98 and a specificity of 0.95 compared with 0.97 and 0.78 for radiography, although the changes with the former antedated radiological alterations, often by months. As emphasized by Gelfand et al,[50] radiological evidence may never appear if, because of early scintigraphic diagnosis, weight bearing is restricted sufficiently soon. Cavailloles et al[54] reported similar sensitivity and specificity for scintigraphy, 0.94 and 0.97 respectively. Danigelis et al[56] suggested that scintigraphy provided evidence of revascularization by identifying a stripe of activity in the most lateral aspect of the femoral capital epiphysis (Fig. 84.20), increased uptake in the growth plate and increased activity in the adjacent

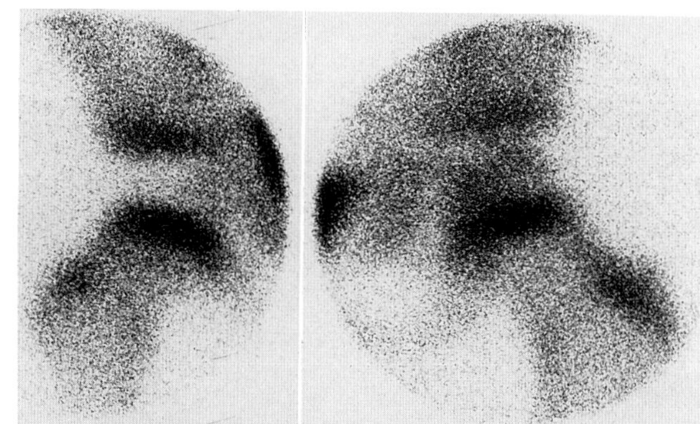

Fig. 84.19 Perthes disease. In a 5-year-old boy the typical appearance of a void of activity in the right proximal femoral epiphysis.

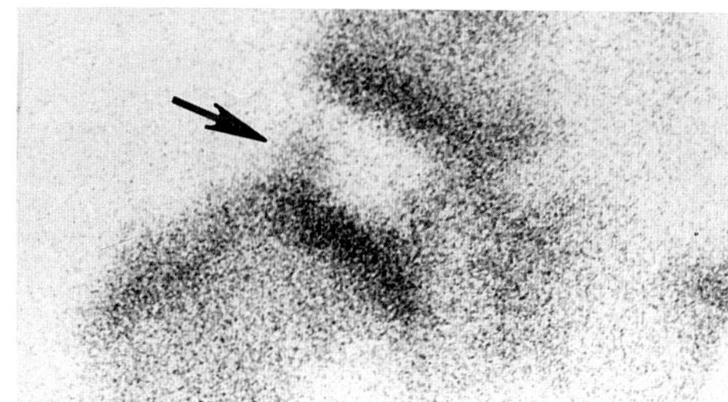

Fig. 84.20 Perthes disease. Characteristic photopenia of the proximal femoral epiphysis, with the 'lateral stripe' (arrow) indicating early revascularization.

metaphysis (Fig. 84.21). Sutherland et al[53] found no correlation of these signs with the Caterall radiographic grading to indicate that they provided evidence of the degree of avascularity of the femoral head. However, a comparison between the initial scan and the time for the appearance of radiological signs of revascularization showed a definite trend, the average interval when the initial scan showed minimal or no revascularization being 6.5 months, but 3.4 months when the scan showed established or late revascularization. Cavailloles et al[54] considered that the scintigraphic changes could permit staging of the abnormality, undertaking serial studies until complete radiological healing. The mean delay for this to occur after normalization of the scan is 11 ± 8 months. Conway[57] has suggested that serial imaging permits no prognosis of the final outcome since this is predictable by the pattern of the revascularization changes. If there is recanalization of the existing vascular channels, the structural integrity of the epiphysis is maintained. This reflects maintenance of blood supply to the epiphysis via the superior capsular arteries arising from the medial circumflex artery and results in the appearance of the 'lateral stripe' of radioactivity. However, if revascularization is via collateral circulation, through the physis from metaphyseal vessels, the process is prolonged, making it probable that there will be complications such as collapse of the head and permanent deformity as a consequence of disruption of the zone of provisional calcification. In these circumstances, scintigraphy will show a gradual widening of the physeal activity and gradual extension from the base of the epiphysis contrasting with the appearance of the 'lateral stripe' and filling in of the radiopharmaceutical accumulation into the anterior aspect which occurs in recanalization.

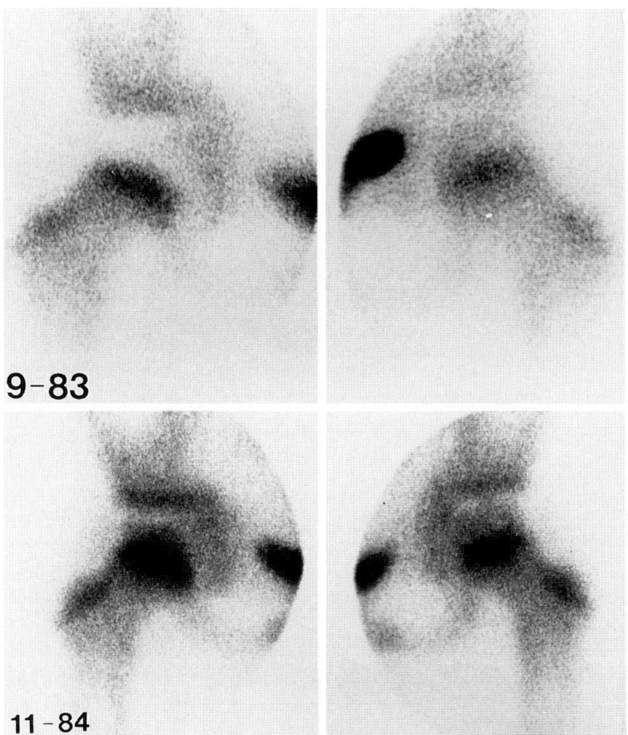

Fig. 84.21 Perthes' disease. Sequential studies in a 19-year-old boy. The initial study (September 1983) demonstrated the characteristic photopenic area in the lateral two-thirds of the proximal femoral epiphysis. Evidence of revascularization 14 months later (November 1984) includes restoration of epiphyseal activity associated with increased accumulation, and also widening and increased uptake in the growth plate.

Avascular necrosis may affect many other bones, a variety of eponyms being attached. Each can readily be identified by bone scanning prior to radiological change. As expected, photopenia may be demonstrable in the early stages and increased accumulation visualized with progressive revascularization. These typical changes were, for example, shown in the second metatarsal head, the site of Freiberg's disease, by Mandell & Harcke[58] and in the navicular, Kohler's disease, by McCauley & Khan.[59]

Reflex sympathetic dystrophy (RSD)

The variety of appellations applied to this syndrome indicate the uncertainty regarding aetiology, but most of them do reflect the clinical evidence of abnormal increased vascularity associated with vasomotor disturbance. In some it occurred following cerebrovascular incidents, but in a significant proportion there is a history of antecedent trauma. However, the mechanism remains uncertain, particularly since a trivial injury can produce pain that far surpasses the magnitude of the initial injury and often persists long after the injury has healed. It is generally agreed that the syndrome is precipitated by nerve injury either to peripheral nerves or to the central nervous system. The consequent tissue responses, inducing release of various substances, initiate a widespread disturbance of autonomic regulation culminating in an abnormal central reflex. The abnormal autonomic nerve flow produces vasodilation and/or vasoconstriction in the affected limb. The clinical presentation, typical of the most common varieties, Sudeck's atrophy and shoulder–hand syndrome, are typically pain, trophic skin changes, oedema and swelling and muscle wasting. Since the radiological changes of bone resorption may be demonstrable only when the condition is well advanced, it is not surprising that three-phase scintigraphy has been widely utilized in both the diagnosis and monitoring of treatment. Increased vascular delivery and hyperaemia in the initial phases may be clear-cut, although McKinnon & Holder[60] believed greater reliance could be placed on observing the typical changes of the delayed images, diffuse uptake in the affected area with an intense periarticular uptake, described by Genant et al[61] (Fig. 84.22). In a study of 23 patients, McKinnon & Holder[60] found a sensitivity of 45% in the perfusion phase, 52% in blood pool phase but a 96% sensitivity for the delayed images. The specificity of the last was 98%.

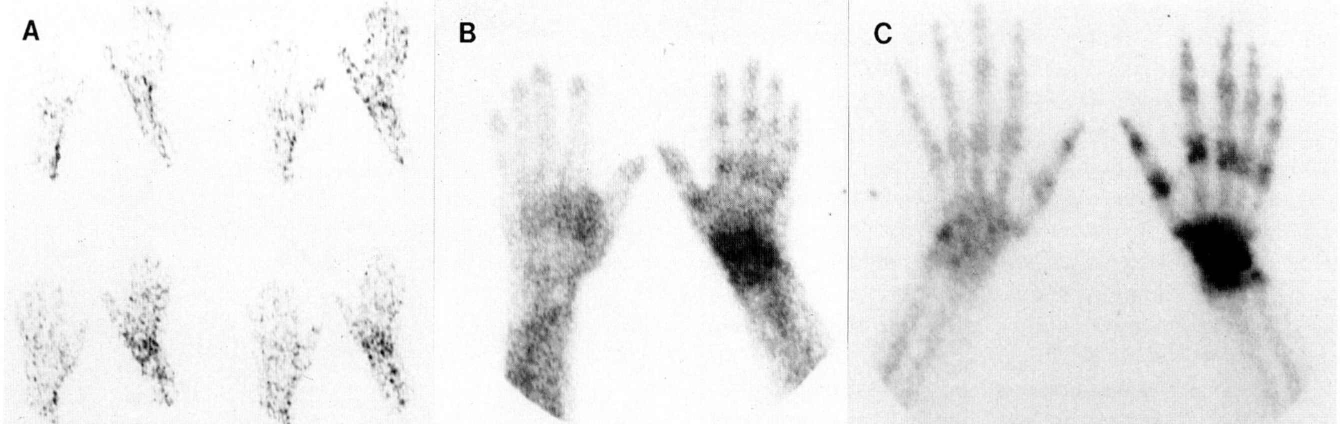

Fig. 84.22 Reflex sympathetic dystrophy. There is a mild asymmetrical delivery in the blood flow images (A) but obvious diffuse hyperaemia of the left wrist and hand in the blood pool phase (B). In the delayed images (C) characteristic juxta-articular uptake is evident.

Although Kosin et al[62] had only found an abnormal study in 60% of their patients, they concluded that the finding indicated a high probability of response to systemic steroid therapy. The complexity of the neurovascular feedback system is, however, exemplified by the observation in both of these series that, even in patients showing the characteristic juxta-articular changes in the delayed images, not only was the typical hyperaemia of the early phases not observed, but in fact decreased activity was demonstrated. Of 25 patients with a cerebrovascular accident studied by Greyson & Tepperman,[63] 21 had the typical increased accumulation in the delayed images. In 13 there was increased flow, but in eight it was decreased, identical to that in 55 cerebrovascular accident patients without reflex sympathetic dystrophy. In their detailed studies of 181 patients suffering from RSD of the hand, Demangeat et al[64] postulated that diminished uptake in the delayed images resulted from severe disuse and/or atrophy. This scan feature was demonstrated in 29% of 108 patients in the period 60–100 weeks from onset, another 29% of the group having normal studies, whereas increased uptake persisted in only 42%. This contrasted with the findings on these patients at earlier stages. In the period 0–20 weeks following onset the characteristic finding was increase in vascularity and in later uptake, while between 20 and 40 weeks the vascularity was no longer demonstrable but the abnormal delayed accumulation persisted. The 'atypical' radionuclide presentation was emphasized by Heck,[65] who reported decreased blood flow in four patients in whom the symptoms of RSD in the feet were related to athletic trauma. In two there was also diminished uptake in the delayed images. This predominantly vasospastic variation was also encountered by Intenzo et al[66] in 23 patients with reflex sympathetic dystrophy. Increased periarticular activity in the early and delayed phases was demonstrable in 19, while decreased activity in the affected limb was observed in three of the remaining four. The scans were, however, normal in eight of the patients who obtained significant relief following nerve block and/or sympathectomy, the response to which was included by Holder et al[67] as one of the diagnostic criteria in their study of 51 patients in whom RSD was a diagnostic consideration. In all 26 patients in whom the condition was proven, the delayed scan showed diffuse accumulation throughout the foot with juxta-articular accentuation of uptake (Fig. 84.23). However, the specificity was only 80% since false-positive images were obtained with infection, diabetes and chronic pain. Nevertheless, normal or decreased uptake has been reported in children during the active stage of RSD,[68, 69]

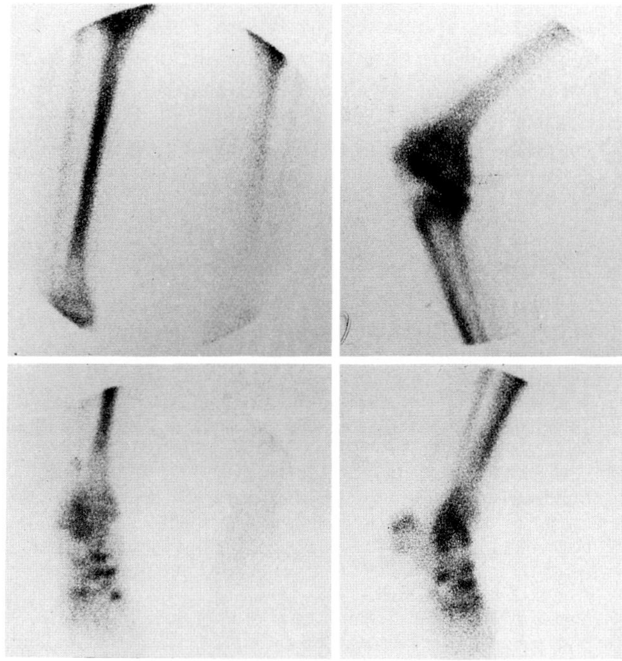

Fig. 84.23 Reflex sympathetic dystrophy. Characteristic alterations in a 16-year-old girl, showing a mild diffuse accumulation in the lower leg and foot but with the typical increased juxta-articular uptake in the knee, ankle and foot.

and in their study of patients with cerebrovascular accidents Greyson & Tepperman[63] had commented that, although hemiparesis and hemiplegia also involved the lower limbs, in only 5 of the 21 patients with reflex sympathetic dystrophy of the upper limbs was there increased uptake in the ipsilateral lower limb on the delayed image. No patient had the typical bone scan changes in an isolated leg. Typical scintigraphic alterations are also of value in diagnosing reflex sympathetic dystrophy of the knee. Athletic injury, often mild, may have occurred but in the majority in most series, previous patello-femoral surgery appeared to be the precipitating trigger. While Cooper et al[70] observed that the radiopharmaceutical uptake was increased in the patella, associated with patello-femoral pain, Ogilvie-Harris & Roscoe[71] observed characteristic bone scan findings of increased blood flow and delayed uptake not merely in the involved knee but, in many patients, in the whole limb, with increased accumulation in the foot and hip as well. Radiological changes of progressive demineralization are identifiable in established cases of the syndrome but Koch et al[72] found magnetic resonance imaging to be of little value.

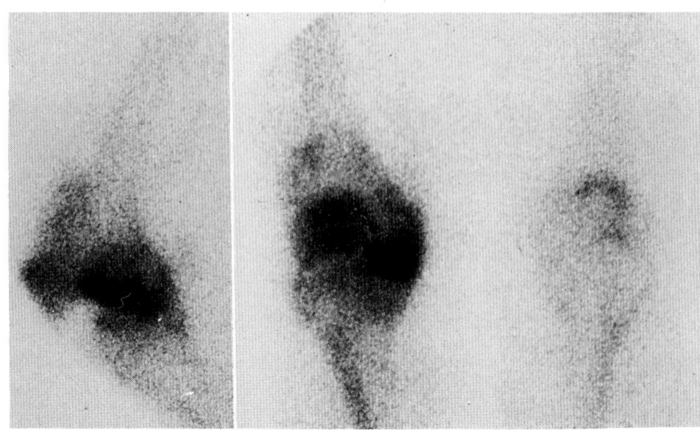

Fig. 84.24 Transient migratory osteoporosis. Characteristic changes include a dominant focus of increased accumulation in the right medial femoral condyle and diffuse periarticular uptake.

Transient osteoporosis

Transient regional osteoporosis is widely considered to be a form of reflex sympathetic dystrophy, differing in that a history of trauma is rare and that frequently there is consecutive involvement of the bones around major joints, especially the hip and knees, although the interval between each incident may vary considerably. The symptoms usually resolve spontaneously within 4–10 months with subsequent remineralization and regression of the radiological changes of localized osteoporosis. The typical changes of three-phase scintigraphy, increased activity in the symptomatic area in perfusion, blood pool and delayed phases, are identifiable prior to radiological alteration.[73] A partial form of this disorder is now recognized, partial transient osteoporosis, for which bone scanning is also critical in identifying the cause of the excruciating pain of rapid onset.[74] The early phases will demonstrate local increased vascularity. The later images differ from most other conditions with somewhat similar symptoms and scan findings, such as osteochondritis dissecans and spontaneous necrosis. There is intense focal uptake but also diffuse accumulation in the surrounding bone (Fig. 84.24). The femoral condyles and the femoral head are typically affected. Radiographs may subsequently show corresponding localized demineralization, which may extend to be widespread around the joints in a pattern typical of transient osteoporosis. Symptoms usually subside within 6 months but may recur in another site. The probability of this migratory pattern may be forecast by the bone scans, revealing changes indicating involvement at other joints before the development of clinical or radiological abnormalities.

REFERENCES

1. Sy W M, Bay R, Camera A 1977 Hand images: normal and abnormal. J Nucl Med 18: 419–424
2. Murray I P C 1978 Bone scanning in occupational acro-osteolysis. Skeletal Radiol 3: 149–154
3. Mazieres B, Jung-Rosenfarb M, Bouteiller G, Fournie A, Arlet T J 1978 La scintigraphie osseuse dans la maladie de Paget. Rev Rhum Mal Osteoartic 45: 311–316
4. Vellenga C J L R, Pauwels E K J, Bijvoet O L M, Frijlink W B, Mulder J D, Helmans J 1984 Untreated Paget's disease of bone studied by scintigraphy. Radiology 153: 799–805
5. Fogelman I, Carr D 1980 A comparison of bone scanning and radiology in the assessment of patients with symptomatic Paget's disease. Eur J Nucl Med 5: 417–421
6. Shirazi P H, Ryan W G, Fordham E W 1974 Bone scanning in evaluation of Paget's disease of bone. CRC Crit Rev Clin Radiol Nucl Med 5: 523–558
7. Smith J, Bodet J F, Yeh S D J 1984 Bone sarcoma in Paget's disease, a study of 85 patients. Radiology 152: 585–590
8. Yeh S D J, Rosen G, Benua R S 1982 Gallium scans in Paget's sarcoma. Clin Nucl Med 7: 546–552
9. Boudreau R J, Lisbone R, Haadijipavlou A 1983 Observations on serial radionuclide blood flow studies in Paget's disease: concise communication. J Nucl Med 24: 880–885
10. Vellenga C J L R, Pauwels E K J, Bijvoet O L M 1984 Comparison between visual assessment and quantitative measurement of radioactivity on the bone scintigram in Paget's disease of bone. Eur J Nucl Med 9: 533–537
11. Smith M L, Fogelman I, Ralston S, Boyce B F, Boyle I T 1984 Correlation of skeletal uptake of 99m-Tc-diphosphonate and alkaline phosphatase before and after oral diphosphonate therapy in Paget's disease. Metab Bone Dis Rel Res 5: 167–170
12. Waxman A D, Ducker S, McKee D, Siemsen J K, Singer F R 1977 Evaluation of sodium etidronate in the treatment of Paget's disease of bone. Clin Orthop 122: 347–358
13. Dunn E K, Vaquer R O, Strashun A M 1988 Paget's disease: a cause of photopenic skeletal defect in Indium-111 WBC scintigraphy. J Nucl Med 29: 561–563
14. Palestro C J, Swyer A J, Kim C K, Vega A, Goldsmith S J 1989 Appearance of Paget's disease on In-111 leukocyte images. J Nucl Med 30: 754

15. Patel U, Gallaher S J, Boyle I T, McKillop J H 1990 Serial bone scans in Paget's disease: development of new lesions, natural variation in bone intensity and nature of changes seen after treatment. Nucl Med Commun 1: 747–760
16. Vellenga C J L R, Pauwels E K J, Bijvoet O L M, Hosking D J, Frijlink W B 1982 Bone scintigraphy in Paget's disease treated with combined calcitonin and diphosphonate (EHDP). Metab Bone Dis Rel Res 4: 103–111
17. Vellenga C J L R, Pauwels E K J, Bijvoet O L M, Hamiek M D, Frijlink W B 1985 Quantitative bone scintigraphy in Paget's disease treated with APD. Br J Radiol 58: 1165–1172
18. Ryan P J, Gibson T, Fogelman I 1992 Bone scintigraphy following intravenous pamidronate for Paget's disease of bone. J Nucl Med 33: 1589–1593
19. Machida K, Nakita K, Nishikawa J, Ohtake T, Lio M 1986 Scintigraphic manifestation of fibrous dysplasia. Clin Nucl Med 11: 422–429
20. Hardoff R, Gips S 1991 Radiographic and scintigraphic demonstration of mono-ostotic fibrous dysplasia of the skull: advantages of SPECT imaging. Clin Nucl Med 16: 869–871
21. Wells R G, Sty J R 1985 Bone scintigraphy in cherubism. Clin Nucl Med 10: 892
22. Pfeffer S, Molina E, Feuillan P, Simon T R 1990 McCune–Albright syndrome: The patterns of scintigraphic abnormalities. J Nucl Med 31: 1474–1478
23. Harris W H, Dudley H R, Barr R J 1962 The natural history of fibrous dysplasia: an orthopaedic, pathological and roentgenographic study. J Bone Joint Surg 44A: 207–233
24. Mankin H J 1992 Nontraumatic necrosis of bone (osteonecrosis). N Engl J Med 326: 1473–1479
25. Turner J H 1983 Post-traumatic avascular necrosis of the femoral head predicted by preoperative technetium-99m antimony-colloid scan. J Bone Joint Surg 65: 787–797
26. Ruland L J, Wang G-J, Teates C D, Gay S, Ruke A 1992 A comparison of magnetic resonance imaging to bone scintigraphy in early traumatic ischemia of the femoral head. Clin Orthol Rel Res 285: 31–34
27. Lutzker L G, Alavi A 1976 Bone and marrow imaging in sickle-cell disease: diagnosis of infarction. Semin Nucl Med 6: 83–91
28. Greyson N D, Kassell E F 1976 Serial bone-scan changes in a current bone infarction. J Nucl Med 17: 184–186
29. Armas R R, Goldsmith S J 1984 Gallium scintigraphy in bone infarction: correlation with bone imaging. Clin Nucl Med 9: 1–3
30. Israel O, Jerushalmi J, Front D 1986 Scintigraphic findings in Gaucher's disease. J Nucl Med 27: 1557–1563
31. Bilchik T R, Heyman S 1992 Skeletal scintigraphy of pseudo-osteomyelitis in Gaucher's disease. Clin Nucl Med 17: 279–282
32. Lisbona R, Rosenthall L 1976 Assessment of bone viability by scintiscanning in frostbite injuries. J Trauma 16: 986–992
33. Lucie R S, Fuller S, Burdick D C, Jonston R M 1981 Early prediction of avascular necrosis of the femoral head following femoral neck fractures. Clin Orthol Rel Res 161: 207–214
34. Stromqvist B, Bismar J, Hansson L I et al 1984 Technetium 99m-methylene diphosphonate scintimetry after femoral neck fracture. A three-year follow-up study. Clin Orthop 182: 177–189
35. Collier B D, Carrera G F, Johnson R P et al 1985 Detection of femoral head avascular necrosis in adults by SPECT. J Nucl Med 26: 979–987
36. Geuen G S, Mears D C, Tauxe W N et al 1987 Distinguishing avascular necrosis from segmental impaction of the femoral head following an acetabular fracture. J Nucl Med 28: 664–665
37. Lee M H, Moon D H, Na H W et al 1992 Diagnosis of femoral head avascular necrosis by triple head high resolution. J Nucl Med 33: 936
38. Myers M H, Teifer D N, Moore T M 1977 Determination of the vascularity of the femoral head with technetium-99m-sulphur colloid. J Bone Joint Surg 59: 658–664
39. Philips T W, Aitken G K, McKenzie R A 1986 Sulphur colloid bone scan assessment of femoral head vascularity following subcapital fracture of the hip. Clin Orthop 208: 52–54
40. Williams A G, Mettler F A Jr, Christie J H 1983 Sulphur colloid distribution in normal hips. Clin Nucl Med 8: 490–492
41. Spencer R P, Lee Y S, Sziklas J J et al 1983 Failure of uptake of radiocolloid by the femoral head: a diagnostic problem. J Nucl Med 24: 116–118
42. Bellmore M C, Cummine J L, Crocker E F, Carseldine D B 1983 The role of bone scans in the assessment of prognosis of scaphoid fractures. Aust NZ J Surg 53: 133–137
43. Reinus W R, Conway W F, Totty W G et al 1986 Carpal avascular necrosis: MRI imaging. Radiology 160: 689–693
44. Shafa M H, Fernandez-Ulloa M, Rost R C, Nyquis T 1983 Diagnosis of aseptic necrosis of the talus by bone scintigraphy. Clin Nucl Med 8: 50–53
45. Conklin J J, Alderson P O, Zizic T M et al 1983 Comparison of bone scan and radiograph sensitivity in the detection of steroid-induced ischaemic necrosis of bone. Radiology 147: 221–226
46. MacLeod M A, McEwan A J B, Pearson R R, Houston A S 1982 Functional imaging in the early diagnosis of dysbaric osteonecrosis. Br J Radiol 55: 497–500
47. Al-Rowaith A, Lindstrand A, Bjorkengren A, Wingstrand H, Thorngren K-G 1991 Osteonecrosis of the knee: Diagnosis and outcome in 40 patients. Acta Orthop Scand 62: 19–23
48. Houpt J B, Alpert B, Lotem M et al 1982 Spontaneous osteonecrosis of the medial tibial plateau. J Rheumatol 9: 81–90
49. Greyson N D, Lotem N M, Gross A E, Houpt J B 1982 Radionuclide evaluation of spontaneous femoral osteonecrosis. Radiology 142: 729–735
50. Gelfand M J, Ball W S, Oestreich A E, Crawford A H, Jolson R, Perlman A 1983 Transient loss of femoral head Tc-99m diphosphonate uptake with prolonged maintenance of femoral head architecture. Clin Nucl Med 8: 347–354
51. Trueta J 1957 The normal vascular anatomy of the human femoral head during growth. J Bone Joint Surg 39B: 358–394
52. Burwell R G 1988 Perthes disease: growth and aetiology. Arch Dis Childh 63: 1408–1412
53. Sutherland A D, Savage J P, Paterson D C, Foster B K 1980 The nuclide bone-scan in the diagnosis and management of Perthes disease. J Bone Joint Surg 62B: 300–306
54. Cavailloles F, Bok B, Bensahel H 1982 Bone scintigraphy and the diagnosis and follow-up of Perthes disease. Eur J Nucl Med 7: 327–330
55. Carty H, Maxted M, Fielding J A et al 1984 Isotope scanning in the 'irritable hip syndrome'. Skeletal Radiol 11: 32–37
56. Dangelis J A 1976 Pinhole imaging in Legg–Perthes disease. Semin Nucl Med 6: 69–82
57. Conway J J 1986 Radionuclide bone scintigraphy in pediatric orthopedics. Pediatr Clin N Am 33: 1313–1334
58. Mandell G A, Harcke H T 1987 Scintigraphic manifestations of infarction of the second metatarsal (Freibert's disease). J Nucl Med 28: 249–251
59. McCauley R G K, Kahn P C 1977 Osteochondritis of the tarsal navicular. Radioisotope appearances. Radiology 123: 705–706
60. Mackinnon S E, Holder S E 1984 The use of three-phase radionuclide bone scanning in the diagnosis of reflex sympathetic dystrophy. J Hand Surg (Am) 9: 556–563
61. Genant H K, Kozin F, Bekerman C, MacCarty D J, Sims J 1975 The reflex sympathetic dystrophy syndrome. Radiology 117: 21–32
62. Kosin F, Soin J S, Ryan L M, Carrera G F, Wortmann R L 1981 Bone scintigraphy in the reflex sympathetic syndrome. Radiology 138: 437–443
63. Greyson N D, Tepperman P S 1984 Three-phase bone scans in hemiplegia with reflex sympathetic dystrophy and the effect of disuse. J Nucl Med 25: 423–429
64. Demangeat J-L, Constantinesco A, Brunot B, Foucher G, Farcot J-M 1988 Three-phase bone scanning in reflex sympathetic dystrophy of the hand. J Nucl Med 29: 26–32
65. Heck L L 1987 Recognition of atypical reflex sympathetic dystrophy. Clin Nucl Med 12: 925–928
66. Intenzo C, Kim S, Millin J, Park C 1989 Scintigraphic pattern of the reflex sympathetic dystrophy of the lower extremities. Clin Nucl Med 14: 657–661
67. Holder L E, Cole L A, Myerson M S 1992 Reflex sympathetic dystrophy in the foot: clinical and scintigraphic criteria. Radiology 184: 531–535
68. Majd M 1979 Bone scintigraphy in children with obscure skeletal pain. Ann Radiol 22: 85–89

69. Laxer R M, Allen R C, Malleson P N, Morrison R T, Petty R F 1985 Technetium-99m-methylene diphosphonate bone scans in children with reflex neurovascular dystrophy. J Pediatr 106: 437–440
70. Cooper D E, DeLee J C, Ramamurthy S 1989 Reflex sympathetic dystrophy of the knee. J Bone Joint Surg 71A: 365–369
71. Ogilvie-Harris D J, Roscoe M 1987 Reflex sympathetic dystrophy of the knee. J Bone Joint Surg 69B: 804–806
72. Koch E, Hofer H O, Sialer G, Marincek B, Von Schulthess G K 1991 Failure of MR imaging to detect reflex sympathetic dystrophy of the extremities. AJR 156: 113–115
73. Bray S T, Partain C L, Teates C D, Guilford W B, Williamson B R J, McLaughlin R C 1979 The value of the bone scan in idiopathic regional migratory osteoporosis. J Nucl Med 20: 1268–1270
74. Lesquesne M, Kerboull M, Bensasson M, Perez C, Dreiser R, Forest A 1977 Partial transient osteoporosis. Skeletal Radiol 2: 1–9

85. Bone scintigraphy in trauma

I. P. C. Murray

The sequence of pathophysiological processes induced by a fracture are all conducive to the preferential localization of the bone-seeking radiopharmaceutical. Such accumulation, therefore, can be visualized soon after a fracture, steadily increasing as the repair occurs and persisting for long periods while remodelling proceeds. Somewhat similar reparative changes occur in response to the failure of bone to adapt to abnormal stress or following injury to the insertional sites of muscle and tendons. These circumstances will also produce radiopharmaceutical uptake at an early stage. Since these scintigraphic alterations can be visualized long before radiographic change, bone scanning has steadily acquired a critical role in the management of trauma. While X-rays remain the modality of choice in demonstrating many traumatic lesions of bone, there is an increasing reliance on scintigraphy. This in part relates to its ability to identify fractures in sites at which radiography encounters difficulties and also the feasibility of diagnosing a variety of injuries which are difficult or even impossible to demonstrate radiographically. Further, the procedure provides a simple means to follow up progress and ascertain whether healing is progressing normally or whether complications such as avascular necrosis, infection or reflex sympathetic osteodystrophy have occurred. In some circumstances the ease with which the degree of metabolic activity can be assessed is invaluable in determining whether the radiographic abnormalities are of clinical significance.

PATHOLOGICAL CONSIDERATIONS

Unlike other tissues which repair by a collagenous scar, fracture healing leads to the formation of a callus which is virtually identical in structure and mechanical strength to the original bone. This reflects the normal growth of bone by apposition with the formation of new bone in layers. The action of osteoclasts in remaining dying osteons and the production of new osteoid by osteoblasts, also derived from the periosteum, are balanced. The osteoid is rapidly mineralized by Ca–P complexes with the development of hydroxyapatite, while the osteoblasts migrate into the lacunae, becoming osteocytes. These processes are accelerated following fracture. The initial reaction is a periosteal response, seen within 48 h of injury. Thickening of periosteum occurs, creating a partial callus of trabecular and cartilaginous tissue, leading to a critical soft-tissue response which results in an early bridging callus associated with angiogenesis and intense cellular activity, particularly of osteoclasts and osteoblasts. Calcification of the cartilage thus formed commences within days. Similar endochondral ossification follows but at a slower rate. These processes are similar to those which take place in the zone of provisional calcification in the growth plate. Over subsequent weeks and months, the trabecular bone gains a mature laminar structure so that, after remodelling into the appropriate shape, the resulting cortical bone possesses the same mechanical strength as the original.

Stress of a lesser degree than that causing a traumatic fracture usually induces a local reaction resulting in more dense bone in order to strengthen the affected site. With such stress, there is deformity of the bone but it returns to the original configuration when stress is discontinued. If, however, the stress is repeated or continuous, resorption may be greater than the reparative reaction so that, as osteons are debonded at the cement line, individual trabeculae collapse, resulting in microfractures. As these increase, cortical cracks occur, producing a stress fracture. The ultimate reaction is progression to structural failure with complete fracture. In a normal individual this sequence, culminating in a fatigue fracture, is the result of muscle activity which is new, strenuous and repetitive. In contrast, normal muscular activity is sufficient to produce an insufficiency fracture when the stress is on bone that is abnormal, particularly when there is reduction of mineral content, as in osteoporosis from any cause. In the latter, compressive forces usually predominate, while the altered biomechanics involved in many fatigue fractures reflect, to a greater extent, the effect of torsion and bending, transmitted through muscular attachments. The consequent altered tension forces reflect not only the abnormally increased use of particular muscles and their fatigue but also the relative weakness of opposing groups not directly involved in the relevant required increase in muscular action. Such abnormal tension forces act primarily on bone cortex, culminating in diaphyseal stress fractures, whereas the compression forces acting on cancellous bone induce metaphyseal fractures.

Muscular overuse is also responsible for the production of 'shin splints'. These reflect the effect of stress along muscle insertions. The muscles are attached to bone by Sharpey's fibres, which are extensions of fibrocartilage anchored in the mineralized matrix. Thus, the stress from abnormal walking or running, for example, can result in changes in metabolism at the insertional sites of the tibialis anterior or posterior on the tibia or on the interosseous membrane. This extended periosteal reaction with increased osteoblastic activity and vascular ingrowth differs from the more localized response to stress which occurs at most musculotendinous or ligamentous insertions, entheses. Also attached by Sharpey's fibres, tendons can act like periosteum at the insertional site. Accordingly, the consequence of abnormal stress, enthesopathies, are those similar to a minor bone injury with osteoblastic response. However, in children and adolescence, the abnormal activity may be such as to cause apophyseal avulsion, most commonly in the pelvis and proximal femur. Healing will involve a considerable osteoblastic response. The associated haematoma may calcify and the end result may be an exostosis.

SCINTIGRAPHIC APPEARANCES

The periosteal reaction can be visualized within hours of the injury but is not of a size or frequency to warrant any reliability being placed on its detection (Fig. 85.1). It has, however, been accepted for years that the vascular and osteoblastic changes integral to the healing process are such as to ensure that marked preferential uptake of the technetium bone-seeking agents occurs within a few days. This intense accumulation, similar to that visualized in the growth plate in children, is readily observed in routine studies, confirming the findings of Matin.[1] He suggested that the scan changes following fracture can be visualized in three phases. The first, an acute stage at an early onset, persists for approximately 2–4 weeks after injury, being characterized by a diffuse area of tracer concentration in which a distinct fracture line might be seen, especially in delayed images. Based on his initial study on 204 patients, reaffirmed with continuing observation in over 1000 patients,[2] he postulated that fractures can be detected within 24 h of injury in approximately 95% of patients, the study being abnormal in 100% within 1 week. The second or subacute phase is characterized by a well-defined linear abnormality at the site of fracture, this being the stage when the fracture is most obvious and lasting for approximately 8–12 weeks. Thereafter the third or healing phase commences and is characterized by gradual diminution in the intensity of the abnormality until the bone scan returns to normal. The time for this return to normality, however, varies considerably and extends well beyond the time for clinical or even radiographic healing. It is only after the passage of some 3 years that 100% of the studies can be considered normal. There was, however, considerable variation and Matin demonstrated that normalization differs markedly in various types of bone.[2] The recent detailed study by Spitz et al[3] suggests that achievement of a high degree of accuracy in early identification of fractures also demands consideration of the likely site. They reviewed the findings in 1369 patients with at least one fresh fracture, calculating a lesion-to-normal bone ratio in each. This permitted the differentiation of a fracture from soft-tissue lesions with reactive hyperaemia, the fractures showing values greater than 1:1. The advent and also the extent and intensity of this accumulation depended on the fracture site. Lesions in the proximity of the joints were demonstrable immediately; lesions of the axial skeleton and the shafts of the long bones were sometimes not demonstrable until after 10–12 days. They suggested that the reasons for these differences could in part be the different extent of callus formation in different bones, reflecting the size of these bones. Also differing from the conclusions of Matin, Spitz et al[3] were unable to demonstrate any influence of age on the time of appearance of these scintigraphic changes. Nevertheless, while such fractures as those in scaphoid will almost certainly be visualized within 72 h, it is prudent not to attempt to identify fractures such as those of the neck of the femur until several days have passed and many indeed consider that any equivocal alteration should warrant a sequential scan a week later.

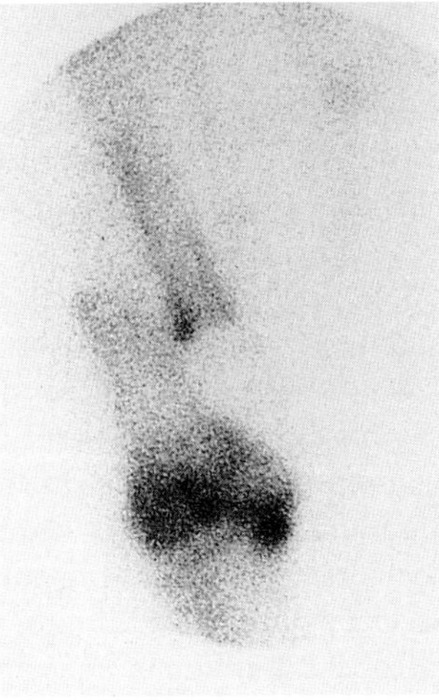

Fig. 85.1 A femoral shaft fracture which occurred less than 4 h previously in an elderly female shows MDP accumulation at the site of the early periosteal reaction.

The scintigraphic changes associated with stress fractures are usually smaller in size than traumatic fractures but, being of similar intensity, are readily identified. Evaluation requires consideration of the site and size. The extent of the scan changes are of such relevance to the management of the patient that grading of the lesion is desirable (Fig. 85.2). That proposed by Zwas et al[4] treats the entire evolutionary process as one continuum of bone overuse injury, reflecting increasing severity which culminates in a complete fracture if untreated. The bone reaction is initially a small, thin, localized, mildly active lesion confined to the cortical bone, grade I. As the process continues to grade II, the focal lesion enlarges and extends along the cortical bone. Further progress leads to a grade III lesion, which extends into the medullary bone, becoming wider, fusiform and occupying about half the width of the bone shaft with highly increased activity. The most extensive lesion, grade IV, occupies the full bone shaft, appearing as a fusiform oval area of intensely increased activity. The staging as suggested by Matin[2] is essentially similar, although dividing the periosteal reaction into two stages. He emphasized that the analysis of this staging does require at least two views of the individual bone in different projections. For example, what might appear to be a complete tranverse abnormality in a tibia in the anterior view may be seen to be much less extensive in a lateral view. Several projections may also be desirable to provide optimal demonstration of the changes occurring as the result of 'shin splints'. The distinctive scintigraphic features reflect the periosteal disruption, appearing as linear, elongated, narrow homogeneous accumulations extending along the bone in a superficial site. It is most unusual for any local hyperaemia to be demonstrated with three-phase studies in 'shin splints', in contrast to the increased local vascularity typically demonstrable in stress fractures shortly after the onset of pain. In evaluating this feature, Rupani et al[5] noted that both the radioangiogram and blood pool images showed local hyperaemia during the first 2–4 weeks, but as healing continues, first the angiogram and subsequently the blood pool images no longer reveal the abnormalities. They commented that the intensity of uptake in the delayed images decreases over 3–6 months, but images can still show a minimal number of abnormalities up to 10 months afterwards, although the configuration of the lesion changes from fusiform to a narrow, less-defined focus. Zwas et al[4] observed that scan changes in 36% of stress fractures of a severity graded I or II disappeared within 3 months and only 12% were unchanged, whereas only 31% of those of grades III and IV were no longer demonstrable. No osseous alteration is demonstrable in patients with compartment syndrome, but in this condition it may be possible to demonstrate decreased blood flow with a consequent reduction of activity in the vicinity of the area of increased pressure, sometimes being associated with some increased concentration both above and below the abnormality.

The sequential scan changes following injury in children are similar, although usually a more exuberant osteoblastic response permits earlier identification of traumatic damage. As always, particular attention to the epiphyses is warranted. When affected by the traumatic insult, increased accumulation and widening of the radioactivity in the growth plate may be apparent while a fracture through the epiphysis can result in decreased metabolic activity readily demonstrable as markedly reduced uptake, inducing concern regarding subsequent cessation of growth. Distortion of the normal shape of growth plate activity may provide evidence of a metaphyseal corner fracture. This lesion, not uncommon in the abused child, can be associated with increased uptake throughout the whole bone, possibly the result of disruption of the periosteal attachment and consequent subperiosteal haematoma formation. Similar generalized increased uptake along the entire length of the injured bone can be observed in occult femoral and tibial fractures in infants and toddlers,[6] masking the oblique mid-shaft abnormality considered by Miller & Sanderson[7] to be typical of the toddler's fracture.

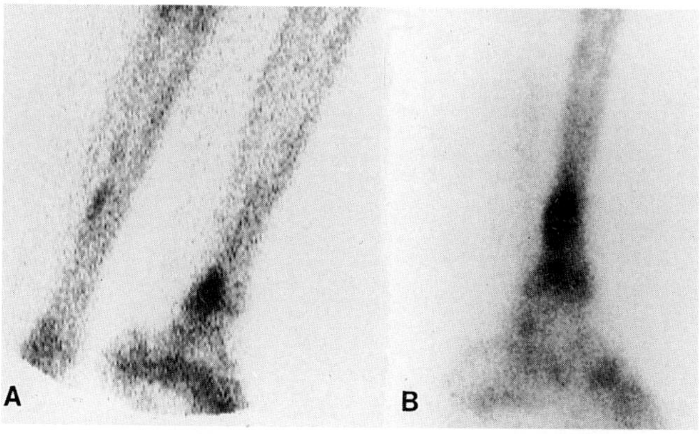

A B

Fig. 85.2 Grades of stress fracture. (A) Grade I lesion in the posterior left tibia in the symptomatic area and unsuspected grade III lesion in the lower right tibia. (B) Grade IV lesion in the lower tibia of a marathon runner.

CLINICAL APPLICATIONS

Traumatic fractures

Following known injury, fractures will be demonstrated by conventional radiography of most sites of trauma. In such circumstances bone scintigraphy has no major role, although unsuspected lesions may be identified (Fig. 85.3). Goldberg et al[8] did observe that, of 119 patients with forearm fractures, bone scans identified a second injury in nine patients with radiological evidence of only an isolated fracture. However, scintigraphy may provide important supplementary information in polytraumatized patients. Spitz et al,[9] using the study as a screening procedure on 162 patients with 1536 radiograph-proven lesions, identified additional fractures in 50%.

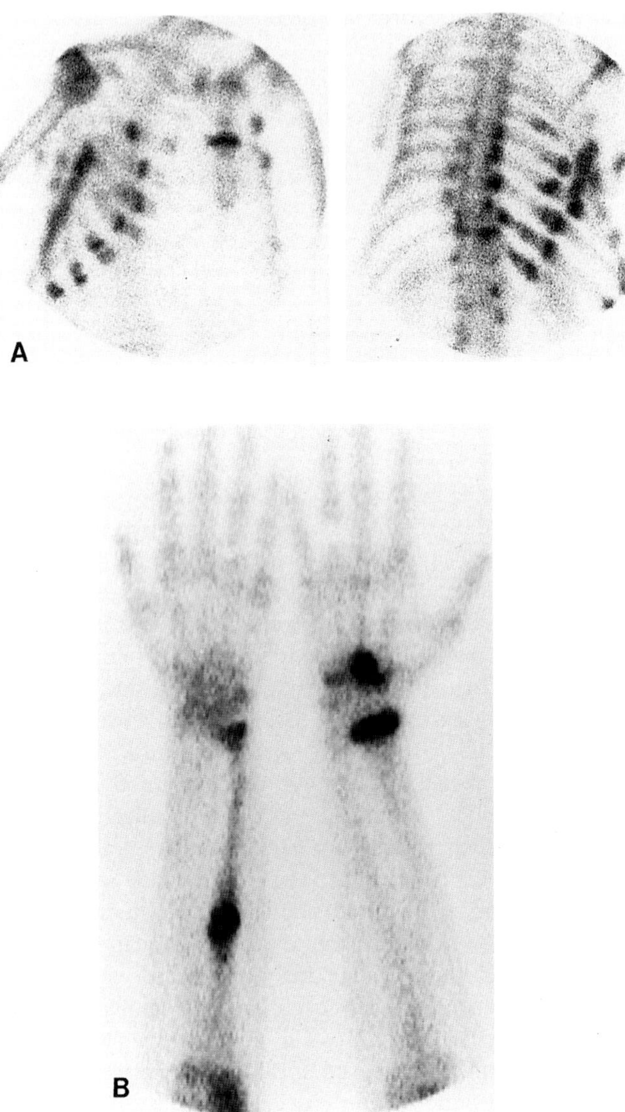

Fig. 85.3 Multiple fractures. (A) Identifiable in the ribs and sternum of a steroid-dependent asthmatic following vigorous physiotherapy. (B) Unsuspected fractures were identified in a woman after a motor vehicle accident.

It is well recognized that the early detection of fractures in some sites cannot be reliably achieved by standard radiography. This difficulty reflects the slow development of radiographic changes. Most common amongst these covert fractures are those of the femoral neck and of the scaphoid. Early detection of hip fractures has assumed increasing importance for a variety of reasons, particularly the social and legal consequences. Bone scintigraphy has been widely advocated as a highly sensitive and specific means for achieving this. Continuing experiences raise some controversy as to its reliability. Thus, for example, whereas the review of 43 patients by Fairclough et al[10] found no false-positive nor false-negative results, a further analysis in the same centre in 1991 did highlight pitfalls which were encountered in scintigraphy of 213 patients suspected of having hip fractures but with normal or equivocal radiographs.[11] They encountered two false-positive and two false-negative radionuclide studies. Both of the latter were in elderly patients and, especially as an avascular femoral head was demonstrable in one without focal uptake or a fracture site, it is possible that imaging at 4 and 7 days was premature. However, no temporal effect on the diagnostic accuracy of detection of hip fractures was found by Holder et al.[12] In 160 studies, the sensitivity for the diagnosis of hip fracture was 93% with a specificity of 95%. Three of seven false-positive studies had trochanteric fractures which were correctly identified in another 33 patients. Although false-negative studies occurred in four patients, all were over 70 years of age and images were obtained within 72 h. Holder et al[12] did not believe that this negated using early studies in order to avoid a delay in diagnosis. Nevertheless, they suggest that, in view of the dependence of MDP uptake on blood flow, the reduction of blood supply in displaced femoral neck fractures and the reduction in skeletal blood flow with increasing age, both 5 and 24 h delayed images are warranted in patients with suboptimal bone-soft tissue studies in the standard study. The experience of Slavin et al,[13] in studying 24 elderly patients with fractures of the femur or pelvis, justifies the opinion that, if an initial scan is equivocal, a repeat study after an interval of several days is required in order to ensure achieving the maximum sensitivity which can be provided by scintigraphy (Fig. 85.4). These problems are not encountered in the identification of scaphoid fractures, which are usually readily visualized within 3 days of trauma. Scintigraphy is therefore of considerable value in identifying this lesion before X-ray change appears, especially as difficulty may be encountered in radiological diagnosis even after 2–3 weeks.[14] In view of the consequences of a misdiagnosis of scaphoid fractures, such as pseudoarthrosis or avascular necrosis of the proximal fragment, confident exclusion of

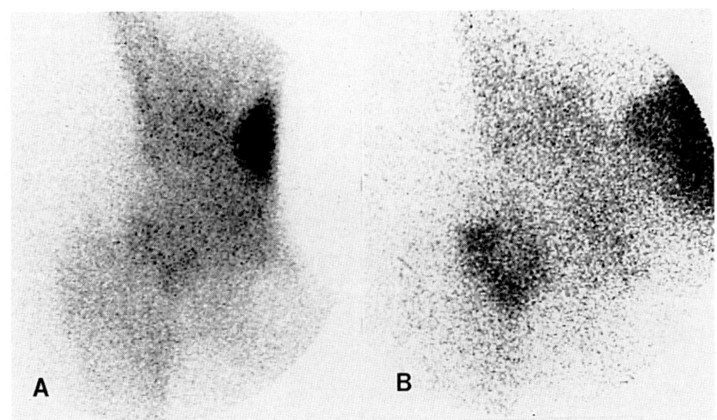

Fig. 85.4 Fractured neck of femur in an elderly osteoporotic female is associated with a minimal abnormality at 5 days (A), whereas increased uptake is readily demonstrable at 16 days (B).

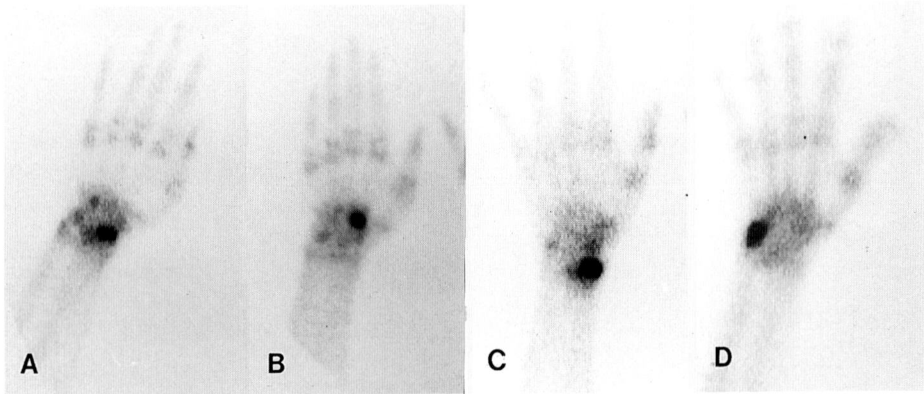

Fig. 85.5 Fractures in the hands and wrists are readily demonstrated by bone scintigraphy. (A) Scaphoid, (B) trapezium. (C) radial styloid, (D) pisiform.

this fracture is essential and can readily be achieved with bone scanning.[15] Indeed, in the study of 50 patients with scaphoid fracture, Bellmore et al[16] noted that, rather than the expected marked increase, a focal area of decreased uptake localized in the proximal pole, compatible with avascular necrosis was present in three patients, two of whom ultimately developed non-union. Premature imaging within 48 h must be avoided, particularly as the osseous scintigraphic changes may be obscured by the diffuse uptake resulting from superficial hyperaemia or traumatic synovitis. Difficulties in identifying the exact anatomical localization of a focus of uptake[17] can be overcome by the technique of a combined display of the scan and the radiograph described by Hawkes et al.[18] Such a display is applicable to scintigraphy of all wrist injuries since routine scintigraphy of the painful wrist frequently identifies fracture in any of the carpal bones (Fig. 85.5) or other results of trauma (Fig. 85.6). Rolfe et al,[19] for example, identified a scaphoid lesion in only 52% of 50 suspected scaphoid fractures, the remaining all having focal increased uptake in other carpal bones or distal radius. The diagnosis may of course be suspected because of a history of trauma or a sporting activity liable to cause fracture, for example the hook of the hamate in golfers. Increased activity in all phases of a three-phase bone scan can occur in an intraosseous ganglion, although because of the radiological appearances this is more likely to be confused with an osteoid osteoma.[20] Maurer et al[21] did advocate the use of three-phase scintigraphy with ^{99}Tc-MDP for evaluation of the hand not merely for the identification of osseous lesions but since such a range of vascular lesions could be observed.

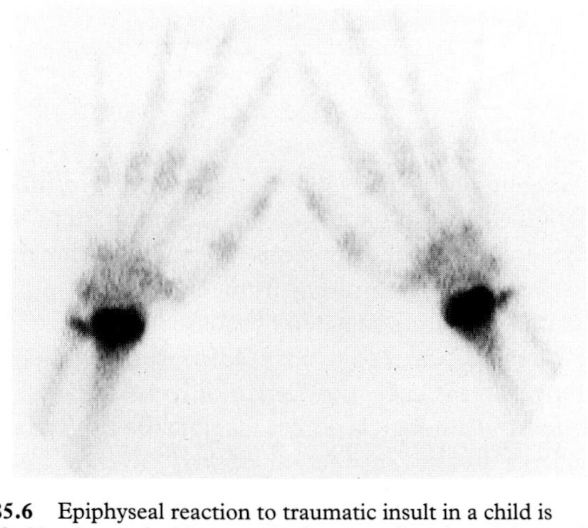

Because of the difficulties in obtaining a history of trauma from a pre-school child or even eliciting a satisfactory description of the location and nature of the pain, bone scintigraphy provides a simple and reliable investigation of the limping toddler and children with obscure lower extremity pain. Thus, focal scan abnormalities were identified by Englaro et al[22] in 30 of 56 children under 5 years of age with leg pain or gait abnormalities. In only nine were alternative imaging studies abnormal. In drawing attention to the incidence of lesions in the feet, they emphasized that nine abnormalities were actually located in the cuboid and only four in the calcaneum, considered a common site of fracture in this age group.[23] Miller & Sanderson[7] demonstrated the role of scintigraphy in identifying the classical toddler's fracture, the spiral lesion in the mid-shaft of the tibia. However, Park et al,[6] studying occult fractures in infants, drew attention to the generalized uptake along the bone which can occur with this fracture as well as in metaphyseal corner fractures, and emphasized the need to exclude infection or vascular occlusive disease. Osseous infection was identified in 20 children by Aronson et al[24] as the cause of a limp in 50 toddlers, and bone trauma as the cause in nine. Abnormal radiographs were present in four of the former group but in none of the latter. The susceptibility of paralysed limbs to trauma can result in occult fractures. As pointed out by Townsend et al,[25] such fractures, especially

Fig. 85.6 Epiphyseal reaction to traumatic insult in a child is identified by the marked increase in the normal preferential growth plate uptake in both distal radii.

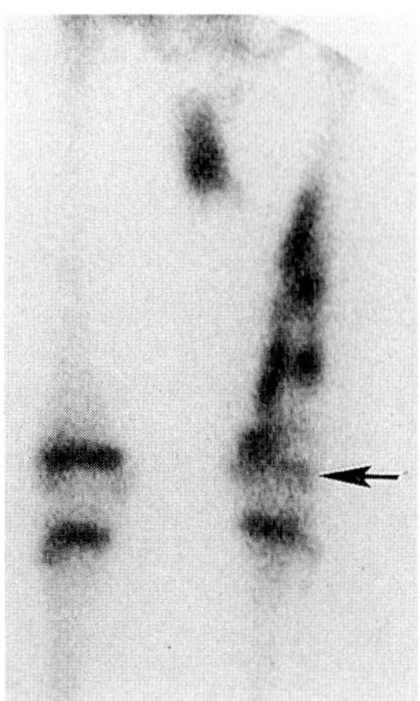

Fig. 85.7 Occult fracture. In a $6\frac{1}{2}$-year-old girl with myelomeningocele, the susceptibility to injury by minimal trauma resulted in epiphyseal fracture and separation. The bone scan showed the marked reduction of normal accumulation is at the site of epiphyseal separation in the distal growth plate of the left femur (arrow), indicating cessation of osteoblastic activity. Extensive uptake surrounded the distal two-thirds of the femur, indicating the cortical hyperostosis resulting from the reaction produced by the periosteal stripping following the injury.

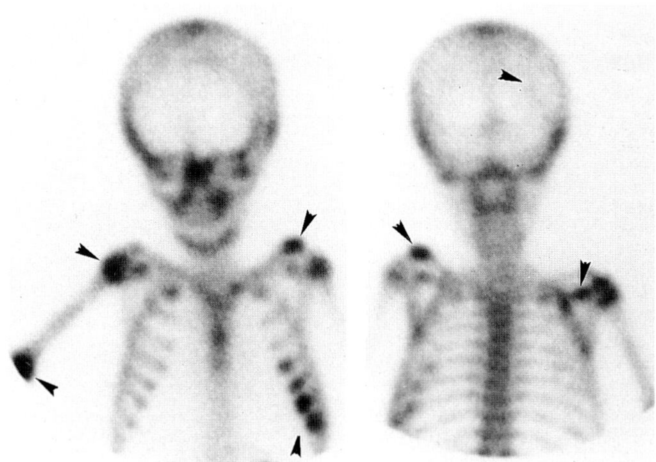

Fig. 85.8 Non-accidental trauma in a $2\frac{1}{2}$-year-old girl is revealed by identification of fractures in four ribs, right humeral, proximal epiphysis and distal metaphysis, left clavicle, left scapula and right parietal skull.

when associated with an epiphyseal separation, may simulate infection. In a study by Kumar et al[26] of 16 children with myelomeningocele, those with diaphyseal or metaphyseal fractures all presented local and systemic features in keeping with an acute infection. Bone scintigraphy, however, can demonstrate the different features which permit identification of the correct diagnosis (Fig. 85.7).

Non-accidental trauma

The sensivity of skeletal scintigraphy allied with the simplicity with which whole surveys may be performed has made the procedure so indispensible in the assessment of the abused child that for medical, social and legal reasons, it is often considered essential whenever such assault is suspected (Fig. 85.8). This role has been identified in numerous studies. Sty & Starshak[27] for example, studying 261 children, found that scintigraphy was positive in 120 with two false-negative studies, whereas radiography was positive in 95 with 32 false-negative results. In 15 patients, one or more of the fractures were demonstrated only in the radionuclide study, while in another 17 it identified additional sites of injury. This reflects, in part, the nature of many of the injuries and, in part, the sites most frequently involved.[28] In addition to the diaphysis, where twisting of the limb induces periosteal reaction, rib fractures, particularly posterior, are the all too common consequence of shaking an infant. Jaudes,[29] comparing modalities in identifying 41 lesions, observed that rib fractures made up eight of the nine fractures not demonstrated by radiographs but positive with scanning. The other common injuries, metaphyseal corner fractures and epiphyseal separations, may be readily visualized by scintigraphy because of the changes in the intensity of uptake and distortion of the shape of the growth plate. However, identification of these changes can be difficult in the infant, particularly when symmetrical. The radionuclide procedure is also less reliable than radiography in identifying skull fractures because of the lesser osteoblastic response in linear fractures and low lesion-to-background ratio. Sty & Starshak[27] did not identify 4 of 11 skull fractures, and Haase et al,[30] while reporting that scans were positive in 39% of abused children with normal radiographs, noted that scintigraphy was normal in two skull fractures. Accordingly, in order to ensure the greatest probability of fracture detection when signs of physical abuse are encountered, complementary scintigraphic and radiographic studies are warranted in the child under 1 year of age and confirmatory radiography employed to examine scintigraphically abnormal areas in the older child. In reviewing the radionuclide studies, other consequences of the trauma may be apparent as extraosseous uptake in sites of cerebral or renal infarction and in haematomas.

Stress injuries

The scintigraphic changes associated with insufficiency and fatigue fractures are essentially similar. The former may be somewhat less obvious because of the reduced delineation of bone resulting from diminished radiopharmaceutical uptake associated with the metabolic disturbance affecting the bone, so predisposing to the injury. Differences in the sites most commonly involved do reflect the differing aetiological forces, weight bearing playing a greater role in the production of insufficiency fractures, whereas the bone insult in fatigue fractures is characteristically the effect of excess muscular action. The latter can result from a variety of activities, each of which may require the use of such particular muscles that the stress injuries occur at sites which are almost specific for various sports.

Compression fractures of a vertebra are probably the most common consequence of severe osteoporosis, readily identified with scintigraphy as the loss of vertebral height and contour with intense linear radiopharmaceutical uptake (Fig. 85.9). Insufficiency fractures of the sacrum also present characteristic images with an H-shaped abnormality (Fig. 85.10).[31] However, much greater difficulty can be experienced in identifying fractures of the pars interarticularis, whether resulting from insufficiency or from a variety of athletic activities. This difficulty is perhaps not surprising in view of the overlapping of the various components of a vertebra when viewed in the standard posterior projection. The ease with which this problem is solved by the use of SPECT exemplifies the virtues of this procedure in providing an accurate image of a body section at a prescribed depth and by separating structures overlapping in planar images. Not only is lesional contrast enhanced but localization is improved, thus providing more exact delineation of the size and extent of a lesion (Fig. 85.11). In view of the feasibility not

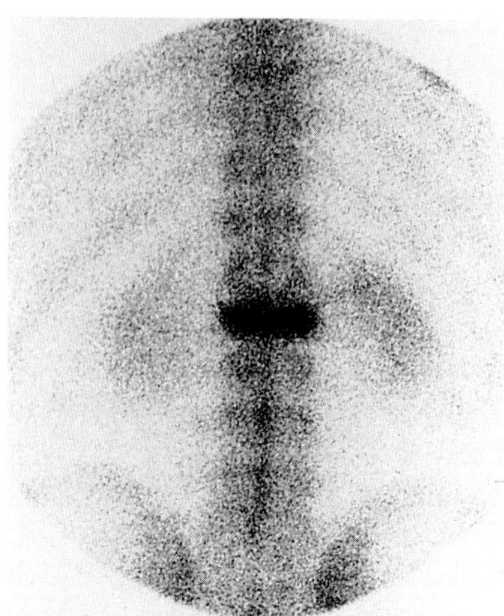

Fig. 85.9 Compression fracture. Typical vertebral insufficiency fracture in an elderly osteoporotic woman, characterized by loss of vertebral contour and linear accumulation throughout the affected vertebral body.

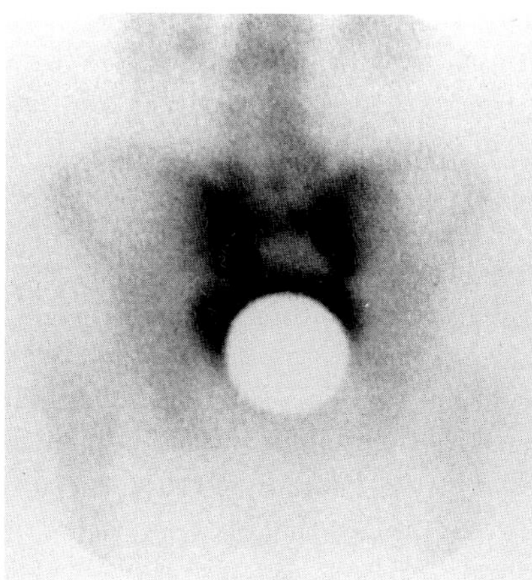

Fig. 85.10 Sacral insufficiency fracture is characterized by H-shaped accumulation identified in both sacroiliac joints and sacrum.

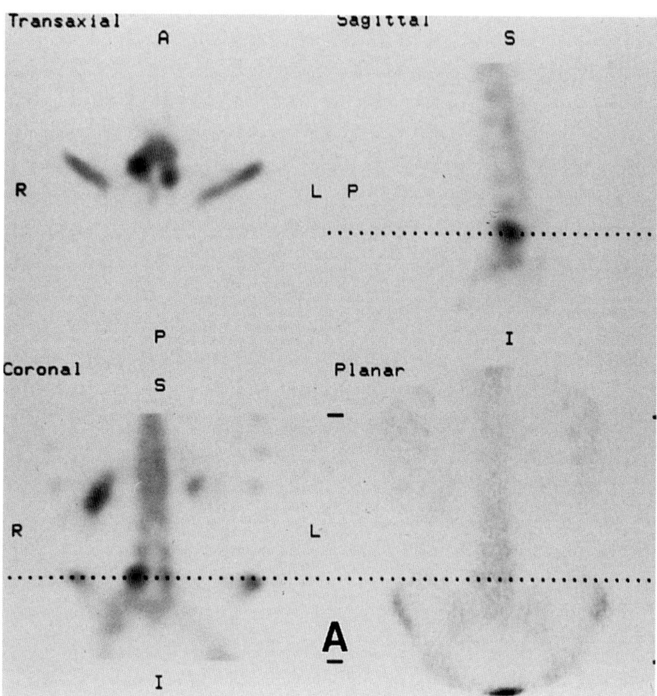

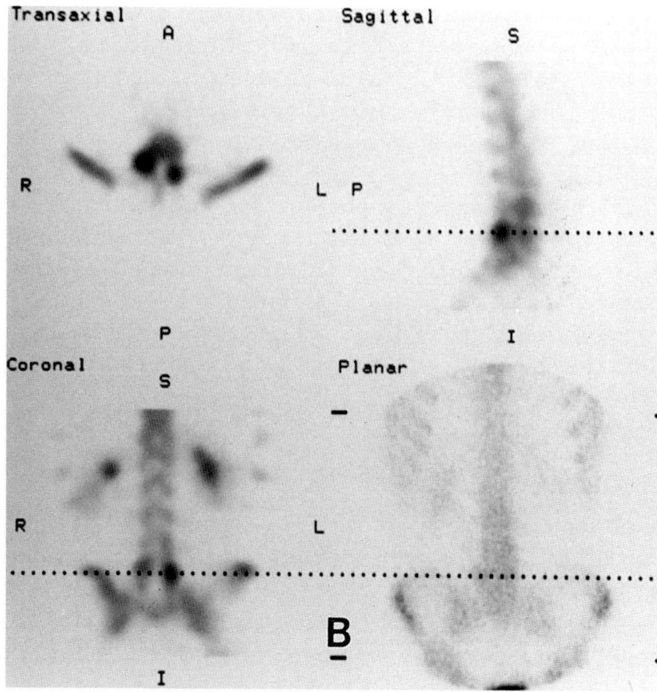

Fig. 85.11 SPECT in evaluation of low back pain. The exact localization which can be achieved with SPECT is demonstrated by the identification at different planes in a patient in whom the same vertebra is the site both of a pars interarticularis stress fracture on the top (A) and osteochondritis in the articular facet on the bottom (B).

only of assessing any alterations in the body of a vertebra but also of identifying the pedicles, laminae and spinous processes separately, SPECT has found a very major role in the investigation of the lumbar spine. This reflects the frequency of the complaint of low back pain and the numerous responsible aetiologies, high amongst which is trauma, both acute and chronic. The value of the procedure has been demonstrated in many series. Ryan et al[32] for example, studying 70 patients with low back pain, detected lesions with planar imaging in 36% and with SPECT in 60%. Additional lesions were found in 39% of the patients with a positive planar scan. Of the lesions detected by SPECT alone, 63% were localized to the posterior element. Radiographs detected 90% of the anterior lesions but only 40% of posterior lesions. In an extensive study by Kanmaz et al[33] of 1390 adult patients with chronic low back pain, abnormal studies were encountered in 1006. Within the lumbosacral spine, 44% of the abnormalities were equally well seen on planar and SPECT, 24% better seen on SPECT but 31% were only seen using SPECT. In the lumbar spine, 36% of the abnormalities were located within the vertebral bodies, but it was possible to identify that 53.8% lay in the laminae or pedicles, 88.7% in the spinous processes and 1.3% in the transverse processes, so clearly demonstrating the feasibility of exact localization. The improved sensitivity conferred by SPECT was elegantly demonstrated by Gates[34] in a study of 100 patients with low back pain, 23 of whom had an abnormality seen only on SPECT. By grading the intensity of the alteration noted in the abnormal planar scans, it was evident that the improved accuracy with SPECT lay in its ability to identify quite readily those lesions with minimal change in planar imaging, 39 (81%) of 48 such lesions being easily detected by SPECT.

The major clinical application for this sensitivity in providing such precise localization again reflects the ability of skeletal scintigraphy to demonstrate the physiological activity of a lesion in bone. This emerges vividly from the work of Collier et al,[35] who studied 19 patients with radiological evidence of spondylolysis and/or spondylolisthesis. The importance of this particular investigation was not merely that SPECT had a sensitivity of 85% compared to 62% with planar scintigraphy but that positive studies only occurred in the 13 patients with pain. Bellah et al[36] undertook lumbar SPECT studies in 162 young athletes with low back pain, the symptoms being referrable to the posterior elements, in most instances suspected to be the result of stress in the pars interarticularis as the result of athletic injury. In 71 patients, lesions were identified with SPECT, whereas the planar study was positive in only 32. In 25 of the individuals in whom SPECT was abnormal, radiological examination was normal, possibly on the basis that spondylolysis resulted from multiple microfractures too small to be seen with radiographs but associated with sufficient osteoblastic activity to accumulate bone-seeking radiopharmaceuticals readily. It was suggested that such discordance between radionuclide and radiological examinations could well be of assistance in deciding whether or not surgery might be required. Further, it was postulated that the patient's management could be assisted by observation of the resolution of the scintigraphic abnormalities in serial examinations (Fig. 85.12). Such resolution certainly can be observed but, as with the evidence of bone remodelling persisting after any trauma, the passage of at least 6 months is usually required before it is possible to identify with confidence a return to normality. Even greater degrees of intensity of accumulation, reflecting osteoblastic response to bone remodelling, is to be expected following surgical trauma with only very gradual reduction as healing is achieved. However, diminution in accumulation should be obvious by 1 year and abnormal persistence of such uptake is clearly of significance as evident in the study by Slizofski et al.[37] Characteristically it will occur in pseudoarthrosis, a complication in up to 56% of patients who have undergone lumbar fusion operations. Lusins et al[38] found similar changes with SPECT in symptomatic patients after fusion, but in patients with persistent pain following laminectomy alone also identified focal increased uptake in the articular facets at levels of maximum instability. It is possible that SPECT could also have a role in the evaluation of continuing symptomatology following surgery in the cervical spine. However, remarkably little attention has been paid to its application in this region, although undoubtedly it can demonstrate abnormalities with a remarkable degree of accumulation compared with those visualized with planar examinations (Fig. 85.13). Boyko et al[39] studied 30 patients with cervical spine trauma with the lateral articular pillar compression deformity on radiography,

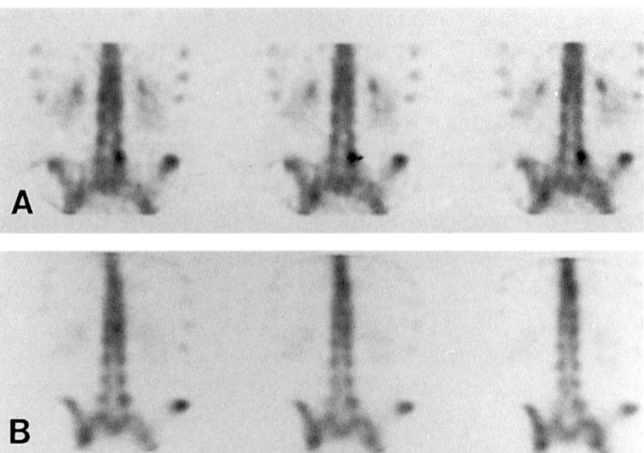

Fig. 85.12 Serial SPECT evaluation of stress fracture. The response to appropriate management in a 12-year-old cricketer who suffered a stress fracture of the pars interarticularis of L5 (A), is readily demonstrated by the marked reduction in the focal osteoblastic activity in the sequential study (B) undertaken 6 months later.

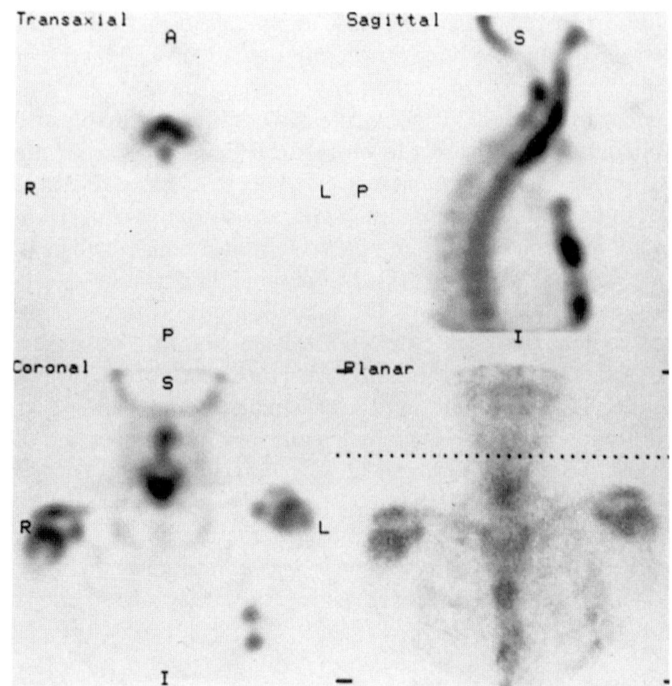

Fig. 85.13 Cervical spine injury. SPECT permits the identification of the extensive abnormal accumulation in the cervical spine following 'whiplash' injury resulting from a motor vehicle accident. In the sagittal view, the sternal fractures are also readily visualized.

concluding that a normal SPECT study negated the diagnosis of recent fracture.

While SPECT can readily enhance the visualization of lesions affecting the sacroiliac region, Onsel et al[40] have drawn attention to the care that must be taken in the evaluation of increased sacroiliac joint uptake visualized with SPECT. Such uptake was demonstrable in 43 (6%) of 753 patients. It was relevant that 15 of the 43 patients had undergone prior lumbar laminectomy and/or spinal fusion. They concluded that such increased sacroiliac joint uptake is usually the result of altered spinal mechanics. These alterations, while occurring in patients with pars interarticularis fractures, will induce mild accumulation, much less delineated and much less intense than in the fracture site, in the contralateral aspect of the posterior element.

Stress fractures

Early detection of stress fractures of the femoral neck is particularly critical. Reflecting the facts that walking exerts forces through the femur approximately six times body weight and that running can increase these to 10–20 times body weight, there is a high probability of progression to complete fracture with the subsequent dire consequences of displacement, whether in the elderly osteoporotic or young military recruit (Fig. 85.14). Differences in the site may be recognized, being in the superior neck in the older patient compared with the inferior neck in young athletes. Stress fractures of the femoral shaft predominantly occur in the proximal third, mainly being visualized on the medial aspect. They do present a different pattern from the focal increased uptake associated with periosteal reaction at the iliopsoas insertion on the lesser trochanter or characteristic alterations of trochanteric bursitis on the upper lateral aspect of the greater trochanter.

The tibia is the most common site of stress fractures, making up more than 50% in almost all series. There is a remarkable disagreement in such series as to the most frequently affected portion of this bone. In some, the mid-shaft has proved to be extremely uncommon, in comparison, for example, to being the location in 164 of 280 tibial stress fractures identified by Zwas et al.[4] However, the posterior aspect of the upper third of the tibia is undoubtedly the most common site in children (Fig. 85.15) and the elderly patient. In contrast, the distal third is typically

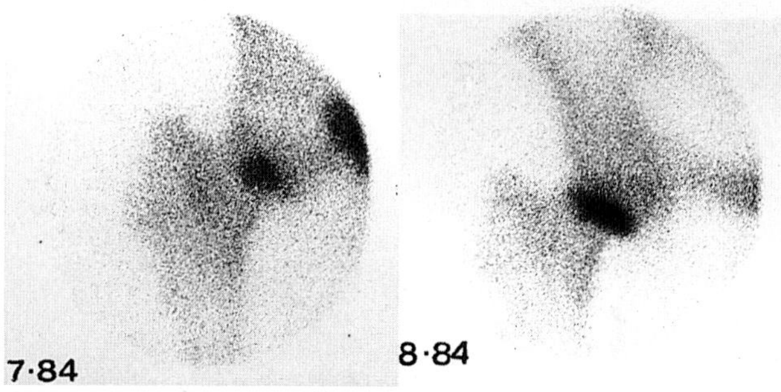

Fig. 85.14 Insufficiency fracture of femoral neck. Serial studies in an 82-year-old woman with osteoporosis: the initial study (July 1984) demonstrated that right hip pain resulted from an insufficiency fracture limited to the lower aspect of the femoral neck which subsequently (August 1984) became much more intense and extended across the entire femoral neck.

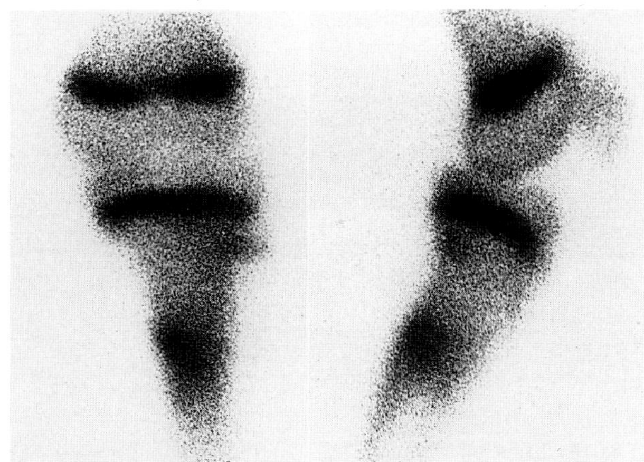

Fig. 85.15 Stress fracture in the upper posterior aspect of the tibia in a 12-year-old boy. The characteristic pattern of uptake identifying the grading as II is best observed in the lateral projection.

affected in marathon runners, in whom the distal fibula may also be the site of stress fractures.

The metatarsals are also a common site for the occurrence of stress fractures, making up 20% of the 1000 consecutive stress fractures in runners reviewed by McBryde.[41] The second and third metatarsals are involved in about 90% (Fig. 85.16). However, any tarsal bone can be affected by trauma and identified as the site of abnormal accumulation by scintigraphy. There may be several areas of increased uptake, in some circumstances the result of the nature of the traumatic insult, for example the anterior impingement syndrome. The injury may be rare, albeit typical of the activity, for example to Lisfranc's joint in kickboxing, or fairly frequently encountered in a variety of sports. Calcaneal stress fractures with a vertical linear band of increased activity in the central portion of the body are associated with activities ranging from parachute jumping to prolonged standing. The latter may induce sesamoiditis visualized with well-delineated small foci of increased uptake, also demonstrable in sesamoid stress fracture, which frequently accompanies other foot injuries. Navicular fractures, usually in the middle third, occur in a variety of sports, usually readily identifiable and distinguishable from the more focal linear uptake of the unstable accessory navicular (Fig. 85.16). While fractures of the neck of the talus can occur, and do cause concern in view of the possibility of subsequent avascular necrosis of the head, the lesion of considerable importance is the subchondral fracture of the talar dome. It is now recognized that this is identical with osteochondritis dissecans of the talus, being traumatic in origin and a not infrequent cause of acute or chronic ankle pain. Bone scanning in different projections readily permits finding the location of the intense localized uptake (Fig. 85.16). Urman et al,[42] for example, studying 102 patients with ankle pain, identified 46 of 48 with talar dome fractures.

Stress fractures are relatively less common in the axial skeleton and upper extremities. These may occur in the

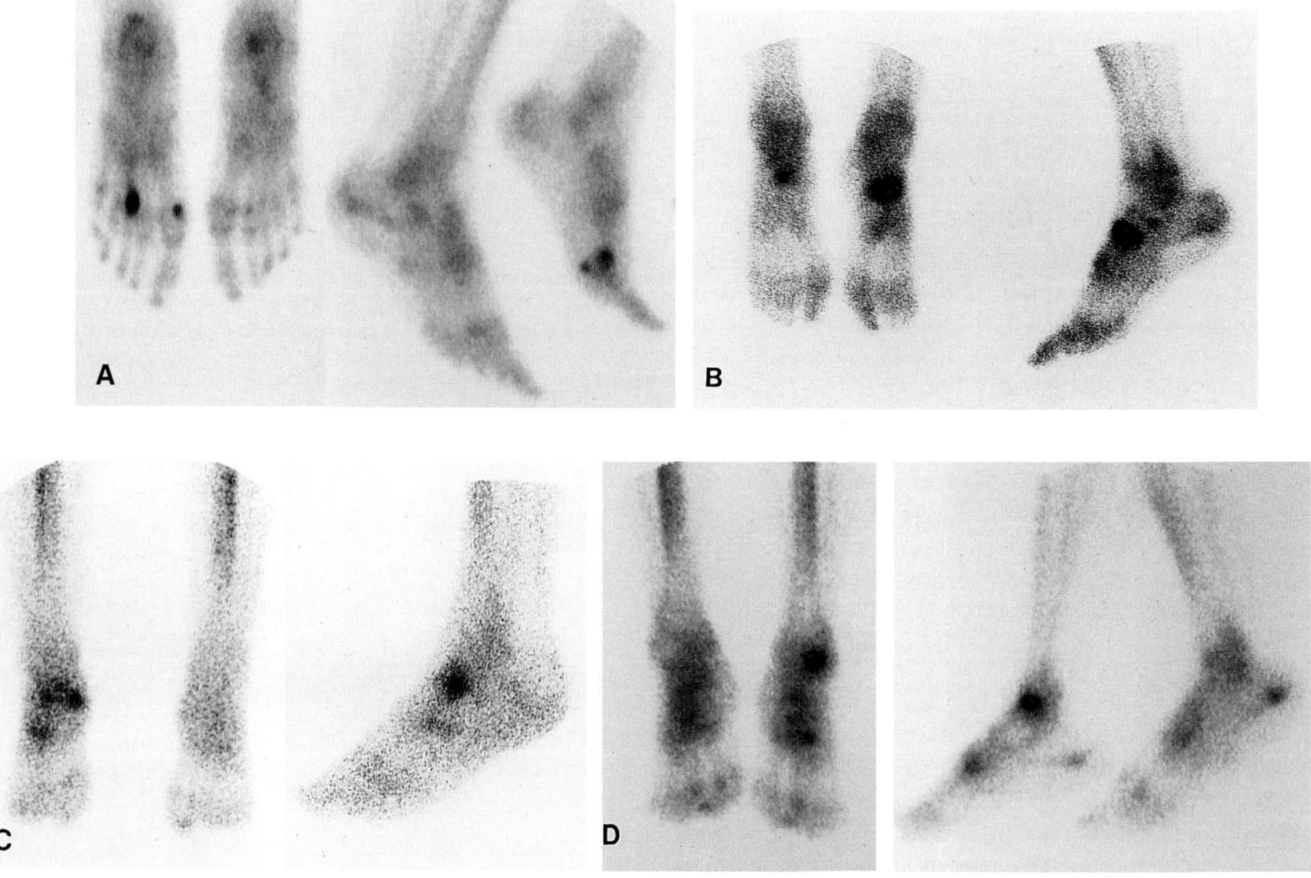

Fig. 85.16 Stress injuries of the feet. (A) Stress fracture of the third metatarsal is demonstrable as a site of intense uptake. A further trauma-related abnormality is noted with the accumulation in the sesamoid. (B) Stress fracture of the navicular. (C) Accessory navicular: focal uptake medial to the navicular identifies traumatic reaction in the accessory navicular and explains the cause of pain in a runner's feet. (D) Talar dome fracture. Focal uptake characteristic of a subchondral fracture on the talar dome. (E) Increased accumulation across the tarsometatarsal joints occurring as the result of injury to Lisfranc's joint in a 16-year-old kickboxer.

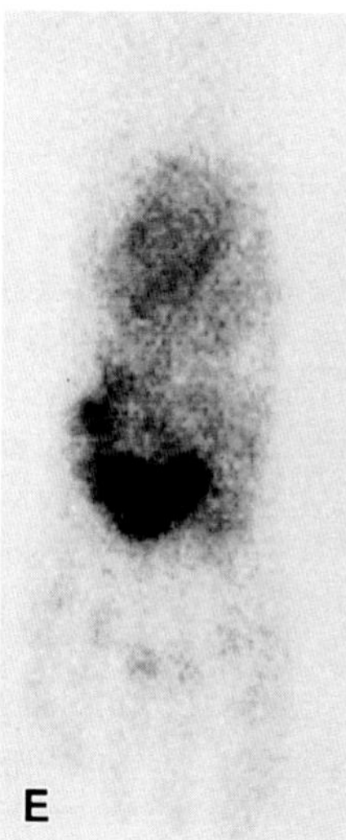

Fig. 85.16E

ribs in golfers and tennis players and have been noted in the humeral shaft, associated with a variety of sports including weightlifting and javelin throwing.

Enthesopathies

The elongated narrow accumulation typical of 'shin splints' is most commonly observed in the posterior aspect of the tibia related to the insertion of the tibialis posterior or soleus (Fig. 85.17). It may be demonstrable anteriorly in the periosteal attachment of the tibialis anterior. Very similar changes have been described as 'thigh splints' as the result of the adductor insertion avulsion syndrome occurring mainly in female military recruits[43] but also demonstrable in ballet dancers. These changes, consistent with periostitis from overuse injury, are seen at the insertion of the large adductor muscles along the proximal and middle third of the femur on the medial aspect, but alterations at the insertion of the gluteus maximus and pectineus have also been observed. The aetiology is similar in the production of scintigraphic alterations at the insertional sites of the pectoralis major on the medial aspect of the proximal humerus, occurring in gymnasts and weightlifters.

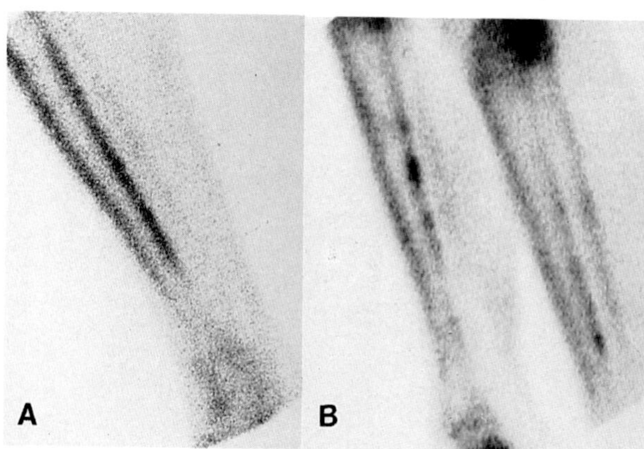

Fig. 85.17 Enthesopathy. (A) Linear increased uptake confined to the cortical surface induced by periosteal reaction to stress, the typical 'shin splints'. (B) More focal areas within the linear uptake indicate that, in this runner, the continuing stress has been such as to initiate the changes of stress fractures.

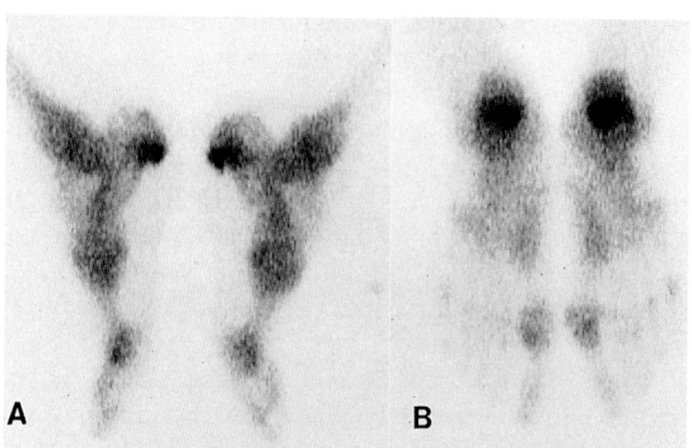

Fig. 85.18 Plantar fasciitis. The insertional reaction is observed as focal uptake in the sites of origin of the plantar fascia on the calcaneum. (A, medial view; B, plantar view)

The intense localized uptake at sites of muscle or ligamentous insertion can be demonstrated at numerous sites throughout the body depending on the nature of the overuse insult. The changes typical of plantar fasciitis[44] (Fig. 85.18) result from overexertion and repeated microtrauma from traction due to dorsiflexion, producing a localized reactive periostitis. Focal uptake is readily demonstrable on the plantar aspect of the calcaneal tuberosity and occasionally at the insertion of the fascia into the bases of the proximal phalanges. It is readily differentiated from Achilles tendonitis, also not visualized radiologically, over the insertion in the upper calcaneal tuberosity. Osteitis pubis is also very readily identified. In the stress context, it represents the effects of overuse of the large adductor muscles, particularly the adductor longus

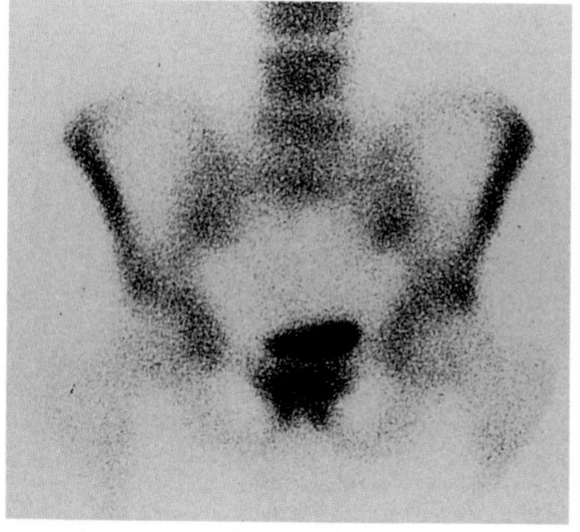

Fig. 85.19 Osteitis pubis in a female runner: characteristic increased accumulation in the symphysis pubis.

and brevis and the gracilis, inducing abnormal shearing forces on the symphysis. Characteristically there is bilateral increased radionuclide accumulation in the pubic rami at the symphysis pubis with sparing of the relatively photopenic cartilagenous symphysis (Fig. 85.19). The evidence of reaction to stress may merely be uptake limited to the insertion of these muscles, but occasionally there may be evidence of frank pelvic stress fracture with increased accumulation extending across the full width of the pubic rami.

Common stress injuries occur at the elbow. Lateral epicondylitis (tennis elbow) (Fig. 85.20) is associated with overuse of the extensive carpi radialis brevis while, on the medial aspect, medial epicondylitis occurs in young baseballers with increased accumulation at the insertions of the flexor and pronator muscle groups. Occasionally abnormal uptake in the radial styloid will identify injury at the insertion of the brachioradialis tendon.

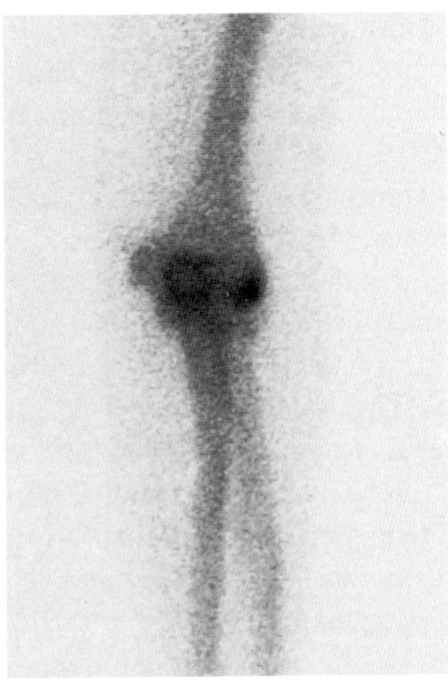

Fig. 85.20 Tennis elbow. Focal abnormal uptake in the lateral epicondyle.

Avulsion injuries

In keeping with the concern regarding excess training of young athletes and the consequent 'big muscles, small bones' increasing the risk of stress injuries, apophyseal avulsion injuries are common in adolescence (Fig. 85.21). The pelvis and hip apophyses are particularly susceptible, fusing later than elsewhere. Early diagnosis is desirable to reduce the continuing displacement of the fragment which occurs, particularly in avulsions of the ischium, the most common injury because of the power of the hamstring muscles. The scintigraphic findings will depend on the displacement and the time of the study since the injury. On occasion the fragment may be clearly demonstrated in its displaced site but, as healing proceeds, localized increased accumulation, often intense and resembling an exostosis, may be demonstrable.

Acute muscle contraction may be responsible for injury to the accessory navicular, which is usually an asymptomatic normal variant. Avulsion of the tibialis posterior can occur or there may be disruption of the fibrocartilaginous union with the navicular itself. These changes induce the characteristic focal accumulation of bone-seeking radiopharmaceuticals. The study therefore has a valuable clinical role in explaining the cause of pain. Lawson et al[45] showed that, even when the radiological variant is bilateral, increased radionuclide activity occurs only on the symptomatic side (Fig. 85.16). Chondro-osseal changes can be shown histologically, compatible with chronic trauma and stress fractures. Similar mechanisms may be responsible for the induction of pain in a bipartite patella, resulting in an unstable synchondrosis. Certainly skeletal scintigraphy can identify preferential accumulation, most

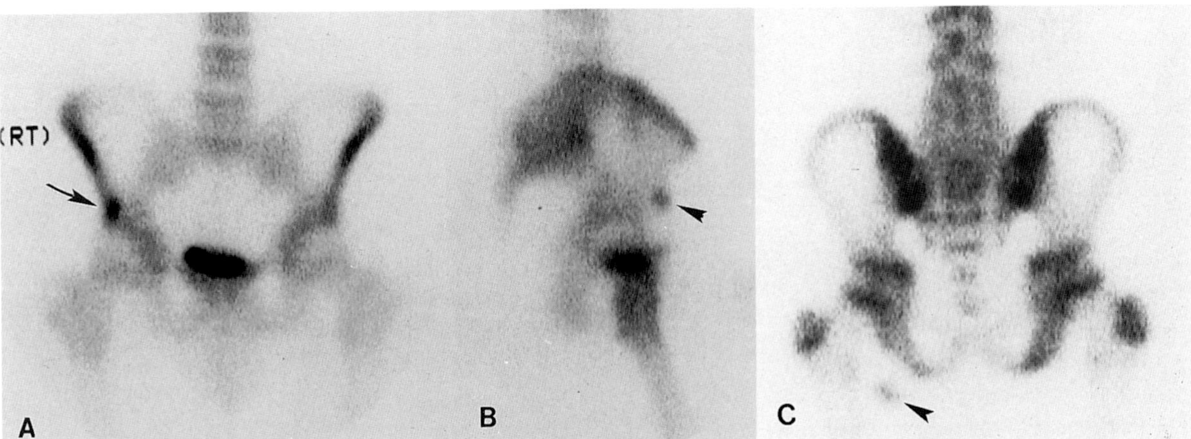

Fig. 85.21 Avulsion injuries. (A and B) Localized increased uptake in the anterior inferior iliac spine indicates avulsive reaction produced by excessive action of the rectus femoris. (C) Avulsion of the ischial tuberosity is shown by identification of the displaced fragment (arrow) and reduced uptake in the ischium compared with the contralateral side.

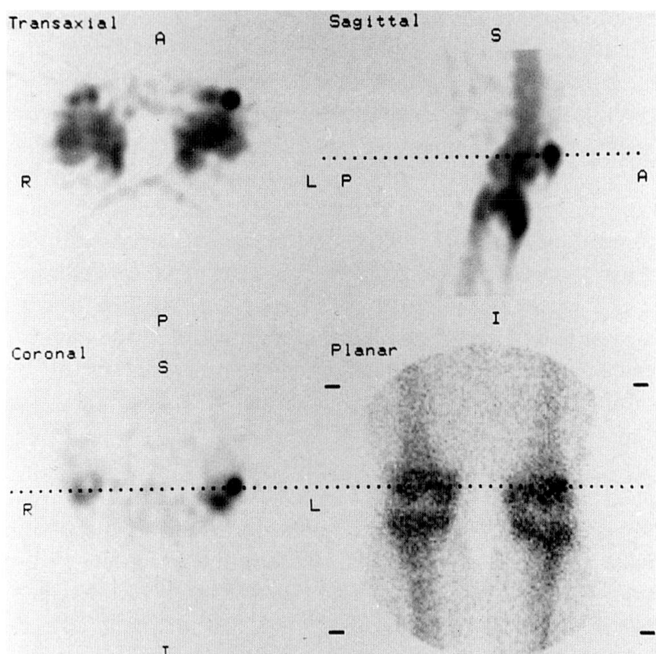

Fig. 85.22 Painful bipartite patellae. Whereas the planar views merely identified an alteration in radiopharmaceutical distribution in the region of the left knee, SPECT permits not only demonstration of the bilateral bipartite patellae but the localization of the intense accumulation in the traumatized lateral fragment on the left, responsible for the knee pain.

commonly in the lateral fragment (Fig. 85.22) and, by demonstrating abnormal metabolic activity, indicate that the radiological abnormality is of clinical significance as the cause of pain.

Intense focal accumulation in the tibial tuberosity is readily demonstrable in the Osgood–Schlatter lesion, in keeping with histological changes similar to those noted in the traumatized accessory navicular or bipartite patella. It is now generally accepted, despite various opinions previously, that the lession is traumatic in origin with microavulsions of the anterior tibial tubercle, although Rosenberg et al[46] have postulated that it is a tendonitis. Preferential accumulation in this tubercle at the insertion of the patellar tendon is a frequent incidental finding in scintigraphic examination of other sports lesions of the knee. The demonstration of such focal accumulation is clearly of clinical significance when associated with local symptomatology, while the scintigraphic demonstration of localized accumulation at the origin of the patellar tendon at the inferior pole of the patella is also of value in establishing the diagnosis of infrapatella tendonitis (jumper's knee, Sinding–Larsen syndrome).[47] On occasion, as in basketball or volleyball players, such foci may be noted at the upper and lower aspects of the patellar tendon (Fig. 85.23). Increased accumulation in both tibial tuberosities has been reported in enthesopathy of the patellar tendon insertion due to chronic isotretinoin therapy.[48]

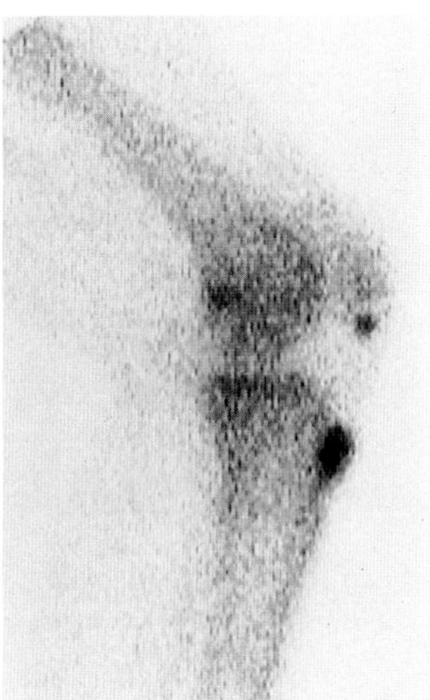

Fig. 85.23 Patellar tendonitis. The changes in 'basketballer's knee': intense focal accumulation at the insertion of the patellar ligament on both the inferior patella and tibial tuberosity is clearly demonstrated.

Other trauma-related lesions

Some of the consequences of trauma may produce scintigraphic alterations not directly attributable to muscle overuse. Indeed, the outcome of some injuries may be post-traumatic arthritis in which the scan will show increased radionuclide activity on both sides of a joint, particularly frequently observed in the ankles (Fig. 85.24).

Impingement syndromes

The posterior impingement syndrome results from repeated plantar flexion such as is employed by ballet dancers, gymnasts and downhill runners. As a consequence the os trigoneum, an accessory ossicle that occasionally forms a synostosis with the posterior aspect of the talus, can be compressed between the calcaneus and the posterior lip of the tibia, eventually creating a fracture. A focal area of

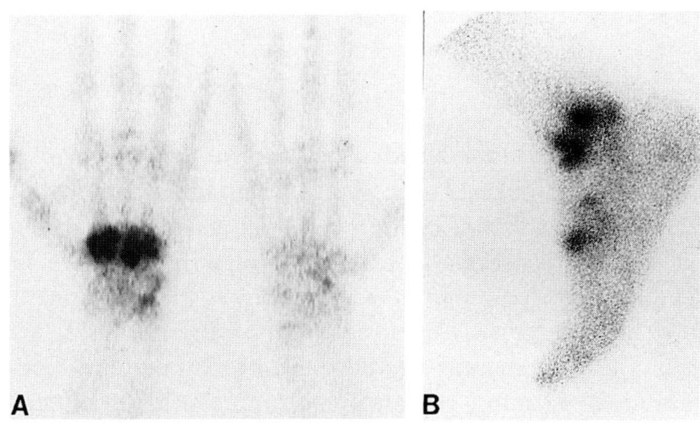

Fig. 85.24 Post-traumatic arthritis. The persistent effect of traumatic injury is visualized as increased uptake on either aspect of the joint. (A) metacarpophalangeal joints, (B) ankle.

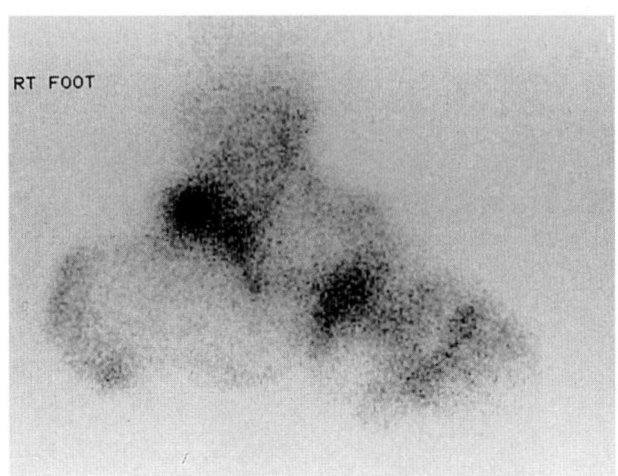

Fig. 85.25 Posterior impingement. As the consequence of repeated plantar flexion and compression of the os trigoneum, intense focal uptake is demonstrable in the posterior aspect of the talus.

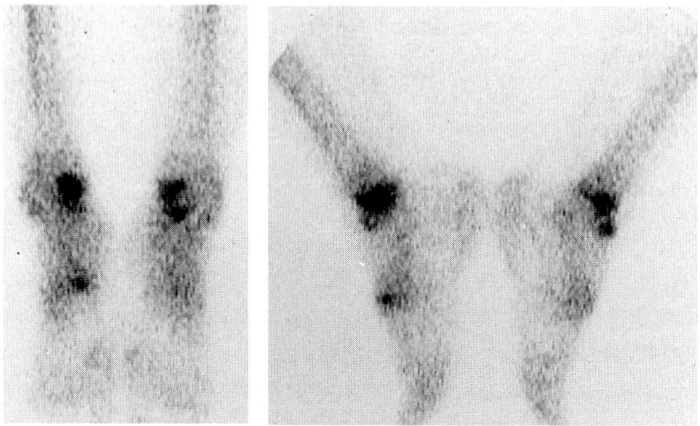

Fig. 85.26 Anterior impingement. At the sites of repetitive contact of the tibia against the talus by repetitive dorsiflexion of the ankle, localized uptake demonstrates the induced osteoblastic reaction.

increased radionuclide activity in the site of the os trigonem is characteristic (Fig. 85.25). Repeated dorsiflexion of the ankle, occurring frequently in ballet dancing, high jumping and basketball, is the underlying mechanism of the anterior impingement syndrome (Fig. 85.26). Repetitive contact of the talus against the tibia induces the growth of hypertrophic spurs on the dorsum of the talus, the tibiotalar joint or the talonavicular joint. These areas of neo-osteogenesis are readily identified in the bone scan.

Subtalar coalitions

Increased radionuclide accumulation in a hypertrophic spur, the talar beak, is a frequent finding in patients with a symptomatic subtalar coalition. It results from the abnormal joint mechanics which produce repetitive trauma on the talar periosteum. Bone scintigraphy is therefore useful in identifying talocalcaneal coalition as the cause of foot pain. These congenital coalitions can be fibrous, fibrocartilaginous or osseous, the most common site being talocalcaneal and involving the middle facet. The talar bar may be very difficult to identify with plain radiography but can be the site of increased accumulation of bone-seeking radiopharmaceuticals.[49] Such uptake was shown by Mandell et al[50] in five of seven non-osseous coalitions and in both osseous coalitions. They advocated the use of pinhole collimation since the magnification views succeeded in separating the talus and the calcaneus. In these studies, increased accumulation, ascribed to physiological activity, was demonstrated in accessory bones, the accessory apophyseal ossification centre of the dorsal process of the talus, the os trigonem tarsi and calcaneus secondarius. These changes are slight in comparison with the intense accumulation associated with stress fracture of the anterior calcaneal process produced by excessive stretching of the bifurcate ligament.

Osteochondritis dissecans

It is now accepted that osteochondritis dissecans of the talus is synonomous with subchondral fracture of the dome and is the result of trauma. Although various alternative causes have been postulated, it is generally considered that trauma, associated with focal avascular necrosis, is also responsible for the disorder at other sites, particularly for the occurrence in the knee. In this joint, there is a predilection for the lateral aspect of the medial femoral condyle, making up 75% of the lesions. The radionuclide study demonstrates focal hyperaemia and intense well-delineated accumulation in the sites of the subchondral fractures, the size reflecting whether separation of the osteochondral fragment has occurred.

The traumatized knee

A variety of lesions in and around the knee can result from both acute and chronic trauma and reflect a number of aetiological mechanisms. Scintigraphic alterations are, therefore, readily induced, but because of the injuries may be multiple, and because of the overlapping anatomical features of the knee difficulties may be experienced in the interpretation. It is not surprising, therefore, that SPECT has been found to be of considerable use in localizing abnormal osteoblastic activity in and around the knee. Its use also exemplifies the role in providing the opportunity to review spatial information in three planes. Thus, in SPECT examinations of the knee, the greatest information may often be obtained from the transaxial images since this plane is, of course, at right angles to the antero-posterior projection of the planar images and only achievable with SPECT. Using planar scintigraphy, Marymont et al[51] reported a high degree of accuracy in the detection of meniscal tears, but their experience was not confirmed and the procedure did not become widely adopted. However, Collier et al[52] used SPECT for the investigation of chronic knee pain and found an overall sensitivity of 90% for the detection of sites of bone pathology. Nevertheless, particularly in the identification of meniscal tears, there was a low specificity, attributed to the long period since the trauma. Scintigraphy does therefore appear to have its greatest value in patients presenting with acute knee pain, particularly those who have recently suffered athletic trauma. In a study of 52 such patients, Murray et al[53] found that the planar images were equivalent to those obtained with SPECT in only 17 patients (33%). In 12 patients the planar was less diagnostic in that the uptake was much less than that obtained with SPECT, whereas in the remaining 23 the accumulation in the region of the knee in the planar studies was too marked and diffuse to allow any localization of the uptake. SPECT, however, readily identified the site and delineated the extent of the different types of injury. Focal accumulation at the site of muscle and ligamentous insertions was clearly localized, indicating reaction to stress such as avulsion of the medial collateral ligament of the medial femoral condyle (Pellegrini–Stieda lesion). Patellar pain, whether due to the stressed bipartite patella, fracture or tendonitis, was usually associated with characteristic scan alterations. While SPECT is useful in locating the abnormality in bipartite patellae, the marked uptake resulting from stress fractures is usually demonstrable with planar scintigraphy.[54] Similar planar studies were adequate for Kohn et al[55] to grade the degree of increased accumulation in 100 patients with chondromalacia and demonstrate a close correlation with the grade observed on

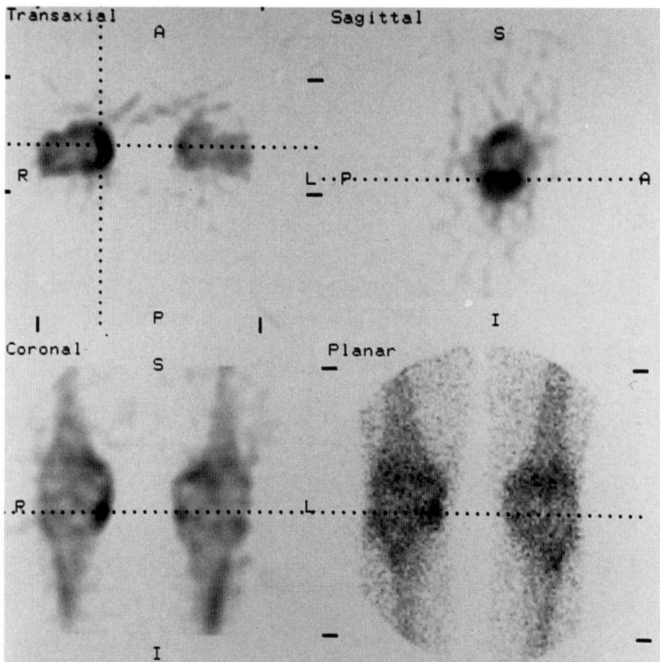

Fig. 85.27 Meniscal damage. Whereas planar imaging merely identified a mild abnormality in the medial aspect of the right knee, SPECT identifies intense accumulation which, particularly in the transaxial view, conforms to the outline of the medial meniscus and is characteristic of a meniscal tear.

arthroscopy. SPECT, however, is particularly valuable in identifying the site and the extent of the damage when meniscal tears are the cause of presenting pain (Fig. 85.27). Finding a sensitivity of 88%, a specificity of 87% and a negative predictive value of 91% for meniscal injuries, Murray et al[53] concluded that a normal SPECT examination indicates that arthroscopy is not required. Dye[56] confirmed the role of SPECT in this extremely common athletic injury and also found that it offers a guide to post-operative prognosis. At follow-up, 6 of 14 (43%) patients with persistent abnormal studies developed overt degenerative changes compared with only 1 of 20 (5%) of those with restoration of normal scintigraphic activity. The sensitivity in these series is certainly similar to that encountered in many series using magnetic resonance imaging, and indeed Miller[57] found an accuracy for MRI diagnosis of meniscal tears of 75% and Kriegsman[58] noted a sensitivity of only 73% for medial meniscal tears and 63.3% for lateral tears. MRI, however, has a very high sensitivity for the detection of cruciate ligament tears, whereas Murray et al[53] encountered a SPECT abnormality in only 5 of 10 patients with this injury, being identified when the tear had resulted in avulsion of the tibial attachment. Other intra-articular abnormalities, such as condylar erosions or separations, can be localized, most commonly in the femoral condyles and trochlea. These alterations, in particular those encountered in osteochondritis dissecans, differ markedly from the scan changes resulting from sub-chondral infarction (Fig. 85.28). In the investigation of 13 patients following acute traumatic haemarthrosis of the knee studied by Marks et al,[59] none showed any abnormality either radiologically or on arthroscopy, whereas both magnetic resonance imaging and SPECT were positive in all patients.

Slipped capital femoral epiphysis

While a variety of factors, predominantly metabolic, predispose to slipping of the capital femoral epiphysis, repetitive trauma may precipitate the event, particularly in inducing acute on chronic slips. The diagnosis is based on anatomical criteria best demonstrated radiologically. Management decision, however, can be greatly influenced by the appearances on skeletal scintigraphy. These changes, in particular the early evidence of widening of the physis with increased radiopharmaceutical avidity described by Gelfand et al,[60] reflect the traumatic consequences of the slip on bone metabolism (Fig. 85.29). It has been suggested that five phases are recognizable (J J Conway, personal communication). The initial phase, representing a stress reaction of the physis, will cause an asymmetrical physeal accumulation which may be seen even when the radiograph is relatively normal. Bilateral early slip may be difficult to recognize, but comparison of the hip with knee activity should be of assistance since the knee should always have greater avidity

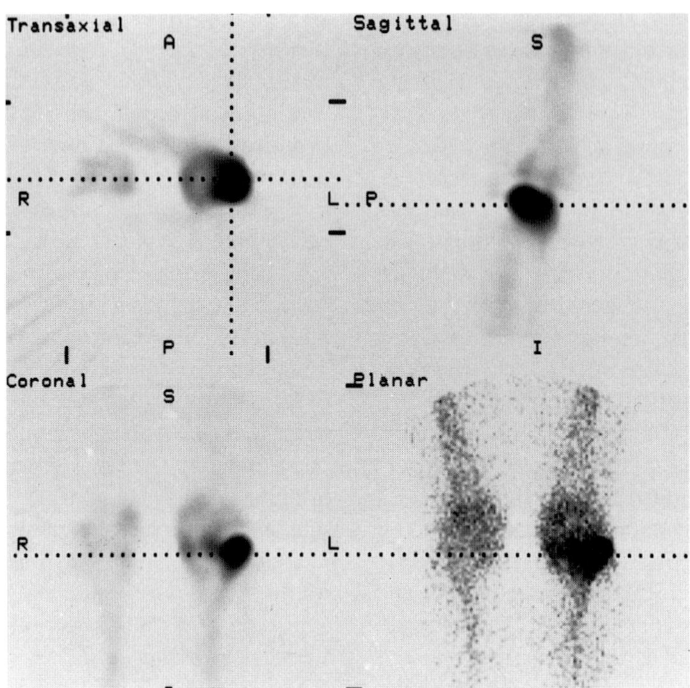

Fig. 85.28 Subchondral infarction is identified by the extensive and very intense accumulation involving the lateral tibial plateau, the extent of the bone bruising being particularly obvious in the transaxial plane. Standard radiographs over a period of 3 months remained entirely normal.

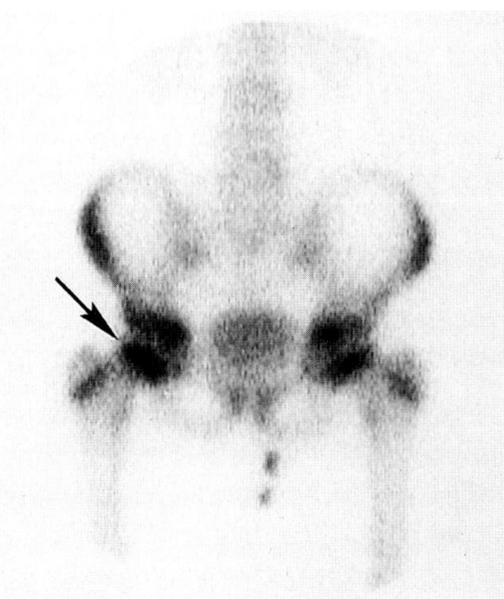

Fig. 85.29 Slipped capital femoral epiphysis. In a 13-year-old male, evidence of an early slip is provided by mild but significant asymmetry of accumulation in the femoral growth plates, that on the right being wider and having relatively increased MDP uptake.

than the hips or ankles. In the second phase there is, in addition, widening or ovaling of the physis because of the posterior angulation which occurs. Later, when the slip is severe, the third phase is demonstrable by the loss of activity in the physis resulting from disruption of the growth plate. The fourth phase is avascular necrosis of the femoral head and the fifth, evidence of chondrolysis, portrayed by an increased localization of the radionuclide in the acetabular roof. Treatment will depend on the degree of slip and whether these complications of avascular necrosis and chondrolysis have already occurred. Mandell et al[61] suggested that serial studies permit observation of reduction of activity in the greater trochanter epiphysis, the 'closing physis sign', as warning the onset of chondrolysis. This scan abnormality was present in 16/16 patients with chondrolysis but not demonstrable in 13 patients with a slipped capital femoral epiphysis but no chondrolysis. The value of observing the scan appearances in modifying management was also described by Smergel et al.[62] The bone scan was used most often to assess the status of the femoral capital growth plate and, by determining if there is evidence of increased and widened uptake, whether continued immobilization or pinning was indicated. Following internal fixation, absence of the normal activity indicates success of the pinning in inducing growth plate closure (Fig. 85.30).

Trochanteric bursitis

Although occurring most frequently in the elderly and obese, the presentation of trochanteric bursitis may lead to a bone scan to exclude a traumatic cause for the pain. A history of frank trauma can usually only be elicited in about 25% of patients, although Allwright et al[63] suggested that it might be caused by inflammation related to gluteal tendon insertion strain and associated periosteal

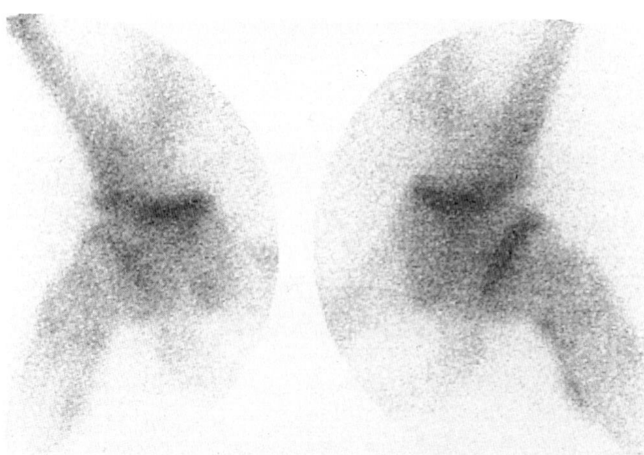

Fig. 85.30 Treated femoral slipped capital epiphyses. There is marked reduction in the uptake by the right femoral growth plate and less than normal in that on the left. These changes, indicating reduction in normal physiological activity, confirmed the success of pinning slipped capital femoral epiphyses 20 months previously on the right and 6 months earlier on the left.

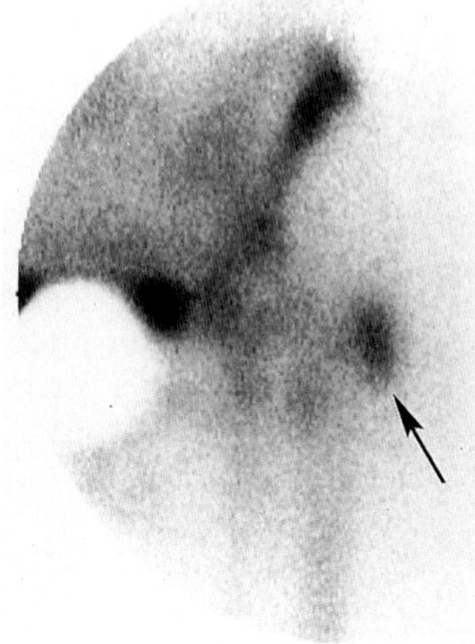

Fig. 85.31 Trochanteric bursitis with typical linear accumulation on the superolateral aspect of the greater trochanter.

reaction. They described the characteristic scintigraphic findings: a short linear band of moderate uptake confined to the superior and lateral aspects of the greater trochanter (Fig. 85.31).

MUSCLE INJURY

Severe intense exertional effort may produce a major insult to muscles and result in rhabdomyolysis. With mechanisms similar to those operating in infarcted myocardium, uptake of the bone-seeking radiopharmaceuticals in ischaemic muscle is usually dramatic, extensive and intense. As shown in a variety of case reports, the involved muscles are those most liable to overuse injury in

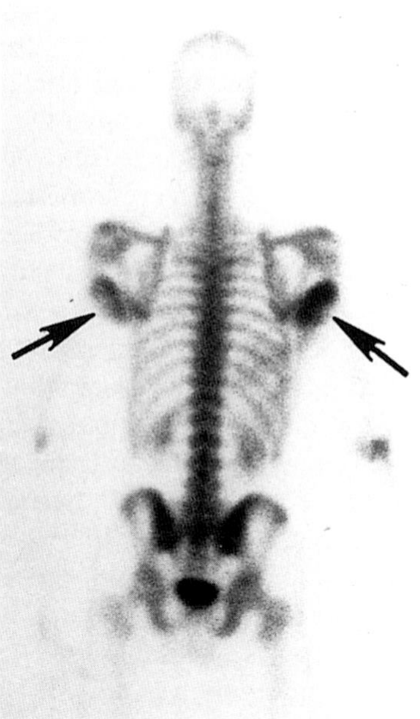

Fig. 85.32 Rhabdomyolysis in each teres minor in a weightlifter, demonstrated by bilateral extraosseous accumulation.

a particular activity (Fig. 85.32). This was demonstrated most conclusively by Matin et al[64] in a study of ultramarathon athletes. Showing that the extraosseous accumulation only occurred in the painful muscles, they identified that the ^{99m}Tc pyrophosphate uptake was confined to the adductor muscles of the thigh in uphill runners, whereas the abnormalities in downhill runners occurred in the hamstring, quadriceps and buttock muscles. In keeping with the chronological pattern which exists in myocardial infarction, follow-up studies at 5 days demonstrated less uptake than in the initial investigations, while later studies at 7–8 days were normal. Delpassand et al[65] reported the observation of soft-tissue uptake resulting from a variety of factors, including child abuse and electrical burns. They suggested that such changes demonstrating the extent of the acute damage of skeletal muscle was valuable in indicating the appropriate treatment. Maurer et al[21] also advocated three-phase skeletal scintigraphy to identify traumatic myositis of the hand in which marked hyperaemia occurs with 'augmented uptake' in adjacent bone in the delayed views.

COMPLICATIONS IN FRACTURE HEALING

The scintigraphic changes reflecting the remodelling of skeletal fractures persist for a considerable period. While diminution or even disappearance of the accumulation is to be expected by 6 months, the rate of change in the alterations is so variable that it is difficult to assess whether there is any significant delay in union. The site of fracture and the age of the patient will influence the rate of return to normality, but many other factors will also be relevant, both systemic and local. Many of these, such as loss of blood supply, failure of immobilization with consequent poor contact of the fracture ends and infection, may be responsible for non-union. Subsequently, a pseudoarthrosis may form at the fracture site. A number of attempts have been made to achieve a method to predict whether or not normal healing would proceed and thus permit early intervention. Most, such as those by Jacobs et al[66] and Smith et al,[67] have shown no predictive pattern, whereas Auchinloss & Watt[68] suggested that a study at 6 weeks was justified in those who might have a healing problem. It may be difficult to separate delayed union from frank non-union, in particular from reactive non-union in which the scan will show persistent intense accumulation at the fragment ends despite the cessation of healing. These appearances differ from those in atrophic non-union in which there may be reduction of accumulation in one or both aspects of the fracture. In particular, visualization of a distinct photopenic gap between the fragment ends indicates a very low probability of union being achieved (Fig. 85.33). These differences have such clinical significance that scintigraphic identification will influence management. Desai et al[69] found that 59 of 62 fractures which showed intense uptake healed successfully with electrical stimulation, whereas no healing could be identified in any of those in which an area of decreased activity was demonstrated. Similar identification of complicated non-union was achieved by Gunalp et al.[70]

Difficulties exist in identifying the presence of complicating infection, mainly because of the vascularity and intense metabolic activity at a fracture site and the consequent uptake, on occasion, of alternative imaging agents. This was confirmed in the experimental studies in rabbits by Bushberg et al.[71] Most attempts to use scintigraphy comparing the congruence of ^{99m}Tc and ^{67}Ga uptake have not been successful.[72] The experience with ^{111}In leucocytes has varied considerably. Esterhai et al,[73] for example, found a sensitivity of 100%, whereas Kim et al[74] reported a sensitivity of only 50% if marked uptake was the diagnostic criterion. Because of the incidence of false positives, the technique does appear most useful in excluding infection by observing a normal study.

Pseudoarthrosis may also be identified by the demonstration of absent accumulation at the site of the false joint. Atrophic pseudoarthrosis, for which bone graft is mandatory, is characterized by the absence of peripheral accumulation in contrast with the intense uptake surrounding a hypertrophic pseudoarthrosis (Fig. 85.34). The complication is a major clinical problem in patients who have undergone lumbar fusion but with continued post-operative low back pain. Slizofski et al[37] studied 26 patients who had undergone a lumbar spinal fusion more than 6 months previously. In 15 who were symptomatic, focal accumulation compatible with pseudoarthrosis was visualized, SPECT identifying a more focal area of intense activity within the area of increased accumulation at the fusion site. Six of 11 asymptomatic patients had focal areas of increased uptake. It was suggested that this might reflect painless pseudoarthrosis, reputed to occur in 50% of patients, although the possibility does exist that a longer period is required before the abnormal uptake becomes significantly reduced.

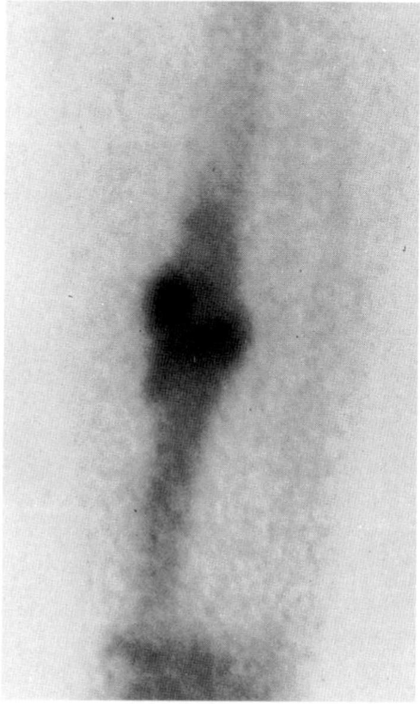

Fig. 85.33 Non-union of a femoral fracture is confirmed by the bone scan evidence of a distinct gap between the fragments with poor callus formation on either aspect.

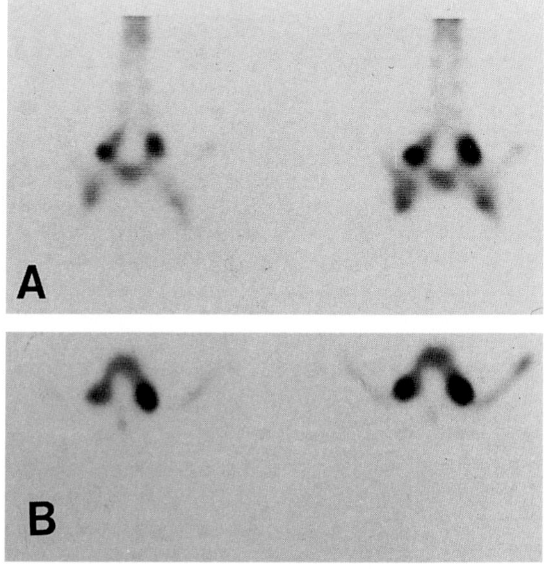

Fig. 85.34 Pseudoarthrosis. Persistence of abnormal focal increased activity within the bony mass 15 months following spinal fusion identifies pseudoarthrosis as the cause of persistent pain.

BONE GRAFT VIABILITY

Although a variety of methods to ascertain the progress of a bone graft can be utilized, radionuclide imaging offers a simple method for the assessment of the graft's physiological status. As initially shown in experimental studies by Stevenson et al,[75] the revascularization of a conventional graft commences at the host–graft junctions so that serial images will demonstrate the extension of the accumulation from these sites throughout the graft until finally coalescing. Velasco et al,[76] for example, utilizing split rib grafts in 10 patients, observed this pattern in nine in whom there was consolidation of the graft, but observed no uptake in the remaining graft which failed. With microvascularized bone

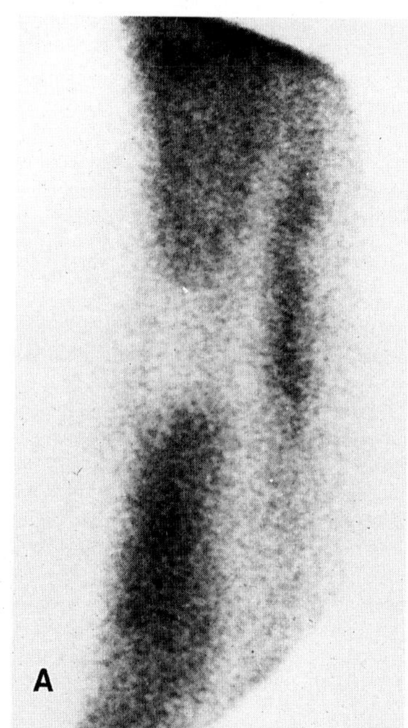

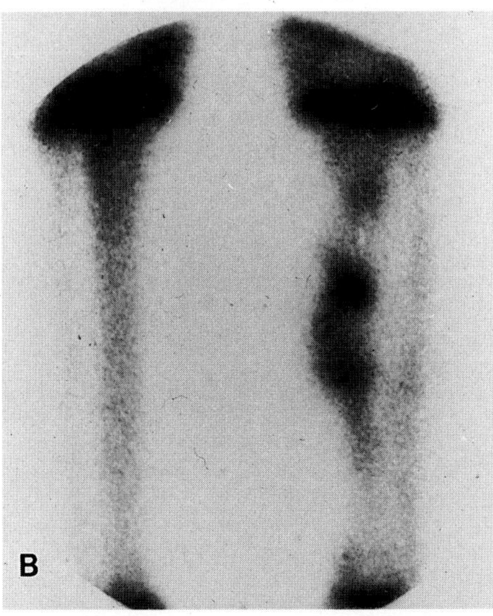

Fig. 85.35 Bone graft assessment. (A) Absent uptake associated with non-viable graft in the mid-tibial shaft. (B) Clearly demonstrable activity lying between two foci of avid uptake indicates the viability of a free vascularized bone graft.

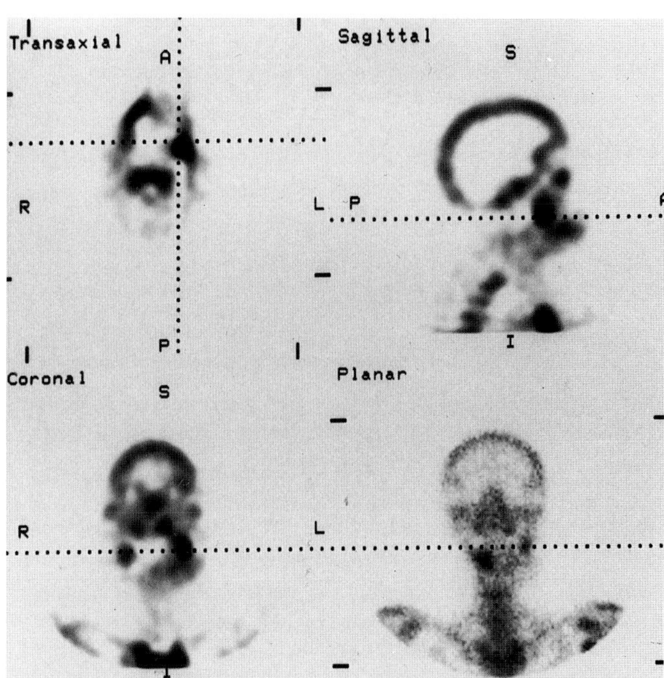

Fig. 85.36 Bone graft non-viability. With SPECT, the total void of activity in a mandibular bone graft indicates non-viability with much greater clarity than planar views because of the elimination of the associated soft tissue hyperaemia.

grafts, three-phase scintigraphy is particularly useful in that it permits assessment both of the integrity of the blood supply to the bone graft and of the viability of the bone demonstrated by functioning osteocytes (Fig. 85.35). Breggren et al[77] emphasized the importance of timing of such studies. If performed more than 1 week post-operatively, there may be a false-positive bone image due to the onset of 'creeping substitution' whereby new bone is formed on the surface of the graft. However, Itoh et al[78] favoured serial three-phase imaging since it not only permitted assessment of the vascular patency at an early stage but also allowed continuing observation of the metabolic status of the graft, so allowing identification of any complications. They also drew attention to a patient with an iliac bone graft in whom, following the demonstration of negative findings in all phases of the scintigraphy, hyperbaric therapy was undertaken with subsequent serial bone images showing an improvement in the vascularity and in the bone uptake in the grafted bone. In some sites it may be difficult to visualize the graft clearly because of the difficulty of separating the overlying soft tissues with hyperaemia in the recent post-operative period from the bone. However, the use of SPECT in studying microvascularized bone grafts in the mandible allowed Moskowitz & Lukash[79] to overcome this problem and also the difficulties arising from 'shine through' of bone structures from the opposite side (Fig. 85.36). It was also possible to identify that the uptake in bone was uniform throughout the entire graft and not only in the surface, as results from 'creeping substitution'.

REFERENCES

1. Matin P 1979 Appearance of bone scans following fractures: including immediate and long-term studies. J Nucl Med 20: 1227
2. Matin P 1988 Basic principles of nuclear medicine techniques for detection and evaluation of trauma in sports medicine injuries. Semin Nucl Med XVIII: 90–112
3. Spitz J, Lancer I, Tittle K, Weigand H 1993 Scintimetric evaluation of remodelling after bone fracture in man. J Nucl Med 34: 1403–1409
4. Zwas S T, Elkanovitch R, Frank G 1987 Interpretation and classification of bone scintigraphic findings in stress fractures. J Nucl Med 28: 452–457
5. Rupani H D, Holder L E, Espinola D A, Engin S I 1985 Three-phase radionuclide bone imaging in sports medicine. Radiology 156: 187–196
6. Park H M, Kernek C B, Robb J A 1988 Early scintigraphic findings of occult femoral and tibial fractures in infants. Clin Nucl Med 13: 271–275
7. Miller J H, Sanderson R A 1988 Scintigraphy of toddler's fracture. J Nucl Med 29: 2001–2003
8. Goldberg H D, Young J W R, Reiner B I, Resnick C S, Gillespie T E 1992 Double injuries of the forearm: a common occurrence. Radiology 185: 223–227
9. Spitz J, Tittel K, Becko, Weigand H 1991 The clinical benefit of bone scanning in polytraumated patients. J Nucl Med 32: 914
10. Fairclough J, Colhoun E, Jolinson D, Williams L A 1987 Bone scanning for suspected hip fracture. J Bone Joint Surg 69: 251–253
11. Lewis S L, Rees J I S, Thomas G V, Williams L A 1991 Pitfalls of bone scintigraphy in suspected hip fractures. Br J Radiol 64: 403–408
12. Holder L E, Schwartz C, Wernicke P G, Michael R H 1990 Radionuclide bone imaging in the early detection of fractures of the proximal femur (hip): multifactorial analysis. Radiology 174: 509–515
13. Slavin Jr J D, Mathews J, Spencer R P 1986 Bone imaging in the diagnosis of fractures of the femur and pelvis in the sixth to tenth decades. Clin Nucl Med 11: 328
14. Dias J J, Thomson J, Barton N J, Gregg P J 1991 Suspected scaphoid fractures: the value of radiographs. J Bone Joint Surg 72B: 98–101
15. Jorgensen T M, Andresen J H, Thommesen P, Hansen H H 1979 Scanning and radiology of the carpal scaphoid bone. Acta Orthop Scand 50: 663–665
16. Bellmore M C, Cummine J L, Crocker E F, Carseldine D B 1983 The role of bone scans in the assessment of prognosis of scaphoid fractures. Aust NZ J Surg 53: 133–137
17. Tiel-van Buul L M, van Beck E J R, van Dongen A, van Royen E A 1992 The reliability of the 3-phase bone scan in suspected scaphoid fracture: an inter- and intraobserver variability analysis. Eur J Nucl Med 19: 848–852
18. Hawkes D J, Robinson L, Crossman J E, Sayman H B, Mistry R, Maisey M N, Spencer J D 1991 Registration and display of the combined bone scan and radiography in the diagnosis and management of wrist injuries. Eur J Nucl Med 18: 752–756
19. Rolfe E B, Gartie N W, Khan M A, Ackery D M 1981 Isotope bone imaging in suspected scaphoid trauma. Br J Radiol 54: 762–767
20. Wardlaw J M, Best J J K 1988 Triple phase bone scanning of an intraosseous ganglion: case report and discussion. Clin Nucl Med 13: 647
21. Maurer A H, Holder L E, Espinola D A, Rupani H D, Wilges E F S 1983 Three-phase radionuclide scintigraphy of the hand. Radiology 146: 761–775
22. Englaro E E, Gelfand M J, Paltiel H J 1991 Bone scintigraphy in pre-school children with lower extremity pain of unknown origin. J Nucl Med 33: 351–354
23. Moss E H, Carty H 1991 Scintigraphy in the diagnosis of occult fractures of the calcaneus. Skeletal Radiol 19: 575–577
24. Aronson L J, Garvin K, Seibert J, Glasier C, Tursky E A 1992 Efficiency of the bone scan for occult limping toddlers. J Pediatr Orthop 12: 38–44
25. Townsend F P, Cowell H R, Steg N L 1979 Lower extremity fractures simulating infection in myelomeningocele. Clin Orthop 144: 255–259
26. Kumar S J, Cowell H R, Townsend P 1984 Physeal, metaphyseal and diaphyseal injuries of the lower extremities in children with myelomeningocele. J Paediatr Orthop 4: 25–27
27. Sty J R, Starshak R J 1983 The role of bone scintigraphy in the evaluation of the suspected abused child. Radiology 146: 369–375
28. Kleinman P K 1990 Diagnostic imaging in infant abuse. AJR 155: 702–712
29. Jaudes P K 1984 Comparison of radiology and radionuclide bone scanning in the detection of child abuse. Pediatrics 73: 166–168
30. Haase G M, Oritz B N, Sfakinakis G N, Morse T S 1980 The value of radionuclide bone scanning in the early recognition of deliberate child abuse. J Trauma 20: 873–875
31. Cooper K L, Beabout J W, Swee R G 1985 Insufficiency fractures of the sacrum. Radiology 156: 15–20
32. Ryan P J, Fogelman, I, Gibson T et al 1991 Scintigraphy with SPECT in chronic low back pain. J Nucl Med 32: 913
33. Kanmaz B, Liu Y, Uzum F, Uygur G et al 1992 SPECT vs planar bone scintigraphy in patients with low back pain. J Nucl Med 33: 868
34. Gates G F 1988 SPECT imaging of the lumbosacral spine and pelvis. Clin Nucl Med 13: 907–914
35. Collier B D, Johnson R P, Carrera G F et al 1985 Painful spondylolysis or spondylolisthesis studied by radiography and single-photon emission computed tomography. Radiology 154: 207–211
36. Bellah R D, Summervilee D A, Treves S T, Micheli L J 1991 Low back pain in adolescent athletes: Detection of stress injury to the pars interarticularis with SPECT. Radiology 180: 509–512
37. Slizofski W J, Collier D B, Flatley T J, Carrera G F, Hellman R S, Isitman A T 1987 Painful pseudoarthrosis following lumbar spinal fusion: detection by combined SPECT and planar bone scintigraphy. Skeletal Radiol 16: 136–141
38. Lusins J O, Danielski E F, Goldsmith S J 1989 Bone SPECT in patients with persistent back pain after lumbar spine surgery. J Nucl Med 30: 490–496
39. Boyko O B, Kreipke D L, Park H M et al 1987 Evaluation with technetium-99m MDP and SPECT of unilateral articular pillar compression deformity in acute cervical spine trauma. J Nucl Med 28: 751
40. Onsel C, Collier B D, Kir K M et al 1992 Increased sacroiliac joint uptake after lumbar fusion and/or laminectomy. Clin Nucl Med 17: 283–287
41. McBryde A M 1985 Stress fractures in runners. Clin Sports Med 4: 737–752
42. Urman I M, Amman W, Sisler J, Lentle B C, Lloyd-Smith R, Loomer R, Risher C 1991 The role of bone scintigraphy in the evaluation of talar dome fractures. J Nucl Med 32: 2241–2244
43. Charkes N D, Siddhivarn N, Schneck C D 1987 Bone scanning in the adductor insertion avulsion syndrome ('thigh splints'). J Nucl Med 28: 1835–1838
44. Intenzo C M, Wapner K L, Park C H, Kim S M 1991 Evaluation of plantar fasciitis by three-phase bone scintigraphy. Clin Nucl Med 16: 325–328
45. Lawson J P, Ogden J A, Sella E, Barwick K W 1984 The painful accessory navicular. Skeletal Radiol 12: 250–262
46. Rosenberg Z S, Kawelblum M, Citeung Y Y, Be Tran J, Lehman W B, Grant A D 1992 Osgood–Schlatter lesion: fracture or tenditis? Scintigraphic, CT + MR imaging features. Radiology 185: 853–858
47. Kahn D, Wilson M A 1987 Bone scintigraphic findings in patellar tendonitis. J Nucl Med 28: 1768–1770
48. Scuderi A J, Datz F L, Valdiva S, Morton K A 1993 Enthesopathy of the patella tendon insertion associated with Isotretinoin therapy. J Nucl Med 34: 455–457
49. Goldman A B, Pavlov H, Schneider R 1981 Radionuclide bone scanning in subtalar coalitions. AJR 138: 427–432
50. Mandell G A, Harcke H T, Hugh J, Kumar S T, Maas K W 1990 Detection of talocalcaneal coalitions by magnification bone scintigraphy. J Nucl Med 31: 1797–1801
51. Marymont J V, Lynch M A, Henning C E 1983 Evaluation of meniscus tears of the knee by radionuclide imaging. Am J Sports Med 11: 432–435

52. Collier B D, Johnson R P, Carrera G F et al 1985 Chronic knee pain assessed by SPECT: comparison with other modalities. Radiology 157: 795–802
53. Murray I P C, Dixon J, Kohan L 1990 SPECT for acute knee pain. Clin Nucl Med 15: 828–840
54. Rockett J F, Freeman B L 1990 Stress fracture of the patella: confirmation by triple-phase bone imaging. Clin Nucl Med 15: 873–875
55. Kohn H S, Guten G N, Collier B D, Veluvolu P, Whalen J P 1989 Chondromalacia of the patella: bone imaging correlated with arthroscopic findings. Clin Nucl Med 13: 96–98
56. Dye S F 1992 Restoration of osseous homeostasis of the knee following meniscal surgery. Proc Am Acad Orthop Surg 348
57. Miller G K 1992 A prospective study comparing the accuracy of clinical diagnosis of meniscal tear to magnetic resonance imaging and its effect on clinical outcome. Proc Am Acad Orthop Surg 346
58. Kriegsman J 1992 Negative magnetic resonance imaging findings in knee injury: clinical implications. Proc Am Acad Orthop Surg 347
59. Marks P H, Goldenberg J A, Vezina W C, Chamberlain M J, Vellet A D, Fowler P J 1992 Subchondral bone infarctions in acute and ligamentous knee injuries demonstrated on bone scintigraphy and magnetic resonance imaging. J Nucl Med 33: 516–520
60. Gelfand M J, Strife J L, Graham E J, Crawford A H 1983 Bone scintigraphy in slipped capital femoral epiphysis. Clin Nucl Med 8: 613–615
61. Mandell G A, Harcke H T 1990 Secondary chondrolysis in slipped epiphysis: detection by bone scintigraphy. J Nucl Med 31: 742
62. Smergel E M, Harcke H T, Pizzutillo P D, Betz R R 1987 Use of bone scintigraphy in the management of slipped capital femoral epiphyses. Clin Nucl Med 12: 349–352
63. Allwright S J, Cooper R A, Nash P 1988 Trochanteric bursitis: bone scan appearance. Clin Nucl Med 13: 561–564
64. Matin P, Lang G, Carretta R F, Simon G 1983 Scintigraphic evaluation of muscle damage following extreme exercise. J Nucl Med 24: 308–311
65. Delpassand E S, Dhekne R D, Barron B J, Moore W H 1991 Evaluation of soft tissue injury by Tc-99m bone agent scintigraphy. Clin Nucl Med 16: 309–314
66. Jacobs R R, Jackson R P, Preston D F, Williamson J A, Gallagher J 1981 Dynamic bone scanning in fractures. Injury 12: 455–459
67. Smith M A, Jones E A, Strachan R K et al 1987 Prediction of fracture healing in the tibia by quantitative radionuclide imaging. J Bone Joint Surg 69: 441–447
68. Auchincloss J M, Watt I 1982 Scintigraphy in the evaluation of potential fracture healing: a clinical study of tibial fractures. Br J Radiol 55: 707–713
69. Desai A, Alavi A, Dalinka M, Brighton C, Esterhai J 1980 Role of bone scintigraphy in the evaluation and treatment of nonunited fractures. J Nucl Med 21: 931–934
70. Gunalp B, Ozguven M, Ozturk E, Ercenk B, Bayhan H 1992 Role of bone scanning in the management of non-united fractures: a clinical study. Eur J Nucl Med 19: 845–847
71. Bushberg J T, Hoffer P B, Schreiber G T, Lawson A J, Lawson J P, Lord P 1985 Comparative uptake of ^{67}Ga and 99m Tc MDP in rabbits with benign noninfected bone lesion (fracture). Invest Radiol 20: 498–503
72. Esterhai J L, Goll S R, McCarthy K et al 1987 Indium-111 leukocyte scintigraphic detection of subclinical osteomyelitis complicating delayed and nonunion long bone fracture. A prospective study. J Orthop Res 5: 1–6
73. Esterhai J L, Brighton C T, Heppenstall R B 1984 Technetium and gallium scintigraphic evaluation of patients with long bone fracture nonunion. Orthop Clin N Am 15: 125–130
74. Kim E E, Pjura G A, Lowry P A, Gobuty A H, Traina J F 1987 Osteomyelitis complicating fracture: Pitfalls of ^{111}In leukocyte scintigraphy. AJR 148: 927–930
75. Stevenson J S, Bright R W, Dunson G L, Nelson F R 1974 Technetium-99m phosphate bone imaging: a method of assessing bone graft healing. Radiology 110: 391–396
76. Velasco J G, Vega A, Leisorek A, Callejas F 1976 The early detection of free bone graft viability with ^{99m}Tc: A preliminary report. Br J Plast Surg 29: 344–346
77. Breggren A, Weiland A J, Ostrup L T 1982 Bone scintigraphy in evaluating the viability of composite bone grafts revascularised by microvascular anastomoses, conventional autogenous bone grafts and free nonvascularised periosteal grafts. J Bone Joint Surg 64A: 799–809
78. Itoh K, Minami A, Sakuma T, Furudate M 1989 The use of three-phase bone imaging in vascularised fibular and iliac bone grafts. Clin Nucl Med 14: 494–500
79. Moskowitz G W, Lukash F 1988 Evaluation of bone graft viability. Semin Nucl Med 18: 246–254

86. Growth and metabolic disorders

I. P. C. Murray

DISORDERS OF GROWTH

In a variety of relatively uncommon congenital disorders skeletal abnormalities are usually obvious radiologically but bone scanning can provide images that are not only of interest but are of value in reflecting the current physiological activity. In some, such as Schmidt's metaphyseal dysplasia, the scan probably only serves to mirror the obvious radiograph changes, whereas in diaphyseal aclasis it differentiates growing osteocartilaginous exostoses from those that are quiescent.[1] Extensive abnormalities are demonstrable in chronic familial hyperphosphataemia[2] and in the diverse disorders classified as craniotubular dysplasia.[3] In the malignant form of osteopetrosis, for example, intense accumulation occurs throughout the skeleton,[4] whereas in the benign form the markedly increased uptake is predominantly in areas of bone growth: the splayed metaphyseal regions of the long bones (Fig. 86.1), the tubular bones of the hands, the facial bones and in the frontal bossing.[5] Similar accumulation in the long bones, predominantly metaphyseal, has been noted in lipid granulomatosis (Erdheim–Chester disease).[6] Shier et al[7] showed the value of bone scanning in differentiating progressive diaphyseal dysplasia (Englemann's disease) from the less extensive changes which occur in multiple diaphyseal sclerosis (Ribbing's disease). The long bone changes in the latter are somewhat similar to the scintigraphic alterations occurring in infantile cortical hyperostosis (Caffey's disease). While these usually occur at multiple sites throughout the body, involvement of a single bone can occur, and the differential diagnosis must include disorders producing similar scintigraphic changes, particularly those indicating the reaction to periosteal trauma including scurvy, congenital syphilis and, in particular, the abused child.[8] The radiographic changes in melorheostosis, another rare dysplasia, are characteristic, but Davis et al[9] considered that the scan alterations are also typical: asymmetrical cortical activity which may cross joints to involve contiguous bones. Normal studies which, by indicating the absence of abnormal metabolic activity, may be of importance if radiographs cause suspicion of metastases, are found in osteopoikolosis and osteopathia striata.[10]

Failure of normal cessation of growth results in mandibular condylar hyperplasia, which is responsible for the development of facial asymmetry. Decision as to whether mandibular osteotomy is preferable to mandibular condylectomy rests on knowledge of the physiological activity in the condylar growth centre. The increased uptake in the condyles seen with scintigraphy provides this assessment (Fig. 86.2). In a study of 17 patients, Allwright et al[11] showed increased sensitivity in its detection with SPECT. Although the clinical context differs, similar asymmetry can be associated with internal derangement of the temporomandibular joint, although often bilateral. The increased uptake is also best demonstrable with SPECT. Collier et al,[12] studying 32 patients with temporomandibular joint dysfunction, noted a sensitivity with SPECT of 94% compared with that of planar scintigraphy of 76%. The former was similar to that achieved with arthrography (96%). However, in studies by both Katzberg et al[13] and Krasnow et al,[14] positive SPECT images were found in patients with pain involving the temporomandibular joint who had no abnormality demonstrable with arthrography, suggesting that scintigraphy may detect functionally significant altered joint mechanics not evident on anatomical imaging.

DISEASES OF METABOLISM

Many metabolic bone disorders are characterized by a high bone turnover, and, as a consequence, generalized alterations in the biological fate of the technetium diphosphonates can be expected. Since the amount of newly mineralizing bone throughout the body is related to the general state of skeletal metabolism, influenced by parathyroid hormones, vitamin D and calcium phosphate availability, an increase in new osteoid will result in increased accumulation of the technetium phosphates on to immature amorphous calcium phosphate. The resulting

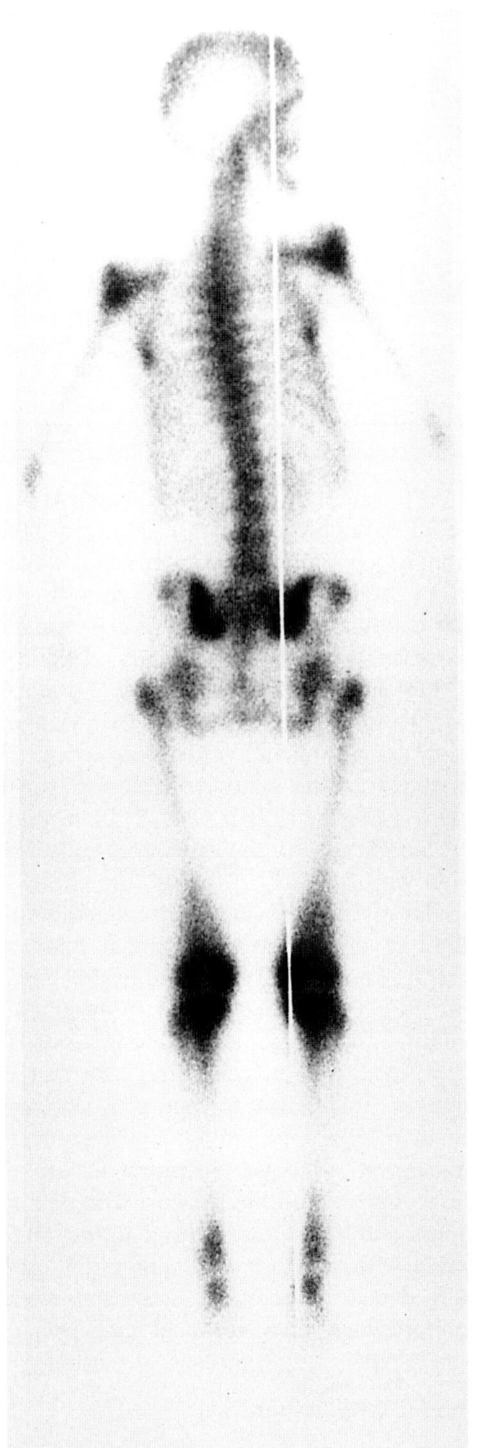

Fig. 86.1 Osteopetrosis ('marble bone disease') with the typical increased uptake in the typical splayed metaphyses of the long bones, particularly obvious at the knees.

increased radiopharmaceutical uptake throughout the entire skeleton, the superscan, is therefore typical of most of these disorders. It is very frequently observed in hyperparathyroidism, particularly secondary, as in renal osteodystrophy, in which there is an increase in both bone resorption and bone formation. The superscan may also be observed in osteomalacia. The high radiopharmaceutical uptake is possibly related to the large volume of the abnormally slow mineralizing areas in the excessive amounts of osteoid which are characteristic of this disorder, thus increasing the area available for chemisorption. However, as the most characteristic scintigraphic changes reflect the profound metabolic effects of advanced disease, a variety of quantitative measurements have been advocated in order to achieve early diagnosis or to monitor treatment. The altered metabolism can, for example, be assessed by measurement of the whole-body retention of the radiopharmaceuticals, as shown by Fogelman et al[15] using a shadow-shield whole-body monitor. An elevated whole body retention is diagnostic of accelerated turnover, albeit non-specific and demonstrable in several disorders. However, it can be used to assess the severity of skeletal involvement in primary hyperparathyroidism and to monitor the response to therapy, and has been advocated as useful in excluding metabolic bone disorders such as osteomalacia.[16] The method is only valid as an index of skeletal metabolism if the serum creatinine is normal and cannot be employed in the investigation of renal osteodystrophy. Availability of the equipment is, of course, limited, and alternative methods to assess whole-body retention, such as 24 h urine collections, are fraught with potential inaccuracy. The increased bone metabolism in hyperparathyroidism and thyrotoxicosis and the anticipated reduction following therapy has been shown with the use of quantitative SPECT by Israel et al.[17] Nevertheless, conventional imaging remains valuable and indeed essential to identify the focal abnormalities which are encountered in these metabolic disorders.

Renal osteodystrophy

Severe renal osteodystrophy is characterized by the demonstration of the superscan in which there is increased uptake throughout the skeleton with marked contrast of bone accumulation to soft-issue activity. In keeping with this the kidneys appear faint and frequently are not visualized. The appearances do reflect the generalized increase in bone turnover and not an increase in bone uptake made possible by the continuing availability of the radiopharmaceutical because of the retention caused by renal failure. Total absence of bladder activity makes it more likely that a superscan is due to renal osteodystrophy than to other metabolic disorders or the other conditions in which it can be seen. These include widespread infiltration by disseminated metastatic disease, in which close examination of the scan will probably permit identification of more focal abnormalities, particularly in the appendicular skeleton. Similarly, it is usually possible to identify that the widespread increased accumulation of radioactivity in diffuse bone marrow diseases tends to be more intense

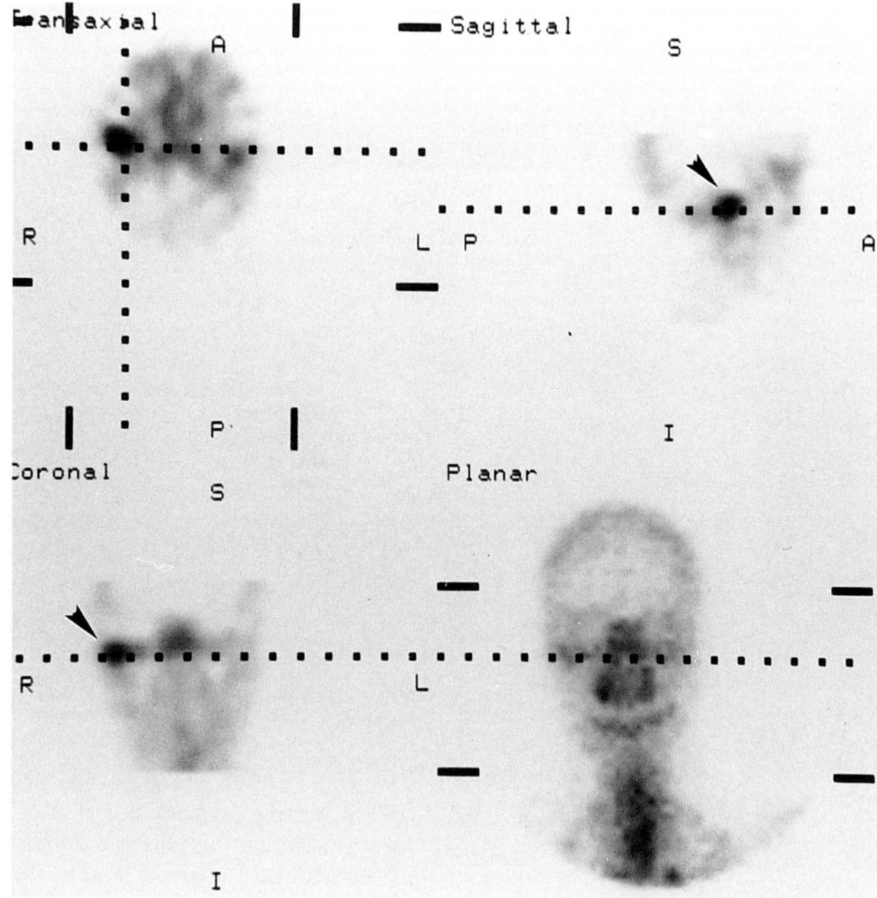

Fig. 86.2 Mandibular condylar hyperplasia. In a comparison of the uptake in the mandibular condyles there was minimal asymmetry in planar views. With SPECT the marked increased uptake localized to the left condyle was obvious in all projections, indicating the abnormal persistence of physiological activity.

peripherally. Close inspection of the scan in renal osteodystrophy is rewarding since it will reveal features which are particularly characteristic (Fig. 86.3) and may indeed indicate the diagnosis of metabolic bone disorders when the generalized uptake is only slightly increased. Diffuse abnormal uptake over the calvarium is usually obvious and frequently associated with undue prominence of the suture lines. In the anterior view of the skull, the mask-like periorbital accumulation, the 'Lone Ranger' sign, is almost pathognomonic, as is the uptake in the mandible and the maxilla. The sternum is usually very prominent, the 'tie' sign, sometimes with horizontal lines of uptake, the 'striped-tie' sign. The costochondral junctions typically demonstrate the 'rosary beads' appearance. Increased uptake in the limbs is often apparent but it is now accepted that the 'hot patella' sign is too non-specific. The effect of the primary renal disease on the skeletal maturation, the 'renal dwarf', may manifest as marked prolongation of the age at which epiphyseal accumulation can still be visualized. These changes are usually readily identifiable, but Fogelman et al[18] defined a metabolic index scoring their presence and severity. An increased index was encountered in 29 patients with renal osteodystrophy, whereas it was normal in all of 50 control patients. In a further study of 24 patients with renal bone disease, all had increased scores but only 14 showed radiological changes.[19] This sensitivity of scintigraphy in comparison with radiography has been shown in many series, in most of which abnormal bone scans have been found in approximately 80–90% of patients with renal osteodystrophy compared with abnormal radiography in less than 50%.[20–22]

The profound disturbances of calcium metabolism result in widespread visceral calcium deposits. In autopsy studies pulmonary calcification has been found in 60–75% of patients, cardiac calcification in 53–58%, gastric in 53–60% and renal in 53–92%. Uptake of diphosphonates is uncommon in these, in contrast with that readily visualized in many organs in which visceral calcification is associated with hypercalcaemia resulting from malignancy and other disorders. This probably reflects differences in the chemical composition since avid radiopharmaceutical accumulation occurs in the hydroxyapatite crystal deposits

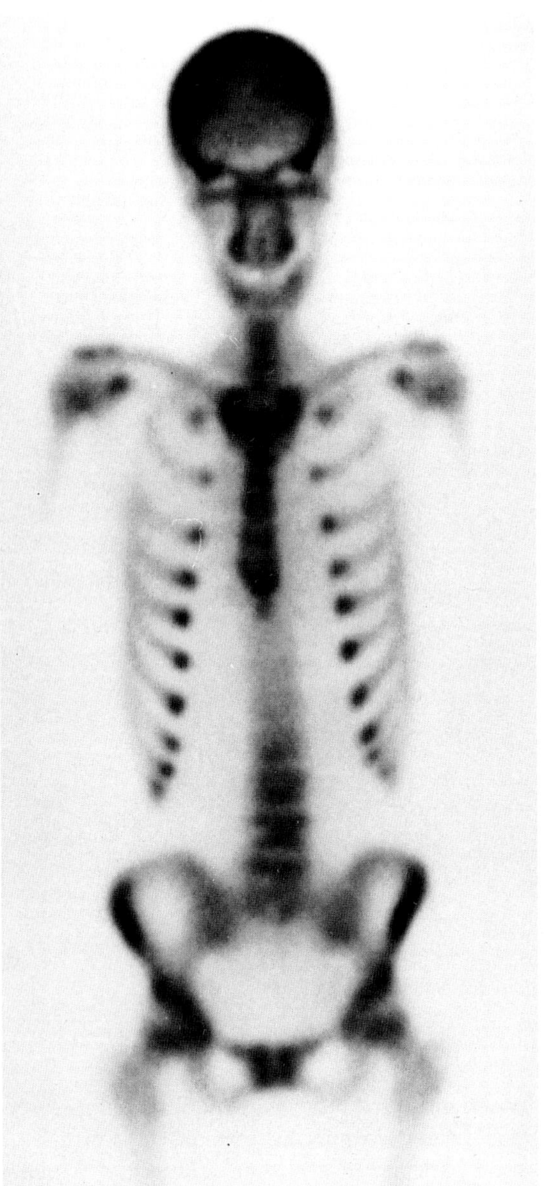

Fig. 86.3 Renal osteodystrophy. Typical alterations in the axial skeleton, characterized by the generalized marked increase in skeletal uptake, also obvious in the long bones. Preferential accumulation is particularly obvious over the calvarium around the orbits and in the maxilla, mandible, sternum and costochondral junctions.

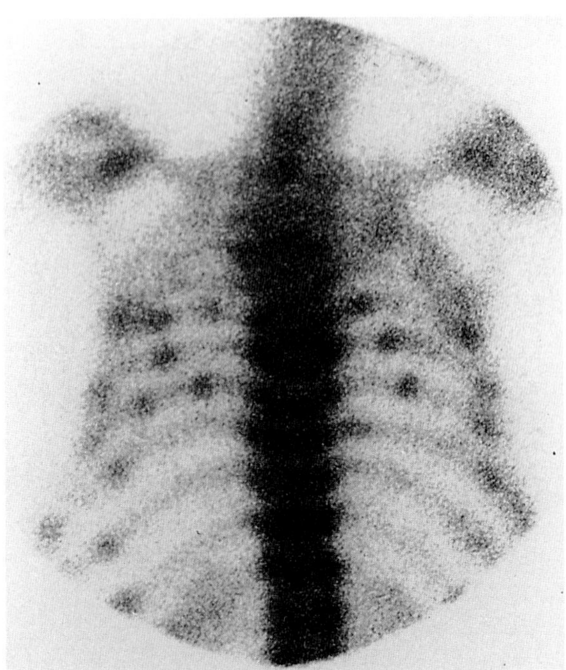

Fig. 86.4 Osteomalacia. Multiple small foci of accumulation indicative of pseudofractures (Looser's zones) in numerous ribs.

in tumoral calcinosis, which may develop to an impressive size in periarticular sites, mainly around the large joints, sometimes multiple and incapacitating.[23] Periarticular uptake may be demonstrable in amyloid deposits developing in chronic dialysis patients.

A variety of localized abnormalities in the skeleton may be visualized as a consequence of renal disease. Some, such as osteonecrosis, are of major clinical significance, as is the increased incidence of osteomyelitis. These lesions usually present the typical scintigraphic changes. More unusual alterations include the subperiosteal bone formation occurring in the long bones and observed as the increased linear uptake surrounding the shafts, typical of periostitis.[24] Osteosclerosis, visualized as increased accumulation on the cortical borders of the vertebrae, has been described by Fogelman and Citrin.[25] Brown tumours indicating areas of intense osteoclastic activity are now also uncommon.

Osteomalacia

The pattern of generalized uptake and the typical features of metabolic bone disease may be obvious but the frequency does vary, being noted in all 11 patients by Rai et al,[26] 9/10 by Fogelman et al[27] and 10/17 by Wilkins et al.[28] The last group obtained histological confirmation of excess osteoid in all the abnormal patients. Looser's zones or pseudofractures, bands of rarefaction in cortical bone occupied by uncalcified or incompletely calcified callus, can be observed at sites of skeletal weakness but are most often noted in the ribs with scintigraphy (Fig. 86.4).

The scan appearances of aluminium-induced osteomalacia occurring in uraemic patients on haemodialysis differ markedly. This reflects the effect of the aluminium in blocking mineralization at the site of its deposition at the calcification front as well as its possible action of suppressing PTH secretion. As a consequence, the images are of poor quality with marked reduction in bone uptake and persistent high background activity. Improvement of quality following desferrioxamine therapy has been identified by Vanherweghem et al.[29]

Primary hyperparathyroidism

The characteristic changes of metabolic bone disease and even the superscan may be observed in primary hyperparathyroidism but not invariably and are usually less pronounced. Thus, in a comparison by Fogelman and Carr[19] between scintigraphy and radiography, even although the latter identified only 3 of 14 patients with primary hyperparathyroidism, the radionuclide imaging merely identified seven. The variability reflects the feasibility of early diagnosis prior to major skeletal change. Scintigraphy has little to offer as a routine diagnostic procedure, and the observation of radiopharmaceutical uptake in visceral calcification, most often manifest in the stomach and lungs,[30] is only of incidental interest. Nevertheless, the alterations in calcium metabolism can be more sensitively identified by measurement of the 24 h retention of diphosphonate[31] or by SPECT quantitation.[17]

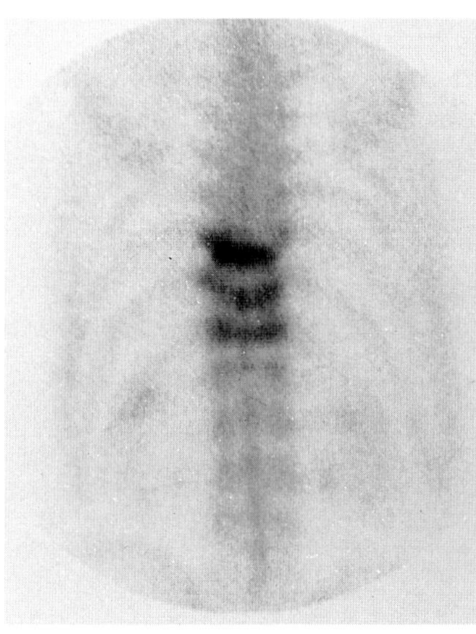

Fig. 86.5 Osteoporosis. The commonly occurring compression fractures of vertebrae with the abnormal accumulation in the linear pattern typical of anatomical distortion. The varying intensity indicates different phases of healing.

Other metabolic disorders

Generalized increased uptake throughout the skeleton, on occasion even producing a superscan, can be demonstrated in severe thyrotoxicosis and in active acromegaly. In neither does there appear to be a clinical role for bone scanning or quantitation of altered bone metabolism. In diabetes mellitus, however, scintigraphy has a major role in view of the frequent occurrence of osteomyelitis. Because of the difficulty in differentiating focal infection from the marked uptake resulting from diabetic arthropathy, the use of additional infection-seeking agents is often indicated.

Widespread features of metabolic bone disease were observed by Fogelman et al[32] in three patients with hypervitaminosis D. The changes in hypervitaminosis A are more localized. Increased uptake along the sutures may be present, but the typical finding is marked accumulation in the diaphyseal regions of the long bones, especially the femurs, tibias and fibulas.[33] This is very similar to the linear diaphyseal uptake of the periostitis which may be demonstrable in scurvy[34] and in congenital syphilis.[35] It is likely that this reflects the effect of these disorders on the metaphysis, particularly affecting the juxtaepiphyseal periosteal attachment and causing susceptibility to periosteal avulsion with subsequent subperiosteal haematoma formation. Periosteal uptake is also demonstrable in Menke's kinky hair syndrome. Marked periarticular accumulation has been described in congenital lipodystrophy.[36]

Osteoporosis

Skeletal scintigraphy has a limited role in osteoporosis since this disorder characteristically results in poor-quality studies because of the lower uptake of the radiopharmaceutical. Against such poorly delineated skeletal images, however, the osteoblastic reaction to insufficiency fractures appears very pronounced. Vertebral collapse typically demonstrates intense linear accumulation with obvious distortion of the anatomical outline. The changes gradually diminish with healing (Fig. 86.5) and, even although some abnormality may persist for 1–2 years, the degree of intensity is of value in ascertaining how recent the collapse may have been. The pattern of the abnormality also assists in differentiation from the changes resulting from a metastasis which tends to be more focal. Insufficiency fractures of the neural arch, however, may merely be observed as localized accumulation, and SPECT is required to differentiate such lesions from metastases in the vertebral body or osteoarthritic changes in the articular facets. Following therapy with fluoride for osteoporosis, various scan alterations have been reported. O'Duffy et al[37] observed multiple focal areas, many compatible with stress fractures. Numerous focal sites were also noted by Weingrad et al,[38] but increased periosteal activity extending along the shafts of the long bones was also present. The abnormal uptake demonstrated by Schulz et al[39] was confined to the metaphyseal areas, but they also suggested the changes might be the result of periosteal periostitis. Similar changes, although also with more generalized uptake, were noted by Thivolle et al[40] in chronic fluorine intoxication.

REFERENCES

1. Epstein D A, Levin E J 1978 Bone scintigraphy in hereditary multiple exostoses. AJR 130: 331–333
2. Iancu T C, Almagor G, Friedman E, Hardoff R, Front D 1978 Chronic familial hyperphosphatemia. Radiology 129: 669–679
3. Leslie W D, Reinhold C, Rosenthall L, Tan C, Glorieux F H 1992 Panostotic fibrous dysplasia: a new craniotubular dysplasia. Clin Nucl Med 17: 556–560
4. Rosenthall L, Lisbona R 1984 Skeletal imaging. Appleton-Century-Crofts, Norwalk, CT, p 294
5. Park H M, Lambertus J 1977 Skeletal and reticuloendothelial imaging in osteopetrosis: case report. J Nucl Med 18: 1091–1095
6. Resnick D, Greenway G, Genant H, Brower A, Haghighi P, Emmett M 1982 Erdheim–Chester disease. Radiology 142: 289–295
7. Shier C K, Krasicky G A, Ellis B I, Kottamasu S R 1987 Ribbing's disease: Radiographic–scintigraphic correlation and comparison with Engelmann's disease. J Nucl Med 28: 244–248
8. Tien R, Barron B J, Dhekne R D 1988 Caffey's disease: nuclear medicine and radiologic correlation: a case of mistaken identity. Clin Nucl Med 13: 583–585
9. Davis D C, Syklawer R, Cole R L 1992 Melorheostosis on three-phase bone scintigraphy. Clin Nucl Med 17: 561–564
10. Whyte M P, Murphy W A, Siegel B A 1988 99m-Tc pyrophosphate bone imaging in osteopoikilosis, osteopathia striata and melorheostosis. Radiology 172: 439–443
11. Allwright S J, Cooper R A, Shuter B, Normal J, Ede B 1988 Bone SPECT in hyperplasia of the mandibular condyle. J Nucl Med 29: 780
12. Collier B D, Carrera G F, Messer E J et al 1983 Internal derangement of the temporo-mandibular joint: detection by single-photon emission computed tomography. Radiology 149: 557–561
13. Katzberg R W, O'Mara R E, Tallents R H 1984 Radionuclide skeletal imaging and single photon emission tomography in suspected internal derangement of the temporomandibular joint. J Oral Maxillofac Surg 42: 782–787
14. Krasnow A Z, Collier B D, Kneeland J B 1987 Comparison of high-resolution MRI and SPECT bone scintigraphy for non-invasive imaging of the temporo-mandibular joint. J Nucl Med 28: 1268–1274
15. Fogelman I, Bessant R G, Turner J G, Citrin D L, Boyle I T, Greig W R 1978 The use of whole-body retention of Tc-99m diphosphonate in the diagnosis of metabolic bone disease. J Nucl Med 19: 270–275
16. Fogelman I 1980 The value of 24 hour skeletal uptake of diphosphonate in the exclusion of metabolic bone disease. Nucl Med Comm 1: 351–356
17. Israel O, Front D, Hardoff R, Ish-Shalom S, Jerushalmi J, Kolodny G M 1991 In vivo SPECT quantitation of bone metabolism in hyperparathyroid and thyrotoxicosis. J Nucl Med 32: 1157–1161
18. Fogelman I, Citrin D L, Turner J G, Hay I D, Bessent R G, Boyle I T 1979 Semi-quantitative interpretation of the bone scan in metabolic bone disease. Eur J Nucl Med 4: 287–289
19. Fogelman I, Carr D 1980 A comparison of bone scanning and radiology in the evaluation of patient with metabolic bone disease. Clin Radiol 31: 321–326
20. Cavalli P L, Camuzzini G F, Ghezzi P, Palanca R, Rovere A, Torture P 1976 Total body gammagraphy in uraemic patients. Minerva Nefrol 23: 142–148
21. Olgaard K, Heerfordj J, Wiadsen S 1976 Scintigraphic skeletal changes in uremic patients or regular hemodialysis. Nephron 17: 325–334
22. De Graaf P, Schicht I M, Pauwels E K J, te Velde J, de Graeff J 1978 Bone scintigraphy in renal osteodystrophy. J Nucl Med 19: 1289–1296
23. Eisenberg B, Tzamaloukas A H, Hartshorne M F, Listrom M B, Arringtov E R, Sherrard D J 1990 Periarticular tumoral calcinosis and hypercalcaemia in a hemodialysis patient without hyperparathyroidism: a case report. J Nucl Med 31: 1099–1103
24. Rosenthall L, Rush C 1986 Radiophosphate disclosure of subperiosteal bone formation in renal osteodystrophy. J Nucl Med 27: 1572–1576
25. Fogelman I, Citrin D C 1981 Bone scanning in metabolic bone disease: a review. Appl Radiol 10: 158–166
26. Rai G S, Webster S G P, Wraight E P 1981 Isotopic scanning of bone in the diagnosis of osteomalacia. J Am Geriat 29: 45–48
27. Fogelman I, McKillop J H, Bessent R G, Boyle I T, Turner J G, Greig W R 1978 The role of bone scanning in osteomalacia. J Nucl Med 19: 245–248
28. Wilkins W E, Chalmers A, Sanerkin N G, Rowe M J 1983 Osteomalacia in the elderly: the value of radio-isotope bone scanning in patients with equivocal biochemistry. Age Ageing 12: 195–200
29. Vanherweghem J L, Schoutens A, Bergmann P 1984 Usefulness of 99m-Tc-pyrophosphate bone scintigraphy in aluminium bone disease. Trace Elements in Medicine 1: 80–83
30. Cooper R A, Riley J W, Middleton W R J, Wiseman J C, Hales I M 1978 Transient metastatic calcification in primary hyperparathyroidism. Aust NZ J Med 8: 285–287
31. Fogelman I, Bessent R G, Beastall G, Boyle I T 1980 Estimation of skeletal involvement in primary hyperparathyroidism. Ann Intern Med 92: 65–67
32. Fogelman I, McKillop J H, Cowden E A, Fine A, Boyce B, Boyle I T, Greig W R 1977 Bone scan findings in hypervitaminosis D: case report. J Nucl Med 18: 1205–1207
33. Miller J H, Hayon I I 1985 Bone scintigraphy in hypervitaminosis A. AJR 144: 767–768
34. Front D, Hardoff R, Levy J, Benderly A 1978 Bone scintigraphy in scurvy. J Nucl Med 19: 916–917
35. Heyman S, Mandell G A 1983 Skeletal scintigraphy in congenital syphilis. Clin Nucl Med 8: 531–534
36. Yip T-C, Houle S, Griffiths H J 1989 Scintigraphic findings – congenital lipodystrophy. Clin Nucl Med 14: 28–31
37. O'Duffy J D, Wahner H W, O'Fallon W M, Johnson K A, Muhs J, Riggs B L 1986 Mechanism of acute lower extremity pain syndrome in fluoride-treated osteoporotic patients. Am J Med 80: 561–566
38. Weingrad T R, Eymontt M J, Martin J H, Steltz M D 1991 Periostitis due to low-dose fluoride intoxication demonstrated by bone scanning. Clin Nucl Med 16: 59–61
39. Schulz E E, Libanati C R, Farley S M, Kirk G A, Baylink D J 1984 Skeletal scintigraphic changes in osteoporosis treated with sodium fluoride: concise communications. J Nucl Med 25: 651–655
40. Thivolle P, Mathieu L, Damideaux J, Houzard C, Mathieu P, Berger M 1986 Bone imaging in a case of chronic fluorine intoxication with mineral water. Clin Nucl Med 11: 771–772

87. Arthritis: current status of scintigraphy and future trends

Marjolein H. W. de Bois   Ernest K. J. Pauwels

Arthritis is a ubiquitous, disabling disease that places substantial demands on health care resources. Patients with rheumatoid arthritis (RA) have a reduced life expectancy with a one in three chance of becoming disabled, depending upon the severity of the disease in the first years. The most characteristic disease manifestation of RA is arthritis, in which joint pain, joint swelling and loss of mobility are the result of inflammation in the synovial tissue. For optimal patient management and, in particular, when choosing disease-modifying anti-rheumatic drugs, the physician has to be informed of the level of synovitis activity. At present, synovitis activity is quantified by means of subjective or non-specific parameters. Investigative tools for the objective detection and measurement of disease activity in RA have still to be fully developed. Radiopharmaceuticals have been used as such tools since the mid-1950s. Initially they were applied intra-articularly, but since the introduction of technetium-99m (^{99m}Tc) many new radiopharmaceuticals for intravenous use have been developed. This chapter reviews the current status of scintigraphy and future trends.

CLASSIFICATION OF THE RHEUMATIC DISEASES

The rheumatic diseases can be classified broadly as inflammatory and non-inflammatory joint diseases (Table 87.1).

Table 87.1 Classification of the rheumatic diseases

Inflammatory joint diseases	Non-inflammatory joint diseases
(a) Diffuse connective tissue diseases	(a) Degenerative joint disease (Osteoarthritis, osteoarthrosis)
1. Rheumatoid arthritis	1. primary (induces erosive osteroarthritis)
2. Juvenile rheumatoid arthritis	2. secondary
3. Systemic lupus erythematosus	
4. Systemic sclerosis	
5. Polymyositis/dermatomyositis	(b) Trauma
6. Necrotizing vasculitis and other vasculopathies	
7. Sjögren syndrome	(c) Neuropathic disorders
8. Overlap syndrome	1. Charcot joints
	2. Compression neuropathies
(b) Spondylarthropathies	3. Reflex sympathetic dystrophy
1. Ankylosing spondylitis	
2. Reiter's syndrome	(d) Non-articular rheumatism
3. Psoriatic arthritis	1. Fibromyalgia, fibrositis
4. Arthritis associated with chronic inflammatory bowel disease	2. Low back pain and intervertebral disc disorders
	3. Tendinitis and/or bursitis
(c) Infections	4. Ganglion cysts
1. Bacterial	5. Fasciitis
2. Viral	6. Vasomotor disorders
3. Fungal	
4. Parasitic	
(d) Crystal-induced arthropathies	
1. Monosodium urate (gout)	
2. Calcium pyrophosphate dihydrate pseudogout	
3. Apatite	
4. Oxalate	

The inflammatory joint diseases include RA and other connective tissue diseases, spondylarthropathies, infection and crystal-induced arthropathies. The most frequently occurring non-inflammatory joint disease is degenerative joint disease (osteoarthritis), but other entities in the group include trauma, neuroarthropathy, and non-articular rheumatism.[1] In non-articular rheumatism, disorders of soft tissues, such as ligaments, tendons and muscles, may be involved.

RA is a chronic systemic inflammatory disease of unknown aetiology characterized primarily by a chronic synovitis of the peripheral joints.[2] It afflicts approximately 1% of the adult population worldwide. The primary manifestations are pain, swelling and limited motion of the joints, but, in addition, a variety of extra-articular manifestations may also occur. The disease may be mild and relapsing, but is chronic in the majority of patients and results in irreversible articular damage with loss of joint function.

Osteoarthritis (OA) is characterized by progressive loss of articular cartilage and by reactive changes at the margins of the joints and in subchondral bone.[2] OA is the most common joint disorder in all populations and its prevalence increases with age.[3] Clinical manifestations include slowly developing joint pain, stiffness and enlargement of the joint by bony proliferation accompanied by limitation of motion. Furthermore, secondary synovitis is common.

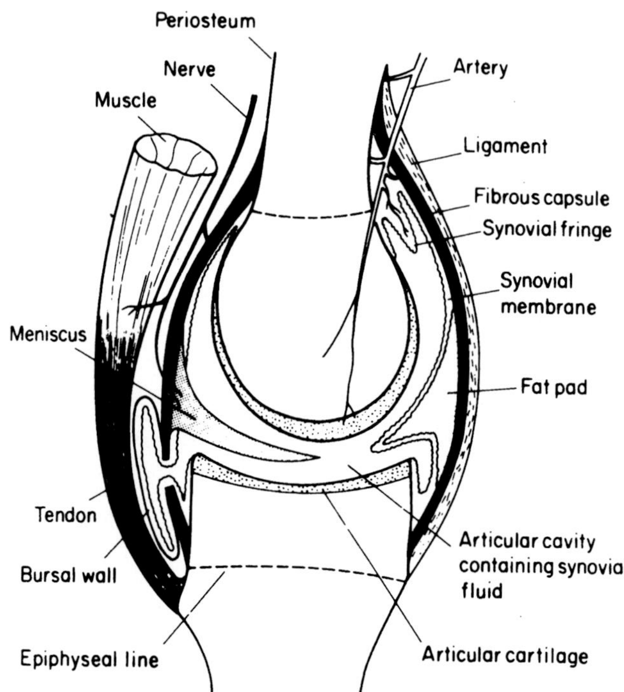

Fig. 87.1 Synovial joint: diagrammatic representation. Redrawn from Scott[4] by courtesy of J.T. Scott and Churchill Livingstone.

HISTOLOGICAL FEATURES

Normal synovium

The pathological changes of RA centre upon the 264 synovial (diarthrodial) joints. The synovial membrane is the tissue that lines the non-cartilaginous surfaces of a synovial joint (Fig. 87.1). The membrane is composed of a synoviocyte layer (intima) and an underlying loose connective tissue (the subsynoviocyte connective tissue) (Fig. 87.2).[5] The synoviocyte layer is normally 1–3 cell layers thick and there is no underlying basement membrane. The principal cells are type A (macrophage-like) and type B (fibroblast-like), and these cells reside in a matrix which is rich in collagen fibrils and proteoglycans. The subsynoviocyte connective tissue can be areolar, adipose or fibrous. The structure of the subsynoviocyte connective tissue varies greatly, ranging from a limited collagen-rich matrix to an abundantly rich vascular matrix. There are many small arteries, arterioles, capillaries, venules and small veins; they are accompanied by lymphatic channels and by periarterial nerve fibres. Mast cells

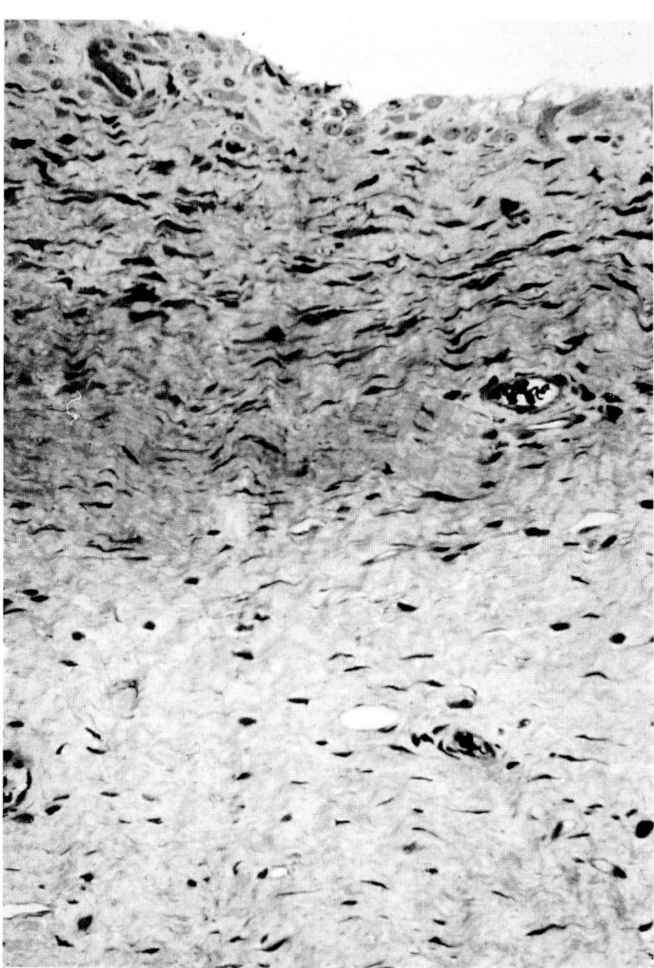

Fig. 87.2 Normal synovial tissue: small lining cell area at top with connective tissue in the subsynovial area (magnitude 400×).

are scattered in the periarterial territories, and the intervening loose connective tissue contains small numbers of histiocytes. The synovial membrane is a complex series of folds which changes in shape as joint movement occurs. The folds may be leaf-shaped, fan-like or villous. The boundary between the synovial membrane and articular cartilage, intra-articular disc or meniscus is a precisely delineated zone in which the synovial capillary arcades turn back towards the parent territory. The synoviochondral interface constitutes the site at which inflammatory arthropathies originate; it is the primary 'attack zone' for common disorders such as RA. The pathological changes in RA joints merge with, and may be indistinguishable from, those of the other connective tissue diseases (such as systemic lupus erythematosus) and from the spondylarthropathies.[5]

Synovitis

Initially, during the acute phase of the inflammation, one can observe hyperaemia followed by a diffuse cell infiltration of polymorphonuclear leucocytes, lymphocytes and, occasionally, plasma cells into the synovial stroma and the joint cavity. The acute phase gradually changes into the chronic phase. This signifies that the diffuse cell infiltration gradually becomes a non-diffuse cellular infiltration, principally consisting of lymphocytes, macrophages and plasma cells (Fig. 87.3). The majority of the lymphocytes in the rheumatoid synovium are T cells. With progression, the characteristic changes appear in the form of a proliferation of the synovial lining cells and of a vascular hyperplasia of the subsynovial connective tissue. Focal or segmental vascular changes are a regular feature of rheumatoid synovitis, with manifestations of venous distension, capillary obstruction and areas of thrombosis and perivascular haemorrhage.[6] The oedematous synovium protrudes into the joint cavity in the form of slender villous projections. The proliferating synovial membrane is referred to as the pannus (granulation tissue). Within the same joint the proportions of the various inflammatory constituents differ considerably. In due time the pannus and the digestant in the synovial fluid cause destruction of the articular cartilage, bone, ligaments and tendons. Eventually, the total articular surface is eroded and the joint space obliterated. These processes, aggravated by mechanical pressure and regular use, result in deformities. In the late stages fibrous adhesions or even bony ankylosis may unite the opposite joint surface.

Characteristic of OA is the deterioration of the cartilage, with leakage of the proteoglycans and also fibrillation as a result of the injured collagen fibres. Proliferative changes are also found in OA. Microscopy of synovium has revealed either no abnormality or only mild, non-specific secondary inflammatory changes, which are often accompanied by hyperplasia of the synovial cells.[7] The aberration of the cartilage is considered the main trigger for secondary inflammatory changes.

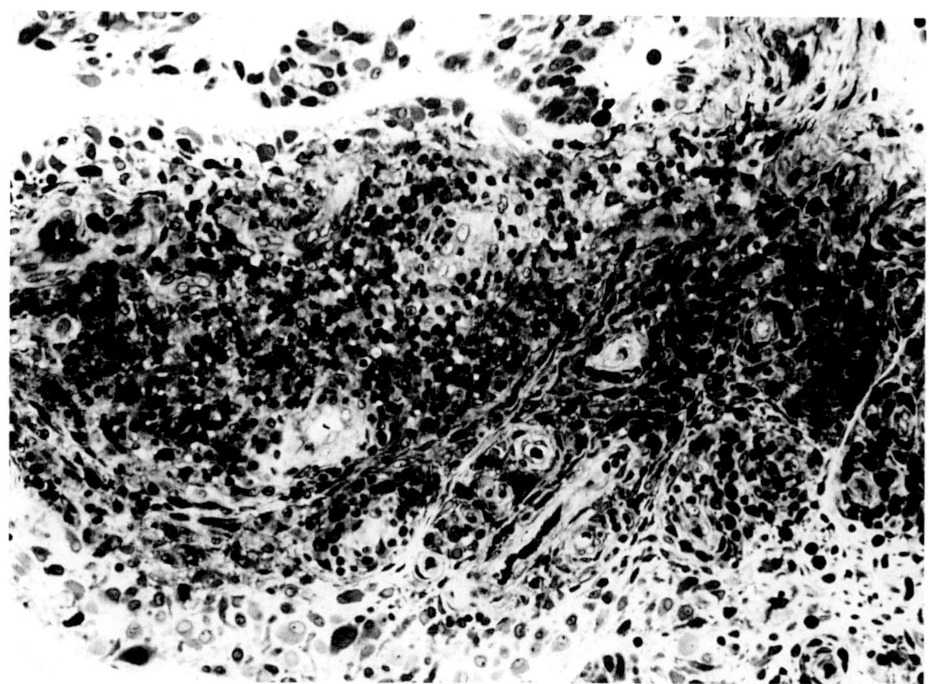

Fig. 87.3 Heavily infiltrated synovial tissue: synovial lining cell hyperplasia (4–5 cell layers) with mononuclear cell infiltration of the subsynoviocyte connective tissue (magnitude 400×).

RADIOPHARMACEUTICALS AND IMAGING

This section reviews the current application of radiopharmaceuticals for imaging arthritis activity. The physical characteristics of the radiopharmaceuticals and their places and mechanism of accumulation in arthritis are summarized respectively in Tables 87.2 and 87.3.

^{99m}Tc-diphosphonates

The most commonly used compounds in imaging bone disorders are methylene diphosphonate (MDP) and hydroxymethylene diphosphonate (HDP). About 50% of the injected dose is taken up by bone, and the rest is excreted in urine. In inflammatory joint disease, the uptake of diphosphonates in bone is either secondary to increased blood flow to periarticular bone, via juxtaepiphyseal and epiphyseal vessels that arise from the increased synovial network; or is related to new bone formation with diphosphonate adsorbed onto the surface of hydroxyapatite crystals; or it is a combination of both factors. The degree of bone uptake of diphosphonate compounds has been reported to correlate with local activity of osteoblasts.[8] In OA it has been shown in animal models that the radiopharmaceutical accumulation occurs in areas of active subchondral bone and in growing osteophytes.[9] Furthermore, it has been demonstrated, in surgically removed human femoral heads with end-stage OA,

Table 87.2 Characteristics of the radiopharmaceuticals

Radiopharmaceutical	Imaging after	Dose equivalent (mSv/MBq)	Recommended dose (MBq)
^{99m}Tc diphosphonates	2–3 min* 2–4 h†	8.0×10^{-3}	500
^{67}Ga citrate	48–65 h	1.2×10^{-1}	100
^{111}In leucocytes	22–24 h	5.9×10^{-1}	10
^{99m}Tc-HMPAO leucocytes	22–24 h	1.7×10^{-2}	200
^{99m}Tc nanocolloids	45 min	1.4×10^{-2}	300
^{99m}Tc-IgG	4 h	4.2×10^{-3}	300
^{111}In chloride	2–3 days	2.6×10^{-1}	75
^{99m}Tc liposomes	20–22 h	1.0×10^{-2}	300
^{99m}Tc anti-CD4 antibodies	4–6 h	?	500

* Blood pool phase.
† Late phase.

Table 87.3 Places and mechanism of accumulation of radiopharmaceuticals in arthritis

	Synovitis			
Radiopharmaceutical	Acute inflammation	Chronic inflammation	Bone	Remarks
^{99m}Tc diphosphonates	Increased vascular pool	Increased bone turnover	Adsorption on hydroxyapatite crystals	Sensitive, but not specific
^{67}Ga citrate	Increased vascular pool Increased vascular permeability Binding to transferrin, ferritin, lactoferrin and leucocytes	Binding to transferrin receptor	–	The presence of iron in synovial tissue is not confined to RA
^{111}In leucocytes ^{99m}Tc-HMPAO leucocytes	Increased vascular pool chemotaxis	–	–	Preparation is time-consuming
^{99m}Tc nanocolloids	Increased vascular pool Increased vascular permeability	–	–	Needs further evaluation
^{99m}Tc-IgG	Increased vascular pool Increased vascular permeability	?	– evaluation	Needs further
^{111}In chloride	Increased vascular pool Increased vascular permeability Binding to transferrin	Binding to transferrin receptor	–	The presence of iron in synovial tissue is not confined to RA
^{99m}Tc liposomes	Increased vascular pool phagocytosis	Phagocytosis	–	Preparation is time-consuming
^{99m}Tc anti-CD4 antibodies	Increased vascular pool Increased vascular permeability	Binding to CD4 lymphocytes	–	Needs further evaluation

that the radiopharmaceutical accumulation is primarily in the subchondral bone and in the wall of cysts.[10] Different scintigraphic patterns of the knee joint, which reflect various aspects of disease process of OA, are reported in a recent study, conducted in 100 patients with OA.[11] Finally, it has been shown that scintigraphy with ^{99m}Tc-diphosphonates can be abnormal in the absence of radiographic changes and that an abnormal scintigram is a predictor of subsequent radiological change compatible with OA[12,13]

Scintigraphy with ^{99m}Tc diphosphonates appears to be a more sensitive method for detecting inflammatory joint disease than radiography and also more sensitive than clinical evaluation in diagnosis of joint inflammation of wrists, hands, ankles and feet.[14] In addition, negative ^{99m}Tc diphosphonate scintigraphy accurately excludes active arthritis in patients with persistent polyarthralgia.[15] ^{99m}Tc diphosphonate scintigraphy is also able to predict the development of erosions in RA.[16] Erosions are most likely to develop in joints showing high radionuclide uptake, particularly when high activity persists. Joints showing no uptake in repeated scintigraphy never erode.[17] In one study, however, no apparent association was found between radionuclide uptake and development of erosions.[17] In this study patients with early RA were not included and ^{99m}Tc diphosphonate scintigraphy was performed just once.

However, a disadvantage of scintigraphy with ^{99m}Tc diphosphonates is their low specificity. Almost all types of articular disorders, and many periarticular conditions that lead to increased local blood flow and/or increased bone turnover, may give increased accumulation of the diphosphonate compounds in the joint.[18–20] Moreover, ^{99m}Tc diphosphonate scintigraphy could not differentiate between different degrees of arthritis activity in RA.[21,22]

Gallium-67 citrate

Upon injection, most gallium-67 citrate (^{67}Ga) is bound immediately to transferrin and ferritin and, in a small percentage, to leucocytes.[23] 10–25% of the injected dose is excreted by the kidneys within 24 h. Gallium–transferrin complex behaves like a macromolecular tracer. Increased vascular permeability,[24–26] binding to lactoferrin and ferritin[27,28] and bacterial uptake[29] have been suggested to explain the accumulation of ^{67}Ga in inflammatory lesions. In rheumatoid synovium a high iron content is present. It has also been shown that transferrin iron is taken up by synovium macrophages in active RA.[30] Only one study has examined the relationship between ^{67}Ga accumulation, clinical assessment and synovial fluid analysis in rheumatoid knee joints.[31] It was demonstrated that the accumulation of ^{67}Ga in the knee joints reflects the level of clinical activity. The increased level of gallium activity increased steadily with increased synovial leucocyte concentration. Another study reported that scintigraphy with ^{67}Ga and ^{99m}Tc-MDP was unable to monitor acute changes in joint inflammation, despite clinical improvement in patients with RA who were receiving non-steroidal anti-inflammatory drug (NSAID) treatment.[32] Furthermore, a study has demonstrated that scintigraphy with both ^{67}Ga and ^{99m}Tc-MDP is unable to identify septic arthritis in patients with RA because of the lack of specificity of both ^{67}Ga and ^{99m}Tc-MDP.[33] The disadvantages of scintigraphy with ^{67}Ga are the physical characteristics of the radiopharmaceutical, the high radiation exposure and the considerable delay between the injection and the moment of imaging.

Radiolabelled leucocytes

For the detection of arthritis, labelling of autologous leucocytes has been performed with either indium-111 (^{111}In)[34,35] or with ^{99m}Tc.[36,37] During the acute phase of synovitis, leucocytes accumulate in the synovial membrane and synovial fluid. The number of leucocytes in synovial fluid approximately parallels the severity of the inflammation of the synovial membrane. Furthermore, it has been shown in RA that this leucocyte accumulation is a specific phenomenon and not just a blood pool effect.[38] Accumulation of ^{111}In-labelled leucocytes has been reported in joints with clinical signs of active inflammation in patients with RA, psoriatic arthritis and, in one case, with pseudogout.[35,39] When using intra-articular triamcinolone hexacetonide injection, scintigraphy with ^{99m}Tc-labelled leucocytes showed a 50–80% reduction of in vivo migration of neutrophils into an RA knee joint.[37] Furthermore, accumulation of ^{99m}Tc-labelled leucocytes has been demonstrated in the synovial membrane of the joints of patients with OA.[40] The need to isolate and label leucocytes from blood samples makes this technique relatively time-consuming, complicated and costly. It takes at least 3 h to prepare the radiopharmaceutical. Moreover, not every nuclear medicine department has the facilities to label leucocytes and to perform the necessary quality control of the final preparation.

^{99m}Tc nanocolloid

During an acute inflammatory reaction nanometre-sized albumin particles can leak through the fenestrations of the basal membrane of the capillary vessel wall.[41] The accumulation of ^{99m}Tc-labelled nanocolloid (^{99m}Tc-Nc) in inflamed joints is a result of the increased vascular permeability of the synovial membrane. In rats with collagen-induced arthritis, scintigraphy with ^{99m}Tc-Nc appeared to be inferior to scintigraphy with ^{99m}Tc human immunoglobulin (^{99m}Tc-IgG) or ^{99m}Tc human serum albumin (^{99m}Tc-HSA).[42] Only a slight accumulation of ^{99m}Tc-Nc in the arthritic joints was found. Furthermore, no correlation could be demonstrated between the objective scores of ankle inflammation and clinical indices of arthritis activity for both ^{99m}Tc-HSA and ^{99m}Tc-Nc. In patients with RA, several studies have demonstrated that ^{99m}Tc-Nc accumulates in both clinically inflamed joints,[43–46] and, also, in clinically uninvolved joints.[45,46] In addition, scintigraphy with ^{99m}Tc-Nc is able to reflect variation in the degree of arthritis activity after local treatment[45,47] and scintigraphy with ^{99m}Tc-Nc correlates better with the degree of arthritis activity than scintigraphy with ^{99m}Tc diphosphonates.[45]

^{99m}Tc human immunoglobulin G

The mechanism of immunoglobulin G (IgG) accumulation at the site of the inflammation has still to be conclusively determined. The following hypotheses have been proposed: increased vascular permeability,[48] binding to bacteria,[49] and specific trapping of IgG by Fc receptors, located on inflammatory cells.[50,51] However, the assignment of a major role for the Fc part of the molecule and the Fc receptor binding was to be rejected in later publications.[48,52,53] Labelling of IgG can be performed with ^{111}In[54] and ^{99m}Tc.[55] The advantages of ^{99m}Tc over ^{111}In are its relatively easy availability, low radiation exposure, short half-life and low price. Recent studies have shown that scintigraphy with ^{99m}Tc-IgG may provide an objective test in detecting synovitis and measuring the activity of RA[21,42,46,56–58] (Fig. 87.4). In contrast to scintigraphy with ^{99m}Tc disphosphonates, ^{99m}Tc-IgG scintigraphy is a more specific method of detecting synovitis[22] (Fig. 87.5) and also shows differentiation between different degrees of arthritis activity in RA[21,22] (Fig. 87.6). In addition, it has been shown that ^{99m}Tc-IgG scintigraphy reflects intra-individual variation in arthritis activity[59] (Fig. 87.7). However, it has been reported that ^{99m}Tc-IgG also accumulated in joints which were clinically uninvolved; it should be noted that the histology of these joints was not reported.[46,57]

Indium-111 chloride

Indium-111 chloride ($^{111}InCl_3$) binds to cells which express transferrin receptors and competes more specifically than ^{67}Ga for the iron binding site of transferrin.[26] Transferrin receptors are abundantly present in inflamed synovium in RA. Experimental studies have indicated that scintigraphy with $^{111}InCl_3$ objectively measures synovial inflammation.[54,60] Only two clinical studies, performed in a limited number of RA patients, have reported that scintigraphy with $^{111}InCl_3$ is able to identify involved joints.[54,61] A disadvantage of this tracer is that $^{111}InCl_3$ is unstable at body pH, and the proportion to which it binds to transferrin is difficult to ascertain.[62,63] High radiation exposure and the delay between the injection and the moment of imaging are other disadvantages.

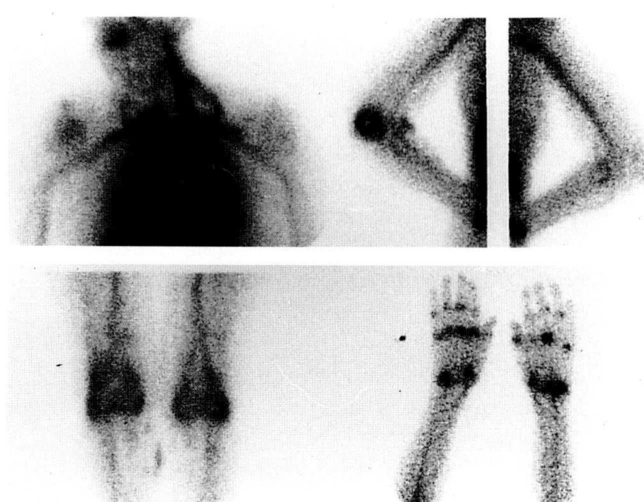

Fig. 87.4 Anterior spot views of technetium-99m immunoglobulin G (^{99m}Tc-IgG) scintigraphy of a patient with rheumatoid arthritis (RA), with arthritis of the right shoulder, right elbow, both knees and wrists, metacarpophalangeal joints (2–5 right; 1, 3, 5 left) and proximal interphalangeal joints (1, 3–5 right; 3, 4 left). The right hand is marked with a dot.

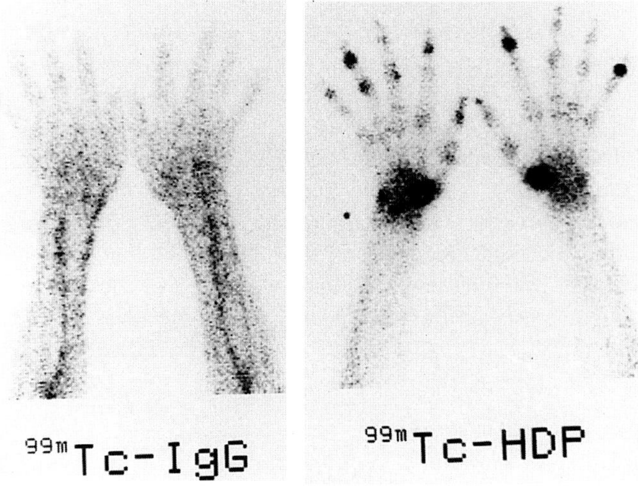

Fig. 87.5 Anterior spot views of the hands of a patient with osteoarthritis with ^{99m}Tc-IgG (left side) and ^{99m}Tc-HDP (right side) scintigraphy. The ^{99m}Tc-IgG scintigraphy shows no accumulation in the joints, whereas ^{99m}Tc-HDP scintigraphy demonstrated accumulation of the radiopharmaceutical in the right wrist, both first carpometacarpal joints, proximal interphalangeal joints (PIP 1, 3, 4 right) and distal interphalangeal joints (DIP 2, 4, 5 right; 2, 5 left).

Liposomes

Liposomes are small microscopic spheres composed of one or more concentric phospholipid bilayers.[64] After being intravenously injected they are taken up by the phagocytic cells of the reticular endothelial system.[65] Increased accumulation of liposomes in the synovium represents endocytosis of liposomes by phagocytic cells.[66,67] Scintigraphy with ^{99m}Tc-labelled liposomes was performed on a limited number of patients with RA[66], psoriatic arthritis[67] and OA.[68] The studies showed that ^{99m}Tc-labelled liposomes accumulated in inflamed joints. In addition, this

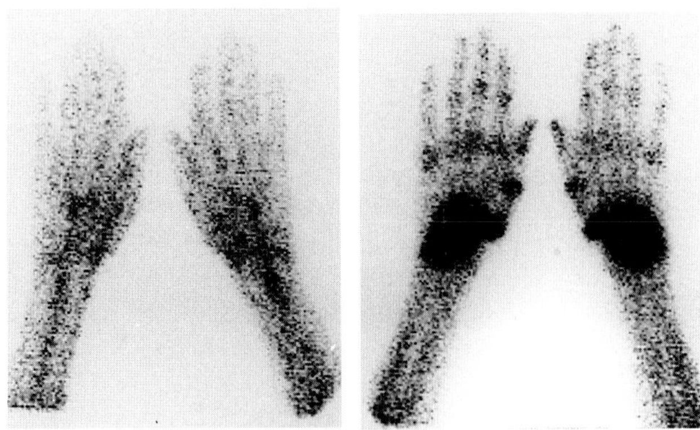

Fig. 87.6 Anterior spot views of the hands of a patient with an erosive RA in remission with ^{99m}Tc-IgG (left side) and ^{99m}Tc-HDP (right side) scintigraphy. The ^{99m}Tc-IgG scintigraphy shows no accumulation in the joints, whereas ^{99m}Tc-HDP scintigraphy demonstrated accumulation of the radiopharmaceutical in the wrists, metacarpophalangeal joints (MCP 1, 2 right; 1 left), and PIP joints (PIP 1–3 right).

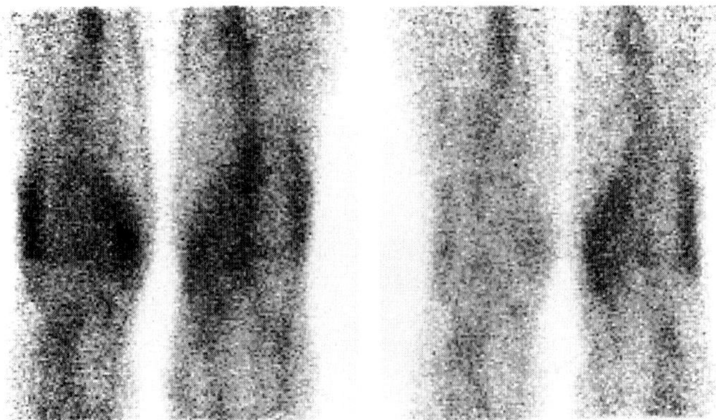

Fig. 87.7 Anterior spot views of ^{99m}Tc-IgG scintigraphy of a patient with RA, with arthritis of both knees before (left side) and 14 days after (right side) intra-articular injection of 20 mg of triamcinolone hexacetonide in the right knee joint. The scintigram shows reduced radiopharmaceutical uptake in the right knee after corticocosteroid treatment and unchanged high uptake in the untreated contralateral knee.

accumulation was most clearly seen in patients with active RA and in patients with psoriatic arthritis. Occasionally accumulation of ^{99m}Tc liposomes was observed in patients with inflammatory OA. A disadvantage of scintigraphy with ^{99m}Tc-labelled liposomes is the preparation procedure, which is technically complicated and time-consuming.

^{99m}Tc anti-CD4 (T-helper) lymphocyte antibodies

CD4-positive T cells, the helper/inducer subset of T lymphocytes, are likely to play a predominant role in rheumatoid synovitis. Recent studies have shown a beneficial effect of anti-CD4 monoclonal antibodies (MAb) in the treatment of RA.[69] A study in RA patients investigated the usefulness of ^{99m}Tc-labelled IgG1 murine anti-CD4 monoclonal antibodies. The localization of the diseased joints with anti-CD4 antibody scintigraphy correlated with the clinical signs of arthritis and with the results of early diphosphonate scintigraphy. There was only a weak correlation between the results of anti-CD4 antibody scintigraphy and late bone scintigraphy.[70] However, an experimental study demonstrated that both anti-CD4 and a control MAb accumulated indistinguishably in the inflamed joints.[71] Thus the sensitivity of ^{99m}Tc anti-CD4 antibody scintigraphy is less than had been theoretically expected. Furthermore, the development of human anti-mouse antibodies, associated with a diminished therapeutic response, is another disadvantage.[72] The question of whether IgG scintigraphy with antibodies, directed at specific antigens present in the joint, is superior to scintigraphy with non-specific polyclonal IgG remains to be determined.

RESPONSE TO TREATMENT

Various reports attest to the value of radiopharmaceuticals in monitoring treatment efficacy in patients with RA (Table 87.4). Certain joint groups, in particular the wrists, small hand joints and knees, were evaluated. The studies mentioned in Table 87.4 were conducted after 1980. Scintigraphy with ^{99m}Tc-MDP and ^{67}Ga was not useful for monitoring therapeutic interventions.[32] In addition, scintigraphy with ^{99m}Tc pertechnetate and ^{99m}Tc pyrophosphate was able to monitor systemic therapeutic intervention in RA patients.[73–76] Scintigraphy with radiolabelled leucocytes, nanocolloid and IgG is able to reflect the local therapeutic intervention, but its capability to monitor systemic therapeutic intervention has yet to be determined.[37,45,47,59]

OTHER IMAGING TECHNIQUES IN RELATION TO SCINTIGRAPHY

Conventional radiographs have been used for many years to measure the progression of joint destruction which is caused by RA and OA. The radiographs image the biological end point of inflammation and enzymatic degradation of cartilage and subchondral bone:[77] but they give hardly any information about current inflammation. Radiographs are less sensitive than other imaging techniques in the detection of early bone erosions.[16,78]

Computed tomography (CT) and the nearly abandoned classical tomography are serving as adjuncts in the evaluation of specific joints. The role of CT in rheumatological imaging is limited primarily to joints that have complex anatomy and those obscured by overlying structures.[79] CT is useful in the evaluation of spinal disorders, arthritis of subtalar joints, talocalcaneal coalition, of abnormalities of the sternoclavicular joint, chondromalacia patellae and patellofemoral joint subluxation and in preoperative assessment of the hip and shoulder. The disadvantages of CT include radiation exposure, limited soft-tissue discri-

Table 87.4 Response to treatment

Radiopharmaceutical	Number of RA patients	Drug	Time	Response	Reference
^{99m}Tc Pertechnetate	12	Cyclophosphamide	12 months	Decrease in CP and RU	73
^{99m}Tc Pertechnetate	6	Piroxicam	4 months	Decrease in CP and RU	74
^{99m}Tc Pertechnetate	10	Tenoxicam	8 weeks	Decrease in CP and RU two patients showed increase in RU	75
^{67}Ga citrate	15	Sulindac	6 weeks	Variable in CP in most cases no change in RU	32
^{99m}Tc MDP	15	Sulindac	6 weeks	Variable in CP, no change in RU	32
^{99m}Tc pyrophosphate	9	Levamisole	8 months	No significant changes in CP and RU	76
^{99m}Tc pyrophosphate	12	Penicillamine	8 months	Decrease in CP and RU	76
^{99m}Tc pyrophosphate	15	Azathioprine	8 months	Decrease in CP and RU	76
^{99m}Tc HMPAO leucocytes	7	Triamcinolone hexacetonide i.a.	5–10 days	Decrease in RU in six patients, no change in one patient	36
^{99m}Tc HMPAO leucocytes	11	Triamcinolone hexacetonide i.a.	5–10 days	Decrease in CP and RU in 10 patients	37
^{99m}Tc MDP	11	Triamcinolone hexacetonide i.a.	5–10 days	Decrease in CP, variable response in RU	37
^{99m}Tc Nanocolloid	16	Liquid nitrogen	10 days	Decrease in CP and RU	47
^{99m}Tc Nanocolloid	11	Triamcinolone hexacetonide i.a.	7 days	Eight joints: decrease in RU, of which four decrease in CP, Two joints: no change in CP and RU One joint: decrease in CP no chance in RU	45
^{99m}Tc IgG	7	Triamcinolone hexacetonide i.a.	14 days	Decrease in CP in all patients Decrease in RU in six patients One patient showed no RU despite clinical and histological inflammation.	59

Abbreviation: RA, rheumatoid arthritis; CP, clinical parameters; RU, radiopharmaceutical uptake; i.a., intra-articular

mination, bone streaking artifacts and limited direct imaging in other than the axial plane.

In the relatively short time since its introduction, magnetic resonance (MR) imaging has had a profound impact on the evaluation of musculoskeletal disorders and has become established as the preferred imaging method when direct visualizaticon of soft-tissue structures is desired. MR imaging offers many advantages over the more traditional techniques: simultaneous evaluation of bone and soft tissues, multiplanar capabilities, unsurpassed contrast resolution and lack of need for ionizing radiation.[80] MR imaging has been found to be more sensitive than radiographs in the early detection of bone erosions and evaluation of the extent of hyaline and fibrous cartilage damage.[77,78] MR imaging also demonstrates small joint effusions, which may be difficult to detect by physical examination, and furthermore has been proved to be useful in differentiating acutely inflamed pannus from joint effusion.[81] However, MR imaging is expensive and time-consuming. In addition, patients with certain metal implants and electrical devices can not be exposed to the electromagnetic fields. The role of MR imaging in staging and following (erosive) arthritis has yet to be determined and needs to be further evaluated.

High-resolution ultrasound is an imaging technique which is useful for the assessment of disruption of the capsule, ligaments and tendons and masses in muscles and to localize fluid collections in tendon sheaths and bursae. This technique is often used for guiding aspiration and biopsy procedures.[82]

ROLE OF SCINTIGRAPHY IN CLINICAL MANAGEMENT

The advantage of the use of radiopharmaceuticals in the detection of arthritis activity, when compared with the other above-mentioned imaging techniques, is the possibility of direct imaging of all the joints by means of whole-body scintigraphy. Furthermore, it may image joints which are difficult to assess clinically or by radiographs; and it may detect joint inflammation in an early phase. However, the disadvantages of the use of radiopharmaceuticals are: intravenous injection, radiation exposure and delay between injection and moment of imaging. When considering the various scintigraphic techniques, scintigraphy with ^{99m}Tc diphosphonates, ^{67}Ga, radiolabelled leucocytes and liposomes is, bearing in mind its disadvantages, not suitable for the detection of arthritis activity. Promising results have been demonstrated in preliminary reports with scintigraphy with ^{99m}Tc-Nc[43–47] and with ^{99m}Tc anti-CD4 antibody.[70] However, because of the small number of RA patients involved in these studies and the lack of control patients, it is not possible, at present, to define the accuracy of both scintigraphic techniques. More data are available concerning ^{99m}Tc-IgG scintigraphy. The advantage of radiolabelled IgG is that it is a well-defined radiopharmaceutical, stable in the circulation and easy to prepare. It has been reported that ^{99m}Tc-IgG scintigraphy detects synovitis in joints and measures the different degrees of synovitis activity in RA, but these reports need further confirmation.[21,42,46,56–58] It has been demonstrated that ^{99m}Tc-IgG also accumulates in joints which are clinically uninvolved.[46,57] Since histological examination of these joints was not available, one cannot decide, with regard to the detection of arthritis, whether the ^{99m}Tc-IgG scintigraphic results have to be considered false positive or whether ^{99m}Tc-IgG scintigraphy is superior to physical examination. Histologically proven inflammation of synovial tissue in the absence of clinical signs of arthritis has been well described in RA.[83]

It is conceivable that scintigraphy with ^{99m}Tc IgG and, possibly, scintigraphy with ^{99m}Tc Nc have opened new ways to objectively assess parameters for the determination of arthritis activity.

REFERENCES

1. Schumacher E 1988 Primer on the rheumatic diseases, 9th edn. Arthritis Foundation, Atlanta
2. McCarty D J, Koopman W J 1993 Arthritis and allied conditions. A textbook of rheumatology, Vols 1 and 2, 12th edn. Lea & Febiger, Philadelphia
3. Saase van J L C M, Romunde van L K J, Cats A, Vandenbroucke J P, Valkenburg H A 1989 Epidemiology of osteoarthritis: Zoetermeer survey. Comparison of radiological osteoarthritis in a Dutch population with that in 10 other populations. Ann Rheum Dis 48: 271–280
4. Scott J T 1986 Copeman's textbook of the rheumatic diseases, Vol 1. Churchill Livingstone, Edinburgh
5. Gardner D L 1992 Pathological basis of the connective tissue diseases. Edward Arnold, London
6. Rothschild B M, Masi A T 1982 Pathogenesis of rheumatoid arthritis. A vascular hypothesis. Semin Arthritis Rheum 12: 11–31
7. Roy S 1967 Ultrastructure of synovial membrane in osteoarthritis. Ann Rheum Dis 26: 517–527
8. Fogelman I 1980 Skeletal uptake of diphosphonate: a review. Eur J Nucl Med 5: 473–476
9. Christensen S B 1983 Localization of bone-seeking agents in developing, experimentally induced osteoarthritis in the knee joint of the rabbit. Scand J Rheumatol 12: 343–349
10. Christensen S B, Arnoldi C C 1980 Distribution of ^{99m}Tc-phosphate compounds in osteoarthritic femoral heads. J Bone Joint Surg 62-A: 90–96
11. McCrae F, Shouls J, Dieppe P, Watt I 1992 Scintigraphic assessment of osteoarthritis of the knee joint. Ann Rheum Dis 51: 938–942
12. Hutton C W, Higgs E R, Jackson P C, Watt I, Dieppe P A 1986 ^{99m}Tc HMDP bone scanning in generalised nodal osteoarthritis. I. Comparison of the standard radiography and four hour bone scan image of the hand. Ann Rheum Dis 45: 617–621
13. Hutton C W, Higgs E R, Jackson P C, Watt I, Dieppe P A 1986 ^{99m}Tc HMDP bone scanning in generalised nodal osteoarthritis. II. The four hour bone scan image predicts radiographic change. Ann Rheum Dis 45: 622–626
14. Desaulniers M, Fuks A, Hawkins D, Lacourciere Y, Rosanthall L 1974 Radiotechnetium polyphosphate joint imaging. J Nucl Med 15: 417–423
15. Shearman J, Esdaile J, Hawkins D, Rosenthall L 1982 Predictive value of radionuclide joint scintigrams. Arthr Rheum 25: 83–86
16. Möttönen T T, Hannonen P, Toivanen J, Rekonen A, Oka M 1988 Value of joint scintigraphy in the prediction of erosiveness in early rheumatoid arthritis. Ann Rheum Dis 47: 183–189
17. Pitt P, Berry H, Clarke M, Foley H, Barratt J, Parsons V 1986 Metabolic activity of erosions in rheumatoid arthritis. Ann Rheum Dis 45: 235–238
18. McCarty D J, Polcyn R E, Collins P A 1970 ^{99m}Technetium scintiphotography in arthritis. II. Its nonspecificity and clinical and roentgenographic correlations in rheumatoid arthritis. Arthr Rheum 13: 21–32
19. Helfgott S, Rosenthall L, Esdaile J, Tannenbaum H 1982 Generalized skeletal response to ^{99m}Technetium methylene diphosphonate in rheumatoid arthritis. J Rheumatol 9: 939–941
20. Esdaile J, Rosenthal L 1983 Radionuclide joint imaging. Compr Ther 9: 54–63
21. Berná L, Torres G, Diez C, Estorch M, Martinez-Duncker D, Carrió I 1992 Technetium-99m human polyclonal immunoglobulin G studies and conventional bone scans to detect active joint inflammation in chronic rheumatoid arthritis. Eur J Nucl Med 19: 173–176
22. Bois de M H W, Arndt J W, van der Velde E A, Pauwels E K J, Breedveld F C 1994 Joint scintigraphy for quantification of synovitis with ^{99m}Tc-labelled human immunoglobulin G compared to late phase scintigraphy with ^{99m}Tc-labelled diphosphonate Br J Rheumatol 33: 67–73
23. Tsan M F, Chen W Y, Scheffel U, Wagner H N 1978 Studies on gallium accumulation in inflammatory lesions. I. Gallium uptake by human polymorphonuclear leukocytes. J Nucl Med 19: 36–43
24. Tzen K Y, Oster Z H, Wagner H N, Tsan M F 1980 Role of iron-binding proteins and enhanced capillary permeability on the accumulation of gallium-67. J Nucl Med 21: 31–35
25. Brunetti A, Blasberg R G, Finn R D, Larson S M 1988 Gallium-transferrin as a macromolecular tracer of vascular permeability. Nucl Med Biol 25: 665–672
26. Otsuki H, Brunetti A, Owens E S, Finn R D, Blasberg R G 1989 Comparison of iron-59, indium-111, and gallium-69 transferrin as a macromolecular tracer of vascular permeability and the transferrin receptor. J Nucl Med 30: 1676–1685
27. Weiner R E, Hoffer P B, Thakur M L 1978 Identification of Ga-67 binding component in human neutrophils. J Nucl Med 19: 732
28. Hoffer P 1980 Gallium: mechanisms. J Nucl Med 21: 282–285
29. Menon S, Wagner H N, Tsan M F 1978 Studies on gallium accumulation in inflammatory lesions. II. Uptake by staphylococcus aureus (concise communication). J Nucl Med 19: 44–47
30. Wilkins M, Williams P, Cavill I 1977 Transferrin iron uptake by human synovium. Ann Rheum Dis 36: 474–475
31. McCall I W, Sheppard H, Haddaway M, Park W M, Ward D J 1983 Gallium 67 scanning in rheumatoid arthritis. Br J Radiol 56: 241–243
32. Tannenbaum H, Rosenthall L, Arzoumanian A 1987 Quantitative scintigraphy using radiophosphate and radiogallium in patients with rheumatoid arthritis. Clin Exp Rheumatol 5: 17–21
33. Coleman R E, Samuelson C O, Baim S, Christian P E, Ward J R 1982 Imaging with Tc-99m MDP and Ga-67 citrate in patients with rheumatoid arthritis and suspected septic arthritis (concise communication). J Nucl Med 23: 479–482
34. Uno K, Matsui N, Nohira K et al 1986 Indium-111 leukocyte imaging in patients with rheumatoid arthritis. J Nucl Med 27: 339–344
35. Rydgren L, Wollmer P, Hultquist R, Gustafson T 1991 ^{111}Indium-labelled leukocytes for measurement of inflammatory activity in arthritis. Scand J Rheumatol 20: 319–325
36. Al-Janabi M A, Jones A K P, Solanki K et al 1988 ^{99}Tc^{m}-labelled leucocyte imaging in active rheumatoid arthritis. Nucl Med Commun 9: 987–991
37. Al-Janabi M A, Sobnack R, Solanki K K et al 1992 The response of ^{99}Tc^{m}-methylene diphosphonate and ^{99}Tc^{m}-hexamatazime-labelled neutrophils to intra-articular steroid injection in rheumatoid arthritis. Nucl Med Commun 13: 528–534
38. Al-Janabi M A, Critchley M, Maltby P, Britton K E 1991 Radiolabelled white blood cell imaging in arthritis. Is it a blood pool effect? Nucl Med Commun 12: 1013–1024
39. Palestro C J, Goldsmith S J 1992 In-111 labeled leukocyte imaging in a case of pseudogout. Clin Nucl Med 17: 366–367
40. Al-Janabi M A, Solanki K, Critchley M, Smith M L, Britton K E,

Huskisson E C 1992 Radioleucoscintigraphy in osteoarthritis. Is there an inflammatory component? Nucl Med Commun 13: 706–712
41. Schrijver de M, Streule K, Senekowitsch R, Fridrich R 1987 Scintigraphy of inflammation with nanometer-sized colloidal tracers. Nucl Med Commun 8: 895–908
42. Breedveld F C, van Kroonenbrugh M J P G, Camps J A J, Feitsma H I J, Markusse H M, Pauwels E K J 1989 Imaging of inflammatory arthritis with technetium-99m-labeled IgG. J Nucl Med 30: 2017–2021
43. Rüther W, Haass F, Schattauer T H 1991 Die Szintigraphie mit ^{99m}Tc-Nanokolloiden in der Diagnostik rheumatischer Synovitiden. NucCompact 22: 4–8
44. Lindhoudt van D, Ott H, Hoeflin F 1991 Nanocolloid scintigraphy for rheumatic diseases of the hands. Ann Rheum Dis 50: 969–970
45. Heijne von A, Seideman P, Dahlborn M 1992 Evaluation of the inflammatory activity in rheumatoid arthritis. Nanocolloid scintigraphy vs. clinical examination and bone scintigraphy. Inflammopharmacology 1: 223–229
46. Liberatore M, Clemente M, Iurilli A P et al 1992 Scintigraphic evaluation of disease activity in rheumatoid arthritis: a comparison of technetium-99m human non-specific immunoglobulins, leucocytes and albumin nanocolloids. Eur J Nucl Med 19: 853–857
47. Campini R, Galante M, Giubbini R 1989 ^{99m}Tc Nanocolloid scintigraphy in the management of rheumatoid arthritis. Eur J Nucl Med 15: 488
48. Morrel E M, Tompkins R G, Fischman A J et al 1989 Autoradiographic method for quantitation of radiolabeled proteins in tissues using indium-111. J Nucl Med 30: 1538–1545
49. Calame W, Feitsma H I J, Ensing G J, Arndt J W, Furth van R, Pauwels E K J 1991 Binding of ^{99m}Tc-labelled polyclonal human immunoglobulin to bacteria as a mechanism for scintigraphic detection of infection. Eur J Nucl Med 18: 396–400
50. Rubin R H, Fischmann A J, Callahan R J et al 1989 ^{111}In-labeled nonspecific immunoglobulin scanning in the detection of focal infection. N Engl J Med 321: 935–940
51. Fischman A J, Rubin R H, White J A et al 1990 Localization of Fc and Fab fragments of nonspecific polyclonal IgG at focal sites of inflammation. J Nucl Med 31: 1199–1205
52. Oyen W J G, Claessens R A M J, Rademakers J M M, Pauw de B E, Meer van der J W M, Corstens F H M 1992 Diagnosing infection in febrile granulocytopenic patients with indium-111 labeled human IgG. J Clin Oncol 10: 61–68
53. Corstens F H M, Claessens R A M J 1992 Imaging inflammation with human polyclonal immunoglobulin: not looked for but discovered. Eur J Nucl Med 19: 155–158
54. De Sousa M, Bastos A L, Dynesius-Trentham R et al 1986 Potential of indium-111 to measure inflammatory arthritis. J Rheumatol 13: 1108–1116
55. Buscombe J R, Lui D, Ensing G, de Jong R, Ell P J 1990 ^{99m}Tc-human immunoglobulin (HIG) –first results of a new agent for the localization of infection and inflammation. Eur J Nucl Med 16: 649–655
56. Lubbe van der P A H M, Arndt J W, Calame W, Ferreira T C, Pauwels E K J, Breedveld F C 1991 Measurement of synovial inflammation in rheumatoid arthritis with technetium-99m labelled human polyclonal immunoglobulin G. Eur J Nucl Med 18: 119–123
57. Bois de M H W, Arndt J W, van der Velde E A et al 1992 ^{99}Tc-human immunoglobulin scintigraphy – a reliable method to detect joint activity in rheumatoid arthritis. J Rheumatol 19: 1371–1376
58. Pons F, Moya F, Herranz R et al 1993 Detection and quantitative analysis of joint activity inflammation with ^{99m}Tc^{m}-polyclonal human immunoglobulin G. Nucl Med Commun 14: 225–231.
59. Bois de M H W, Arndt J W, Tak P P et al 1993 Technetium-99m labelled polyclonal human immunoglobulin G scintigraphy before and after intra-articular knee injection of triamcinolone hexacetonide in patients with rheumatoid arthritis. Nucl Med Commun 14: 880–887
60. Zalutsky M R, de Sousa M, Venkatesan P, Shortkroff S, Zuckerman J, Sledge C 1987 Evaluation of Indium-111 chloride as a radiopharmaceutical for joint imaging in a rabbit model of arthritis. Invest Radiol 22: 733–740
61. Shmerling R H, Parker A J, Johns W D, Trentham D E 1990 Measurement of joint inflammation in rheumatoid arthritis with indium-111 chloride. Ann Rheum Dis 49: 88–92
62. Desai A G, Thakur M L 1985 Radiopharmaceuticals for spleen and bone marrow studies. Semin Nucl Med XV: 229–238
63. Kulprathipanja S, Hnatowich D J, Evans H 1978 The effect of pH on the in vitro and in vivo behaviour of complex-free ^{68}Ga and ^{113}In^{m}. Int J Nucl Med Biol 5: 140–144
64. Gregoriadis G 1967 The carrier potential of liposomes in biology and medicine. N Engl J Med 295: 704–710
65. Richardson V J, Ryman B E, Jewkes R F et al 1979 Tissue distribution and tumour localization of 99m-technetium-labelled liposomes in cancer patients. Br J Cancer 40: 35–43
66. Williams B D, O'Sullivan M M, Saggu G S, Williams K E, Williams L A, Morgan J R 1987 Synovial accumultion of technetium labelled liposomes in rheumatoid arthritis. Ann Rheum Dis 46: 314–318
67. O'Sullivan M M, Powell N, French A P, Williams K E, Morgan J R, Williams B D 1988 Inflammatory joint disease: a comparison of liposome scanning, bone scanning, and radiography. Ann Rheum Dis 47: 485–491
68. Williams B D, O'Sullivan M M, Saggu G S, Williams K E, Williams L A, Morgan J R 1986 Imaging in rheumatoid arthritis using liposomes labelled with technetium. Br Med J 293: 1143–1144
69. Herzog Ch, Walker Ch, Pichler W et al 1987 Monoclonal anti-CD4 in arthritis. Lancet 2; 1461–1462
70. Becker W, Emmrich F, Horneff G et al 1990 Imaging rheumatoid arthritis specifically with technetium 99m CD4-specific (T-helper lymphocytes) antibodies. Eur J Nucl Med 17: 156–159
71. Kinne R W, Becker W, Simon G et al 1993 Joint uptake and body distribution of a technetium-99m-labeled anti-rat-CD4 monoclonal antibody in rat adjuvant arthritis. J Nucl Med 34: 92–98
72. Kroonenburgh van M J P G, Pauwels E K J 1988 Human immunological response to mouse monoclonal antibodies in the treatment or diagnosis of malignant diseases. Nucl Med Commun 9: 919–930
73. Grimaldi M G 1981 Long-term cyclophosphamide treatment in rheumatoid patients: effects on serum sulphydryl levels, technetium index, ESR and clinical response. Br J Clin Pharmacol 12: 503–506
74. Katona G, Burgos R, Zimbron A 1983 Sequential quantitative joint scintigraphy in the investigation of anti-inflammatory effects of piroxicam. Eur J Rheum Inflam 6: 63–72
73. Berg D, Scholz H J 1989 The efficacy of tenoxicam in patients suffering from rheumatoid arthritis (including assessments of quantified articular scintigraphic data). Scand J Rheumatol 80 (suppl): 41–47
76. Olsen N, Halberg P, Halskov O, Bentzon M W 1988 Scintimetric assessment of synovitis activity during treatment with disease modifying antirheumatic drugs. Ann Rheum Dis 47: 995–1000
77. Fries J F, Block D A, Sharp J T et al 1986 Assessment of radiologic progression in rheumatoid arthritis: a randomized, controlled trial. Arthr Rheum 29: 1–9
78. Gilkeson G, Polisson R, Sinclair H et al 1988 Early detection of carpal erosions in patients with rheumatoid arthritis. A pilot study of magnetic resonance imaging. J Rheumatol 166: 1361–1366
79. Winlski C S, Shapiro A W 1991 Computed tomography in the evaluation of arthritis. Rheum Dis Clin N Am 17: 543–557
80. Berquist T H 1991 Magnetic resonance techniques in musculoskeletal disease. Rheum Dis Clin N Am 17: 599–615
81. Weissman B N, Hussain S 1991 Magnetic resonance imaging of the knee. Rheum Dis Clin N Am 17: 637–668
82. Benson C B 1991 Sonography of the musculoskeletal system. Rheum Dis Clin N Am 17: 487–504
83. Soden M, Rooney M, Cullen A, Whelan A, Feighery C, Bresnihan B 1989 Immunohistological features in the synovium obtained from clinically uninvolved knee joints of patients with rheumatoid arthritis. Br J Rheumatol 28: 287–292

88. Radiation synovectomy

F. T. A. Lovegrove

Radiation synovectomy (synoviolysis, synoviorthesis) was developed in the 1950s as an adjuvant treatment in rheumatoid arthritis. In a study involving 24 patients (30 injections), Ansell et al[1] described a good response in 16, and some benefit in seven knee joints 1 year following intra-articular injection of gold-198 colloid (^{198}Au). The list of radionuclides used (Table 88.1) expanded later to include yttrium-90 (^{90}Y),[2,3] erbium-169 (^{169}Er),[4] rhenium-186 (^{186}Re),[5] and dysprosium-165 (^{165}Dy).[6,7] Other forms of joint disease (Table 88.2) were also reported successfully treated, and the treatment, initially applied to the knee joint, was used in other joints.

Table 88.1 Physical properties of radionuclides in radiation synovectomy

Radionuclide	Half-life (days)	Beta-energy (Mev)	Gamma-energy (Mev)	Mean tissue penetration (mm)
Gold-198	2.7	0.96	0.41 (96%)	0.8
Yttrium-90	2.7	2.25	Nil	3.8
Dysprosium-165	0.1	1.28	0.09 (4%)	1.4
Rhenium-186	9.4	1.07	0.14 (9%)	0.9
Erbium-169	3.7	0.34	0.03	0.3
Samarium-153	1.95	0.8	0.10 (28%)	0.7
Holmium-166	1.13	1.84	0.08 (13%)	2.2

Table 88.2 Conditions treated with radiation synovectomy

Rheumatoid arthritis
Psoriatic arthritis
Ankylosing spondylitis
Osteoarthritis
Chronic pyrophosphate arthropathy
Haemophilia–haemosiderin arthropathy
Pigmented villonodular synovitis
Baker's cyst

INDICATIONS FOR RADIATION SYNOVECTOMY

Radiation synovectomy is best suited to the treatment of an individual joint or a few joints which remain swollen and painful with failure to respond to systemic or localized anti-inflammatory therapy, including intra-articular corticosteroids. The best results have been reported when articular damage is minimal. Irradiation of the synovium destroys the pathological tissue, but does not influence the articular surface.

The clinical spectrum of arthritis (Fig. 88.1) includes patients with inflammatory synovitis, in which pain, stiffness and swelling are caused by a combination of proliferation of the inflamed synovium and recurrent or persistent inflammatory effusion, and those with non-inflammatory synovial proliferation or chronic effusion. Pain associated with articular damage alone is not likely to respond to radiation synovectomy.

Rheumatoid arthritis, with the variant forms of seronegative rheumatoid arthritis and juvenile chronic arthritis, and psoriatic arthritis make up the majority of the group with inflammatory synovitis, for whom medical treatment includes the non-steroidal anti-inflammatory drugs (NSAIDs), disease-modifying agents (gold, anti-malarials, anti-metabolites), systemic corticosteroids and intra-articular corticosteroid injection. Ankylosing spondylitis and other HLA B27-associated spondyloarthropathies are associated with the development of acute synovitis of peripheral joints.

The Clinical Spectrum of Arthritis

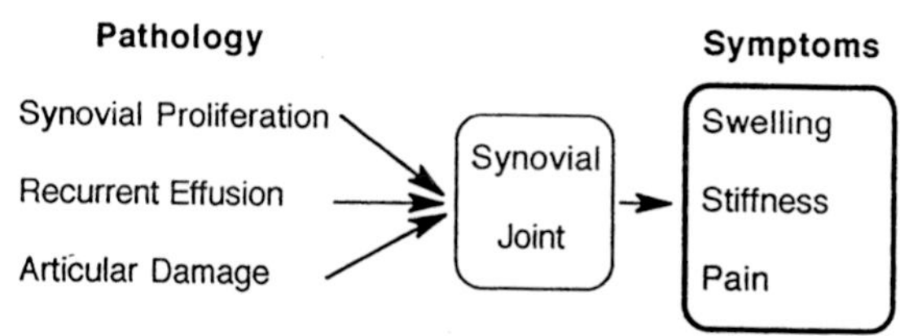

Fig. 88.1 The clinical spectrum of arthritis.

In osteoarthritis, the development of recurrent non-inflammatory effusion contributes to the pain and instability of the joint damage, which is primarily articular. Patients with any of these conditions may develop an excessive popliteal extension of the synovial cavity in the knee, a popliteal or Baker's cyst.

In gout and pseudogout, the presence of crystals in the synovial tissue evokes an intense inflammatory reaction, proliferative engorgement of the synovial tissue and acute or subacute effusion. Chronic pyrophosphate arthropathy is associated with a destructive arthritis which may result from a crystal-induced synovitis.

Two other less common forms of joint disease which are associated with synovial proliferation deserve particular mention. Haemophilia (and occasionally therapeutic anticoagulation) is a cause of recurrent intra-articular haemorrhage. As a result of the haemorrhage, a reactive synovitis develops, causing increased bulk of synovium and increased risk of minor trauma to the synovium, and recurrent haemorrhage. In pigmented villonodular synovitis, proliferation of the synovium causes a similar increased risk of minor trauma and recurrent sanguinous effusion.

Because of the increasing availability of arthroscopy, twisting injuries of the knee are often examined and treated with arthroscopic surgery. In a proportion of patients with these injuries, despite the correction of internal derangements (meniscal tears, cartilaginous abrasion), persistent synovitis is noted. The mechanism is often uncertain, although an underlying inflammatory synovitis may be revealed by further investigation.

RADIOPHARMACEUTICALS

The radiopharmaceuticals used (Table 88.3) in radiation synovectomy deliver a high radiation absorbed dose to a thin layer of synovial cells distributed in the lining of the joint capsule.[8] The disadvantage of ^{198}Au colloid is the presence of a high-energy gamma emission as well as the beta-particle, and relatively small particle size, leading to increased lymphatic migration from the joint. Williams et al[9] showed that some patients had high uptake in regional lymph nodes after injection with ^{198}Au colloid, resulting in unnecessary radiation; the expected increase in whole-body dose from the gamma emission was accentuated by loss of activity from the joint and uptake in the draining lymph nodes.[9] ^{90}Y colloids are preferred because of the pure beta emission and 64 h half-life of this isotope. Yttrium silicate has a mean particle size of 0.1 μm, about 50 times larger than gold colloid, and has been shown to have low joint leakage[3] and a low incidence of radiation damage to circulating lymphocytes.[10]

^{165}Dy, which has a beta emission of maximum energy 1.28 Mev, a low-yield gamma and a half-life of 139 min, has been used successfully as hydroxide macroaggregates[11] and as ferric hydroxide macroaggregates,[6] and has been shown by McLaren et al to have negligible leakage in an animal model.[7] The larger mean particle size (5 μm) and a short half-life reduces the duration of immobilization, and therefore of hospital confinement. The reduced leakage was confirmed in an Australian trial comparing ^{165}Dy-HMA with yttrium silicate colloid.

Table 88.3 Radiopharmaceuticals in radiation synovectomy

	Particle size (average)(μm)	pH
Gold-198 colloid	0.02	7
Yttrium-90 silicate	0.1	10
Dysprosium-165		
Ferric hydroxide macroaggregates (FHMA)	5	10
Hydroxide macroaggregates (HMA)	5	10.5
Erbium-169 silicate	0.01	7

Other radiopharmaceuticals have been developed in animal models but not yet used in human subjects. The ideal agent would have negligible joint leakage, pure beta emission and a half-life of about 12 h. Samarium 153 (beta 0.8 Mev, 1.95 days) and holmium 166 (beta 1.84 Mev, 1.13 days) have been proposed as suitable isotopes.[12,13]

By far the greatest published experience is in the treatment of knee arthritis, but the mechanism of action is the same for all synovial joints. Since the absorbed dose depends on the surface area of the synovium, which is difficult to calculate, a standard dose (Table 88.4) is injected for each joint. For the knee joint, a dose of ^{90}Y of 185 MBq delivers approximately 10 000 cGy.[14] To achieve an equivalent synovial dose requires injection of 10 GBq of ^{165}Dy for the knee.[15]

Uptake in the superficial layer of the synovium results in synovial irradiation, with the major dose delivered to a depth of 1–2 mm.[16] ^{90}Y beta-energy is higher than other radionuclides used, and is suited to the large and medium-sized joints – knee, hip, ankle, shoulder and elbow. For injection of small joints like the finger, a softer beta-emitter such as ^{169}Er has been recommended.[4] However, Ruotsi et al[17] found that radiation synovectomy in the digital joints had no advantage over local corticosteroid injection.

The technique of radiation synovectomy differs slightly from arthrocentesis, and this discussion is confined to

Table 88.4 Yttrium-90 average doses

Joint	Dose (MBq)
Knee	185
Ankle	185
Hip	185
Shoulder	110
Elbow	95

highlighting these differences. The complications of intra-articular injection include sepsis, and an aseptic technique is mandatory. The position of the needle in the synovial cavity must be confirmed before injection of the therapeutic dose. This may be done by aspirating synovial fluid, by injecting contrast using radiograph screening, or by injecting ^{99m}Tc colloid and gamma-camera imaging. A non-infective synovitis and pain from the physical properties of colloid may be reduced by the concomitant injection of a long-acting corticosteroid such as triamcinolone hexacetonide or methylprednisolone, and this also reduces the underlying inflammatory synovitis and improves retention of the radiopharmaceutical in the joint. Immobilization of the injected joint should also improve retention and, although this has not been demonstrated in clinical trials,[18] in most cases the joint is immobilized for 2–3 days to limit lymphatic spread. Radionuclide leakage back along the needle track is rare,[19] but is associated with localized radiation burns, and this problem is potentially greatest in small-capacity joints, the ankle, elbow and shoulder. If the overlying skin is displaced a few millimetres at the time of injection, a discontinuous track will be left as the tissue layers reposition on withdrawing the needle.

RESULTS OF RADIATION SYNOVECTOMY

Rheumatoid arthritis and inflammatory synovitis

Improvement in symptoms ranging from complete remission of synovitis to subjective reduction in pain follows radiation synovectomy in 70–80% of patients at 6–12 months following injection. In most cases the improvement in pain and reduction of swelling is present immediately after injection, and this is attributed to rest and to the concomitant injection of corticosteroid. Immediate relief may persist until the irradiated synovium is resorbed, but in a significant proportion of cases the effusion recurs and requires further aspiration at 1–2 months, and further corticosteroid injection is usually administered at this aspiration. Ansell et al[1] described a good result at 1 year in 16 (53%) and some benefit in seven (23%) of 30 knees treated with ^{198}Au colloid. Results at 3 weeks were disappointing. Bridgman et al[2] compared ^{90}Y resin against placebo (saline) in a double-blind trial and found a significant improvement in joint range and circumference in the treated group. Transient increase in pain and swelling of the injected joint followed ^{90}Y in 8 of 23 cases, but these settled with supportive therapy. No intra-articular steroid was used in these series, and the prevalence of this paradoxical reaction is reduced to less than 10% with simultaneous injection of triamcinolone hexacetonide. In a controlled trial with a mean follow-up of 2 years, the efficacy of treating persistent synovitis of the knee with surgical synovectomy or ^{90}Y colloid was compared by Gumpel & Roles.[20] No significant difference in relapse rate was shown, with 2 of 10 knees relapsing after radiation synovectomy and 3 of 10 relapsing after surgery during the 2-year follow-up. Hospital stay, physiotherapy requirement and return of knee flexion after treatment favoured radiation synovectomy, which also appeared more likely to offer protection to the treated knee during general 'flare-ups' of disease. Where the indications for radiation synovectomy (persistent effusion or synovitis) remain 6 months after initial treatment with ^{90}Y colloid, repeat treatment further increases the remission rate. Winfield & Gumpel[21] reported on 30 patients (46 knees) 6 months after repeat injection and found complete remission in six patients (nine knees), and symptomatic improvement in 19 patients (28 knees). The remaining nine knees (17%) showed no improvement.

An attempt to compare ^{90}Y with triamcinolone hexacetonide in rheumatoid arthritis in a multicentre trial was inconclusive.[22] Dwindling recruitment has been cited as a problem in similar trials (G R Carroll, personal communication). Patients for whom there are clinical indications for synovectomy are unwilling to be confined to a hospital bed for 4 days when the alternative treatment of intra-articular steroid alone requires a shorter period of detention. Grant et al[23] studied the long-term result of ^{90}Y silicate and triamcinolone hexacetonide and at 6 years were unable to show a significant difference in a small group of patients with rheumatoid arthritis. They concluded that the co-administration of intra-articular corticosteroid contributes to the response to ^{90}Y synovectomy.

The shorter half-life and larger particle size of ^{165}Dy ferric hydroxide macroaggregate leads to reduced leakage from the injected joint so that the whole-body and liver radiation dose are reduced. Sledge et al[6] demonstrated that 86% (49 of 53 knees) of injected patients, all of whom had significant effusion at the time of radiation synovectomy, had absent or diminished joint effusion 6 months later. Inflammation was assessed by measuring the synovitis index of the treated knee using ^{99m}Tc pertechnetate flow studies and a computerized ratio, and this showed good correlation. In a trial comparing yttrium silicate colloid with dysprosium hydroxide macroaggregate, Edmonds et al[24] confirmed improved retention in the knee of the latter agent, and showed no significant difference in the clinical response in 59 patients with either rheumatoid arthritis or osteoarthritis.

Results in other forms of joint disease

Osteoarthritis is often associated with persistent effusion, and may be complicated by the development of popliteal cyst. Progressive enlargement of the cyst reduces mobility and ruptured popliteal (Baker's) cyst causes acute calf pain. Radiation synovectomy is successful in reducing the development of effusion and prevents recurrence of the

Baker's cyst.[1,25] Moderate radiological abnormalities do not exclude satisfactory control of effusion.

Pigmented villonodular synovitis is also effectively treated with radiation synovectomy, and the best results were obtained by Gumpel & Shawe[26] when there had been no prior surgery.

In haemophilic arthropathy, recurrent haemarthroses occur because of the bleeding disorder initially, but repeated bleeds also cause a chronic arthropathy in which the hypertrophied, inflamed synovium further predisposes the tissue to trauma and haemorrhage. Ahlberg[27] studied the effect of ^{198}Au injection after suitable anti-haemophilic preparation, and reported results similar to those in rheumatoid arthritis and other forms of inflammatory arthritis; in about 60% the symptoms of synovitis and the haemorrhage ceased, and in about 25% they improved.

Chronic pyrophosphate arthropathy causes a progressive destructive arthritis particularly afflicting elderly women. In a double-blind randomized trial of this condition involving the knees, treatment with ^{90}Y and triamcinolone hexacetonide was significantly superior in relieving pain and stiffness to triamcinolone hexacetonide and saline (control group) with the maximal benefit at 6 months.[28]

CONCLUSION

Radiation synovectomy, when used to destroy pathological synovium which is resistant to or unsuitable for treatment with anti-inflammatory medications, is often effective and is free of significant complications. Improvement is present within 6 months and retreatment should be considered if the indications for radiation synovectomy persist or recur after this time.

REFERENCES

1. Ansell B A, Crook A, Mallard J R, Bywaters E G L 1963 Evaluation of intra-articular colloidal gold 198 in the treatment of persistent knee effusions. Ann Rheum Dis 22: 435–439
2. Bridgman J F, Bruckner F, Bleehen N M 1971 Radioactive yttrium in the treatment of rheumatoid knee effusions. Ann Rheum Dis 30: 180–182
3. Gumpel J M, Beer T C, Crawley J C W, Farren H E A 1975 Yttrium 90 in persistent synovitis of the knee – a single centre comparison. The retention and extra-articular spread of four ^{90}Y radiocolloids. Br J Radiol 48: 377–381
4. Menkes C J, Le Gô A, Verrier P, Aignam M, Delbarre F 1977 Double blind study of Erbium 169 injection (synoviorthesis) in rheumatoid digital joints. Ann Rheum Dis 36: 254–256
5. Bowring C S, Keeling D H 1978 Absorbed radiation dose in radiation synovectomy. Br J Radiol 51: 836–837
6. Sledge C B, Atcher R W, Shortkroff S, Anderson R J, Bloomer W D, Hurson B J 1984 Intra-articular radiation synovectomy. Clin Orthopaed Rel Res 182: 37–40
7. McLaren A, Hetherington E, Maddalena D, Snowden G 1990 Dysprosium (^{165}Dy) hydroxide macroaggregates for radiation synovectomy – animal studies. Eur J Nucl Med 16: 627–632
8. Webb F W S, Lowe J, Bluestone R 1969 Uptake of colloidal radioactive yttrium by synovial membrane. Ann Rheum Dis 28: 300–302
9. Williams E D, Caughey D E, Hurley P J, John M B 1976 Distribution of yttrium 90 ferric hydroxide colloid and gold 198 colloid after injection into knee. Ann Rheum Dis 35: 516–520
10. Daker M G 1979 Prospective chromosomal study of 30 patients undergoing ^{90}Y synovectomy. Rheum Rehab 18: 41–44
11. Laurent R, Edmonds J 1992 Dysprosium-165 and yttrium-90 in radiation synovectomy – a multi-centre double blind clinical trial. Aust NZ J Med 22: 733
12. Chinol M, Vallabhajosula S, Zuckerman J D, Gordon R E, Klein M J, Goldsmith S J 1990 Radiation synovectomy using Ho-166-FHMA in rabbits with antigen induced arthritis. J Nucl Med 31: 780–781
13. Shortkroff S, Mahmood A, Sledge C B et al 1992 Studies on Ho-166-labelled hydroxyapatite: a new agent for radiation synovectomy. J Nucl Med 33: 937
14. Johnson L S, Yanch J C 1991 Absorbed dose profiles for radionuclides of frequent use in radiation synovectomy. Arthritis Rheum 34: 1521–1530
15. Hnatowich D J, Kramer R I, Sledge C B, Noble J, Shortkroff S 1978 Dysprosium 165 ferric hydroxide mcroaggregates for radiation synovectomy. J Nucl Med 19: 303–308
16. Bridgman J F, Bruckner F, Eisen V, Tucker A, Bleehen N M 1973 Irradiation of the synovium in the treatment of rheumatoid arthritis. Q J Med 42: 357–367
17. Ruotsi A, Hypén M, Reconen A, Oka M 1979 Erbium 169 versus triamcinoline hexacetanide in the treatment of rheumatoid finger joints. Ann Rheum Dis 38: 45–47
18. Winfield J, Crawley J C W, Hudson E A, Fisher M, Gumpel J M 1979 Evaluation of two regimes to immobilize the knee after injections of yttrium 90. Br Med J 1: 986–987
19. Gumpel J M 1979 ^{90}Y Colloids in chronic synovitis of the knee. Rheum Rehab 18: 38–41
20. Gumpel J M, Roles N C 1975 A controlled trial of intra-articular radiocolloids versus surgical synovectomy in persistent synovitis. Lancet 1: 488–489
21. Winfield J, Gumpel J M 1979 An evaluation of repeat intra-articular injections of yttrium-90 colloids in persistent synovitis of the knee. Ann Rheum Dis 38: 145–147
22. Arthritis and Rheumatism Council Multicentre Radiosynoviorthesis Trial Group 1984 Intra-articular radioactive yttrium and triamcinolone hexacetonide: an inconclusive trial. Ann Rheum Dis 43: 620–623
23. Grant E N, Bellamy N, Fryday-Field K, Disney T, Dreidger A, Hobby K 1992 Double-blind randomized controlled trial and six-year open follow-up of yttrium-90 radiosynovectomy versus triamcinolone hexacetonide in persistent rheumatoid knee synovitis. Immunopharmacology 1: 231–238
24. Edmonds J, Smart R, Laurent R et al 1993 A comparative study of the safety and efficacy of dysprosium-165 hydroxide macroaggregate and yttrium-90 silicate colloid in radiation synovectomy – a multicentre double blind clinical trial. Arthr Rheum (in press)
25. Spooren P F M J, Rasker J J, Arens R P J H 1985 Synovectomy of the knee with ^{90}Y. Eur J Nucl Med 10: 441–445
26. Gumpel J M, Shawe D J 1991 Diffuse pigmented villonodular synovitis: non-surgical management. Ann Rheum Dis 50: 531–533
27. Ahlberg Å 1971 Radioactive gold in the treatment of chronic synovial effusion in haemophilia. Proceedings of the VII World Congress of the Federation of Haemophilia, Teheran, 1971. Exerpta Medica, Amsterdam
28. Doherty M, Dieppe P A 1981 Effect of intra-articular yttrium-90 on chronic pyrophosphate arthropathy of the knee. Lancet ii: 1243–1246

SECTION 7

Nuclear cardiology

PART A

Techniques

89. Radiopharmaceuticals for the study of the heart

P. Rigo   S. Braat

HISTORICAL PERSPECTIVE

The first cardiovascular nuclear medicine studies resulted from the use by Blumgart & Weiss of intravenous radon to measure circulation times in vivo.[1] Vascular transit and cardiac functional studies remained at the forefront of development with the introduction of technetium-labelled blood pool agents and of the Anger camera culminating in the equilibrium gated cardiac blood pool and first pass studies.[2–5] Perfusion imaging was slower to develop starting with rubidium,[6,7] caesium,[8,9] potassium, and finally thallium.[6–13] During the 1970s imaging of myocardial necrosis was demonstrated and the fate of labelled substrates, principally radiolabelled fatty acids, was also investigated.[14,15] In the 1980s the development of SPECT and PET provided the impetus for the introduction of new technetium-labelled perfusion tracers and of a wide variety of positron labelled flow tracers, substrates, ligands and mediators. This chapter will review the currently available cardiovascular radiopharmaceuticals and analyse their physical characteristics and biological behaviour.

MYOCARDIAL PERFUSION TRACERS

Types of tracer

Freely diffusible tracers

The use of freely diffusible tracers such as oxygen-15 labelled water, carbon-11 butanol, xenon-133 and krypton-85 requires kinetic modelling and either positron emission tomography or selective intracoronary injection to focus analysis to the myocardium and separate it from tracer activity present in surrounding tissues and the ventricular cavities.

Oxygen-15 is a positron-emitter with a half-life of 2.04 min. It is primarily produced by the $^{14}N(d,n)^{15}O$ reaction. The oxygen-15 tracer can be converted to $CO^{15}O$ by passing through an on-line charcoal system at 400°C. Alternatively, direct production by irradiation of 2% carbon dioxide in nitrogen is more commonly employed. $H_2{}^{15}O$ is commonly prepared from oxygen-15 by reaction with hydrogen using a palladium catalyst.[16] Oxygen-15 labelled water can be injected as such or obtained by the inhalation of $C^{15}O_2$ rapidly transformed into $H_2{}^{15}O$ by means of carbonic anhydrase.[17,18] Oxygen-15 labelled water diffuses freely across membranes and is highly extracted by myocardial tissue over a wide range of flow. It is not retained in the myocardium but diffuses back rapidly into the vascular compartment. Quantification of flow is usually performed using a two compartment model (a vascular and an extravascular compartment) and dynamic data acquisition. Measurement of the rate constants describing the exchange between these two compartments allows estimation of flow in regions of interest defined over the myocardium. Use of this technique, however, does not provide an adequate image of the myocardium as the vascular activity needs to be subtracted. Carbon monoxide labelled with ^{15}O has been proposed for that purpose but the distribution of $C^{15}O$ in the central blood pool is different from that of $H_2{}^{15}O$ leading to other problems. In addition, blood pool images should theoretically be recorded at stress as well as at rest. Widespread application of oxygen-labelled water has been hampered by the need to handle high count rates and by the lack of images but renewed interest in the technique might result from analysis of the volume of distribution of water, the so-called tissue fraction.[19] Indeed, this approach might provide a way to derive combined information on blood flow and viability from a single tracer.

Fully extracted tracers

Labelled microspheres of adequate size are fully extracted in the first encountered capillary bed and therefore require left atrial or left ventricular injection for homogeneous distribution into the systemic circulation (selective intra-arterial injection does not allow perfusion quantification). Their use according to the Sapirstein principle has been well validated in animals.[20] Regional blood flow to any organ can be computed as the ratio of the activity accumulated in the organ or fraction of the organ divided by the total arterial concentration accumulated over time (i.e. the integrated arterial concentration curve). In practice, this latter determination is obtained by arterial sampling at a given rate.

Human experience has been acquired with microspheres labelled with carbon-11 (PET), or technetium or indium (SPECT).[21,22] Microspheres labelled with single photon emitters do not allow determination of absolute myocardial blood flow especially when injected into the coronary arteries. Carbon-11 labelled microspheres however, provide the reference method for absolute myocardial blood flow determination and have been used to verify the overall accuracy of the technique.

Partially extracted tracers

Most tracers currently used for the assessment of myocardial perfusion belong to this category. Evaluation of blood flow with these tracers requires kinetic modelling or application of a modification of the microsphere formula with separate evaluation of the extraction fraction, because the ratio of myocardial uptake over the integral of the input function measures the product of flow and net extraction, rather than flow alone.

*The ideal perfusion tracer

The ideal tracer for the assessment of myocardial perfusion should have the following characteristics. It should be distributed in the myocardium in proportion to blood flow over the range of values experienced in health and disease. It should be extracted efficiently from the blood by the myocardium on its first passage through the heart. It should remain within the myocardium for the period of data acquisition. After acquisition, rapid elimination from the body should allow repeat studies under different conditions. Other desirable properties are that it should have a high photon flux at an energy between 100 and 200 keV, a low radiation burden to the patient, it should be easily available, and it should be cheap. Needless to say, no tracer possesses all these properties.

Single photon tracers

*Thallium-201

Thallium-201 is the most commonly used radionuclide for myocardial perfusion studies. Compared with the ideal tracer outlined above, it has a number of unfavourable properties but, because of the large experience with its use, it is the standard against which other tracers must be judged. Thallium is a metallic element of Group IIIA in the periodic table. Thallium-201 is produced by the $^{203}Tl(p,3n)^{201}Pb \rightarrow {}^{201}Tl$ reaction. It decays by electron capture to mercury-201 with a physical half-life of 73 h. Gamma photons of 135 and 167 keV are emitted (12% abundance) but the main emission is the mercury X-ray of 69–80 keV (88% abundance).[13–23]

Thallium is administered intravenously as thallous chloride and the usual dose is 80 MBq. Higher doses have become popular in some countries although the high radiation burden associated with such doses is a problem. Uptake is rapid and the half-life in the blood is only 30 s. Following intravenous injection, approximately 85% is cleared from the blood after the first circulation but because the myocardium receives only 5% of the cardiac output, only 4% of the total dose is taken up within 10–20 min after injection.[24–26] The hydrated thallium ion is similar in size to the hydrated potassium ion and a proportion (approximately 60%) enters the cardiac myocyte by active transport using the sodium–potassium ATPase-dependent exchange mechanism. The remainder enters passively probably along the electropotential gradient. The extraction efficiency is reduced by acidosis and hypoxaemia although these are only small effects and may not reduce extraction significantly until close to cell death.[27]

Distribution within the myocardium is proportional to myocardial blood flow over a wide range of values although at high rates of flow, extraction may become rate limiting.[28] In animal experiments, this proportionality to flow is maintained in non-viable tissue (TTC negative) 60 min after reperfusion following prolonged (3 h) occlusion.[29] In humans it has been recommended to delay studies aimed at assessing reperfusion to avoid underestimating infarct size.[30] The half-life of elimination from the heart is 1–1½ h after intracoronary injection, although this is prolonged to 4–5 h after intravenous injection because of equilibration with the blood pool and with the activity released by other organs. It is mainly excreted by the kidneys and the whole-body biological half-life is around 10 days.[13]

After stress injection or during ischaemia, thallium undergoes progressive redistribution with gradual normalization of the images reflecting the haemodynamic conditions. The mechanism of redistribution has been debated.[28–31] It could result from differential washout as washout is proportional to flow. This alone should not lead to activity equilibration even if the lesion contrast would diminish with time. Redistribution is more importantly related to secondary tracer uptake related to persistent thallium blood activity. Although thallium leakage from the whole body is usually sufficient to provide enough circulating thallium, lack of redistribution in ischaemic non-infarcted tissue has been reported, and it is now recommended to use thallium reinjection or injection at rest to differentiate ischaemia from scar.[32] Redistribution in hibernating myocardium is more difficult to understand, however, as flow remains abnormal. Evidence

*Modified from Pennell et al 1994 Thallium myocardial perfusion tomography in clinical cardiology. Springer-Verlag, London, pp 5–6

for a non-flow related component of thallium redistribution, has, however, been presented.[33] It could reflect progressive equilibration of the intracellular to extracellular concentration gradient among regions with different exchange kinetics. Alternatively, redistribution in hibernating myocardium could be used as an argument favouring the hypothesis that this phenomenon results from frequent recurrent episodes of severe flow reductions alternating with periods of flow improvement.

Thallium has been used routinely as a tracer of myocardial perfusion for almost two decades and the experience collected over this time is considerable. Normal appearances of both planar and tomographic images are well established and the protocols for acquisition and image processing have been standardized. The radiopharmaceutical is widely available at short notice and its cost is low. It does, however, have some limitations. First, because of the relatively long half-life within the body, radiation exposure to the patient is high. Eighty megabecquerels deliver an effective dose equivalent of 20 mSv and this is more than the average exposure during coronary arteriography, which is 5–10 mSv. Second, because of the desire to limit radiation exposure the injected dose is kept low and, to compound the problem, only 4% of the injected dose is taken up by the myocardium. The count density of the myocardial images is therefore low with high background levels. Third, the low energy emission at 69–80 keV leads to low resolution images with significant attenuation by soft tissues. Technetium-99m compounds do not suffer all these problems which has encouraged their development.

Technetium-labelled tracers

Several classes of technetium-labelled perfusion tracers have emerged: the isonitriles, the diphosphines, the substituted oximes. Some of these tracers are under development and are not yet available commercially.[34–36]

Technetium-labelled isonitriles A number of early technetium-99m isonitriles suffered from high lung and liver uptake, but 2-methoxy-isobutyl-isonitrile (sestamibi) has the best myocardium to background ratio.[37] Its advantages over thallium are its lower radiation burden to the patient and the higher resolution images that it provides. In clinical practice, it gives at least the same sensitivity and specificity for the detection of coronary artery disease.

The blood clearance of ^{99m}Tc sestamibi is very rapid with $t_{\frac{1}{2}}$ of a few minutes both at rest and exercise.[38] It diffuses passively through the capillary membrane, although less readily than thallium resulting in a lower immediate extraction.[39] It crosses the myocardial cell membrane along the electropotential gradient with a higher permeability than thallium. Within the cell it is localized in the mitochondria where its concentration can reach 140 times that of the blood.[40] It remains trapped in the mitochondria of living cells with slow secondary release, so that its net extraction is almost equivalent to thallium at around 40%. Despite slow myocardial release (half-life of 5–6 h) significant redistribution does not occur within 3-4 h, probably because the blood activity decreases very rapidly while tracer taken up by the liver and kidneys is eliminated rather than being secondarily released back into the blood as for thallium. The 24 h urinary excretion is 27% and the 48 h fecal excretion is 37%. Sestamibi does not appear to be metabolized.[41]

Images of ^{99m}Tc sestamibi have higher spatial resolution and higher count densities than those of thallium because of the higher energy photon produced by ^{99m}Tc (140 keV) and the shorter half-life (6 h), allowing larger doses to be given for the same radiation burden. The maximum dose recommended for routine use in the UK is 300 MBq for planar imaging and 400 MBq for tomography with total doses of 800 MBq and 1000 MBq respectively if stress and rest studies are performed on the same day. 1000 MBq corresponds to an effective dose equivalent of 10 mSv. The count density allows the tomograms to be electrocardiographically gated, and hence regional wall motion and thickening can be assessed.[42] An alternative method of assessing ventricular function is to record the first passage of the tracer through the heart in an identical fashion to conventional first-pass radionuclide ventriculography.[43]

Technetium-99m diphosphine complexes The potential of ^{99m}Tc diphosphine complexes for myocardial perfusion imaging has been explored.[34] The Tc-(DMPE)2 Cl_2+ complex had significant heart uptake but imaging was impaired by high liver uptake and poor blood and liver clearance characteristics in man while animal data in most species had been encouraging. Functionalized diphosphine complexes have met greater success.[44] One such complex, ^{99m}Tc tetrofosmin, is the ether functionalized diphospine ligand 1,2-bis bis (2-ethoxy-ethylphosphine) ethane. After intravenous administration, this compound is rapidly cleared from the blood (<5% by 10 min). It is taken up by the heart, liver, spleen, kidneys and skeletal muscles. Its distribution appears proportional to blood flow. Once in the myocardium there is little if any redistribution over at least 3 h. The mechanism of uptake is probably similar to that of ^{99m}Tc sestamibi, being related to diffusion along an electropotential gradient. Clearance is primarily through the hepatobiliary and urinary route, each contributing approximately 35% of injected activity by 48 h.[45,46]

A non-reducible Tc(III) cationic phosphine ligand, Q12, also provides favourable characteristics for myocardial imaging. Its clearance from the blood is biexponential with an initial half-life in the dog of 11 min and a late half-life of 221 min. The relationship of Q12 myocardial activity to microsphere myocardial flow is linear up to flow of 2 ml/g/min. Myocardial uptake is 2.3% of the injected dose, no evidence of redistribution is observed and clearance is both hepatobiliary and renal (33%).[47,48]

Technetium-99m teboroxime Another group of compounds that has shown promise for myocardial perfusion imaging are the boronic acid adducts with technetium dioxime.[49] Teboroxime has seven coordinate covalent bonds to the ^{99m}Tc central atom, two of each from three dioxime molecules and one from the chlorine atom. It has been introduced in the USA but no similar compounds are available in Europe at the time of writing. It is a neutral lipophilic compound which passively diffuses rapidly into the cardiac myocyte. The proportion of the injected dose taken up by the myocardium is relatively high (more than 3% at 1 min), and the first-pass extraction is greater than 70%.[50] The net extraction after five min is similar to thallium, however, because of a rapid clearance from the myocardium, with a $t_{\frac{1}{2}}$ of 5–15 minutes.[51,52] Because of the rapid washout, imaging must be started immediately after clearance of the tracer from the blood pool and preferably completed within 5 min. Differential washout occasionally provides the equivalent of some 'redistribution'. Blood clearance of this agent is fast but follows a biexponential mode with the first $t_{\frac{1}{2}}$ being less than a minute (88%) and the second, 154 min (12%).[50] Excretion is mainly through the liver and the mean 24 h urinary excretion is 22%.

Tc N-NOET Bis (N ethoxy, N ethyl dithiocarbamate) nitride ^{99m}Tc (V) (Tc N-NOET) is a new neutral myocardial imaging agent. This complex possesses a very small overall net charge with a distorted square pyramidal geometry. Tc N-NOET has high first-pass extraction (0.89) but slow blood washout (15 and 90 min activity of 37% and 18% respectively). Redistribution is observed in models of coronary ligation followed by reperfusion while optimal myocardial images are recorded 60 min after tracer injection.[53]

PET blood flow tracers

Rubidium-82

Rubidium-82 has a half-life of 75 s and is available from the ^{82}Sr/^{82}Rb generator. The parent ^{82}Sr ($t_{\frac{1}{2}}$ 25 d) is produced by high energy cyclotron or linear accelerator[54] and decays to ^{82}Rb by electron capture. Rubidium-82 is eluted from the generator as RbCl and administered directly with an infusion pump. Its short half-life allows repeated myocardial blood flow measurements at short intervals.[55] The disadvantages of rubidium-82 include the high energy of its positron (3.3 MeV) and a rather low extraction fraction (65%).

62Cu-PTSM

The zinc 62/copper 62 generator offers the possibility to use ^{62}Cu-PTSM, a newly introduced flow tracer.[56,57] Despite some attractive characteristics the usable period of that generator is only 1 day, while images are degraded by a high hepatic uptake. Compounds labelled with generator produced gallium-68 have also been reported.[58]

Nitrogen-13 ammonia

13N ammonia has a physical half-life of 10 min, is avidly taken by the myocardium and clears rapidly from the blood pool.[59] It is fixed in the myocardium by metabolic incorporation into ^{13}N-glutamine.[60,61] Myocardial clearance is slow and high myocardial contrast is generally obtained despite increased lung uptake in patients with pulmonary congestion and in smokers. It is also concentrated in the liver and this sometimes interferes with evaluation of the inferior wall. $^{13}NH_3$ extraction fraction is high at low and normal flows (extraction fraction of 79% at coronary blood flow of 100 ml/min/g in the dog) while net extraction fraction drops to 49% at flow of 500 ml/min/g. Changes in extraction fraction related to changes in metabolic conditions appear less significant although they are difficult to exclude.[62] Knowledge of the relationship between flow and extraction, use of a compartmental model[63] or graphical analysis using a Patlak plot provide the means to assess regional myocardial blood flow in quantitative terms using ^{13}N ammonia.[63–64]

Potassium-38

Potassium-38 is a cyclotron produced cation.[65] Although ^{38}K can only be produced by a relatively large cyclotron using the ^{35}Cl (α,n) reaction, it has desirable physical and biological features. It is the reference tracer on which other flow tracers have been modelled, its mechanism of uptake through the NaK ATPase is well known and characterized, and potassium extraction fraction is high, although lower than that of ammonia. Concern has been raised in the past regarding secondary potassium release in ischaemic or infarcted myocardium. Current data, however, indicate that potassium extraction fraction increases at low flow including in ischaemic myocardium, while accelerated secondary release is indicative of non-viable myocardium.[66] The longer half-life of ^{38}K ($t_{\frac{1}{2}}$ 7 min) makes it a more attractive tracer than 82Rb ($t_{\frac{1}{2}}$ 75 s) to evaluate tracer leakage as images of adequate statistical values are maintained longer, and the overall count rates are higher. These studies show that in the absence of non-viable myocardium, potassium leakage is minimal. Serial evaluation of myocardial perfusion to monitor the effect of interventions is easily performed with potassium as the duration of irradiation and processing (30 min) adequately matches the interval necessary for decay of the previous dose (approximately 4 half-lives) and for physical recovery from exercise to rest. Overall myocardial imaging of perfusion tracers at rest and stress displays relative or absolute (using quantitative PET) perfusion reserve, useful measures of overall coronary function.[67]

BLOOD POOL AGENTS

First-pass ventriculography

The first-pass technique requires a tracer that transits rapidly through the lungs and is not trapped into the lung capillaries or lung tissue and reaches the left ventricular cavity without excessive dispersion. Most technetium-labelled compounds fulfil these requirements but Tc pertechnetate or Tc-DTPA are usually preferred for the sake of simplicity (ease of preparation/or because DTPA is rapidly cleared from the blood allowing repeat injection at stress or in another projection).[68] Despite this, escalating doses (400–600 then 750–1000 MBq) are usually used for serial protocols.

The use of a short-lived, generator produced tracer for first-pass ventriculography allows flexible serial first-pass protocols with a limited patient dose. $^{195m}Hg/^{195m}Au$ generators[69] ($t_{\frac{1}{2}}$ of 41.6 h and 30.5 s respectively), $^{191}Os/^{191m}Ir$ generators[70] ($t_{\frac{1}{2}}$ 14 days and 4.7 s) and $^{178}W/^{178}Ta$ generators[71] ($t_{\frac{1}{2}}$ 22 days and 9.3 min) have been produced and investigated. None of these approaches, however, had durable success due to high cost, production difficulties or the suboptimal energy of the tracer.

The $^{81}Rb/^{81m}Kr$ generator remains available, however, as it is used in Europe for pulmonary ventilation imaging. Perfusion of a sterile generator with isotonic glucose solution elutes krypton dissolved in water. By intravenous infusion the krypton-81m has unique features, as it is readily eliminated during the lung first transit and activity does not accumulate or reach the left ventricle. It therefore provides excellent visualization of the right ventricle as well as of the venous circulation. Right ventriculography during krypton infusion appears to be the best technique to study the effect of intervention on right ventricular function.[72]

Equilibrium gated ventriculography

Equilibrium gated studies require agents that label the blood pool. Tc-labelled human serum albumin was first used but has largely been abandoned because of lack of stability and high hepatic uptake. New methods of labelling human serum albumin modified by the introduction of a new mercapto group might remove these limitations.[73] Red cell labelling, however, is in common use. Labelling can be performed in vivo[74], in vitro[75] or by combined methods. The in vivo method requires pre-injection of Sn^{2+} ion (10 µg/kg body weight) using kits of stannous pyrophosphate or tartrate. After intravenous injection, stannous ion is cleared from the plasma but penetrates red cells and subsequent injection of pertechnetate after an optimal interval of 20 min leads to labelling as technetium is transported into the red cell probably through an anion transport enzyme (the band 3 transport protein[76] is reduced from the 7+ state to a lower value and binds to the beta chain of haemoglobin). Labelling efficiency increases with time over 10–15 min as technetium, having initially migrated to the interstitial space, equilibrates back into the plasma to be trapped into red cells. An alternative approach, the combined in vivo/vitro method, adds technetium to a pre-tinned anticoagulated blood sample but delays reinjection 10 or 15 min to allow completion of labelling and to diminish the amount of extracellular technetium. The in vitro technique requires red cell centrifugation and separation prior to addition of pertechnetate, followed by resuspension and washing to remove the unbound ^{99m}Tc prior to reinjection.

Using these techniques more than 95% of the ^{99m}Tc is bound to red cells and contrast beween the cardiac blood pool and the surrounding tissues is about 3:1. The effective half-life in the blood is 6 h. Activity in the liver is low but activity in the spleen is high, reflecting red cell concentration. The radiation burden to the spleen is about 1 mSv per 37 MBq.

Combined perfusion and function studies

Recently, the opportunity to use technetium-labelled perfusion tracers to study perfusion and function simultaneously has attracted attention.[77] Indeed, these tracers can be used to study right and left global ventricular function where there is good correlation with reference techniques despite initial lung uptake and concurrent myocardial uptake, as in the case of ^{99m}Tc sestamibi, for instance. Evaluation of regional left ventricular function is more difficult with first-pass, but gating of the perfusion image obtained through planar or tomographic technique can also be used for global and regional functional evaluation.

METABOLIC SUBSTRATES AND ANALOGUES

The myocardium has a high energy demand with 80% of myocardial oxygen consumption (6–8 ml per min per 100 g at rest) devoted to mechanical work, and 20% used for maintenance of cellular integrity. Under fasting conditions, the heart derives up to 70% of its energy from free fatty acid oxidation (mainly palmitate),[78,79] but depending on plasma substrate level, hormonal factors, myocardial oxygen demand and availability, glucose, lactate, pyruvate, ketone bodies or amino acids are also used.

Carbohydrate loading increases glucose oxidation as plasma insulin rises and free fatty acid levels decrease. Lactate is an important alternate energy source during exercise. However, the oxidative metabolism of these substrates (and their tracers) is largely interrelated as the tricarboxylic acid cycle is their final common pathway. Ischaemia alters the balance of substrate metabolism as beta-oxidation of free fatty acids is impaired. Energy production then relies on an accelerated glycolytic flux with increased glycogen breakdown. In severe ischaemia, however, accumulation of metabolites such as lactate inhibits glycolysis. The principal substrate groups have been labelled with positron emitting tracers which allows evaluation of regional substrate utilization. The fate of these tracers can be followed, but analysis requires knowledge of cardiac metabolism and the application of kinetic data modelling, as it is not possible with PET at a given time to determine with which chemical species the radiolabel is associated.[80]

^{18}F fluorodeoxyglucose (FDG)

The use of substrate analogues such as FDG, which only in part follows the metabolism of glucose, is sometimes preferable. ^{18}F has a $t_{\frac{1}{2}}$ of 110 min and decays by $\beta+$ emission. It is produced in the cyclotron by the ^{18}O(p,n)^{18}F reaction on ^{18}O water targets.[81–82] F ion is then used to produce the 2-fluoro-2-D-glucose.[83] After intravenous injection, FDG competes with glucose for transmembranous transport and phosphorylation by the hexokinase reaction to FDG-6-phosphate. This is not metabolized as it is not a substrate for glycolysis, the pentose shunt or glycogen synthesis and it remains trapped in the myocardium because of low membrane permeability for back-diffusion. Measurement of FDG incorporation into the myocardium together with the input function, use of a mathematical model and correction for the difference in affinity for transport and phosphorylation between FDG and glucose allow qualitative and quantitative estimation of exogeneous glucose utilization.[84,85] Myocardial imaging is usually performed 40–60 min after IV administration of 10 mCi ^{18}F-FDG. The single pass extraction fraction is low and variable but the cumulative uptake of 1–4% of the injected dose is adequate. The uptake and myocardial metabolic rates vary widely between the fasting and non-fasting states (2.8 times increase in the glycolytic state). Heart to lung, heart to blood and heart to liver ratios are above 10. Blood clearance is multiexponential with a $t_{\frac{1}{2}}$ of 0.2–0.3 min, followed by a $t_{\frac{1}{2}}$ of 11.6 min and a small longer third component.

The primary clinical application of FDG in the heart is to identify jeopardized but viable myocardium using the FDG/flow mismatch patterns. Unfortunately, no single photon labelled tracer with biological characteristics analogous to FDG has yet been described.

Fatty acid tracers

Other substrates can be labelled using heteroatoms such as ^{18}F or ^{123}I to yield analogues available for conventional nuclear medicine studies. A large variety of fatty acid analogues have been labelled to study their uptake and utilization by the heart, and results are promising. Caution is important in this field considering the complexity of fatty acid metabolism and the experience with ^{11}C palmitate. ^{11}C palmitate is synthesized from pentadecyl magnesium bromide and $^{11}CO_2$.[86] Palmitate comprises approximately 25–30% of the circulating fatty acids in the blood and it circulates bound to albumin. It diffuses into the myocyte and is transferred to the intracellular carrier proteins to be thioesterified. As a result of high extraction, the initial distribution is proportional to blood flow. It clears from the myocardium in biexponential fashion, the early rapid phase clearance represent beta oxidation which correlates with changes in cardiac workload and substrate utilization, while the slow second phase reflects incorporation in the lipid pool. However, the clinical application of this tracer has been limited by its complexity and by recognition of back-diffusion of unmetabolized tracer contaminating the early clearance phase and data interpretation.[87]

^{11}C acetate is highly extracted and metabolized only by the TCA cycle and has been proposed as a more direct alternative to study myocardial oxidative metabolism. The rate constant of the early rapid clearance of acetate correlates with MVO2 and is only minimally influenced by myocardial substrate availability.[88–90] Correction of acetate kinetics for ^{11}C metabolite contamination[91] allows quantitative assessment of acetate utilization and a non-invasive approach for the quantitative assessment of myocardial oxygen consumption.

^{18}F fatty acid analogues have been evaluated for myocardial metabolic imaging but their metabolic characteristics are different from normal fatty acid substrates so that interpretation of the PET images is difficult.[92] 1-^{11}C-β-methylheptadecanoic acid has been found to metabolize only partially in the myocardium.

Other fatty acid analogues are those labelled with ^{123}I but the size of the heteroatom probably modifies the metabolic behaviour of these analogues. Iodo penta, hexa and heptadecanoic acids (IHA) have been prepared. Their initial kinetics are comparable to ^{11}C palmitate indicating that IHA follows the natural metabolism of free fatty acids.[93] Clearance of IHA is modified by metabolic or haemodynamic intervention known to influence substrate utilization (glucose administration, pacing, beta-blockade or catecholamines).[94]

A major problem with the use of iodinated fatty acids, however, is dehalogenation with rapid increase in the free iodine background activity. Use of iodophenylpentadecanoic analogues circumvents this.[95] In man, ortho and para IPPA have very different behaviours as ortho IPPA is bound to coenzyme-A and is retained in the cytosolic lipid pool in the myocardium whereas para IPPA is metabolized by mitochondrial oxidation.[96,97]

Iodine-labelled betamethyl heptadecanoic acid is another analogue, which has prolonged myocardial retention but appears useful in studying viability in patients with recent myocardial infarction in comparison with a blood flow tracer.[98] Mismatch of fatty acid uptake and flow (low fatty acid uptake with relatively preserved flow) may indicate a jeopardized but viable segment while matched defects indicate necrosis.[99]

Radiolabelled amino acids

Radiolabelled amino acids have not found significant application in the heart. ^{13}N glutamate initially proposed as an agent to indicate ischaemia in fact behaves like a blood flow tracer due to its very high extraction in man (in contrast to dogs).[100]

INFARCT AVID AGENTS

Tetracycline derivatives, bone seeking agents and dicarboxylic derivatives localize in areas of myocardial infarction but of these, only technetium pyrophosphate has been studied extensively.[101] Recently, antibodies to cardiac myosin have been developed as a more specific marker of myocyte necrosis.[102]

Pyrophosphate accumulates in myocardial infarction within a few hours of the acute event if the infarct related vessel is patent, or somewhat later (12 h) if the artery remains occluded. Maximum infarct uptake is obtained 24–72 h after infarction, and remains detectable for 6–10 days.[103] Pyrophosphate accumulation parallels the development of myofibrillar degeneration, a histological picture characterized by the development of mitochondrial calcium deposition suggestive of necrosis with reperfusion. It is probable that the pyrophosphate binds to a calcium phosphate crystalline structure even though some studies[101] have not confirmed the subcellular localization of pyrophosphates within the mitochondria but have shown a diffuse deposition even in tissues with calcified mitochondria. Consistent with this mechanism of uptake, pyrophosphate concentration is maximal in areas with moderate reduction of myocardial blood flow (20–40% of maximum) while uptake is low in regions of severely reduced flow. This may result in the so-called doughnut pattern in large infarcts, a situation when uptake is maximal at the periphery of the infarct.

Myosin is one of the myofibrillar proteins. It is composed of light and heavy chain subunits. Isotypes of cardiac origin display some cross reactivity with corresponding skeletal isotypes. Myosin represents a large target within the myocardium as it comprises 40–50 mg/g of cardiac muscle. It is not normally exposed to circulating antibodies, as the intact sarcolema will not permit macromolecules to enter the cell. This barrier fails following myocyte necrosis because of cell membrane disruption and anti-myosin antibodies to attach to the exposed myosin filaments. The available clinical tracer is now labelled with indium,[104] although progress with technetium labelling has been made. The uptake is highly specific for myocyte necrosis. Tracer accumulation is greatest in regions of lowest myocardial blood flow, and although positive images may be seen 12 h after injection, optimal images require 24–48 h to develop. Infarct size demonstrated by quantitative imaging correlates with the peak CK-MB values and the extent of akinesia.

Patients requiring anti-myosin imaging for infarct evaluation should be injected as soon as possible with imaging 24–48 h later. In the days following infarction, cardiac myosin disappears gradually and the uptake becomes less intense. No uptake is usually seen at the site of an old infarct but positive images have occasionally been reported up to 9 months after the acute event.

Comparative studies of anti-myosin and pyrophosphate show improved results with anti-myosin with smaller infarct size. This might reflect the lower specificity of pyrophosphates or a technical problem related to the increased uptake at the periphery of the infarct. Myocyte necrosis is not limited to patients with acute myocardial infarction. Indeed, cellular necrosis also occurs in patients with myocarditis as well as in cardiac allograft rejection.[105–107]

TRACERS FOR EVALUATION OF CARDIAC INNERVATION

Both the sympathetic and parasympathetic nervous systems innervate the heart and radiopharmaceuticals have been developed to map the presynaptic nerve terminals and the postsynaptic receptors. The sympathetic system has been most studied. Radiopharmaceuticals have been developed with a high affinity for the uptake nerve terminal transport mechanism. These false neurotransmitters have structural analogy to noradrenaline and their retention reflects neuronal uptake and vesicular storage. ^{18}F fluorometaraminol, ^{11}C metahydroxyephedrine and ^{123}I-MIBG have been used. Their retention is altered by desipramine or reserpine pretreatment, by sympathetic denervation or injury, as well as in dilated cardiomyopathic heart.[108]

In addition to these, ^{11}C-CGP 12177, a hydrophilic beta-blocker, has been found to map myocardial beta-receptors adequately both in animal and in human studies,[109] and the muscarinic receptor distribution in the human heart can be imaged using ^{11}C methyl QNB.[110]

VARIA

Cardiovascular imaging can also benefit from labelling of various circulating cells and proteins. Indium-labelled leucocytes or ^{99m}Tc-HM PAO labelled leucocytes are routinely used in nuclear medicine for the detection of foci of infection. However, cardiac infections are only infrequently associated with abcesses while valve vegetations contain more platelets and fibrin than leucocytes. Uptake of leucocytes can, however, be observed in some patients with ring abcesses, prosthetic valve endocarditis as well as in cases of purulent pericarditis.[111] Indium-labelled platelets and monoclonal antibodies against platelets have been used to image arterial thrombi both in the ventricular cavities and in the great vessels. Although the sensitivity of this technique appears lower than that of echo, detected thrombi can be demonstrated to accumulate platelets actively.[112] Indium, iodine or technetium-labelled LDL have been shown to be cleared by the liver as a function of the density of LDL receptors. Accumulation of LDL in atherosclerotic plaques has been observed, principally in lipid rich lesions, but due to persisting blood activity, the target to background ratio is too low to permit imaging and further research appears necessary.[113] ^{123}Iodine-labelled serum amyloid protein (SAP) is a normal plasma constituent. ^{123}Iodine-labelled SAP accumulates in amyloid deposits in most target organs of the disease. It remains unclear, however, why cardiac deposition has not usually been observed in patients with cardiac amyloidosis.[114]

REFERENCES

1. Blumgart H L, Weiss S 1927 Studies on the velocity of blood flow: VI. The method of collecting the active deposits of radium and its preparation for intravenous injection. J Clin Invest 4: 389–398
2. Strauss H W, Zaret B L, Hurley P J, Natarajan T K, Pitt B 1971 A scintiphotographic method for measuring left ventricular ejection fraction in man without cardiac catheterisation. Am J Cardiol 28: 575–580
3. Chervu H R 1979 Radiopharmaceuticals in cardiovascular nuclear medicine. Semin Nucl Med 9: 241–256
4. Van Dyke D, Anger H O, Sullivan R W et al 1972 Cardiac evaluation from radioisotope dynamics. J Nucl Med 13: 585–592
5. Schelbert H R, Verba J W, Johnson A D et al 1975 Non traumatic determination of left ventricular ejection fraction by radionuclide angiography. Circulation 51: 902–909
6. Donato L, Bartolomei G, Giordani R 1964 Evaluation of myocardial blood perfusion in man with radioactive potassium or rubidium and precordial counting. Circulation 29: 195–203
7. Love W D, Burch G E 1969 Interference of the rate of coronary plasma flow on the extraction of Rb-86 from coronary blood. Circ Res 7: 24–30
8. Poe N D 1975 Comparative myocardial uptake and clearance characteristics of potassium and cesium. J Nucl Med 13: 557–560
9. Rigo P, Gach J, Mengeot P 1975 Pre- and post-operative myocardial and blood pool scans in a case of left ventricular aneurysm. J Nucl Med 16: 1024–1026
10. Rigo P, Strauss H W, Pitt B 1975 The combined use of gated cardiac blood pool scanning and myocardial imaging with potassium-43 in the evaluation of patients with myocardial infarction. Radiology 115: 387–391
11. Lebowitz E, Green M W, Fairchild R et al 1975 Thallium-201 for medical use. J Nucl Med 16: 151–155
12. Grunwald A M, Watson D D, Holzgrefe H H et al 1981 Myocardial thallium-201 kinetics in normal and ischemic myocardium. Circulation 64: 610–618
13. Atkins H L, Budinger T F, Lebowitz E et al 1977 Thallium-201 for medical use. Part 3 : Human distribution and physical imaging properties. J Nucl Med 18: 133–140
14. Bonte F J, Parkey R W, Graham K D et al 1974 A new method for radionuclide imaging of myocardial infarcts. Radiology 110: 473–474
15. Evans J R, Gunton R, Baker R W et al 1965 Use of radioiodinated fatty acid for photoscan of the heart. Circ Res 16: 1–10
16. Clarke J C, Crouzel C, Meyer G J, Strijckmans K 1987 Current methodology for oxygen 15 production for clinical use. Appl Radiat Isot 38: 597–600
17. Lammertsma A A, De Silva R, Araujo L I, Jones T 1992 Measurement of regional myocardial blood flow using C15O2 and positron emission tomography: comparison of tracer models. Clin Phys Physiol Meas 13: 1–20
18. Bergmann S R, Herrero P, Markham J et al 1989 Noninvasive quantitation of myocardial blood flow in human subjects with oxygen-15 labelled water and positron emission tomography. J Am Coll Cardiol 14: 639–652
19. De Silva R, Yamamoto Y, Rhodes C G et al 1992 Preoperative prediction of the outcome of coronary revascularization using positron emission tomography. Circulation 86: 1738–1742
20. Heymann M A, Payne B D, Hoffman J I E, Rudolph A M 1977 Blood flow measurements with radionuclide-labeled particles. Prog Cardiovasc Dis 20: 55–79
21. Selwyn A P, Shea M J, Foale R et al 1986 Regional myocardial and organ blood flow after myocardial infarction. Application of the microsphere principle in man. Circulation 73: 433–443
22. Parodi O, Sambuceti G, Roghi A et al 1993 Residual coronary reserve despite decreased resting blood flow in patients with critical coronary lesions. Circulation 87: 330–344
23. Beller G A, Watson D D 1982 Quantitative thallium-201 imaging. Am J Cardiol 49: A20–A21
24. L'Abbate A, Biagini A, Michelassi C, Maseri A 1979 Myocardial kinetics of thallium and potassium in man. Circulation 60: 776–785
25. Pohost G M, Alpert N M, Ingwall J S, Strauss H W 1980 Thallium redistribution: mechanisms and clinical utility. Sem Nucl Med 10: 70–93
26. Weich H, Strauss H W, Pitt B 1977 The extraction of thallium-201 by the myocardium. Circulation 56: 188–191
27. Ingwall J S, Kramer M, Kloner N M et al 1979 Thallium accumulation: differentiation between reversible and irreversible myocardial injury. Circulation 59: 678
28. Okada R D, Leppo J A, Strauss H W, Boucher Ca, Pohost G M 1982 Mechanisms and time course for the disappearance of thallium-201 defects at rest in dogs. Am J Cardiol 49: 699–706
29. Melin J A, Becker L C, Healy Bulkley B 1983 Differences in thallium-201 uptake in reperfused and nonreperfused myocardial infarction. Circ Res 53: 414–419
30. De Coster P M, Melin J A, Detry J M, Brasseur L A, Beckers C, Col J 1985 Coronary artery reperfusion in acute myocardial infarction: assessment by pre- and postintervention thallium-201 myocardial perfusion imaging. Am J Cardiol 55: 889–895

31. Pohost G M, Zir L M, Moore R H, McKusick K A, Guiney T, Beller G A 1977 Differentiation of transiently ischemic from infarcted myocardium by serial imaging after a single dose of thallium-201. Circulation 55: 294–302
32. Dilzizian V, Rocco T P, Freedman N M T, Leon M B, Bonow R O 1990 Enhanced detection of ischemic but viable myocardium by the reinjection of thallium after stress redistribution imaging. N Engl J Med 323: 141–146
33. Gerry Jl Jr, Becker L C, Flaherty J T, Weisfeldt M L 1980 Evidence for a flow-independent contribution to the phenomenon of thallium redistribution. Am J Cardiol 45: 58–61
34. Deutsch E A, Glavan K A, Sodd V J et al 1981 Cationic Tc-99m complexes as potential myocardial imaging agents. J Nucl Med 22: 897–907
35. Gerson M C, Deutsch E A, Nishiyama X et al 1983 Myocardial perfusion imaging with 99mTc-DMPE in man. Eur J Nucl Med 8: 371–374
36. Jones A G, Abrams M J, Davidson A et al 1984 Biological studies of a new class of technetium complexes: the hexakis (alkylisonitrile) technetium (I) cation. Int J Nucl Med Biol 23: 1093–1101
37. Holman B L, Jones A G, Lister-James J et al 1984 A new Tc-99m labeled myocardial imaging agent, hexakis (t-butylisonitrile)-technetium(I) (Tc-99m TBI): initial experience in the human. J Nucl Med 25: 1350–1355
38. Wackers F J T, Berman D S, Maddahi J et al 1989 Technetium-99m hexakis 2-methoxyisobutyl isonitrile: human biodistribution, dosimetry, safety and preliminary comparison to thallium-201 for myocardial perfusion imaging. J Nucl Med 30: 301–311
39. Leppo J A 1993 Cardiac transport of single photon myocardial perfusion agents. In: Zaret B L, Beller G A, eds. Nuclear cardiology, state of the art and future direction. Mosby, St Louis. pp 35–44
40. Piwnica-Worms D, Kronauge J F, Chiu M L 1990 Uptake and retention of hexakis (2-methoxyisobutyl isonitrile) technetium (I) in cultured chick myocardial cells. Mitochondrial and plasma membrane potential dependence. Circulation 82: 1826–1838
41. Okada R D, Glover D, Gaffney T et al 1988 Myocardial kinetics of technetium-99m-hexakis-2-methoxy-2-methylpropyl-isonitrile. Circulation 77: 491–498
42. Iskandrian A S, Heo J, Kong B, Lyons E, Marsch E 1989 Use of technetium-99m isonitrile (RP-30) in assessing left ventricular perfusion and function at rest and during exercise in coronary artery disease, and comparison with coronary angiography and exercise thallium-201 thallium SPECT imaging. Am J Cardiol 64: 270
43. Larock M P, Cantineau R, Legrand V, Kulbertus H, Rigo P 1990 99mTc-MIBI (RP-30) to define the extent of myocardial ischemia and evaluate ventricular function. Eur J Nucl Med 16: 223–230
44. Highley B, Lahiri A, Kelly D J 1992 Technetium-99m complexes of functionalized diphosphines for myocardial perfusion imaging in man. In: van der Wall E E, ed. What's new in cardiac imaging. Kluwer Academic Publishers, Dordrecht, The Netherlands. pp 93–109
45. Jain D J, Wackers F J Th, Mattera J, McMahon M, Sinusas A J, Zaret B L 1993 Biokinetics of technetium-99m-tetrofosmin: myocardial perfusion imaging agent: implications for a one-day imaging protocol. J Nucl Med 34: 1254–1259
46. Kelly D J, Forster A M, Higley B et al 1993 Technetium-99m-tetrofosmin as a new radiopharmaceutical for myocardial perfusion imaging. J Nucl Med 34: 222–227
47. Rossetti C, Best T, Paganelli G et al 1990 A new, nonreducible Tc-99m(III) myocardial perfusion tracer: human biodistribution and initial clinical experience. J Nucl Med 31: 834
48. Gerson M C, Millard R W, Roszell N et al 1992 Relationship of Tc-99m Q12 activity to myocardial blood flow in the canine heart. J Nucl Med 33: 993
49. Nunn A D, Treher E N, Feld T 1986 Boronic acid adducts of technetium oxime complexes (BATO's): a new class of neutral complexes with myocardial imaging capabilities. J Nucl Med 27: 893
50. Narra R K, Nunn A D, Kuczynki B L et al 1989 A neutral technetium-99m complex for myocardial imaging. J Nucl Med 30: 1830–1837
51. Leppo J A, Meerdinck D J 1990 Comparative myocardial extraction of two technetium labeled BATO derivatives (SQ30217, SQ 32014) and thallium. J Nucl Med 31: 67–74
52. Johnson L L, Seldin D W 1990 Clinical experience with technetium-99m Teboroxime, a neutral, lipophilic myocardial perfusion imaging agent. Am J Cardiol 66: 63E–67E
53. Ghezzi C, Arvieuw C C, Fagret D et al 1994 Myocardial kinetics of TcN-NOET: a new neutral lipophilic complex of 99mTc. In press
54. Yano Y, Chu P, Budinger T F et al 1977 82Rb generators for imaging studies. J Nucl Med 18: 46–50
55. Saha G B, Go R T, MacIntyre W J et al 1990 Use of 82Sr/82Rb generator in clinical PET studies. Nucl Med Biol 17: 763–768
56. Green M A, Mathias C J, Welch M J et al 1990 Copper-62-labeled pyruvaldehyde bis(N4methylthiosemicarbazonato)-copper(II): synthesis and evaluation as a positron emission tomography tracer for cerebral and myocardial perfusion. J Nucl Med 31: 1989–1996
57. Melon P, Schwaiger M 1992 Imaging of metabolism and autonomic innervation of the heart by positron emission tomography. Eur J Nucl Med 19: 453–464
58. Green M A, Mathias C J, Neumann W L, Fanwick P E, Janik M, Edward A 1993 Potential gallium-68 tracers for imaging the heart with PET: Evaluation of four gallium complexes with functionalized tripodal Tris(salicylaldimine) ligands. J Nucl Med 34: 228–233
59. Krizek H, Lembares N, Dinwoodie R et al 1973 Production of radiochemically pure 13NH3 for biomedical studies using the 16O(p,α)13N reaction. J Nucl Med 14: 629–630
60. Schelbert H R, Phelps M E, Hoffman E J et al 1979 Regional myocardial perfusion assessed with ammonia and positron emission computerized axial tomography. Am J Cardiol 43: 209–218
61. Schelbert H R, Phelps M E, Huang S C et al 1981 N-13 ammonia as an indicator of myocardial blood flow. Circulation 63: 1259–1272
62. Nienaber C A, Ratib O, Gambhir S S et al 1991 A quantitative index of regional blood flow in canine myocardium derived noninvasively with N-13 ammonia and dynamic positron emission tomography. J Am Coll Cardiol 17: 260–269
63. Hutchins G, Schwaiger M, Rosenspire K, Krivokapich J, Schelbert H, Kuhl D 1990 Noninvasive quantification of regional myocardial blood flow in the human heart using (13N) ammonia and dynamic PET imaging. J Am Coll Cardiol 15: 1032–1042
64. Choi Y, Huang S C, Hawkins R A et al 1993 A simplified method for quantification of myocardial blood flow using nitrogen-13-ammonia and dynamic PET. J Nucl Med 34: 488–497
65. Guillaume M, De Landsheere C, Rigo P et al 1988 Automated production of potassium-38 for the study of myocardial perfusion using positron emission tomography. J Appl Radiat Isot 39: 97–107
66. Wijns W, Baudhuin Th, Bol A et al 1993 Myocardial perfusion and necrosis estimates with potassium-38 in experimental canine myocardial infarction. Eur Heart J 14 (Suppl Augustus): 187
67. Gould K L 1991 Coronary artery stenosis. Elsevier, New York
68. Ashburn W L, Schelbert H R, Verba J W 1978 Left ventricular ejection fraction: a review of several radionuclide angiographic approaches using the scintillation camera. Prog Cardiovasc Dis 20: 267–284
69. Mena I, Narahara K A, deJong R et al 1983 Gold-195m, an ultrashort-lived generator-produced radionuclide: clinical application in sequential first pass ventriculography. J Nucl Med 24: 139–144
70. Brihaye C, Knapp F F, Butler T A, Guillaume M 1985 A new osmium-191/iridium-191 generator system. J Nucl Med 26: P27
71. Lacey J L, Verani M S, Ball M E, Boyce T M, Gibson R W, Roberts R 1988 First-pass radionuclide angiography using a multiwire gamma camera and tantalum-178. J Nucl Med 29: 293–301
72. Sugrue D D, Kamal S, Deanfield J E et al 1983 Br J Radiol 56: 657–663

73. Verbeke K A, Vanbilloen H P, De Roo M J, Verbruggen A M 1993 Technetium-99m merceptoalbumin as a potential substitute for technetium-99m labelled red blood cells. Eur J Nucl Med 20: 473–482
74. Pavel D G, Zimmer A M, Patterson V W 1977 In vivo labeling of red blood cells with 99mTc: a new approach to blood pool visualization. J Nucl Med 18: 305–308
75. Smith T D, Richards P 1976 A simple kit for the preparation of 99mTc red blood cells. J Nucl Med 17: 126–132
76. Callahan R J, Rabito C A, McKusick K A, Leppo J, Strauss H W 1982 J Nucl Med 23: 315–318
77. Jones R H, Boreges-Neto S, Potts J 1990 Simultaneous measurement of myocardial perfusion and ventricular function during exercise from a single injection of technetium-99m Sestamibi in coronary artery disease. Am J Cardiol 66: 68E–71E
78. Bing R J, Ginsburg R, Minobe W et al 1982 Decreased catecholamine sensitivity and *-adrenergic receptor density in failing human hearts. N Engl J Med 30: 205–211
79. Neely J R, Morgan H E 1974 Relationship between carbohydrate and lipid metabolism and the energy balance of heart muscle. Ann Rev Physiol 36: 413–459
80. Rigo P, De Landsheere C, Melon P, Kulbertus H 1990 Imaging of myocardial metabolism by positron emission tomography. Cardiovasc Drugs and Therapy 4: 847–852
81. Kilbourn M R, Hood J T, Welch M J 1984 A simple 18O water target for 18F production. Appl Radiat Isot 37: 599–602
82. Guillaume M, Luxen A, Nebeling B, Argentini M, Clark J C, Pike V W 1991 Recommendations for fluorine-18 production. Appl Radiat Isot 42: 749–762
83. Hamacher K, Coenen H H, Stocklin G 1986 Efficient stereospecific synthesis of no-carrier-added 2-18F-fluoro-2-deoxy-D-glucose using aminopolyether supported nucleophilic substitution. J Nucl Med 27: 235–283
84. Phelps M E, Hoffman E J, Selin C et al 1978 Investigation of F-18-fluoro-2-deoxyglucose for the measure of myocardial glucose metabolism. J Nucl Med 19: 1311–1319
85. Ratib O, Phelps M E, Huang S C, Henze C, Selin C E, Schelbert H R 1982 Positron tomography with deoxyglucose for estimating local myocardial glucose metabolism. J Nucl Med 23: 577–586
86. Weiss E S, Ahmed S A, Welch M J et al 1977 Quantification of infarction in cross sections of canine myocardium in vivo with positron emission transaxial tomography and 11C-palmitate. Circulation 55: 66–73
87. Fox K A, Abendschein D R, Ambos H D, Sobel B E, Bergmann S R 1985 Efflux of metabolized and nonmetabolized fatty acid from canine myocardium. Implications for quantifying myocardial metabolism tomographically. Circ Res 57: 232–243
88. Brown M A, Myears D W, Bergmann S R 1989 Validity of estimates of myocardial oxidative metabolism with carbon-11 acetate and positron emission tomography despite altered patterns of substrate utilization. J Nucl Med 30: 187–193
89. Brown M A, Myears D W, Bergmann S R 1988 Noninvasive assessment of canine myocardial oxidative metabolism with carbon-11 acetate and positron emission tomography. J Am Coll Cardiol 12: 1054–1063
90. Buxton D B, Schwaiger M, Nguyen A, Phelps M E, Schelbert H R 1988 Radiolabeled acetate as a tracer of myocardial tricarboxylic acid cycle flux. Circ Res 63: 628–634
91. Buck A, Wolpers G, Hutchins G et al 1991 Effect of carbon-11 acetate recirculation on estimates of myocardial oxygen consumption by PET. J Nucl Med 32: 1950–1957
92. Knust E J, Kupfernagel C, Stocklin G 1979 Long-chain F-18 fatty acids for the study of regional metabolism in heart and liver: odd-even effects of metabolism in mice. J Nucl Med 20: 1170–1175
93. Lerch R A, Bergman S R 1985 Assessment of myocardial metabolism with C-14-palmitate. Comparison with I-123-heptadecanoic acid. Eur Heart J 6 (Suppl B): 21–27
94. Dudczak R, Kletter K, Frischauf H et al 1985 The use of I-123-labeled heptadecanoic acid (HDA) as metabolic tracer: preliminary report. Eur J Nucl Med 9: 81–85
95. Machulla H J, Dutschka K, Van Beuningen D 1981 Development of 15-(p-I-phenyl)-pentadecanoic acid for in vivo diagnosis of the myocardium. J Radioanalyt Chem 65: 279–286
96. Kaiser K P, Geunting B, Grossman K et al 1990 Tracer kinetics of 15-(ortho-123/131I-phenyl)-pentadecanoic acid (oPPA) and 15-(para-123/131I-phenyl)-pentadecanoic acid (pPPA) in animals and man. J Nucl Med 31: 1608–1616
97. Antar M A, Spohr G, Herzog H H et al 1986 15-(ortho-123I-phenyl)-pentadecanoic acid – a new myocardial imaging agent for clinical use. Nucl Med Commun 7: 683–696
98. Knapp F F, Kropp J, Goodman M M et al. The development of iodine-123-methyl-branched fatty acids and their applications in nuclear cardiology. In: Proceedings of the third international symposium on radioiodinated free fatty acids, Kyoto, Japan, 10–11 February, 1993. Ann Nucl Med In press
99. Franken P R, De Geeter F, Dendale P, Block P, Bossuyt A 1993 Regional distribution of 123I-(ortho-iodophenyl)-pentadecanoic acid and 99mTc-MIBI in relation to wall motion after thrombolysis for acute myocardial infarction. Nucl Med Com 14: 310–317
100. Krivokapich J, Barrio J R, Huang S C et al 1990 Dynamic positron tomographic imaging with nitrogen-13 glutamate in patients with coronary artery disease: comparison with nitrogen-13 ammonia and fluorine-18 fluorodeoxyglucose imaging. J Am Coll Cardiol 16: 1158–1167
101. Dewanjee M K, Kahn P C 1976 Mechanisms of localisation of 99m-Tc labelled pyrophosphate and tetracycline in infarcted myocardium. J Nucl Med 17: 639–646
102. Khaw B A, Fallon J T, Strauss H W, Haber E 1980 Myocardial infarct imaging of antibodies to canine cardiac myosin with indium-111-diethylenetriamine pentaacetic acid. Science 209: 295–297
103. Buja L M, Tofe A J, Kulkarni P V et al 1977 Sites and mechanisms of localisation of technetium-99m phosphorus radiopharmaceuticals in acute myocardial infarcts and other tissues. J Clin Invest 60: 724–740
104. Khaw B A, Gold H K, Yasuda T et al 1986 Scintigraphic quantification of myocardial necrosis in patients after intravenous injection of myosin-specific antibody. Circulation 74: 501–508
105. Alavi A, Gupta N, Berget H, Palevsky H, Jatlow A, Kelley M 1988 Detection of venous thrombolysis with In-111 labeled antifibrin (59D8) antibody imaging. J Nucl Med 29: 825
106. Dec G W, Palacios I, Yasuda T et al 1990 Antimyosin antibody cardiac imaging. Its role in the diagnosis of myocarditis. J Am Coll Cardiol 16: 97–104
107. Ballester-Rodes M, Carrio-Gasset I, Abadal-Berini L et al 1988 Patterns of evolution of myocyte damage after human heart transplantation detected by indium-111 monoclonal antimyosin. Am J Cardiol 62: 623–627
108. Schwaiger M, Kalff V, Rosenspire K et al 1990 The noninvasive evaluation of the sympathetic nervous system by PET in the human heart. Circulation 82: 457–464
109. Merlet P, Delforge J, Syrota A et al 1993 Positron emission tomography with 11C CGP-12177 to assess *-adrenergic receptor concentration in idiopathic dilated cardiomyopathy. Circulation 87: 1169–1178
110. Syrota A, Comar D, Paillotin G et al 1985 Muscarinic cholinergic receptor in the human heart evidenced under physiological conditions by positron emission tomography. Proc Nation Acac Sci USA 82: 584–588
111. Spies S M, Meyers S N, Barresi C et al 1977 A case of myocardial abscess evaluated by radionuclide techniques: case report. J Nucl Med 18: 1089–1090
112. Ezekowitz M D 1991 Imaging of intracardiac thrombi in cardiac nuclear medicine. In: Gerson M C, ed. Cardiac nuclear medicine. McGraw Hill, New York, pp 591–602
113. Sinzinger H, Virgolini I 1990 Nuclear medicine and atherosclerosis. Eur J Nucl Med 17: 160–178
114. Hawkins P N, Lavender J P, Myers M J, Pepys M B 1988 Diagnostic radionuclide imaging of amyloidosis: biological targeting by circulating human serum amyloid P component. Lancet 25: 1413–1418

90. Radionuclide ventriculography

S. Walton

INTRODUCTION

In this chapter the techniques of first pass and equilibrium radionuclide ventriculography will be described. Their application to the measurement of ventricular contraction and relaxation and to the evaluation of valvular regurgitation will be discussed. Although the basic physics of imaging and non-imaging detectors, computer systems and radiopharmaceuticals are described elsewhere, they will be considered in so far as there are special implications for radionuclide ventriculography. Also included are brief reviews of the relevance of some of the measurements which can be made. An effort has been made throughout to highlight those areas of particular importance, in which strict observation of correct technique is vital if accurate and reproducible results are to be obtained.

It is possible to image the intracardiac blood pools either during the initial transit through the central circulation of a peripherally injected bolus of a radionuclide, or when a blood pool tracer has reached equilibrium concentration. These two approaches, subsequently referred to as the first pass and equilibrium respectively, have particular advantages and disadvantages. They are not mutually exclusive; it is certainly possible, although not necessarily ideal, to perform a first pass study during the initial injection of a blood pool tracer which is intended for subsequent equilibrium imaging.

INSTRUMENTATION

General comments

There is a direct relationship between, on the one hand, the number of detected scintillations or 'counts' in the image and, on the other, temporal and spatial resolution. The amount of tracer which can be administered is usually limited by dosimetry and so there is also a limitation on the number of scintillations coming from the region of interest within the heart per unit time. With a static organ, it is relatively simple to extend data collection until the acquired image has a satisfactory number of counts, but the heart poses special problems. During a first pass study, data collection is limited to the transit time of the tracer through the chamber of interest – usually only a few cardiac cycles. It is of crucial importance to collect as many counts as possible during this period. Subsequently, during analysis, there is a direct choice between temporal and spatial resolution, as the total number of counts is fixed. For a resting equilibrium study, data collection is limited to that time for which a patient can remain still enough to avoid motion artefact. Count rates from the heart are, however, relatively low and the data are usually divided into a number of images each of which represents a particular portion of the cardiac cycle, thus further diminishing the number of counts available for each image. During stress studies, it may not be reasonable to maintain a particular stage of exercise or other intervention for more than 2–3 min; tomography requires multiple images to be collected in a series of projections around a 180° or 360° degree arc.

Non-imaging probes

The simplest, and by far the least expensive, approach to radionuclide ventriculography entails the use of non-imaging probes. These devices are usually very sensitive, so much so that they can provide data about cardiac contraction[1] and relaxation on a beat by beat basis. This high sensitivity necessitates only small doses of radioactive tracer for each study; either the radiation burden to the patient can be reduced or serial studies can be carried out with radiation dosage equivalent to a single conventional study. Probes respond well to high count rates, and so they are suitable for first pass as well as equilibrium studies. Their disadvantage is, of course, extremely limited spatial resolution. They must be placed over the region of interest (usually the left ventricle, but occasionally the lungs) either by a trial and error method, in which the probe is moved over the praecordium until a characteristic count profile is detected, or using a gamma camera study. They are available either as a free-standing probe which is connected to a mobile unit containing facilities for basic data processing or as miniature devices which can be applied to the chest wall as part of a special vest. The latter can perform prolonged measurements of ejection fraction and ventricular volumes whilst the subject is fully mobile, in a manner analagous to Holter recording of the electrocardiogram.

Imaging detectors

The versatility, intrinsic resolution and wide availability of the standard Anger gamma camera makes it a very popular device for radionuclide ventriculography. However, such investigations can place severe demands on the imaging system, and Anger cameras are not ideal in every application. During first pass studies, for example, count rates may reach 400 000/s. Many of the older cameras respond to increasing count rate in a linear manner only up to about 40 000/s, although it is claimed that the latest generation of single crystal cameras can handle higher count rates more reliably. At equilibrium, count rates are much lower and much more suitable for single crystal cameras.

More recently, the gas-filled, wire chamber detector has become available. This device does not depend on a sodium iodide crystal for scintillation detection and both high count rate capacity and high spatial resolution are claimed. Unfortunately, it requires ^{178}Ta, a radionuclide with a short half-life which is produced by a special generator.

RADIOPHARMACEUTICALS

The chief requirement is that the tracer should remain within the vascular compartment during data collection.

For a first pass study, this requirement is far less prohibitive than for an equilibrium study; almost any radioactive tracer will remain intravascular during the initial transit and other considerations become paramount. First amongst these is that the radionuclide should have decay characteristics which are suitable for the imaging device to be employed. For both single and multicrystal gamma cameras, ^{99m}Tc is widely available and its imaging characteristics are almost ideal, but for the gas-filled wire chamber detector ^{178}Ta is required.[2] Another important factor in first pass studies is the half-life of the radiopharmaceutical. Serial studies should, ideally, be performed with a short-lived tracer, both to lessen total radiation burden and also to prevent the progressive build up of background activity with successive injections. ^{178}Ta has already been mentioned. ^{81m}Kr (half-life 13 s),[3] ^{195m}Au (30.5 s)[4] and ^{191m}Ir (4.9 s)[5] are all suitable for imaging by conventional gamma cameras and are obtainable as portable generators.

Blood pool labelling

For equilibrium studies, a tracer is required which remains within the vascular compartment at relatively stable concentration during data collection. In intervention studies, this may mean imaging over a period of several hours. Although there are a variety of tracers which would fulfill this requirement, ^{99m}Tc labelling of erythrocytes is almost universally employed.[6–9]

In vitro labelling of erythrocytes requires a 10–15 ml sample of blood. A small dose of stannous ion is then added as a reducing agent and the blood is incubated with ^{99m}Tc pertechnetate in the laboratory. The principle behind this technique is that technetium, in its normal oxidized form, diffuses freely into and out from red blood cells, eventually reaching an equilibrium concentration across the cell membrane. In its reduced form, it binds tightly to the beta chain of haemoglobin, resulting in effective labelling of the red blood cells. An excellent labelling efficiency (98%) can be acheived by this technique. The red blood cells are then reinjected for subsequent imaging.

A similar result can be achieved in vivo. In this approach, ^{99m}Tc is injected i.v. 10–15 min after stannous pyrophosphate. Sufficient stannous ion must be administered to reduce all the ^{99m}Tc, otherwise background levels will be raised by free ^{99m}Tc, but too much will reduce some of the ^{99m}Tc before it can enter the erythrocyte. This results in a reduced efficiency of labelling (80–90%) compared to the in vitro method, but the whole procedure is simpler, requiring merely two intravenous injections a few minutes apart. Labelling is at its least reliable using the in vivo method in very ill patients; certain drugs can also interfere with the efficiency of labelling.

A somewhat improved labelling efficiency (90–93%) is claimed for the modified in vivo method in which stannous pyrophosphate is administered to the patient as in the in vivo method. A small sample of blood is withdrawn from the patient into a shielded syringe containing Tc. The red cells are then incubated within the syringe but outside the body for approximately 10 min. Heparin is one of the drugs that will interfere with erythrocyte labelling (v.i.), yet some anticoagulation is required. A small amount of acid–citrate–dextrose solution can be employed for this purpose.

DATA ACQUISITION AND STORAGE

The data from radionuclide ventriculography can be collected and stored in either list mode or frame mode.

List mode acquisition

In list mode acquisition the *x* and *y* coordinates of each scintillation are stored, along with ECG R wave and time markers as sequential words in the computer memory.

This approach provides for maximum flexibility in subsequent data processing. The exact relationship of each scintillation to particular time and R wave markers is known and the data can consequently be framed at any desired rate. If irregularity of the heart rate results in significant variability of R–R interval, then data from those cycles with an unacceptibly short or long R–R interval can be excluded before data analysis begins. List mode acquisition is particularly popular for first pass studies, but it is less widely used for equilibrium studies when the amount of data to be stored is much greater.

Frame mode acquisition

A frame is a portion of computer memory which corresponds to a number of display elements. In turn, these represent the field of view of the gamma camera. In frame mode acquisition, the x and y coordinates of each scintillation define a particular display element within the frame and for each scintillation at a particular location the word in the computer memory corresponding to that display element is incremented by one. After a certain preset time interval each frame is stored and collection into a new frame commences. The sequence of frames does contain temporal information, although the exact relationship of each scintillation to time and ECG R wave markers, which is a feature of list mode acquisition, is lost. Frame mode can be used for first pass studies, when framing durations of 50 ms or less are often necessary, but it is more typically applied, in a somewhat modified form described below, to equilibrium studies.

Electrocardiographic triggering

In a standard equilibrium study, continuous ECG monitoring allows each R wave to be detected. For each R wave, a pulse is produced which triggers data acquisition in frame mode. It is particularly important, if data collection is to commence at the very onset of systole, that this process is completed very rapidly. Problems occur, occasionally, when the R wave morphology is unusual, as in left bundle branch block for example. Each R–R interval is divided into a preset number of time slices, typically 16, 24, 32 or 64. The R wave pulse triggers data acquisition into a frame corresponding to the first of these time slices. At the end of each time slice, data collection is switched to a frame corresponding to the next time slice. A new R wave pulse will restart the cycle with data collection into the first frame of the series. In this way, data can be summed from a number of cardiac cycles – several hundred for the average equilibrium study – to produce a series of images which represents a single, average cycle. Such a series is referred to as a representative cine cycle.

This method of data collection assumes that all cardiac cycles from which data are collected are of identical length. Problems arise when the R–R interval varies.[10–12] If the R–R interval of a particular beat is short, then the data acquisition into the later frames of the cine cycle will be cut short by the subsequent R wave pulse; if it is too long, then the series of time slices will terminate before the next R wave pulse starts the sequence again and data will be discarded. As heart rate varies, the duration of systole is relatively constant; a change in heart rate being brought about largely by a change in the length of diastole. Furthermore, except at high heart rates, systole is confined to the early part of the cardiac cycle. Thus, a slight variation in R–R interval will affect, predominantly, the latter part of diastole; systolic measurements should be reliable. Techniques are available to correct for the effect of occasional extrasystoles and sinus arrhythmia. However, when the heart rhythm is grossly irregular, as in atrial fibrillation or when extrasystoles are multiple and frequent, this approach is questionable. For diastolic measurements, it is possible to record a study in list mode and to analyse the data in such a way that the early, systolic part of the curve is produced by gating forward from the R wave in the usual way, but the diastolic portion of the curve is produced by gating backwards from the R wave.

Projections

First pass studies are usually performed in the right anterior oblique projection, a view which is normally parallel to the long axis of the left ventricle. The right ventricle overlies the left but, with a good bolus, there is temporal separation between right and left heart phases of bolus transit. High count rates, progressively increasing background levels with sequential injections and relatively poor spatial resolution have limited the popularity of this approach, but there is no doubt that with a multicrystal camera, gas-filled wire chamber detector or a modern single-crystal camera, particularly if short-lived tracers are employed, this is a very powerful tool. Measurements of left ventricular contraction can be made in any projection with an excellent temporal resolution, low background activity and a low radiation dose to the patient.

Correct injection technique is very important for an accurate first pass study. The bolus of tracer must be as compact as possible. When the left ventricle is the object of the investigation, various factors cannot be controlled; even a compact bolus will be spread out by the time that it passes through a dilated right heart, a regurgitant tricuspid or pulmonary valve or congested lungs. However, unless the bolus is compact to start with, there is no chance at all of it arriving compact. It is best to have a bolus small in volume, but with a high specific activity, say 740 MBq ^{99m}Tc pertechnetate in 0.1 ml. This bolus should be loaded into a cannula, itself inserted into a large, medial vein in the right antecubital fossa, and flushed in as quickly as possible using a bolus of saline. The right arm should be abducted at the shoulder, to allow direct access to the superior vena cava.

Equilibrium studies are usually performed in a modified left anterior oblique projection, because of the necessity to obtain spatial separation between right and left ventricles. The exact projection is chosen which provides optimal visualization of the interventricular septum. Cranio-caudal tilt will then separate the left ventricle from the left atrium in most cases. The right atrium cannot be separated from the right ventricle quite so easily and difficulties may be experienced with continuing left atrial overlap in those subjects with left atrial enlargement. The left ventricle is considerably foreshortened along its long axis in the left anterior oblique projection. Due to absorption of radiation from deeper, inferior regions of the ventricle by more superficial regions, inferior wall motion abnormalities may be poorly represented in a standard, left anterior oblique study. For this reason, many centres routinely perform imaging in a second projection, either a steep left anterior oblique, an anterior or a left posterior oblique view.[13,14] None achieves the necessary spatial differentiation of left and right ventricles, but they do provide a glimpse of the inferior wall which may be sufficient to detect an inferior abnormality. Background levels are high at equilibrium compared to first pass studies (approximately 60% *vs.* 30%). Nevertheless, equilibrium studies are very popular. Count rates are relatively low, bringing them easily within the scope of a standard Anger camera; data collection can usually be extended until sufficient counts have been collected for satisfactory statistical accuracy; and multiple measurements can be made after a single injection of tracer.

Tomographic acquisition

Blood pool tomography imposes special difficulties. If the heart were merely a static organ there would still be problems associated with its size and its situation (eccentric within a medium of variable thickness and absorptive properties). Add to this the requirement for the several images of a representative cine cycle at multiple positions around the imaging arc and it is easy to appreciate why blood pool tomography is not widely employed.

Most tomographic studies are carried out by using a rotating gamma camera, an approach which provides for excellent spatial resolution. However, a high degree of mechanical stability is also necessary. With the introduction of multi-headed gamma camera systems, this seems to be the way in which blood pool tomography will develop. However, there are advantages to the alternative, which is to employ a series of static detectors arranged around the patient. Data collection and manipulation can be markedly simplified.

With a rotating gamma camera, it is usual to employ a 180° rotation, with imaging between right anterior oblique and left posterior oblique projections, although some centres use 360°. A compromise is necessary between imaging time, temporal resolution and the number of counts in each image. Data collection can be shortened by using the multidetector arrays and multi-headed cameras. Such devices theoretically allow attenuation correction, by the simultaneous performance of transmission and emission imaging.

DATA ANALYSIS AND DISPLAY

Before data analysis commences some preliminary assessment is required of the reliability of the recorded data. For a first pass study, this will involve a measure of bolus quality.[15] For equilibrium studies a histogram of R–R intervals and some information about which beats were actually accepted are essential steps. It may be necessary to modify the data in some way, for example to correct for slight variations in R–R interval, before processing continues. One popular approach assumes that the total counts from the field of view from each image in the representative cine cycle is constant, and corrects the data accordingly. Other, more complex algorithms are also available.

First pass radionuclide ventriculography

A useful starting point for the analysis of a first pass study is the reconstruction of a series of images representing bolus transit throughout the central circulation. This will provide basic data about the timing of right and left heart phases of bolus transit, and a preliminary assessment of chamber size and shape. Regions of interest can then be defined, for which curves of activity against time can be plotted (Figs 90.1–90.3). At low temporal resolution, say 1 s, these curves can be used to define transit times, to quantify intracardiac shunts and to measure flow. At high

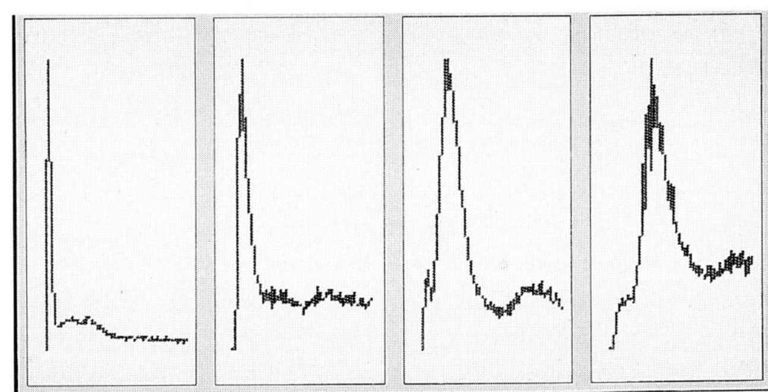

Fig. 90.1 First pass radionuclide angiocardiography. Activity time curves from a normal subject. (A) Superior vena cava. (B) Right ventricle. (C) Lung. (D) Left ventricle. Note the shape of the SVC curve, which reflects a compact bolus injection, and the progressive spread of the distribution as the bolus passes through the central circulation. (Reproduced with permission from *Nuclear Cardiology*.)

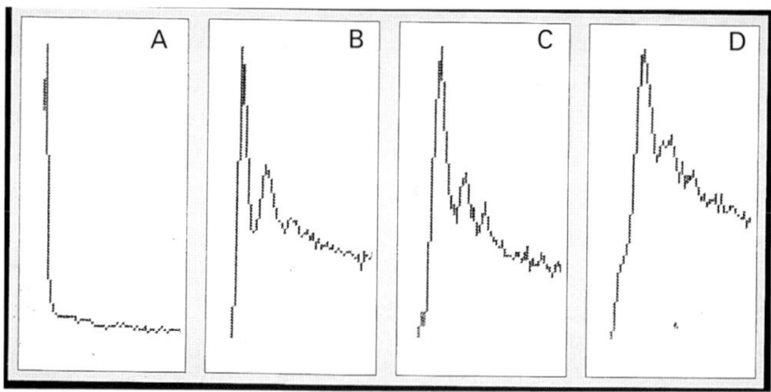

Fig. 90.2 First pass radionuclide angiocardiography. Activity time curves from a subject with a left-to-right shunt at ventricular level (A) Superior vena cava. (B) Right ventricle. (C) Lung. (D) Left ventricle. Note the good bolus injection and the effect of recirculation on all curves downstream from the site of the shunt. (Reproduced with permission from *Nuclear Cardiology*.)

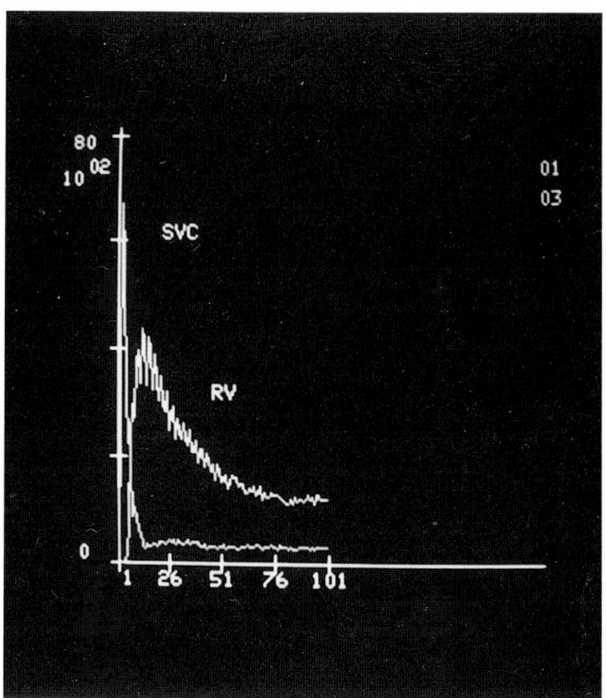

Fig. 90.3 First pass radionuclide angiocardiography. Activity time curves from a subject with tricuspid regurgitation. Top = Right ventricle. Bottom = Superior vena cava. After a satisfactory bolus injection, the effect of the tricuspid regurgitation is to spread out the bolus. (Also shown in colour on Plate 23.)

temporal resolution, curves from ventricular regions of interest will be seen to be composed of two components, the low frequency component which reflects bolus transit and superimposed high frequency fluctuations corresponding to the variations of activity within the ventricle during individual cardiac cycles. These fluctuations can themselves be used to identify those cycles – so-called 'intrinsic' gating. Data from several cardiac cycles can then be summed to produce a representative cine cycle. Rather more reliable, however, when data have been recorded in list mode is 'extrinsic' gating, whereby individual cardiac cycles are identified by the R wave markers stored within the list mode data. Once a representative cine cycle has been produced it can be analysed for ejection fraction and regional wall motion as described below for the equilibrium study.

Intracardiac shunting may be apparent on the original series of images which represent bolus transit. In tricuspid atresia, for example, the bolus will be seen to pass from right to left atrium without entering the right ventricle. If there is a left to right shunt then recirculation through the lungs of tracer which has returned to the right heart via the shunt will be apparent as a secondary deflection on the downslope of the pulmonary activity–time curve. Various mathematical techniques exist which use these curves to obtain an estimate of systemic to pulmonary flow and, hence, the magnitude of the shunt.[16–21] In general, they use the relative heights or areas of the initial and recirculation deflections to calculate the inital flow and that due to recirculation through the shunt. These two measurements can be used to arrive at the pulmonary-to-systemic flow ratio. Data recording is simple; indeed, a non-imaging probe is able to provide an excellent pulmonary activity–time curve from a relatively small dose of radionuclide. However, a good, compact bolus is essential and great care must be taken with curve fitting during subsequent analysis.

Cardiac output can be calculated by a modification of the Stewart–Hamilton formula. As generally applied to any indicator dilution curve, this states that cardiac output is given by

$$\text{Cardiac output} = \frac{\text{Total amount of indicator injected}}{\text{Area beneath the concentration time curve}}$$

In its application to first pass radionuclide ventriculography, which furnishes activity–time curves and not concentration–time curves, the formula becomes

$$\text{Cardiac output} = \frac{\text{Total blood volume} \times \text{counts at equilibrium}}{\text{Area beneath the activity time curve}}$$

In order to obtain activity at equilibrium, a tracer which remains within the vascular compartment must be used.

Equilibrium radionuclide ventriculography

Preliminary inspection of the representative cine cycle provides a qualitative analysis of chamber size and volume. If the images are displayed sequentially in real time it is possible to make a subjective analysis of cardiac contraction.

For quantitative analysis it is usual to employ both temporal and spatial smoothing of the images at this stage[22,23] and then to correct for background activity. This comprises radiation which arises from tracer present in tissues above, below and around the heart, and a variety of techniques has been employed to correct for it.[24,25] Their number and variety is testimony to the fact that none is ideal. In general, most methods attempt to sample background activity around the heart and to assume that that behind the heart is identical. Cardiac background activity is heterogeneous, however, and choice of sampling region can be crucial. Other algorithms look at the variation of activity around the heart in both x and y axes and from this variation they extrapolate behind the heart. Some techniques assume a constant background throughout the cardiac cycle, whereas others calculate different backgrounds at both end systole and end diastole.

At equilibrium, tracer is, by definition, uniformly mixed with blood. After background correction, therefore, activity should be proportional to chamber volume. Regions of interest can be assigned to both ventricles but if the end-diastolic image alone is used for this it can be difficult to identify the exact limits of the ventricular chambers.[26-28] More accurate and reproducible results are achieved if the regions are defined simultaneously on several images which include, in addition to the end-diastolic image, one or more of the various functional, or parametric, images described below (Fig. 90.4). Once the ventricular regions of interest are defined, a plot of activity for each frame of the representative cine cycle results in ventricular volume curves. These curves are expressed in counts, although correction to absolute volumes is possible. Ejection fraction is a relative measurement and so, if measurement of this parameter is the sole purpose of the study, such conversion, which may itself introduce artefact, is not necessary. Similarly, in serial studies, it may be sufficient to detect a percentage change in end-diastolic, end-systolic or stroke volumes. If absolute volumes are necessary, then a blood sample must be taken and the activity per unit volume measured. The depth of the heart from the anterior chest wall is then measured from an image at right angles to the original study and the activity per unit volume corrected for attenuation by assuming an average absorption per unit thickness of tissue.[29-31]

Analysis of the ventricular volume curve

Ejection fraction, the percentage of ventricular contents ejected with each beat, is by no means ideal as an index of ventricular contraction. In common with other such measurements made during contraction, it is a function of the loading conditions of the ventricle. 'Load' includes ventricular volume, shape, pressure and wall thickness. There are, therefore, two issues: First, how accurately and reproducibly can the measurement be made; second, what is the correct interpretation of the measurement once made? Here we will be concerned chiefly with the former; with regard to the latter, suffice it to say that ejection fraction is widely used as an index of ventricular contraction and prognosis.

From the background corrected ventricular activity time curve, ejection fraction is simply calculated as

$$\text{Ejection fraction} = \frac{\text{End-diastolic counts} - \text{End systolic counts}}{\text{End-diastolic counts}}$$

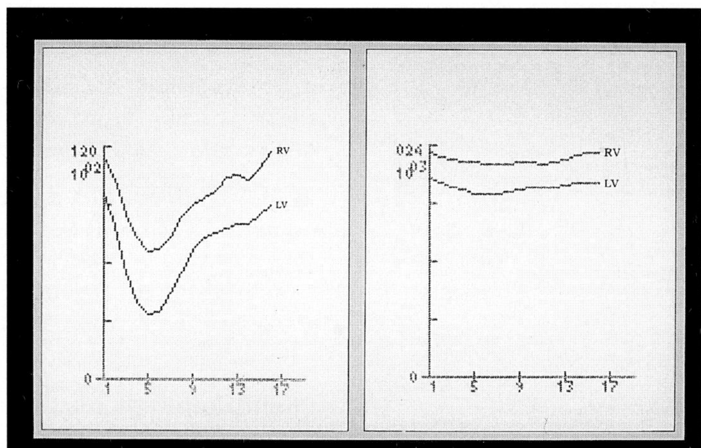

Fig. 90.4 Equilibrium radionuclide angiocardiography. Ventricular volume curves from a normal subject (left) and a subject with dilated cardiomyopathy (right). RV = right ventricle; LV = left ventricle. In both subjects, the end-diastolic counts of the right and left ventricles are similar, suggesting similar volumes. Ejection fraction is easily calculated from such background corrected curves as the percentage of ventricular contents ejected with each beat. The ratio of right-to-left ventricular stroke counts reflects the ratio of right-to-left ventricular stroke volume. It can be used to detect valvular regurgitation. (Reproduced with permission from *Nuclear Cardiology*.)

When ejection fraction is measured at cardiac catheterization it is necessary to assume that the ventricle conforms to a particular geometric shape. Theoretically a nuclear, counts-based approach should be independent of ventricular shape. To a certain extent this is true but, because of the foreshortening of the left ventricle in the left anterior oblique projection there is considerable absorption of radiation from the inferior left ventricular surface by the more superficial regions of the ventricle.[32] Thus, the ejection fraction calculation will tend to be unduly influenced by events occurring near the anterior wall. In inferior infarction, the ejection fraction may be normal or only slightly depressed; conversely, in the presence of a large, anterior, left ventricular aneurysm the contractile segment of the ventricle may be obscured and ejection fraction may be underestimated.

Accurate background correction is crucial to ejection fraction estimation. There is no ideal method for background correction; each manufacturer favours a different approach. Largely because of this, there is little agreement between centres about the limits of the normal range, and differences exist within centres when different items of equipment are employed. Background levels are relatively high during equilibrium studies; measured ejection fractions from such studies tend to be somewhat lower than those measured at cardiac catheterization. A combination of these two factors – lower than expected values and considerable variation from centre to centre – poses significant problems for the technique. Each centre must, at the very least, establish its own normal range for comparison of experimental and clinical results. Background levels are lower in first pass studies and ejection fractions do tend to be rather higher than those measured at equilibrium.

Whichever approach is used, and despite doubts about absolute accuracy, the reproducibility of ejection fraction measurement is excellent, at least in the short term, making this a most appealing approach for serial measurement of left ventricular contraction in intervention studies.

Measurement of right ventricular ejection fraction is problematical. At equilibrium[33,34] in the left anterior oblique projection, there is considerable overlap between right atrium and right ventricle, an overlap which cannot be totally corrected by cranio-caudal angulation. Thus, the right ventricular volume curve always contains a contribution from the right atrial volume curve, resulting in a reduction of measured ejection fraction. Techniques are available to select background regions which contain significant amounts of right atrium, but such corrections are only partially successful. During a first pass, right heart study,[35–38] background levels are extremely low and the right ventricle can be imaged in the right anterior oblique projection. However, bolus transit through the right ventricle is very rapid, allowing only two or three cardiac cycles for data collection, count rates are very high and there are theoretical doubts about adequate mixing in the right heart.

Valvular regurgitation and the left-to-right stroke volume ratio (L/RSV)

Although there may be small variations from beat to beat, over the period of time necessary for data collection during an equilibrium study the outputs of the right and left ventricles must be equal. Heart rate is the same for both ventricles and, as output is the product of rate and stroke volume, stroke counts should also be equal. This is not to say that the volumes and ejection fractions of the ventricles are necessarily the same; it is possible to have a particular stroke output with either a large volume and small ejection fraction or with a small volume and large ejection fraction. This concordance between stroke volumes is the basis for a technique which is designed to assess the severity of valvular regurgitation.[39–42] The measurement L/RSV is simply taken as the ratio of the stroke counts from the volume curves of the left and right ventricles. In normals, the ratio should theoretically be unity, although in practice underestimation of right ventricular stroke volume (v.s.) leads to values up to 1.7. Left sided valvular regurgitation, be it mitral or aortic, results in an increase in the ratio; pulmonary or tricuspid regurgitation will result in a ratio < 1. Considerable caution must be taken if there is regurgitation on both sides of the heart. A combination of severe right- and left-sided regurgitation may result in a normal value if the regurgitation is of equal severity.

L/RSV can be used both to detect and to quantify the severity of the regurgitation; as with most techniques, it is more reliable in the former than the latter.

Diastolic measurements

Diastole consists of several phases which include isovolumic relaxation, a period of rapid ventricular filling and a period of somewhat slower filling which in its latter stages is augmented by atrial contraction in those patients who are in sinus rhythm. If these stages are to be recognized on a ventricular volume curve and measurements to be made during them, then considerable attention to data collection and analysis is essential.[43–45]

First, temporal resolution must be adequate,[46] probably of the order of 40 ms. Second, great care must be taken in construction of the diastolic portion of the curve, as artefact can easily be introduced by R–R interval variation.

The intention is an analysis of ventricular relaxation and compliance. Unfortunately, those measurements which can be made from the ventricular volume curve bear only a partial relationship to these variables. As with ejection, filling is markedly affected by loading conditions. Any variation in filling rates or times may equally well reflect changes in ventricular size, shape, filling pressure and wall thickness. Considerable caution is necessary in interpretation of the results which can be obtained.

Assessment of regional ventricular contraction patterns

Some subjective appreciation of regional wall motion can be obtained by observing the images of the representative cine cycle played in order in real time. This sequence can be replayed over and over if necessary and this approach is a reasonable starting point in any evaluation of regional contraction patterns. However, spatial resolution is not one of the strengths of radionuclide ventriculography and when attempts are made by an objective technique to quantify wall motion, which is of the order of 1 cm or less, problems arise.

A variety of methods have been tried for edge definition.[47] Isocount contours have the advantage of simplicity. More sophisticated operations, such as the use of the second derivative of the counts profile, have also been advocated but none work reliably in all ventricles. To a large extent, wall motion measurements have been superseded by the functional images described below.

Functional (or parametric) imaging of the heart

So far, we have considered images which represent the actual distribution of radioactive tracer and have used a series of such images to describe variations of that tracer distribution with time. It is also possible to produce images which represent the distribution not of a tracer but of a particular functional variable.[48–51]

The simplest functional image to produce is the stroke volume image. This is produced by the subtraction of the end–systolic image of the representative cine cycle from the end–diastolic image. In effect for each pixel, end–systolic counts are being subtracted from end–diastolic counts. The resulting image will reflect regional stroke volume: those pixels in regions with good contraction showing high values of stroke counts and those from regions with poor contraction low stroke counts. All regions with no apparent contraction as well as those with negative stroke counts (atria, for example, will have higher counts at end systole than at end-diastole) are set to zero. Subtraction of the end–diastolic image from end–systolic – the so-called paradox image–highlights regions such as atria, great vessels and ventricular aneurysms, with higher counts at end-systole than end-diastole.

Dividing the stroke volume image by the end-diastolic image results in the regional ejection fraction image.[52,53]

The major problem with the stroke volume, paradox and regional ejection fraction images is that they all require an end-diastolic and an end-systolic frame to be identified. End-diastole is defined by the R wave, but end-systole is rather more difficult to identify. In the presence of impaired contraction, different parts of the ventricle may even reach maximum contraction at different times and no one image can describe end-systole satisfactorily. Thus, on the stroke volume and regional ejection fraction images it is possible for a region with delayed contraction (tardokinesis) to appear akinetic, even if the eventual extent of contraction is normal.

A more sophisticated approach involves mathematical manipulation of activity–time curves from individual pixels. The ventricular volume curve is a background-corrected plot of activity against time for all pixels within a selected ventricular region of interest. Each of those pixels, indeed all pixels in the image, will have an activity–time curve of its own which is produced by plotting the activity for that individual pixel for each frame of the representative cine cycle. Fourier analysis is a mathematical operation which can be used to characterize any periodic function as combination of sine and cosine waves of different frequencies. Each of these frequencies is characterized by a particular amplitude and phase. Fourier analysis can be applied to the activity–time curves of individual pixels. The activity–time curve for each pixel is analysed and the phase and amplitude of the Fourier transform of the fundamental frequency is determined. These values are then used to produce a phase and an amplitude image (Figs 90.5–90.11). The fundamental frequency of the variation is the heart rate. Of course, these curves are far more complex than a single sine or cosine wave, but the addition of extra harmonics to achieve a more lifelike curve does not seem to produce much more in the way of useful clinical information. In general, a 15% cut-off is used on the amplitude image to

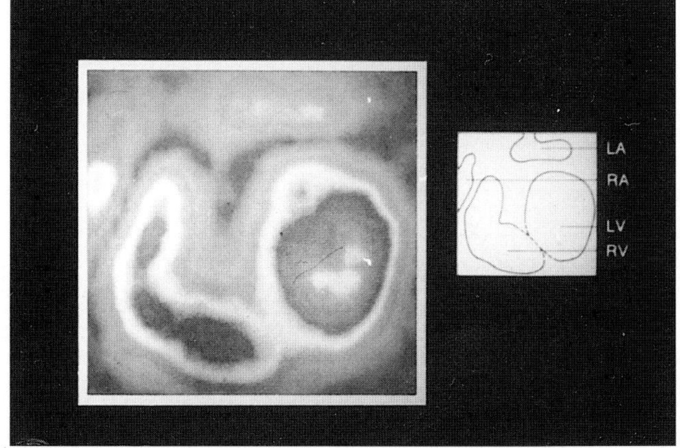

Fig. 90.5 Equilibrium radionuclide angiocardiography. Amplitude image; normal subject. Each pixel is colour coded according to the Fourier amplitude of its time activity curve. Ventricular regions with good contraction manifest high values of amplitude and are shown in red. In this example, there are high values of amplitude across both left and right ventricles. (Also shown in colour on Plate 23.) (Reproduced with permission from *Nuclear Cardiology*.)

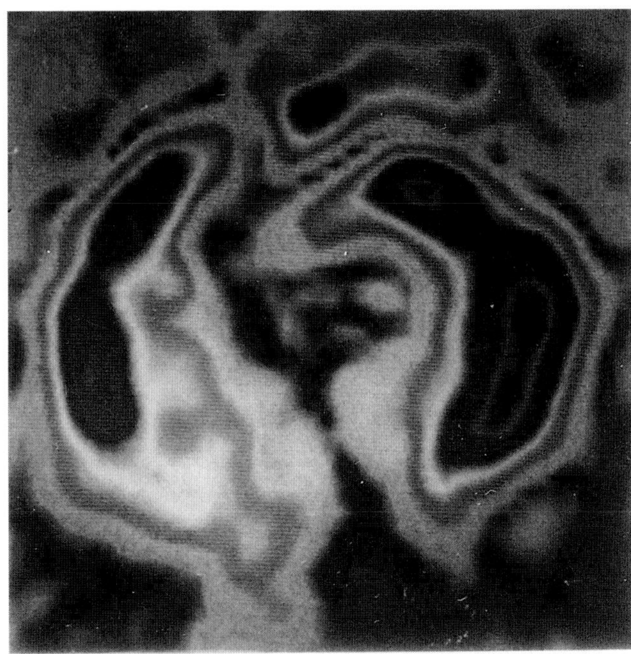

Fig. 90.6 Equilibrium radionuclide angiocardiography. Amplitude image; septal infarction. High values of amplitude are apparent in the lateral region of the left ventricle and throughout the right ventricle. The interventricular septal and apical regions of the left ventricle have very low values of amplitude, suggesting akinesis. (Also shown in colour on Plate 23.)

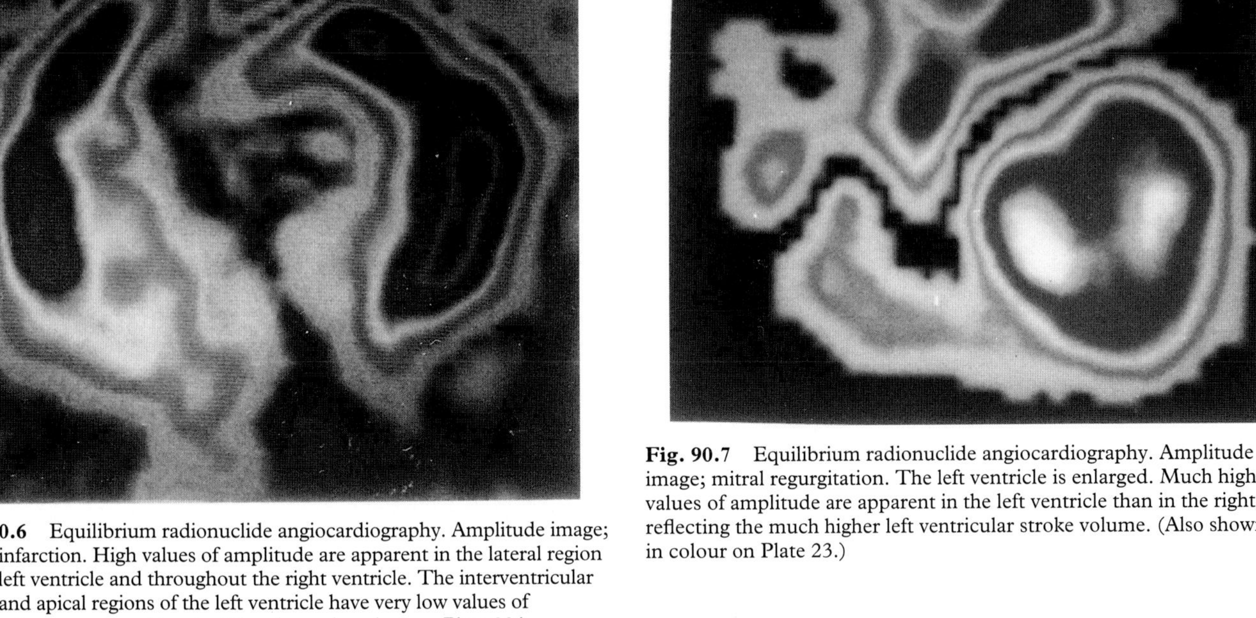

Fig. 90.7 Equilibrium radionuclide angiocardiography. Amplitude image; mitral regurgitation. The left ventricle is enlarged. Much higher values of amplitude are apparent in the left ventricle than in the right, reflecting the much higher left ventricular stroke volume. (Also shown in colour on Plate 23.)

Fig. 90.8 Equilibrium radionuclide angiocardiography. Phase image; normal subject. Each pixel is colour coded according to the Fourier phase of its time activity curve. Regions, such as normal ventricles, which empty relatively early in the cardiac cycle have low phase values and are coloured blue or green; regions, such as atria and great vessels, which empty relatively late during the cardiac cycle are coloured red. (Also shown in colour on Plate 24.)

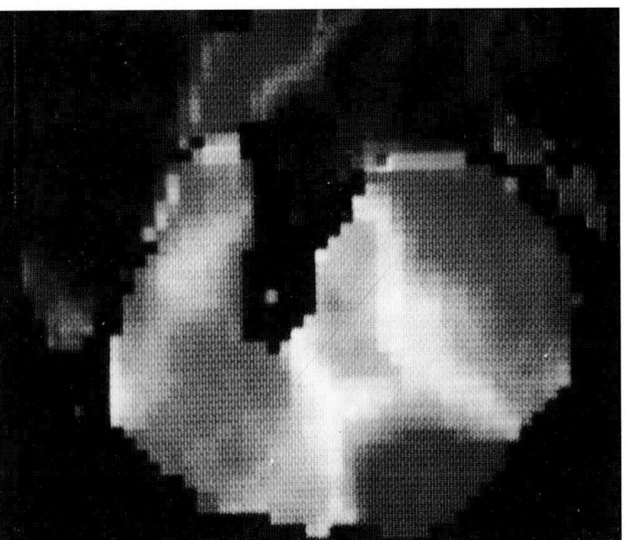

Fig. 90.9 Equilibrium radionuclide angiocardiography. Phase image; septal infarction and apical aneurysm. Intermediate (yellow) and high (red) phase values are seen within the left ventricle. The high values at the left ventricular apex reflect paradoxical emptying typical of an aneurysm. In such cases, it is possible to calculate an ejection fraction from that portion of the ventricle which contracts normally as well as the left ventricle as a whole. In this case the left ventricular ejection fraction was 19% and that of the contractile segment 36%. After removal of the aneurysm, left ventricular ejection fraction was 33%. (Also shown in colour on Plate 24.)

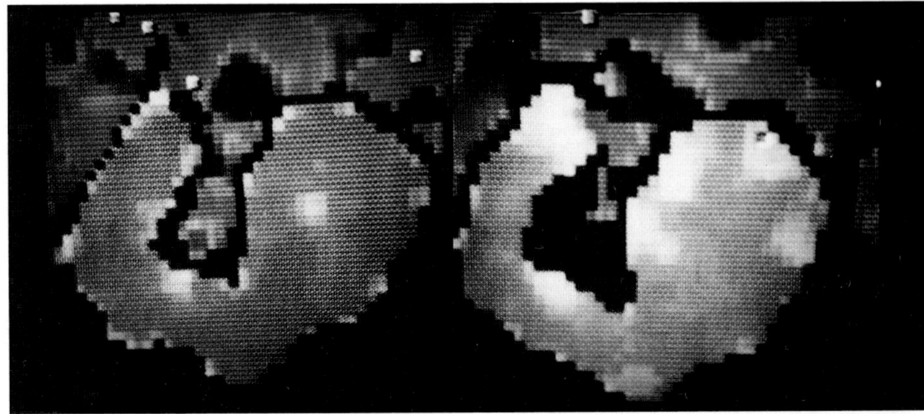

Fig. 90.10 Equilibrium radionuclide angiocardiography. Phase image; pre-excitation. Phase images are shown from the same subject with Wolff-Parkinson-White syndrome during normally conducted sinus rhythm (left) and pre-excitation (right). When the by-pass is conducting, two areas of very early activation of the left ventricle (light blue) can be seen high on the lateral wall. (Also shown in colour on Plate 24.)

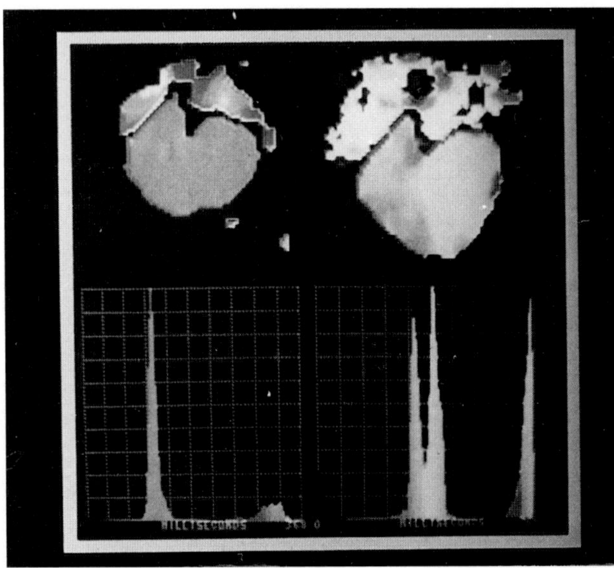

Fig. 90.11 Equilibrium radionuclide angiocardiography. Phase image; quantitative analysis. Phase images (top) are shown from a normal subject (left) and from one with left bundle branch block (right). Below each phase image is a histogram of phase values from that image. In the normal subject there is a narrow peak at low values of phase, reflecting uniform, early emptying of both ventricles. A minor peak of high values reflects atrial emptying. In left bundle branch block, intermediate values of phase are apparent throughout the left ventricle, reflecting delayed emptying. On the histogram, there are two peaks within the low phase values, the lowest corresponding to right and the higher to left ventricular phase values. Once again, high phase values corresponding to atrial emptying are easily distinguished. Such histograms can be used to analyse the distribution of phase values within a particular ventricle. (Also shown in colour on Plate 25.) (Reproduced with permission from *Nuclear Cardiology*.)

mask the phase image, i.e. pixels with an amplitude of <15% are assumed to have no phase.

The phase image provides information about the timing of contraction.[54,55] Ventricular regions with normal contraction have relatively low values of phase. Atria and great vessels fill and empty paradoxically to the ventricles, and they have high values of phase. In patients with abnormalities of wall motion, delayed contraction leads to intermediate values of phase, akinesis to absent phase and paradoxical expansion to high values of phase within the ventricles themselves. The sensitivity of the technique can be illustrated by the demonstration of differences between the ventricles in bundle branch block and abnormal patterns of phase within a particular ventricle when there is hemiblock or when a pacemaker is present.[56] In pre-excitation it is possible to demonstrate early emptying in the region of insertion of the bypass into the ventricles, as these regions manifest low values of phase. In ventricular tachycardia, one can detect the site of origin of the tachycardia as the site of lowest phase values and to compare this location to that of any wall motion abnormalities which may be present. One word of warning is appropriate, however. If regions with different phase overlap, then the phase value calculated will be a composite value from the two regions, weighted by various factors. Thus, with an inferior infarction, it is often found that normal phase values are found throughout the left ventricle, because of the overwhelming contribution from overlying, normally contracting myocardium.

The amplitude image provides information about the extent of contraction. In normal ventricles, there are high values of amplitude across both ventricles. Hypokinesis results in reduced and akinesis in absent amplitude. Conversely, valvular regurgitation increases amplitude values in the ventricle which is primarily affected by the regurgitant valve.[57] The information provided by the amplitude image is similar to that obtained from the stroke volume and regional ejection fraction image, except that it is independent of the timing of end-systole.

Phase and amplitude images provide an excellent description of ventricular contraction, in terms of both its timing and its extent, in a form which is readily understandable and easily filed in the hospital notes. Further analysis is also possible. A histogram of phase values[58,59] can be used to describe the heterogeneity of contraction within a ventricle.

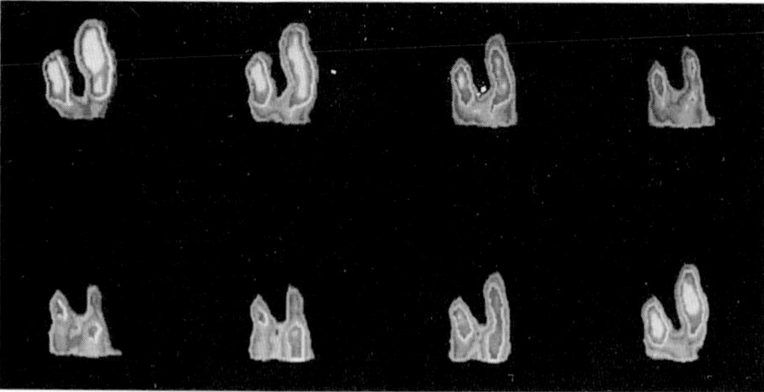

Fig. 90.12 Gated blood pool tomography. Reconstructed tomogram in the horizontal long axis view; normal subject. In each of the 8 views shown, the projection is the same. The series of images starts at end-diastole and represents a single cardiac cycle. The left ventricle lies on the left and it is separated from the right by a space which corresponds to the interventricular septum. Emptying of both ventricles is normal. (Also shown in colour on Plate 25.)

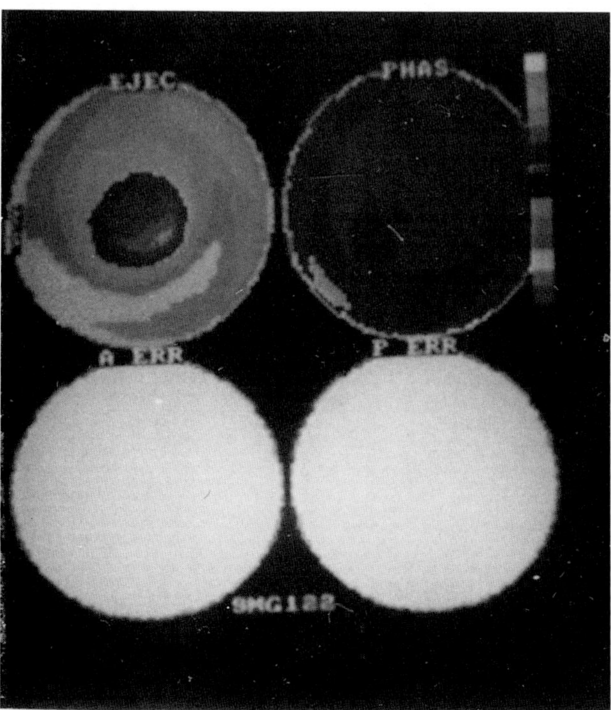

Fig. 90.13 Gated blood pool tomography. 'Bull's eye' display of wall motion; normal subject. In the 'Bull's eye' display, the left ventricle is represented as if its apex were at the centre of the display and as if its base were around the periphery. The upper portion of each display represents the anterior wall, the left portion the interventricular septum, the right portion the lateral wall and the lower portion the inferior wall. Here, Fourier amplitude and phase have been used to describe wall motion. The top left image shows the distribution of amplitude values, maximal at the apex (red), and the top right phase values. Below, these amplitude and phase values have been compared to the normal range; the uniform blue colour confirms that all values of amplitude and phase are normal. (Also shown in colour on Plate 26.)

Blood pool tomography

Many of the problems associated with planar studies, such as background correction and attenuation artefacts, could, theoretically, be overcome by tomographic imaging. However, relatively few centres perform this technique routinely. Two major reasons for this relative unpopularity are the length of time required to generate sufficient projections for the tomograms and the enormous quantity of data which needs to be condensed into a suitable display format.

Once the basic data are collected, images of slices through the heart in the transverse plane can be produced (Figs 90.12–90.16). Subsequent reconstruction enables multiple slices to be taken through the blood pools both parallel and at right angles to the long axis of the left ventricle. Ejection fraction measurement is made from estimates of end-diastolic and end-systolic volumes.[60] Wall motion[61–64] can be observed from the end-diastolic and end-systolic outlines or from the 'beating' 3-D image and, with sufficiently sophisticated data processing, this process can be observed as the 3-D image is rotated through to any projection. Finally, phase and amplitude values can be calculated for each portion of the ventricles and displayed either as 'target' or 'bull's-eye' polar maps or as colours on the 3-D, blood pool image.[64]

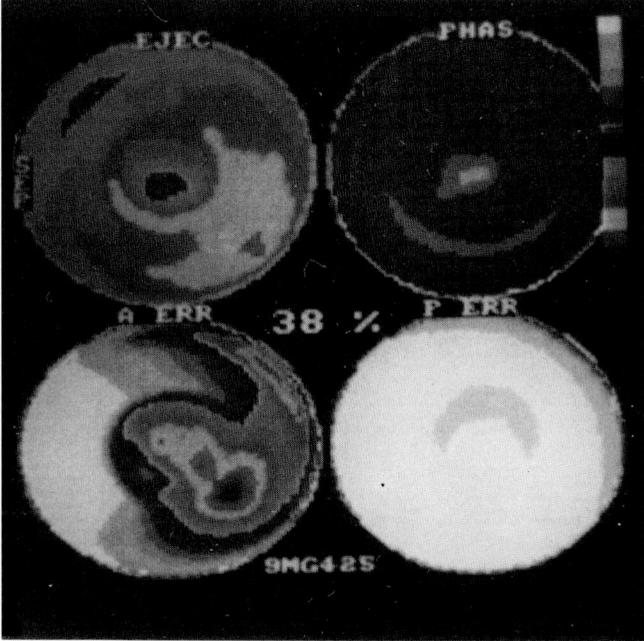

Fig. 90.14 Gated blood pool tomography. 'Bull's eye' display of wall motion; inferolateral infarction. The format is the same as that of Fig. 90.13. There is some heterogeneity of amplitude values in particular. Comparison with the normal range shows abnormal amplitude, corresponding to akinesis, in the inferolateral region of the left ventricle. In this case, phase values are relatively normal. (Also shown in colour on Plate 26.)

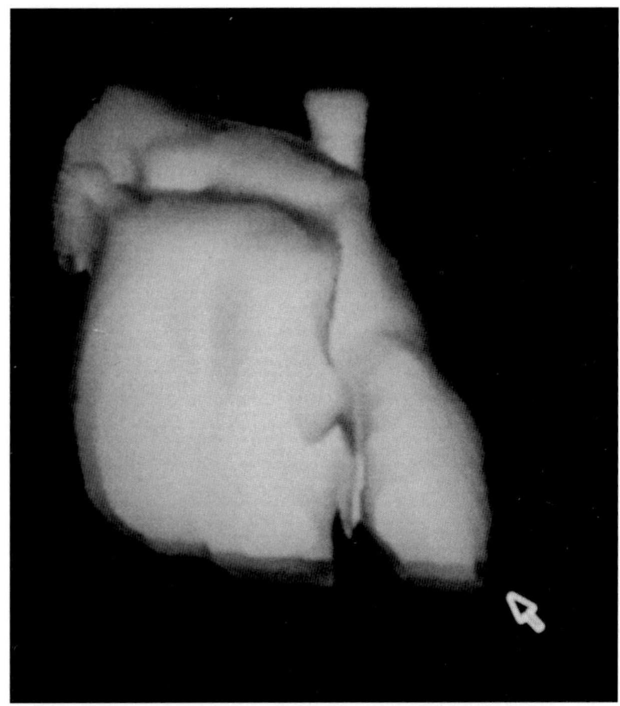

Fig. 90.15 Gated blood pool tomography. Three dimensional reconstruction; normal subject. The 'Bull's eye' display is a useful way of showing three dimensional information in a ready format, but it does lead to a certain degree of distortion. The tomographic data can also be reconstructed into the type of solid body display shown here. Motion can be superimposed and the display can be rotated, permitting observation of the beating heart in any orientation. Here, the heart is viewed in the right anterior oblique projection. The right ventricle is seen on the left and the left ventricle (arrowed) on the right of the image. (Also shown in colour on Plate 26.)

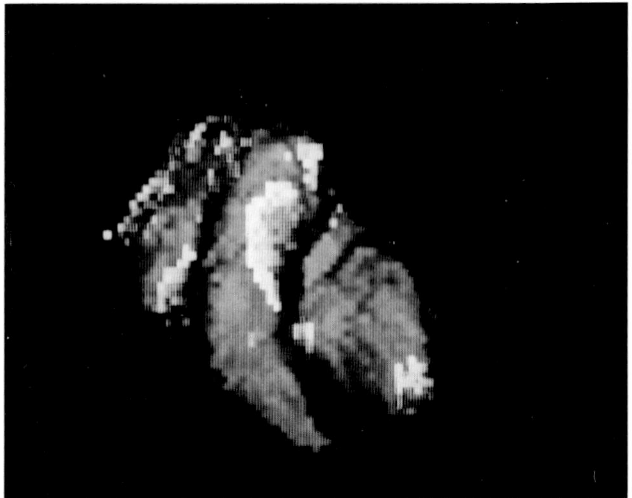

Fig. 90.16 Gated blood pool tomography. Three dimensional reconstruction; phase display – left ventricular infarction. The left anterior oblique projection has been chosen and phase values have been superimposed. In this colour scale, low phase values are seen red or green and high phase values blue. High phase values are apparent within the right atrium and at the apex of the left ventricle, the latter representing infarction and possibly a small aneurysm. (Also shown in colour on Plate 26.)

With respect to the right ventricle,[65] tomography offers the possibility of imaging, including phase and amplitude detection of wall motion, without complications from right atrial overlap and the irregular shape of the chamber.

REFERENCES

1. Bacharach S L, Green M V, Borer J S et al 1977 ECG gated scintillation probe measurement of left ventricular function. J Nucl Med 18: 1176–1183
2. Holman B, Neirinckx R D, Treves S, Tow D E 1979 Cardiac imaging with tantalum-178. Radiology 131: 525–526
3. Horn M, Wiztum K, Neveu C et al 1985 Krypton 81m imaging of the right ventricle. J Nucl Med 26: 33–36
4. Wackers F J, Giles R W, Hoffer P B et al 1982 Gold-195m: a new generator produced short lived radionuclide for sequential assessment of ventricular performance by first pass radionuclide angiocardiography. Am J Cardiol 50: 89–94
5. Treves S, Cheng C, Samuel A et al 1980 Iridium-191 angiocardiography for the detection and quantitation of left to right shunting. J Nucl Med 21: 1151–1157
6. Hamilton R G, Alderson P O 1977 A comparative evaluation of techniques for rapid and efficient labelling of red cells with TC 99m pertechnetate. J Nucl Med 18: 1010–1017
7. Thrall J H, Freitas J E, Swanson D P et al 1978 Clinical comparison of cardiac blood pool visualisation with technetium 99m red blood cells labelled in vivo and with technetium 99m human serum albumin. J Nucl Med 19: 796–803
8. Callahan R J, Froelich J W, McCusick K A et al 1982 A modified method for the in vivo labelling of red blood cells with Tc-99m: Concise communication. J Nucl Med 23: 315–318
9. Hladik W B, Nigg K K, Rhodes B A 1982 Drug induced changes in the biologic distribution of radiopharmaceuticals. Semin Nucl Med 12: 184–218
10. Brash Hm, Wraith P K, Hamman W J et al 1980 The influence of ectopic heart beats in gated ventricular blood pool studies. J Nucl Med 21: 391–393
11. Bacharach S L, Green M V, Borer J S et al 1980 Beat by beat validation of ECG gating. J Nucl Med 21: 307–311
12. Bacharach S L, Green M V, Bonow R O et al 1981 Measurement of ventricular function by ECG gating during atrial fibrillation. J Nucl Med 22: 226–231
13. Kelly M J, Giles R W, Simon T R et al 1981 Multigated equilibrium radionuclide angiocardiography: Improved detection of left ventricular wall motion abnormalities and aneurysms by the addition of the left lateral view. Radiology 139: 167–173
14. Freeman M R, Berman S, Staniloff H M et al 1981 Improved assessment of inferior segmental wall motion by the addition of a 70-degree left anterior oblique view in multiple gated equilibrium scintigraphy. Am Heart J 101: 169–173
15. Dymond D A, Elliot A, Stone D et al 1982 Factors that affect the reproducibility of measurements of left ventricular function from first pass radionuclide ventriculograms. Circulation 65: 311–322
16. Folse R, Braunwald E 1962 Pulmonary vascular dilution curves recorded by external detection in the diagnosis of left to right shunts. Br Heart J 24: 166–172
17. Flaherty J T, Canent R V, Boineau J P et al 1967 Use of external recorded radioisotope dilution curves for quantitation of left to right shunts. Am J Cardiol 20: 341–345
18. Maltz D L, Treves S 1973 Quantitative radionuclide

angiocardiography: determination of Qp:Qs in children. Circulation 47: 1049–1056

19. Askenazi J, Ahnberg DS, Korngold E et al 1976 Quantitative radionuclide angiography: Detection and quantitation of left to right shunts. Am J Cardiol 37: 382–387
20. Parker J A, Treves S 1977 Radionuclide detection, localisation and quantitation of intracardiac shunts and shunts between the two great arteries. Prog Cardiovasc Dis 20: 121–150
21. Baker E J, Ellam S V, Lorber A et al 1985 Superiority of radionuclide over oximetric measurement of left to right shunts. Br Heart J 53: 535–540
22. Makler P T, Pizer S M, Todd-Pokropek A E 1978 Improvement of scintigrams by computer processing. Semin Nucl Med 8: 125–146
23. Miller T R, Sampathkumaran K S 1982 Digital filtering in nuclear medicine. J Nucl Med 23: 66–72
24. Goris M L, Daspit S G, McLaughlin P, Kriss J P 1976 Interpolative background subtraction. J Nucl Med 17: 744–747
25. Slutsky R, Pfisterer M, Verba J et al 1980 Influence of different background and left ventricular assignments on the ejection fraction in equilibrium radionuclide angiography. Radiology 135: 725–730
26. Goris M L, Wallington J, Baum D, Kriss J P. Nuclear angiocardiography: Automated selection of regions of interest for the generation of time activity curves and parametric image display and interpretation. Clin Nucl Med 1976; 1: 99–106
27. Goris M L, McKillop J H, Briandet P A 1981 A fully automated determination of the left ventricular region of interest in nuclear angiocardiography. Cardiovasc Interven Radiol 4: 117–123
28. Sorensen S G, Caldwell J, Ritchie J et al 1981 'Abnormal' responses of ejection fraction to exercise, in healthy subjects, caused by region of interest selection. J Nucl Med 22: 1–7
29. Links J M, Becker L C, Shindledecker J G et al 1982 Measurement of absolute left ventricular volume from gated blood pool studies. Circulation 65: 82–91
30. Burns R J, Druch M N, Woodward D S et al 1983 Repeatability of estimates of left ventricular volume from blood pool counts: Concise communication. J Nucl Med 24: 775–781
31. Seiderer M, Bohn I, Buell U et al 1983 Influence of background and absorption correction on nuclear quantification of left ventricular end diastolic volume. Br J Radiol 56: 183–187
32. Schneider R M, Jaszczak R J, Coleman R E et al 1984 Disproportionate effects of regional hypokinesis on radionuclide ejection fraction: Compensation using attenuation corrected ventricular volumes. J Nucl Med 25: 747–754
33. Legrand V, Chevigny M, Foulon J et al 1983 Evaluation of right ventricular function by gated blood pool scintigraphy. J Nucl Med 24: 886–893
34. Morrison D A, Turgeon J, Ovitt T 1984 Right ventricular ejection fraction measurement: Contrast ventriculography versus gated blood pool and gated first pass radionuclide methods. Am J Cardiol 54: 651–653
35. Reduto L A, Berger H J, Cohen I S et al 1978 Sequential radionuclide assessment of left and right ventricular performance after transmural myocardial infarction. Ann Int Med 89: 441– 447
36. Tobinick E, Schelbert H R, Henning H et al. Right ventricular ejection fraction in patients with acute anterior and inferior infarction assessed by radionuclide angiography. Circulation 57: 1078–1084
37. Walton S, Rowlands D J, Shields R A, Testa H J 1979 Study of right ventricular function in ischaemic heart disease using radionuclide angiocardiography. Intens Care Med 5: 121–126
38. Knapp W H, Helus F, Lambrecht R M et al 1980 Kr-81m for determination of right ventricular ejection fraction. Eur J Nucl Med 5: 487–492
39. Rigo P, Alderson P O, Robertson R M et al 1979 Measurement of aortic and mitral regurgitation by gated blood pool scans. Circulation 60: 306–312
40. Lam W, Pavel D, Byrom E et al 1981 Radionuclide regurgitant index: Value and limitations. Am J Cardiol 47: 292–298
41. Nicod P, Corbett J R, Firth B G et al 1982 Radionuclide techniques for valvular regurgitation index: Comparison in patients with normal and depressed ventricular function. J Nucl Med 23: 763–779
42. Berthout P, Cardot J C, Baud M et al 1984 Factors influencing the quantification of valvular regurgitation by gated equilibrium radionuclide angiography. Eur J Nucl Med 9: 112–114
43. Polak J F, Kemper A J, Bianco J A et al 1982 Resting early peak diastolic filling rate: A sensitive index of myocardial dysfunction in patients with coronary disease. J Nucl Med 23: 471–478
44. Shaffer P, Bashore T, Magorien D 1983 Do normalised filling rates measured by radionuclide ventriculography actually represent ventricular filling rates? J Nucl Med 24: P89 (abstr)
45. Miller T R, Goldman K S, Sampathkumaran K S et al 1983 Analysis of cardiac diastolic function: application in coronary artery disease. J Nucl Med 24: 2–7
46. Bacharach S L, Green M V, Borer J S et al 1979 Left ventricular peak ejection rate, filling rate and ejection fraction – frame rate requirements at rest and exercise. Concise communication. J Nucl Med 20: 189–193
47. Chang W, Henkin R E, Hale D J et al 1980 Methods for detection of ventricular edges. Semin Nucl Med 10: 39–53
48. Geffers H, Adam W E, Bitter F et al 1977 Data processing and functional imaging in radionuclide ventriculography. In: Information in medical processing. Oak Ridge Biological Computing Technology Information Centre, p 322
49. Schad N 1977 Nontraumatic assesment of left ventricular wall motion and regional stroke volume after myocardial infarction. J Nucl Med 18: 333–341
50. Goris M L 1982 Functional or parametric images. J Nucl Med 23: 360
51. Links J M, Douglass K H, Wagner H J Jr 1980 Patterns of ventricular emptying by Fourier analysis of gated blood pool studies. J Nucl Med 21: 978–982
52. Bodenheimer M M, Banka V S, Fooshee C M et al 1979 Comparison of wall motion and regional ejection fraction at rest and during isometric exercise. Concise communication. J Nucl Med 20: 724–732
53. Maddox D E, Holman B L, Wynne J et al 1978 Ejection fraction image: a non-nvasive index of regional left ventricular wall motion. Am J Cardiol 41: 1230–1238
54. Walton S, Yiannikas J, Jarritt P H et al 1981 Phasic abnormalities of left ventricular emptying in coronary artery disease. Br Heart J 46: 245–253
55. Botvinick E, Dunn R, Frais M et al 1982 The phase image: its relationship to patterns of contraction and conduction. Circulation 65: 551–560
56. Underwood S R, Walton S, Lamming P J et al 1984 Patterns of ventricular contraction in patients with conduction abnormality studied by radionuclide angiocardiography. Br Heart J 51: 568–574
57. Makler P T Jr, McCarthy D M, Velchik M G et al 1982 Fourier amplitude ratio: a new way to assess valvular regurgitation. J Nucl Med 24: 204–207
58. Mancini G B J, Peck W W, Slutsky R A et al 1985 Analysis of phase angle histograms from equilibrium radionuclide studies: correlation with semiquantitative grading of wall motion. Am J Cardiol 15: 535–540
59. Underwood S R, Walton S, Lamming P J et al 1989 Quantitative phase analysis in the assessment of coronary artery disease. Br Heart J 61: 14–22
60. Stadius M L, Williams D L, Harp G et al 1985 Left ventricular volume determination using single photon emission computed tomography. Am J Cardiol 55: 1185–1191
61. Corbett J R, Jansen D E, Lewis S E et al 1985 Tomographic gated blood pool radionuclide ventriculography: Analysis of wall motion and left ventricular volumes in patients with coronary artery disease. J Am Coll Cardiol 6: 349–358
62. Underwood S R, Walton S, Laming P J et al 1985 Left ventricular volume and ejection fraction determined by gated blood pool emission tomography. Br Heart J 53: 216–222
63. Nakajima K, Bunko H, Tada S et al 1985 Nuclear tomographic phase analysis: Localisation of accessory pathway in patients with Wolff Parkinson White syndrome. Am Heart J 109: 809–815
64. Norton M Y, Walton S, Evans N T S 1988 Gated cardiac tomography. Eur J Nucl Med 14: 472–476
65. Cross S J, Lee H S, Norton M Y et al 1992 Three dimensional imaging of the right ventricle using blood pool tomography. Eur J Radiol 2: 95–98

91. Myocardial perfusion scintigraphy techniques using single photon radiotracers

Rodney J. Hicks

INTRODUCTION

Having choice is sometimes more difficult than not. In the case of myocardial perfusion scintigraphy, many options confront the practitioner of nuclear cardiology. How myocardial perfusion scintigraphy is performed in a given clinical setting is often determined by the combination of personal preference, previous experience, and the availability of equipment, analysis software and radiotracers, as much as by research and expert opinion.

In establishing the methodology to perform myocardial perfusion scintigraphy, it is important to recognize that all reviewers have biases, and that the experience, training, equipment and technical resources available to them may not be widely available. The methodology used in an individual laboratory necessarily reflects the expertise and technology available. It is, however, important that studies should be tailored where possible to the clinical problem presented by the patient.

CHOICE OF RADIOPHARMACEUTICAL AND IMAGING PROTOCOL

^{201}Tl or ^{99m}Tc perfusion agents?

The superior imaging characteristics of ^{99m}Tc compared with ^{201}Tl have led to a search for Tc-labelled myocardial perfusion tracers. Of the potential agents, [^{99m}Tc] hexakis-2-methoxy-2-isobutyl-isonitrile (MIBI) (Cardiolite, Dupont) and ^{99m}Tcteboroxime (Cardiotec, Squibb Diagnostics) have been most intensively evaluated and are both licensed in the United States. Another agent, ^{99m}Tc tetrofosmin (Myoview, Amersham) is also now licensed.

There are several studies directly comparing ^{201}Tl and the ^{99m}Tc myocardial perfusion agents,[1–10] which generally report improved subjective image quality with the latter, but no improved diagnostic performance. There are significant differences in the biological behaviour of ^{201}Tl compared with the ^{99m}Tc-labelled compounds and these differences may be an important factor in the better performance of ^{201}Tl in clinical practice than might be expected purely by its suboptimal imaging and physical characteristics. Studies comparing the ^{99m}Tc-labelled myocardial perfusion tracers have been limited,[9] but these tracers have markedly different biological characteristics requiring different imaging methods to be used for each.

The choice of radiopharmaceutical can logically be made by considering the clinical information required, the stress used and the imaging equipment available. The ability of the myocardium to concentrate ^{201}Tl over time provides a sensitive means to detect myocardial viability and this suggests that a protocol involving delayed imaging after a resting injection of ^{201}Tl would be a good choice in patients with known advanced coronary disease.[11,12] The uniformity of perfusion under stress conditions can probably be similarly assessed by all agents,[1–10,13] and therefore all would be suitable for the detection of coronary disease in patients without prior myocardial infarction. The decreased extraction fraction of ^{99m}Tc MIBI at high flow rates[14,15] may render it a less suitable agent for stress studies using potent vasodilating drugs such as adenosine.[16] The rapid myocardial loss of ^{99m}Tc teboroxime[17] requires multi-detector gamma-camera systems for single photon emission computed tomography (SPECT),[18] while the higher radiation dose rates to hospital staff from the ^{99m}Tc agents than with ^{201}Tl may make them less suitable for studies on inpatients requiring high dependency nursing care. Conversely, in patients with symptoms of exertional dyspnoea and in whom assessment of left ventricular function during exercise is of interest, the ability to assess the function of the heart by gated, first pass radionuclide ventriculography with ^{99m}Tc labelled radiopharmaceuticals may be desirable. Whilst this is possible with both ^{99m}Tc MIBI and ^{99m}Tc teboroxime, the former is preferable because of its substantially lower first pass lung retention.[19]

The time taken to complete a study may also be an important factor in the choice of radiotracer. Prolonged studies cause patient inconvenience and may impair efficient time-tabling of a busy nuclear medicine practice.

Thus, 24 h delayed ^{201}Tl imaging and 2 day MIBI protocols may not be ideal. The rapid myocardial loss of ^{99m}Tc teboroxime may provide a means to assess myocardial ischaemia with a short and convenient imaging series.[17] In patients with a relatively low pretest likelihood of coronary artery disease, a normal stress study with any of the radiotracers would obviate the need for a resting perfusion study. Therefore, protocols in which stress imaging precedes the resting phase studies would be appropriate in such patients. ^{201}Tl- or ^{99m}Tc teboroxime or the 2 day ^{99m}Tc MIBI study with initial stress study[20] would meet these needs.

It may be that a composite study utilizing the strengths of ^{201}Tl- and ^{99m}Tc-labelled compounds would provide the greatest possible information about the heart in specific patients with advanced cardiac disease. For example, a resting injection of ^{201}Tl with the patient returning for imaging several hours later could be used to provide analysis of the distribution of viable myocardium.[21–23] During subsequent exercise or pharmacological stress, first pass radionuclide ventriculography could be performed using i.v administration of ^{99m}Tc MIBI to assess left ventricular function.[6,19] Assessment of the distribution of perfusion during stress could then be compared with the distribution of viable myocardium as identified by ^{201}Tl uptake in order to determine the extent of ischaemically jeopardized myocardium. Gated SPECT assessment of the perfusion study could also be used to analyse regional and global left ventricular function under resting conditions. The acquisition of separate rest ^{201}Tl and stress ^{99m}Tc MIBI protocols appears to be a practicable approach.[24]

Two day or same day ^{99m}Tc MIBI studies?

Unlike ^{201}Tl, ^{99m}Tc MIBI does not redistribute significantly in the myocardium after stress imaging.[25] There may, however, be some early fill-in of stress perfusion abnormalities if there is sufficient persisting circulating ^{99m}Tc levels after reversal of ischaemia,[26] suggesting that maintenance of stress for an adequate period after the administration of radiotracer is important for the detection of stress perfusion defects. This lack of redistribution necessitates the administration of separate stress and rest doses of ^{99m}Tc MIBI. Dosimetry allows for administration of up to 1110 MBq (30 mCi) of this radiopharmaceutical in divided doses.[27] Various protocols have been evaluated for the timing of resting and stress studies. Evaluation of both same and 2-day protocols has been performed by Taillefer and coworkers[1] with comparable diagnostic results by both but with greater convenience with the same day protocol.

The same day protocol involves administration of 200–250 MBq of ^{99m}Tc MIBI at rest followed by imaging 30–60 min later. By allowing time for hepatobiliary excretion, the delay in imaging decreases liver activity which otherwise limits evaluation of the inferior wall.[27] After rest imaging, the patient is stressed and given 600–750 MBq of ^{99m}Tc MIBI. Stress imaging is also performed 30–60 min after radiotracer administration. The 2 day protocol is performed with an initial stress study using 300–400 MBq of radiotracer followed, if required, several days later by a resting study using a similar dose. Either study protocol allows for evaluation of first pass radionuclide ventriculography under stress conditions,[6,19,28–32] but the low activity used for the rest study of the same day protocol, while feasible, may limit the statistical quality of a first pass study.

The prolonged retention of ^{99m}Tc MIBI in the myocardium and high count rates makes this radiopharmaceutical ideally suited to SPECT imaging. It is possible to perform SPECT studies gated to the cardiac cycle and thereby assess regional wall thickening.[33]

Separate rest and stress ^{99m}Tc teboroxime or is a single stress-redistribution study adequate?

Comparison of ^{99m}Tc teboroxime with ^{201}Tl has shown similar diagnostic efficacy with both agents.[5] The protocol used involved rapid planar imaging commencing within 2 min of stress and with 3, 6 and 9 min images obtained in the upright anterior, LAO 30° and LAO 60° projections. The longer imaging times for the later images related rapid wash-out of activity from the heart after stress. A dose of 15 mCi of ^{99m}Tc teboroxime was given at stress and around 2 h later for resting imaging. The resting image acquisition protocol was identical to that used in the stress study.

Subsequent experimental data suggested that delayed wash-out of activity from the myocardium may be a marker of ischaemia,[34] and human studies have suggested that rapid teboroxime redistribution may be an ischaemic marker, being present in 48% of ischaemic segments compared with only 13% of normal segments.[17] The early normalization of activity in ischaemic territories suggests the possibility for single injection studies and reinforces the need for rapid imaging protocols with this agent.[35] Without a multi-detector system, the need for rapid acquisition of data would probably preclude SPECT. This tracer also appears to be less suitable than ^{99m}Tc MIBI for first pass radionuclide ventriculography studies due to significant pulmonary retention on initial lung transit.[19]

SELECTION OF ACQUISITION METHODOLOGY

Planar or SPECT imaging?

Validation studies with ^{201}Tl myocardial perfusion scintigraphy in the 1970s used planar imaging in several orthogonal projections, whilst a decade later, the development of SPECT led to studies comparing the performance of these two imaging techniques. Comparative studies performed in patients with infarction showed substantially higher sensitivity with SPECT for the detection of perfusion abnormalities.[36-38] Subsequently, similar comparisons documented greater sensitivity for the detection of coronary artery disease and of individual vessel disease by SPECT in patients without myocardial infarction.[4,39,40] Multivessel disease was also more accurately predicted by SPECT.[40] The higher sensitivity of SPECT has also been documented for with ^{99m}Tc MIBI.[4]

Review of published series has been performed for planar[41] and SPECT[42] acquisition protocols. Average sensitivity and specificity for planar scanning with visual analysis were 78% and 91%, and with quantitative analysis, 91% and 88%.[41] A review of more than 1000 patients undergoing exercise ^{201}Tl SPECT showed a sensitivity of 90% and specificity of 70%.[42] However, because of differing referral biases, and perhaps differing levels of experience and expertise in the performance and interpretation of planar and SPECT scintigrams, it is difficult to compare accurately the relative sensitivity and specificity of each technique in this way. The number of studies directly comparing these techniques in the same patient have been relatively few. One such study showed a significantly greater area under a receiver operating characteristics curve for SPECT than planar imaging implying superior diagnostic ability for SPECT.[43]

Despite its apparently lower sensitivity compared with SPECT, the prognostic power of a normal planar ^{201}Tl scan is excellent,[44-46] and is similar to SPECT imaging.[47] Recognition of the presence of non-critical coronary disease may be an important impetus for risk factor modification, and may direct appropriate symptomatic management without recourse to further investigations.

180° or 360° SPECT acquisition?

While it is possible to reconstruct tomographs of the heart following either 180° or 360° acquisitions, most institutions currently perform 180° acquisition from the 45° RAO projection to the 45° LPO projection.[48] There has, however, been controversy over whether 180° or 360° acquisition is preferable. Using heart phantom and patient studies, Coleman et al[38] compared 180° data collection without attenuation correction against 360° acquisition with attenuation correction.[49] The 180° and 360° data collection studies were performed using a dual head system but with analysis of only the RAO to LPO data from one head in the 180° study. The imaging time and total counts of the 180° study were thus only half those for the 360° study. The ability to perform attenuation correction with 360° of data decreased variations in count density introduced by photon scatter and yielded similar, albeit slightly lower, image contrast than for a 180° acquisition. The authors thus supported use of 360° acquisitions for a dual head camera system. Similar studies comparing 180° and 360° acquisitions with a single head rotating gamma-camera were also performed at around the same time and documented superior image contrast with the 180° acquisition despite halving of the total imaging time.[50] Not surprisingly the 180° acquisition was felt to be preferable. It should, however, be noted that no attenuation correction was performed for either SPECT acquisition protocol in this study. Go et al[51] subsequently evaluated both 180° and 360° acquisitions in patients with documented coronary artery anatomy and found a 36% incidence of false positive segmental perfusion abnormalities and a 24% incidence of moderate to severe image distortion with 180° acquisition. Despite also documenting improved image contrast, the authors concluded that despite decreased imaging times the spatial distortions associated with 180° acquisition were unacceptable and that 180° acquisition should be abandoned.

Further evaluation of this issue was performed by Eisner and coworkers who systematically assessed the accuracy of reconstructed data from 180° and 360° circular and elliptical orbits using complex computer simulations and experimental results from point source reconstructions.[48] This important paper demonstrated similar distortions for both 180° and 360° acquisitions but, as previously observed, improved contrast resolution with 180° acquisition. Furthermore, for fixed patient acquisition times, significantly more counts were acquired with studies of the anterior chest alone. With these data it became widely accepted that 180° acquisition is the method of choice for ^{201}Tl myocardial SPECT studies using single detector rotating gamma-camera systems. While not specifically addressed in the studies discussed above, reduction of imaging time associated with 180° acquisition also potentially decreases the likelihood of patient movement during the study and associated imaging artefacts and is an additional potential benefit of 180° acquisition.

The effect of scatter and attenuation which poses major problems with 360° ^{201}Tl studies may, however, be less important for the ^{99m}Tc-labelled myocardial perfusion agents.[52] With the wider availability of multi detector gamma cameras, improved attenuation correction algorithms including measured attenuation by transmission studies,[53,54] 360° acquisition may allow more accurate quantification of the distribution and severity of perfusion abnormality associated with coronary artery disease if ^{99m}Tc myocardial perfusion agents are used. A clinical comparison of 180° and 360° data collection in a small number of patients studied using [^{99m}Tc]MIBI, however, demonstrated no particular advantage with 360° acquisition.[55]

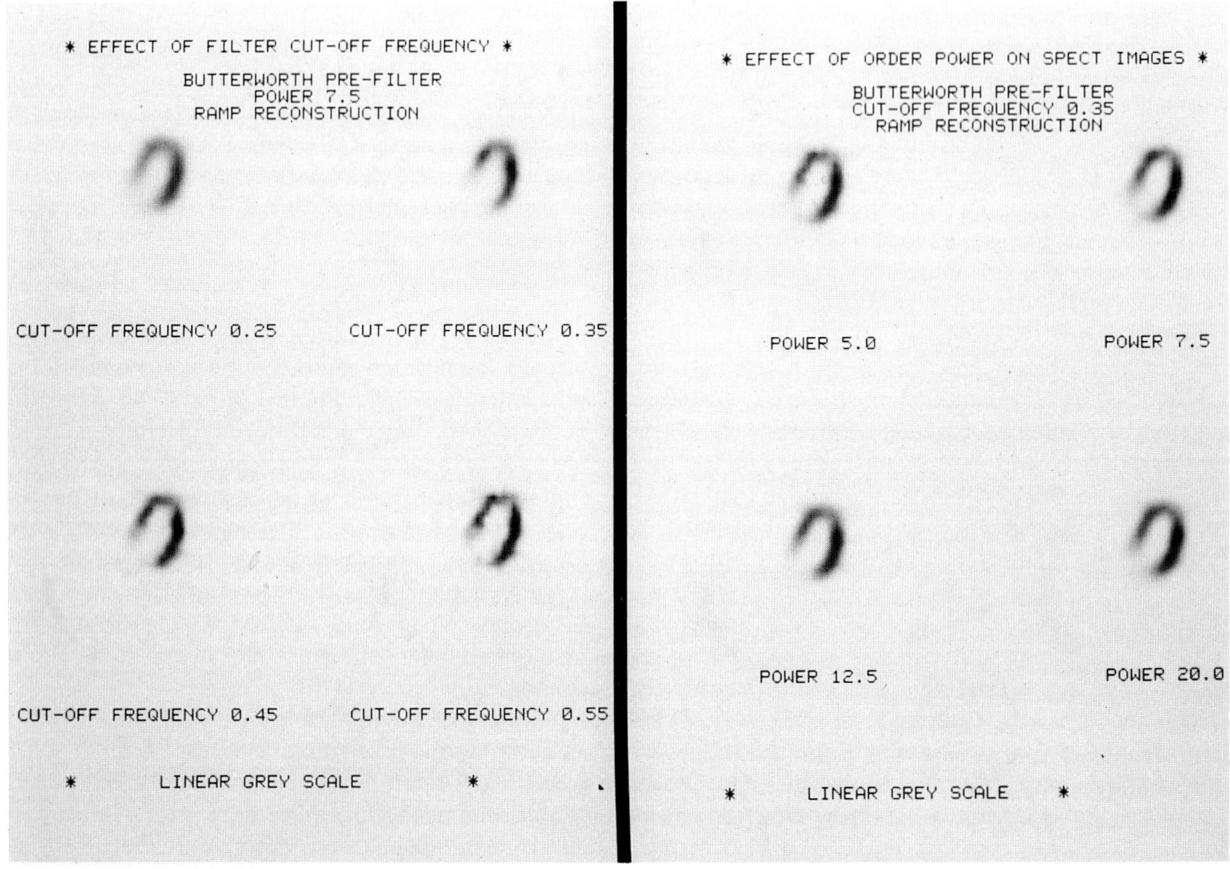

Fig. 91.1 The effect of varying reconstruction filters can be seen on this series of reconstructions of the same transaxial slice. Varying the order and cut-off of the Butterworth filter can provide a range of final image qualities. Although highly filtered data may be pleasing to the eye, the potential loss of physiological signal means that images should retain some of the 'noise' which is an integral part of a scintigraphic study. The left panel demonstrates the effect of altering cut-off frequency while maintaining a constant power. The right panel demonstrates the effect of altering the power with a set cut-off frequency.

SELECTION OF ANALYSIS AND DISPLAY METHODOLOGY

Data filtering

The data used to reconstruct tomographic images of the heart is obtained from a series of planar images. The three-dimensional distribution of activity is established by back-projection of data from each planar image along the radii of the circle of acquisition. The noise contained in the planar images substantially degrades the appearances of the reconstructed tomographs and the back-projection process itself introduces distortion of the regional distribution of radioactivity. To improve the appearance of the final images it is usual to filter the data. Most gamma camera systems come with a series of reconstruction filter options or allow reconstruction of a sample tomogram using a range of user-defined filters (Fig. 91.1).

Realignment of images

The oblique and variable orientation of the heart in the thorax makes evaluation of the distribution of activity in the standard anatomical planes quite difficult. To standardize the display of tomographic data, the images are reoriented to the long axis of the left ventricle which extends from the centre of the mitral valve plane to the cardiac apex (Fig. 91.2). After definition of this axis, images are reoriented cutting the cardiac volume from superior to inferior parallel to the long axis creating vertical long axis slices, and from the septum to the lateral wall creating horizontal long axis images. Images reconstructed perpendicular to the long axis create short-axis slices. Misalignment of the cardiac long axis can create significant distortions of both the reconstructed tomograms and polar-coordinate maps used in quantitative evaluation of myocardial perfusion by SPECT (Figs 91.2 and 91.3).

Qualitative or quantitative analysis?

As a result of scatter, attenuation, and the non-uniform thickness of the myocardium, there is a normal variation

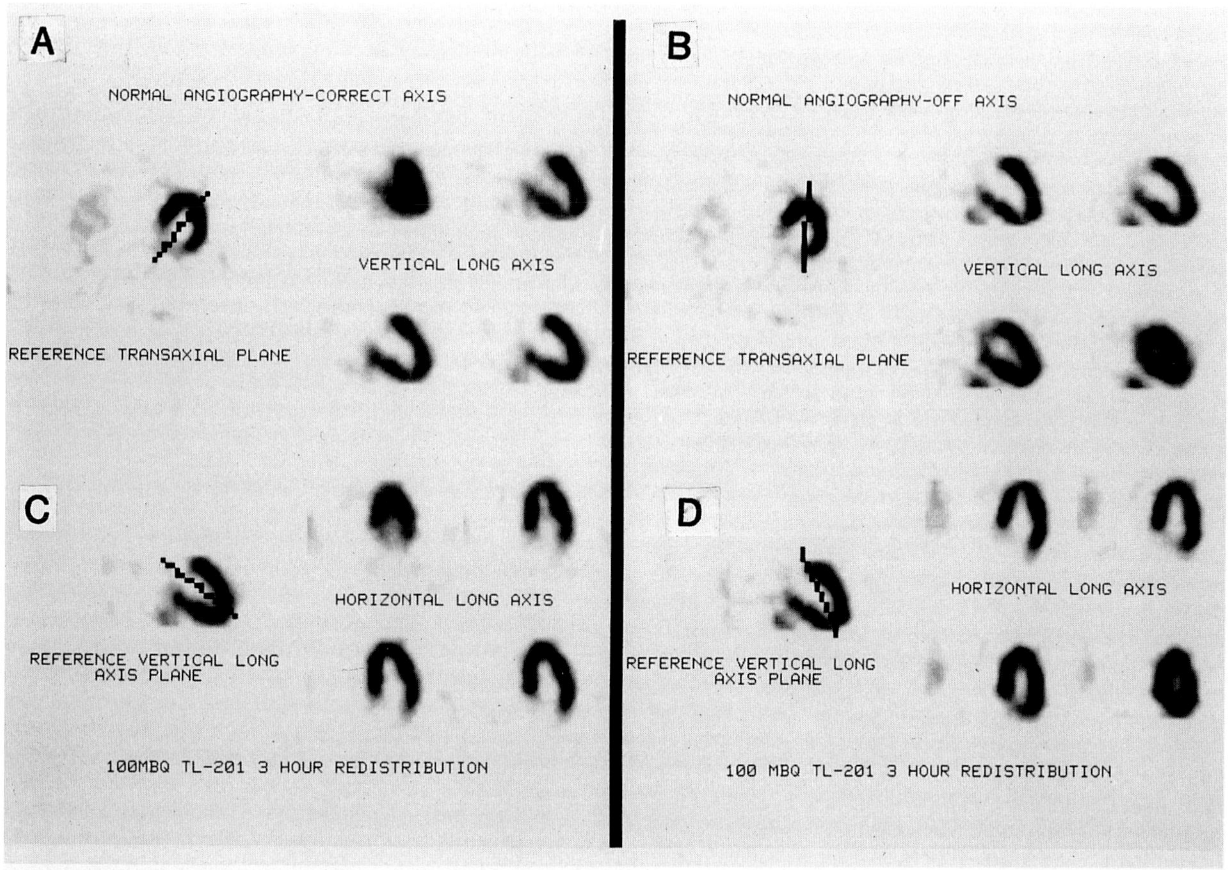

Fig. 91.2 A The angulation of the vertical long axis images in relationship to the sagittal plane of the body is determined by reviewing the series of transaxial reconstruction slices. Having selected a plane which passes roughly through the mid-level of the mitral valve plane, the axis is defined by passing from a point equidistant from the basal septal and basal lateral walls of the left ventricle to the left ventricular apex. Due to the curvilinear course of the lateral wall, it is helpful to use the septum as a guide to the appropriate angle. B Inappropriate selection of this angle will lead to oblique vertical axis slices which can be identified as ovoid rather than U-shaped slices. **C** The angulation of the horizontal long axis images in relationship to the true transaxial plane of the body is determined by reviewing the series of vertical long axis reconstruction slices. Having selected a plane which passes roughly through the mid-level of the mitral valve plane, the axis is defined by a line passing from a point equidistant from the basal anterior and basal inferior walls of the left ventricle to the left ventricular apex. Due to the more curvilinear course of the anterior wall, it is helpful to use the inferior wall as a guide to the appropriate angle. **D** Inappropriate selection of this angle will lead to oblique horizontal axis slices which can be identified as ovoid rather than the expected U-shaped slices.

in the apparent activity in various regions of the heart.[56,57] Qualitative interpretation of myocardial perfusion scintigrams requires pattern recognition which incorporates the possible effects of attenuating structures such as the breast. These skills take time to develop. To provide a more objective means of analysis, various quantitative software analysis systems have been developed for both planar and SPECT studies. In general, these studies have reported an improvement in the diagnostic performance of myocardial perfusion scintigraphy. However, these quantitative methods are in fact semi-quantitative in that they are determining relative rather than absolute radioactivity levels in each region of the heart. Thus, changes in attenuation characteristics, such as altered breast position, are poorly dealt with by quantitative analysis but can be readily perceived by qualitative analysis.

For planar imaging the major problem for quantitative analysis is background activity, which is particularly different in the stress and resting studies when ^{201}Tl is used as the radiotracer, and the commonest approach has been to use an interpolative method.[58] All quantitative analysis programs also involve alignment of initial and delayed images, and determination of regional myocardial activity, the latter generally involving circumferential count profile analysis.[59] When compared with a normal database or normalized to each other, these profiles allow detection of the severity and extent of perfusion abnormality, and the degree of redistribution. The problems associated with developing a robust quantitative analysis program have led to some laboratories favouring qualitative analysis. It is, however, clear that when a well-validated quantitative analysis is combined with expert

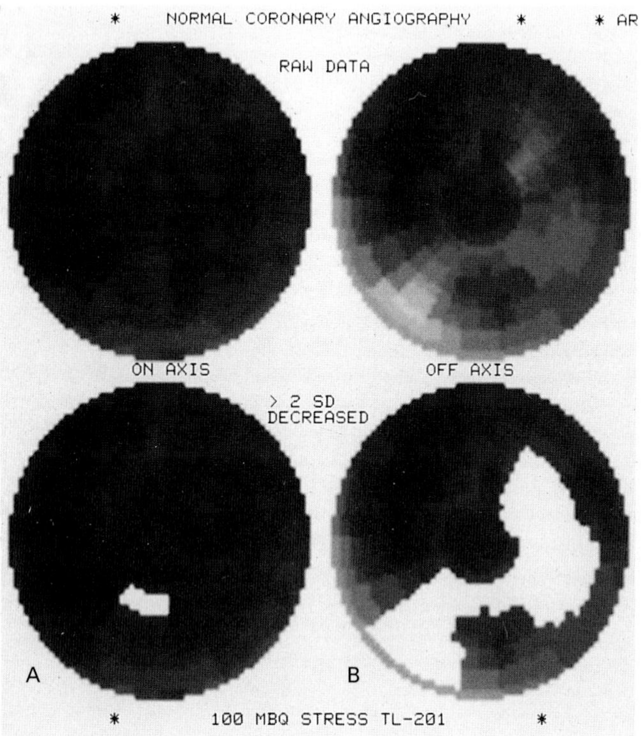

Fig. 91.3 The polar map involves display of circumferential profile data in a standardized format. Information from apical slices is displayed in the centre of the polar map, while information from basal slices is displayed peripherally. The lateral wall is to the right, the inferior wall below, the septum to the left, and the anterior wall above. Thus, data from the three-dimensional information contained in short-axis and vertical long-axis images is mapped onto a two-dimensional plane. Misalignment of the cardiac axes can create substantial artefactual 'perfusion abnormalities' on polar coordinate maps. A The appropriately aligned data reconstruction set in this patient with a normal coronary angiogram has no significant perfusion abnormalities. B Rotation of the assigned cardiac axis creates a semi-lunar artefact peripherally and an apical perfusion defect. The raw data presented (top) along with those pixels with values >2 standard deviations below normal based on age- and sex-matched controls (bottom).

interpretation of planar ^{201}Tl scintigrams, additional diagnostic accuracy can be achieved.[60,61]

Quantitative analysis has also been used to enhance the diagnostic information provided by SPECT.[38,62–64] The Cedars–Sinai group have described,[63] validated[64,65] and made available an analysis program which uses the polar-map format to display circumferential profile data from the slice reconstructions (Fig. 91.3). A similar program has been developed at Emory University.[66] Background activity is not a problem for quantitative SPECT analysis but the effects of attenuation and varying wall thickness are. Thus, quantitative analysis of myocardial perfusion defects by SPECT must include comparison of the uniformity of distribution of activity in the myocardium with that in a control population. Because of differences in the distribution of attenuation characteristics,[57] it is important that such programs allow for gender.

None of these quantitative programs currently include factors such as a pretest assessment of the likelihood of coronary artery disease, the adequacy of cardiovascular stress, the presence of evidence of ischaemia during the stress study, or allowance for patients of differing body habitus. As outlined below, these are critical pieces of information in interpreting myocardial perfusion studies. Quantitative ^{201}Tl SPECT analysis should only be used as an additional help. Where qualitative and quantitative interpretations are discordant, attempts should be made to reconcile them by analysis of other information available, and if no explanation for the differences can be determined, the equivocal nature of the findings emphasized.

REPORTING OF MYOCARDIAL PERFUSION STUDIES

General principles

Interpretation of clinical myocardial perfusion scintigraphic stress tests should include not only evaluation of the perfusion images, but also such factors as the pretest likelihood of disease[67,68] the exercise performance including electrocardiographic findings,[69] the patient's sex,[57,70] and the patient's body habitus.[71,72] Using these approaches, the clinical performance of this technique is likely to be superior to that achieved by blinded, experimental reading of the imaging data alone as used in clinical evaluation trials. However, diagnostic efficacy cannot be simply regarded as the ability to determine the presence or absence of disease (sensitivity and specificity), but also encompasses the ability to determine the severity of that disease, the prognosis, and the appropriate management strategy. As discussed in more detail in subsequent chapters, myocardial perfusion scintigraphy can potentially provide much of this information.

Reporting of planar scintigrams

A knowledge of the typical distributions of perfusion abnormalities in the left anterior descending artery (Fig. 91.4), right coronary artery (Fig. 91.5) and circumflex artery (Fig. 91.6) on planar imaging[73,74] and common soft-tissue artefacts[71] is important for the interpretation of planar ^{201}Tl scintigrams. However, the location of perfusion abnormality is not the only important piece of scintigraphic information. The severity and extent of myocardial perfusion abnormalities allow evaluation of the functional significance of the stenosis within a vascular territory in a manner not possible by anatomical evaluation by coronary angiography.[75,76] The degree of reversibility of perfusion abnormalities identified on stress studies, compared with those demonstrated on subsequent delayed images at rest, also allows documentation of the extent of ischaemically jeopardized myocardium

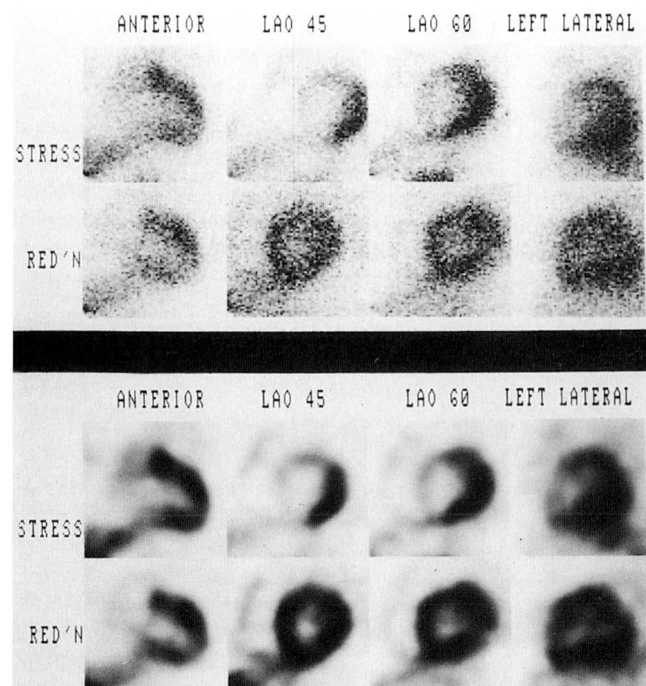

Fig. 91.4 The typical distribution of perfusion abnormality in the presence of flow-limiting coronary artery disease in the left anterior descending coronary artery includes abnormalities in the septum, anterior wall and apical segments. Extension around the apex into the infero-apical segment need not imply coexistent disease in the posterior descending artery. Row data (top) and Metz-filtered images (below) demonstrates an extensive, severe and almost completely reversible anterior, anteroseptal and apical perfusion abnormality.

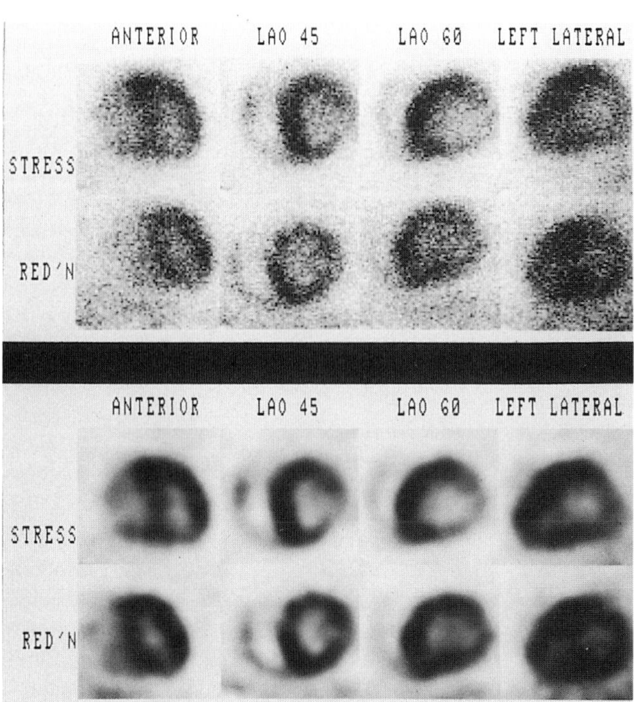

Fig. 91.6 Circumflex cononary artery disease can be difficult to identify on planar ^{201}Tl scintigrams. The combination of a shallow (30–45°) and steep (60–70°) may improve the sensitivity of planar scanning for the detection of circumflex artery perfusion abnormalities. In this example raw data (upper) and Metz-filtered images (lower) demonstrate a reversible inferolateral perfusion abnormality, best characterized in the LAO 60° projection, with relatively little involvement of the true inferior wall suggesting a non-dominant circumflex artery.

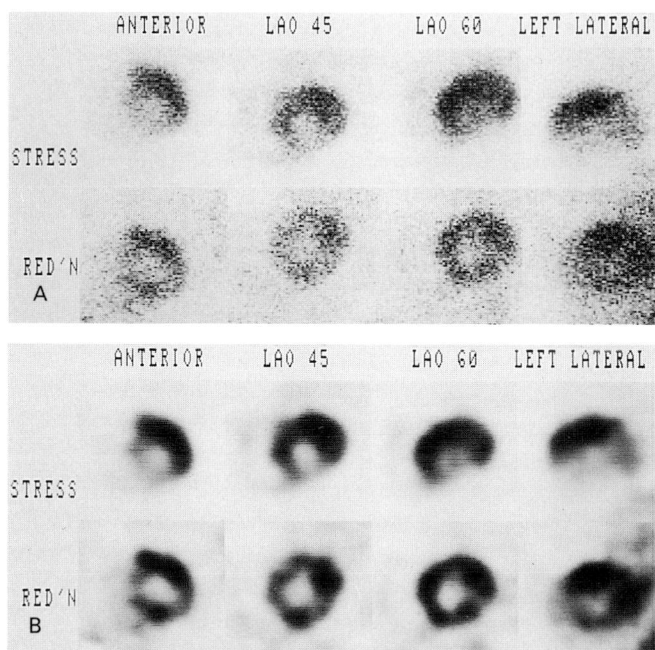

Fig. 91.5 Disease in the right coronary artery causes perfusion abnormalities in the inferior septum and inferior walls. Raw data (A) and images following Metz-filtering (B) are used to assess the extent, severity and location of perfusion abnormalities and to determine the degree of reversibility between stress and redistribution (RED'N).

and of prior myocardial infarction. Additional important scintigraphic parameters include the presence of ischaemic left ventricular dilatation with stress, which is a recognized indicator of multi vessel coronary disêase,[77] and increased thallium activity in the lungs[78–80] (Fig. 91.7), reflecting elevated left ventricular end diastolic pressure. Both these findings are adverse prognostic indicators.[81] Comparison of myocardial activity in the stress and delayed image may also provide diagnostic information.[82]

As discussed in Chapter 95, there is a substantial body of literature detailing the prognostic significance of ^{201}Tl results.[79,83–87] These data are additional to the basic pathophysiological data relating to the location and severity of likely coronary artery disease and should be communicated to the referring physician above and beyond the pure description of the scintigraphic findings.

Reporting SPECT studies

Evaluation of the three-dimensional extent and severity of perfusion abnormalities is enhanced by tomographic imaging. Direct slice by slice comparison of stress

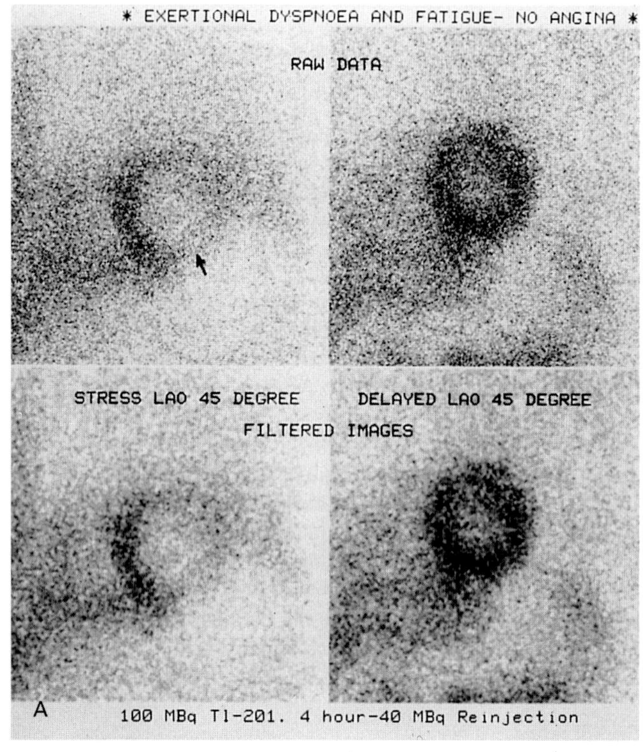

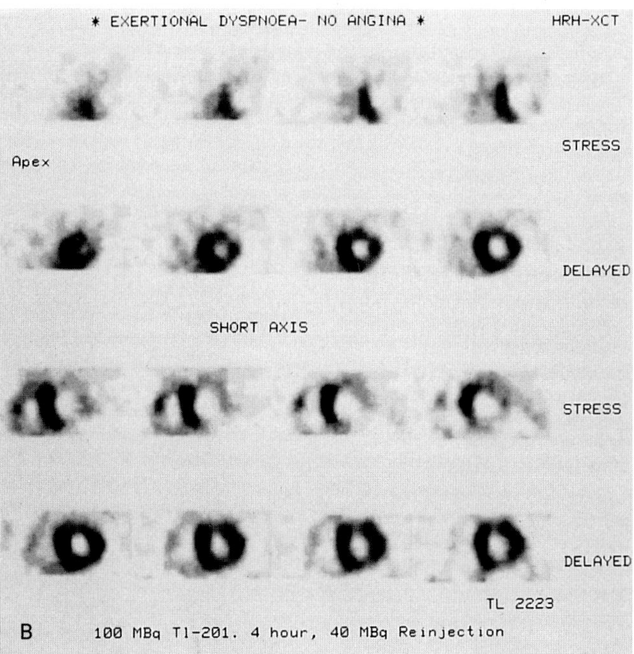

Fig. 91.7 A Increased lung uptake and left ventricular dilation on the preliminary planar images in this patient indicate an adverse prognosis. B SPECT images demonstrate substantial reversible perfusion abnormalities in the anterior, lateral and inferiolateral walls, suggesting coronary disease affecting both the left anterior descending (LAD) and circumflex coronary artery distributions. This patient had left main, LAD and circumflex disease.

and delayed images, also allows for assessment of the degree of reversibility in observed perfusion abnormalities. Assessment of lung uptake is less useful on the SPECT data than it is on early planar imaging, although attempts have been made to obtain these data from the planar projection data acquired during the SPECT study.[88] Typical examples of SPECT perfusion abnormalities in the left anterior descending artery (Fig. 91.8), right coronary artery (Fig. 91.9) and circumflex artery (Fig. 91.10) need to be recognized. As with planar

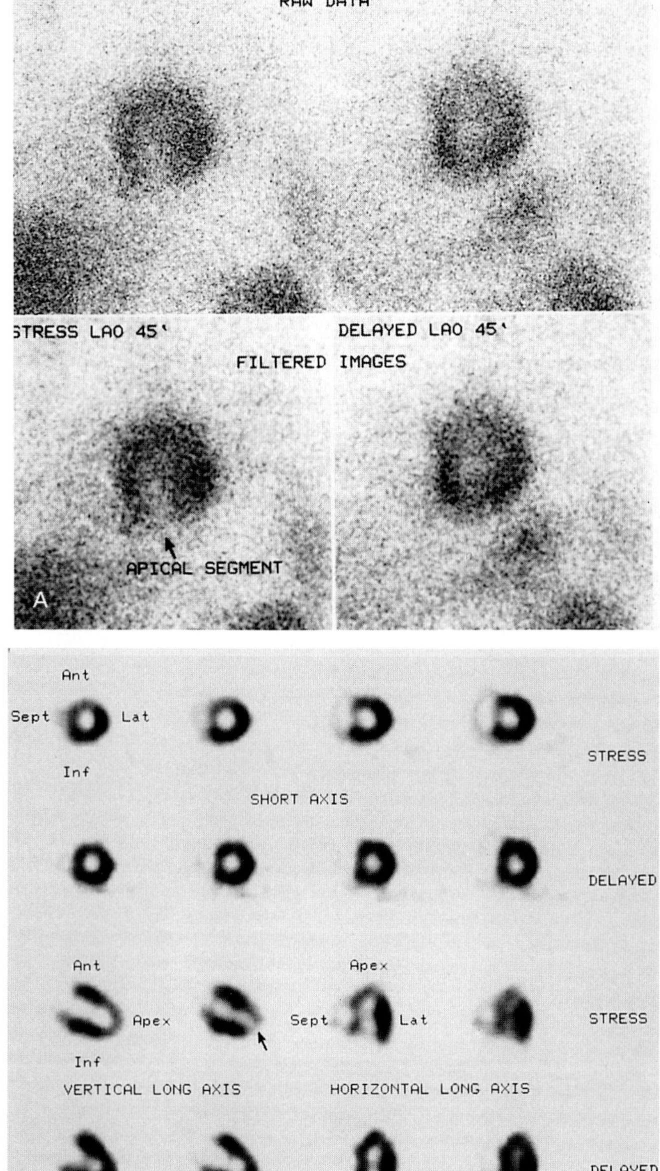

Fig. 91.8 Functionally significant coronary artery disease involving the left anterior descending artery causes reversible perfusion abnormalities in the anterior, anteroseptal and apical walls and may extend into the infero-apical region.

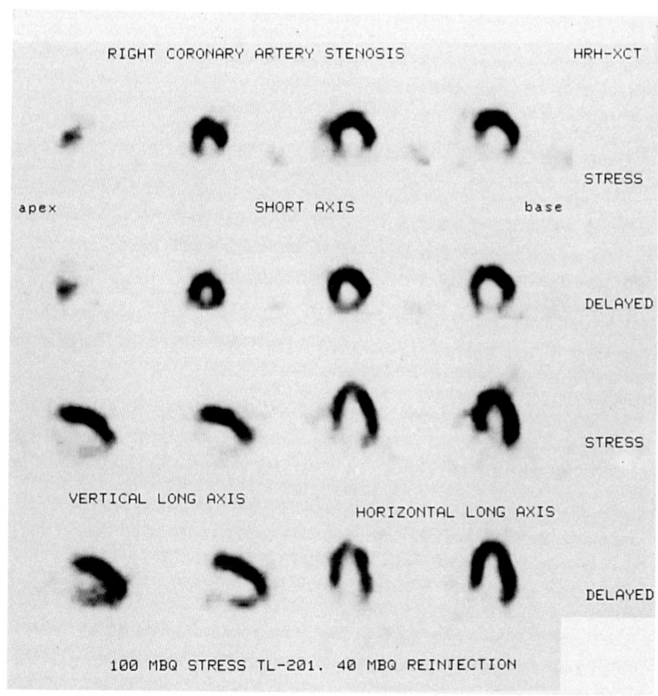

Fig. 91.9 Isolated right coronary artery disease causes perfusion abnormalities in the inferior septum and inferior wall. The extent of true posterior perfusion abnormality is dependent on whether the right coronary or circumflex artery supplies the posterior descending coronary artery.

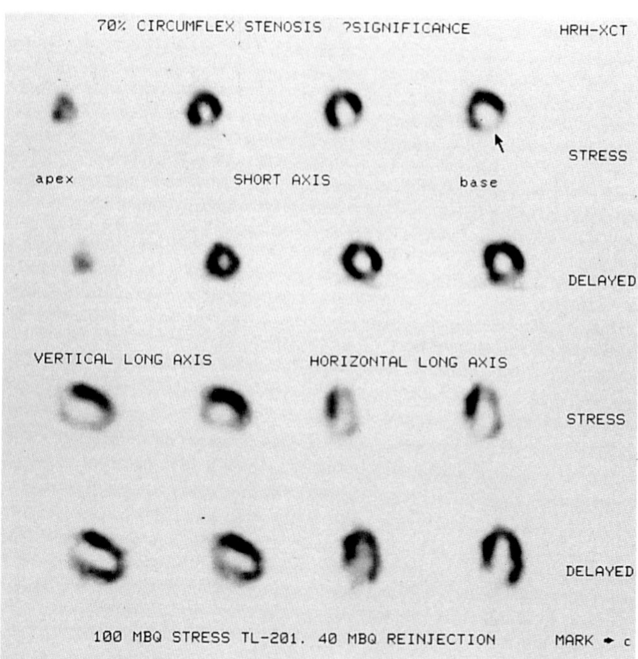

Fig. 91.10 Circumflex coronary artery disease has a variable distribution depending on the size and dominance of the vessel and the site of involvement. High obtuse marginal branch or intermediate ramus stenoses tend to involve the anterolateral wall, while most perfusion abnormalities due to stenoses in the circumflex trunk tend to occur in the lateral, inferolateral and inferior walls.

imaging, recognition of imaging artefacts and patterns associated with prognostically significant disease is important[89] (Fig. 91.7).

Artefacts and quality control

Since false positive studies are more likely to proceed to investigation than are false negative studies, a lack of specificity can be an important cause of decreased confidence in test results by referring clinicians. Many of these false positive results can, however, be recognized by experienced observers who are aware of common imaging artefacts. Recognition of scintigraphic abnormalities which are likely to be artefactual can reduce the number of unnecessary angiograms.[90] In addition to the distribution of scintigraphic abnormality, important factors that allow differentiation between significant and artefactual scintigraphic abnormalities include assessment of the likelihood of coronary artery disease based on clinical history and response to the stress component of the test, a knowledge of the sex and body habitus of the patient, and interpretation of the electrocardiograph.

Planar imaging artefacts

Possible causes of false positive results on planar imaging can be divided into normal variants, soft-tissue attenuation artefacts, overlying visceral activity, physiological alteration in coronary blood flow, and non-coronary cardiac disease.

Normal variants include apical thinning, and upper septal thinning. Activity in both these regions is partially dependent on the cardiac orientation. For example, the apex of a vertically oriented heart will tend to move superiorly during systole, leading to undersampling of apical counts in the planar image which is a composite of the entire cardiac cycle. Conversely, in a horizontally oriented heart, the 'apical' segment may be superimposed on the inferior wall, increasing apparent apical counts. The membranous septum, which does not contain myocardium and hence does not take up perfusion tracers, may also appear as a perfusion abnormality in the upper septum if the heart is vertically oriented.

Soft-tissue artefacts are a common cause of imaging artefact on planar myocardial perfusion scintigrams.[71] In women, the left breast is the most common soft-tissue attenuator. The severity of the abnormality is not only related to the size of the breast but also to its density. Small but firm breasts can create more marked and focal perfusion abnormalities than large pendulous breasts. Review of the raw data planar images will usually demonstrate a clear demarcation line of a breast attenuation artefact crossing both cardiac and background activity (Fig. 91.11). By obtaining a left lateral planar image with the patient's right side in the decubitus position, the left breast is projected away from the heart and allows further

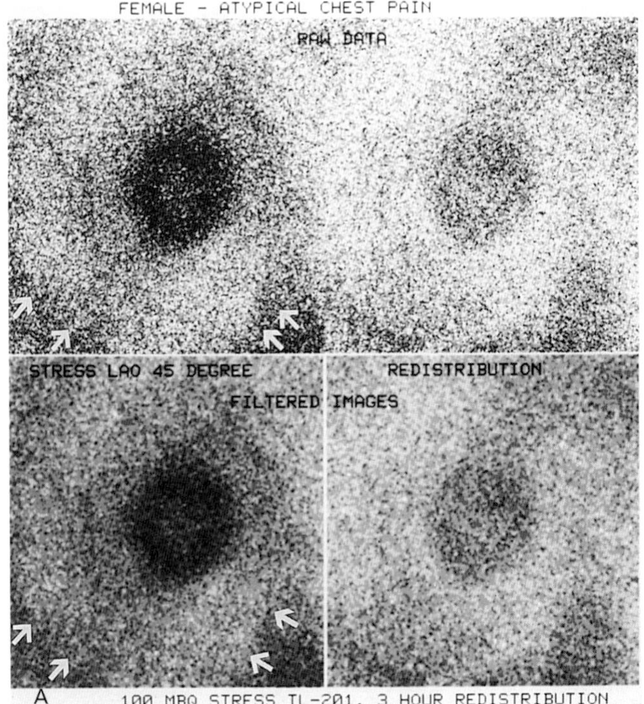

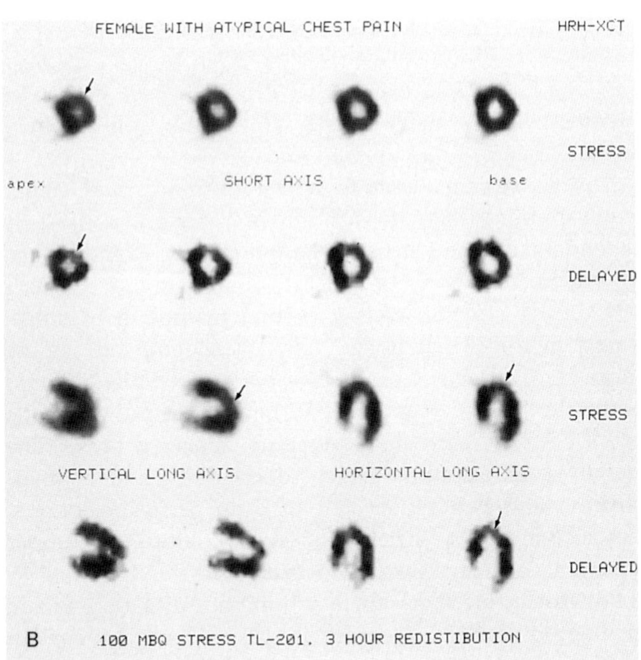

Fig. 91.11 Breast attenuation artefacts can be identified by knowledge of the patient's body habitus, review of a preliminary planar image (A) on which an attenuation shadow may be seen crossing the cardiac borders (arrows), and by the typical apicolateral distribution on SPECT imaging (B). Comparison with a normal female database will further decrease suspicion that the scintigraphic abnormality is significant.

documentation of the true nature of myocardial perfusion distribution. If in doubt, further images can be obtained with the breast outlined by radioactive markers or in differing positions.

In obese individuals, adipose tissue in the lateral thoracic wall can attenuate activity in the lateral wall.[71] Diaphragmatic attenuation of the inferior wall can also cause problems with planar imaging. This problem may also be reduced by obtaining a left lateral planar image with the patient's right side in the decubitus position.[91] Overlying visceral activity can be a problem in conditions such as diaphragmatic hernia but can usually be readily appreciated. Additional planar images can help to further characterize the distribution of myocardial perfusion tracers in the heart. In ^{99m}Tc MIBI images where activity in the liver can compromise evaluation of the inferior wall; delaying imaging to allow time for hepatobiliary clearance of activity may overcome this problem.[27]

Physiological alteration in myocardial perfusion tracer distribution may occur with left bundle branch block, which is a recognized cause of reversible perfusion abnormalities in the septum[92,93] (Fig. 91.12). Asynchrony of myocardial contraction, with impaired diastolic coronary flow during tachycardia is probably the mechanism for this abnormality. Review of the resting and stress electrocardiographs is important to recognize left bundle branch block as a potential cause of false positive imaging results. Abnormalities confined to the septum and sparing the anterior wall are more likely to be artefactual than defects also involving the anterior wall.[93] Right bundle branch block appears to be less likely to cause perfusion abnormalities,[93] although perfusion abnormalities have been described with this conduction abnormality.[94] An important cause of apparently false positive results is the presence of a coronary stenosis, which is functionally significant in terms of flow limitation while not fulfilling classic angiographic criteria for significant disease.[75,76]

Various cardiac diseases can cause perfusion abnormalities mimicking coronary artery disease. These include both dilated[23,95-98] and hypertrophic[99,100] cardiomyopathy, sarcoidosis,[101] and lymphoma.[102]

SPECT imaging artefacts

The same categories of artefacts that apply to planar imaging are also seen in SPECT studies. In addition, there are sources of artefact which are specific to tomographic imaging.

While attenuation of activity in the anterolateral wall by the left breast is common in women, such abnormalities can be identified with increased certainty on SPECT by comparing ^{201}Tl distribution on tomographic imaging with a normal database.[58,66] On qualitative analysis of tomographic slices, breast attenuation artefacts typically involve the apicolateral wall of the ventricle and are fixed

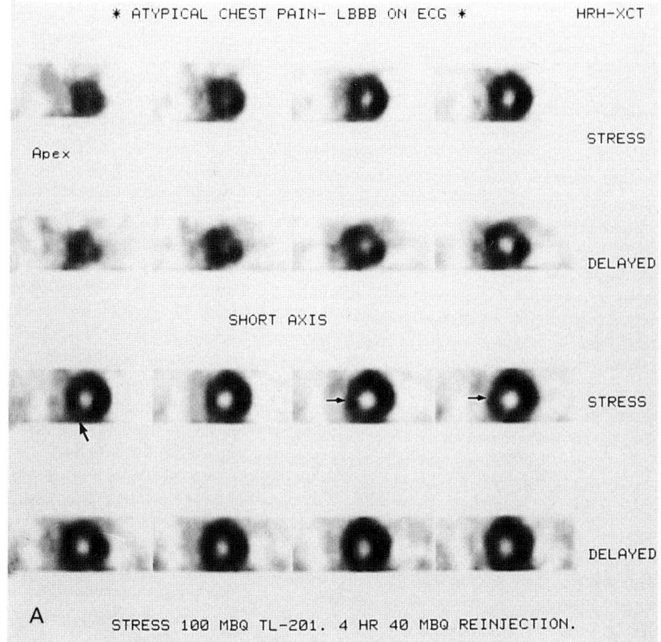

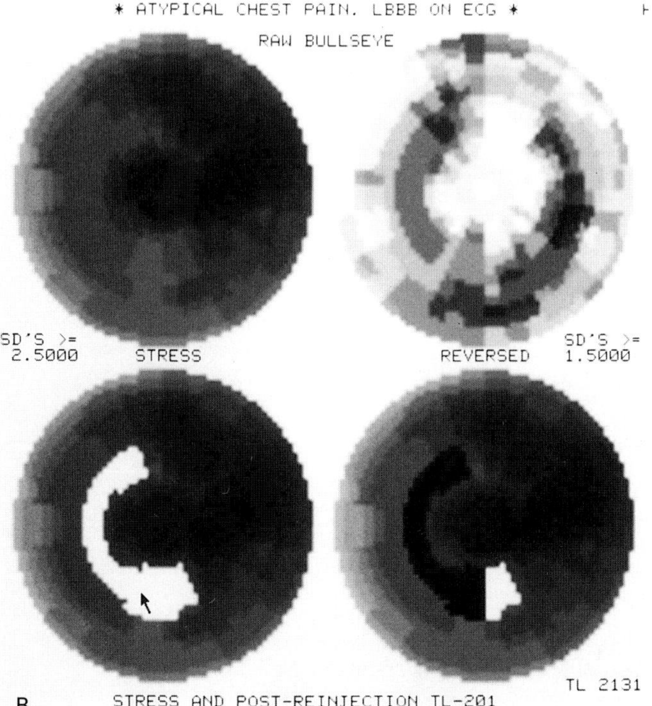

Fig. 91.12 Left bundle branch block is a recognized cause of reversible perfusion abnormalities in the septum. The SPECT study can be helpful to diagnose this artefact with extensive septal perfusion abnormality involving both the anteroseptal and inferoseptal walls but sparing the true anterior and inferior walls. This distribution is unusual with coronary disease, although 'balanced' LAD and PDA disease could create such an abnormality. (A) Short axis SPECT images, and (B) the polar maps of raw data (above left), of extent of stress abnormality (below left) and of reversibility (blackened area) (below right).

(Fig. 91.11). Since the breast moves across the heart during tomographic acquisition, review of the raw projection data may be helpful.[72] It is not uncommon for breast attenuation artefacts to be more noticeable on planar imaging than on SPECT studies due to this blurring of breast attenuation over the heart in multiple angles.

Fixed lateral wall scintigraphic abnormalities can occur in obese patients. Again, review of the medical history and resting electrocardiograph for evidence of prior infarction, and a knowledge of the patient's body habitus, are helpful in recognizing these artefacts. Liver and diaphragmatic attenuation of activity in the inferior wall are the most common causes of SPECT imaging artefacts in males.[57,66] These artefacts are seldom of clinical importance since they tend to be mild and fixed. The absence of other evidence of inferior infarction and review of the planar projection data to assess the relative relationships of the dome of the liver and the inferior wall of the left ventricle may aid the recognition of these artefacts. Prone imaging protocols[103–105] have been reported to decrease the occurrence of such abnormalities. However, even with specifically designed,cut-away imaging beds and quantitative analysis, this approach may trade defects in the inferior wall for artefacts in the anterior wall.[106] Given the clinicalimportance of disease in the left anterior coronaryartery, false positive results in this distribution, evenif mild, are more likely to lead to unnecessary coronary angiography. Thus, it is difficult to support this approach. All the attenuation artefacts discussed above could potentially be eliminated by performing measured attenuation correction using transmission studies.[53,54]

However, attenuation correction will not compensate for physiological variation in myocardial perfusion. Just as left bundle branch block is a cause of perfusion abnormalities, SPECT studies with both ^{201}Tl[107] and ^{99m}Tc MIBI[108] have demonstrated reversible septal perfusion abnormalities which are unrelated to the presence of coronary artery disease (Fig. 91.12). The lack of involvement of the anterior wall and apex despite extensive involvement of the anteroseptal and inferoseptal regions in patients with a left bundle block pattern on stress electrocardiography should provide a clue to the non-obstructive nature of this abnormality. In patients with coexistence of reversible anterior perfusion abnormality and left bundle branch block, the extent of reversible septal perfusion abnormality may not be an accurate guide to the extent of left anterior descending artery territory ischaemia.

The non-coronary cardiac diseases mentioned in the section on planar imaging artefacts also affect SPECT images. Hypertensive heart disease can alter the distribution of ^{201}Tl to create appearances which may suggest prior lateral wall myocardial infarction.[89]

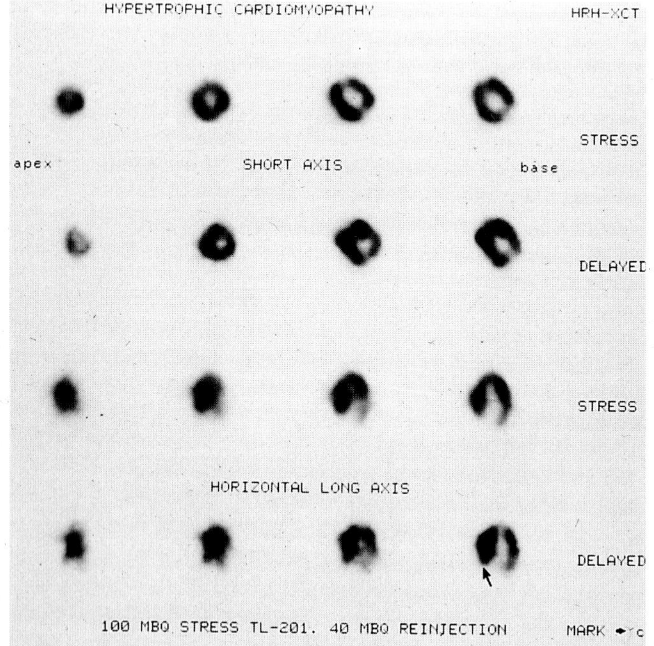

Fig. 91.13 In this patient with atypical chest pain and a family history of hypertrophic cardiomyopathy, stress SPECT images revealed an apparent inferolateral perfusion abnormality and only slight prominence of the interventricular septum. The delayed images demonstrated marked septal uptake. The lower septal uptake during stress can reflect relative ischaemia of the interventricular septum which may be an important mechanism in the subsequent development of left ventricular dysfunction.

Review of the medical history and electrocardiograph will facilitate recognition of this artefact. Hypertrophic cardiomyopathy creates unusual SPECT appearances[100] (Fig. 91.13).

The imaging artefacts which are specific to SPECT include patient and cardiac motion during the study,[109–112] and reconstruction errors related to incorrect assignment of the cardiac axis, centre-of-rotation malalignment, or flood field non-uniformity.[72] 'Hot spot' artefacts are also peculiar to SPECT imaging (Fig. 91.14). Although the cause of these abnormalities is not clearly defined, it may relate to the variable point-spread function of activity depending on the distance from the centre of rotation of SPECT acquisition.[48]

'Upward creep' of the heart due to a decreasing respiratory excursion of the heart after exercise stress is a common cause of artefacts in the inferior and inferoseptal walls of the left ventricle if imaging is commenced too soon after exercise.[111] A delay in the commencement of SPECT acquisition can be constructively utilized to acquire a planar image to assess left ventricular size and lung uptake, which are important prognostic indicators.[79,80,113,114] A preliminary planar image can also provide a useful correlative image to compare with the SPECT data in differentiating between attenuation

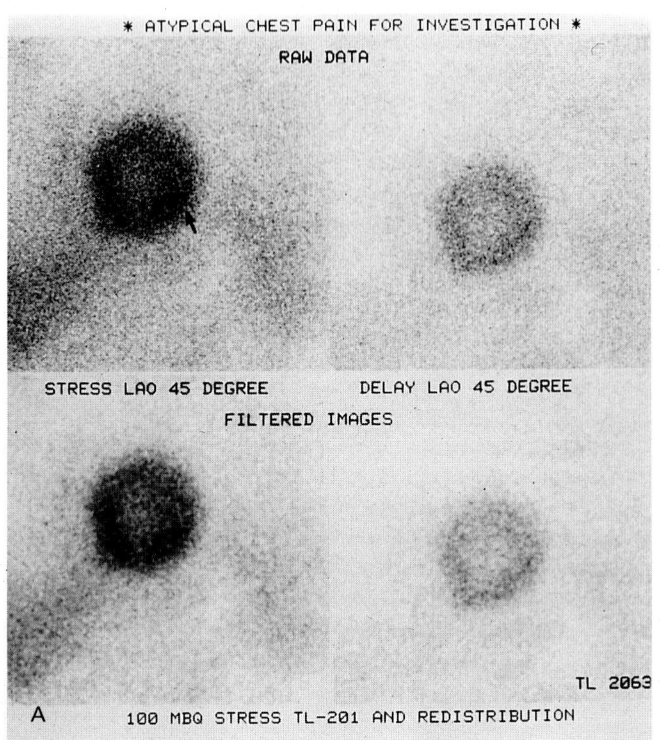

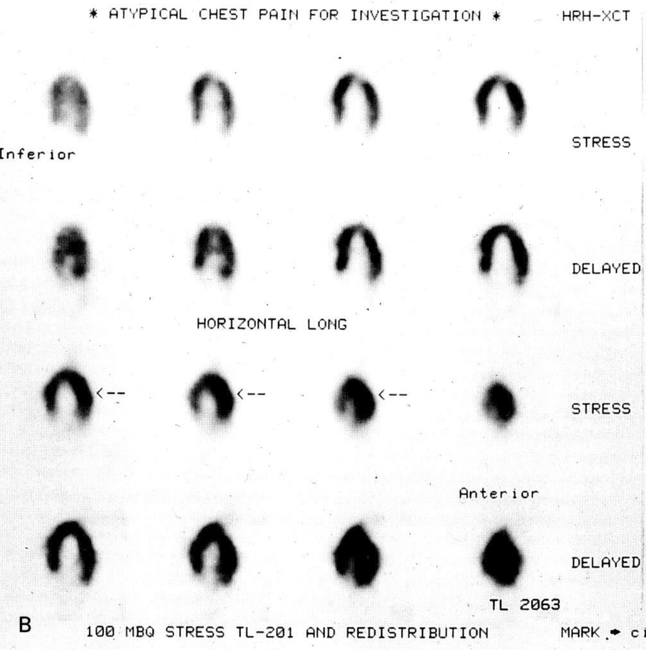

Fig. 91.14 Lateral wall 'hot spot' artefacts may give the false impression of widespread perfusion abnormalities. Lack of other objective evidence of ischaemia should aid in recognition of the phenomenon. In this example the planar image revealed no significant abnormality, but the SPECT images had an apparent perfusion abnormality in the interventricular septum due to rescaling on the lateral 'hot spot' (arrow).

artefacts and true perfusion defects. Although there may be theoretical concerns regarding a delay in commencing SPECT imaging,[115] important diagnostic and prognostic information is being acquired during the planar study[113,114] and any defect that would redistribute in the time taken to acquire the planar study would have been likely to redistribute significantly during SPECT acquisition also. Early redistribution would also appear to be relatively unlikely to occur with significantly flow-limiting coronary disease.[116]

Movement of the heart during SPECT acquisition can also create significant artefacts. Various approaches have been applied to the detection and correction of such movements.[109,110,117] None of these programs can hope to compensate completely for the complex translational and rotational reorientation of the heart that can occur in some patient movements. Time taken to ensure patient comfort and to limit imaging time to that required to obtain an adequate study will minimize the likelihood of patient movement during the study. Misalignment of the cardiac axis can create significant artefactual abnormalities on polar coordinate maps (Fig. 91.3). These can be detected by simple review of the tomographic slices and reconstruction axes. Centre-of-rotation and flood non-uniformity should not occur with appropriate quality control. Centre-of-rotation artefacts extend through the myocardium as linear defects with misalignment of opposing walls being most apparent on the long axis images. On polar maps, such artefacts appear as comma-shaped defects.[72] Flood field non-uniformity can create ring-artefacts, although these are often difficult to perceive amongst the noise intrinsic to myocardial perfusion tomograms.

Quality control

A detailed discussion of the multiple levels of quality control which are necessary for optimum diagnostic performance of myocardial perfusion scintigraphy is beyond the scope of this chapter. However, it should involve all levels of the study from adequate clinical appraisal of the patient prior to study, through maintenance of detector performance by regular centre-of-rotation calibration and flood uniformity analysis, to review of the reconstruction parameters used in each individual patient. Factors as seemingly inconsequential as grey-scale selection or film processing variation can degrade the diagnostic information available.

CONCLUSION

Myocardial perfusion scintigraphy has become a powerful diagnostic tool in clinical cardiology. To extract the multiple levels of information that are available from this modality, attention to detail and planning are required to design the test to suit the clinical problem and to obtain the most accurate data possible.

REFERENCES

1. Taillefer R, Laflamme L, Dupras G, Picard M, Phaneuf D C, Leveille J 1988 Myocardial perfusion imaging with 99mTc-methoxy-isobutyl-isonitrile (MIBI): comparison of short and long time intervals between rest and stress injections. Preliminary results. Eur J Nucl Med 13: 515–522
2. Kahn J K, McGhie I, Akers M S et al 1989 Quantitative rotational tomography with 201Tl and 99mTc 2-methoxy-isobutyl-isonitrile. A direct comparison in normal individuals and patients with coronary artery disease. Circulation 79: 1282–1293
3. Taillefer R, Lambert R, Dupra S G et al 1989 Clinical comparison between thallium-201 and Tc-99m-methoxy isobutyl-isonitrile (hexamibi) myocardial perfusion imaging for detection of coronary artery disease. Eur J Nucl Med 15: 280–286
4. Kiat H, Maddahi J, Roy L T et al 1989 Comparison of technetium 99m methoxy isobutyl isonitrile and thallium 201 for evaluation of coronary artery disease by planar and tomographic methods. Am Heart J 117: 1–11
5. Seldin D W, Johnson L L, Blood D K et al 1989 Myocardial perfusion imaging with technetium-99m SQ30217: comparison with thallium-201 and coronary anatomy. J Nucl Med 30: 312–319
6. Iskandrian A S, Heo J, Kong B, Lyons E, Marsch S 1989 Use of technetium-99m isonitrile (RP-30A) in assessing left ventricular perfusion and function at rest and during exercise in coronary artery disease, and comparison with coronary arteriography and exercise thallium-201 SPECT imaging. Am J Cardiol 64: 270–275
7. Cuocolo A, Pace L, Ricciardelli B, Chiariello M, Trimarco B, Salvatore M 1992 Identification of viable myocardium in patients with chronic coronary artery disease – Comparison of thallium-201 scintigraphy with reinjection and technetium-99m-methoxyisobutyl isonitrile. J Nucl Med 33: 505–511
8. Oshima M, Ishihara M, Sano H et al 1992 Comparison of thallium-201 and technetium-99m teboroxime myocardial single photon emission tomography with coronary arteriography. Eur J Nucl Med 19: 522–526
9. Taillefer R, Lambert R, Essiambre R, Phaneuf D C, Leveille J 1992 Comparison between thallium-201, technetium-99m-sestamibi and technetium-99m-teboroxime planar myocardial perfusion imaging in detection of coronary artery disease. J Nucl Med 33: 1091–1098
10. Serafini A N, Topchik S, Jimenez H, Friden A, Ganz W I, Sfakianakis G N 1992 Clinical comparison of technetium-99m-teboroxime and thallium-201 utilizing a continuous SPECT imaging protocol. J Nucl Med 33: 1304–1311
11. Bonow R O, Dilsizian V 1992 Assessing viable myocardium with thallium-201. Am J Cardiol 70: E10–E17
12. Maublant J C, Lipiecki J, Citron B et al 1993 Reinjection as an alternative to rest imaging for detection of exercise-induced ischemia with thallium-201 emission tomography. Am Heart J 125: 330–335
13. Wackers F J T 1992 Comparison of Thallium-201 and Technetium-99m Methoxyisobutyl Isonitrile. Am J Cardiol 70: E30–E34
14. Leppo J A, Meerdink D J 1989 Comparison of the myocardial uptake of a technetium-labeled isonitrile analogue and thallium. Circ Res 65: 632–639
15. Marshall R C, Leidholdt E M J, Zhang D-Y, Barnett C A 1990 Technetium-99m hexakis 2-methoxy-2-isobutyl isonitrile and

thallium-201 extraction, washout and retention at varying flow rates in rabbit heart. Circulation 82: 998–1007
16. Allman K C, Berry J, Sucharski L A et al 1992 Determination of extent and location of coronary artery disease in patients without prior myocardial infarction by thallium-201 tomography with pharmacologic stress. J Nucl Med 33: 2067–2073
17. Weinstein H, Dahlberg S T, McSherry B A, Hendel R C, Leppo J A 1993 Rapid redistribution of teboroxime. Am J Cardiol 71: 848–852
18. O'Connor M K, Cho D S 1992 Rapid radiotracer washout from the heart – effect on image quality in SPECT performed with a single-headed gamma-camera system. J Nucl Med 33: 1146–1151
19. Williams K A, Taillon L A, Draho J M, Foisy M F 1993 First-pass radionuclide angiographic studies of left ventricular function with technetium-99m-teboroxime, technetium-99m-sestamibi and technetium-99m-DTPA. J Nucl Med 34: 394–399
20. Worsley D F, Fung A Y, Coupland D B, Rexworthy C G, Sexsmith G P, Lentle B C 1992 Comparison of stress-only vs stress/rest with technetium-99m methoxyisobutylisonitrile myocardial perfusion imaging. Eur J Nucl Med 19: 441–444
21. Berger B C, Watson D D, Burwell L R et al 1979 Redistribution of thallium at rest in patients with stable and unstable angina and the effect of coronary artery bypass graft surgery. Circulation 60: 1114–1125
22. Gerwirtz H, Beller G A, Strauss H W et al 1979 Transient defects of resting thallium scans in patients with coronary artery disease. Circulation 59: 707–713
23. Iskandrian A S, Hakki A-H, Kane A S 1986 Resting thallium-201 myocardial perfusion patterns in patients with severe left ventricular dysfunction: differences between patients with primary cardiomyopathy, chronic coronary artery disease, or acute myocardial infarction. Am Heart J 111: 760–767
24. Berman D S, Kiat H, Wang F P et al 1992 Separate rest thallium-201/stress technetium-99m sestamibi dual isotope myocardial perfusion SPECT: results of a larger clinical trial. (Abstract). J Am Coll Cardiol 19
25. Taillefer R, Dupras G, Sporn V et al 1989 Myocardial perfusion imaging with a new radiotracer, technetium-99m-hexamibi (methoxy isobutyl isonitrile): comparison with thallium-201 imaging. Clin Nucl Med 14: 89–96
26. Mousa S A, Cooney J M, Stevens S 1992 Kinetics of technetium-99m-sestamibi and thallium-201 in a transient ischemic myocardium animal model – insight into the redistribution phenomenon. Cardiology 81: 157–163
27. Wackers F J, Berman D S, Maddahi J et al 1989 Technetium-99m hexakis 2-methoxyisobutyl isonitrile: human biodistribution, dosimetry, safety, and preliminary comparison to thallium-201 for myocardial perfusion imaging. J Nucl Med 30: 301–311
28. Sporn V, Perez Balino N, Holman B L et al 1988 Simultaneous measurement of ventricular function and myocardial perfusion using the technetium-99m isonitriles. Clin Nucl Med 13: 77–81
29. Baillet G Y, Mena I G, Kuperus J H, Robertson J M, French W J 1989 Simultaneous technetium-99m-MIBI angiography and myocardial perfusion imaging. J Nucl Med 30: 38–44
30. Larock M P, Cantineau R, Legrand V, Kulbertus H, Rigo P 1990 Technetium-99m-MIBI (RP30) to define the extent of myocardial ischemia and evaluate ventricular function. Eur J Nucl Med 16: 223–230
31. Jones R H, Borges-Neto S, Potts J M 1990 Simultaneous measurement of myocardial perfusion and ventricular function during exercise from a single injection of ^{99m}Tc-sestamibi in coronary artery disease. Am J Cardiol 66: 68E–71E
32. Boucher C A, Wackers F J, Zaret B L, Mena I G 1992 Technetium-99m sestamibi myocardial imaging at rest for assessment of myocardial infarction and first-pass ejection fraction. Multicenter Cardiolite Study Group. Am J Cardiol 69: 22–27
33. Pace L, Betocchi S, Piscione F, Stefano M L M D, Chiariello M, Salvatore M 1993 Evaluation of myocardial perfusion and function by technetium-99m methoxy isobutyl isonitrile before and after percutaneous transluminal coronary angioplasty – preliminary results. Clin Nucl Med 18: 286–290
34. Gray W A, Gerwirtz H 1991 Comparison of 99mTc-teboroxime with thallium for myocardial imaging in the presence of a coronary stenosis. Circulation 84: 1796–1807
35. Hendel R C, McSherry B, Karimeddini M, Leppo J A 1990 Diagnostic value of a new myocardial perfusion agent, teboroxime (SQ30217), utilizing a rapid planar imaging protocol; preliminary results. J Am Coll Cardiol 16: 855–861
36. Maublant J, Cassagnes J, Le Jeune J J et al 1982 A comparison between conventional scintigraphy and emission tomography with thallium-201 in the detection of myocardial infarction: concise communication. J Nucl Med 23: 204–208
37. Ritchie J L, Williams D L, Harp G, Stratton J L, Caldwell J H 1982 Transaxial tomography with thallium-201 detecting remote myocardial infarction. Comparison with planar imaging. Am J Cardiol 50: 1236–1241
38. Tamaki S, Nakajima H, Murakami T et al 1982 Estimation of infarct size by myocardial emission computed tomography with thallium-201 and its relation to creatine kinase-MB release after myocardial infarction in man. Circulation 66: 994–1001
39. Kirsch C M, Doliwa R, Buell U, Roedler D 1983 Detection of severe coronary heart disease with Tl-201: comparison of resting single photon emission tomography with invasive arteriography. J Nucl Med 24: 761–767
40. Nohara R, Kambara H, Suzuki Y et al 1984 Stress scintigraphy using single-photon emission computed tomography in the evaluation of coronary artery disease. Am J Cardiol 53: 1250–1254
41. Kaul S 1989 A look at 15 years of planar thallium-201 imaging. Am Heart J 118: 581–601
42. Mahmarian J J, Verani M S 1991 Exercise thallium-201 perfusion scintigraphy in the assessment of ischemic heart disease. Am J Cardiol 67: 2D–11D
43. Fintel D J, Links, Brinker J A, Frank T L, Parker M, Becker L C 1989 Improved diagnostic performance of exercise thallium-201 single photon emission computed tomography over planar imaging in the diagnosis of coronary artery disease: A receiver operating characteristic analysis. J Am Coll Cardiol 13: 600–612
44. Pamelia F X, Gibson R S, Watson D D, Craddock G B, Sirowatka J, Beller G A 1985 Prognosis with chest pain and normal thallium-201 exercise scintigrams. Am J Cardiol 55: 920–926
45. Wackers F J, Russo D S, Russo D, Clements J P 1985 Prognostic significance of normal qualitative planar thallium-201 stress scintigraphy in patients with chest pain. J Am Coll Cardiol 6: 27–32
46. Brown K A, Rowen M 1993 Prognostic value of a normal exercise myocardial perfusion imaging study in patients with angiographically significant coronary artery disease. Am J Cardiol 71: 865–867
47. Ladenheim M L, Pollock B H, Rozanski A et al 1986 Extent and severity of myocardial hypoperfusion as predictors of prognosis in patients with suspected coronary artery disease. J Am Coll Cardiol 7: 464–471
48. Eisner R L, Nowak D J, Pettigrew R, Fajman W 1986 Fundamentals of 180 degree acquisition and reconstruction in SPECT imaging. J Nucl Med 27: 1717–1728
49. Coleman R E, Jaszczak R J, Cobb F R 1982 Comparison of 180° and 360° data collection in thallium-201 imaging using single-photon emission computerized tomography (SPECT): concise communication. J Nucl Med 23: 655–660
50. Tamaki N, Mukai T, Ishii Y et al 1982 Comparative study of thallium emission myocardial tomography with 180° and 360° data collection. J Nucl Med 23: 661–666
51. Go R T, MacIntyre W J, Houser T S et al 1985 Clinical evaluation of 360 degrees and 180 degrees data sampling techniques for transaxial SPECT thallium-201 myocardial perfusion imaging. J Nucl Med 26: 695–706
52. Hoffman E J 1982 180° compared with 360° sampling in SPECT. J Nucl Med 23: 745–747
53. Tsui B M, Gullberg G T, Edgerton E R et al 1989 Correction of nonuniform attenuation in cardiac SPECT imaging. J Nucl Med 30: 497–507
54. Bailey D L, Hutton B F, Walker P J 1987 Improved SPECT using

simultaneous emission and transmission tomography. J Nucl Med 28: 844–851
55. Maublant J C, Peycelon P, Kwiatkowski F, Lusson J-R, Stanke R H, Veyre R 1989 Comparison between 180° and 360° data collection in technetium-99m MIBI SPECT of the myocardium. J Nucl Med 30: 295–300
56. Clausen M, Bice A N, Civelek A C, Hutchins G M, Wagner H N J 1986 Circumferential wall thickness measurements of the human left ventricle: reference data for thallium-201 single-photon emission computed tomography. Am J Cardiol 58: 827–831
57. Eisner R L, Tamas M J, Cloninger K et al 1988 Normal SPECT thallium-201 bull's-eye display: gender differences. J Nucl Med 29: 1901–1909
58. Goris M L, Daspit S G, McLaughlin P, Kriss J P 1976 Interpolative background subtraction. J Nucl Med 17: 744–747
59. Burow R D, Pond M, Schefer A W, Becker L 1979 'Circumferential profile': a new method for computer analysis of thallium-201 myocardial perfusion images. J Nucl Med 20: 771–777
60. Wackers F J T, Bodenheimer M, Fleiss J L, Brown M 1993 Factors affecting uniformity in interpretation of planar thallium-201 imaging in a multicenter trial. J Am Coll Cardiol 21: 1064–1074
61. Kaul S, Chesler D A, Okada R D, Boucher C A 1987 Computer versus visual analysis of exercise thallium-201: a critical analysis in 325 patients with chest pain. Am Heart J 114: 1129–1137
62. Caldwell J H, Williams D L, Harp G D, Stratton J R, Ritchie J L 1984 Quantitation of size of relative myocardial perfusion defect by single-photon emission computed tomography. Circulation 70: 1048–1056
63. Garcia E V, Van Train K, Maddahi J et al 1985 Quantification of rotational thallium-201 myocardial tomography. J Nucl Med 26: 17–26
64. Van Train K, Maddahi J, Berman D S et al 1990 Quantitative analysis of tomographic stress thallium-201 myocardial scintigrams: a mulitcenter trial. J Nucl Med 31: 1168–1179
65. Maddahi J, van Train K, Pringent F et al 1989 Quantitative single photon emission computed tomography for detection and localization of coronary artery disease: optimization and prospective validation of a new technique. J Am Coll Cardiol 14: 1489–1499
66. DePasquale E H, Nody A C, DePuey E G et al 1988 Quantitative rotational thallium-201 tomography for identifying and localizing coronary artery disease. Circulation 77: 316–327
67. Melin J A, Piret L J, Vanbutsele R J M et al 1981 Diagnostic value of exercise electrocardiography and thallium myocardial scintigraphy in patients without prior myocardial infarction: a Bayesian approach. Circulation 5: 1019–1024
68. Melin J A, Wijns W, Vanbutsele R J et al 1985 Alternative strategies for coronary artery disease in women; demonstration of the usefulness and efficiency of probability analysis. Circulation 3: 535–542
69. Iskandrian A S, Heo J, Kong B, Lyons E 1989 Effect of exercise level on the ability of thallium-201 tomographic imaging in detecting coronary artery disease: analysis of 461 patients. J Am Coll Cardiol 14: 1477–1486
70. Fagan L F, Shaw L, Kong B A, Caralis D G, Wiens R D, Chaitman B R 1992 Prognostic value of exercise thallium scintigraphy in patients with good exercise tolerance and a normal or abnormal exercise electrocardiogram and suspected or confirmed coronary artery disease. Am J Cardiol 69: 607–611
71. Dunn R F, Wolff L, Wagner S, Botvinick E H 1981 The inconsistent pattern of thallium defects: a clue to the false positive perfusion scintigram. Am J Cardiol 48: 224–232
72. DePuey E G, Garcia E V 1989 Optimal specificity of thallium-201 SPECT through recognition of imaging artifacts. J Nucl Med 30: 441–449
73. Ritchie J L, Albro P J, Caldwell J H, Trobaugh G B, Hamilton G W 1979 Thallium-201 myocardial imaging: a comparison of the redistribution and rest images. J Nucl Med 20: 477–483
74. Wainwright R J 1981 Scintigraphic anatomy of coronary artery disease in digital thallium-201 myocardial images. Br Heart J 46: 465–477
75. Kalff V, Kelly M J, Soward A et al 1985 Assessment of the haemodynamic significance of isolated stenoses of the left anterior descending coronary artery using thallium-201 myocardial scintigraphy. Am J Cardiol 55: 342–347
76. Wijns W, Serruys P W, Reiber J H C et al 1985 Quantitative angiography of the left anterior descending coronary artery; correlations with pressure gradient and results of exercise thallium scintigraphy. Circulation 71: 273–279
77. Chouraqui P, Rodrigues E A, Berman D S, Maddahi J 1990 Significance of dipyridamole-induced transient dilation of the left ventricle during thallium-201 scintigraphy in suspected coronary artery disease. Am J Cardiol 66: 689–694
78. Boucher C A, Zir L M, Beller G A et al 1980 Increased lung uptake of thallium-201 during exercise myocardial imaging: clinical hemodynamic and angiographic implications in patients with coronary artery disease. Am J Cardiol 46: 189–196
79. Gill J B, Ruddy T D, Newell J B, Finkelstein D M, Strauss H W, Boucher C A 1987 Prognostic importance of Tl uptake by the lungs during exercise in coronary artery disease. N Engl J Med 317: 1485–1489
80. Jain D, Lahiri A, Raferty E B 1990 Clinical and prognostic significance of lung thallium uptake on resting imaging in acute myocardial infarction. Am J Cardiol 65: 154–159
81. Christian T F, Miller T D, Bailey K R, Gibbons R J 1992 Noninvasive identification of severe coronary artery disease using exercise tomographic thallium-201 imaging. Am J Cardiol 70: 14–20
82. Pieri P, McKusick K A, Fischman A J, Alpert N, Bopugas C, Strauss H W 1993 Characterization of the thallium image. J Nucl Med 34: 879–884
83. Eagle K A, Boucher C A 1989 Cardiac risk of noncardiac surgery. N Engl J Nucl Med 321: 1330–1332
84. Brown K A 1991 Prognostic value of thallium-201 myocardial perfusion imaging: a diagnostic tool comes of age. Circulation 83: 363–381
85. Blackburn T, Beller G 1992 Scintigraphic assessment of myocardial perfusion using thallium-201 and technetium-99m imaging. Coronary Artery Dis 3: 274–280
86. Brown K A 1992 Prognostic value of thallium-201 myocardial perfusion imaging in three primary patient populations. Am J Cardiol 70: E23–E29
87. Travin M I, Boucher C A, Newell J B, Laraia P J, Flores A R, Eagle K A 1993 Variables associated with a poor prognosis in patients with an ischemic thallium-201 exercise test. Am Heart J 125: 335–344
88. Kahn J K, Carry M M, McGhie I, Pippin J J, Akers M S, Corbett J R 1989 Quantitation of postexercise lung thallium-201 uptake during single photon emission computed tomography. J Nucl Med 30: 288–294
89. DePuey E G, Guertler-Krawczynska E, Perkins J V, Robbins W L, Whelchel J D, Clements S D 1988 Alterations in myocardial thallium-201 distribution in patients with chronic systemic hypertension undergoing single-photon emission computed tomography. Am J Cardiol 62: 234–238
90. Desmarais R L, Kaul S, Watson D D, Beller G A 1993 Do false positive thallium-201 scans lead to unnecessary catheterization? – outcome of patients with perfusion defects on quantitative planar thallium-201 scintigraphy. J Am Coll Cardiol 21: 1058–1063
91. Johnstone D E, Wackers F J T, Berger H J et al 1979 Effect of patient positioning on left lateral thallium-201 myocardial images. J Nucl Med 20: 183–188
92. Hirzel H O, Senn M, Buttner C, Pfeiffer A, Hess O M, Krayenbuhl H P 1984 Thallium-201 scintigraphy in complete left bundle branch block. Am J Cardiol 53: 764–769
93. Delonca J, Camenzind E, Meier B, Righetti A 1992 Limits of thallium-201 exercise scintigraphy to detect coronary disease in patients with complete and permanent bundle branch block – a review of 134 cases. Am Heart J 123: 1201–1207
94. Shih W J, Berk M R, Mills B J A 1992 Reversible thallium-201 perfusion defects of the septal and inferoapical segments in a patient with incomplete right bundle branch block and normal coronary angiogram. J Nucl Med 33: 1556–1557

95. Dunn R F, Uren R F, Sadick N et al 1982 Comparison of thallium-201 scanning in idiopathic dilated cardiomyopathy and severe coronary artery disease. Circulation 66: 804–810
96. Juilliere Y, Gillet C, Danchin N et al 1990 Abstention from alcohol in dilated cardiomyopathy: complete regression of clinical disease but persistence of myocardial perfusion defects on exercise thallium-201 tomography. Eur J Nucl Med 15: 279–281
97. Chikamori T, Doi Y L, Yonezawa Y, Yamada M, Seo H, Ozawa T 1992 Value of dipyridamole thallium-201 imaging in noninvasive differentiation of idiopathic dilated cardiomyopathy from coronary artery disease with left ventricular dysfunction. Am J Cardiol 69: 650–653
98. Tamura T, Shibuya N, Hashiba K, Oku Y, Mori H, Yano K 1993 Evaluation of myocardial damage in Duchenne's muscular dystrophy with thallium-201 myocardial SPECT. Jpn Heart J 34: 51–61
99. Sakuma H, Takeda K, Tagami T et al 1993 P-31 MR spectroscopy in hypertrophic cardiomyopathy – comparison with Tl-201 myocardial perfusion imaging. Am Heart J 125: 1323–1328
100. Nishimura T 1993 Approaches to identify and characterise hypertrophic myocardium. J Nucl Med 34: 1013–1019
101. Makler P T, Lavine S J, Denenberg B S, Bove A A, Idell S 1981 Redistribution on the thallium scan in myocardial sarcoidosis: Concise communication. J Nucl Med 22: 428–432
102. McDonnel T J, Becker L C, Bulkley B H 1981 Thallium imaging in cardiac lymphoma. Am Heart J 101: 809–814
103. Segall G M, Davis M J, Goris M L 1988 Improved specificity of prone versus supine thallium SPECT imaging. Clin Nucl Med 13: 915–916
104. Esquerre J P, Coca F C, Martinez S J, Guirand R F 1989 Prone decubitus: a solution to inferior wall attenuation in thallium-201 myocardial tomography. J Nucl Med 30: 398–401
105. Segall G M, Davis M J 1989 Prone versus supine thallium myocardial SPECT: a method to decrease artifactual inferior wall defects. J Nucl Med 30: 548–555
106. Kiat H, van Train K F, Friedman J D et al 1992 Quantitative stress-redistribution thallium-201 SPECT using prone imaging – methodologic development and validation. J Nucl Med 33: 1509–1515
107. DePuey E G, Guertler-Krawczynska E, Robbins W L 1988 Thallium-201 SPECT in coronary artery disease patients with left bundle branch block. J Nucl Med 29: 1479–1485
108. Knapp W H, Bentrup A, Schmidt U, Ohlmeier H 1993 Myocardial scintigraphy with thallium-201 and technetium-99m-hexakis-methoxyisobutylisonitrile in left bundle branch block – a study in patients with and without coronary artery disease. Eur J Nucl Med 20: 219–224
109. Eisner R, Churchwell A, Noever T et al 1988 Quantitative analysis of the tomographic thallium-201 myocardial bullseye display: critical role of correcting for patient motion. J Nucl Med 29: 91–97
110. Friedman J, Berman D S, Van Train K et al 1988 Patient motion in thallium-201 myocardial SPECT imaging. An easily identified frequent source of artifactual defect. Clin Nucl Med 13: 321–324
111. Friedman J, Van Train K, Maddahi J et al 1989 'Upward creep' of the heart: a frequent source of false-positive reversible defects during thallium-201 stress-redistribution SPECT. J Nucl Med 30: 1718–1722
112. Eisner R L, Aaron A M, Worthy M R et al 1993 Apparent change in cardiac geometry during single-photon emission tomography thallium-201 acquisition – a complex phenomenon. Eur J Nucl Med 20: 324–329
113. Miller D D, Kaul S, Strauss H W, Okada R D, Boucher C A 1988 Increased exercise thallium-201 lung uptake: a prognostic index n two-vessel coronary artery disease. Can J Cardiol 4: 270–276
114. Al-Khwaja I, Lahiri A, Rodrigues E A, Heber M E, Raferty E B 1988 Clinical significance of exercise-induced pulmonary uptake of thallium-201 in uncomplicated myocardial infarction. Am J Cardiac Imaging 2: 135–141
115. Rothendler J A, Okada R D, Wilson R A et al 1985 Effect of a delay in commencing imaging on the ability to detect transient thallium defects. J Nucl Med 26: 880–883
116. Gutman J, Berman D S, Freeman M, Rozanski A, Swan H J C 1983 Time to completed redistribution of thallium-201 in exercise myocardial scintigraphy: relationship to the degree of coronary artery stenosis. Am Heart J 106: 989–995
117. Geckle W J, Frank T L, Links J M, Becker L C 1988 Correction for patient and organ movement in SPECT: application to exercise thallium-201 cardiac imaging. J Nucl Med 29: 441–450
118. Taillefer R, Lambert R, Dupras G et al 1989 Clinical comparison between thallium-201 and Tc-99m-methoxy isobutyl isonitrile (hexamibi) myocardial perfusion imaging for detection of coronary artery disease. Eur J Nucl Med 15: 280–286

92. Positron emission tomography

Paolo G. Camici   Terence J. Spinks

INTRODUCTION

The great potential of positron emission tomography (PET) to elucidate tissue function is reflected in the increasing number of centres being established. Not only does the technique offer greater accuracy in the measurement of regional radioactivity concentration but it also enables the use of true biological tracers. PET is still seen as an expensive tool, principally because of the need of a cyclotron to produce the short-lived isotopes. However, much development has been carried out in recent years into compact, self-shielding cyclotrons which do not need a team of engineers for their maintenance. In addition, automated kits for the production of commonly used tracers are now available. In some cases, central cyclotron facilities are being installed to distribute tracers (principally ^{18}F-labelled compounds) to nearby centres. Parallel innovations in tomographic scanner design continue to blossom. These are providing greater efficiency of photon detection and improved image resolution. New detector and electronic designs are bringing with them greater reliability.

There has been much discussion about the dual roles of 'research' and 'clinical' PET.[1] A number of centres, particularly in the United States, have installed PET systems purely for clinical diagnosis, mainly in the determination of myocardial viability but also for applications in oncology and neurology. Diagnostic testing of this kind is clearly derived from original work carried out at research establishments. The terms 'research' and 'clinical' should therefore be regarded as complementary. PET centres devoted to medical research will, by their very nature, not become widespread. They rely on close connection with clinicial research institutes and the collaboration between clinicians, radiochemists, tracer modellers, physicists and radiographers. Naturally, this will be an expensive undertaking, but the survival of such centres and, just as importantly, collaboration between them, is vital for the survival of PET in general. This chapter deals with current trends in instrumentation and advances in myocardial PET research.

COINCIDENCE DETECTION

Positrons (positively-charged electrons) are emitted from atoms which are unstable because their proton/neutron ratio is 'too high'. For example, ^{15}O, in releasing a positron, turns into stable ^{15}N:

$$^{15}\text{O} \longrightarrow \beta^{+} + {}^{15}\text{N}$$

(8 protons 7 neutrons)   (positron)   (7 protons 8 neutrons)

The 'anti-matter' positron cannot exist for long. Within a mm or so in tissue the positron collides with an electron resulting in the disappearance (annihilation) of both and the emission of two gamma-rays in opposite directions. The energy of each gamma-ray is 511 keV (the same for all positrons) and the 'back-to-back' emission is a result of conservation of momentum, which is zero or close to zero for the electron–positron pair just before annihilation. These properties greatly facilitate the accurate measurement of positron-emitting tracer distribution within the body. The gamma-rays must be detected in a certain way, known as coincidence detection.[2] Detectors are placed on opposite sides of the body [Fig. 92.1(a)] and a 'count' is only registered when interactions are recorded simultaneously in the two detectors. Figure 92.1(a) shows the two gamma-rays being emitted from an annihilation (A) within the myocardium. The term 'simultaneous' is, of course, not strictly correct because of the finite speed of response of the detectors. Current systems operate with a 'time window' of ~ 12×10^{-9} s (or 12 ns). Coincidence detection provides a natural collimation of the emitted radiation (often termed electronic collimation) because it has directional information. In contrast, with tracers that only emit one gamma-ray per disintegration (single photon), lead collimation in front of the detectors is needed to give the directional information and hence improve resolution. This in turn reduces efficiency relative to coincidence detection.

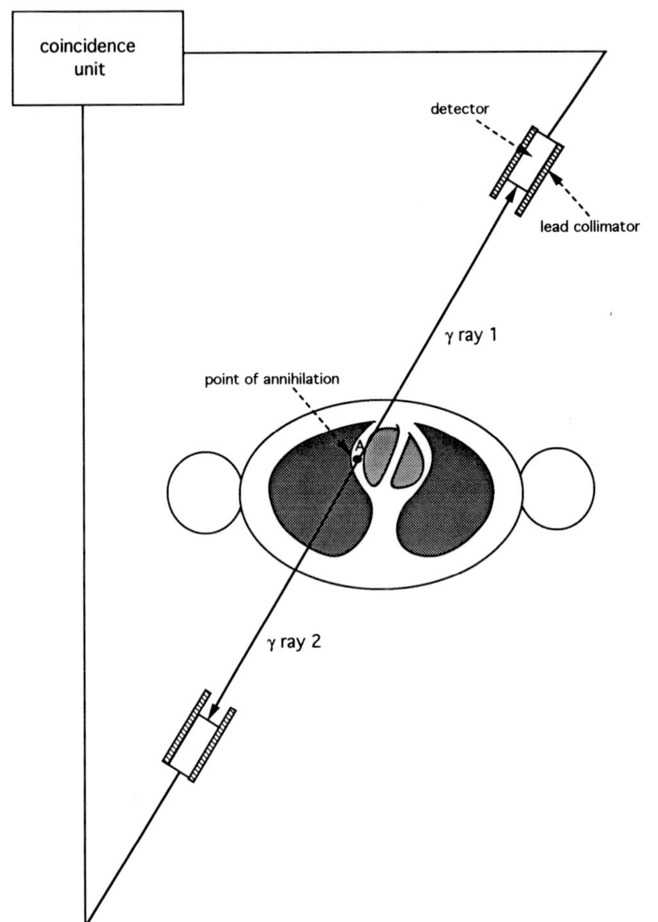

Fig. 92.1a Scheme for coincidence detection of annihilation gamma-rays from positron decay (at point A). Typical time window is 12 ns.

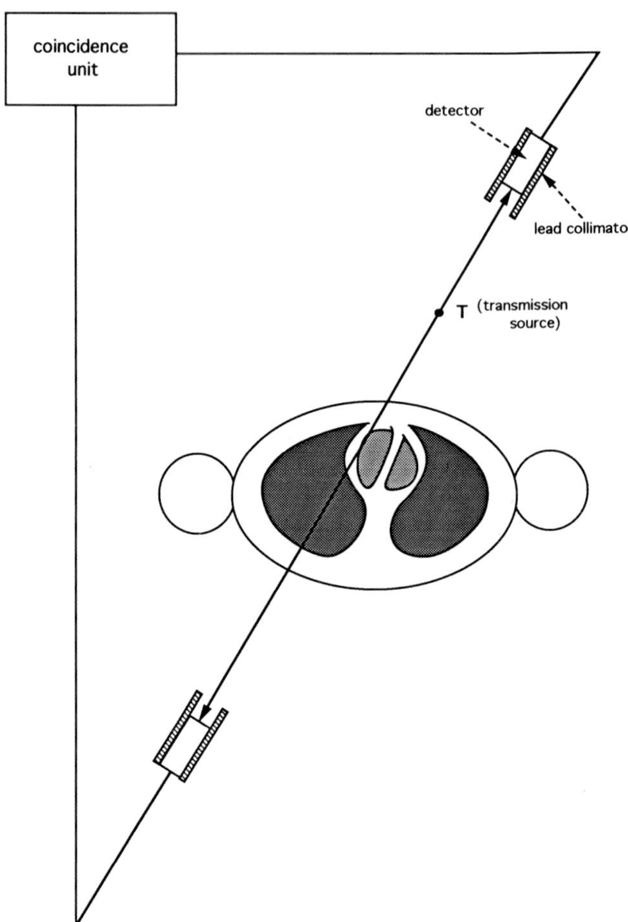

Fig. 92.1b Scheme for attenuation correction using an external transmission source (T) usually ^{68}Ge. This can take the form of ring sources or rotating rod sources.

When a coincidence event occurs as in Figure 92.1(a) the device assumes that the annihilation event took place somewhere along the line joining the two detectors. This 'line-of response' (LOR) of course has finite width limited by the width of the detectors, which determines the fundamental (or 'intrinsic') spatial resolution of the image produced. The other important advantage of coincidence detection is that the total path length travelled through the patient for the two gamma-rays along the LOR is independent of the location of the annihilation. A large proportion of the emitted gamma-rays are scattered or absorbed by electron collisions (attenuation) and so are removed from the LOR. This effect must be corrected for and is conveniently done in PET by placing a source outside the patient [T in Fig. 92.1(b)] and measuring the events recorded in the LOR with (transmission scan) and without (blank scan) the patient in place. The attenuation correction factor is simply the ratio of counts (blank/transmission). The source can be either a continuous ring of long-lived activity (^{68}Ge, $t_{1/2}$ 9 months) or, as in most new machines, rotating rod sources.[3]

SCATTER AND RANDOM CORRECTIONS

Inevitably, there are drawbacks to any technique and those associated with coincidence detection are demonstrated in Figure 92.2. First, two gamma-rays (γ_B and γ_C) from different annihilations (B and C) could, by chance, be recorded in an LOR within the time window. The probability of this occurring increases with activity in the field-of-view (FOV) and with the window width. Second, as mentioned above, many gamma-rays are scattered, changing in energy and direction, and a proportion of these are detected. A 'scatter' event ($\gamma_D - \gamma_D'$) is a true coincidence but gives false positional information. If not corrected for, scatter and random events lead to reduced image contrast and inaccurate quantification. Randoms are monitored and subtracted during data acquisition in modern tomographs. Scatters can be reduced by excluding events below a certain energy threshold but they cannot be entirely excluded and must be corrected for once the data have been acquired.[4]

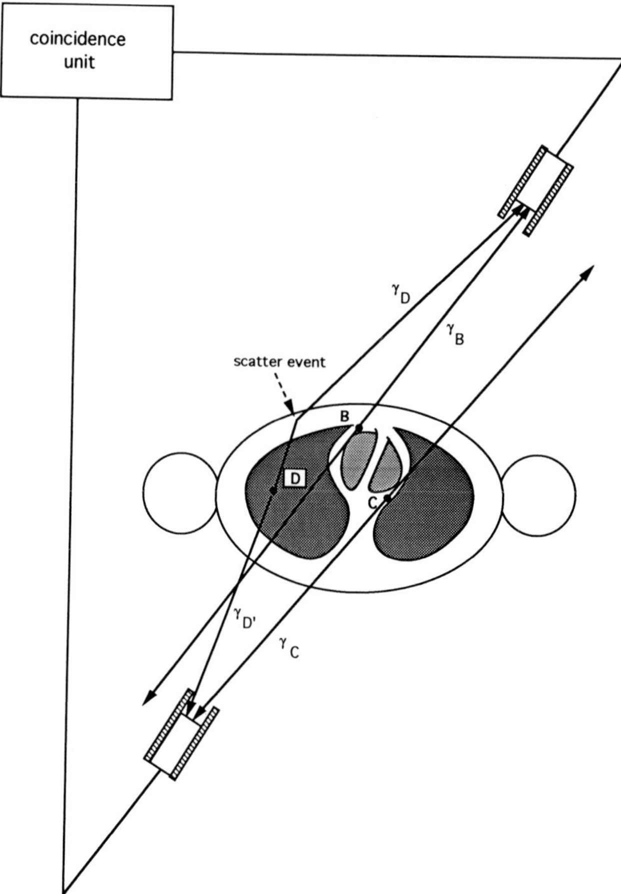

Fig. 92.2 Registration of random (γ_B and γ_C) and scatter ($\gamma_D - \gamma_D{}'$) coincidence events which are mispositioned and cause loss of contrast and accuracy.

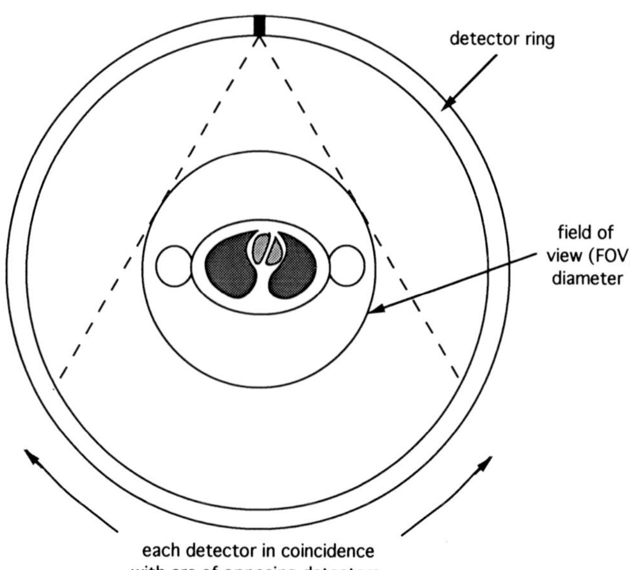

Fig. 92 3a Detection field of view for a single detector. Each detector is connected in coincidence with an arc of detectors on the opposite side of the same ring and, in the latest configurations, with all other rings.

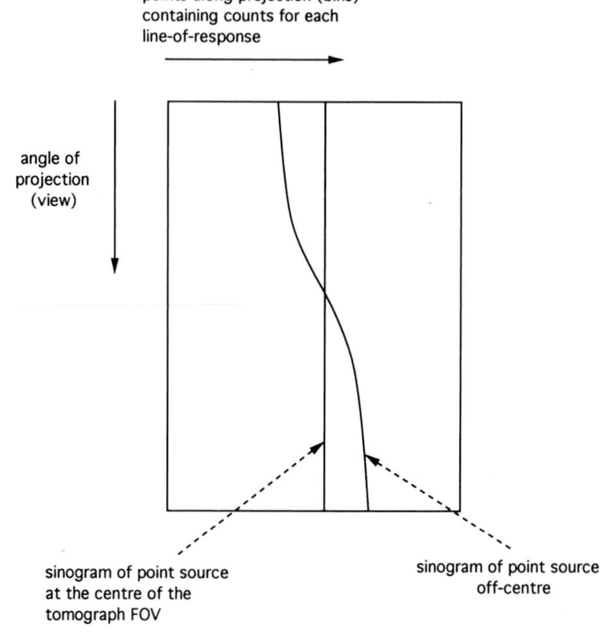

Fig. 92.3b Schematic representation of a sinogram which is a two dimensional array of counts per projection elements vs angle of projection. A point source in the centre of the tomograph's field of view is a vertical line while that for an off-centre source shows a sine wave variation.

TOMOGRAPH DESIGN AND IMAGE RECONSTRUCTION

In order to produce an image, the patient must be viewed from different directions and thus surrounded by detectors. The latest tomographs consist of several circular rings (up to 24) with many hundreds of detectors in each ring. The axial FOV now extends up to about 15 cm. Each detector is connected in coincidence with an arc of detectors on the opposite side of the same ring [Fig. 92.3(a)] and, in the latest configurations, with all other rings. There can therefore be several million LORs. The total counts collected in each of these are stored separately, which gives rise to very large data sets (up to about 70 megabytes for a single scan or 'time-frame'). Sets of parallel LORs are termed 'projections' or 'views'. The complete set of views around the patient for coincidences within a ring or between two rings is termed a 'sinogram' [Fig. 92.3(b)] since the count density from a point source (S) describes a sine wave.

The basic process in forming an image from the projections is termed 'back-projection'.[5] Since the location of an annihilation along an LOR is unknown, back-projection places counts proportional to the LOR counts in volume elements (voxels) which form a grid encompassing the object to be imaged. Typically, these have a square cross-section in the transverse plane and dimension in the axial direction related to the axial detector width. Voxel size is arbitrary but if made too large, resolution will be impaired. It is clear that back-projection will blur the image of a spatially concentrated source and so the projections are filtered prior to back-projection. The filtering suppresses the low frequency blur and amplifies the relatively high frequency signal, leading to an accurate representation of tracer distribution provided the number of views and LORs per view is adequate.[6] Filtered back-projection (FBP) is the most common method of image generation although iterative methods are becoming popular. In these, iterative adjustments of the image are made until it is consistent with the projection data according to a given 'stopping criterion'.[7] This process is slow compared with FBP but can give more satisfactory results with data of poor statistical quality (low acquired counts) as well as giving resolution close to the intrinsic detector resolution. With poor statistics, the attempt to yield high resolution can lead to poor images due to the amplification of high frequency noise. The slowness of iterative methods is increasingly less of an impediment with modern computers.

Tomograph development is directed towards improved resolution and efficiency, two interdependent parameters. Good resolution will give a sharp image but only if sufficient counts are recorded. Most tomographs today use bismuth germanate (BGO) scintillation detectors. BGO is very dense (7.1 g/ml) and thus is highly efficient at stopping gamma-rays. An interaction causes the emission of light (scintillation) which is recorded by photomultipliers (PMTs). The dominant configuration is the block detector where a number of detector elements are viewed by a smaller number of PMTs. A recent design, shown schematically in Figure 92.4, has 56 (7 × 8) elements of dimension 2.9 mm × 4 mm × 30 mm which are viewed by four PMTs. Identification of the element within which an event has taken place is achieved by calculating the ratios of signals between the PMTs.

The block detector has made multiple ring tomographs commercially viable but also has better spectroscopic characteristics than individual small detectors. Energy resolution in the gamma-ray spectrum is dependent on the number of scintillation photons collected. In the block design, the PMT outputs are also summed to maximize energy resolution (and, with it, time resolution), allowing better discrimination against lower energy scattered and random events. A disadvantage of the block detector is that, because it can only process one event at a time, the proportion of events that go unrecorded is higher than for individual detector : PMT arrangements. It is said to have relatively high 'dead time'. Accurate on-line correction schemes are now provided but dead time still represents a loss of efficiency and care should be exercised to limit administered radioactivity such that it is not excessive.

It has been the convention, since multi-ring tomographs were introduced, to place lead or tungsten septa between detector rings. These are tapered or parallel-sided annuli (about 1–3 mm thick) which extend from the detector face towards the centre of the FOV, their radial length depending on tomograph design.[8] As a consequence, data has been acquired as a set of independent 'slices' through the patient. The role of septa is to reduce random and scatter events from activity outside the slice. Only coincidences within a ring or between closely adjacent rings are possible due to septa geometry.[9] This is termed the 2D mode nominally because events are assigned to individual, nominally two-dimensional, slices.

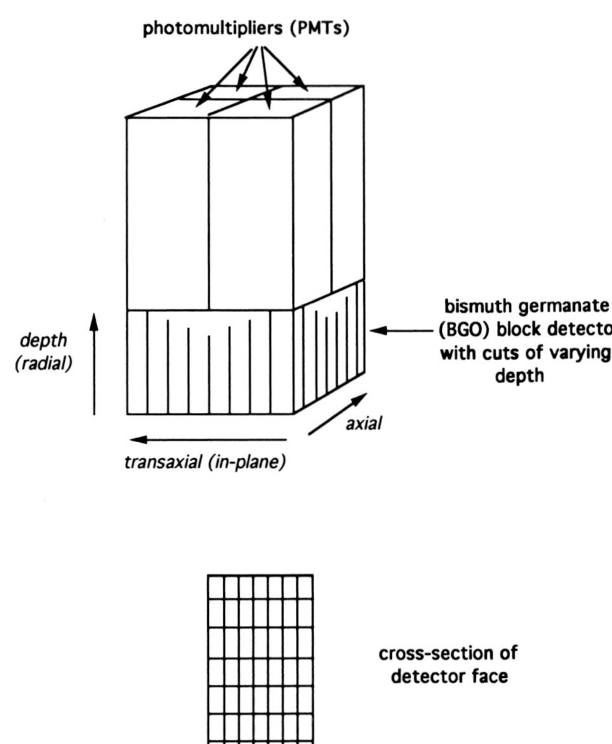

Fig. 92.4 Schematic representation of block detector in latest generation scanner (CTI/Siemens Exact HR) with 56 elements of approximate dimensions 3 × 4 × 30 mm.

However, it is clear that while randoms and scatters are reduced, so are true (unscattered) events. Septa, to some degree, shield the detectors but also prohibit acquisition of coincidence data between any two rings. This represents a very significant loss of efficiency. Recent trends have therefore been towards removal of septa and '3D' acquisition where the data are treated on a volume rather than a slice basis. Automatic septa retraction and 3D acquisition are now standard features in commercial scanners. The more difficult task of reconstructing a 3D image has gone through considerable developments but is now routine in a number of centres.[10] At low count rates, 3D efficiency is some five times higher than that for 2D, allowing for the fraction of scatters.[9] At higher rates, where an increasing statistical penalty is paid for subtraction of randoms,[11] the effective gain is still around a factor of three.[12] The higher efficiency of 3D PET gives greater scope for following time-activity curves of ^{11}C-labelled compounds (half-life 20.4 min) for instance in studies of receptor binding. In contrast, higher count rate procedures, such as the measurement of blood flow with $H_2{}^{15}O$, can be carried out with reduced dose relative to the 2D mode. Scatter correction algorithms are still being developed[13] for 3D and although promising solutions have been found for brain imaging, there is at present very little experience in cardiology. Nevertheless, it is anticipated that the maximal detection efficiency of 3D and therefore optimum use of the resolution now available (about 3 mm) will greatly enhance the potential of PET in cardiology research.

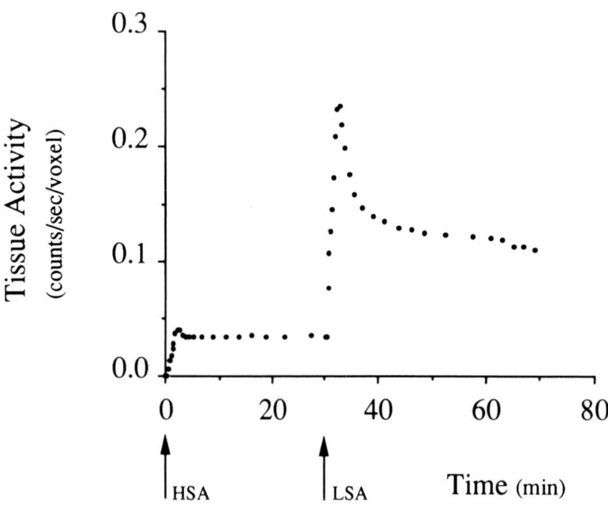

Fig. 92.5 A typical myocardial time–activity curve obtained following a high specific activity (HSA) and a second low specific activity (LSA) injection of S-[^{11}C]CGP 12177, a ligand for the measurement of β-adrenoceptors, in a normal subject. The myocardial tracer time–activity curves are corrected for radioactive decay and for vascular activity. The sections of the curve corresponding to the two slow phases (plateau), which represent S-[^{11}C]CGP 12177 bound to β-adrenoceptors, are exponentially extrapolated on the y axis back to the start of the infusions. The β-adrenoceptor density is derived from the maximum number of available specific S-[^{11}C]CGP 12177 binding sites per g of tissue (B_{max}) in the region of interest.

FROM TISSUE COUNTS TO PHYSIOLOGICAL PARAMETERS

After the corrections to the raw PET data outlined above have been made, the reconstructed image represents the radioactivity concentration per unit mass. The content of radioactivity in tissue and blood can be simultaneously assessed by appropriate placement of regions of interest (ROI). Generally, the data set consist of many time-frames (dynamic acquisition) which are used to measure the rate of change of radioactivity with time. ROIs defined in one plane can be automatically copied onto sequential frames. To convert these measurements of radioactivity into physiological parameters, a tracer model for the system needs to be applied. The conventional approach is to divide the system into one or more compartments and to calculate the rates of entrance and clearance of the tracer from these compartments. Specific models have been developed and validated for the measurements of myocardial blood flow,[14] metabolism,[15] and, more recently, receptor function[16] (Fig. 92.5).

APPLICATIONS IN CARDIOLOGY

Current applications of PET imaging in cardiology can be divided into three main categories: studies of regional myocardial blood flow, metabolism and pharmacology.

Myocardial blood flow

Radionuclide imaging techniques, e.g. thallium-201, have enabled the assessment of nutritive tissue perfusion as opposed to measurements of epicardial coronary flow as measured by either thermodilution[17] or Doppler catheter techniques.[18,19] Prior to the advent of PET imaging technology, only directional changes of regional myocardial blood flow could be assessed using either planar gamma scintigraphy or single photon emission computerized tomography with different single photon emitters.[20] Quantification of myocardial blood flow using these techniques was rendered impossible due to the physical limitations of the imaging systems and the tracers available. PET overcomes the physical limitations of previously available imaging systems by providing the means for accurate attenuation correction, thus enabling absolute quantification of the concentration of radiolabelled tracer in the organ of interest.[21] As PET technology has advanced and rapid dynamic imaging has become possible, quantification of myocardial blood flow has been achieved following the development of suitable tracer kinetic models.

A number of tracers have been used for measurement of myocardial blood flow using PET, in particular, oxygen-15 labelled water ($H_2{}^{15}O$),[22–25] nitrogen-13 labelled ammonia ($^{13}NH_3$),[15,26–28] the cationic potassium analogue rubidium-82 (^{82}Rb)[29] and carbon-11 and gallium-68 labelled albumin microspheres.[30,31] Early PET studies used $^{13}NH_3$[26] and ^{82}Rb[32] to provide qualitative assessments of myocardial blood flow. Although kinetic models have been proposed for quantification of myocardial blood flow using ^{82}Rb,[33] these are limited by the dependence of the myocardial extraction of this tracer on the prevailing flow rate and myocardial metabolic state.[34] Therefore, quantification of myocardial blood flow, either under hyperaemic conditions or in metabolically impaired myocardium, is inaccurate. Furthermore, the high positron energy of this radionuclide results in relatively poor image quality and in a reduced spatial resolution due to the relatively long positron track of ^{82}Rb.[34] Although positron-labelled albumin microspheres can provide accurate estimates of myocardial blood flow, they require intraventricular injection which renders their use impractical. Currently, $H_2{}^{15}O$ and $^{13}NH_3$ are the most widely used tracers used for the quantification of regional myocardial blood flow with PET (Figs 92.6 and 92.7). Tracer kinetic models for quantification of myocardial blood flow have been successfully validated in animals against the radiolabelled microsphere method over a wide flow range for both $H_2{}^{15}O$[22–25] and $^{13}NH_3$[15,26,35] The values of myocardial blood flow determined in normal human volunteers using both tracers either at rest or during pharmacologically-induced coronary vasodilatation are similar.[22,28] The use of $H_2{}^{15}O$ for quantification of regional myocardial blood is theoretically superior to $^{13}NH_3$ in that $H_2{}^{15}O$ is a metabolically inert and freely diffusible tracer[36] which has

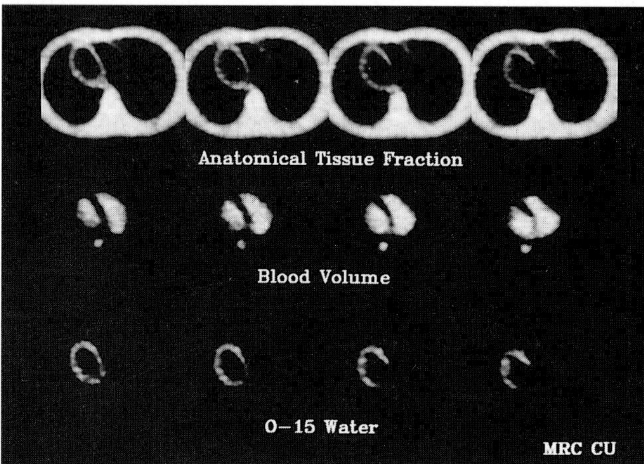

Fig. 92.6 Transaxial images of the chest of a normal volunteer illustrating extravascular tissue density (top row) and tissue $H_2{}^{15}O$ (bottom row) which were both obtained by subtraction of the blood pool scan using $C^{15}O$ (middle row) from the transmission scan and total $H_2{}^{15}O$, respectively.

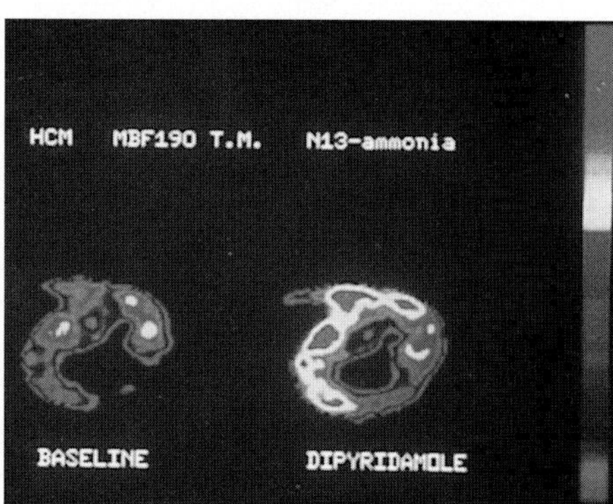

Fig. 92.7 Transaxial images of the heart obtained with $^{13}NH_3$ in a patient with hypertrophic cardiomyopathy at baseline and following i.v. dipyridamole (0.56 mg/kg). The extraordinary thickness (39 mm) of the interventricular septum (9 to 1 o'clock position) allowed the assessment of transmural flow distribution. The subendocardial/subepicardial flow ratio which was 1.01 at baseline, decreased to 0.69 following dipyridamole suggesting subendocardial underperfusion. (Also shown in colour on Plate 27.)

a virtually complete myocardial extraction which is independent of both flow rate[37] and myocardial metabolic state.[24] This makes $H_2{}^{15}O$ a particularly suitable tracer for measurements of absolute perfusion also under circumstances where metabolic abnormalities, which could affect myocardial trapping of $^{13}NH_3$,[38] may be present. On the other hand, the quality of myocardial $^{13}NH_3$ images is superior to that of $H_2{}^{15}O$ images. Both $H_2{}^{15}O$ and $^{13}NH_3$ have short physical half-lives (2 and 10 min respectively) which allow repeat measurements of myocardial blood flow in the same session.

Prior to the advent of PET technology, investigations of regional coronary blood flow in man were restricted to the level of the epicardial coronary artery. However, it is well established that the major regulatory site of tissue perfusion is at the level of the arterioles which are not amenable to catheterization. With the development of quantitative myocardial blood flow measurement using PET, it is becoming possible to challenge the function of the coronary microvasculature by measuring the coronary vasodilator reserve (CVR) which is generally calculated as the ratio of the maximal flow following pharmacological challenge to the resting flow level. This definition of CVR is, however, dependent on the coronary perfusion pressure and also assumes that maximal vasodilatation has been achieved.[39] PET studies in healthy human volunteers have established that the normal CVR in response to a standard intravenous dose of dipyridamole (0.56 mg/kg over 4 min) is approximately 3.5–4.0 (Fig. 92.8).[22,28] These data are similar to those reported using the Doppler catheter technique for measuring epicardial coronary flow velocity.[41] The measurement of CVR is useful for the assessment of the functional significance of coronary stenoses in patients with coronary artery disease.[41] In addition, PET is particularly helpful in those circumstances where the CVR is diffusely (and not regionally) blunted, e.g. in patients with hypertrophic cardiomyopathy,[42] due to a widespread abnormality of the coronary microcirculation.

Myocardial metabolism

In 1947 Bing and coworkers[43] started to use coronary sinus catheterization for the study of myocardial metabolism in man. This procedure is based on the combined catheterization of the coronary sinus and an artery with measurement of substrate concentrations in simultaneously drawn blood samples. This approach, however, has several limitations: the spatial resolution is very crude and temporal resolution modest; regional information is limited to the territory of distribution of the left anterior descending coronary artery (i.e. the anterolateral wall of the left ventricle) if the catheter tip is placed in the distal portion of the great cardiac vein which drains blood from this region; right atrial reflux into the coronary sinus, but

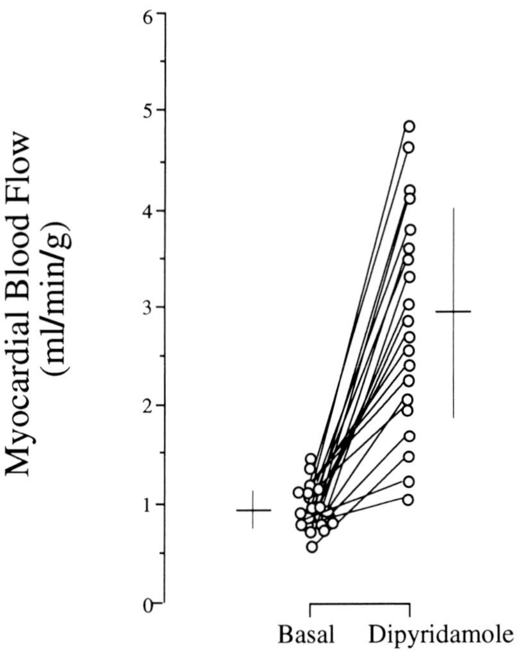

Fig. 92.8 Individual values of average left ventricular myocardial blood flow in 20 normal subjects at baseline and following i.v. dipyridamole (0.56 mg/kg) measured by $H_2{}^{15}O$.

not into the great cardiac vein, may interfere with the measurements particularly when atrial pacing is employed.[44]

The introduction of PET has made it possible to study regional myocardial metabolism in humans non-invasively. Studies have been performed using labelled amino acids to measure amino acid metabolism and protein turnover rates.[45] However, the majority of PET metabolic studies have focused upon investigation of the pathways involved in energy metabolism and the alterations which occur in disease.

Oxidative metabolism

In the postabsorptive state the normoxic heart relies mainly upon oxidation of free fatty acid (FFA) as its main source of high energy phosphates while the uptake and oxidation of carbohydrates (glucose + lactate + pyruvate) is low. In the fed state, the uptake of carbohydrate is high and accounts for virtually all of the concurrent oxygen uptake.[46] This change from predominantly carbohydrate to predominantly lipid usage is explained by the glucose-FFA cycle of Randle. An important observation was that the oxidation of glucose by the isolated rat heart was markedly inhibited by concurrent provision of FFA.[46] The factors that regulate myocardial substrate utilization are complex and depend, in addition to substrate concentration, upon the action of different hormones. Insulin which stimulates myocardial glucose uptake and utilization also inhibits adipose tissue lipolysis, so that the circulating levels of FFA are low.[46] Catecholamine decreases rather than increases glycolysis in the heart together with a greatly increased uptake and oxidation of FFA.[46] Myocardial utilization of carbohydrates is also affected by cardiac workload and oxidation of carbohydrates accounts for more than 50% of energy produced during conditions of maximal stress.[47] Finally, glucose utilization is increased during conditions of reduced oxygen supply; under these circumstances exogenous glucose uptake and glycogen breakdown are increased, glycolysis is stimulated and ATP can be produced from the anaerobic catabolism of glucose with concomitant formation of lactate.[46]

In order to measure the flux through this pathway during normoxic and ischaemic conditions, PET imaging has been performed after intravenous administration of the natural free fatty acid palmitate labelled with carbon-11 (^{11}C-palmitate).[48] These studies indicated that the clearance of ^{11}C-palmitate from the myocardium was related to the degree of oxidative metabolism, though absolute quantification of utilization rates was not possible due to the over-complexity of the model required to explain the behaviour of ^{11}C-palmitate in tissue.[48] Interpretation of myocardial uptake and clearance of ^{11}C-palmitate is further complicated by the dependence of these two parameters on the prevailing blood flow and dietary state.

Carbon-11 labelled acetate (^{11}C-acetate) has been advocated as a tracer of tricarboxylic acid cycle activity[49] and has been used as an indirect marker of myocardial oxygen consumption (MVO_2) by PET in both experimental animals[50–52] and humans.[53–54] A number of studies have shown that the rate constant describing the clearance of ^{11}C-acetate from the myocardium correlates well with catheter measurements of oxygen extraction fraction (OEF) from analysis of arteriovenous differences of blood oxygen content using the Fick Principle.[52–54] However, the lack of appropriate models which describe the complex tissue kinetics of ^{11}C-acetate accurately have prevented absolute quantification of MVO_2 using this tracer. Furthermore, measurements of MVO_2 using this tracer will be subject to blood flow and dietary constraints similar to those encountered during measurements made using labelled FFAs. Therefore, it has been suggested that standardization of metabolic status is important to make meaningful assessments of MVO_2 using this tracer.[55]

A new method to quantify MVO_2 by inhalation of oxygen-15 labelled molecular oxygen gas ($^{15}O_2$) has been developed recently.[56] The accuracy of this approach to quantify OEF and MVO_2 has been successfully validated over a wide range of values in experimental animal studies

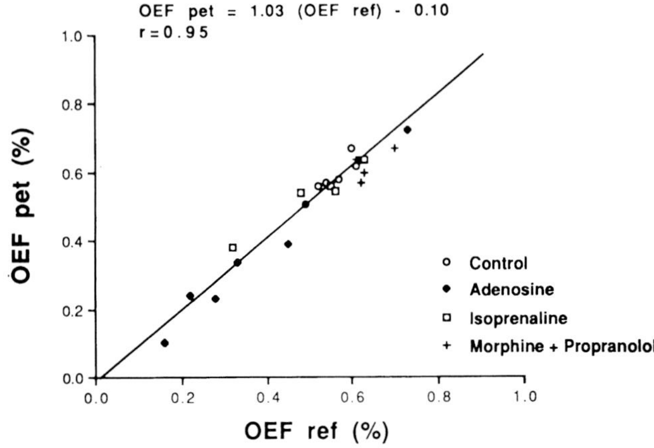

Fig. 92.9 Comparison of the oxygen extraction fraction (OEF) measured in dogs using conventional arteriovenous sampling (x axis) and PET with $^{15}O_2$ (y axis). Different pharmacological agents (adenosine, isoprenaline, morphine and propranolol) were administered to vary cardiac workload and myocardial blood flow.

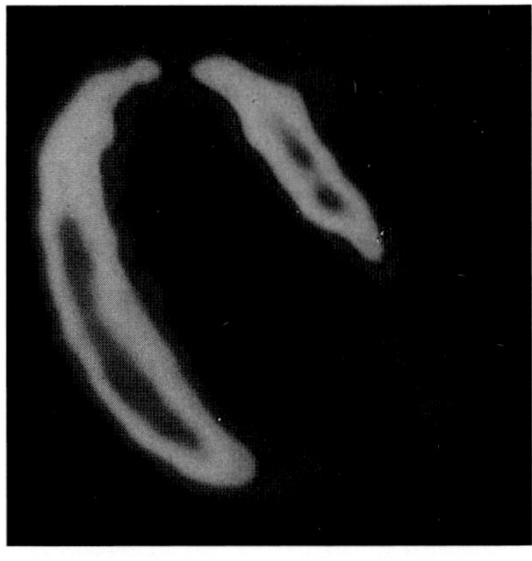

Fig. 92.10 An example of transaxial image of the heart in a patient with coronary artery disease obtained with 18F-fluorodeoxyglucose and PET during euglycaemic-hyperinsulinaemic clamp. (Also shown in colour on Plate 27). (Reprinted with permission from Knuuti et al 1992 J Nucl Med 33: 1255–1262)

(Fig. 92.9).[57] Preliminary studies in human subjects yielded mean OEF and MVO_2 values of 61 ± 1.8% and 9.4 ± 1.8 ml/min/100 g, respectively,[56] which are consistent with those values previously reported for man obtained from invasive catheterization studies.

Glucose utilization

The utilization of exogenous glucose by the myocardium can be assessed using PET with ^{18}F-2-fluoro-2-deoxyglucose (FDG) as a tracer.[58] FDG is transported into the myocyte by the same trans-sarcolemmal carrier as glucose and is then phosphorylated to FDG-6-phosphate by the enzyme hexokinase. This is essentially a unidirectional reaction and results in FDG-6-phosphate accumulation within the myocardium, as no glucose-6-phosphatase (the enzyme that can hydrolyze FDG-6-phosphate back to free FDG + free phosphate) has yet been identified in cardiac muscle.[59] Thus, measurement of the myocardial uptake of FDG is proportional to the overall rate of trans-sarcolemmal transport and hexokinase-phosphorylation of exogenous (circulating) glucose by heart muscle. Measurement of myocardial FDG uptake by PET, however, does not provide any information about the further intracellular disposal of glucose (i.e. glycogen synthesis–glycolysis–pentose shunt).

A number of kinetic modelling approaches have been used for the quantification of glucose utilization rates using FDG.[59] The major limitation of these approaches is that quantification of glucose metabolism requires the knowledge of the lumped constant (LC), a factor which relates the kinetic behaviour of FDG to naturally occurring glucose in terms of the relative affinity of each molecule for the trans-sarcolemmal transporter and for hexokinase. Unfortunately, the value of the lumped constant in humans under different physiological and pathophysiological conditions is not known, thus making true in vivo quantification of myocardial metabolic rates of glucose very difficult. Still the quantification of the uptake of this glucose analogue (particularly if obtained under standardized dietary conditions as during insulin clamp[60]) allows comparison of absolute values from different individuals and may help to establish the absolute rates of glucose utilization (in FDG units) in normal and pathologic myocardium (Fig. 92.10).

Myocardial pharmacology

Several beta blocker drugs have been labelled with carbon-11 for imaging by PET.[61] The most promising of these is CGP 12177. This is a non-selective beta adrenoceptor antagonist which is particularly suited for PET studies due to its high affinity and low lipophilicity, thus enabling the functional receptor pool on the cell surface to be studied.[62] Initially, racemic (R,S)-CGP 12177 was successfully labelled with carbon-11 and used to produce images in dogs.[61] However, it became clear that better quality data could be obtained by using the pure active enantiomer, (S)-CGP 12177, labelled with carbon-11. Studies in both greyhounds and rats[63] demonstrated significantly improved myocardial uptake using the labelled (S)-enantiomer compared to the racemic compound. Analysis of plasma samples by high performance liquid chromatography taken up to 1 h after intravenous injection of both (RS)- and (S)-CGP 12177 labelled with carbon-11 indicated the presence of 30% radiolabelled metabolites in rats and virtually none in greyhounds.[64] These animal studies indicated that ^{11}C-(S)-CGP 12177 should be an ideal ligand for human PET studies. A graphical method for quantification of β-adrenoceptor density (β_{max}, pmol/g) from the PET data has been developed.[65] This approach requires two injections of ^{11}C-(S)-CGP 12177, one at a high specific activity followed by a second at a lower specific activity (Fig. 92.5). This analytical approach is particularly attractive for clinical studies as it does not require an input function and thus obviates the need for arterial cannulation. Studies in our institution in a group of young healthy subjects have yielded β_{max} values of 10.4±1.7 pmol/g, using a modified version of the above graphical analysis, a figure which is comparable with the values measured using in vitro binding.[66]

Attempts have been made to study α-1 adrenoceptors in vivo using carbon-11 labelled prazosin and PET,[61] but to date human studies have not been performed. Investigations of the α-adrenergic system would be of interest as their levels have been found to alter as a result of myocardial ischaemia[67] and they have also been implicated in arrhythmogenesis.[68]

In addition to postsynaptic receptor studies, PET has also been used to investigate the integrity of presynaptic sympathetic innervation of the heart. Three tracers have been used for this purpose: fluorine-18 labelled fluorometaraminol,[69] fluorine-18 labelled fluorodopamine,[70] and carbon-11 labelled hydroxyephedrine.[71] These tracers compete with endogenous noradrenaline for the transport into the presynaptic nerve terminal via the neuronal uptake-1 transport system. Once within the neurone these compounds are metabolized and trapped and hence serve as markers of sympathetic innervation. Recent studies have demonstrated decreased retention of carbon-11 labelled hydroxyephedrine in patients after cardiac transplant which is consistent with the heart being denervated.[72] However, with time, some sympathetic re-innervation occurred particularly in the anteroseptal region of the heart. This has recently been correlated with the recovery of sensation of angina pectoris in these patients.[73]

In addition to studies of the sympathetic nervous system, PET studies using carbon-11 labelled MQNB have been used to quantify the density of myocardial muscarinic cholinergic receptors in both experimental animals[74] and in man.[75] These studies should be extended to patient groups given the possible pathophysiological role of muscarinic receptors in arrhythmogenesis and control of sympathetic nerve function.

REFERENCES

1. Coleman R E, Robbins M S, Siegel B A 1992 The future of PET in clinical medicine and the impact of drug regulation. Semin Nucl Med 12: 193
2. Hoffman E J, Phelps M E 1986 Positron emission tomography: principles and quantitation. In: Phelps M E, Mazziotta J, Schelbert H, eds. Positron emission tomography and autoradiography: principles and applications for the brain and heart. Raven Press, New York. Chapter 6
3. Huesman R H, Derenzo S E, Cahoon J L et al 1988 Orbiting transmission source for positron tomography. IEEE Trans Nucl Sci NS-35: 735
4. Hoverath H, Kuebler W K, Ostertag H J et al 1993 Scatter correction in the transaxial slices of a whole-body positron emission tomograph. Phys Med Biol 38: 717
5. Brooks R A, DiChiro G 1976 Principles of computer assisted tomography (CAT) in radiographic and radioisotopic imaging. Phys Med Biol 24: 689
6. Huesman R H 1977 The effects of a finite number of projection angles and finite lateral sampling of projections on the propagation of statistical errors in transverse section reconstruction. Phys Med Biol 22: 511
7. Shepp L A, Vardi Y 1982 Maximum likelihood reconstruction for emission tomography. IEEE Trans Med Imaging MI-1: 113
8. Spinks T J, Jones T, Gilardi M-C, Heather J D 1988 Physical performance of the latest generation of commercial positron scanner. IEEE Trans Nucl Sci NS-35: 721
9. Spinks T J, Jones T, Bailey D L et al 1992 Physical performance of a positron tomograph for brain imaging with retractable septa. Phys Med Biol 37: 1637
10. Townsend D W, Geissbuhler A, Defrise M et al 1991 Fully three-dimensional reconstruction for a PET camera with retractable septa. IEEE Trans Med Imaging 10: 505
11. Spinks T J, Araujo L I, Rhodes C G, Hutton B H 1991 Physical aspects of cardiac scanning with a block detector whole body tomograph. J Comput Assist Tomogr 15: 893
12. Bailey D L, Jones T, Spinks T J, Gilardi M-C, Townsend D W 1991 Noise equivalent count measurements in a neuro-PET scanner with retractable septa. IEEE Trans Med Imaging 10: 256
13. Grootoonk S, Spinks T J, Kennedy A M, Bloomfield P M, Sashin D, Jones T 1992 The practical implementation and accuracy of dual window scatter correction in a neuroPET scanner with the septa retracted. IEEE Medical Imaging Conference Record (Orlando, FL) 2: 942
14. Bellina C R, Parodi O, Camici P et al 1990 Simultaneous in vitro and in vivo validation of nitrogen-13-ammonia for the assessment of regional myocardial blood flow. J Nucl Med 31: 1335
15. Camici P, Araujo L I, Spinks T J et al 1986 Increased uptake of ^{18}F-fluorodeoxyglucose in postischemic myocardium of patients with exercise-induced angina. Circulation 74: 81
16. Syrota A 1991 Positron emission tomography: evaluation of cardiac receptors. In Marcus M L, Schelbert H R, Skorton D J, Wolf G L, eds. Cardiac imaging. A companion to Braunwald's heart disease. W B Saunders Company, Philadelphia. p 1256
17. Ganz W, Tamura K, Marcus H S, Donoso R, Yoshida S, Swan H J C 1971 Measurement of coronary sinus blood flow by continuous thermodilution in man. Circulation 44: 181
18. Hartley C J, Cole J S 1974 An ultrasonic pulsed Doppler system for measuring blood flow in small vessels. J Appl Physiol 37: 626
19. Cole J S, Hartley C J 1977 The pulsed Doppler coronary artery catheter. Preliminary report of a new technique for measuring rapid changes in coronary artery flow velocity in man. Circulation 56: 1
20. van der Waal E E 1992 Nuclear cardiology and cardiac magnetic resonance. Hans Soto Production, The Netherlands
21. Hoffman E J, Phelps M E 1986 Positron emission tomography: principles and quantitation. In: Phelps M E, Mazziotta J C, Schelbert H R eds. Positron emission tomography and autoradiography: principles and applications for the brain and the heart. Raven Press, New York. pp 113–148
22. Araujo L I, Lammertsma A A, Rhodes C G et al 1991 Non-invasive quantification of regional myocardial blood flow in normal volunteers and patients with coronary artery disease using oxygen-15 labeled carbon dioxide inhalation and positron emission tomography. Circulation 83: 875–885
23. Iida H, Kanno I, Takahashi A et al 1989 Measurement of absolute myocardial blood flow with $H_2{}^{15}O$ and dynamic positron emission

tomography: strategy for quantification in relation to the partial-volume effect. Circulation 78: 104–115
24. Bergmann S R, Fox K A A, Rand A L et al 1984 Quantification of regional myocardial blood flow in vivo with $H_2{}^{15}O$. Circulation 70: 724–733
25. Bergmann S R, Herrero P, Markham J, Weinheimer C J, Walsh M N 1989 Noninvasive quantification of myocardial blood flow in human subjects with O-15 labelled water and positron emission tomography. J Am Coll Cardiol 14: 639–652
26. Schelbert H R, Phelps M E, Hoffman E J, Huang S C, Selin C E, Kuhl D E 1979 Regional myocardial perfusion assessed by N-13 labelled ammonia and positron computerized axial tomography. Am J Cardiol 43: 209–218
27. Krivokapich J, Smith G T, Huang S C et al 1989 Nitrogen-13 ammonia myocardial imaging at rest and with exercise in normal volunteers: quantification of coronary flow with positron emission tomography. Circulation 80: 1328–1337
28. Hutchins G D, Schwaiger M, Rosenspire K C, Krivokapich J, Schelbert H, Kuhl D E 1990 Noninvasive quantification of regional blood flow in the human heart using N-13 ammonia and dynamic positron emission tomographic imaging. J Am Coll Cardiol 15: 1032–1042
29. Herrero P, Markham J, Shelton M E, Weinheimer C J, Bergmann S R 1990 Noninvasive quantification of regional myocardial perfusion with rubidium-82 and positron emission tomography. Exploration of a mathematical model. Circulation 82: 1377–1386
30. Beller G A, Alten W J, Cochavi S, Hnatowich D, Brownell G L 1979 Assessment of regional myocardial perfusion by positron emission tomography after intracoronary administration of Ga-68 labeled albumin microspheres. J Comput Assist Tomogr 3: 447–452
31. Wilson R A, Shea M J, De Landsheere C H et al 1984 Validation of quantification of regional myocardial blood flow in vivo with 11C-labeled human albumin microspheres and positron emission tomography. Circulation 70: 717–723
32. Selwyn A P, Allan R M, L'Abbate A et al 1982 Relation between regional myocardial uptake of rubidium-82 and perfusion: absolute reduction of cation uptake in ischemia. Am J Cardiol 50: 112–121
33. Huang S C, Williams B A, Krivokapich J, Araujo L I, Phelps M E, Schelbert H R 1989 Rabbit myocardial ^{82}Rb kinetics and a compartmental model for blood flow estimation. Am J Physiol 256: H1156–H1164
34. Araujo L I, Schelbert H R 1984 Rubidium-82: dynamic positron emission tomography in ischaemic heart disease. Am J Cardiac Imag 1: 117–124
35. Shah A, Schelbert H R, Schwaiger M, Hansen H, Selin C 1985 Measurement of regional myocardial blood flow with N-13 ammonia and positron emission tomography in intact dogs. J Am Coll Cardiol 5: 92 –100
36. Johnson J A, Cavert H M, Lifson N 1952 Kinetics concerned with distribution of isotopic water in isolated dog heart and skeletal muscle. Am J Physiol 171: 687–693
37. Yipintsoi T, Bassingthwaite J B 1970 Circulatory transport of iodoantipyrine and water in the isolated dog heart. Circ Res 27: 461–467
38. Bergmann S R, Hack S, Tewson T, Welch M J, Sobel B E 1980 The dependence of accumulation of $^{13}NH_3$ by myocardium on metabolic factors and its implications for the quantitative assessment of perfusion. Circulation 61: 34–43
39. Hoffman J I E 1984 Maximal coronary flow and the concept of coronary vascular reserve. Circulation 70: 153–159
40. Rossen J D, Simonetti I, Marcus M L, Winniford M D 1989 Coronary dilatation with standard dose dipyridamole and dipyridamole combined with handgrip. Circulation 79: 556–572
41. Gould K L, Kirkeeide R L, Buchi M 1990 Coronary flow reserve as a physiologic measure of stenosis severity. J Am Coll Cardiol 15: 459–474
42. Camici P G, Chiriatti G, Lorenzoni R et al 1991 Coronary vasodilation is impaired in both hypertrophied and nonhypertrophied myocardium of patients with hypertrophic cardiomyopathy: a study with nitrogen-13 ammonia and positron emission tomography. J Am Coll Cardiol 17: 879–886
43. Bing R J 1954 The metabolism of the heart. Fla, Orlando, Academic Press, Inc., New York. Harvey Lecture Series 50. pp 27–70
44. Camici P G, Marraccini P, Lorenzoni R et al 1991 Metabolic markers of stress-induced myocardial ischemia. Circulation 83 (Suppl III): III-8–III13
45. Schelbert H R, Schwaiger M 1986 PET studies of the heart. In: Phelps M E, Mazziotta J C, Schelbert H R, eds. Positron emission tomography and autoradiography. Principles and applications for the brain and the heart. Raven Press, New York. pp 581–662
46. Camici P G, Ferrannini E, Opie L H 1989 Myocardial metabolism in ischemic heart disease: basic principles and applications to imaging by positron emission tomography. Prog Cardiovasc Dis 32: 217–238
47. Camici P G, Marraccini P, Marzilli M et al 1989 Coronary hemodynamics and myocardial metabolism during and after pacing stress in normal humans. Am J Physiol 257: E309–E317
48. Schelbert H R, Henze E, Schon H R et al 1983 C-11 Palmitic acid for the noninvasive evaluation of regional myocardial fatty acid metabolism with positron computed tomography. IV. In vivo demonstration of impaired fatty acid oxidation in acute myocardial ischemia. Am Heart J 106: 736–750
49. Buxton D B, Schwaiger M, Nguyen A, Phelps M E, Schelbert H R 1988 Radiolabeled acetate as a tracer of myocardial tricarboxylic acid cycle flux. Circ Res 63: 628–634
50. Armbrecht J J, Buxton D B, Schelbert H R 1990 Validation of [1-^{11}C]acetate as a tracer for noninvasive assessment of oxidative metabolism with positron emission tomography in normal, ischemic, postischemic, and hyperemic canine myocardium. Circulation 81: 1594–1605
51. Brown M A, Myears D W, Bergmann S R 1988 Noninvasive assessment of canine myocardial oxidative metabolism with carbon-11 acetate and positron emission tomography. J Am Coll Cardiol 12: 1054–1063
52. Buxton D B, Nienaber C A, Luxen A et al 1989 Noninvasive quantitation of regional myocardial oxygen consumption in vivo with [1-^{11}C]acetate and dynamic positron emission tomography. Circulation 79: 134–142
53. Armbrecht J J, Buxton D B, Brunken R C, Phelps M E, Schelbert H R 1989 Regional myocardial oxygen consumption determined noninvasively in humans with [1-^{11}C] acetate and dynamic positron tomography. Circulation 80: 863–872
54. Walsh M N, Geltman E M, Brown M A et al 1989 Noninvasive estimation of regional myocardial oxygen consumption by positron emission tomography with carbon-11 acetate in patients with myocardial infarction. J Nucl Med 30: 1798–1808
55. Hicks R J, Herman W H, Kalff V et al 1991 Quantitative evaluation of regional substrate metabolism in the human heart by positron emission tomography. J Am Coll Cardiol 18: 101–111
56. Iida H, Rhodes C G, Yamamoto Y, Jones T, De Silva R, Araujo L I 1990 Quantitative measurement of myocardial metabolic rate of oxygen ($MMRO_2$) in man using positron emission tomography. Circulation 82: III–614 (Abstract)
57. De Silva R, Yamamoto Y, Rhodes C G, Iida H, Maseri A, Jones T 1992 Non-invasive quantification of regional myocardial oxygen consumption in anaesthetized greyhounds. J Physiol 446: 219P (Abstract)
58. Gallagher B M, Fowler J S, Gutterson N I, MacGregor R R, Wan C-N, Wolf A P 1978 Metabolic trapping as a principle of radiopharmaceutical design: some factors responsible for the biodistribution of [^{18}F] 2-deoxy-2-fluoro-D-glucose. J Nucl Med 19: 1154–1161
59. Huang S C, Phelps M E 1986 Principles of tracer kinetic modeling in positron emission tomography and autoradiography. In: Phelps M E, Mazziotta J C, Schelbert H R, eds. Positron emission tomography and autoradiography. Principles and applications for the brain and heart. Raven Press, New York. pp 287–346
60. Ferrannini E, Santoro D, Bonadonna R, Natali O, Parodi O, Camici P G 1993 Metabolic and hemodynamic effects of insulin on human hearts. Am J Physiol 264: E308–E315
61. Syrota A 1991 Positron emission tomography: evaluation of cardiac receptors. In: Marcus M L, Schelbert H R, Skorton D J, Wolf G L, eds. Cardiac imaging. A comparison to Braunwald's HEART DISEASE. W B Saunders Company, Philadelphia. pp 1256–1270
62. Staehelin M, Hertel C 1983 [^{3}H]CGP12177: a β-adrenergic

ligand suitable for measuring cell surface receptors. J Recent Res 3: 35–43
63. Araujo L I, Rhodes C G, Hughes J M B et al 1991 Assessment of myocardial beta receptors in vivo using C-11 (S) CGP12177 and positron emission tomography (PET). J Nucl Med 32: S927 (Abstract)
64. Jones H A, Rhodes C G, Law M P et al 1991 Rapid analysis for metabolites of ^{11}C-labelled drugs: fate of [^{11}C]-S-4-(tert.-butylamino-2-hydroxypropoxy)-benzimidaz ol-2-one in the dog. J Chromat 570: 361–370
65. Delforge J, Syrota A, Lançon J-L et al 1991 Cardiac beta-adrenergic receptor density measured in vivo using PET, CGP12177, and a new graphical method. J Nucl Med 32: 739–748
66. Brodde O-E 1991 β_1 and β_2-adrenoceptors in the human heart: properties, function, and alterations in chronic heart failure. Pharmacol Rev 43: 203–242
67. Corr P B, Crafford W A 1981 Enhanced alpha-adrenergic responsiveness in ischemic myocardium: role of alpha-adrenergic blockade. Am Heart J 102: 605–612
68. Sheridan D J, Penkoske P A, Sobel B E, Corr P B 1980 Alpha-adrenergic contributions to dysrhythmias during myocardial ischemia and reperfusion in cats. J Clin Invest 65: 161–171
69. Wieland D, Rosenspire K, Hutchins G et al 1990 Neuronal mapping of the heart with 6-[F-18]-Fluorometaraminol. J Med Chem 33: 956–964
70. Goldstein D S, Chang P C, Eisenhofer G et al 1990 Positron emission tomographic imaging of cardiac sympathetic innervation and function. Circulation 81: 1606–1621
71. Schwaiger M, Kaliff V, Rosenspire K et al 1990 Noninvasive evaluation of the sympathetic nervous system in the human heart by PET. Circulation 82: 457–464
72. Schwaiger M, Hutchins G D, Kalff V et al 1991 Evidence for regional catecholamine uptake and storage sites in the transplanted human heart by positron emission tomography. J Clin Invest 87: 1681–1690
73. Stark R P, McGinn A L, Wilson R F 1991 Chest pain in cardiac-transplant recipients. Evidence for sensory reinnervation after cardiac transplantation. N Engl J Med 324: 1791–1794
74. Delforge J, Janier M, Syrota A et al 1990 Noninvasive quantification of muscarinic receptors in vivo with positron emission tomography in the dog heart. Circulation 82: 1494–1504
75. Delforge J, Le Guludec D, Syrota A, Crouzel C, Merlet P 1991 In vivo quantification of myocardial muscarinic receptors in humans with PET. Circulation 84 (Suppl. II):II–423 (Abstract)

93. Cardiac stress testing

D. J. Pennell

INTRODUCTION

The use of exercise for stress of the heart has been practised for over 60 years and clinicians are both familiar and comfortable with its use during exercise electrocardiography. It has also been widely used for nuclear medicine studies of the heart. However, no matter how well validated a technique, newer alternatives arise to challenge its use as has happened with the pharmacological stress agents. A large number of cardiac patients are unable to exercise to their full potential because of non-cardiac reasons, and a standard exercise stress test is then a suboptimal means of assessing them. The pharmacological stress agents largely remove the need for patient cooperation and motivation, and enable a confident assessment of cardiac function in virtually all cases. This has led to a great increase in their popularity, and numerous studies have now validated their use, particularly for myocardial perfusion imaging. This chapter examines the role of exercise and pharmacological stress for the assessment of the heart by nuclear medicine methods with detail on the physiological changes provoked by stress, the types of protocols in common use, the rationale behind them, when to use each technique and their important contraindications.

DYNAMIC EXERCISE STRESS

Dynamic exercise stress protocols

The earliest exercise protocols used steps,[1] but today the treadmill or the bicycle ergometer are in common use. The treadmill belt speed and slope incline can both be altered and the most commonly applied protocol uses progressive increases in both every 3 min to provide an intense workload over a relatively short period of time (Table 93.1).[2] For patients with lower exercise capacity a modified Bruce protocol or the Naughton-Balke protocol are available.[3] The bicycle ergometer is more difficult to use for elderly patients but has the advantages of providing a stable base for producing electrocardiographic tracings without motion artefact and the exercise is independent of the patient's weight which allows the ready assessment of the actual work performed. The usual protocol is for 2 min stages starting at a workload of 25 watts with 25 watt increments (Table 93.2). There is no definitive evidence that either the bicycle ergometer or the treadmill is superior for assessment of exercise tolerance. Whilst walking is a more physiological form of exercise that is commonly associated with the patient's symptoms, the bicycle is smaller, less expensive and much better suited to imaging techniques. Arm exercise protocols have been devised but are less well tolerated and are not in common use.

Table 93.1 The standard Bruce protocol for dynamic treadmill exercise

Stage	Duration	Speed (miles/h)	Grade (%)
1	3 min	1.7	10
2	3 min	2.5	12
3	3 min	3.4	14
4	3 min	4.2	16
5	3 min	5.0	18
6	3 min	5.5	20
7	3 min	6.0	22

Table 93.2 Typical supine bicycle exercise protocol

Stage	Revs/min	Watts	Duration (perfusion)	Duration (RNV)
1	50	25	2 min	3 min
2	50	50	2 min	3 min
3	50	75	2 min	3 min
4	50	100	2 min	3 min
5	50	125	2 min	3 min
6	50	150	2 min	3 min
7	50	175	2 min	3 min
8	50	200	2 min	3 min

Safety of dynamic exercise stress

The safety of exercise testing has been reported in five major studies of over 1.6 million patient tests. The complication rates vary widely according to the population under examination, from no complications in 385 000 tests in healthy student athletes,[4] to 0.23% in patients with arrhythmias.[5] In the largest retrospective survey of 1 356 168 exercise tests from outpatient cardiology clinics, the overall complication rate was 0.011% whilst in the largest prospective survey of 50 000 tests the complication rate was 0.048%.[6] The mortality rate has been reported as 0.094%[7] to 0.0014%.[8]

Contraindications to dynamic exercise stress

These have been summarized in detail,[9] but essentially dynamic exercise should normally be avoided during active inflammation or infection of the heart (endocarditis, myocarditis, pericarditis); when unstable cardiac conditions are present (unstable angina, severe left main stem stenosis, severe aortic stenosis, uncontrolled heart failure, severe systemic or pulmonary hypertension); and when malignant rhythm disorders may be provoked.

Normal physiological responses to dynamic exercise

Many haemodynamic variables have been studied during exercise in normal subjects and patients with coronary artery disease. There are substantial variations in the results for some variables because of differences in stress technique, measurement technique, posture, age of the subjects and severity of arterial disease. In general the published data is more complete for the bicycle ergometer because of the difficulties of some invasive measurements during upright treadmill exercise.

With treadmill exercise the systolic blood pressure rises almost linearly with the level of exercise until the maximum level of oxygen consumption (mVO_2) is reached. At peak exercise the blood pressure may fall slightly with the onset of predominantly anaerobic work. The peak systolic blood pressure is higher in men, older patients and in well-trained athletes. The diastolic blood pressure falls slightly during upright exercise due to decreased systemic vascular resistance but this is often difficult to determine during high levels of exercise.[10] During sitting bicycle ergometry, there is a similar response except that the diastolic blood pressure rises slightly.[11,12] The heart rate increases approximately linearly during treadmill exercise,[10] and during sitting bicycle ergometry.[11] The maximum heart rate is inversely related to age.[13,14] Women achieve a higher heart rate at each level of exercise,[10] but a lower maximum heart rate.[13,14] The rate-pressure or double product is the product between systolic blood pressure and the heart rate. It is the best non-invasive index of myocardial oxygen consumption, although the most significant component is the heart rate.[15] During treadmill exercise and sitting bicycle ergometry the double product rises approximately linearly with workload.[16] Coronary blood flow is closely related to the double product (Fig. 93.1).[17]

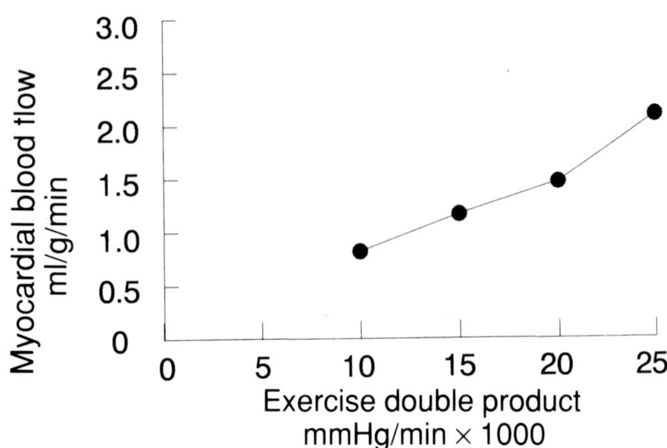

Fig. 93.1 The coronary flow rises approximately linearly as the exercise double product increases. The increase observed is generally lower than with the vasodilators. (Adapted from reference 17).

The cardiac output rises approximately linearly with exercise.[18] Both the resting and the maximal level with exercise is attenuated with increasing age.[19] The response of the stroke volume to exercise is less well defined however, with poor consensus in the early literature because of the large variation between individuals and the substantial changes caused by posture, different levels of exercise achieved between studies and the effects of heart rate. As the body adopts a more upright position more blood is distributed into the periphery from the thorax and the heart becomes smaller. The reduced diastolic filling causes a fall in stroke volume. Exercise in the upright position rapidly re-establishes venous return by muscle activity and the stroke volume rises and is maintained, whilst in the supine position the resting stroke volume is initially much higher and during exercise the stroke volume remains constant and at a higher level than that which occurs with the upright position. Individual responses, however, are unpredictable.[20] The increase in the cardiac output during exercise is mainly caused by the heart rate increase and relatively little part is played by the stroke volume increase.[21] Non-invasive studies by Doppler echocardiography have confirmed this pattern during supine and sitting bicycle ergometry and suggested that at peak supine exercise a small fall in the stroke volume may occur.[22]

The change in end-diastolic volume with exercise is disputed, with some studies showing an increase,[23,24] and others a decrease.[25,26] This may be the result of variation in normal subjects but in addition, increases in the maximum exercise end-diastolic volume occur after a period of physical training which supports a greater maximum cardiac output.[27] The end-systolic volume decreases with exercise and therefore the ejection fraction increases.[24,25]

Regional wall motion (excursion of the endocardium from end-diastole to end-systole) and contraction (change in myocardial thickness between epicardium to endocardium from end-diastole to end-systole) vary widely at rest between individuals and throughout the myocardium.[28] Despite this normal variation, the response to exercise is an increase in regional ejection fraction (regional wall motion) with a reduction in regional variation.[29] The response of wall thickening to exercise in humans is not well documented because of the technical difficulties of acquiring good quality echocardiographic images of the left ventricle during exercise and problems in surveying the whole left ventricle, but experiments in dogs using pharmacological stress during ultrafast X-ray computerized tomography show that thickening increases with this form of stress.[30] Echocardiography may be used to examine parameters of ascending aortic flow during systole as indices of global systolic function, but the results depend on the position of the patient prior to exercise. The peak flow velocity and the peak flow acceleration rise in normal subjects with supine and upright exercise but the increase in both cases is higher for upright exercise. This is because a significant reduction in these parameters occurs on rising from the supine position at rest, though during maximal exercise the peak values are the same.[31] Men and women respond similarly but the increases are attenuated with advancing age.[32] A reduction in these parameters also occurs at rest with advancing age,[33] and this may be due to an increase in aortic root diameter,[34] a confounding factor that is not corrected during Doppler studies.[35]

Flow in the coronary arteries occurs predominantly in diastole when the myocardial wall stress is low and it can be measured in a number of ways. During exercise the coronary flow (Q) increases and the ratio Q_{max}/Q_{basal} is known as the coronary flow reserve, which is a useful physiological measure of the disturbance to increased flow caused by stenoses irrespective of their number and anatomical appearance. In humans the typical coronary flow reserve in normal arteries is approximately 5.0.[36] The increase in coronary flow during exercise is difficult to measure because of the invasive techniques required and the first reported attempt to measure it used an ^{131}I-albumin technique during leg raising and coronary flow increased by only a factor of 1.4.[37] More modern techniques, during maximal supine bicycle ergometry in normal subjects, have demonstrated an increase in coronary flow from 2.6 using the ^{133}Xe washout technique,[17] to between 2.1[38] and 3.9[39] using coronary sinus thermodilution.

Abnormal haemodynamic responses to dynamic exercise

Patients who develop myocardial ischaemia during exercise have an impaired haemodynamic response, but the specificity of these responses is poor for detecting coronary artery disease. The systolic blood pressure may fail to rise or even fall and a reduction of more than 10 mmHg is regarded as an indication to stop the exercise test. The heart rate at peak exercise limited by symptoms may be below 85% of the maximum predicted for age, which is regarded as the level at which satisfactory maximum exercise has been achieved, but this is affected by the physical condition of the patient and the limiting symptoms may be non-cardiac in origin. Regional abnormalities in contraction may lead to an increase in the end-diastolic and end-systolic volumes which cause the ejection fraction to decrease. The changes in stroke volume and cardiac output with myocardial ischaemia are not well documented although the maximum stroke volume and cardiac output at peak exercise is reduced in patients with angina or infarction, though it is not clear if this is simply related to reduced exercise tolerance.[19] Doppler-derived parameters of aortic flow have been measured in patients with coronary artery disease during exercise and significantly lower responses of peak flow velocity have been found by some[40,41] but not others,[42] whilst the lower response of aortic flow acceleration was found useful in one study.[42] Unfortunately because the normal and ischaemic responses were qualitatively similar, the differences were difficult to distinguish in individuals.

ALTERNATIVE STRESS TECHNIQUES TO DYNAMIC EXERCISE

A number of stress techniques other than dynamic exercise have been used in coronary artery disease (Table 93.3). Other than the pharmacological techniques, none has gained significant popularity in the clinical setting. This section concentrates on the physiological actions, results in the clinical setting, and safety and contraindications to the use of the pharmacological stress agents. Each

Table 93.3 Forms of cardiovascular stress

Exercise	Dynamic isometric	Treadmill bicycle Handgrip
Pharmacological	Vasodilator	Dipyridamole Adenosine
	Vasoconstrictor	Ergonovine Vasopressin Angiotensin
	Beta agonists	Adrenaline Isoprenaline Dopamine Dobutamine
Thermal	Cold pressor	
Pacing	Atrial	
Neural	Mental stress	

produces different physiological and haemodynamic changes and the suitability of each for stress depends on the imaging technique being used.

ADENOSINE

Physiology

The use of adenosine for the detection of coronary artery disease is increasing and in time may supplant dipyridamole. Adenosine is a naturally occurring purine (Fig. 93.2) which mediates the cellular action of dipyridamole and can be given intravenously for a direct effect. It causes vasodilation by binding to the A2 receptor and increasing intracellular cyclic AMP (Fig. 93.3). Its main attraction is the very short half-life of between 4[43] and 10s,[44] which affords rapid control of the vasodilatation and any side-effects. The typical haemodynamic response to infusion of adenosine is a mild increase in heart rate, probably mediated by reflex response to peripheral vasodilatation, and a modest fall in systolic and diastolic blood pressure. The double product rises by a small amount. No significant difference has been demonstrated between the coronary hyperaemic response to adenosine and dipyridamole.[45,46]

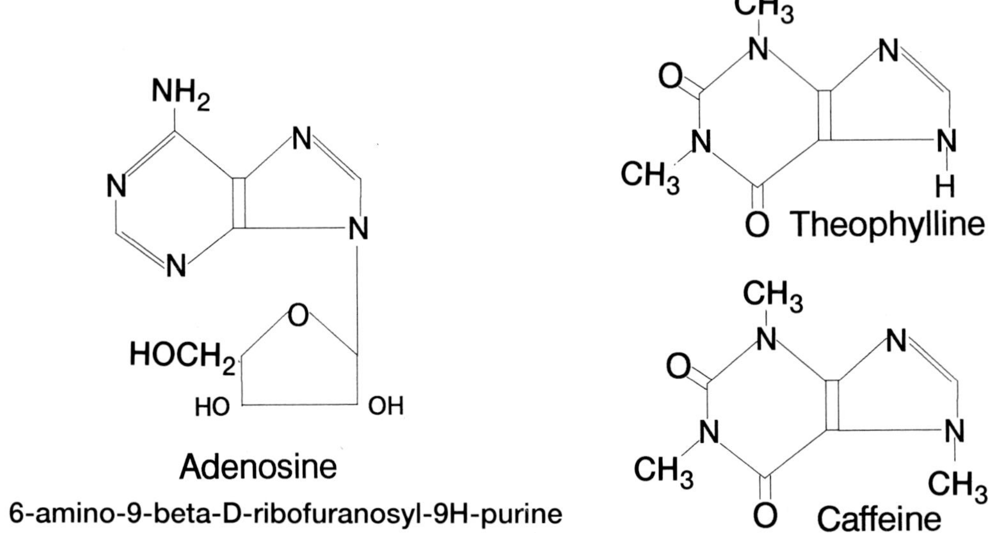

Fig. 93.2 The structural formula of adenosine. Note the similarity with the structure of the methylxanthines which competitively antagonize the action of adenosine.

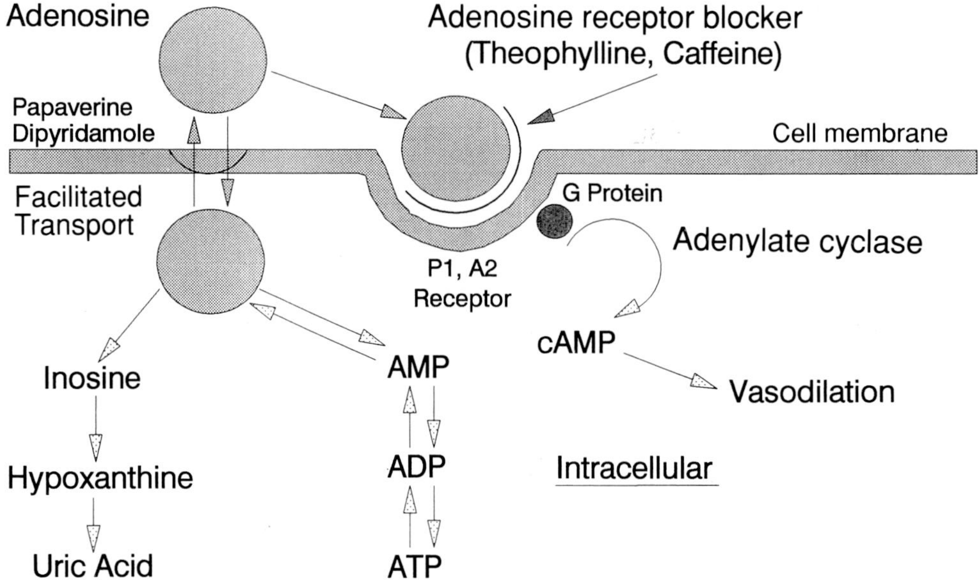

Fig. 93.3 The action of adenosine on the A2 receptor. The intracellular mediator is cyclic AMP.

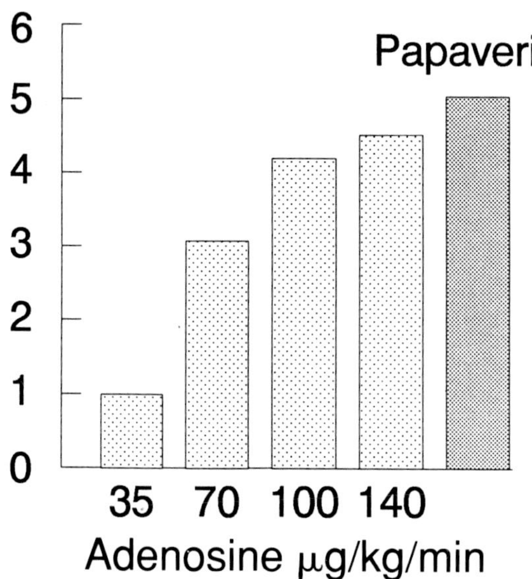

Fig. 93.4 Adenosine dose ranging in humans using coronary blood flow velocity (CBFV) measured by Doppler catheter. In comparison with a maximal dilatory response to papaverine, 92% of patients achieve near maximal coronary hyperaemia at an intravenous dose of 140 μg/kg/min. (Adapted from reference 36).

Clinical imaging infusion protocol

Near maximal coronary vasodilatation is achieved in 92% of patients with an intravenous dose of 140 μg/kg/min (Fig. 93.4) and the increase in coronary flow in humans at this dose is 4.4 times baseline.[36] A myocardial perfusion agent is injected in the third or fourth minute of the infusion.

Symptoms caused by adenosine infusion

Symptoms are very common (80%) with adenosine infusion,[47] but they are very short lived and it is unusual to need to resort to intravenous aminophylline, which competitively inhibits the action of adenosine on the purinoceptor.[48] The pattern of side-effects is very similar to those seen with dipyridamole, but because of the rapid onset of action and the higher plasma adenosine levels seen with direct infusion, the patient experiences more intense effects. Thus the facial flushing which occurs in 35% of patients is particularly profound, and this may cause anxiety or occasionally even morbid fear. Chest pain also occurs in one third of patients but it is of limited diagnostic value because of its frequent occurrence in normal subjects.[49,50] Other symptoms include headache (21%), dyspnoea (19%), throat and epigastric pain (9% each), nausea (5%), dizziness (5%), sour taste (3%) and pains in other sites.[47]

Side effects, and contraindications to adenosine

Adenosine exerts electrophysiological effects on the heart

Open potassium channels – hyperpolarization
Block calcium channels – inhibitory effects

SA node	Increased cycle length
	SA exit block
	Shift of pacemaker to crista terminalis
Atrium	Reduction in atrial refractoriness
AV node	Slows conduction (prolonged AH interval)
	AV block
WPW	Little effect
Ventricle	Little effect

Fig. 93.5 The actions of adenosine on the A1 receptor mediate the adverse electrophysiological events which occur during adenosine stress testing.

by binding to the A1 receptor (Fig. 93.5). This causes inhibition of atrioventricular conduction and thus heart block (1° in 9%, 2° in 3%, and 3° in 0.1%). Pre-existing high degree heart block without a pacemaker is therefore a contraindication to adenosine, although this is unlikely to occur in clinical practice. Pre-existing first degree heart block is not a contraindication as there is no evidence that this progresses to higher grade block with adenosine.[47] If first degree heart block occurs de novo during the adenosine infusion, however, 25% will progress to higher degree of block. Most cases of heart block during adenosine infusion are asymptomatic and respond to stopping of the infusion,[51] but patients with sinoatrial disease are at risk. These patients have unusual sensitivity to the action of adenosine on sinoatrial function,[52] and sinus bradycardia[53] may result which can progress to sinus arrest.[54] This results from hyperpolarization of atrial cells as a result of increased potassium conductance.[55] A greatly exaggerated response to adenosine is also seen in patients receiving treatment with dipyridamole, because of inhibition of adenosine deaminase. Ideally dipyridamole should be avoided for at least 12 h prior to the use of adenosine, otherwise very low doses with titration to patient symptoms must be used. Other drugs such as the benzodiazepines potentiate the effects of adenosine.[56]

Adenosine is also contraindicated in asthma. Inhaled adenosine is a potent bronchoconstrictor of asthmatic but not normal airways.[57] Adenosine may be a bronchoconstrictor mediator of asthma[58] because it is released from the lung in response to hypoxia[59] and antigen challenge.[60] After inhalation of adenosine, specific airways conductance (sGaw) falls reaching a nadir of −45% at 5 min with a slow recovery.[57] The kinetics of bronchoconstriction are similar in allergic and non-allergic asthmatic subjects though non-allergic subjects appear less sensitive.[57] Intravenous injection of adenosine has also been reported to cause severe bronchospasm.[61] Therefore, if asthmatic patients are unable to exercise, the correct alternative is to use dobutamine which has been shown to be very safe in asthma.[62]

Caffeine[63–65] and treatment with methylxanthines[66] also interfere with the action of adenosine for coronary vasodilation. This is because of competitive inhibition at the A2 receptor which occurs with low normal doses of these compounds.[67] Caffeine has a half-life of 5–7 h and should be avoided for at least 12 h prior to the study, and methylxanthines should be avoided for at least 24 h.

Safety of adenosine

Single centre studies and clinical experience suggest a good safety record for adenosine. There are no published myocardial infarctions or deaths directly associated with adenosine infusion in the literature in over 2400 patient studies, although cardiac arrest has occurred in two patients with clandestine sinoatrial disease.[54]

Clinical imaging results with adenosine

Adenosine has been studied mainly for use with thallium myocardial perfusion imaging and has shown excellent results compared with coronary angiography.[68–71] There is also an excellent correlation between exercise and adenosine stress in the assessment of coronary artery disease.[72–75] However, the induction of wall motion abnormalities by adenosine is disputed with evidence that adenosine has little effect on wall motion,[76] and clinical results show a large variation with sensitivity values from 10%[72] to 85%.[77] Adenosine has also proved useful in the assessment of left bundle branch block, by improving the specificity of perfusion imaging in the detection of coronary artery disease when compared with exercise stress.[78] This is probably because of the lower heart rate during stress compared with exercise, which allows longer diastolic filling of the coronary arteries which is impaired during tachycardia by the late septal contraction. Adenosine has not been much used in conjunction with the electrocardiogram because of a low sensitivity for detection of coronary disease. Only one third of patients with coronary artery disease demonstrate ST depression during adenosine infusion, and this bears no relationship to the severity of the ischaemia but is related to the presence of collateral vessels.[79]

DIPYRIDAMOLE

Physiology

Dipyridamole (Fig. 93.6) increases interstitial levels of adenosine by the combined effects of inhibition of the facilitated uptake of adenosine and inhibition of its breakdown by adenosine deaminase.[80] The increase in coronary flow in humans using Gould's original canine regime of 0.56 mg/kg intravenous dipyridamole over 4 min[81] (Fig. 93.7) is between 2.5[186] and 6.0 times baseline.[82] The flow reserve is reduced in arteries with fixed stenoses[83] and the heterogeneous flow produced produces defects of myocardial thallium activity. Ischaemia may also be provoked and the mechanisms for this are complex: first, the increased flow causes a fall in distal perfusion pressure which may be sufficient to cause subendocardial ischaemia;[81] second, flow is redirected from the subendocardium to the subepicardium (Fig. 93.8);[83,84] third, flow in high resistance collateral vessels may be reduced because of the generalized vasodilation and fall in perfusion pressure;[85] fourth, dipyridamole increases the rate

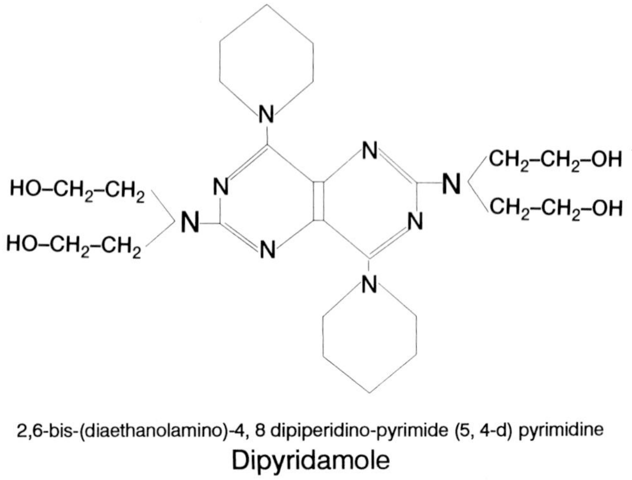

2,6-bis-(diaethanolamino)-4, 8 dipiperidino-pyrimide (5, 4-d) pyrimidine

Dipyridamole

Fig. 93.6 The structural formula of dipyridamole.

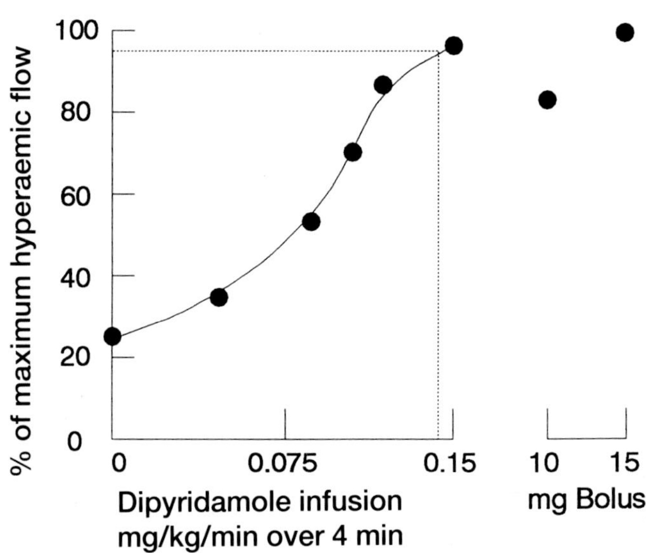

Fig. 93.7 Dipyridamole dose ranging in dogs. The dose of 0.142 mg/kg/min for 4 min caused 95% of the peak hyperaemic response. (Adapted from reference 81).

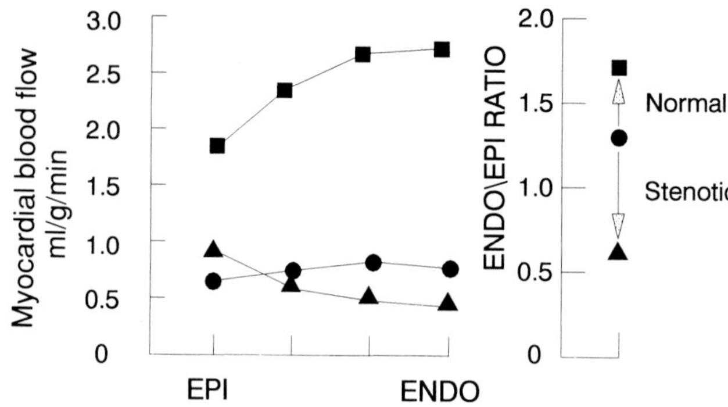

Fig. 93.8 Changes in transmural flow with dipyridamole infusion (the same principles apply to adenosine). At baseline (circles), the transmural blood flow (measured by microspheres in this dog model) is even throughout. After dipyridamole in a myocardial territory supplied by a normal coronary artery (squares), flow increases by up to 5 times baseline with preferential supply to the subendocardium. Therefore the ratio of endocardial to epicardial flow (Endo/Epi) increases. In a myocardial territory supplied by a stenosed coronary artery (triangles), the change in flow is very different. Epicardial flow increases slightly whilst endocardial flow actually decreases in absolute terms. Therefore the Endo/Epi ratio falls. The shunting of blood flow from the endocardium to the epicardium may be termed transmural steal, and endocardial hypoperfusion may lead to ischaemia. (Adapted from reference 84).

pressure product, which raises myocardial oxygen demand.

The increase in coronary flow after dipyridamole reaches its zenith approximately 2 min after the end of the 4 min infusion,[82,86] and it is at this time that a myocardial perfusion agent should be given. The hyperaemic response is prolonged and the half-life of reduction in coronary flow is in the order of 30 min,[186] therefore side-effects and ischaemia may be prolonged. These can be readily reversed using intravenous aminophylline, but in some patients the effect of the dipyridamole outlasts the aminophylline reversal and side-effects can re-emerge later. Caffeine[87,88] and treatment with methylxanthines[89] has been shown to interfere with the coronary hyperaemia induced by dipyridamole and thallium scans after caffeine become falsely negative. Thus, caffeine and methylxanthines should be avoided before dipyridamole injection in the same way as for adenosine studies.

Clinical imaging infusion protocol

Dipyridamole can either be given orally (400 mg) or intravenously at a standard dose (0.56 mg/kg), or at higher doses when used with echocardiography (0.84–1 mg/kg). Because gastric absorption of dipyridamole is very variable, plasma levels after an oral dose are unpredictable and the time of maximum coronary flow is unknown.[90] This makes oral administration unreliable for the production of perfusion abnormalities and it leads to a higher incidence of unpleasant gastrointestinal side-effects.[91] Intravenous administration is therefore preferred.

Symptoms caused by dipyridamole

The non-cardiac side-effects of dipyridamole are very similar to those described for adenosine, though they tend to be less intense because of the slower onset of hyperaemia. Following intravenous dipyridamole, chest pain occurs in 20% of patients, headache in 12%, dizziness in 12% and nausea in 5%.[92] Other side-effects are less common and mild.

Side-effects and contraindications to dipyridamole

Minor dysrhythmias after dipyridamole are common with the incidence of ventricular premature beats reported as ranging from 5%[92] to 20%.[100] Other dysrhythmias are very rare with reports of symptomatic bradycardia,[93] atrial fibrillation,[94] ventricular tachycardia[104] and ventricular fibrillation,[95,104] although one case was complicated by the use of high dose aminophylline.[95]

Bronchospasm after dipyridamole is recognized in asthmatic patients.[96,97] One severe case and six less serious cases of bronchospasm after dipyridamole were reported in one series,[92] and eight cases in another,[104] with some of these patients and others[98] requiring intubation. Existing treatment with steroids does not appear to protect patients.[104] Therefore a history of asthma should be considered a contraindication to the use of dipyridamole, and dobutamine has been shown to be an effective alternative.[62] Other rare but serious complications with dipyridamole stress include stroke[99] and transient ischaemic attacks[104] which may be related to reduced cerebral perfusion from hypotension or steal.

Safety of dipyridamole

The safety of intravenous dipyridamole in patients with coronary artery disease has been the subject of close scrutiny and it has a good record.[92,100–102] In the largest published study of 3911 patients, one patient (0.026%) with chronic stable angina suffered myocardial infarction within 24 h of the dipyridamole infusion. A further three patients (0.077%) with unstable angina also had a myocardial infarction and two of the patients (0.051%) died. In another study, 170 patients with known or suspected unstable angina were studied by thallium imaging using dipyridamole infusion and two small infarctions (1.2%) but no deaths resulted.[103] Because of the high incidence of infarction in patients with unstable angina, it is not possible to conclude that the infarctions were a direct effect of dipyridamole but it suggested that the use of dipyridamole in such patients was associated with increased risk. A follow-up study of 64 000 patients undergoing dipyridamole testing has recently been presented in abstract form and this throws further light on the incidence of serious complications from the use of dipyridamole.[104] The incidence of cardiac deaths was 0.01% and non-fatal myocardial infarction 0.02%.

The safety of dipyridamole infusion protocols other than the standard intravenous dose of 0.56 mg/kg has also been examined. The higher dose dipyridamole protocol (0.84 mg/kg) has been reviewed in 10 451 studies.[105] Major complications occurred in seven patients (0.07%) and included one death, two myocardial infarctions, and prolonged ventricular tachycardia, pulmonary oedema and ventricular asystole in one patient each. Hypotension or bradycardia requiring aminophylline treatment was seen in 0.4%. These figures are not substantially different from those published for the standard dose dipyridamole protocol. The other route of dipyridamole administration has been oral. Again no increase in serious complications has been reported compared to the intravenous route.[102]

Clinical imaging results with dipyridamole

The action of dipyridamole as a coronary vasodilator suggested a possible role in the treatment of angina, but subsequent experience showed that it frequently exacerbated chest pain particularly when given intravenously, and double blind trials confirmed its lack of efficacy.[106,107] It was later shown to reduce subendocardial blood flow,[108] and a study using it in the diagnosis of coronary artery disease by provocation of chest pain was published.[109] Subsequently dipyridamole has been widely used in conjunction with imaging techniques. The first of these used intravenous dipyridamole with thallium myocardial perfusion imaging,[110] and comparisons with coronary angiography[111–113] have shown excellent results, with diagnostic equivalence in comparison with exercise stress.[114–116] Oral dipyridamole has also been used successfully.[117–120] Comparison of the diagnostic potential of the intravenous and oral protocols show similar results,[121] but in general, the intravenous protocol is preferred. Comparison of submaximal stress against dipyridamole for thallium imaging has shown improved results with dipyridamole, suggesting that vasodilators should be used instead of exercise where adequate suspicion of poor exercise tolerance exists.[122] Dipyridamole has been less successful when used with radionuclide ventriculography,[123–126] which suggests that perfusion defects may occur without accompanying wall motion abnormality. This has also been found with echocardiography[127,128] and higher doses are commonly used to provoke ischaemia.[129–131] These results have also been reproduced using magnetic resonance imaging.[132–135] Dipyridamole thallium imaging has also been shown to be useful in defining prognosis in stable angina,[136] before non-cardiac surgery,[137,138] after myocardial infarction[139,140] in the elderly,[141] and in renal disease.[142] Dipyridamole echocardiography may also be useful in defining prognosis.[143]

DOBUTAMINE

Choice of β-agonist and physiology

The β-agonists (Fig. 93.9) increase myocardial oxygen demand through a combined inotropic and chronotropic action with varying actions on the adrenergic receptors (Fig. 93.10). There are a number of differences between the drugs in route of administration, safety, and efficacy in the provocation of myocardial ischaemia for study. Epinephrine should be given by a central line because of venous constriction from α-agonist effects and the same is true of dopamine, though its constricting action is less intense. Isoprenaline has no α-agonist effects but is

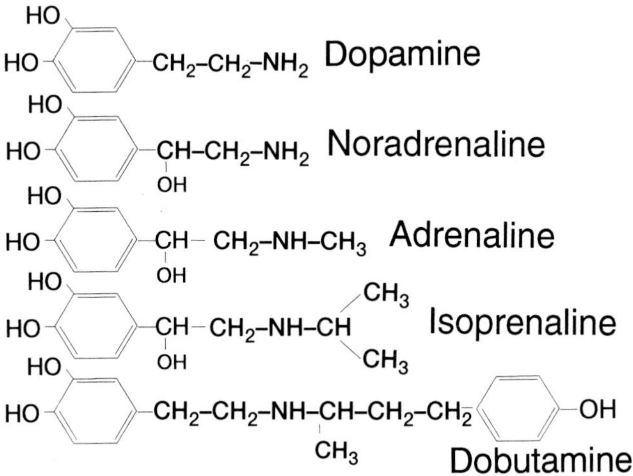

Fig. 93.9 The structural formulae of the commonly available β-agonists. Dobutamine is the most complex molecule and, like isoprenaline, is synthetic.

	Alpha	Beta-1	Beta-2
Dopamine	++	+++	++
Noradrenaline	++++	++++	0
Adrenaline	++++	++++	++
Isoprenaline	0	++++	++++
Dobutamine	+	++++	++

Fig. 93.10 Actions of the common β-agonists on the adrenergic receptors. Agents with high α activity are not suitable for peripheral infusion because of the induction of venospasm.

maintained in a solution of pH 2, which causes intense irritation to small veins. It raises the heart rate with no action on the blood pressure and therefore does not mimic the physiological changes of dynamic exercise. Dobutamine however is produced in a neutral non-irritant solution and its mild α-agonist effects make it the only commonly available inotrope for safe infusion in peripheral veins (Fig. 93.11). Dobutamine also causes significantly less dysrhythmia than the other inotropes in the ischaemic heart (Fig. 93.12),[144] a property also described in the human ischaemic heart.[145,146]

Dobutamine increases myocardial oxygen demand by virtue of its inotropic and chronotropic actions, and in the setting of acute ischaemia it has been shown to increase oxygen demand above availability.[147] But it also has other effects which contribute to the provocation of myocardial ischaemia. It dilates the distal coronary vessels which leads to an increase in coronary flow,[148–150] and a fall in perfusion pressure distal to coronary stenoses. Flow therefore becomes heterogeneous[151] and may be redirected to the subepicardium.[148] In this respect dobutamine is similar to adenosine and dipyridamole. Dobutamine may also increase flow resistance at the site of a stenosis.[148] The increase in coronary flow with dobutamine is not well studied but has been reported as 2.1 times baseline for an intermediate dose of 10 μg/kg/min.[148] A recent PET study suggests an increase of 2.9 times baseline at 40 μg/kg/min.[152] Dobutamine has a rapid onset and cessation of action (plasma half-life 120 s) allowing easy control of blood levels over any duration of imaging.

	Vasospasm	Inflammation
Epinephrine	++++	-
Norepinephrine	++++	-
Dopamine	++	-
Isoproterenol	0	+++
Dobutamine	0	0

Fig. 93.11 Actions of the β-agonists on the peripheral veins. Vasospasm occurs because of α effects but, in addition, isoprenaline is maintained in highly acidic solution which causes intense venous inflammation. Therefore, dobutamine is the only commonly available β agonist which may be infused safely in peripheral veins. This is a major advantage for routine non-invasive clinical usage.

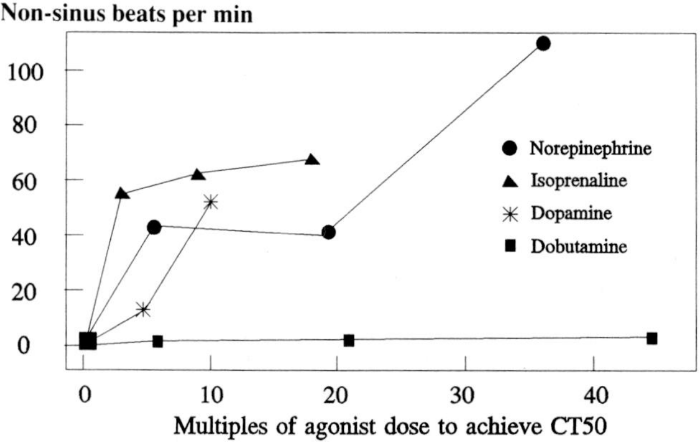

Fig. 93.12 The arrhythmogenicity of the β-agonists. The dose given is expressed in terms of the number of multiples of dose required to induce a 50% maximum contractile response in an isolated muscle strip. When non-sinus beats are used as the criterion for propensity to induce arrhythmia, dobutamine was the safest drug. (Adapted from reference 144.)

Imaging infusion protocol

Dobutamine has proved very useful as an alternative to both exercise and the vasodilators. Dobutamine is given as an infusion and there is no accepted protocol for this at present. Doses up to 40 μg/kg/min have been used safely and a possible protocol compromising between allowing equilibrium at each stage of stress and the length of the stress might be to commence at 10 μg/kg/min and proceed in 10 μg/kg/min steps every 3 min. The longest duration of stress would then be approximately 12 min.

Symptoms caused by dobutamine

Non-cardiac symptoms caused by dobutamine include tingling, flushing, nausea, headache, shaking and light-headedness,[157] which, in general, are related to activation of the sympathetic nervous system.

Side-effects and contraindications to dobutamine

Non-sustained ventricular tachycardia occurs in about 4% of patients but is usually well tolerated.[153] Supraventricular tachycardia and atrial fibrillation may also occur. Ventricular and atrial premature beats are common, occurring in approximately 15 and 10% respectively. Other cardiac related symptoms include pounding, palpitation and dyspnoea. Hypotension may occur during dobutamine infusion, but this may relate to intraventricular obstruction[154] and is not associated with the same adverse prognosis as when it is seen during dynamic exercise.[155] Dobutamine is contraindicated in the same conditions that apply to dynamic exercise, but is safe in asthma.[62]

Safety of dobutamine

The safety of dobutamine stress for thallium imaging has not been assessed but one study of its use for echocardiography in over 1000 patients with known or suspected coronary artery disease was not associated with myocardial infarctions, deaths or other serious sequelae.[153]

Clinical imaging results

Dobutamine has been used for thallium,[62,156–159] and MIBI[160] myocardial perfusion imaging, with excellent results in comparison with coronary angiography and exercise stress. There has been little experience with the use of dobutamine for radionuclide ventriculography[161–163] and the results have been mixed. This does not concur with the excellent results in the detection of wall motion abnormalities seen by echocardiography,[164–168] and magnetic resonance imaging.[169,170] If patients have a poor chronotropic response to the dobutamine stress, atropine in doses from 0.25 to 1 mg has been shown to improve the diagnostic accuracy by provoking a tachycardia.[171] Dobutamine has also been used with thallium imaging[172] and echocardiography[173] to determine the risk of surgery, and at low dose levels it may identify viable myocardium by increasing wall thickening in asynergic areas.[174]

COMPARISONS BETWEEN THE PHARMACOLOGICAL STRESS AGENTS

There are few direct comparisons of the stress agents involving nuclear medicine studies. A recent comparison of adenosine and dobutamine for both MIBI SPECT and echocardiography showed equivalence for the two agents for MIBI, but poor sensitivity using adenosine for echocardiography.[175] A comparison of adenosine, dipyridamole and dobutamine for echocardiography showed the best sensitivity for dobutamine but the best specificity for adenosine.[176]

COMBINED VASODILATOR AND EXERCISE STRESS

The vasodilators have an excellent record in assessing coronary artery disease but suffer from several minor disadvantages. These include the very common level of troublesome side-effects and the high splanchnic thallium uptake which may interfere with image interpretation. It has been shown that both of these problems can be resolved with the addition of moderate exercise to the vasodilator protocol. This would typically be 50–75 W on the bicycle ergometer. This has been demonstrated both for dipyridamole[177–179] and adenosine,[180] and for both drugs a trend towards improved diagnostic performance may be seen when the additional exercise is used. In the case of adenosine, it has also been shown that there is a significant reduction in dysrhythmias such as heart block with the added exercise.[180]

OTHER STRESS TECHNIQUES

Vasoconstrictors

There is little reported use of vasoconstrictors in the detection of coronary artery disease, though vasopressin,[181] ergonovine[182] and angiotensin[183] have been tried. These agents increase myocardial oxygen demand by increasing the blood pressure with little change in heart rate. Their value is limited except for ergonovine which has been used more recently during cardiac catheterization in the diagnosis of coronary artery spasm.

Handgrip isometric exercise

Isometric exercise raises systolic and diastolic blood pressure with only a small increase in heart rate and cardiac output. The hand dynamometer is commonly used to allow monitoring of the degree and duration of the effort. Electrocardiographic changes can be produced in patients with coronary artery disease but with a low sensitivity[184] that is improved by the demonstration of a decrease in regional ejection fraction by radionuclide ventriculography.[185] However, the results are not impressive and handgrip exercise is probably most useful following dipyridamole infusion to augment coronary vasodilation.[186] It is also unsuited for prolonged imaging techniques because of muscle fatigue.

Atrial pacing

Atrial pacing has been used successfully in the catheter laboratory and has proved valuable for invasive stress studies. The development of ST-segment depression has a similar sensitivity to exercise electrocardiography[187] but it also has a poor specificity, although this can be improved by combining pacing with thallium imaging,[188] echocardiography,[189] and radionuclide ventriculography.[190] Because of the need for intracardiac electrodes, the technique is not suitable for routine use outside the catheter laboratory.

Cold pressor stress

The cold pressor test causes vasoconstriction of the epicardial arteries with reflex coronary resistance vessel dilatation, whilst raising the blood pressure without tachycardia. It rarely produces abnormalities in patients with coronary artery disease when combined with electrocardiography,[191] but improved results are seen with the use of echocardiography[192] or thallium-201 myocardial perfusion imaging.[193] The reasons for the difficulty of combining the cold pressor test with imaging techniques have been demonstrated by first pass radionuclide ventriculography which showed that the time course of ejection fraction depression was highly variable and often delayed or short lived.[194] Capricious results with equilibrium radionuclide ventriculography are therefore inevitable.[195] The technique is not pleasant and is rarely favourably received by patients.

Mental stress

Mental stress (arithmetic, word testing, public speaking) causes significant ejection fraction changes which have been documented using radionuclide blood pool monitoring and a non-imaging probe.[196] Such stress increases the double product, but by a relatively small amount. Ejection fraction changes can be observed within 1 min and they persist until the end of stress with a rapid recovery. Unfortunately it requires considerable patient cooperation and an imaging technique capable of registering rapid changes in ejection fraction.

CONCLUSION

Exercise stress remains the technique of choice for evaluation of the cardiovascular system by nuclear medicine techniques, because it provides extra information such as the exercise duration and symptoms. In addition the electrocardiographic changes may be useful. However, there are a large number of patients whose exercise tolerance is suboptimal and, in clinical practice, patients who are difficult to assess because of physical or psychological limitations are commonly referred for nuclear medicine procedures. The stress agent of first choice in all these cases will be adenosine if it is available, and infusion should be coupled with mild to moderate exercise to limit side-effects and dysrhythmias. This technique is fast and requires little patient cooperation. It is also reasonable to use adenosine with exercise stress in all patients when the exercise tolerance has already been established by exercise electrocardiography. Dobutamine should be used in patients with asthma.

REFERENCES

1. Master A M, Oppenheimer E T 1929 A simple exercise tolerance test for circulatory efficiency with standard tables for normal individuals. Am J Med Sci 177: 223–242
2. Bruce R A 1972 Multi-stage treadmill test of submaximal and maximal exercise. In: Exercise testing and training of apparently healthy individuals: A handbook for physicians. The American Heart Association, New York. Appendix B.
3. Fox S M, Naughton J P, Haskell W L 1971 Physical activity and the prevention of coronary heart disease. Ann Clin Res 3: 404–432
4. Wendt T, Scherer W D, Kaltenbach M 1984 Life threatening complications in 1,741,106 ergometries. Dtsch Med Wochenschr 109: 123–127
5. Young D Z, Lampert S, Graboys T B, Lown B 1984 Safety of maximal exercise testing in patients at high risk for ventricular arrhythmia. Circulation 70: 184–191
6. Atterhog J H, Jonsson B, Samuelsson R 1979 Exercise testing: a prospective study of complication rates. Am Heart J 98: 572–579
7. Rochmis P, Blackburn H 1971 Exercise tests. A survey of procedures, safety and litigation experience in approximately 170,000 tests. JAMA 217: 1061–1066
8. Gibbons L, Blair S N, Kohl H W, Cooper K 1989 The safety of maximal exercise testing. Circulation 80: 846–852
9. Sheffield L T 1984 Exercise stress testing. In: Braunwald E, ed. Heart disease: a textbook of cardiovascular medicine. 2nd edn. Saunders, Philadelphia
10. Wolthuis R A, Froelicher V F, Fischer J, Triebwasser J H 1977 The response of healthy men to treadmill exercise Circulation 55: 153–157
11. Gleichmann U 1984 In: Blutdruck unter körperlicher Belastung. Steinkopf, Darmstadt. p 62
12. Heck H 1984 In: Blutdruck unter körperlicher Belastung. Steinkopf, Darmstadt. p 49
13. Sheffield L T 1972 In: Exercise testing and training of apparently healthy individuals: a handbook for physicians. American Heart Association, New York p 35
14. Sheffield L T, Maloof J A, Sawyer J A, Roitman D 1978 Maximal heart rate and treadmill performance of healthy women in relation to age. Circulation 57: 79–84
15. Nelson R R, Gobel F L, Jorgensen C R, Wang K, Wang Y, Taylor H L 1974 Hemodynamic predictors of myocardial oxygen consumption during static and dynamic exercise. Circulation 50: 1179–1189
16. Kariv I, Kellerman J J 1969 Effects of exercise on blood pressure. Mal Cardiovasc 10: 247–252
17. Holmberg S, Serysko W, Varnauskas E 1971 Coronary circulation during heavy exercise in control subjects and patients with coronary heart disease. Act Med Scand 190: 465–480
18. Rühle K H, Fischer J, Matthys H 1983 Sollwerte für die Spiroergometrie. Atemw U Lungenkr 9: 157–173
19. Hossack K F, Bruce R A, Green B, Kusumi F, DeRouen T A, Trimble S 1980 Maximal cardiac output during upright exercise: approximate normal standards and variations with coronary heart disease. Am J Cardiol 46: 204–212
20. Bevegård S, Holmgren A, Jonsson B 1960 The effect of body position on the circulation at rest and during exercise, with special reference to the influence on the stroke volume. Acta Physiol Scand 49: 279–298
21. Hossack K F 1987 Cardiovascular responses to dynamic exercise. Cardiol Clin 5: 147–156
22. Rassi A, Crawford M H, Richards K L, Miller J F 1988 Differing mechanisms of exercise flow augmentation at the mitral and aortic valves. Circulation 77: 543–551
23. Horwitz L D, Atkins J M, Leshin S J 1972 Role of Frank-Starling mechanism in exercise. Circ Res 31: 868–875
24. Poliner L R, Dehmer G J, Lewis S E et al 1980 Left ventricular performance in normal subjects: a comparison of the responses to exercise in the upright and supine positions. Circulation 62: 528–534
25. Wyns W, Melin J A, Vanbutsele R J et al 1982 Assessment of right and left ventricular volumes during upright exercise in normal men. Eur Heart J 3: 529–536
26. Higginbotham M B, Morris K G, Coleman R E et al 1984 Sex related differences in the normal cardiac response to upright exercise. Circulation 70: 357–366
27. Revyck S K, Scholz P M, Sabiston D C et al 1980 Effects of exercise training on left ventricular function in normal subjects. A longitudinal study by radionuclide angiography. Am J Cardiol 45: 244–252
28. Pandian N G, Skorton D J, Collins S M, Falsetti H L, Burke E R, Kerber R E 1983 Heterogeneity of left ventricular segmental wall thickening and excursion in 2-dimensional echocardiograms of normal human subjects. Am J Cardiol 51: 1667–1673
29. Roig E, Chomka E V, Castaner A et al 1989 Exercise ultrafast computed tomography for the detection of coronary artery disease. J Am Coll Cardiol 13: 1073–1081
30. Lanzer P, Garrett J, Lipton M J et al 1986 Quantitation of regional myocardial function by cine computed tomography: pharmacologic changes in wall thickness. J Am Coll Cardiol 8: 682–692
31. Daley P J, Sagar K B, Wann L S 1985 Doppler echocardiographic measurement of flow velocity in the ascending aorta during supine and upright exercise. Br Heart J 54: 562–567
32. Lazarus M, Dang T, Gardin J M, Henry W L 1988 Evaluation of age, gender, heart rate and blood pressure changes and exercise conditioning on Doppler measured aortic blood flow acceleration

and velocity during upright treadmill testing. Am J Cardiol 62: 439–443
33. van Dam I, Heringa A, de Boo T et al 1987 Reference values for pulsed Doppler signals from the blood flow on both sides of the aortic valve. Eur Heart J 8: 1221–1228
34. Krovetz J 1975 Age related changes in size of the aortic valve annulus in man. Am Heart J 90: 569–574
35. Gardin J M, Davidson D M, Rohan M K et al 1987 Relationship between age, body size, gender, and blood pressure and Doppler flow measurements in the aorta and pulmonary artery. Am Heart J 113: 101–109
36. Wilson R F, Wyche K, Christensen B V, Zimmer S, Laxson D D 1990 Effects of adenosine on human coronary arterial circulation. Circulation 82: 1595–1606
37. Messer J V, Wagman R J, Levine H J, Neill W A, Krasnow N, Gorlin R 1962 Patterns of human myocardial oxygen extraction during rest and exercise. J Clin Invest 41: 725–742
38. Gertz E W, Wisneski J A, Stanley W C, Neese R A 1988 Myocardial substrate utilisation during exercise in humans. J Clin Invest 82: 2017–2025
39. Bertrand M E, Carre A G, Ginestet A P, Lefebvre J M, Desplanque L A, Lekieffre J P 1977 Maximal exercise in normal subjects. Eur J Cardiol 5: 481–491
40. Bryg R J, Labovitz A J, Mehdirad A, Williams G A, Chaitman B R 1986 Effects of coronary artery disease in Doppler derived parameters of aortic flow during upright exercise. Am J Cardiol 58: 14–19
41. Mehdirad A A, Williams G A, Labovitz A J, Bryg R J, Chaitman B R 1987 Evaluation of left ventricular function during upright exercise: correlation of exercise Doppler with postexercise two dimensional echocardiographic results. Circulation 75: 413–419
42. Harrison M R, Smith M D, Friedman B J, DeMaria A N 1987 Uses and limitations of exercise Doppler echocardiography in the diagnosis of ischaemic heart disease. J Am Coll Cardiol 10: 809–817
43. Möser G H, Schrader J, Deussen A 1989 Turnover of adenosine in plasma of human and dog blood. Am J Physiol 256: C799–806
44. Klabunde R E 1983 Dipyridamole inhibition of adenosine metabolism in human blood. Eur J Pharmacol 93: 21–26
45. Rossen J D, Quillen J E, Lopez A G, Stenberg R G, Talman C L, Winniford M D 1991 Comparison of coronary vasodilation with intravenous dipyridamole and adenosine. J Am Coll Cardiol 18: 485–491
46. Chan S Y, Brunken R C, Czernin J et al 1992 Comparison of maximal myocardial blood flow during adenosine infusion with that of intravenous dipyridamole in normal men. J Am Coll Cardiol 20: 979–985
47. Abreu A, Mahmarian J J, Nishimura S, Boyce T M, Verani M S 1991 Tolerance and safety of pharmacologic coronary vasodilation with adenosine in association with thallium-201 scintigraphy in patients with suspected coronary artery disease. J Am Coll Cardiol 18: 730–735
48. Curnish R R, Berne R M, Rubio R 1972 Effect of aminophylline on myocardial reactive hyperemia. Proc Soc Exp Biol Med 141: 593–598
49. Sylven C, Beermann B, Jonzon B, Brandt R 1986 Angina pectoris like pain provoked by intravenous adenosine in healthy volunteers. Br Med J 293: 227–230
50. Sylven C, Borg G, Brandt R, Beermann B, Jonzon B 1988 Dose effect relationship of adenosine provoked angina pectoris like pain – a study of the psychophysical power function. Eur Heart 9: 87–91
51. Lee J, Heo J, Ogilby J D, Cave V, Iskandrian B, Iskandrian A S 1992 Atrioventricular block during adenosine thallium imaging. Am Heart J 123: 1569–1573
52. Watt A H 1985 Sick sinus syndrome: an adenosine mediated disease. Lancet i: 786–788
53. Benedini G, Cuccia C, Bolognesi R et al 1984 Value of purinic compounds in assessing sinus node dysfunction in man: a new diagnostic method. Eur Heart J 5: 394–403
54. Pennell D J, Mahmood S, Ell P J, Underwood S R 1994 Bradycardia progressing to cardiac arrest during adenosine thallium myocardial perfusion imaging in covert sino-atrial disease. Eur J Nucl Med 21: 170–172
55. Belardinelli L, Isenberg G 1983 Isolated atrial myocytes: adenosine and acetylcholine increase potassium conductance. Am J Physiol 244: H734–737
56. Kenakin T P 1982 The potentiation of cardiac responses to adenosine by benzodiazepines. J Pharmacol Exp Ther 222: 752–758
57. Cushley M J, Tattersfield A E, Holgate S T 1983 Inhaled adenosine and guanosine on airway resistance in normal and asthmatic subjects. Br J Clin Pharmac 15: 161–165
58. Holgate S T, Mann J S, Cushley M J 1984 Adenosine as a bronchoconstrictor mediator in asthma and its antagonism by methylxanthines. J Allergy Clin Immunol 74: 302–306
59. Mentzer R M, Rubio R, Berne R M 1975 Release of adenosine by hypoxic canine lung tissue and its possible role in pulmonary circulation. Am J Physiol 229: 1625–1631
60. Fredholm B B 1981 Release of adenosine from rat lung by antigen and compound 48/80. Acta Physiol Scand 111: 507–508
61. Taviot B, Pavheco Y, Coppere B, Pirollet B, Rebaudet P, Perrin-Fayolle M 1986 Bronchospasm induced in an asthmatic by the injection of adenosine. Presse Med 15: 1103
62. Pennell D J, Underwood S R, Ell P J 1993 Safety of dobutamine stress for thallium myocardial perfusion tomography in patients with asthma. Am J Cardiol 71: 1346–1350
63. Smits P, Boekema P, de Abreu R, Thien Th, Laar van't A 1987 Evidence for an antagonism between caffeine and adenosine in the human cardiovascular system. J Cardiovasc Pharmacol 10: 136–143
64. Fredholm B B, Persson C G A 1982 Xanthine derivatives as adenosine receptor antagonists. Eur J Pharmacol 81: 673–676
65. Smits P, Schouten J, Thien Th 1989 Cardiovascular effects of two xanthines and the relation to adenosine antagonism. Clin Pharm Ther 45: 593–599
66. Alfonso S 1970 Inhibition of coronary vasodilating action of dipyridamole and adenosine by aminophylline in the dog. Circ Res 26: 743–752
67. Sollevi A, Ostergren J, Fagrell B, Hjendahl P 1984 Theophylline antagonises cardiovascular responses to dipyridamole in man without affecting increases in plasma adenosine. Acta Physiol Scand 121: 167–171
68. LaManna M M, Mohama R, Slavich I L et al 1990 Intravenous adenosine (Adenoscan) versus exercise in the noninvasive assessment of coronary artery disease by SPECT. Clin Nucl Med 15: 804–805
69. Verani M S, Mahmarian J J, Hixson J B, Boyce T M, Staudacher R A 1990 Diagnosis of coronary artery disease by controlled coronary vasodilation with adenosine and thallium-201 scintigraphy in patients unable to exercise. Circulation 82: 80–87
70. Nishimura S, Mahmarian J J, Boyce T M, Verani M S 1992 Equivalence between adenosine and exercise thallium-201 myocardial tomography: a multicenter, prospective, crossover trial. J Am Coll Cardiol 20: 265–275
71. Mahmarian J J, Pratt C M, Nishimura S, Abreu A, Verani M S 1993 Quantitative adenosine T1-201 single photon emission computed tomography for the early assessment of patients surviving acute myocardial infarction. Circulation 87: 1197–1210
72. Nguyen T, Heo J, Ogilby D, Iskandrian A S 1990 Single photon emission computed tomography with thallium-201 during adenosine induced coronary hyperaemia: correlation with coronary arteriography, exercise thallium imaging and two-dimensional echocardiography. J Am Coll Cardiol 16: 1375–1383
73. Coyne E P, Belvedere D A, Van de Streeke P R, Weiland F L, Evans R B, Spaccavento L J 1991 Thallium-201 scintigraphy after intravenous infusion of adenosine compared with exercise thallium testing in the diagnosis of coronary artery disease. J Am Coll Cardiol 17: 1289–1294
74. Nishimura S, Mahmarian J J, Boyce T M, Verani M S 1991 Quantitative thallium-201 single photon emission computed tomography during maximal pharmacologic vasodilation with adenosine for assessing coronary artery disease. J Am Coll Cardiol 18: 736–745

75. Gupta N C, Esterbrooks D J, Hilleman D E, Mohiuddin S M 1992 Comparison of adenosine and exercise thallium-201 single photon emission computed tomography (SPECT) myocardial perfusion imaging. J Am Coll Cardiol 19: 248–257
76. Ogilby J D, Iskandrian A S, Untereker W J, Heo J, Nguyen T N, Mercuro J 1992 Effect of intravenous adenosine infusion on myocardial perfusion and function. Hemodynamic/angiographic and scintigraphic study. Circulation 86: 887–895
77. Zoghbi W A, Cheirif J, Kleiman N S, Verani M S, Trakhtenbroit A 1991 Diagnosis of ischemic heart disease with adenosine echocardiography. J Am Coll Cardiol 18: 1271–1279
78. O'Keefe J H, Bateman T M, Silvestri R, Barnhart C 1992 Safety and diagnostic accuracy of adenosine thallium-201 scintigraphy in patients unable to exercise and those with left bundle branch block. Am Heart J 124: 614–621
79. Nishimura S, Kimball K T, Mahmarian J J, Verani M S 1993 Angiographic and hemodynamic determinants of myocardial ischemia during adenosine thallium-209 scintigraphy in coronary artery disease. Circulation 87: 1211–1219
80. Szegi J, Szentmiklosi A J, Cseppento A 1987 On the action of specific drugs influencing the adenosine induced activation of cardiac purinoceptors. In: Papp J Gy, ed. Cardiovascular pharmacology 1987: results, concepts and perspectives. Akademiai Kiado, Budapest. pp 591–599
81. Gould K L 1978 Noninvasive assessment of coronary stenoses by myocardial perfusion imaging during pharmacologic coronary vasodilatation. 1 Physiologic basis and experimental validation. Am J Cardiol 41: 267–278
82. Wilson R F, Laughlin D E, Ackell P H et al 1985 Transluminal, subselective measurement of coronary artery blood flow velocity and vasodilator reserve in man. Circulation 72: 82–92
83. Feldman R L, Nichols W W, Pepine C J, Conti C R 1981 Acute effects of intravenous dipyridamole on regional coronary haemodynamics and metabolism. Circulation 64: 333–344
84. Mays A E, Cobb F R 1984 Relationship between regional myocardial blood flow and thallium-201 distribution in the presence of coronary artery stenosis and dipyridamole induced vasodilatation. J Clin Invest 73: 1359–1366
85. Chambers C E, Brown K A 1988 Dipyridamole induced ST segment depression during thallium-201 imaging in patients with coronary artery disease: angiographic and haemodynamic determinants. J Am Coll Cardiol 12: 37–41
86. Wilson R F, White C W 1986 Intracoronary papaverine: an ideal coronary vasodilator for studies of the coronary circulation in conscious humans. Circulation 73: 444–451
87. Smits P, Aengevaeren W R M, Corstens F H M, Thien T 1989 Caffeine reduced dipyridamole induced myocardial ischaemia. J Nucl Med 30: 1723–1726
88. Smits P, Corstens F H M, Aengevaeren W R M, Wackers F J, Thien T 1991 False negative dipyridamole thallium-201 myocardial imaging after caffeine infusion. J Nucl Med 32: 1538–1541
89. Daley P J, Mahn T H, Zielonka J S, Krubsack A J, Akhtar R, Bamrah V S 1988 Effect of maintenance oral theophylline on dipyridamole thallium-201 myocardial imaging using SPECT and dipyridamole induced hemodynamic changes. Am Heart J 115: 1185–1192
90. Segall G M, Davis M J 1988 Variability of serum drug level following a single oral dose of dipyridamole. J Nucl Med 29: 1662–1667
91. Askut S V, Port S, Collier D et al 1988 Dipyridamole thallium-201 imaging. Complications associated with oral and intravenous routes of administration. Clin Nuc Med 13: 786–788
92. Ranhosky A, Rawson J 1990 The safety of intravenous dipyridamole thallium myocardial perfusion imaging. Circulation 81: 1205–1209
93. Pennell D J, Underwood S R, Ell P J 1990 Symptomatic bradycardia complicating the use of intravenous dipyridamole for thallium-201 myocardial perfusion imaging. Int J Cardiol 27: 272–274
94. Pennell D J, Ell P J 1992 Atrial fibrillation after intravenous dipyridamole for thallium-201 myocardial perfusion imaging. Eur J Nucl Med 19: 1064–1065
95. Bayliss J, Pearson M, Sutton G C 1983 Ventricular dysrhythmias following intravenous dipyridamole during stress myocardial imaging. Br J Radiol 56: 686
96. Cushley M J, Tallant N, Holgate S T 1985 The effect of dipyridamole on histamine and adenosine induced bronchoconstriction in normal and asthmatic subjects. Eur J Respir Dis 67: 185–192
97. Crimi N, Palermo F, Oliveri R et al 1988 Enhancing effect of dipyridamole inhalation on adenosine induced bronchospasm in asthmatic patients. Allergy 43: 179–183
98. Lette J, Cerino M, Laverdier M, Tremblay J, Prenovault J 1989 Severe bronchospasm followed by respiratory arrest during dipyridamole-thallium imaging. Chest 95: 1345–1347
99. Whiting J H, Datz F L, Gabor F V, Jones S R, Morton K A 1993 Cerebrovascular accident associated with dipyridamole thallium-201 myocardial imaging: case report. J Nucl Med 34: 128–130
100. Homma S, Gilliland Y, Guiney T E, Strauss H, Boucher C A 1987 Safety of intravenous dipyridamole for stress testing with thallium imaging. Am J Cardiol 59: 152–154
101. Lam J Y T, Chaitman B R, Glaenzer M et al Safety and diagnostic accuracy of dipyridamole-thallium imaging in the elderly. J Am Coll Cardiol 11: 585–589
102. Askut S V, Port S, Collier D et al 1988 Dipyridamole thallium-201 myocardial imaging: complications associated with oral and intravenous routes of administration. Clin Nucl Med 13: 281–287
103. Zhu Y Y, Chung W S, Botvinick E H et al 1991 Dipyridamole infusion scintigraphy: the experience with its application in one hundred seventy patients with known or suspected unstable angina. Am Heart J 121: 33–43
104. Lette J and the multicenter dipyridamole safety study 1993 Safety of dipyridamole testing in 64,000 patients. J Am Coll Cardiol 21 (Suppl A): 207 (Abstract)
105. Picano E, Marini C, Pirelli S et al 1992 Safety of intravenous high-dose dipyridamole echocardiography. Am J Cardiol 70: 252–258
106. Foulds T, Mackinnon J 1960 Controlled double blind trial of Persantin in treatment of angina pectoris. Br Med J 241: 835–838
107. Kinsella D, Troup W, McGregor M 1962 Studies with a new coronary vasodilator drug: persantin. Am Heart J 63: 146–151
108. Flameng W, Wusten B, Schaper W 1974 On the distribution of myocardial blood flow II. Effects of arterial stenosis and vasodilatation. Basic Res Cardiol 69: 435–446
109. Tauchert M, Behrenbreck D W, Hoetzel J, Hilger H H 1976 Ein neuer pharmakologischer Test zur diagnose der Koronarinsuffizienz. Dtsch Med Wochenschr 10: 37–42
110. Albro P C, Gould K L, Westcott R J et al 1978 Noninvasive assessment of coronary stenoses by myocardial imaging during pharmacological coronary vasodilation. III. Clinical trial. Am J Cardiol 42: 751–760
111. Leppo J, Boucher C A, Okada R D, Newell J B, Strauss W, Pohost G M 1982 Serial thallium-201 myocardial imaging after dipyridamole infusion: diagnostic utility in detecting coronary stenoses and relationship to regional wall motion. Circulation 66: 649–657
112. Schmoliner R, Dudczak R, Kronik G et al 1983 Thallium-201 imaging after dipyridamole in patients with coronary multivessel disease. Cardiology 70: 145–151
113. Fransisco D A, Collins S M, Co R T, Ehrhardt J C, van Kirk O C, Marcus M L 1982 Tomographic thallium-201 myocardial perfusion scintigrams after maximal coronary artery vasodilation with intravenous dipyridamole. Circulation 66: 370–379
114. Josephson M A, Brown B G, Hecht H S, Hopkins J, Pierce C D, Petersen R B 1982 Noninvasive detection and localisation of coronary stenoses in patients: comparison of resting dipyridamole and exercise thallium-201 myocardial perfusion imaging. Am Heart J 103: 1008–1018
115. Varma S K, Watson D D, Beller G A 1989 Quantitative comparison of thallium-201 scintigraphy after exercise and dipyridamole in coronary artery disease. Am J Cardiol 64: 871–877
116. Wilde P, Walker P, Watt I, Rees J R, Davies E R 1982 Thallium myocardial imaging: recent experience using a coronary vasodilator. Clin Radiol 33: 43–50

117. Homma S, Callahan R J, Ameer B et al 1986 Usefulness of oral dipyridamole suspension for stress thallium imaging without exercise in the detection of coronary artery disease. Am J Cardiol 57: 503–508
118. Gould K L, Sorenson S G, Albro P, Caldwell J H, Chaudhuri T, Hamilton G W 1986 Thallium-201 myocardial imaging during coronary vasodilation induced by oral dipyridamole. J Nucl Med 27: 31–36
119. Borges-Neto S, Mahmarian J J, Jain A, Roberts R, Verani M S 1988 Quantitative thallium-201 single photon emission tomography after oral dipyridamole for assessing the presence, anatomic location and severity of coronary artery disease. J Am Coll Cardiol 11: 962–969
120. Beer S, Heo J, Kong B, Lyons E, Iskandrian A 1989 Use of oral dipyridamole SPECT thallium-201 imaging in detection of coronary artery disease. Am Heart J 118: 1022–1027
121. Taillefer R, Lette J, Phaneuf D C, Léveillé J, Lemire F, Essiambre R 1986 Thallium-201 myocardial imaging during pharmacological coronary vasodilation: comparison of oral and intravenous administration of dipyridamole. J Am Coll Cardiol 8: 76–83
122. Young D Z, Guiney T E, McKusick K A, Okada R D, Strauss H W, Boucher C A 1987 Unmasking potential myocardial ischemia with dipyridamole thallium imaging in patients with normal submaximal exercise thallium tests. Am J Noninvas Cardiol 1: 11–14
123. Harris D, Taylor D, Condon B, Ackery D, Conway N 1982 Myocardial imaging with dipyridamole: comparison of sensitivity and specificity of Tl-201 versus MUGA. Eur J Nucl Med 7: 1–5
124. Sochor H, Pachinger O, Ogrist E, Probst P, Kaindl F 1984 Radionuclide imaging after coronary vasodilation: myocardial scintigraphy with thallium-201 and radionuclide angiography after administration of dipyridamole. Eur Heart J 5: 500–509
125. Tono-Oka I, Meguro M, Takeishi Y et al 1989 Relationship of thallium-201 defect and left ventricular function after dipyridamole infusion. Jpn Circ J 53: 707–715
126. Cates C U, Kronenberg M W, Collins H W, Sandler M P 1989 Dipyridamole radionuclide ventriculography: a test with high specificity for severe coronary artery disease. J Am Coll Cardiol 13: 841–851
127. Picano E, Distante A, Masini M, Morales M A, Lattanzi F, L'Abbate A 1985 Dipyridamole-echocardiography test in effort angina pectoris. Am J Cardiol 56: 452–456
128. Margonato A, Chierchia S, Cianflone D et al 1986 Limitations of dipyridamole-echocardiography in effort angina pectoris. Am J Cardiol 59: 225–230
129. Picano E, Lattanzi F, Masini M, Distante A, L'Abbate A 1986 High dose dipyridamole-echocardiography test in effort angina pectoris. J Am Coll Cardiol 8: 848–854
130. Masini M, Picano E, Lattanzi F, Distante A, L'Abbate A 1988 High dose dipyridamole-echocardiography test in women: correlation with exercise-electrocardiography test and coronary arteriography. J Am Coll Cardiol 12: 682–685
131. Mazeika P, Nihoyannopoulos P, Joshi J, Oakley C M 1992 Uses and limitations of high dose dipyridamole stress echocardiography for evaluation of coronary artery disease. Br Heart J 67: 144–149
132. Pennell D J, Underwood S R, Longmore D B 1990 The detection of coronary artery disease by magnetic resonance imaging using intravenous dipyridamole. J Comput Assist Tomogr 14: 167–170
133. Pennell D J, Underwood S R, Ell P J, Swanton R H, Walker J M, Longmore D B 1990 Dipyridamole magnetic resonance imaging: a comparison with thallium-201 emission tomography. Br Heart J 64: 362–369
134. Baer F M, Smolarz K, Jungehulsing M et al 1992 Feasibility of high dose dipyridamole magnetic resonance imaging for detection of coronary artery disease and comparison with coronary angiography. Am J Cardiol 69: 51–56
135. Casolo G C, Bonechi F, Taddei T et al 1991 Alterations in dipyridamole induced LV wall motion during myocardial ischaemia studied by NMR imaging. Comparison with Tc-99m-MIBI myocardial scintigraphy. G Ital Cardiol 21: 609–617
136. Hendel R C, Layden J J, Leppo J A 1990 Prognostic value of dipyridamole thallium scintigraphy for evaluation of ischemic heart disease. J Am Coll Cardiol 109–116
137. Leppo J, Plaja J, Gionet M, Tumolo J, Paraskos J A, Cutler B S 1987 Noninvasive evaluation of cardiac risk before elective vascular surgery. J Am Coll Cardiol 9: 269–276
138. Lette J, Waters D, Lapointe J et al 1989 Usefulness of the severity and extent of reversible perfusion defects during thallium dipyridamole imaging for cardiac risk assessment before noncardiac surgery. Am J Cardiol 64: 276–281
139. Leppo J A, O'Brien J, Rothendler J A, Getchell J D, Lee V W 1984 Dipyridamole thallium-201 scintigraphy in the prediction of future cardiac events after acute myocardial infarction. New Engl J Med 310: 1014–1018
140. Gimple L W, Hutter A M, Guiney T E, Boucher C A 1989 Prognostic utility of predischarge dipyridamole thallium imaging compared to predischarge submaximal exercise electrocardiography and maximal exercise thallium imaging after uncomplicated acute myocardial infarction. Am J Cardiol 64: 1243–1248
141. Shaw L, Chaitman B R, Hilton T C et al 1992 Prognostic value of dipyridamole thallium-201 imaging in elderly patients. J Am Coll Cardiol 19: 1390–1398
142. Derfler K, Kletter K, Balcke P, Heinz G, Dudczak R 1991 Predictive value of thallium-201 dipyridamole myocardial stress scintigraphy in chronic haemodialysis patients and transplant recipients. Clin Nephrol 36: 192–202
143. Picano E, Severi S, Michelassi C et al 1989 Prognostic importance of dipyridamole-echocardiography test in coronary artery disease. Circulation 80: 450–457
144. Tuttle R R, Mills J 1975 Dobutamine, development of a new catecholamine to selectively increase cardiac contractility. Circ Res 36: 185–196
145. Sakamoto T, Yamada T 1977 Haemodynamic effects of dobutamine in patients following open heart surgery. Circulation 55: 525–533
146. Leier C V, Heban P T, Huss P et al 1978 Comparative systemic and regional haemodynamic effects of dopamine and dobutamine in patients with cardiomyopathic heart failure. Circulation 58: 466–475
147. Willerson J T, Hutton I, Watson J T, Platt M R, Templeton G H 1976 Influence of dobutamine on regional myocardial blood flow and ventricular performance during acute and chronic myocardial ischemia in dogs. Circulation 53: 828–833
148. Warltier D C, Zyvlowski M, Gross G J, Hardman H F, Brooks H L 1981 Redistribution of myocardial blood flow distal to a dynamic coronary arterial stenosis by sympathomimetic amines. Comparison of dopamine, dobutamine and isoproterenol. Am J Cardiol 48: 269–279
149. Vasu M A, O'Keefe D D, Kapellakis G Z et al 1978 Myocardial oxygen consumption: effects of epinephrine, isoproterenol, dopamine, norepinephrine and dobutamine. Am J Physiol 235: 237–241
150. Fowler M B, Alderman E L, Oesterle S N et al 1984 Dobutamine and dopamine after cardiac surgery: greater augmentation of myocardial blood flow with dobutamine. Circulation 70 (Suppl I): 103–111
151. Meyer S L, Curry G C, Donsky M S, Twieg D B, Parkey R W, Willerson J T 1976 Influence of dobutamine on haemodynamics and coronary blood flow in patients with and without coronary artery disease. Am J Cardiol 38: 103–108
152. Krivokapich J, Huang S C, Schelbert H R 1993 Assessment of the effects of dobutamine on myocardial blood flow and oxidative metabolism in normal human subjects using nitrogen-13 ammonia and carbon-11 acetate. Am J Cardiol 71: 1351–1356
153. Mertes H, Sawada S G, Ryan T et al 1993 Symptoms, adverse effects and complications associated with dobutamine stress echocardiography. Experience in 1118 patients. Circulation 88: 15–19
154. Pellikke P A, Oh J K, Bailey K R, Nichols B A, Monahan K H, Tajik A J 1992 Dynamic intraventricular obstruction during dobutamine stress echocardiography: a new observation. Circulation 86: 1429–1432

155. Rosamund T L, Vacek J L, Hurwitz A, Rowland A J, Beauchamp G D, Crouse L J 1992 Hypotension during dobutamine stress echocardiography: initial description and clinical relevance. Am Heart J 123: 403–407
156. Mason J R, Palac R T, Freeman M L et al 1984 Thallium scintigraphy during dobutamine infusion: nonexercise dependent screening test for coronary disease. Am Heart J 107: 481–485
157. Pennell D J, Underwood S R, Swanton R H, Walker J M, Ell P J 1991 Dobutamine thallium myocardial perfusion tomography. J Am Coll Cardiol 18: 1471–1479
158. Wallbridge D R, Tweddel A C, Martin W, Hutton I 1993 A comparison of dobutamine and maximal exercise as stress for thallium scintigraphy. Eur J Nucl Med 20: 319–323
159. Hays J T, Mahmarian J J, Cochran A J, Verani M S 1993 Dobutamine thallium-201 tomography for evaluating patients with suspected coronary artery disease unable to undergo exercise or vasodilator pharmacologic stress testing. J Am Coll Cardiol 21: 1583–1590
160. Forster T, McNeill A J, Salustri A et al 1993 Simultaneous dobutamine stress echocardiography and technetium-99m isonitrile single photon emission computed tomography in patients with suspected coronary artery disease. J Am Coll Cardiol 21: 1591–1596
161. Freeman M L, Palac R, Mason J et al 1984 A comparison of dobutamine and supine bicycle exercise for radionuclide cardiac stress testing. Clin Nuc Med 9: 251–255
162. Konishi T, Koyama T, Aoki T et al 1990 Radionuclide assessment of left ventricular function during dobutamine infusion in patients with coronary artery disease: comparison with ergometer exercise. Clin Cardiol 13: 183–188
163. Mohaved A, Reeves W C, Rose G C, Wheeler W S, Jolly S R 1990 Dobutamine and improvement of regional and global left ventricular function in coronary artery disease. Am J Cardiol 66: 375–377
164. Cohen J L, Greene T O, Ottenweller J et al 1991 Dobutamine digital echocardiography for detecting coronary artery disease. Am J Cardiol 67: 1311–1318
165. Sawada S G, Segar D S, Ryan T et al 1991 Echocardiographic detection of coronary artery disease during dobutamine infusion. Circulation 83: 1605–1614
166. Salustri A, Fioretti P M, Pozzoli M M A, McNeill A J, Roelandt J R T C 1992 Dobutamine stress echocardiography: its role in the diagnosis of coronary artery disease. Eur Heart J 13: 70–77
167. Mazeika P K, Nadazdin A, Oakley C M 1992 Dobutamine stress echocardiography for detection and assessment of coronary artery disease. J Am Coll Cardiol 19: 1203–1211
168. Segar D S, Brown S E, Sawada S G, Ryan T, Feigenbaum H 1992 Dobutamine stress echocardiography: correlation with coronary lesion severity as determined by quantitative angiography. J Am Coll Cardiol 19: 1197–1202
169. Pennell D J, Underwood S R, Manzara C C et al 1992 Magnetic resonance imaging during dobutamine stress in coronary artery disease. Am J Cardiol 70: 34–40
170. Pennell D J, Underwood S R, Manzara C C et al 1991 Magnetic resonance imaging of aortic flow during dobutamine stress predicts extent of myocardial ischaemia. Br Heart J 66: 105 (Abstract)
171. McNeil A J, Fioretti P M, El-Said M E-S, Salustri A, Forster T, Roelandt J R T C 1992 Enhanced sensitivity for detection of coronary artery disease by addition of atropine to dobutamine stress echocardiography. Am J Cardiol 70: 41–46
172. Elliott B M, Robinson J G, Zellner J L, Hendrix G H 1991 Dobutamine T1-201 imaging: assessing cardiac risks associated with vascular surgery. Circulation 84 (Suppl III): 54–60
173. Poldermans D, Fioretti P M, Forster T et al 1993 Dobutamine stress echocardiography for assessment of perioperative cardiac risk in patients undergoing major vascular surgery. Circulation 87: 1506–1512
174. Piérard L A, de Landsheere C M, Berthe C, Rigo P, Kulbertus H E 1990 Identification of viable myocardium by echocardiography during dobutamine infusion in patients with myocardial infarction after thrombolytic therapy: comparison with positrom emission tomography. J Am Coll Cardiol 15: 1021–1031
175. Marwick T, Willemart B, D'Hondt A M et al 1993 Selection of the optimal nonexercise stress for the evaluation of ischemic regional myocardial dysfunction and malperfusion: comparison of dobutamine and adenosine using echocardiography and Tc-99m-MIBI single photon emission computed tomography. Circulation 87: 345–354
176. Martin T W, Seaworth J F, Johns J P, Pupa L E, Condos W R 1992 Comparison of adenosine, dipyridamole and dobutamine in stress echocardiography. Ann Intern Med 116: 190–196
177. Casale P N, Guiney T E, Strauss W, Bocher C 1988 Simultaneous low level treadmill exercise and intravenous dipyridamole stress thallium imaging. Am J Cardiol 62: 799–802
178. Stern S, Grenberg D I, Corne R 1991 Effect of exercise supplementation on dipyridamole thallium-201 image quality. J Nucl Med 32: 1559–1564
179. Verzijlbergen F J, Vermeersch P H M J, Laarman G J, Ascoop C A P L 1991 Inadequate exercise leads to suboptimal imaging. Thallium-201 myocardial perfusion imaging after dipyridamole combined with low-level exercise unmasks ischemia in symptomatic patients with non-diagnostic thallium-201 scans who exercise submaximally. J Nucl Med 32: 2071–2078
180. Pennell D J, Mavrogeni S, Forbat S M, Karwatowski S P, Underwood S R 1993 Adenosine combined with exercise for Tl-201 myocardial tomography improves imaging and reduces side-effects. Br Heart J 62 (Abstract)
181. Ruskin A 1947 Pitressin test of coronary insufficiency. Am Heart J 36: 569–579
182. Stein I 1949 Observations on the action of ergonovine on the coronary circulation and its use in the diagnosis of coronary artery insufficiency. Am Heart J 37: 36–45
183. Payne R M, Horowitz L D, Mullins C M 1973 Comparison of isometric exercise and angiotensin infusion as stress test for evaluation of left ventricular function. Am J Cardiol 31: 428–435
184. Kerber R E, Miller R A, Najjar S M 1975 Myocardial ischaemic effects of isometric, dynamic and combined exercise in coronary artery disease. Chest 67: 388–394
185. Bodenheimer M M, Banka V S, Fooshee C M, Gillespie J A, Helfant R H 1978 Detection of coronary heart disease using radionuclide determined regional ejection fraction at rest and during handgrip exercise: correlation with coronary arteriography Circulation 58: 640–648
186. Brown G, Josephson M A, Petersen R D et al 1981 Intravenous dipyridamole combined with isometric handgrip for near maximal coronary flow in patients with coronary artery disease. Am J Cardiol 48: 1077–1085
187. Stratmann H G, Aker U T, Vandormael M, Ischinger T, Wiens R, Kennedy H L 1987 Atrial pacing during percutaneous coronary angioplasty: results and comparison with exercise treadmill testing. Angiology 38: 663–671
188. Stratmann H G, Mark A L, Walter K E, Fletcher J W, Williams G A 1987 Atrial pacing and thallium-210 scintigraphy: combined use for dignosis of coronary artery disease. Angiology 38: 807–814
189. Chapman P D, Doyle T P, Troup P J, Gross C M, Wann L S 1984 Stress echocardiography with transoesophageal atrial pacing: preliminary report of a new method for detection of ischaemic wall motion abnormalities. Circulation 70: 445–450
190. Dehmer G J, Firth B G, Nicod P, Lewis S E, Hills L D 1983 Alterations in left ventricular volumes and ejection fraction during atrial pacing in patients with coronary artery disease: assessment with radionuclide ventriculography. Am Heart J 106: 114–124
191. Verani M S, Zacca N M, DeBauche T L, Miller R R, Chahine R A 1982 Comparison of cold pressor and exercise radionuclide angiocardiography in coronary artery disease. J Nucl Med 23: 770–776
192. Goldi B, Nanda N C 1984 Cold pressor test during 2D-echocardiography: usefulness in detection of patients with coronary disease. Am Heart J 107: 278–285
193. Ahmad M, Dubiel J P, Haibach H 1982 Cold pressor thallium-201 myocardial scintigraphy in the diagnosis of coronary artery disease. Am J Cardiol 50: 1253–1257

194. Dymond D S, Caplin J L, Flatman W, Burnett P, Banim S, Spurrell R 1984 Temporal evolution of changes in left ventricular function induced by cold pressor stimulation. An assessment with radionuclide angiography and gold 195m. Br Heart J 51: 557–564
195. Northcote R J, Cooke M B D 1987 How useful are the cold pressor test and sustained handgrip exercise with radionuclide ventriculography in the evaluation of patients with coronary artery disease. Br Heart J 57: 319–328
196. LaVeau P J, Rozanski A, Krantz D S et al 1989 Transient left ventricular dysfunction during provocative mental stress in patients with coronary artery disease. Am Heart J 118: 1–8

PART B

Diagnosis

94. Single photon myocardial perfusion imaging and exercise radionuclide angiography in the detection of coronary artery disease

James E. Udelson   Jeffrey A. Leppo

INTRODUCTION

The fact that more Americans die from ischaemic heart disease (IHD) than any other disease demands that better methods be developed to diagnose IHD and to determine the response to therapy.[1] The World Health Organization Task Force on Nomenclature defines myocardial ischaemia as a diminished supply of blood in respect to cellular demands caused by coronary perfusion changes (Fig. 94.1).[2] This definition is used to describe any patients with IHD caused by coronary artery disease (CAD) with all other possible causes of 'ischemia' placed in another category. As graphically displayed in Fig. 94.1, non-catheterization methods to detect IHD depend upon determinations of the consequences of altered regional coronary blood flow such as reduction in ventricular function or electrocardiographic (ECG) changes from rest to stress. Traditional objective methods used to determine the presence of IHD include the measurement of metabolic products in the coronary venous drainage and contrast coronary angiography. Non-invasive methods for the evaluation of IHD have traditionally included ECG at rest and stress but, over the past decade, nuclear imaging techniques have also been added to the evaluation of patients with IHD.

Since the objective demonstration of ischaemia by ECG or radionuclide imaging in patients with either chronic CAD,[3–5] or after a recent myocardial infarction,[6–9] is associated with a significantly higher morbidity and mortality, we will review the cellular basis of ischaemia and then outline both the invasive and non-invasive techniques currently available for evaluating patients with possible IHD. Finally, an overall approach to the evaluation of the patient with ischaemia will be outlined.

The detection of myocardial ischaemia relies on measurements at the cellular level, because it is at this level that energy supply and demand meet. In the heart, increased oxygen demands must be met almost entirely by increased coronary flow. As a result, myocardial function and myocardial flow are tightly coupled.[10–15] Excellent reviews of normal and abnormal myocardial cell metabolism have been published by Opie,[16–18] Neely & Morgan,[19] and others.[20–23] Ischaemia in myocardial cells is a highly dynamic process because of the heavy dependence on oxidative metabolism. The contractile function of myocardial cells becomes impaired during an ischaemic insult lasting as little as 1–2 s, because anaerobic metabolism cannot adequately satisfy the metabolic demands of heart cells and the heart cannot incur an oxygen debt.[24–26] The detrimental effects of ischaemia are usually reversible, but after periods of ischaemia as short as 20–40 min, necrosis of myocardial tissue results.[27,28]

Most of the myocardial cell's energy utilization goes to maintain the contractile state. If energy is not constantly

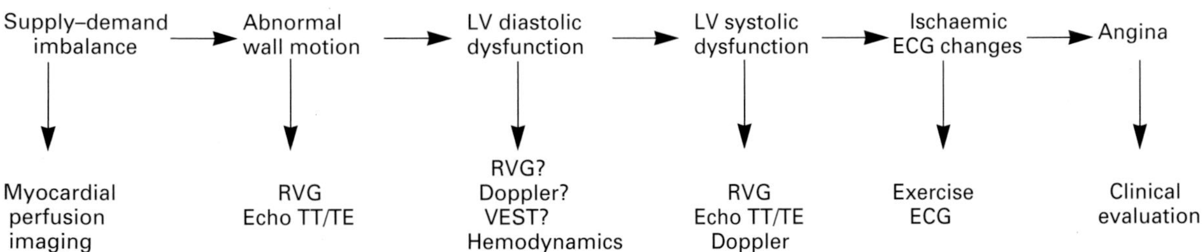

Fig. 94.1 Schematic diagram illustrating the sequence of events during reduction in coronary flow or during demand ischaemia beginning with relative reduction in flow with no sequelae, through diastolic then systolic dysfunction, ischaemic electrocardiographic (ECG) changes and angina. Different imaging modalities will investigate different points on the spectrum. LV = left ventricular, RVG = radionuclide ventriculogram, TT = trans-thoracic, TE = trans-oesophageal.

replenished by oxidative metabolism, energy stores will fall, metabolic byproducts accumulate, and contractile activity decline.[29] Therefore, direct serial tissue measurements or myocardial energy stores (creatine phosphate and adenosine triphosphate) can provide a sensitive guide to the presence or absence of ischaemia,[30,31] although technically this is extremely difficult. Other less direct metabolic measures of ischaemia include local pCO_2,[32,33] lactate production,[34] lactate pyruvate ratio,[35] potassium,[36] or phosphate release.[37] However, all measurements that require myocardial sampling can be used only in experimental animals. Clinically, measurements of metabolites in coronary sinus blood require cardiac catheterization, and these measurements can be altered by conditions other than IHD. Coronary sinus determinations also suffer from the problem that while myocardial ischaemia is usually regional, these measurements reflect total myocardial, not regional myocardial energy balance.[38,39] This is a particular problem when stress is employed in order to exaggerate supply–demand imbalance. In this circumstance, changes in regional flow and metabolism occur that will be masked by the larger volume of normal metabolic washout products found in coronary sinus blood. Therefore, these difficulties with myocardial biopsy and coronary sinus sampling make direct evaluation of myocardial metabolism generally impractical in humans.

NON-INVASIVE EVALUATION

Exercise and ECG

The pioneering work started by Master[40,41] has led to an established role for the ECG-monitored exercise–stress test in the evaluation of IHD. There are reports[42–45] that question the usefulness of exercise testing, especially in populations where IHD would be expected to have a low prevalence. Nevertheless, dynamic exercise–stress testing supplies information useful for evaluating the predisposition to ischaemia during normal daily activity. Most of the published reports in this field support the conclusion that IHD is present when typical angina and reversible ST depression occur during a stress test.[3–5,46–53] In addition, a multifactor analysis of the entire stress test findings can improve the overall accuracy of an exercise evaluation.[54]

The sensitivity of ECG testing for CAD has in large part been based on the findings noted on coronary angiography. There are several potential problems with this analysis:

1. The presence of arterial stenoses do not necessarily imply that a region of myocardial tissue is ischaemic, but rather that there is a potential for the attenuation of regional coronary reserve capacity.
2. Scheuer & Brachfeld[55] have shown that electrochemical changes (ST depression) may not occur until the contractile state is already impaired, which suggests that a certain level of cellular ischaemia must be reached prior to clinically apparent ECG changes.
3. The effect of coronary collateral flow supply to the myocardium distal to a stenosis and the extent of small vessel disease is difficult to interpret.

Therefore, one can conclude that in patients with angiographic coronary stenoses, the sensitivity of ECG evidence of ischaemia ranges from 49% to 80% and the specificity of this test is 41–95% (when 1 mm of ST depression was defined as a positive result).[3–5,47–54]

There are certain factors such as abnormal resting ECG,[55] prior myocardial infarction,[57] hyperventilation,[58] neurasthenia changes,[59,60] drug intake,[61,62] and left ventricular hypertrophy[63,64] that can make interpretation difficult. It is especially in these more difficult cases that radionuclide imaging can provide much greater diagnostic significance.

CONTRIBUTION OF PERFUSION IMAGING, RADIONUCLIDE VENTRICULOGRAPHY AND POSITRON EMISSION TOMOGRAPHY TO THE DIAGNOSIS OF CAD

The sequence of events occurring during the genesis of regional myocardial ischaemia (as outlined in Fig. 94.1) emphasizes the concept that regional abnormalities in myocardial perfusion comprise a continuum from minor relative differences in flow without metabolic or regional functional consequences, to the full expression of myocardial ischaemia with systolic and diastolic dysfunction, ECG signs, and angina.[55,65,66] Seminal studies of coronary blood flow in the early 1970s demonstrated that while a stenosis of approximately 80–90% was necessary to induce a detectable regional coronary flow abnormality at rest, a stenosis of approximately 50% would result in regional flow disturbances during pharmacologically induced hyperaemia.[67] At about the same time, radionuclide imaging of myocardial perfusion was first being reported.[68] These radionuclide techniques evaluating myocardial perfusion, subsequently using ^{201}Tl, were then widely applied in the study of coronary blood flow in humans during stress. The concepts derived in animal models regarding the degree of stenosis required to induce a physiological flow abnormality during hyperaemic stress[67] were applied to these studies, such that a 50% stenosis on a coronary angiogram became the 'gold standard' against which myocardial perfusion imaging was often tested.

Shortly thereafter, the ability to evaluate regional and global systolic ventricular function became available with the use of exercise radionuclide angiography (RNA).[69] This technique was also applied to the study of patients with known or suspected CAD in order to find a non-invasive diagnostic test that would be theoretically more effective than exercise ECG, by measuring a physiological parameter which is affected earlier by ischaemia than the ECG.

Conceptually, if a regional flow disturbance associated with an epicardial coronary stenosis in the presence of an increased myocardial demand represents a continuum from a mild regional flow abnormality to a severe supply–demand imbalance,[55,65,66] then myocardial perfusion imaging should be the most sensitive technique to detect the presence of an epicardial coronary stenosis, with the study of stress regional wall motion by RNA the next most sensitive, and exercise ECG the least sensitive. To some degree, this is reflected in numerous studies evaluating the sensitivities for detecting CAD, and particularly the findings in several studies that myocardial perfusion imaging detects CAD more efficiently at lower work loads than functional imaging or exercise ECG.[70–73] Furthermore, positron emission tomographic (PET) techniques are likely to be the most sensitive technique, as absolute values of regional coronary flow reserve can be measured, presumably detecting more modest heterogeneities in regional flow during a hyperaemic stress.[74–76]

RADIONUCLIDE TECHNIQUES FOR DETECTION OF CAD

Myocardial perfusion imaging

Throughout the late 1970s and early 1980s, many studies examined the use of myocardial perfusion imaging with ^{201}Tl and planar techniques to detect the presence of CAD in comparison with exercise ECG. As summarized by Rozanski & Berman,[77] these studies generally showed that myocardial perfusion imaging had higher sensitivity for detecting disease (80%), as well as a higher specificity for ruling out the presence of disease (92%), compared to exercise ECG (64% and 82% respectively). These early studies generally used a 50% stenosis as the angiographic gold standard for comparison. The initial series of reports thus suggested that myocardial perfusion imaging, as technically performed in these studies (predominantly with visual analysis of planar images), is better than the exercise ECG in detecting the presence of CAD.[77]

Myocardial perfusion imaging has matured considerably since these early studies. There have been advances in imaging acquisition and analysis, as well as advances in the radioisotopes available to trace myocardial perfusion.

Influence of image acquisition technique upon the detection of CAD

The development of single photon emission computerized tomography (SPECT) of myocardial perfusion[78] led to the expectation of improved diagnosis of CAD. This expectation was based on the improved resolution SPECT, and the absence of overlap of myocardial territories which plagues planar imaging, particularly for the left circumflex coronary artery territory. SPECT imaging is technically more demanding than planar imaging, however, and artefacts such as patient motion, non-uniformity of the image detector, or inappropriate centre of rotation, may appear as opponent perfusion defects in the final image.[79] In planar imaging, artefacts such as breast tissue overlying the anterior wall, or diaphragm overlying the inferior wall or apex, are readily apparent from review of the raw and final processed data. In SPECT imaging, these artefacts may be misinterpreted as perfusion defects unless the raw projection data are inspected as a cine-loop display.[79]

How do planar and SPECT imaging compare for the overall diagnosis of CAD? Henkin et al[80] have recently compiled a survey of studies evaluating ^{201}Tl imaging using either planar or SPECT techniques for the diagnosis of angiographically confirmed CAD. A subset was selected for final analysis on the basis of valid experimental design and clearly defined criteria for normal or abnormal images, as well as patient group >50 subjects. The average sensitivity for planar imaging was 85% compared with 93% for SPECT without any loss of specificity: specificity for planar imaging averaged 78% compared to 77% for SPECT. It is important to note that these studies compare planar imaging and SPECT on a study-by-study basis and are not composed of patients undergoing both tests. In addition, the definition of 'coronary disease' varied; some studies used an angiographic cut-off of 50% while others used 70% as the gold standard. Despite these caveats, this survey suggests that SPECT is more sensitive for detecting CAD than is planar imaging, without loss of specificity. Taken together, these studies reflect the information that is available from the few studies in which both modalities have been compared in the same patient population.

In a well-designed study, Fintel et al[81] compared SPECT and planar ^{201}Tl imaging in 112 patients undergoing catheterization and 23 normal volunteers. The studies were performed in random order to obviate the problem of early redistribution of ^{201}Tl following stress which might result in lower sensitivity for the second set of images. In a receiver operating characteristic analysis, SPECT was more powerful than planar imaging. In subgroup analysis, SPECT was particularly accurate for the detection of disease in individual vessel territories, in men, and in those patients with more moderate coronary stenoses (lesion severity $\geq$ 50%, but < 70%). A clinically important difference between the two was the enhanced ability of SPECT to detect multivessel disease in patients with prior myocardial infarction.

Thus, data, both from studies examining the individual modalities,[80] as well as studies comparing these modalities in the same patients,[81–84] suggest that SPECT is more sensitive in detecting CAD, as well as more powerful in detecting the extent of disease, with little or no loss in specificity compared with planar imaging.

Normal variations in planar and SPECT imaging. In planar myocardial perfusion imaging, camera positions are relatively standard. Thus, the reader must allow for anatomical variation (horizontal or vertical heart, clockwise or counterclockwise apical rotation). Because the position of the heart within the thorax is variable, anatomical structures such as the valve planes and the membranous portion of the upper septum are viewed in different projections. These variations, if not appreciated, can be an important source of false positive studies.

With SPECT, the heart is oriented in a standard fashion during the reconstruction process so that with image display, there is more standardization of anatomical landmarks. In some patients, however, normal variations such as the 'drop-out' of the upper septum due to the muscular septum merging with the membranous upper septum, particularly as viewed in the more basal short-axis slices, as well as the normal variations of apical thinning, may be quite prominent (Figs 94.2 and 94.3). A careful review of a series of normal volunteers or subjects with a low probability of CAD with one's own equipment is an important step in minimizing the influence of these normal variations on the sensitivity and specificity for detecting CAD disease in an individual laboratory.

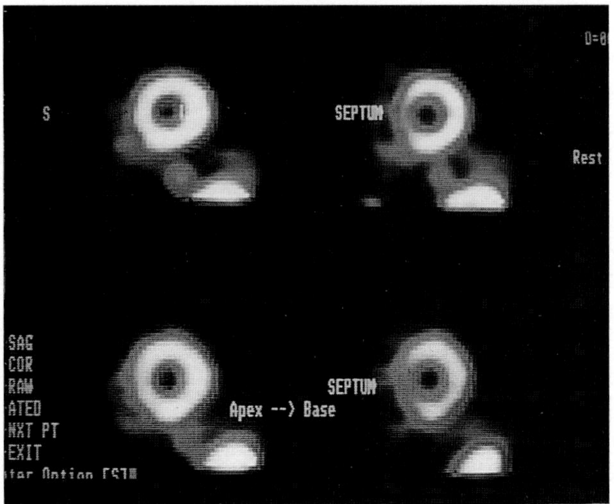

Fig. 94.2 SPECT ^{99m}Tc sestamibi images from a subject with a very low probability of coronary artery disease. This short-axis tomogram demonstrates the normal variation of the membranous portion of the upper septum in the most basal short-axis slice. (Also shown in colour on Plate 28.)

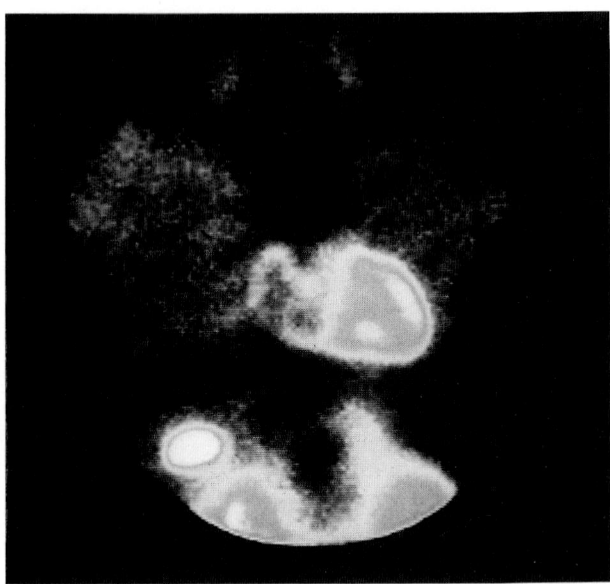

Fig. 94.3 Normal variation apical thinning in a large field-of-view anterior planar ^{99m}Tc sestamibi image from a subject with a low probability of coronary artery disease. Apical thinning may at times be quite prominent. (Also shown in colour on Plate 28.)

Breast attenuation. Attenuation of anterior wall tracer activity by overlying breast tissue has plagued the interpretation of myocardial perfusion imaging studies in women. While gender-matched quantitative databases have had a favourable though modest impact these normal databases generally consist of subjects who are of average body size and breast size. In large-breasted patients significant attenuation will occur, creating artefacts which vary considerably in appearance and location (Fig. 94.4). With planar imaging, it is more readily apparent that breast attenuation is the cause of an anterior or anterolateral defect on the processed images, as the raw data are more easily appreciated. With SPECT, a review of the cine-display of all of the raw projection images will often reveal possible breast attenuation, but the effect on the final images are more difficult to predict. The problem of breast attenuation has been ameliorated to some degree, by ^{99m}Tc-labelled myocardial perfusion agents such as sestamibi or teboroxime; the degree of tissue attenuation is generally less than that of ^{201}Tl.

Several approaches have been taken towards minimizing the impact of breast attenuation in order to try to improve diagnosis in women. These include breast markers to outline the external contour of the breast for better appreciation of its location, particularly relevant for planar imaging, as well as taping or 'flattening' breast tissue such that the attenuation is more homogeneously spread across the anterior and lateral walls of the myocardium. Some labs have also used prone imaging in such patients. No approach has completely obviated this problem.

Inferior wall attenuation. This artefact may be

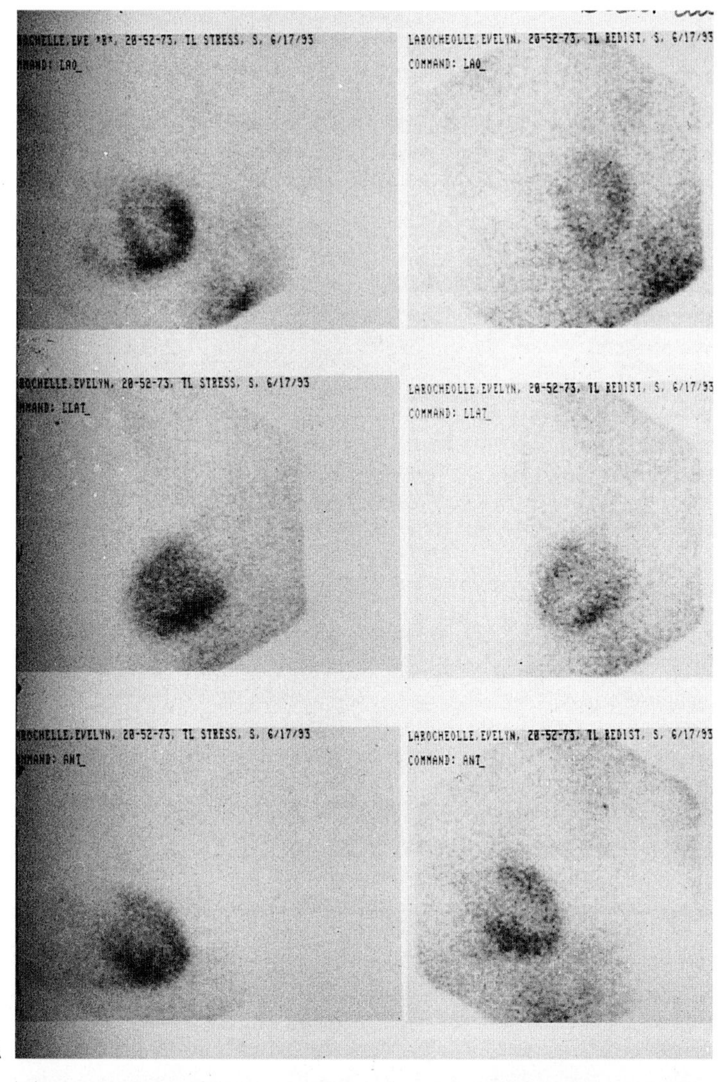

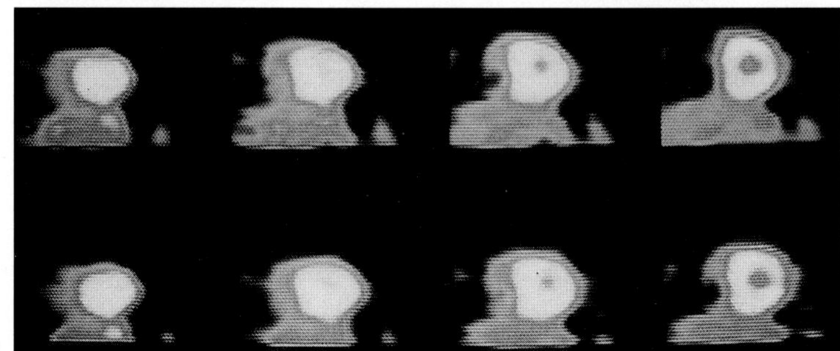

Fig. 94.4 A Breast attenuation in planar imaging. The overlying attenuation by breast tissue is readily noted in the planar data in both the stress ^{201}Tl study (left column) and the redistribution study (right column). B An apparent anterolateral wall mild irreversible defect caused by breast attenuation. With SPECT imaging, breast attenuation is more difficult to recognize in the final processed images, and a review of the cine-projection data is important. (B also shown in colour on Plate 28.)

caused by several underlying factors: overlap of the inferior wall by the diaphragm, attenuation of counts from the inferior wall by the overlying cardiac structures, and, in SPECT imaging, the longer distance from the inferior wall to the camera in all locations throughout the semicircular orbit, as well as the phenomenon of 'upward creep'.

This latter phenomenon is related to the change in orientation of the heart from very early after exercise to the end of the SPECT acquisition (approximately 20 min).[85] If the acquisition is started very early after a high level of exercise, the depth of respiration is generally larger; thus the diaphragm is, on the average, lower and the position of the heart is more vertical. Over the time of the acquisition, as the depth of respiration becomes more shallow, the average position of the diaphragm shifts upward, and the heart becomes more horizontal. This 'upward creep' of the heart leads to a relative paucity of counts in the inferior wall which can appear as an inferior wall defect. Delaying the beginning of the acquisition for approximately 10 min can often avoid this problem. In addition, since the ^{99m}Tc-labelled tracers with a long retention time, such as sestamibi or tetrofosmin, are not imaged until approximately 20–30 min after stress, the phenomenon of 'upward creep' would not be expected to occur.

Attenuation of the inferior wall, particularly in stress studies, can be quite apparent (Fig. 94.5). This problem has also not been completely alleviated by ^{99m}Tc-labelled agents.

Influence of quantification of myocardial perfusion images in the detection of CAD

There is significant inherent intra- and inter-observer variability in the visual analysis of planar myocardial perfusion images, particularly with ^{201}Tl. Agreement is generally highest (though still variable) for determining whether an image is normal or abnormal, and is significantly more variable for determining the location defect.[86,87] Several methods of quantification have been developed.[88,89] The goals of this type of analysis are to reduce the variability in reading, to allow comparison of regional uptake with a normal database, and to investigate tracer kinetics.

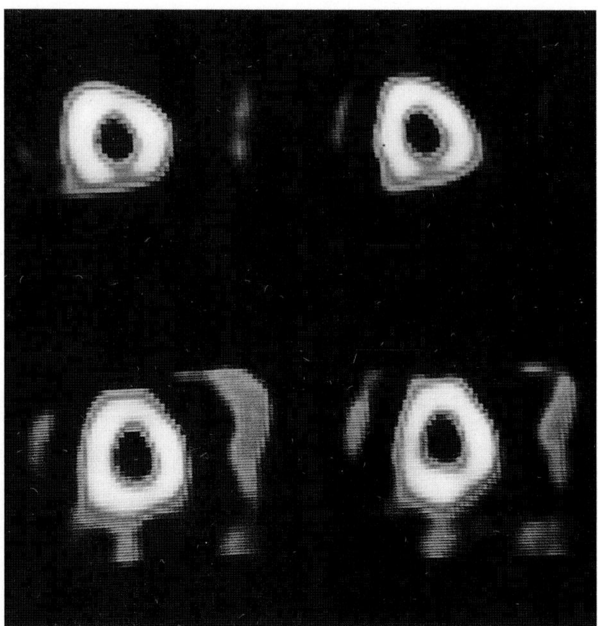

Fig. 94.5 Short-axis SPECT ^{201}Tl images from a young, highly trained normal subject demonstrating an apparent reversible inferior defect, due to inferior attenuation in the stress images (top row) and possible 'upward creep'. See text for details. (Also shown in colour on Plate 28.)

The most commonly employed method of quantitative analysis in planar imaging is the circumferential profile method developed by Garcia et al.[88] A second method involves the use of linear count activity profiles across the myocardium in the different planar images, developed by Watson et al.[89] In general, the sensitivity and specificity for detecting CAD have been modestly, though consistently, improved by quantitative analysis of planar images when images from the same patients have been analysed both visually and quantitatively.[88,90–93]

Perhaps the most important use of quantitative analysis involves the improved recognition of the extent of disease. Maddahi et al[91] demonstrated that the addition of circumferential profile quantitative assessment of ^{201}Tl wash-out kinetics could identify the presence of CAD remote from the segment with the most obvious visual defect. Thus, quantitative analysis in planar imaging improves the assessment of the extent of CAD, confirming data from Berger et al[90] using linear profiles.

There are significant quality control issues that accompany the use of quantitative assessment in planar imaging, and these are particularly important for the use of wash-out analysis. The rate of myocardial ^{201}Tl wash-out can be affected by a number of factors unrelated to the presence of epicardial CAD, particularly the level of exercise and the heart rate achieved during exercise.[94,95] If these and other technical factors are carefully controlled and optimized, quantitative analysis may add an important dimension to planar myocardial perfusion imaging in the evaluation of disease extent. However, widespread confirmation of the findings of these two laboratories[90,91] are not yet forthcoming.

The circumferential profile method of quantitative analysis has also been applied to tomographic imaging.[96] In contrast to the results of quantitative analysis of planar images, there seems to be only minimal (if any) improvement in the overall discrimination between the presence and absence of CAD when comparing quantitative and visual analysis with SPECT (Fig. 94.6).[97,98] Quantification with SPECT is also associated with only marginally better determination of the site and extent of disease, as well as the overall extent of disease. Several studies comparing quantitative and visual analysis of tomographic ^{201}Tl imaging have been concordant in this respect.[97–100]

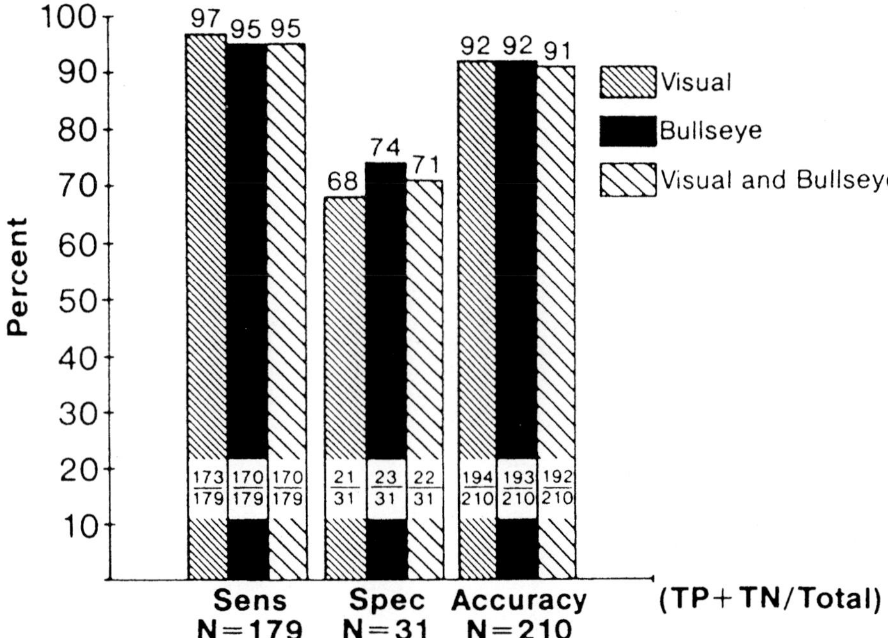

Fig. 94.6 The influence of quantitative analysis compared with visual analysis on performance characteristics of SPECT for detection of coronary artery disease (CAD). In this study, quantitative analysis (bull's-eye) performed as well as visual analysis in terms of sensitivity (sens), specificity (spec), or overall accuracy. TN=true negative, TP=true positive. (Reprinted with permission from DePasquale E E, Nody A C, DePuey E G et al 1988 Quantitative rotational thallium-201 tomography for identifying and localizing coronary artery disease. Circulation 77: 316.)

Influence of the type of perfusion tracer on detection of CAD

The majority of studies concerning the detection of CAD using myocardial perfusion imaging have used ^{201}Tl. Throughout the early 1980s, the research and development into ^{99}Tc as a perfusion tracer was driven in part by the expectation of improved diagnosis. ^{99m}Tc has many favourable attributes as a radioisotope for gamma camera imaging compared with ^{201}Tl. Theoretically, the diminished attenuation of ^{99m}Tc, as well as the potential for using higher doses based on the shorter half-life, promised higher count rates and improved resolution.

Studies comparing ^{201}Tl, ^{99m}Tc sestamibi, and ^{99m}Tc teboroxime have not shown significant improvement in sensitivity or specificity with the ^{99m}Tc-labelled agents however. In a multicentre trial involving several hundred patients, a stress and redistribution ^{201}Tl protocol was compared with a stress–rest sestamibi protocol using both planar imaging and SPECT. Sensitivity for detecting CAD was similar between the two agents using either imaging technique.[101] The normalcy rate (the specificity in a low prevalence, non-catheterized population) was also similar between the two agents.[101] Other studies comparing these two tracers have confirmed these findings.[102–106]

In general, there has been less experience with comparing ^{201}Tl ^{99m}Tc teboroxime. Hendel et al[107] compared teboroxime images to thallium images in 30 patients. These investigators found concordant information regarding normality or abnormality of the scans in 94% of the patients (Fig. 94.7). Other investigators have found similar sensitivity and specificity for detecting angiographically proven CAD.[108–110]

In a comprehensive study comparing all three of the agents in the same group of patients, Taillefer et al[111] examined 18 patients using exercise stress testing with ^{201}Tl, ^{99m}Tc sestamibi and ^{99m}Tc teboroxime. This investigation demonstrated no significant differences in the sensitivity nor in the specificity for detecting CAD between the three agents.

Thus, the available literature suggests that the choice of radiotracer for perfusion imaging does not greatly affect the ability to diagnose CAD. It is important to recognize, however, that such studies are often comprised of subjects who are likely to be relatively straightforward to image; the ^{99m}Tc-labelled agents may have better performance in obese and large-breasted patients.

Pharmacological stress testing with myocardial perfusion imaging for the diagnosis of CAD

For patients unable to perform treadmill or bicycle

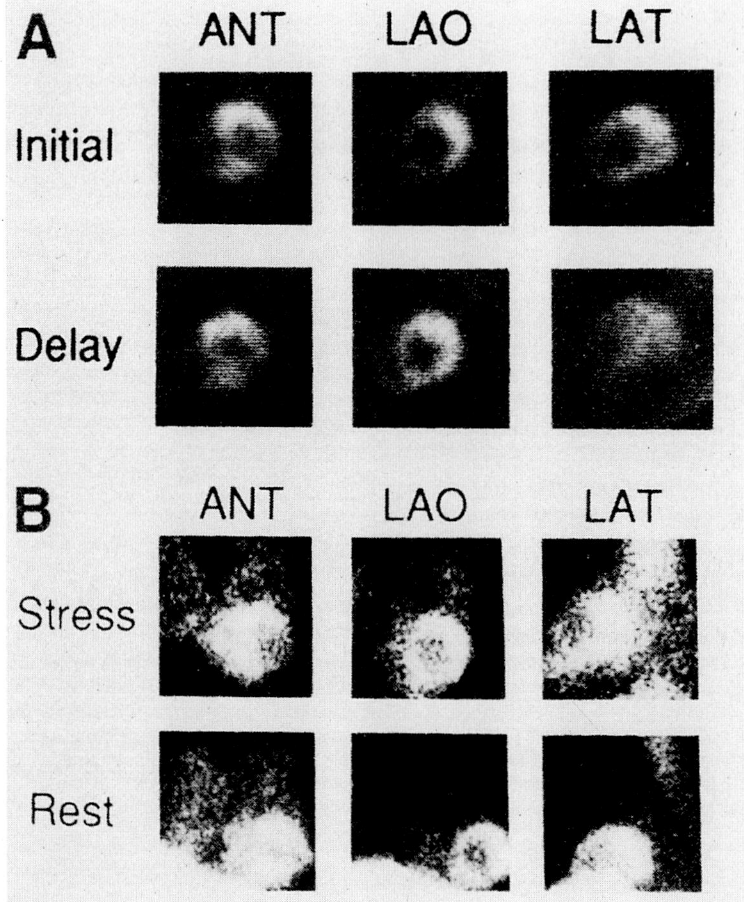

Fig. 94.7 ^{201}Tl and ^{99m}Tc teboroxime planar images in the same patient with coronary artery disease. The studies with the two different isotopes provide generally concordant information. (Reprinted with permission from Hendel R C et al 1990. Diagnostic value of a new myocardial perfusion agent, teboroxime (SQ 30,217) utilizing a rapid planar imaging protocol: preliminary results. J Am Coll Cardiol 16: 855.)

exercise, pharmacological stress testing, particularly with dipyridamole or adenosine as vasodilator stressors, has come into widespread use for detecting CAD in conjunction with myocardial perfusion imaging.[112]

Physiologically, these agents dilate of the coronary resistance vessels, and reduce coronary vascular resistance. This results in an increase in coronary flow greater than that seen with treadmill exercise. Theoretically, the greater hyperaemic response associated with pharmacological agents might also result in a greater degree of flow disparity in regional perfusion, which could improve the detection of CAD. This could be particularly important in the presence of moderate stenoses (50–70%), when compared with exercise perfusion imaging.[113]

However, as reviewed by Verani,[114] most reports examining the sensitivity and specificity of vasodilator pharmacological stress combined with myocardial perfusion imaging for the detection of CAD have revealed data quite similar to those seen with exercise as the stressor. In addition, several studies have compared pharmacological vasodilation and exercise myocardial perfusion imaging in the same patients for the detection of angiographic CAD. These studies have confirmed that vasodilators (the majority of these studies done with dipyridamole) and exercise produce similar stress perfusion scans.[112,114]

To some degree, these data run counter to the notion that a more powerful hyperaemic stress should be associated with better detection of CAD using perfusion tracers. This phenomenon is likely related to the 'roll off' property of diffusable tracers (particularly ^{201}Tl and ^{99m}Tc sestamibi), which is caused by reduced extraction at high blood levels.[115,116] Thus, the more favourable hyperaemic stress, which presumably should create more heterogeneity of flow with underlying moderate coronary stenosis, is offset by the lack of linear tracer uptake in the areas with the highest flow. ^{99m}Tc Teboroxime has exhibited the most linear relationship of uptake at high blood flow levels compared with ^{201}Tl and ^{99m}Tc sestamibi.[117,118] Thus, there was the expectation that ^{99m}Tc teboroxime in association with vasodilator stress might provide improved

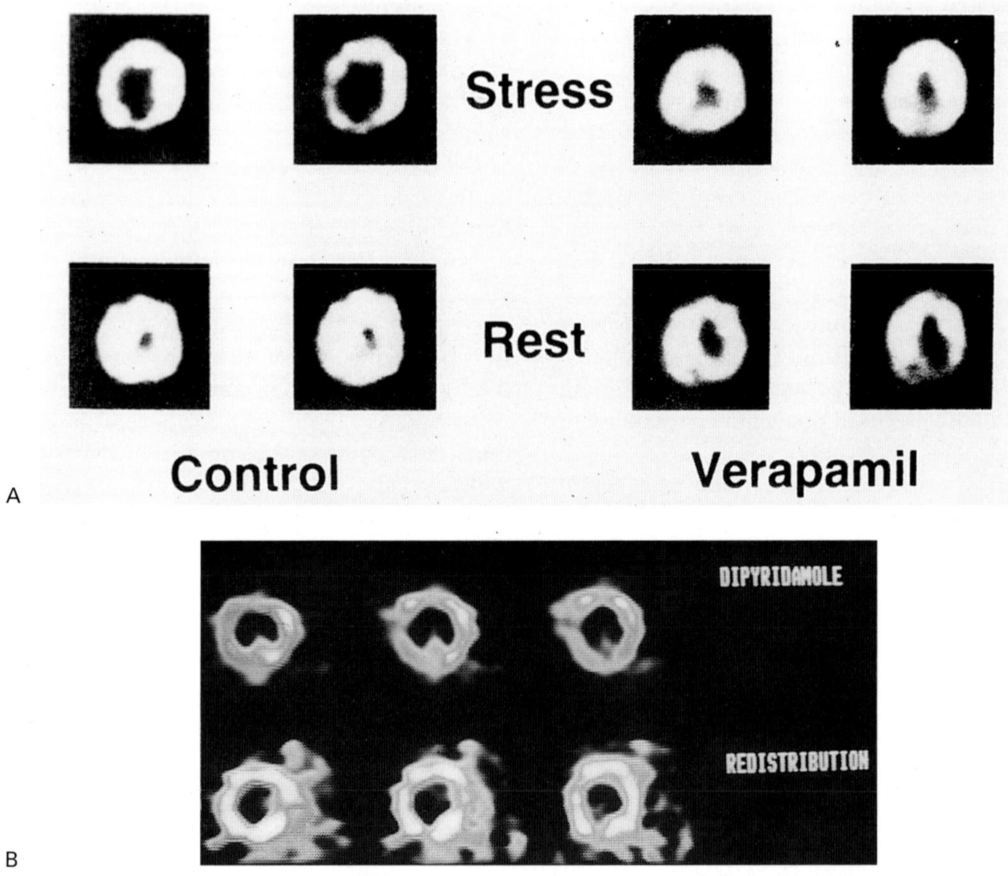

Fig. 94.8 Abnormal myocardial perfusion images in patients with structural heart disease in the absence of epicardial coronary artery disease. A SPECT ^{201}Tl imaging at stress (top) and at rest (4 h redistribution, bottom) in a young asymptomatic patient with hypertrophic cardiomyopathy. Anterior and septal reversible perfusion defects are apparent, as is transient cavity dilatation (control, left panel). These abnormalities are prevented by pre-treatment with verapamil despite a similar exercise time (verapamil, right panel). (Reprinted with permission from Udelson J E et al 1989 Verapamil prevents silent myocardial perfusion abnormalities during exercise in asymptomatic hypertrophic cardiomyopathy. Circulation 79: 1052.) B Short-axis ^{201}Tl SPECT images following dipyridamole (top) and redistribution (bottom) in a patient with idiopathic dilated cardiomyopathy and normal epicardial arteries. Multiple reversible defects are apparent. (B also shown in colour on Plate 29.)

diagnostic sensitivity. This has not been established, possibly because of the technical difficulties inherent in ^{99m}Tc teboroxime imaging as well as the significant hepatic uptake and short myocardial retention time. These factors may offset the more favourable extraction properties of ^{99m}Tc teboroxime during pharmacologically induced hyperaemia.

The sympathomimetic agent dobutamine has also been used as a pharmacological stress agent for myocardial perfusion imaging.[119] Although the experience is small, publications have suggested that the diagnostic ability of dobutamine stress imaging is generally similar to that of other pharmacological and exercise–stress modalities for the detection of CAD.[119,120] There are several unresolved issues related to the use of dobutamine in conjunction with perfusion imaging for detecting CAD. These include the most appropriate upper dose at which to inject tracer in the absence of symptoms, the use of atropine in conjunction with dobutamine to enhance the heart rate response, and the diagnostic ability of dobutamine imaging in the presence of beta blockers.

Myocardial perfusion abnormalities unrelated to CAD

There are several categories of underlying heart disease in which myocardial perfusion imaging has demonstrated stress-induced perfusion abnormalities in the absence of epicardial CAD. In some settings, such as hypertrophic cardiomyopathy, pathophysiological correlates of myocardial ischaemia have been consistently demonstrated. In other settings, the evidence that perfusion abnormalities demonstrated by planar or SPECT imaging truly represent myocardial ischaemia is more circumstantial.

Left bundle branch block (LBBB). Many laboratories have reported isolated perfusion defects of the interventricular septum in patients with LBBB.[121–126] In a dog model of LBBB created by right ventricular pacing, Hirzel et al[121] demonstrated that this phenomenon probably represents true heterogeneity of flow between the left anterior descending and left circumflex territories. Flow probes placed on the left anterior descending and left circumflex arteries were used to demonstrate blunting of the coronary flow reserve in the left anterior descending coronary arterial bed at increasing heart rates in the presence of right ventricular pacing (creating LBBB). The aetiology for this phenomenon may be due to delayed tension decay within the late contracting interventricular septum, resulting in more resistance to coronary flow during early diastole, or lessened oxygen demand based on the late contraction of the septum during the later phase of systole when wall stress is decreasing.

Thus, the specificity and predictive value of a septal defect for true CAD of the left anterior descending artery are low. However, studies have demonstrated that concomitant apical or anterior involvement in septal perfusion defects considerably increases the specificity of this finding for CAD.[124] As a septal defect in left bundle branch block is most commonly seen at high heart rates, some investigators have proposed using dipyridamole imaging, with its diminished heart rate rise compared with exercise stress, to improve the specificity of detecting left anterior descending CAD. Preliminary studies support this contention.[127,128]

Hypertrophic cardiomyopathy (HCM) Many reports using both planar and SPECT imaging have demonstrated the significant prevalence of inducible myocardial perfusion abnormalities in patients with HCM.[129–132] Such findings appear to have important pathophysiological significance: patients with fixed perfusion defects are far more likely to have thinned akinetic walls on echocardiography and diminished ejection fractions by radionuclide angiography, while those with reversible perfusion defects are more likely to have hyperdynamic left ventricles.[132] Even in asymptomatic HCM patients, approximately 50% will have reversible perfusion abnormalities during myocardial perfusion imaging in the absence of epicardial CAD (Fig. 94.8A).[133] Such patients have more abnormal indexes of diastolic function,[133] demonstrate haemodynamic and metabolic abnormalities consistent with ischaemia during atrial pacing tachycardia,[134] and these perfusion abnormalities are, for the most part, prevented by verapamil,[133] which supports the concept that the defects truly represent inducible myocardial ischaemia.

Left ventricular hypertrophy (LVH). Many studies have demonstrated the presence of inducible perfusion abnormalities in patients with pressure overload LVH due to either hypertension or aortic stenosis.[135–137] Often, these patients do not have epicardial CAD, and it is presumed that these abnormalities represent regional myocardial ischaemia caused by abnormalities of the microcirculation. Coronary flow studies have demonstrated limited vasodilator reserve in patients with LVH.[138,139] Thus, the value of myocardial perfusion imaging to detect epicardial CAD in the presence of LVH accurately is diminished; however, the negative predictive value remains high.[135–137]

Dilated cardiomyopathy (DCM). Similar to the findings in patients with left ventricular hypertrophy, numerous investigators have reported abnormalities in myocardial scintigraphy in patients with DCM (Fig. 94.8B).[140–142] An important diagnostic consideration in patients presenting with DCM involves distinguishing those patients whose cardiomyopathy may be primarily due to CAD (potentially reversible IHD) from those whose disease is idiopathic. Several studies have shown that those patients with more extensive perfusion abnormalities are more likely to have CAD as the aetiology.[140–142] However, there is often a great deal of overlap between the CAD and non-CAD groups, thus the predictive value of perfusion imaging for accurate detection of underlying epicardial CAD in the presence of dilated cardiomyopathy is diminished. Again, it is likely that the perfusion abnormalities, even in dilated cardiomyopathy patients with normal epicardial arteries, truly represent regional myocardial ischaemia, as several studies have demonstrated abnormalities in coronary flow reserve in these patients.[143,144] The prognostic and therapeutic significance of such findings have not been well described.

Myocardial perfusion imaging for detecting the extent of CAD

In formulating a management strategy for patients with chest pain and suspected CAD, it is often more important for non-invasive testing to determine the extent of disease rather than just the presence or absence of disease.

In this regard, it is important when reviewing the literature to distinguish studies that document the sensitivity of myocardial perfusion imaging in patients with three-vessel disease, from those studies examining the sensitivity of perfusion imaging for accurately detecting three-vessel or left main disease. In the former case, the question being asked is how often the scan is positive or abnormal in patients with multivessel disease. Most studies demonstrate that 95–98% of patients with three-vessel disease will have an abnormal scan; however the abnormality will not necessarily reflect the presence of three-vessel disease. In the latter case, myocardial perfusion imaging with single-photon agents is limited by its spatial relativity; if all areas are hypoperfused in the presence of three-vessel CAD, the least hypoperfused area will look relatively normal, thus the extent of disease may be underestimated. In fact, many reports have observed a low (25–60%) sensitivity for accurately detecting the presence of three-vessel disease using visual analysis of ^{201}Tl imaging (predominantly planar).[145–149]

Several reports have examined whether quantitative

analysis may aid in the detection of the extent of CAD, using the ability to determine abnormalities in ^{201}Tl kinetics in territories that appear visually normal. Maddahi et al[149] and Abdulla et al[150] found that the sensitivity for detecting three-vessel or left main CAD was significantly improved by combined analysis of an exercise-induced perfusion defect and a remote abnormality in ^{201}Tl wash-out kinetics. The sensitivity for detecting left main or three-vessel disease was increased from 16% to 63% with the addition of analysis of quantitative abnormalities in ^{201}Tl kinetics, at a similar specificity.[149] Incorporating the clinical response to treadmill exercise testing further increased the sensitivity for detecting this type of patient.[149]

An infrequent but potentially important finding using quantitative analysis is the patient with visually normal images, but abnormalities in ^{201}Tl wash-out kinetics in all coronary territories, the 'diffuse slow wash-out' pattern.[151] In one database survey, Bateman et al[151] found that only approximately 1% of patients demonstrated this pattern; however, it was a very important finding as the majority of such patients were found to have left main or three-vessel disease.[151] It was hypothesized that because all territories were hypoperfused at stress in a relatively homogeneous manner, the visual images appeared relatively normal, and that only analysis of ^{201}Tl wash-out kinetics using count-based quantitative analysis properly identified these patients with very important underlying disease. As noted above, however, it is important when quantifying abnormalities in ^{201}Tl kinetics to bear in mind that the measured parameters reflecting percentage of ^{201}Tl wash-out may be significantly affected by heart rate achieved and other factors.[94,95]

SPECT, with its better contrast resolution and ability to allow visual analysis of all coronary regions without significant overlap (particularly the left circumflex territory), should be better in determining the extent of CAD compared with planar imaging. Fintel et al[81] demonstrated this to be the case: visual analysis of SPECT was significantly more likely to be correct in identifying the number of vessels with significant epicardial stenoses than planar imaging.

As the physiology of the pharmacological 'stress' induced by dipyridamole and adenosine is distinct from the demand stress of exercise, the ability to detect the extent of CAD might also be different with pharmacological stress. Few studies have addressed this issue. Chambers & Brown[151] found that the strongest correlate of dipyridamole-induced ischaemic ST depression was multivessel CAD with jeopardized collaterals.[152] Thus, myocardial perfusion imaging with pharmacological stress can also suggest the extent of CAD, despite the lack of enhanced oxygen demand.

Several scintigraphic signs other than regional perfusion abnormalities reflect extensive CAD and its physiological consequences during stress myocardial perfusion imaging. These include pulmonary uptake of tracers, as well as apparent transient ischaemic dilatation of the left ventricle.

In early studies using visual analysis of planar imaging, pulmonary uptake of ^{201}Tl was significantly increased in patients with an extensive degree of myocardial ischaemia.[153,154] Studies in animal models confirmed this to be the case and also demonstrated that prolonged transit time across the pulmonary vascular bed (resulting either from elevated left atrial pressure or from an increase in pulmonary vascular resistance) resulted in enhanced pulmonary ^{201}Tl extraction.[153] Thus, the appearance of excessive pulmonary uptake of ^{201}Tl following stress is indicative of left ventricular dysfunction and an elevation in left-sided filling pressures (Fig. 94.9). In patients with normal resting left ventricular function, this implies that a large mass of myocardium has become ischaemic, and correlates with extensive CAD. Such findings have been reported using either visual[154] or quantitative analysis of pulmonary ^{201}Tl uptake.[155,156] Little work has been done in this area regarding the newer myocardial perfusion agents, ^{99m}Tc sestamibi and ^{99m}Tc teboroxime, so that the implications and angiographic correlates of increased pulmonary uptake of these agents if imaged soon after stress testing is as yet unclear.

There is an important caveat in the analysis of pulmonary uptake of ^{201}Tl for detecting extensive CAD: as this scintigraphic sign is most closely related to the presence of left ventricular dysfunction during exercise and an elevation in left-sided filling pressures, any structural heart disease that results in such a haemodynamic abnormality will result in pulmonary ^{201}Tl uptake. Thus, patients with ischaemic or non-ischaemic cardiomyopathy may demonstrate pulmonary uptake of ^{201}Tl even in the absence of extensive CAD. In addition, the angiographic correlates of pulmonary ^{201}Tl uptake during pharmacological stress testing are not as clear as during treadmill testing. The physiology of the haemodynamic stress is distinct during pharmacological stress testing, and myocardial ischaemia is induced much less often. While some investigators have demonstrated some correlation of pulmonary ^{201}Tl uptake and severe CAD in patients receiving dipyridamole,[157,158] others have noted a great deal of overlap in the magnitude of pulmonary uptake among patients with varying extents of disease.[159]

Analogous to the concepts of significant exercise-induced ischaemia of the left ventricle resulting in elevated left-sided filling pressures and pulmonary ^{201}Tl uptake, data have also suggested that enhanced hepatic ^{201}Tl activity is associated with significant right CAD;[160] this finding is presumably related to exercise-induced ischaemia of the right ventricle. As with pulmonary uptake of ^{201}Tl, this scintigraphic finding may

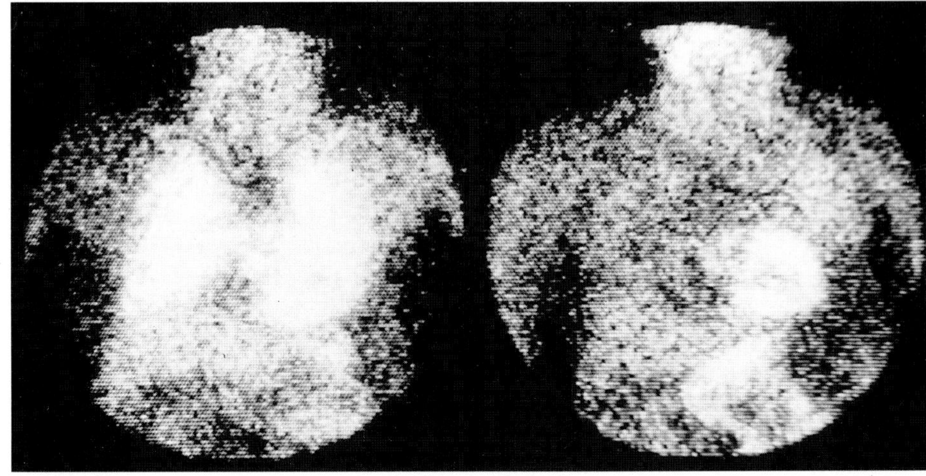

Fig. 94.9 Large field of view anterior planar images immediately following treadmill exercise (left) and 4 h later for comparison (right) demonstrating marked pulmonary uptake of ^{201}Tl in a patient ultimately found to have three-vessel coronary artery disease. (Also shown in colour on Plate 29.)

also result in enhanced diagnosis of multivessel disease, suggesting the presence of right CAD when only regional perfusion abnormalities of the left coronary system are visually evident.[160]

Transient ischaemic dilatation of the left ventricle refers to an apparent increase in the size of the left ventricular cavity during stress imaging that is no longer apparent on rest imaging. Several groups of investigators have correlated this finding with the presence of extensive CAD using either treadmill testing[161] or pharmacological stress (Fig. 94.10).[159,162] The aetiology of this finding may involve diffuse subendocardial hypoperfusion, although this concept has not been formally tested. In fact, the quantitative methods for analysing this finding vary considerably: in the method used by Weiss et al[161], the outer edge of the entire left ventricle was traced, suggesting that transient ischaemic dilatation represents an increase in total cardiac volume. Other investigators have traced the apparent endocardial border,[162] more consistent with the concept that this finding represents subendocardial hypoperfusion. With both methods, however, this sign has been significantly correlated to the presence of three-vessel or left main disease.[159,161–163]

RADIONUCLIDE ANGIOGRAPHY FOR DETECTION OF CAD

Following the application of radionuclide studies of

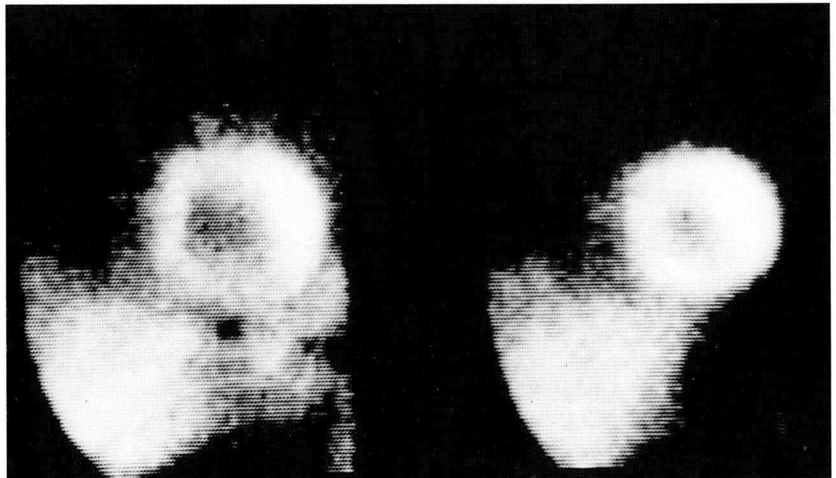

Fig. 94.10 Anterior planar ^{201}Tl images obtained following infusion of dipyridamole (left) and 4 h later (right), demonstrating septal and inferior reversible perfusion abnormalities as well as transient ischaemic dilatation of the ventricle, manifest as apparent dilatation of the left ventricular cavity.

regional and global left ventricular function to the physiology of exercise in addition to resting imaging,[69] many studies investigated the ability of exercise radionuclide angiography (RNA), using either first pass or gated equilibrium techniques, to detect or rule out the presence of significant CAD accurately. Using this technique, changes in both regional and global ventricular function are analysed during exercise and compared with findings at rest, in order to detect the functional consequences of regional myocardial ischaemia associated with the presence of an epicardial stenosis.

Table 94.1 summarizes the performance characteristics (sensitivity and specificity) of exercise RNA from a series of reports published through the late 1970s and early 1980s.[164–181] The earliest reports demonstrated very high sensitivity and specificity, while in later reports the results were less good. These differences illustrate the principles of pre- and post-test referral bias inherent in the determination of the performance of a non-invasive modality to detect CAD, as will be discussed later.

The very high sensitivity of the earlier reports may well be related to the selection of patients for study with either extensive CAD or a history of a myocardial infarction. Determination of sensitivity in a population with a high prevalence of previous infarction will result in high values, as patients with a history of myocardial infarction are likely to have a regional wall motion abnormality even at rest.[77] Moreover, as subsequent studies in large numbers of patients clearly demonstrated, the magnitude of an abnormal ejection fraction response is significantly related to the extent of CAD (Fig. 94.11).[182] Thus, early reports predominantly including patients with extensive disease would also result in high sensitivity. In later reports, as the test was more widely applied and as it was applied to populations with less extensive disease and lower prevalence of myocardial infarction, sensitivity values began to decrease. However, while the ejection fraction response to exercise may be a relatively insensitive index to detect CAD, particularly among patients with less extensive disease, many studies have shown that there is powerful prognostic information inherent in the global ejection fraction response to exercise.[183–185]

As the left ventricular ejection fraction response to exercise may be normal in many patients with less extensive CAD,[182] the finding of a regional wall motion abnormality during exercise theoretically may be more sensitive for identifying the presence of a coronary stenosis. Technical limitations in the acquisition of the radionuclide data, however, limit the sensitivity of the finding of a regional wall motion abnormality. In most laboratories using either the first pass or the gated equilibrium technique, the radionuclide ventricular function data during exercise are acquired in only one view, the LAO 'best septal' view; the limited time available for acquisition during exercise obviates the ability to acquire multiple views. While some preliminary reports have used two view exercise RNA,[186,187] and some newer camera systems are capable of acquiring biplanar first pass data, most data in the literature are reported from studies using a single LAO view during exercise. Thus, since the view of the inferior wall is limited, the development of a new regional wall motion abnormality is relatively insensitive for right CAD.

In several initial reports of exercise RNA, the specificity for ruling out significant CAD was reported as 100%.[164,166,167,169,170,173] Subsequent studies over time, however, documented an apparent decline in specificity.[188] This phenomenon has been ascribed to several factors. In the initial reports, the normal range for an exercise ejection fraction response was defined by a group of relatively young normal volunteers with no

Table 94.1 Exercise radionuclide angiography (RNA) and detection of coronary artery disease (CAD)

First author	Ref.	'Normals' n	CAD n	Method	RWMA Sens	RWMA Spec	ΔEF Sens	ΔEF Spec
Borer	164	64	63	GE	94	100	89	100
Slutsky	165	10	25	GE			76	80
Berger	166	13	60	FP	47	100	73	100
Pfisterer	167	20	40	GE			88	100
Verani	168	17	35	FP	51	94		
Brady	169	19	70	GE	74	100	90	100
Jengo	170	8	11	FP	100	100	100	100
Okada	171	12	42	GE	19	92	64	83
Hecht	172	12	35	GE	63	100		
Iskandrian	173	12	24	FP			83	100
Elkayam	174	8	56	GE	89	75		
Kirshenbaum	175	11	50	GE	54	73	72	55
Freeman	176	15	22	GE	95	93		
Austin	177	63	158	FP	61	79		
DePace	178	18	47	FP			70	72
Bodenheimer	179	20	28	FP	75	65	82	30
Osbakken	180	21	32	GE			53	62
Manyari	181	22	20	GE	90	95	75	91

Abbreviations: ΔEF=change in ejection fraction from rest to exercise, FP=first pass technique, GE=gated equilibrium technique, RWMA=regional wall motion abnormality, Sens=sensitivity, spec=specificity. A 'normal' EF response to exercise is defined as a ≥ 5% increase from rest to exercise.

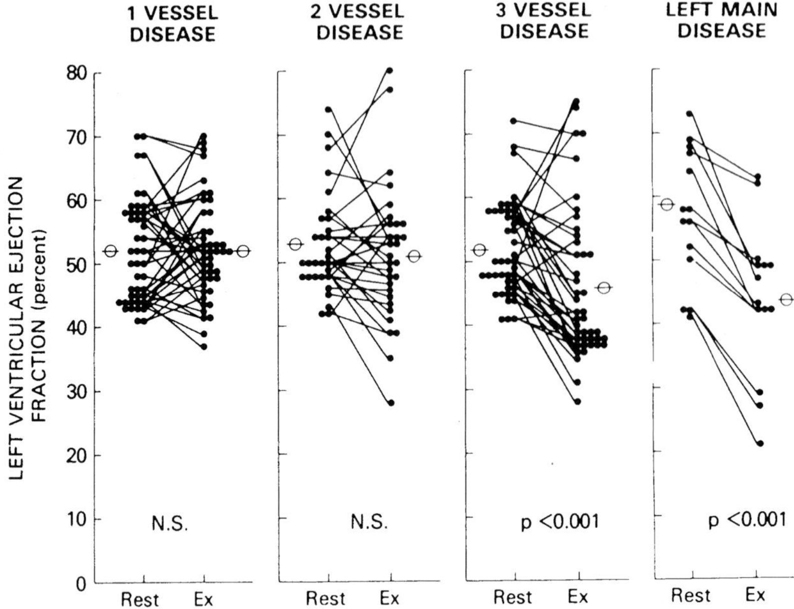

Fig. 94.11 The relation between the angiographic extent of coronary artery disease (CAD) and the ejection fraction response to exercise, as determined by rest and exercise radionuclide angiography. With increasing extent of CAD, the magnitude of the abnormal ejection fraction response to exercise increases. However, there is significant overlap between groups, reflecting the varying mass of ischaemic myocardium within any angiographic subgroup. (Reprinted with permission from Bonow R O et al 1987 Prognostic implications of symptomatic vs. asymptomatic (silent) myocardial ischemia induced by exercise in mildly symptomatic and in asymptomatic patients with angiographically documented coronary artery disease. Am J Cardiol 60: 778.)

clinical evidence of CAD. Subsequent reports documented that this population differs significantly from the population of patients with chest pain and normal coronary arteriograms.[189] Both Cannon et al[190] as well as Gibbons et al[191] have demonstrated that patients with chest pain and normal coronary arteries may have an abnormal ventriculographic response to exercise and thus are a heterogeneous group, some having inducible abnormalities in coronary flow reserve[190] and consequent limitations in left ventricular functional reserve. A subpopulation of these patients has been found, when followed serially, to develop resting left ventricular dysfunction.[192] The phenomenon of post-test referral bias has also been invoked to explain the apparent decline in specificity in exercise RNA over time.[188] As discussed in more detail below, this refers to the bias inherent when patients with a normal ventriculographic response to exercise are not referred for catheterization. These subjects, who probably represent a large group of 'true negatives' in terms of test performance characteristics, will then not be included in equations calculating specificity, resulting in an apparent lower specificity for the test in question. Thus, the true specificity of exercise RNA is difficult to define. However, in a similar manner to normal myocardial perfusion scintigraphy, a preserved ventricular response to exercise is associated with a good prognosis[183–185] despite the presence of CAD. This implies that the information provided by exercise RNA is a powerful management tool for patients with chest pain and suspected CAD.

Further confounding the determination of specificity of the exercise ejection fraction response is the influence of numerous other variables on this parameter such as age,[193–195] gender,[195–197] and the presence of underlying hypertension.[198–200] In young normals, there is almost uniformly a rise in left ventricular ejection fraction with exercise, while elderly normal subjects may manifest no change in ejection fraction with exercise. Thus, the normal response varies significantly with age.[164,193–195]

Patients with systemic hypertension may also manifest an abnormal ejection fraction response to exercise in the absence of CAD.[198–200] While excessive afterload during exercise may contribute to this phenomenon, other mechanisms may also be in play. Cuocolo et al[200] studied two groups of hypertensive patients with exercise RNA: one group with a normal ejection fraction response to exercise, and a second group with an abnormal response. Both groups had similar blood pressure and end-systolic volume responses to exercise, thus it is unlikely that differences in afterload during exercise could have significantly affected the exercise response. In contrast, the group with an abnormal ejection fraction response had significantly impaired parameters of diastolic filling: peak filling rate at rest was lower, and the ability to recruit preload reserve (the increment in left ventricular end-diastolic volume with exercise) was also impaired. Thus, these data provide evidence that diastolic mechanisms in the absence of CAD may contribute importantly to systolic dysfunction during exercise.[200]

The specificity of the global ejection fraction response to exercise for determining the absence of CAD may also be influenced by other types of structural heart disease. An 'abnormal' response has been reported in asymptomatic[201] and symptomatic[202] patients with aortic stenosis. Furthermore, patients with valvular heart disease have also been reported to have a significant prevalence of abnormal regional wall motion responses to exercise, assessed by RNA.[203]

Resting left ventricular function also has an important influence on the ejection fraction response to exercise. Subjects with high resting ejection fraction may not manifest the expected increase with exercise, even in the absence of CAD.[191,204,205] At the other end of the spectrum, the ejection fraction response to exercise in patients with resting left ventricular dysfunction is a complex physiological phenomenon incorporating the changes in preload and afterload as well as inducible ischaemia. In light of these issues, Gibbons et al[206] found that the absolute value of the exercise ejection fraction is a more significant diagnostic variable than the change from rest to exercise, particularly when incorporated with other exercise data.

However, in patients with left ventricular dysfunction at rest, the ejection fraction response to exercise (albeit mediated by multiple factors unrelated to CAD) can provide significant diagnostic[207,208] and prognostic[209] information.

Exercise RNA and the extent of CAD

It would be expected that the left ventricular ejection fraction response to exercise would be a reflection of the mass of stress-induced ischaemic myocardium, and as such, would be a significant indicator of the extent of CAD. Several publications have confirmed this concept (Fig. 94.11), although there is a significant degree of overlap in the exercise ejection fraction responses among patients in various angiographic subgroups.[178,182,210] This reflects the variability in the mass of ischaemic myocardium among each individual angiographic group. In a multivariate analysis examining clinical, exercise, haemodynamic, and exercise RNA variables, Gibbons et al[206] formulated a model in which the probability of three-vessel or left main disease could be estimated with more accuracy than with the use of the exercise RNA data alone.

In addition to the magnitude of the fall in ejection fraction from rest to exercise,[178,182,252] other parameters that may be observed in exercise RNA reflecting more extensive CAD include the extent of regional wall motion abnormality with exercise,[187] and transient ventricular chamber dilatation.[211]

Effect of exercise workload on results of RNA detection of CAD

In contrast to studies of myocardial perfusion imaging demonstrating little change in the prevalence of perfusion defects or the ability to detect CAD at submaximal workloads[70–72] (see below), several studies have shown that the sensitivity for detecting CAD by exercise RNA is significantly impaired at submaximal workloads.[73,169] Seaworth et al[73] studied a group of patients at varying workloads with first pass exercise RNA. These investigators found that the prevalence of an abnormal RNA response to exercise, either an abnormal ejection fraction response or an abnormal regional wall motion response, were significantly lower at submaximal than at maximal workload (Fig. 94.12). Thus, achieving a maximal workload and acquiring the RNA data at that high workload are important components in optimizing the results of this technique for the detection of CAD.

PERFUSION OR FUNCTION FOR DIAGNOSIS?

In reviewing the large amount of literature available on the efficacy of radionuclide imaging of either myocardial perfusion or regional and global ventricular function for detection of CAD, it is clear that both techniques are capable of providing important diagnostic information. Conceptually, the concept of the ischaemic cascade,[65,66] as described earlier, would suggest that techniques which are capable of detecting regional heterogeneities in myocardial perfusion should be more sensitive in detecting CAD, particularly stenoses of more modest calibre.

In practice, applications of these physiological concepts are limited by the ability of perfusion imaging with single-photon agents to resolve modest degrees of regional perfusion heterogeneity, as well as the confidence factor in attempting to determine whether a mild regional difference in photon activity is due to a true perfusion abnormality or an imaging artefact related to attenuation, acquisition, or reconstruction. The sensitivity of regional wall motion analysis by exercise RNA, in turn, is most importantly limited by the single view acquisition that is performed in most laboratories. PET, with its better spatial resolution, and ability to measure regional flow reserve differences, is likely to be the most sensitive technique for detecting the earliest onset of CAD,[74–76] based on the inherent limitations of single photon perfusion imaging and functional imaging with exercise RNA.

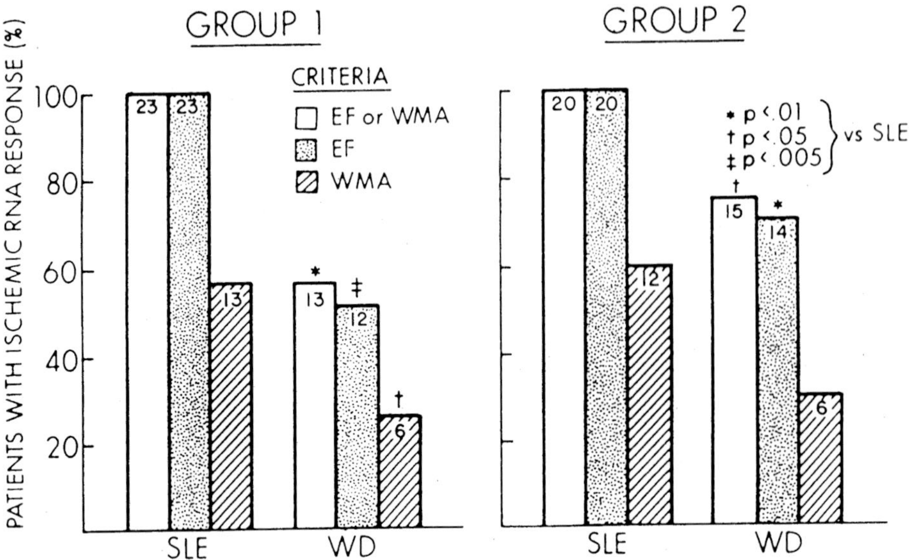

Fig. 94.12 The influence of exercise workload on the prevalence of abnormal exercise radionuclide angiographic responses to exercise. With workload reduction (WD), the prevalence of an abnormal regional wall motion response (WMA) or an abnormal ejection fraction response (EF) to exercise are diminished compared with symptom-limited exercise (SLE), thus suggesting that a maximal workload is important for maintaining the sensitivity of an abnormal RNA response to exercise for detecting coronary artery disease. Group 1=50% workload reduction, group 2=more moderate workload reduction. (Reprinted with permission from Seaworth J F et al 1983 Effect of partial decreases in exercise work load on radionuclide indexes of ischemia. J Am Coll Cardiol 2: 522.)

On practical grounds, however, all of these techniques have been demonstrated to provide not only important diagnostic information related to the presence or absence of CAD, but a significant ability to discriminate extensive from less extensive disease to aid in management decisions, and the ability to yield important prognostic information which can then be incorporated into patient management decisions. The decision to analyse regional perfusion or regional function will thus be based on many factors, perhaps the most important of which are local experience and expertise.

Based on these concepts, the combined analysis of regional perfusion as well as regional and global function at rest as well as during exercise using ^{99m}Tc-labelled agents with long retention times is attractive and potentially quite cost-efficient.[212] For instance, for the same apparent inferior wall inducible perfusion abnormality seen on an exercise myocardial perfusion scan in two patients, the patient with a normal ejection fraction response to exercise assessed with the first pass technique using ^{99m}Tc-labelled agents would be presumed to have a good prognosis, and thus managed medically. A different patient with the same inferior perfusion defect but a drop in ejection fraction during exercise would be considered to have a worse prognosis[183–185] and would potentially be managed more aggressively, with consideration of cardiac catheterization. While these concepts have not been formally tested, the large amount of data on changes in regional and global function with exercise as they relate to diagnosis[164–181] and prognosis[183–186] could only add more powerful information to that already inherent in the analysis of regional myocardial perfusion by single photon tracers. These combination techniques also have the potential to simplify and streamline imaging protocols. The analysis of stress perfusion and resting function using gated planar or SPECT imaging following one injection of ^{99m}Tc sestamibi or ^{99m}Tc tetrafosmin, for example, may demonstrate the presence of preserved regional wall thickening in the territory of a stress perfusion defect, thus identifying that segment as ischaemic and viable, and obviating the need for rest imaging. Recent data have suggested that the finding of preserved regional wall thickening at the site of a stress perfusion defect is highly predictive of reversibility or 'fill-in' of that defect on rest imaging.[213,214]

THE INCREMENTAL VALUE OF RADIONUCLIDE IMAGING FOR DETECTION OF CAD

The usefulness of any imaging modality is only as important as the non-redundant information it supplies compared with more easily available and less expensive clinical or non-invasive data.

As Rozanski & Berman[77] have pointed out, a compilation of early reports comparing exercise planar ^{201}Tl imaging to exercise ECG demonstrated the superior sensitivity and specificity of the former. However, this incremental value in the detection of CAD comprises a spectrum of values depending on patient subgroups and specific clinical situations.

The subset of patients in whom radionuclide imaging provides significant incremental diagnostic information includes those in whom exercise ECG is known to be imprecise: left bundle branch block, pre-excitation, or left ventricular hypertrophy and secondary ST and T wave changes on the resting ECG. Other important clinical situations in which radionuclide imaging will provide significant incremental information compared with exercise ECG include those patient groups with non-diagnostic exercise ECGs, as well as in women.

In many studies comparing radionuclide imaging with exercise ECG for the detection of CAD, the techniques are operating at an optimal level, in that adequate exercise endpoints are reached. A major incremental improvement in diagnosis is provided by radionuclide techniques compared with exercise ECG when adequate exercise endpoints and cardiac workload are not reached, as demonstrated by a number of studies.

Effect of exercise workload on detection of CAD

As discussed above, the onset of heterogeneity of regional perfusion in the presence of an epicardial stenosis will occur prior to the onset of regional functional abnormality, ischaemic ECG changes, or clinical symptoms related to ischaemia.[65,66] This implies that changes in regional perfusion may be evident at lower heart rates during exercise than will regional or global functional abnormalities or ECG changes, and it follows that myocardial perfusion imaging should be more sensitive than wall motion imaging or exercise ECG in detecting the presence of CAD at lower heart rates and workloads.

Several studies support this concept. In reviewing a large database of exercise myocardial perfusion studies, Esquivel et al[70] found that perfusion abnormalities were significantly more common among patients exercising to submaximal (86% of maximum predicted heart rate for age) workloads than were ischaemic ECG or clinical symptoms of angina. Other studies have confirmed these findings.[71] Such database investigations are limited, however, by the fact that different patients are being studied at the various workloads. One study has examined the same patients at both a submaximal and a maximal workload to investigate potential difference of symptom response, ECG changes, and ^{201}Tl imaging to detect CAD. Heller et al[72] studied a group of patients with known coronary disease at both a maximal and then later at a submaximal workload using planar ^{201}Tl imaging. The prevalence of an exercise-induced thallium perfusion abnormality was similar at both the submaximal and maximal workload (Fig. 94.13). In contrast, the prevalence of ischaemic ECG changes was lower at the submaximal workload, as was the presence of angina. Taken together, all of these studies support the concept that myocardial perfusion imaging retains its sensitivity at submaximal heart rates compared with exercise ECG, thus providing significant incremental information with regard to the detection of underlying CAD compared with exercise ECG.

Based on the concept of the ischaemic cascade, one would expect that functional wall motion imaging may not provide as much incremental data as perfusion imaging during submaximal exertion. Seaworth et al[73] examined exercise RNA for its sensitivity in detecting CAD at various workloads during graded bicycle exercise testing. As predicted, the angiograms obtained at lower workloads provided less diagnostic information relating to changes in regional or global left ventricular function than did those acquired at maximum exercise. These concepts regarding functional imaging at submaximal workloads obviously apply to exercise echocardiography as well, and investigators have reported a significantly reduced sensitivity of this technique for detecting CAD at submaximal workloads.[215]

INFLUENCE OF DISEASE PREVALENCE, IMAGE INTERPRETATION, AND REFERRAL BIAS IN THE DETECTION OF CAD BY RADIONUCLIDE TECHNIQUES

Performance characteristics of a test to detect disease are often expressed in terms of the sensitivity and specificity to detect or rule out disease, particularly in the initial reports of a new testing modality. These performance characteristics, however, fail to take into account numerous influences on the test itself. These influences include the prevalence of the disease in the population being studied, the 'conservativeness' or 'aggressiveness' with which the images are interpreted as normal or abnormal, and finally, the selection of patients from among those undergoing the non-invasive imaging test to have the 'gold standard' test, particularly when it involves an invasive procedure such as coronary arteriography.

Bayes' Theorem and the prevalence of disease

When a test having a certain sensitivity and specificity to detect or rule out disease is applied to a population, the predictive value of a positive or negative result for correctly identifying the disease in question is related to the prevalence of the disease in the population being studied. This statistical principle was first described by Bayes in 1763.[216] This concept can be illustrated by a diagram relating the probability of CAD following testing (the post-test likelihood of disease) to the pre-test probability of CAD in an individual (based on age, gender, and symptoms) (Fig. 94.14).[217] The sensitivity and specificity of the test in question will influence the

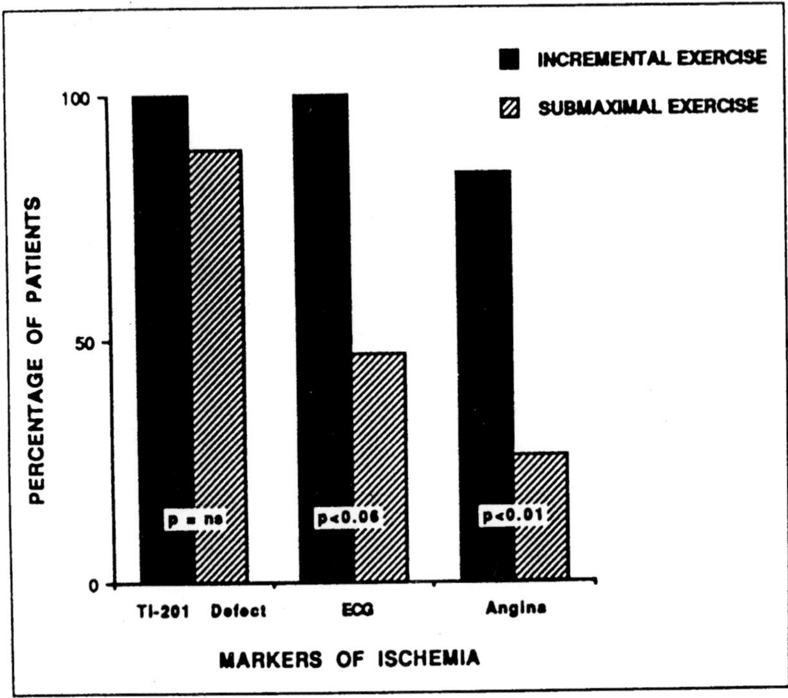

Fig. 94.13 The influence of exercise workload on the prevalence of myocardial perfusion abnormalities (^{201}Tl defect), ischaemic electrocardiographic (ECG) abnormalities, and anginal symptoms in a group of patients with coronary artery disease. At a submaximal workload, the prevalence of ^{201}Tl abnormalities with exercise is similar to that during maximal treadmill exercise (incremental, Bruce protocol). In contrast, the prevalence of ischaemic ECG changes or symptoms of angina fall markedly at submaximal workload. (Reprinted with permission from Heller G V, Ahmed I, Tilkemeier P L et al 1991 Comparison of chest pain, electrocardiographic changes and thallium-201 scintigraphy during varying exercise intensities in men with stable angina pectoris. Am J Cardiol 68: 569.)

positive and negative predictive value curves, such that for any pre-test likelihood of CAD (in essence the assumed prevalence of disease in a population) the post-test probability of disease given a positive or negative test can then be estimated. As is clear from Fig. 94.14, the predictive value of a positive test is relatively low in the lower prevalence range, and similarly, the predictive value of a negative test for ruling out disease is low at a high prevalence of disease. Figure 94.16 illustrates this type of analysis for a test with both a low sensitivity and high specificity (A) as well as a test with a high sensitivity and low specificity (B).[218] A measure of the utility of the test in any pre-test probability range can be expressed as the 'post-test probability difference.' This refers to the difference between the post-test probability of a positive and a negative test.[218] The maximum value of this measure indicates the prevalence at which the discriminatory ability of the test is highest.

This type of analysis can be used to incorporate all of the elements of testing such as the results of the exercise ECG and the scintigraphic results. In this way, a pre-test probability is determined from the clinical data, and a post-test probability is formulated from the results of the exercise ECG data. To interpret the probability of disease based upon the scintigraphic data, the determined probability from the clinical evaluation as well as the exercise ECG results then becomes the pre-test probability of disease when interpreting the scintigraphic results.[77,217]

Thus, the use of Bayesian analysis suggests that the results of scintigraphic testing for the determination of the presence or absence of CAD results in a spectrum or continuum of probabilities rather than a correct or incorrect decision that CAD is present or absent.

Receiver operating characteristic (ROC) curve analysis

The sensitivity and specificity various scintigraphic tests as well as the above discussion relating to Bayes' theorem imply that scintigraphic tests may be read as either 'positive' or 'negative'. While some images truly appear 'normal' or 'abnormal', others are more ambiguous, and it is clear that there is no absolute delineation between a positive scan and a normal scan; rather, a continuum of image interpretation exists from clearly normal, through

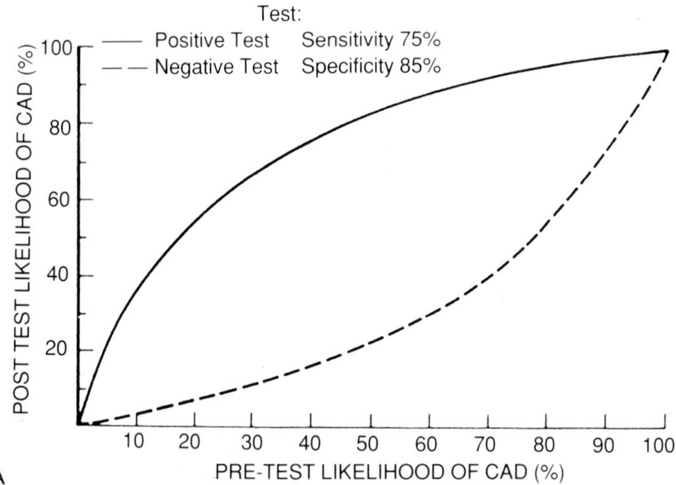

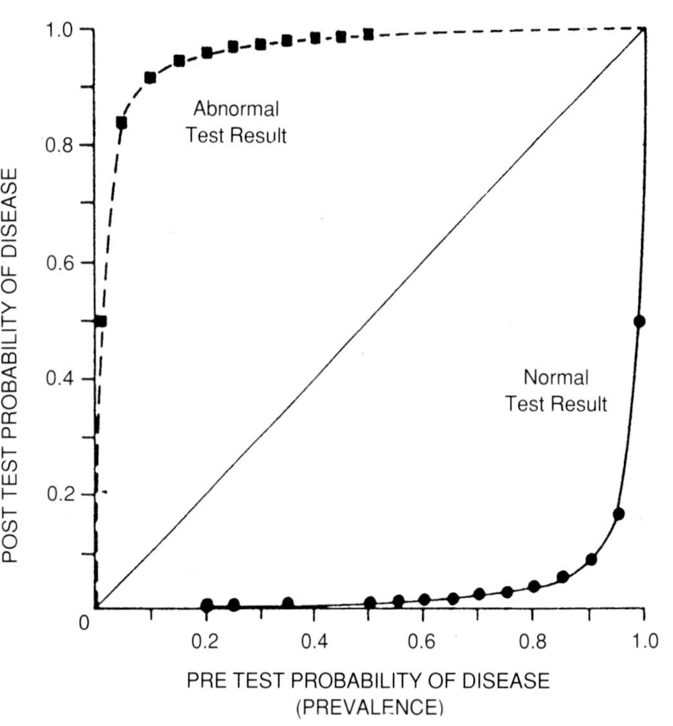

Fig. 94.14 A Diagram illustrating the principles of Bayes' theorem on the influence of disease prevalence on the predictive values of tests. For this test in question, a sensitivity of 75% with a specificity of 85% results in the positive and negative predictive curves (post-test likelihood of coronary artery disease, *y*-axis) for any given pre-test likelihood (*x*-axis). (Reprinted with permission from Epstein S E 1980 Implications of probability analysis on the strategy used for noninvasive detection of coronary artery disease. Am J Cardiol 46: 491.) B If the sensitivity and specificity of the tests are increased to 99% and 99% respectively, the predictive value curves change accordingly such that the predictive value of a positive test is higher across all disease prevalences, as is the predictive value of a negative test. (Reprinted with permission from Hamilton G W et al 1978 Myocardial imaging with thallium-201: an analysis of clinical usefulness based on Bayes' theorem. Semin Nucl Med 8: 358.)

normal variations, through mild abnormalities, to unambiguous abnormalities. In any particular laboratory, the readers will implicitly set their own thresholds for the conservativeness or aggressiveness of the reading. How can the performance characteristics of a test be analysed given the potential variability in thresholds for determining abnormality?

The ROC curve analysis incorporates this concept of varying thresholds into determining testing performance characteristics. The reader is referred to an excellent review on this topic for full discussion.[219] Briefly, however, the ROC analysis plots the true positive fraction (the sensitivity of disease in question) against the false positive fraction (1 – the specificity). Varying the thresholds for determining abnormality with the test will result in a family of points relating the true positive fraction to the false positive fraction (Fig. 94.15). Curve fitting methods are used to create a curve relating the true to the false positive fraction across the entire range of potential decision thresholds.[219] The area under the curve represents the overall utility of the test in discriminating the presence from the absence of disease at all ranges of decision thresholds. Thus, the ROC analysis is thought to be independent of the prevalence of disease in a particular population, and represents test performance at all levels of decision threshold. Fig. 94.17 demonstrates an example of

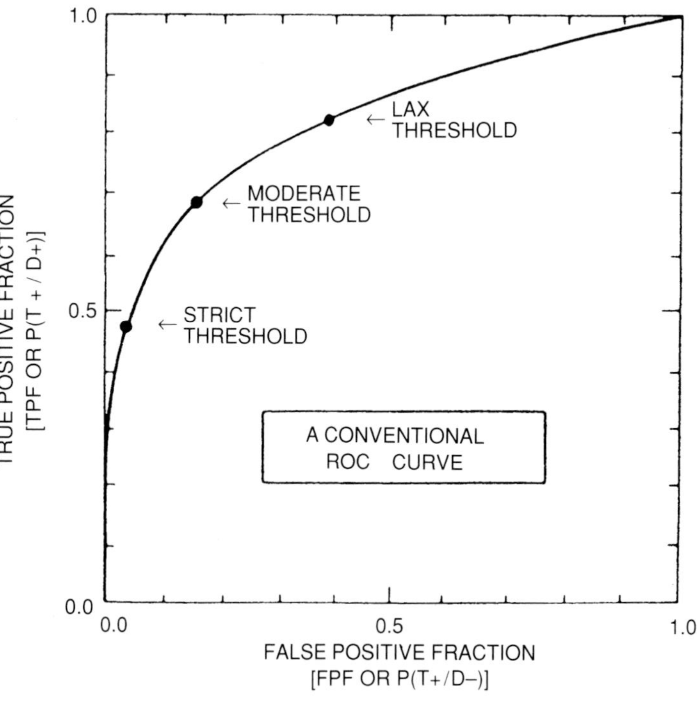

Fig. 94.15 Hypothetical receiver operating characteristic (ROC) curve relating the true positive fraction of a test (sensitivity) to the false positive fraction (1 minus specificity). The test is interpreted at varying thresholds of abnormality and curve fitting methods are used to create the ROC curve, relating the true to the false positive fraction. D– =absence of disease, D+ = presence of disease, P = probability, T– = negative test, T+ = positive test. (Reprinted with permission from Metz C E 1978 Basic principles of ROC analysis. Semin Nucl Med 8: 283.)

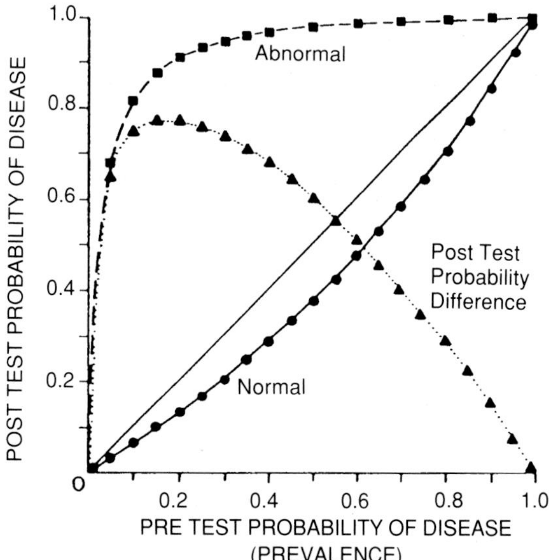

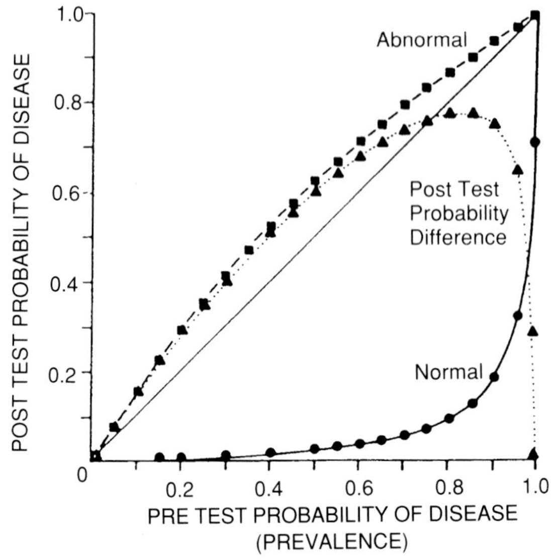

Fig. 94.16 Predictive value curves for tests with varying sensitivity and specificity. In the left panel are predictive value curves for a test with a low sensitivity (40%) and a high specificity (99%), as well as the post-test probability difference representing the difference between the positive (abnormal) and negative (normal) predictive curves at each level of pre-test probability. In this setting, an abnormal test carries a very high predictive value for coronary artery disease (CAD) at most levels of pre-test probability of CAD, while a normal test is less useful for ruling out disease. The peak point on the post-test probability curve (here at approximately 20% pre-test probability) represents the disease prevalence at which the test being evaluated provides the greatest degree of discrimination between the presence and absence of disease. In the right panel are predictive value curves for an abnormal or a normal test, given for a test with a high sensitivity (99%) and a low specificity (40%). Here, a negative or normal test is quite useful for ruling out disease across the whole range of disease prevalence, while a positive test has a relatively low predictive value for disease. (Reprinted with permission from Hamilton G W et al 1978 Myocardial imaging with thallium-201: An analysis of clinical usefulness based on Bayes' theorem. Semin Nucl Med 8: 358.)

ROC analysis in the literature, wherein Fintel et al[81] compared SPECT and planar imaging for the detection of CAD. Because the curve for SPECT imaging lies upwards and to the left of the curve for planar imaging (thus the area under the curve is greater), the ability of SPECT imaging to discriminate the presence from the absence of CAD was determined to be greater than planar imaging.

For an individual reader, the ROC analysis can illustrate the trade-offs implicit in varying the decision thresholds in reading a particular type of image. For instance, if one is operating at a strict reading threshold (that is, requiring a scan abnormality to be unambiguous before calling it abnormal, and calling all other defects within the normal range), that reader will have a relatively low true positive fraction (sensitivity) but also a very low false positive fraction (high specificity). This trade-off might be acceptable if the unfavourable implications or consequences of a 'false positive' decision outweigh the implications of a 'false negative' decision. This in fact may be the case for myocardial perfusion imaging. As a wealth of data suggests that a normal myocardial perfusion study carries with it a very low risk prognosis,[220] the implications of a false negative scan (when 'false' refers to missing CAD by angiography) may not be precipitous in terms of patient management. On the other hand, operating at a much less strict threshold where even minor perturbations in the perfusion pattern are read as 'positive' will result in an operating point on the ROC curve at a high true positive fraction associated with a high false positive fraction (lax threshold in Fig. 94.15). As many patients with a 'positive' myocardial perfusion scan will subsequently undergo coronary arteriography, this type of reading threshold will probably result in a significant subset of patients undergoing angiography who will ultimately be found to have normal coronary arteries.

Thus, ROC analysis can provide a comprehensive description of test performance characteristics, independent of disease prevalence and reading thresholds, incorporating the performance characteristics of the test as well as the observer, and provides a powerful method for evaluating testing modalities.[219]

Pre- and post-test referral bias

Pre-test referral bias describes the effect of disease prevalence on the determination of the performance characteristics of a test, particularly sensitivity and specificity. Most initial studies of a new testing procedure will compare the results of the test in a very 'sick' population with a very 'healthy' population, thus potentially artificially inflating both the sensitivity and specificity.[77] For instance, if exercise myocardial perfusion imaging is performed in a population of patients in whom a high percentage have had a prior myocardial infarction, the sensitivity of the test

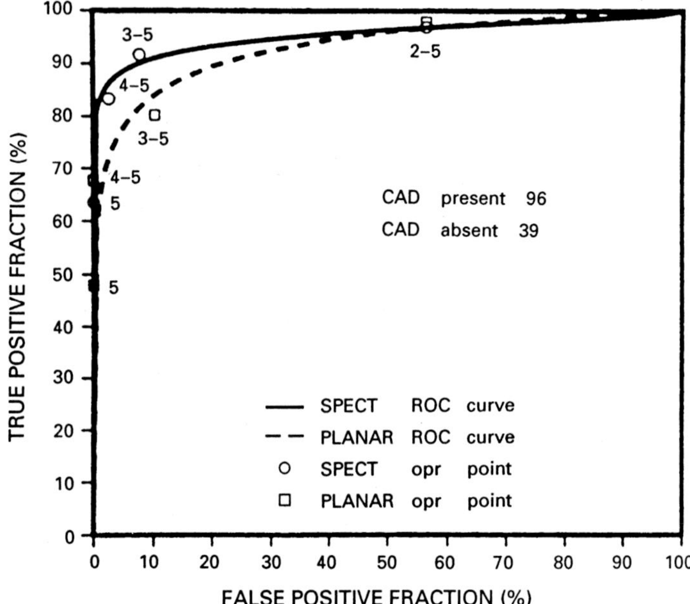

Fig. 94.17 An example of superimposed ROC curves comparing SPECT imaging (solid line) and planar imaging (dashed line) using ^{201}Tl for detecting artery disease (CAD). Because the curve for SPECT imaging lies above and to the left of the curve for planar imaging, the area under the curve is greater for SPECT imaging, and it is concluded that SPECT imaging allows better discrimination of the presence or absence of CAD than planar imaging. The open circles and squares represent different operating (opr) points of abnormality threshold (for SPECT and planar imaging, respectively) on which the curves are based. (Reprinted with permission from Fintel D J, Links J M, Brinker J A et al 1989 Improved diagnostic performance of exercise thallium-201 single photon emission computed tomography over planar imaging in the diagnosis of coronary artery disease: a receiver operating characteristic analysis. J Am Coll Cardiol 13: 600.)

will be quite high, as many of these patients have defined CAD even prior to testing. In evaluating test sensitivity and comparing various reports in the literature, it is important to assess this type of characteristic of the population being reported.

Post-test referral bias describes a phenomenon whereby a test that has been initially compared to a gold standard subsequently becomes the test to screen patients in order to determine the need to go on to the next level of testing, i.e. the gold standard. For instance, a decline over time in the specificity of both exercise RNA[188] and exercise ^{201}Tl scintigraphy[221] has been ascribed to the fact that after the promising initial reports for both techniques, these imaging modalities become screening techniques to determine who did or did not need to go on to coronary angiography.[188] Thus, very few of the large pool of normal test responders subsequently were sent to coronary arteriography. In later reports evaluating the efficacy of these tests, the result was an apparent decline in specificity, as many of the 'true negative' subjects were not included in the analysis because they did not undergo coronary arteriography. In an attempt to determine specificity of a test once this phenomenon has occurred, some have advocated the concept of a normalcy rate,[77,189] which is the specificity in a low prevalence, non-catheterized population. Others have argued that normalcy rate artificially inflates the specificity values.[222] The 'true' specificity of a test, if that can ever be determined, probably lies somewhere between the apparent specificity and the normalcy rate.

THE ASYMPTOMATIC PATIENT AND SCREENING FOR CAD

The discussion regarding the performance characteristics and predictive values of a test in a low prevalence population would suggest that screening an asymptomatic population for the presence of CAD in order to consider early intervention would result in many false positive examinations. In a population with low prevalence of disease, it is possible that of all the positive test results, a much higher percentage would be false positive than true positive. For the general population, then, screening with radionuclide tests is likely to be a cost-ineffective procedure. In the future, should aggresive lipid lowering therapy be shown to induce regression of CAD and significantly reduce subsequent morbid and mortal outcomes, then the cost-effectiveness of screening could be carefully evaluated in terms of ultimate outcome.

There are important subpopulations of subjects, however, in whom the detection of potential underlying asymptomatic CAD is compelling, including airline pilots and military personnel. As would be expected, the predictive values for exercise testing with ECG alone or exercise myocardial perfusion imaging are relatively low in an asymptomatic low prevalence population. However, Uhl et al[223] have shown that exercise ^{201}Tl imaging using quantitative analysis performed well as a 'second line' screening procedure. In a series of airmen who had undergone initial screening with exercise ECG, those with abnormal exercise ECGs subsequently underwent exercise ^{201}Tl imaging and coronary angiography. The predictive value of a positive myocardial perfusion scan was 74%, compared to 21% for the exercise ECG. These results again reflect the workings of Bayes' theorem, as the pre-test probability of CAD in the population undergoing ^{201}Tl imaging was higher than the whole population undergoing exercise ECG; once the asymptomatic air crewmen had a positive ECG, their prior probability of CAD rose accordingly, and ^{201}Tl imaging was applied in a more selected, higher prevalence population.[224] Thus, screening an asymptomatic population for disease with scintigraphic techniques is likely to result in a relatively low predictive value, but a more favourable predictive value when compared to exercise ECG. In populations in whom there is a compelling reason to screen for CAD, it appears that exercise radionuclide techniques may be best applied in a sequential fashion following risk factor analysis and exercise ECG.[224]

Interestingly, Uhl et al[223] also demonstrated that the majority of patients with 'mild' CAD (<50% stenosis) had abnormal scans. How these scan results are classified obviously has a significant impact on the determination of sensitivity and specificity,[97] and illustrates the difficulties inherent in evaluating these performance characteristics with regard to an arbitrary angiographic cut-off point, particularly when the ability to read that cut-off point reproducibly is variable.

DISCORDANT RESULTS BETWEEN EXERCISE ECG, RADIONUCLIDE TECHNIQUES, AND ANGIOGRAPHY

Because an epicardial coronary atherosclerotic plaque is only one aspect of the complex anatomical–physiological substrate that contributes to regional myocardial perfusion abnormalities and regional myocardial ischaemia, discordant results in testing with exercise ECG examining regional ischaemia, myocardial perfusion imaging investigating regional myocardial flow, and coronary arteriography examining the fixed characteristics of an atherosclerotic plaque can often be explained in terms of the different points on the anatomical–physiologic spectrum which these tests are examining.

For instance, myocardial perfusion imaging tests the ability of the entire vessel to deliver flow to the myocardial bed. This involves the degree of luminal obstruction by the atherosclerotic plaque, as well as the dynamic characteristics of vasomotion the vessel wall. Complicating the picture is the dynamic nature of arteriolar resistance as well as the degree of collateralization. Thus, a 90% stenosis supplying a heavily collateralized myocardial bed may demonstrate only a very mild or perhaps no perfusion defect during stress. While this may minimize the ability to detect the 90% stenosis, the perfusion image will accurately reflect the perfusion status (from all sources) of the myocardial region at risk. These studies may also reflect the risk of infarction of the territory at risk, since an unstable plaque could evolve into total obstruction; but the presence of collaterals, as identified by normal or near-normal myocardial perfusion imaging, would imply that little or no myocardium is at risk of infarction. Thus, angiography and perfusion imaging provide complimentary information regarding the overall status of myocardial perfusion and the risk of infarction.

While many studies investigating performance characteristics of myocardial perfusion imaging and exercise RNA use a 50% stenosis as the angiographic cut-off point for 'positive disease', this is a relatively arbitrary value which is subject to a great deal of inter-observer variability.[225] The 50% figure is based on the seminal studies of coronary flow by Gould & Lipscomb[67] in which a 50% stenosis in a dog model was found to reduce regional coronary flow reserve. In humans, however, based on the difficulty in determining the exact percentage stenosis in that range, the dynamic aspects of vasomotor tone during stress, as well as the presence or absence of collateralization, that range of stenosis may or may not be associated with a perfusion abnormality. Complicating the analysis of the performance characteristics of an imaging modality is the fact that, currently, perfusion imaging is often used clinically to define the physiological significance of a moderate stenosis. Thus, one cannot justifiably classify such images as either true or false positives based on the associated angiographic result.

When studies of myocardial perfusion imaging are reanalysed in terms of classifying a more modest stenosis as 'disease', the performance characteristics of testing improve, whether it is in planar imaging[223] or with SPECT.[97] Thus, apparently discordant results (such as a 40% stenosis and a positive perfusion scan in that territory) can be classified as physiologically meaningful based on an understanding of the anatomical–physiological characteristics which are being examined by each testing modality.

In this regard, even in the presence of significant multivessel CAD, a normal or near-normal perfusion pattern identifies an underlying coronary vascular physiology which appears to protect the patient from adverse major coronary events over long-term follow-up.[226] Similar findings have been reported when a CAD patient is noted to have a preserved left ventricular ejection fraction response to exercise.[183]

Thus, once artefacts and normal variants potentially responsible for positive imaging results, as well as workload and other characteristics which may contribute to an apparently normal image, have been considered, apparent discordance between angiography and perfusion or functional imaging usually have important clinical implications.

CONCLUSION

Single photon techniques used to image myocardial perfusion, as well as exercise ventricular functional imaging, have matured considerably since their introduction in the mid-1970s. Technical advances involving hardware and software, as well as newer imaging agents, have expanded the use of these techniques into populations of patients that were difficult to image in the earlier years of their use. While this review has concentrated on the ability of these imaging modalities to discriminate between the presence and absence of CAD in an individual patient, as well as to determine the extent of disease for management purposes, a major focus of more recent research has emphasized the powerful risk stratification and prognostic implications inherent in the perfusion or functional images, as well as the physiological correlation with the anatomical substrate visualized on angiography. While cameras, software, imaging protocols and imaging agents will continue to be evaluated, future directions will probably revolve around early detection of moderate CAD. In addition, a careful evaluation of the optimal application of these techniques to early detection and management strategies with regard to cost-effectiveness will be of great importance.

REFERENCES

1. American Heart Association 1979 Heart Facts, 1980
2. Report of the Joint International Society and Federation of Cardiology, World Health Organization Task Force on Standardization of Clinical Nomenclature 1979 Nomenclature and criteria for diagnosis of ischemic heart disease. Circulation 59: 607
3. Robb G P, Marks M H 1974 Latent coronary artery disease: Determination of its presence and severity by the exercise electrocardiogram. Am J Cardiol 13: 603
4. Ellestad M H, Wan M K C 1975 Predictive implications of stress testing follow-up of 2700 subjects after maximum treadmill stress testing. Circulation 51: 363
5. Goldschlager N, Selzer A, Cohn K 1976 Treadmill stress tests as indications of presence and severity of coronary artery disease. Ann Intern Med 85: 277
6. Schulze R A, Rouleau J, Rigo P et al 1975 Left ventricular function and ventricular arrhythmias in the late hospital phase of acute myocardial infarction. Circulation 52: 1006
7. Schulze R A, Strauss H W, Pitt B 1977 Sudden death in the year following myocardial infarction: Relation to ventricular premature contractions in the late hospital phase and left ventricular ejection fraction. Am J Med 62: 192
8. Pulido J I, Doss J, Tweig D et al 1978 Submaximal exercise testing in patients after acute myocardial infarction: Myocardial scintigraphic and electrocardiographic observations. Am J Cardiol 42: 19
9. Paine T D, Dye L E, Roitman D I et al 1978 Relation of graded exercise test findings after myocardial infarction to extent of coronary artery disease and left ventricular dysfunction. Am J Cardiol 42: 716
10. Messer J V, Wagman R J, Levine M J et al 1962 Patterns of human myocardial oxygen extraction during rest and exercise. J Clin Invest 41: 725
11. Sarnoff S J, Gilmore J P, Skinner N S Jr et al 1963 Relation between coronary blood flow and myocardial oxygen consumption. Circ Res 13: 522
12. Haddy F J 1969 Physiology and pharmacology of the coronary circulation and myocardium, particularly in relation to coronary artery disease. Am J Med 47: 274
13. Braunwald E B 1971 Control of myocardial oxygen consumption. Am J Cardiol 27: 416
14. Knoebel S B, Elliott W C, McHenry P L et al 1971 Myocardial blood flow in coronary artery disease. Am J Cardiol 27: 51
15. Weber K T, Janicki J S 1979 The metabolic demand and oxygen supply of the heart: Physiologic and clinical considerations. Am J Cardiol 44: 722
16. Opie L H 1968 Metabolism of the heart in health and disease. I. Am Heart J 76: 685
17. Opie L H 1969 Metabolism of the heart in health and disease. II. Am Heart J 77: 100
18. Opie L H 1969 Metabolism of the heart in health and disease. III. Am Heart J 77: 383
19. Neely J R, Morgan H E 1974 Relationship between carbohydrate and lipid metabolism and the energy balance of heart muscle. Annu Rev Physiol 36: 413
20. Scheuer J 1967 Myocardial metabolism in cardiac hypoxia. Am J Cardiol 19: 385
21. Katz A M 1970 Contractile proteins of the heart. Physiol Rev 50: 63
22. Katz A M 1973 Effects of ischemia on the contractile process of the heart muscle. Am J Cardiol 32: 456
23. Schwartz A M, Wood J M, Allen J C et al 1973 Biochemical and morphologic correlates of cardiac ischemia. Am J Cardiol 32: 46
24. Braasch W, Gudbjarnason S, Puri P S 1968 Early changes in energy metabolism in the myocardium following acute coronary artery occlusion in anesthetized dogs. Circ Res 23: 429
25. Sayen J J, Sheldon W F, Peirce G et al 1958 Polorographic oxygen, the epicardial electrogram and muscle contraction in experimental acute regional ischemia of the left ventricle. Circ Res 6: 779
26. Harden W R, Barlow C H, Simson M B et al 1979 Temporal relation between onset of cell anoxia and ischemic contractile failure. Am J Cardiol 44: 741
27. Jenning R B, Gantole C E, Reimer K A 1975 Ischemic tissue injury. Am J Pathol 81: 179
28. Herdson P, Sommers H M, Jennings R B 1965 A comparative study of the fine structures of normal and ischemic dog myocardium with special reference to early changes following temporary occlusion of a coronary artery. Am J Pathol 46: 367
29. Wyatt H L, Forrester J S, Tyberg J V et al 1975 Effect of graded reductions in regional coronary perfusion on regional and total cardiac function. Am J Cardiol 36: 185
30. Kubler W, Katz A M 1977 Mechanisms of early pump failure of the ischemic heart: Possible role of adenosine triphosphate depletion and inorganic phosphate accumulation. Am J Cardiol 40: 467
31. Hearse D J 1979 Oxygen deprivation and early myocardial contractile failure: A reassessment of the possible role of adenosine triphosphate. Am J Cardiol 44: 1115
32. Neely J R, Whitman J T, Rovetto M J 1975 Effect of coronary blood flow on glycolytic flux and intracellular pH in isolated rat hearts. Circ Res 37: 733
33. Scheuer J, Berry M N 1967 Effect of alkalosis on glycolysis in the isolated rat heart. Am J Physiol 213: 1143
34. Opie L, Owen P, Thomas M et al 1973 Coronary sinus lactate measurements in assessment of myocardial ischemia. Am J Cardiol 32: 295
35. Huckabee W E 1958 Relationship of pyruvate and lactate during anaerobic metabolism. J Clin Invest 37: 244
36. Parker J O, Chiong M A, West R O et al 1970 The effect of ischemia and alterations of heart rate on myocardial potassium balance in man. Circulation 42: 205
37. Opie L U, Thomas M, Owen P et al 1972 Increased coronary venous phosphate concentrations during experimental myocardial infarction. Am J Cardiol 30: 503
38. Brachfeld N 1976 Characterization of the ischemic process by regional metabolism. Am J Cardiol 37: 467
39. Apstein C S, Gravino F, Hood W B Jr 1979 Limitations of lactate production as an index of myocardial ischemia. Circulation 60: 887
40. Master A M, Jaffe H L 1941 Electrocardiographic changes after exercise in angina pectoris. J Mount Sinai Hosp 7: 629
41. Master A M 1950 Two-step exercise electrocardiogram: Test for coronary insufficiency. Ann Intern Med 32: 842
42. Borer J S, Brensik J F, Redwood D R et al 1975 Limitations of the electrocardiographic response to exercise in predicting coronary artery disease. N Engl J Med 293: 367
43. Redwood D R, Borer R S, Epstein S E 1976 Whither the ST segment during exercise? Circulation 54: 703
44. Epstein S E 1978 Value and limitations of the electrocardiographic response to exercise in the assessment of patients with coronary artery disease. Am J Cardiol 42: 667
45. Weiner D A, Ryan T J, McCabe C H et al 1978 Exercise stress testing: Correlations among history of angina, ST-segment response and prevalence of coronary artery disease in the coronary artery surgery study (CASS). New Engl J Med 301: 230

46. Selzer A, Cohn K, Goldschlager N 1978 On the interpretation of the exercise test. Circulation 58: 193
47. Mason R E, Likar I, Biern R O et al 1967 Multiple-lead exercise electrocardiography: Experience in 107 normal subjects and 67 patients with angina pectoris, and comparison with coronary cinearteriography in 84 patients. Circulation 36: 517
48. Kassebaum D G, Sutherland K L, Judkins M P 1968 A comparison of hypoxemia and exercise electrocardiography in coronary artery disease. Am Heart J 75: 759
49. McHenry P L, Phillips J F, Knoebel S B 1972 Correlation of computer quantitated treadmill exercise electrocardiogram with arteriographic location of coronary artery disease. J Cardiol 30: 747
50. Martin C M, McConahay D R 1972 Maximal treadmill exercise electrocardiography. Circulation 46: 956
51. Kaplan M A, Harris C N, Aronow W S et al 1973 Inability of the submaximal treadmill stress test to predict the location of coronary disease. Circulation 47: 250
52. Keleman M H, Gillilan R E, Bouchard R J et al 1973 Diagnosis of obstructive coronary disease by maximal exercise and atrial pacing. Circulation 48: 1227
53. Bartel A J, Behar V S, Peter R H et al 1974 Graded exercise stress tests in angiographically documented coronary artery disease. Circulation 49: 348
54. Cohn K, Kamm B, Feteih N et al 1979 Use of treadmill score to quantify ischemic response and predict extent of coronary disease. Circulation 59: 2886
55. Scheuer J, Brachfeld N 1966 Coronary insufficiency: Relations between hemodynamic, electrical and biochemical parameters. Circ Res 18: 178
56. Linhart J W, Turnoff M B 1974 Maximum treadmill exercise test in patients with abnormal control electrocardiograms. Circulation 49: 667
57. Castellanet M J, Greenberg P S, Ellestad M H 1978 Comparison of ST segment changes on exercise testings with angiographic findings in patients with prior myocardial infarction. Am J Cardiol 42: 29
58. Lary D, Goldschlager N 1974 Electrocardiographic changes during hyperventilation resembling myocardial ischemia in patients with normal coronary arteriograms. Am Heart J 87: 383
59. Friesinger G C, Biern R O, Liker I et al 1972 Exercise ECG and vasoregulatory abnormalities. Am J Cardiol 30: 733
60. Holmgren A, Jonsson B, Linderholm H et al 1959 ECG changes in vasoregulatory asthenia and the effect of physical training. Acta Med Scand 165: 259
61. Soloff L, Fewell J 1961 Abnormal ECG responses to exercise in subjects with hypokalemia. Am J Med Sci 242: 724
62. Nordstrom-Ohrberg G 1964 Effect of digitalis glycosides on ECG and exercise test in healthy subjects. Acta Med Scand 176: 1
63. Roitman D, Jones W B, Sheffield L T 1970 Comparison of submaximal exercise ECG test with coronary cineangiocardiogram. Ann Intern Med 72: 641
64. Harris C, Aronow W, Parker D et al 1973 Treadmill stress test in left ventricular hypertrophy. Chest 63: 353
65. Sigwart U, Grbic M, Payot M et al 1984 Ischemic events during coronary artery balloon obstruction. In: Rutishauser W, Roskamm H (eds) Silent myocardial ischemia. Springer-Verlag, Berlin, p 29
66. Nesto R W, Kowalchuk G J 1987 The ischemic cascade: temporal sequence of hemodynamic electrocardiographic and symptomatic expressions of ischemia. Am J Cardiol 57: 23C
67. Gould K L, Lipscomb K 1974 Effects of coronary stenoses on coronary flow reserve and resistance. Am J Cardiol 34: 50
68. Zaret B L, Strauss H W, Martin N D et al 1973 Noninvasive regional myocardial perfusion with radioactive potassium: study of patients at rest, exercise and during angina pectoris. N Engl J Med 288: 809
69. Borer J S et al 1977 Real-time radionuclide cineangiography in the noninvasive evaluation of global and regional left ventricular function at rest and during exercise in patients with coronary artery disease. N Engl J Med 296: 839
70. Esquivel L et al: Effect of the degree of effort on the sensitivity of the exercise thallium-201 stress test in symptomatic coronary artery disease. Am J Cardiol 63: 160
71. Iskandrian A S, Heo J, Kong B, Lyons E 1989 Effect of exercise level on the ability of thallium-201 tomographic imaging in detecting coronary artery disease: Analysis of 461 patients. J Am Coll Cardiol 14: 1477
72. Heller G V, Ahmed I, Tilkemeier P L et al 1991 Comparison of chest pain, electrocardiographic changes and thallium-201 scintigraphy during varying exercise intensities in men with stable angina pectoris. Am J Cardiol 68: 569
73. Seaworth J F et al 1983 Effect of partial decreases in exercise work load on radionuclide indexes of ischemia. J Am Coll Cardiol 2: 522
74. Schelbert H R, Wisenberg G, Phelps M E et al 1982 Noninvasive assessment of coronary stenosis by myocardial imaging during pharmacologic coronary vasodilation. VI. Detection of coronary artery disease in man with intravenous NH3 and positron computed tomography. Am J Cardiol 49: 1197
75. Tamaki N, Yonekura Y, Senda M et al 1985 Myocardial positron computed tomography with N-13 ammonia at rest and during exercise. Eur J Nucl Med 11: 246
76. Demer L L, Gould K L, Goldstein R A, Kirkeeide R L 1989 Diagnosis of coronary artery disease by positron emission tomography: Comparison to quantitative coronary arteriography in 193 patients. Circulation 79: 825
77. Rozanski A, Berman D S 1987 The efficacy of cardiovascular nuclear medicine exercise studies. Sem Nucl Med 27: 104
78. Holman B, Hill T, Wynee J et al 1984 Single photon transaxial emission computed tomography of the heart in normal subjects and in patients with infarction. J Nucl Med 25: 893
79. DePuey E G, Garcia E V 1989 Optimal specificity of thallium-201 SPECT through recognition of imaging artifacts. J Nucl Med 30: 441
80. Henkin R E, Kikkawz R M, Kemel A 1993 Thallium myocardial perfusion imaging utilizing single photon emission computed tomography (SPECT). Diagnostic and therapeutic technology assessment. Monograph, American Medical Association
81. Fintel D J, Links J M, Brinker J A et al 1989 Improved diagnostic performance of exercise thallium-201 single photon emission computed tomography over planar imaging in the diagnosis of coronary artery disease: A receiver operating characteristic analysis. J Am Coll Cardiol 13: 600
82. Kasabali B, Woodard M L, Bekerman C et al 1989 Enhanced sensitivity and specificity of thallium-201 imaging for the detection of regional ischemic coronary disease by combining SPECT with 'Bull's Eye' analysis. Clin Nucl Med 14: 484
83. Mendelson M A, Spies S M, Spies W G et al 1992 Usefulness of single-photon emission computed tomography of thallium-201 uptake after dipyridamole infusion for detection of coronary artery disease. Am J Cardiol 69(14): 1150
84. Nohara R, Kambara H, Suzuki Y et al 1984 Stress scintigraphy using single-photon emission computed tomography in the evaluation of coronary artery disease. Am J Cardiol 53: 1250
85. Friedman J, VanTrain K, Maddahi J et al 1986 "Upward creep" of the heart: a frequent source of false-positive reversible defects on Tl-201 stress-redistribution SPECT. J Nucl Med 27: 899
86. Atwood J E, Jensen D, Froelicher V et al 1981 Agreement in human interpretation of analog thallium myocardial perfusion images. Circulation 64: 601
87. Trobaugh G B, Wackers F J T, Busemann S E et al 1978 Thallium-201 myocardial imaging: An interinstitutional study of observer variability. J Nucl Med 19: 359
88. Garcia E, Maddahi J, Berman D S et al 1981 Space/time quantitation of thallium-201 myocardial scintigraphy. J Nucl Med 22: 309
89. Watson D D, Campbell N P, Read E K et al 1981 Spatial and temporal quantitation of plane thallium myocardial images. J Nucl Med 22: 577
90. Berger B C, Watson D D, Taylor G J et al 1981 Quantitative thallium-201 exercise scintigraphy for detection of coronary artery disease. J Nucl Med 22: 585
91. Maddahi J, Garcia E V, Berman D S et al 1981 Improved noninvasive assessment of coronary artery disease by quantitative analysis of regional stress myocardial distribution and washout of thallium-201. Circulation 64: 924
92. Maddahi J, Abdulla A, Garcia E V et al 1986 Noninvasive

identification of left main and triple vessel coronary artery disease: improved accuracy using quantitative analysis of regional myocardial stress distribution and washout of thallium-201. J Am Coll Cardiol 7: 53
93. Wackers F J T, Fetterman R C, Mattera J A, Clements J P 1985 Quantitative planar thallium-201 stress scintigraphy: A critical evaluation of the method. Semin Nucl Med 15: 46
94. Kaul S, Chesler D A, Pohost G M et al 1986 Influence of peak exercise heart rate on normal thallium-201 myocardial clearance. J Nucl Med 27: 26
95. Becker L C, Rogers W J, Links J M, Corn C 1989 Limitations of regional myocardial thallium clearance for identification of disease in individual coronary arteries. J Am Coll Cardiol 14: 1491
96. Gorcia E V 1985 Quantitation of rotational thallium201 myocordial tomography. J Nucl Med 26: 17
97. DePasquale E E, Nody A C, DePuey E G et al 1988 Quantitative rotational thallium-201 tomography for identifying and localizing coronary artery disease. Circulation 77: 316
98. Mahmarian J J, Boyce T M, Goldberg R K et al 1990 Quantitative exercise thallium-201 single photon emission computed tomography for the enhanced diagnosis of ischemic heart disease. J Am Coll Cardiol 15: 318
99. Tamaki N, Yonekura Y, Mukai T et al 1984 Stress thallium-201 transaxial emission computed tomography: Quantitative versus qualitative analysis for evaluation of coronary artery disease. J Am Coll Cardiol 4: 1213
100. Nishimura S, Mahmarian J J, Boyce T M, Verani M S 1991 Quantitative thallium-201 single photon emission computed tomography during maximal pharmacologic coronary vasodilation with adenosine for assessing coronary artery disease. J Am Coll Cardiol 18: 736–745
101. Maddahi J et al 1990 Myocardial perfusion imaging with technetium-99m sestamibi SPECT in the evaluation of coronary artery disease. Am J Cardiol 66: 55E
102. Wackers F J et al 1989 Technetium-99m hexakis 2-methoxyisobutyl isonitrile: Human biodistribution, dosimetry, safety, and preliminary comparison to thallium-201 for myocardial perfusion imaging. J Nucl Med 30: 301
103. Maisey M N et al 1990 European multi-centre comparison of thallium-201 and technetium-99m methoxyisobutylisonitrile in ischemic heart disease. Eur J Nucl Med 16: 869
104. Iskandrian A S et al 1989 Use of technetium-99m isonitrile (RP-30A) in assessing left ventricular perfusion and function at rest and during exercise in coronary artery disease, and comparison with coronary arteriography and exercise thallium-201 SPECT imaging. Am J Cardiol 64: 270
105. Kahn J K et al 1989 Quantitative rotational tomography with Tl-201 and Tc-99m 2-methoxy-isobutyl-isonitrile: A direct comparison in normal individuals and patients with coronary artery disease. Circulation 79: 1282
106. Hassan I M et al 1990 Segmental analysis of SPECT 99m-Tc-methoxy isobutyl isonitrile and 201 Tl myocardial imaging in ischaemic heart disease. Eur J Nucl Med 16: 705
107. Hendel R C et al 1990 Diagnostic value of a new myocardial perfusion agent, teboroxime (SQ 30,217) utilizing a rapid planar imaging protocol: Preliminary results. J Am Coll Cardiol 16: 855
108. Seldin D W et al 1989 Myocardial perfusion imaging with technetium-99m SQ 30217: Comparison with thallium-201 and coronary anatomy. J Nucl Med 30: 312
109. Maddahi J, Kiat H, Berman D S 1991 Myocardial perfusion imaging with technetium-99m-labeled agents. Am J Cardiol 67: 27D
110. Fleming R M et al 1991 Comparison of technetium-99m teboroxime tomography with automated quantitative coronary arteriography and thallium-201 tomographic imaging. J Am Coll Cardiol 17: 1297
111. Taillefer R et al 1992 Comparison between thallium-201-technetium-99m-sestamibi and technetium-99m-teboroxime planar myocardial perfusion imaging in detection of coronary artery disease. J Nucl Med 33: 1091
112. Leppo J A 1989 Dipyridamole-thallium imaging: The lazy man's stress test. J Nucl Med 30: 281
113. Gould K L 1978 Noninvasive assessment of coronary stenoses by myocardial perfusion imaging during pharmacologic coronary vasodilatation. I. Physiologic basis and experimental validation. Am J Cardiol 41: 267
114. Verani M S 1993 Pharmacologic stress myocardial perfusion imaging. Current Problems in Cardiology 18: 483
115. Beller G A, Sinusas A J 1990 Experimental studies of the physiologic properties of technetium-99m isonitriles. Am J Cardiol 66: 72E
116. Glover D K, Okada R D 1990 Myocardial kinetics of Tc-MIBI in canine myocardium after dipyridamole. Circulation 81: 628
117. Coleman R E et al 1986 Imaging of myocardial perfusion with Tc-99m SQ 30217: Dog and human studies. J Nucl Med 27: 893
118. Leppo J A Cardiac transport of single photon myocardial perfusion agents. In: Zaret B L, Beller G A (eds) Nuclear cardiology: state of the art and future directions. CV Mosby, St Louis
119. Pennell D J, Underwood S R, Swanton R H et al 1991 Dobutamine thallium myocardial perfusion tomography. J Am Coll Cardiol 18: 1471
120. Hays J T, Mahmarian J J, Cochran A J et al 1993 Dobutamine thallium-201 tomography for evaluating patients with suspected coronary artery disease unable to undergo exercise or vasodilatory pharmacologic testing. J Am Coll Cardiol 21: 1583
121. Hirzel H O, Senn M, Nuesch K et al 1984 Thallium-201 scintigraphy in complete left bundle branch block. Am J Cardiol 53: 764
122. DePuey E G, Guertler-Krawczynska E, Robbins W L 1988 Thallium-201 SPECT in coronary artery disease patients with left bundle branch block. J Nucl Med 29: 1479
123. Jazmati B, Sadaniantz A, Emaus, S P, Heller G V 1991 Exercise thallium-201 imaging in complete left bundle branch block and the prevalence of septal perfusion defects. Am J Cardiol 67: 46
124. Matzer L, Kiat H, Friedman J D et al 1991 A new approach to the assessment of tomographic thallium-201 scintigraphy in patients with left bundle branch block. J Am Coll Cardiol 17: 1309
125. Braat S H, Brugada P, Barr F W et al 1985 Thallium-201 exercise scintigraphy and left bundle branch block. Am J Cardiol 55: 224
126. Marin H E, Rodriguez P L, Castro B J M et al 1987 Thallium-201 exercise scintigraphy in patients having complete left bundle branch block with normal coronary arteries. Int J Cardiol 16: 43
127. Burns R J, Galligan L, Wright L M et al 1991 Improved specificity of myocardial thallium-201 single-photon emission computed tomography in patients with left bundle branch block with dipyridamole. Am J Cardiol 68: 504
128. Jukema J W, van der Wall E E, van der Vis-Melsen M J et al 1993 Dipyridamole thallium-201 scintigraphy for improved detection of left anterior descending coronary artery stenosis in patients with left bundle branch block. Eur Heart J 14(1): 53
129. Rubin K A et al 1979 Idiopathic hypertrophic subaortic stenosis: Evaluation of anginal symptoms with thallium-201 myocardial imaging. Am J Cardiol 44: 1040
130. Pitcher D et al 1980 Assessment of chest pain in hypertrophic cardiomyopathy using exercise thallium-201 myocardial scintigraphy. Br Heart J 44: 650
131. Hanrath P et al 1981 Myocardial thallium-201 imaging in hypertrophic obstructive cardiomyopathy. Eur Heart J 2: 177
132. O'Gara P T et al 1987 Myocardial perfusion abnormalities in patients with hypertrophic cardiomyopathy: Assessment with thallium-201 emission computed tomography. Circulation 76: 1214
133. Udelson J E et al 1989 Verapamil prevents silent myocardial perfusion abnormalities during exercise in asymptomatic hypertrophic cardiomyopathy. Circulation 79: 1052
134. Cannon R O et al 1991 Myocardial metabolic, hemodynamic and electrocardiographic significance of reversible thallium-201 defects in hypertrophic cardiomyopathy. Circulation 83: 1660
135. DePuey E G et al 1988 Alterations in myocardial thallium-201 distribution in patients with chronic systemic hypertension undergoing single-photon emission computed tomography. Am J Cardiol 62: 234
136. Schulman D S, Francis C K, Black H R, Wackers F J T 1987 Thallium-201 stress imaging in hypertensive patients. Hypertension 10: 16
137. Tubau J F, Szlachcic J, Hollenberg M, Massie B M 1989 Usefulness of thallium-201 scintigraphy in predicting the

development of angina pectoris in hypertensive patients with left ventricular hypertrophy. Am J Cardiol 64: 45

138. Pichard A D et al 1981 Coronary flow studies in patients with left ventricular hypertrophy of the hypertensive type. Am J Cardiol 47: 547
139. Bache R J, Arentzen C E, Simon A B, Vrobel T R 1984 Abnormalities in myocardial perfusion during tachycardia in dogs with left ventricular hypertrophy: Metabolic evidence of ischemia. Circulation 69: 409
140. Bulkley B H, Hutchins G M, Bailey I et al 1977 Thallium-201 imaging and gated cardiac blood pool scans in patients with ischemic and idiopathic congestive cardiomyopathy: a clinical and pathologic study. Circulation 55: 753
141. Dunn R F, Uren R F, Sadick N et al 1982 Comparison of thallium-201 scanning in idiopathic dilated cardiomyopathy and severe coronary artery disease. Circulation 66: 804
142. Yamaguchi S, Tsuiki K, Hayasaka M, Yasui S 1987 Segmental wall motion abnormalities in dilated cardiomyopathy: hemodynamic characteristics and comparison with thallium-201 myocardial scintigraphy. Am Heart J 113: 1123
143. Pasternac A, Noble J, Streulens Y et al 1982 Pathophysiology of chest pain in patients with cardiomyopathies and normal coronary arteries. Circulation 65: 778
144. Nitenberg A, Foult J M, Blanchet F, Zouioueche S 1985 Multifactorial determinants of reduced coronary flow reserve after dipyridamole in dilated cardiomyopathy. Am J Cardiol 55: 748
145. Dash H, Massie B M, Botvinick E H, Brundage B H 1979 The noninvasive identification of left main and three-vessel coronary artery disease by myocardial stress perfusion scintigraphy and treadmill exercise electrocardiography. Circulation 60: 276
146. McKillop H J, Murray R G, Turner J G et al 1979 Can the extent of coronary artery disease be predicted from Tl-201 myocardial images? J Nucl Med 20: 715
147. Rigo P, Bailey I K, Griffith L S C et al 1980 Value and limitations of segmental analysis of stress thallium myocardial imaging for localization of coronary artery disease. Circulation 61: 973
148. Rehn T, Griffith L S C, Aschuff S C et al 1981 Exercise Tl-201 myocardial imaging in left main coronary artery disease: Sensitive but not specific. Am J Cardiol 48: 217
149. Maddahi J, Abdulla A, Garcia E et al 1986 Noninvasive identification of left main and triple vessel coronary artery disease: improved accuracy using quantitative analysis of regional myocardial stress distribution and washout of Tl-201. J Am Coll Cardiol 7: 53
150. Abdulla A, Maddahi J, Garcia E et al 1985 Slow regional clearance of myocardial thallium-201 in the absence of perfusion defect: its contribution to detection of individual coronary artery stenoses and mechanisms for its occurrence. Circulation 71: 72
151. Bateman T M, Maddahi J, Gray R J et al 1984 Diffuse slow washout of myocardial thallium-201: A new scintigraphic indicator of extensive coronary artery disease. J Am Coll Cardiol 4: 55
152. Chambers C E, Brown K A 1988 dipyridamole-induced ST segment depression during thallium-201 imaging in patients with coronary artery disease: Angiographic and hemodynamic determinants. J Am Coll Cardiol 12: 37
153. Bingham J B, McKusick K A, Strauss H W et al 1980 Influence of coronary artery disease on pulmonary uptake of thallium-201. Am J Cardiol 46: 821
154. Boucher C A, Zir L M, Beller G A et al 1980 Increased lung uptake of thallium-201 during exercise myocardial imaging: clinical, hemodynamic and angiographic implications in patients with coronary artery disease. Am J Cardiol 46: 189
155. Levy R, Rozanski A, Berman D S et al 1983 Analysis of the degree of pulmonary thallium washout after exercise in patients with coronary artery disease. J Am Coll Cardiol 2: 719
156. Kushner F G, Okada R D, Kirschenbaum H D et al 1981 Lung Tl-201 uptake after stress testing in patients with coronary artery disease. Circulation 63: 341
157. Okada R D, Dai Y H, Boucher C A, Pohost G M 1984 Significance of increased lung thallium-201 activity on serial cardiac images after dipyridamole treatment in coronary artery disease. Am J Cardiol 53: 470
158. Villenueva F S, Watson S S, Smith W H et al 1989 Significance of increased lung/heart ratio on dipyridamole thallium-201 scintigraphy. Circulation 80: II-201
159. Udelson J E, Metherall J, Oates E, Konstam M A 1990 Transient left ventricular dilatation during dipyridamole thallium scintigraphy: specific and predictive for multivessel coronary artery disease. J Nucl Med 31: 723
160. Chuttani K et al 1992 Hepatic uptake of thallium-201 chloride in patients with right coronary artery disease. Circulation 86: I-579
161. Weiss A T, Berman D S, Lew A S et al 1987 Transient ischemic dilation of the left ventricle on stress thallium-201 scintigraphy: A marker of severe and extensive coronary artery disease. J Am Coll Cardiol 9: 752
162. Iskandrian A S et al 1990 Left ventricular dilation and pulmonary thallium uptake after single-photon emission computed tomography using thallium-201 during adenosine induced coronary hyperemia. Am J Cardiol 66: 807
163. Chouraqui P, Rodrigues E A, Berman D S et al 1990 Significance of dipyridamole-induced transient dilatation of left ventricle during thallium-201 scintigraphy in suspected coronary artery disease. Am J Cardiol 66: 689
164. Borer J S, Kent K M, Bacharach S L et al 1979 Sensitivity, specificity and predictive accuracy of radionuclide cineangiography during exercise in patients with coronary artery disease: comparison with exercise electrocardiography. Circulation 60: 572
165. Slutsky R, Karliner J, Ricci D et al 1979 Response of left ventricular volume to exercise in man assessed by radionuclide equilibrium angiography. Circulation 60: 565
166. Berger H J, Reduto L A, Johnstone D E et al 1979 Global and regional left ventricular response to bicycle exercise in coronary artery disease: Assessment by quantitative radionuclide angiography. Am J Med 66: 13
167. Pfisterer M E, Slutsky R A, Schuler G et al 1979 Profiles of radionuclide left ventricular ejection fraction changes induced by supine bicycle exercise in normal and patients with coronary heart disease. Catheterization and Cardiovasc Diagn 5: 305
168. Verani M S et al 1979 Radionuclide ventriculograms during dynamic and isometric exercise in coronary artery disease: comparisons with exercise thallium201 scintigrams. Clin Res 27: 211
169. Brady T J, Thrall J H, Clare J M et al 1979 Exercise radionuclide ventriculography: Practical considerations and sensitivity of coronary artery detection. Radiology 132: 697
170. Jengo J A, Oren V, Conant R et al 1979 Effects of maximal exercise stress on left ventricular function in patients with coronary artery disease using first pass radionuclide angiocardiography: a rapid, noninvasive technique for determining ejection fraction and segmental wall motion. Circulation 59: 60
171. Okada R D, Pohost G M, Kirshenbaum H D et al 1979 Radionuclide-determined change in pulmonary blood volume with exercise. N Engl J Med 301: 569
172. Hecht H S, Hopkins J M 1981 Exercise-induced regional wall motion abnormalities on radionuclide angiography: lack of reliability for detection of coronary artery disease in the presence of valvular heart disease. Am J Cardiol 47: 861
173. Iskandrian A S, Hakki A, Kane S A, Segal B L 1981 Quantitative radionuclide angiography in assessment of hemodynamic changes during upright exercise: Observations in normal subjects, patients with coronary artery disease, and patients with aortic regurgitation. Am J Cardiol 48: 239
174. Elkayam U, Weinstein M, Berman D et al 1981 Stress thallium-201 myocardial scintigraphy and exercise technetium ventriculography in the detection and location of chronic coronary artery disease: Comparison of sensitivity and specificity of these noninvasive tests alone and in combination. Am Heart J 101: 657
175. Kirshenbaum H D, Okada R D, Boucher C A et al 1981 Relationship of thallium-201 myocardial perfusion pattern to regional and global left ventricular function with exercise. Am Heart J 101: 734
176. Freeman M R, Berman D S, Staniloff H et al 1981 Comparison of upright and supine bicycle exercise in the detection and evaluation

of extent of coronary artery disease by equilibrium radionuclide ventriculography. Am Heart J 102: 182
177. Austin E H, Cobb F R, Coleman R E, Jones R H 1982 Prospective evaluation of radionuclide angiocardiography for the diagnosis of coronary artery disease. Am J Cardiol 50: 1212
178. DePace N L, Iskandrian A S, Hakki A et al 1983 Value of left ventricular ejection fraction during exercise in predicting the extent of coronary artery disease. J Am Coll Cardiol 1(4): 1002
179. Bodenheimer M W et al 1979 Comparative sensitivity of the exercise electrocardiogram, thallium imaging, and stress radionuclide angiography to detect the presence and severity of coronary artery disease. Circulation 60: 1279
180. Osbakken M D, Boucher C A, Okada R D et al 1983 Spectrum of global left ventricular responses to supine exercise: limitation in the use of ejection fraction in identifying patients with coronary artery disease. Am J Cardiol 51: 28
181. Manyari D E, Kostuk W J 1983 Left and right ventricular function at rest and during bicycle exercise in the supine and sitting positions in normal subjects and patients with coronary artery disease: Assessment by radionuclide ventriculography. Am J Cardiol 51: 36
182. Bonow R O et al 1987 Prognostic implications of symptomatic vs asymptomatic (silent) myocardial ischemia induced by exercise in mildly symptomatic and in asymptomatic patients with angiographically documented coronary artery disease. Am J Cardiol 60: 778
183. Bonow R O et al 1984 Exercise-induced ischemia in mildly symptomatic patients with coronary artery disease and preserved left ventricular function: identification of subgroups at risk of death during medical therapy. N Engl J Med 311: 1339
184. Pryor D B et al 1984 Prognostic indicators from radionuclide angiography in medically treated patients with coronary artery disease. Am J Cardiol 53: 18
185. Lee K L et al 1990 Prognostic value of radionuclide angiography in medically treated patients with coronary artery disease: a comparison with clinical and catheterization variables. Circulation 82: 1705
186. Pantaleo N et al 1981 Comparative ability of quantitative Tl-201 analysis and two-view exercise ventriculography to accurately assess the extent of coronary artery disease. IEEE Comput Cardiol
187. Morris D D et al 1984 Noninvasive prediction of the angiographic extent of coronary artery disease following myocardial infarction. Circulation 70: 192
188. Rozanski A et al 1988 The declining specificity of exercise radionuclide ventriculography. N Engl J Med 318: 1005
189. Rozanski A et al 1984 Alternative referent standards for cardiac normality: Implications for diagnostic testing. Ann Intern Med 101: 164
190. Cannon R O et al 1985 Left ventricular dysfunction in patients with angina pectoris, normal epicardial coronary arteries, and abnormal vasodilator reserve. Circulation 71: 218
191. Gibbons R J et al 1981 Ejection fraction response to exercise in patients with chest pain and normal coronary arteriograms. Circulation 64: 952
192. Cannon R O et al 1991 Chronic deterioration in left ventricular function in patients with microvascular angina. J Am Coll Cardiol 17: 28A
193. Port S et al 1980 Effect of age on the response of the left ventricular ejection fraction to exercise. N Engl J Med 303: 1133
194. Rodeheffer R J et al 1984 Exercise cardiac output is maintained with advancing age in healthy human subjects: cardiac dilatation and increased stroke volume compensate for a diminished heart rate. Circulation 69: 203
195. Bonow R O Gated equilibrium blood pool imaging: Current role for diagnosis and prognosis in coronary artery disease. In: Zaret B L, Beller G A (eds) Nuclear cardiology. CV Mosby Publishers. St Lous
196. Hanley P C et al 1989 Gender-related differences in cardiac response to supine exercise assessed by radionuclide angiography. J Am Coll Cardiol 13: 624
197. Higginbotham M B et al 1984 Sex-related differences in the normal cardiac response to upright exercise. Circulation 70: 357
198. Miller D D et al 1987 Left ventricular ejection fraction response during exercise in asymptomatic systemic hypertension. Am J Cardiol 59: 409
199. Wasserman A G et al 1984 Exercise radionuclide ventriculographic responses in hypertensive patients with chest pain. N Engl J Med 311: 1276
200. Cuocolo A et al 1990 Left ventricular hypertrophy and impaired diastolic filling in essential hypertension: Diastolic mechanisms for systolic dysfunction during exercise. Circulation 81: 978
201. Choi B W, Barbour D, Leon M B et al 1990 Left ventricular end diastolic volume response to exercise in patients with aortic stenosis. J Am Coll Cardiol 15: 7A
202. Clyne C A, Arrighi J A, Maron B J et al 1991 Systemic and left ventricular responses to exercise stress in asymptomatic patients with valvular aortic stenosis. Am J Cardiol 68: 1469
203. Hecht H S, Hopkins J M 1981 Exercise-induced regional wall motion abnormalities on radionuclide angiography: lack of reliability for detection of coronary artery disease in the presence of valvular heart disease. Am J Cardiol 47: 861
204. Port S et al 1981 Influence of resting left ventricular function on the left ventricular response to exercise in patients with coronary artery disease. Circulation 63: 856
205. Gibbons R J et al 1982 Ejection fraction response to exercise in patients with chest pain, coronary artery disease and normal resting ventricular function. Circulation 66: 643
206. Gibbons R J et al 1988 Noninvasive identification of severe coronary artery disease using exercise radionuclide angiography. J Am Coll Cardiol 11: 28
207. Schoolmeester W L et al 1981 Radionuclide angiographic assessment of left ventricular function during exercise in patients with a severely reduced ejection fraction. Am J Cardiol 47: 804
208. Higginbotham M B et al 1984 Mechanisms and significance of a decrease in ejection fraction during exercise in patients with coronary artery disease and left ventricular dysfunction at rest. J Am Coll Cardiol 3: 88
209. Mazzotta G et al 1989 Relation between exertional ischemia and prognosis in mildly symptomatic patients with single or double vessel coronary artery disease and left ventricular dysfunction at rest. J Am Coll Cardiol 13: 567
210. Jones R H et al 1981 Accuracy of diagnosis of coronary artery disease by radionuclide measurement of left ventricular function during rest and exercise. Circulation 64: 586
211. Weiss T A et al Persistent ischemic dilatation of the left ventricle following exercise radionuclide ventriculography: a sign of severe coronary artery disease. J Am Coll Cardiol 3: 570
212. Iskandrian A S et al 1989 Use of technetium-99m isonitrile (RP-30A) in assessing left ventricular perfusion and function at rest and during exercise in coronary artery disease, and comparison with coronary arteriography and exercise thallium-201 SPECT imaging. Am J Cardiol 64: 270
213. Kahn J K et al 1989 Assessment of myocardial viability with technetium-99m 2-methoxyisobutyl isonitrile (MIBI) and gated tomography in patients with coronary artery disease. J Am Coll Cardiol 13: 31A
214. Snapper H J, Shea N L, Konstam M A et al 1993 Combined analysis of regional wall motion and perfusion using gated SPECT sestamibi imaging: prediction of stress defect reversibility. Circulation 88: 1–582
215. Marwick T H et al 1992 Accuracy and limitations of exercise echocardiography in a routine clinical setting. J Am Coll Cardiol 19: 74
216. Bayes T 1763 An essay toward solving a problem in the doctrine of chance. Phil Trans R Soc Lond 53: 370
217. Epstein S E 1980 Implications of probability analysis on the strategy used for noninvasive detection of coronary artery disease. Am J Cardiol 46: 491
218. Hamilton G W et al 1978 Myocardial imaging with thallium-201: An analysis of clinical usefulness based on Bayes' theorem. Semin Nucl Med 8: 358
219. Metz C E 1978 Basic principles of ROC analysis. Semin Nucl Med 8: 283
220. Brown K A 1991 Prognostic value of thallium-201 myocardial perfusion imaging: A diagnostic tool comes of age. Circulation 83: 363

221. Van Train K F et al 1990 Quantitative analysis of tomographic stress thallium-201 myocardial scintigrams: a multicentre trial. J Nucl Med 31: 1168
222. Gould K L 1989 How accurate is thallium exercise testing for the diagnosis of coronary artery disease? J Am Coll Cardiol 14: 1487
223. Uhl G S, Kay T N, Hickman J R 1981 Computer-enhanced thallium scintigrams in asymptomatic men with abnormal exercise tests. Am J Cardiol 48: 1037
224. Uhl G S, Froelicher V 1983 Screening for asymptomatic coronary artery disease. J Am Coll Cardiol 1: 946
225. Detre K M, Wright P H, Murphy M L, Takaro T 1975 Observer agreement in evaluating coronary angiograms. Circulation 52: 979
226. Brown K A, Rowen M 1993 Prognostic value of a normal exercise myocardial perfusion imaging study in patients with angiographically significant coronary artery disease. Am J Cardiol 71: 865

PART C

Management

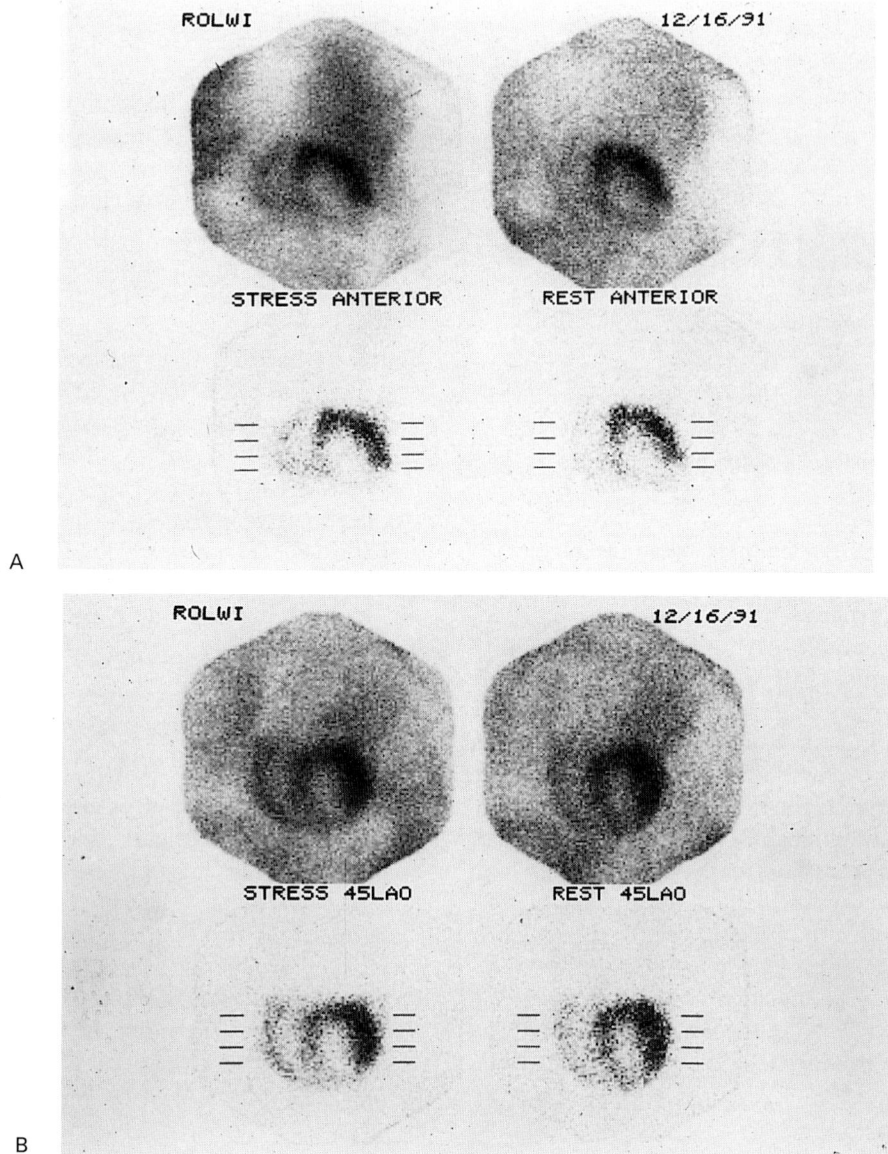

Fig. 95.4 High-risk exercise ^{201}Tl scintigrams showing a persistent defect in the inferior wall (A) and a redistribution defect in the septum (B). Increased lung ^{201}Tl uptake can be seen on the initial post-exercise anterior view image (A).

the exercise ECG for detecting left main CAD. Nygaard et al[21] found that 67% of patients with left main CAD (50% stenosis) had a multivessel CAD scan pattern with perfusion defects in the distribution of two or more coronary supply regions (Fig. 95.5). Also, 42% of patients with left main CAD had abnormal lung ^{201}Tl uptake (Fig. 95.5). The prevalence of a multivessel disease scan pattern was greater than observed in patients with three-vessel CAD in this study. Seventy-seven per cent of the patients with left main disease had either a multivessel disease scan pattern or abnormal lung ^{201}Tl uptake (Fig. 95.5). In the study of Nygaard et al,[21] a high-risk exercise ECG was defined as presence of two or more of the following findings: (1) 2.0 mm ST depression; (2) ST depression of 1.0 mm or greater persisting for 5 min or longer during recovery; (3) appearance of ST depression at 5 METS; and (4) a decrease in systolic blood pressure of 10 mm Hg or more during exercise. The prevalence of a high-risk ECG stress test was 58% in the patients with left main CAD, a value that was considerably lower than the prevalence of a high-risk ^{201}Tl scintigram. The combination of the high-risk ^{201}Tl variables and the high-risk ECG stress test variables was no better than scintigraphy alone in increasing the overall detection rate of left main disease, but the combination did improve the detection rate relative to exercise ECG testing alone (85% vs 58%). This study was performed using quantitative planar ^{201}Tl imaging.

Iskandrian et al[22] sought to determine the value of exercise SPECT ^{201}Tl for predicting extensive CAD in

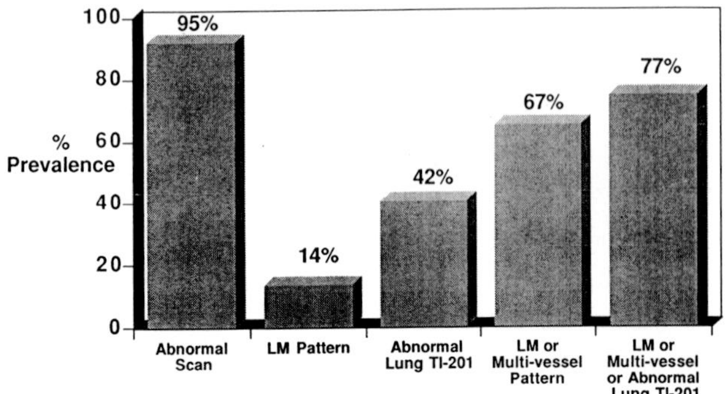

Fig. 95.5 Prevalence of an abnormal exercise ^{201}Tl scan, a left main scan pattern, abnormal lung ^{201}Tl uptake, a left main or a multivessel disease scan pattern and a left main or multivessel disease scan pattern or abnormal lung ^{201}Tl uptake in 43 patients with ≥50% stenosis of the left main coronary artery. (Reproduced with permission from Nygaard et al[21].)

617 men and 217 women of whom 229 had three-vessel or left main disease. Using stepwise logistic regression analysis, only three variables were found to be independent predictors of extensive CAD. These were a multivessel thallium abnormality ($\chi^2 = 107$), exercise heart rate ($\chi^2 = 27$) and ST segment depression ($\chi^2 = 8$). These data indicate that the information from the exercise ^{201}Tl scan using SPECT is more powerful than exercise ECG test data alone for predicting high-risk CAD.

Pollock et al[23] found that only the number of initial post-exercise ^{201}Tl defects, exercise ST depression and age were independent predictors of multivessel CAD. They found a joint effect of these variables in predicting extensive CAD. The lowest rate of angiographic multivessel CAD (5%) was seen in patients less than 58 years of age, with no initial defects and no ST depression. The highest prevalence of multivessel CAD (80%) was seen in patients greater than 58 years of age with greater than one ^{201}Tl defect and associated ischaemic ST depression. Figure 95.6 illustrates the interaction of these three variables in a more continuous fashion. Christian et al[24] utilizing SPECT ^{201}Tl imaging reported that the magnitude of exercise ST depression, the number of defects on short-axis views post-exercise, presence or absence of diabetes and the change in blood pressure during exercise were the independent variables predictive of left main or three-vessel disease.

Thus, these studies show that with either quantitative planar or SPECT ^{201}Tl scintigraphy, left main or three-vessel disease can be predicted with greater accuracy than with exercise ECG testing alone. In most of the studies cited above, the number of defects, particularly when involving greater than a single coronary supply zone, was the best non-invasive stress test variable for predicting high-risk CAD. The probability of extensive CAD rises when mutliple defects are observed in conjunction with ST depression in the elderly patient.

^{201}Tl EXERCISE SCINTIGRAPHY FOR PREDICTING CARDIAC EVENTS

Not only does exercise perfusion imaging assist in the identification of patients with functionally important anatomic CAD, but the test has value for identifying patient subsets at high, intermediate and low risk of experiencing future cardiac events (e.g. death, non-fatal infarction, late bypass surgery). One of the first published reports of the prognostic value of exercise ^{201}Tl imaging by Brown et al[25] revealed that the number of reversible ^{201}Tl defects was the best predictor of death or non-fatal infarc-

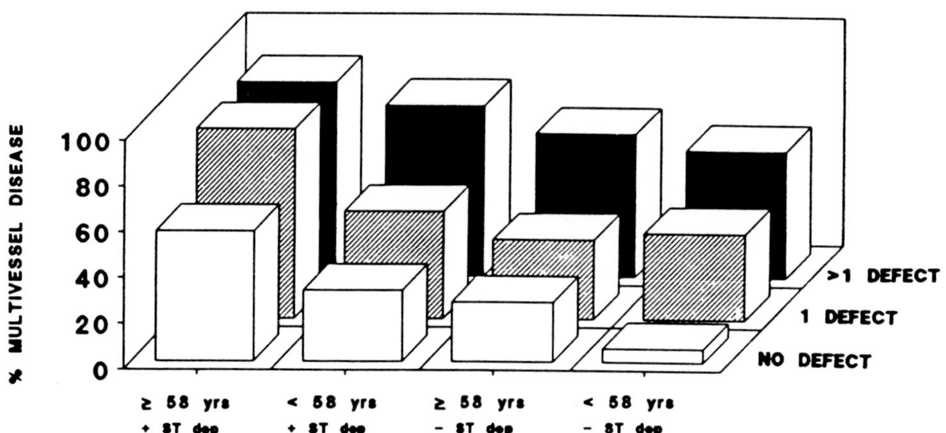

Fig. 95.6 The additive value of including information regarding age (either less than or older than 58 years of age) and presence or absence of exercise-induced ST segment depression on the exercise electrocardiogram (x-axis) to each level of abnormality on initial ^{201}Tl imaging (no defect, 1 defect, >1 defect) (z-axis) on the detection of multivessel coronary artery disease (y-axis). (Reproduced with permission from Pollock et al[23].)

tion in 100 patients without prior infarction (Table 95.6). In that study, neither the number of stenotic arteries nor ST depression on the exercise ECG provided additive prognostic information to the scintigraphic data. In a similar study from Ladenheim et al,[26] stepwise logistic regression analysis identified the number of myocardial segments with redistribution ^{201}Tl defects and the exercise heart rate as the only independent predictors of future cardiac events in 1689 CAD patients without prior infarction. Iskandrian et al[27] found that the total number of ^{201}Tl defects (reversible and persistent) was the single best predictor of subsequent event, and both extent and severity of hypoperfusion were exponentially correlated with event rate. The same group found that presence of redistribution, extent of initial defects and defects observed in a multivessel scan pattern each had significant univariate predictive value for death and infarction in a group of patients 65 years or older. Multivariate analysis identified abnormal ^{201}Tl images and a multivessel scan abnormality as independent predictors of events. Hilton et al[28] found that the combination of peak exercise stage 1 and any ^{201}Tl scan abnormalities the most powerful predictor of subsequent events (relative risk: 5.3 at 1 year) in a group of patients 70 years of age. Patients with a normal scan had a 2% cardiac event rate compared with 18% when a perfusion defect was present.

With respect to the University of Virginia experience, Kaul et al[29] reported the results of a follow-up study of 382 patients who underwent exercise ^{201}Tl scintigraphy and coronary angiography for the evaluation of chest pain. A subset of 83 patients were excluded because they had bypass surgery within 3 months of testing. Of the 299 remaining patients, 210 had no events treated medically and 89 had events (41 deaths, 9 non-fatal infarctions, and 39 late revascularization procedures) during a 4–8 year follow-up. As shown in Table 95.7, when all clinical, exercise, scintigraphic and catheterization variables were analyzed by Cox regression analysis, the number of stenotic vessels on angiography was the single most important predictor of recurrent events. However, when the number of diseased vessels was excluded from analysis, the number of scan segments became the single best variable for predicting future cardiac events. Other variables which contributed independent prognostic information were the change in heart rate from rest to exercise, exercise-induced ST segment depression and ventricular ectopy observed during the stress test. Although the number of stenotic vessels was the single most significant predictor of events (χ^2 = 38.1), the combination of the exercise test and scintigraphic variables when considered as a whole was equally powerful (χ^2 = 41.6). Combination of both non-invasive and catheterization data was superior to either alone (χ^2 = 57) for prognostication. This study also showed that patients demonstrating ^{201}Tl redistribution in any segment had a significantly worse event-free survival during follow-up compared to patients with no redistribution on their exercise scan (Fig. 95.7). The separation of high- and low-risk subgroups was better achieved employing the ^{201}Tl scintigraphic data than using ECG stress test data alone.

Table 95.6 Predictors of cardiac death or non-fatal myocardial infarction in 100 patients without prior myocardial infarction

Predictor	χ^2	*p* value
No. of transient ^{201}Tl defects	6.66	<0.01
Total ^{201}Tl defects	4.83	<0.05
No. of diseased vessels	3.57	<0.10
Ejection fraction	0.86	NS
No. of persistent ^{201}Tl defects	0.03	NS
+ exercise ECG	0.01	NS

(Reproduced with permission from Brown et al[25].)

Table 95.7 Cox regression analysis of clinical, exercise test, ^{201}Tl scintigraphic and cardiac catheterization variables for prediction of future cardiac events in 299 patients treated medically

Variables selected	χ^2	*p* value
All variables used		
No. of stenoses ≥50%	38.1	<0.001
No. of diseased vessels excluded		
No. of ^{201}Tl redistribution segments		16.3 < 0.0001
Change in heart rate from rest to exercise	10.3	0.01
ST depression on exercise	9.1	0.003
Exercise arrhythmias	4.9	0.026

(Reproduced with permission from Kaul et al[29].)

The data from the study of Kaul et al was re-analysed by Pollock et al[30] to determine the incremental prognostic value of clinical, stress test, scintigraphic and angiographic variables when these are entered into the model in a hierarchical order (Fig. 95.8). The inclusion of the number of scan segments showing redistribution significantly added to the prognostic information provided by the combination of clinical and stress test variables. The increment in prognostic information was less when the number of stenotic vessels was added to the combination of clinical, stress test and scintigraphic variables (Fig. 95.8).

In the clinical studies cited above, abnormal ^{201}Tl uptake was not systematically evaluated utilizing the lung/heart ratio as determined quantitatively. Gill et al[31] evaluated the lung/heart ^{201}Tl activity ratio as a predictor of future cardiac events in 525 consecutive patients referred for exercise testing. Of the 105 cardiac events recorded over a 5 year period, there were 25 deaths, 33 non-fatal myocardial infarctions and 47 late bypass operations. Cox survival analysis revealed that an increased lung/heart ^{201}Tl ratio was the best predictor of events (relative risk: 3.5). The next most important predictors were a history of typical angina, prior myocardial infarction and ST segment depression during

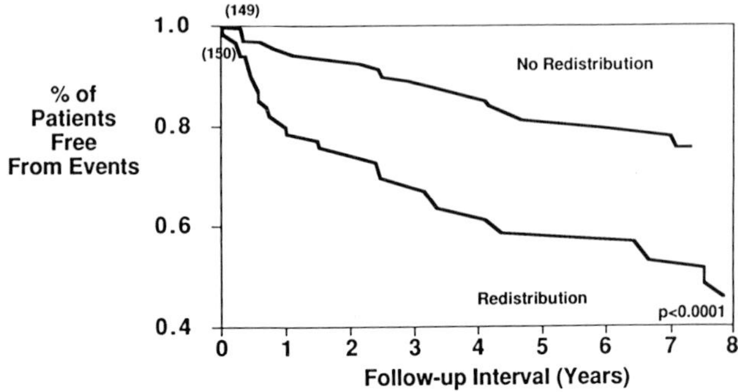

Fig. 95.7 Difference in survival of patients with and without ^{201}Tl redistribution on serial exercise ^{201}Tl scintigrams. (Reproduced with permission from Kaul et al[29].)

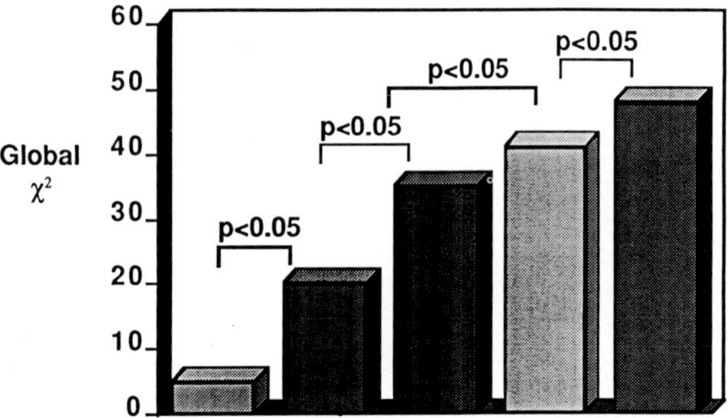

Fig. 95.8 Incremental prognostic value of tests performed in a hierarchical order. First bar: clinical information; 2nd bar: clinical plus ECG stress test data; 3rd bar: clinical, ECG stress test and number of ^{201}Tl redistribution defects; 4th bar: clinical, ECG stress test and cardiac catheterization data; and 5th bar: clinical, ECG stress test, number of ^{201}Tl redistribution defects and cardiac catheterization data. The inclusion of the number of ^{201}Tl defects significantly added to the prognostic information provided by the combination of clinical and stress test variables. (Reproduced with permission from Pollock et al[30].)

exercise. Coronary angiographic variables were not analysed in this study. In a subsequent study from the same institution, Kaul et al[32] analysed data only from patients who underwent both exercise ^{201}Tl scintigraphy and coronary angiography. A lung/heart ^{201}Tl ratio of 0.52 was considered abnormal. A total of 293 patients were followed up from 4–9 years after testing. As shown in Table 95.8, an abnormal lung/heart ^{201}Tl ratio was the single best predictor of subsequent events, even better than the number of diseased vessels on angiography.

Table 95.8 Cox regression analysis of clinical, exercise test, ^{201}Tl scintigraphic variables for prediction of cardiac events in 293 patients

All variables used	χ^2	*p* value
Lung/heart ^{201}Tl ratio	40.21	<0.0001
No. of diseased vessels	17.11	<0.0001
Patient gender	9.43	0.002
Change in heart rate from rest to exercise	4.19	0.04

(Reproduced with permission from Kaul et al[32].)

Pollock et al[30] in re-analysing these data with respect to the increment in prognostic information obtained by multiple tests, found that the angiographic information did not provide additive information over the combination of clinical, stress test and ^{201}Tl scintigraphic data. Finally, in a more recent report from the Massachusetts General Hospital by Travin et al,[33] myocardial infarction during follow-up after testing in 268 patients with unequivocal ^{201}Tl redistribution was most closely related to the extent and severity of ^{201}Tl ischaemia ($p = 0.0086$), whereas cardiac death was significantly associated with abnormal lung ^{201}Tl uptake ($p = 0.0082$) and an inability to exercise to 9.6 METS ($p = 0.014$). The difference in survival curves in patients with and without an increased lung/heart ratio was highly significant ($p = 0.0075$).

SPEC ^{201}Tl imaging also has been shown to provide independent and incremented prognostic information in patients with chest pain.[30A,30B] In both of these studies, defect size as reflected by the number of abnormal scan segments was the best prognostic variable. Iskandrian et al[30A] found that patients with a large defect had an 11-fold higher event rate than that of patients with no or a small perfusion abnormality.

Several reports have indicated that patients with chest pain who have a totally normal myocardial perfusion scan have an excellent prognosis during follow-up.[26,34–36] In a study from the University of Virginia, Pamelia et al[34] found that the yearly mortality rate was 0.5% in 345 patients with chest pain and a normal quantitative ^{201}Tl planar scan. The yearly non-fatal infarction rate was 0.6% in this study. Brown[37] undertook a pooled analysis of studies published in the literature and found a 0.9%/year cardiac death/myocardial infarction rate in 3594 patients with normal ^{201}Tl scans who were followed for an average of 29 months. Steinberg et al reported a 1% cardiac mortality at 10 years in 309 patients with normal stress ^{201}Tl perfusion scans. These authors concluded that a normal exercise perfusion study retains its high negative predictive value for death up to 10 years after testing.

Taken together, the results of the studies cited above suggest that even when cardiac catheterization variables are known, scintigraphic information acquired from exercise SPECT or planar imaging provides useful supplementary prognostic information valuable for risk stratification and selection of therapeutic strategies. The extent of myocardial hypoperfusion reflected by the number of myocardial regions with stress-induced ^{201}Tl defects, particularly the redistribution type, and abnormal lung ^{201}Tl uptake reflecting stress-induced left ventricular dysfunction and transient left ventricular cavity dilation are the most important variables predictive of an adverse outcome with medical therapy. Patients manifesting such high-risk variables most often have underlying multivessel CAD. The presence of anginal chest pain during the

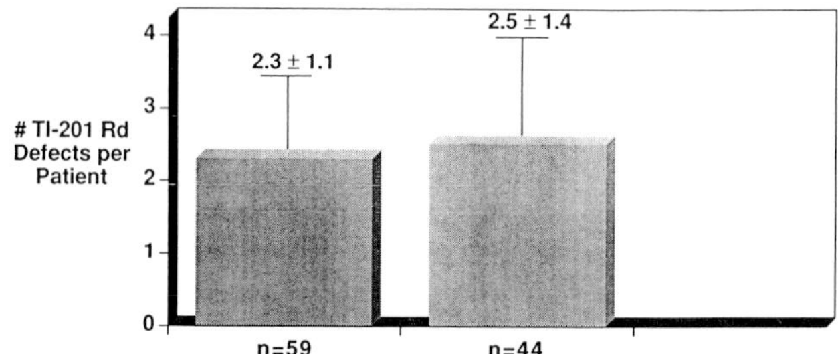

Fig. 95.9 Number (#) of redistribution (Rd) ^{201}Tl defects per patient in 59 patients with silent ischaemia and 44 patients with angina on exercise treadmill testing. Note the number of defects was comparable between the two groups. The patient cohort was a consecutively enrolled group, and the criteria for a positive test was any redistribution on serial imaging. (Reproduced with permission from Gasperetti et al.[38])

exercise test does not provide additional prognostic information. This may be because the ischaemic burden is comparable in patients with and without chest pain during exercise testing (Fig. 95.9).[38] In contrast, patients with normal regional perfusion during exercise stress have an excellent prognosis even if angiographic CAD is present. Patients with evidence of ischaemia in the distribution of a single coronary supply region and no increase in lung ^{201}Tl uptake at an adequate exercise heart rate (>120/min) and workload (>7 METS) have a high probability of angiographic single-vessel CAD and may be excellent candidates for angioplasty. Patients with multiple defects in >1 vascular supply regions with accompanying increased lung ^{201}Tl uptake at a low exercise heart rate or workload have a high probability of functionally significant multivessel or left main CAD and are candidates for early referral for cardiac catheterization.

PROGNOSTIC VALUE OF ^{99m}Tc PERFUSION AGENTS

Little data is available concerning the prognostic utility of ^{99m}Tc myocardial perfusion imaging. No doubt the same principles hold as for ^{201}Tl imaging in that the greater the number of defects observed on ^{99m}Tc sestamibi SPECT images, the greater the probability of multivessel CAD and the greater the risk of a future cardiac event. Preliminary data demonstrate that a normal ^{99m}Tc perfusion scan is associated with a low event rate similar to what was observed employing ^{201}Tl imaging.[39,39A] One potential limitation of this technique compared with ^{201}Tl is the inability to utilize lung tracer uptake as a prognostic variable. Substantial lung activity is seen in normal individuals up to 30 min after ^{99m}Tc sestamibi administration, thereby precluding use of a lung/heart ratio as an index of stress-induced pulmonary congestion. Perhaps the enhanced ability to identify areas of hypoperfusion with ^{99m}Tc sestamibi compared with ^{201}Tl will make up for the lack of lung tracer uptake information.

EXERCISE RADIONUCLIDE ANGIOGRAPHY AND DETECTION OF HIGH-RISK CAD

Exercise radionuclide angiography can also provide useful prognostic information in patients with known or suspected CAD. The LVEF and regional wall motion can be adequately assessed both at rest and during exercise using either equilibrium-gated or first-pass methods. Patients with left main or three-vessel disease manifest a lower ejection fraction at peak exercise and more inducible wall motion abnormalities compared with patients without CAD and patients with a lesser angiographic extent of disease.[40] Additionally, such high-risk patients tend to be older, male, have a lower exercise heart rate and rate-pressure product, have a lower exercise workload and demonstrate more stress-related ST segment depression. Gibbons et al[40] found that by logistic regression analysis, the most important variables predictive of high-risk coronary anatomy were the magnitude of ST depression followed by the peak exercise ejection fraction, peak exercise rate-pressure product and patient gender.

Patients with a proximal LAD stenosis will demonstrate a greater fall in the exercise ejection fraction as a group compared with patients with more distal disease in that vessel.[41] A fall in LVEF of >10% or more is highly suggestive of extensive CAD. Bonow et al[42] reported that in patients with three-vessel CAD who had both ischaemic ST depression and an abnormal LVEF response to exercise, associated with achieving a workload of <120 W, the probability of survival at 4 years was only 71%. No patient with three-vessel CAD who demonstrated an unchanged or increased LVEF with exercise or a negative ST segment response (or both) died while on medical therapy. Other studies published in the literature have confirmed these observations and have shown that the exercise LVEF is an important prognostic variable for predicting outcome.[43–45] Pryor et al[43] found that the exercise LVEF was the variable most closely associated with future cardiac events in 386 patients with symptomatic CAD. Subsequent published studies from the Duke group provide further evidence for this association in a larger number of patients.[44,45] In one such study comprising 571 patients, followed for a mean of 5.4 years, the most important radionuclide angiographic predictor of mortality was the exercise LVEF ($\chi^2 = 81$).[44] Neither the rest LVEF or the change in ejection fraction from rest to exercise contributed supplementary prognostic information. Also in that study, the radionuclide variables contained 84% of the prognostic information provided by clinical and catheterization descriptors combined. Radionuclide angiography contributed significant additional prognostic information to the combination of clinical and catheterization data. Figure 95.10 depicts survival curves in patients with three-vessel disease and a resting LVEF of <45% in this study based upon an exercise ejection fraction

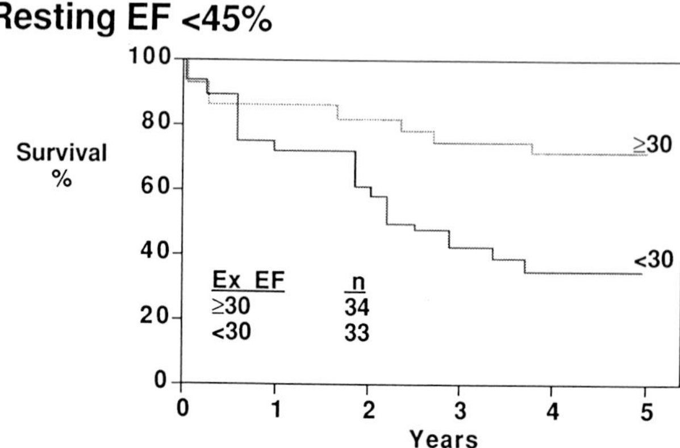

Fig. 95.10 Survival in patients with three-vessel coronary artery disease and a resting left ventricular ejection fraction (EF) of <45% related to the exercise (Ex) EF response. Note that within this group of patients with a depressed resting EF, the exercise EF could further stratify patients into high- and low-risk subsets. (Reproduced with permission from Lee et al.[44])

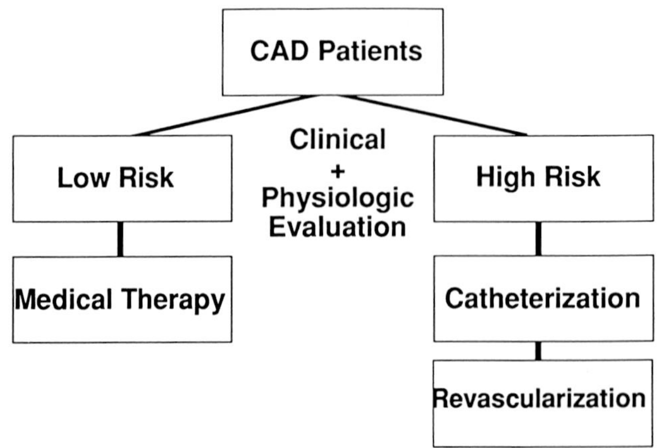

Fig. 95.11 Decision-making algorithm for the noninvasive physiologic assessment of patients with suspected or known coronary artery disease.

≥ 30% or <30%. Note that in patients with a depressed resting LVEF, the exercise LVEF could separate further high- and low-risk subsets.

SUMMARY

The non-invasive assessment of either regional myocardial perfusion or global and regional function certainly appears to yield useful information for risk stratification in patients undergoing exercise testing. Figure 95.11 depicts a decision-making algorithm for the physiologic assessment of patients with suspected or known CAD. Patients with low-risk findings on exercise testing with radionuclide imaging can be spared further invasive evaluation and, if symptoms are minimum, can be treated medically. Conversely, patients demonstrating high-risk findings such as extensive perfusion abnormalities or increased lung ^{201}Tl uptake, or both, or exhibiting an abnormal LVEF response to exercise, would be candidates for angiography and subsequent revascularization if coronary anatomy was suitable. Further clinical research studies are warranted to determine if the ^{99m}Tc-labelled perfusion agents such as sestamibi or tetrafosmin are as predictive as ^{201}Tl imaging for prognostication.

REFERENCES

1. Hammermeister K E, DeRouen T A, Dodge H T 1979 Variables predictive of survival in patients with coronary disease. Selection by univariate and multivariate analyses from the clinical, electrocardiographic, exercise, arteriographic, and quantitative angiographic evaluations. Circulation 59: 421–430
2. Harris P J, Harrell F E Jr, Lee K L, Behar V S, Rosati R A 1979 Survival in medically treated coronary artery disease. Circulation 60: 1259–1269
3. Gohlke H, Samek L, Betz P, Roskamm H 1983 Exercise testing provides additional prognostic information in angiographically defined subgroups of patients with coronary artery disease. Circulation 68: 979–985
4. Froelicher V F, Perdue S, Pewen W, Risch M 1987 Application of meta-analysis using an electronic spread sheed to exercise testing in patients after myocardial infarction. Am J Med 83: 1045–1054
5. McNeer J F, Margolis J R, Lee K L et al 1978 The role of the exercise test in the evaluation of patients for ischemic heart disease. Circulation 57: 64–70
6. Mark D B, Shaw L, Harrell F E Jr et al 1991 Prognostic value of a treadmill exercise score in outpatients with suspected coronary artery disease. N Engl J Med 325: 849–853
7. Morrow K, Morris C K, Froelicher V F et al 1993 Prediction of cardiovascular death in men undergoing noninvasive evaluation for coronary artery disease. Ann Intern Med 118: 689–695
8. Morris C K, Morrow K, Froelicher V G et al 1993 Prediction of cardiovascular death by means of clinical and exercise test variables in patients selected for cardiac catheterization. Am Heart J 125: 1717–1726
9. Beller G A 1991 Current status of nuclear cardiology techniques. Curr Probl Cardiol 16: 451–535
10. Brown K A 1991 Prognostic value of thallium-201 myocardial perfusion imaging. A diagnostic tool comes of age. Circulation 83: 363–381
11. Esquivel L, Pollock S G, Beller G A, Gibson R S, Watson D D, Kaul S 1989 Effect of the degree of effort on the sensitivity of the exercise thallium-201 stress test in symptomatic coronary artery disease. Am J Cardiol 63: 160–165
12. Varnauskas E and the European Coronary Surgery Study Group 1988 Twelve-year follow-up of survival in the randomized European Coronary Surgery Study. N Engl J Med 319: 332–337
13. Boucher C A, Zir L M, Beller G A et al 1980 Increased lung uptake of thallium-201 during exercise myocardial imaging: clinical, hemodynamic and angiographic implications in patients with coronary artery disease. Am J Cardiol 46: 189–196
14. Mannting F 1990 Pulmonary thallium uptake: correlation with systolic and diastolic left ventricular function at rest and during exercise. Am Heart J 119: 1137–1146
15. Kurata C, Tawarahara K, Taguchi T, Sakata K, Yamazaki N, Naitoh Y 1991 Lung thallium-201 uptake during exercise emission computed tomography. J Nucl Med 32: 417–423
16. Homma S, Kaul S, Boucher C A 1987 Correlates of lung/heart

ratio of thallium-201 in coronary artery disease. J Nucl Med 28: 1531–1535

17. Lahiri A, O'Hara M J, Bowles M J, Crawley J C, Raftery E B 1984 Influence of left ventricular function and severity of coronary artery disease on exercise-induced pulmonary thallium-201 uptake. Int J Cardiol 5: 475–490
18. Haines D E, Beller G A, Watson D D, Kaiser D L, Sayre S L, Gibson R S 1987 Exercise-induced ST segment elevation 2 weeks after uncomplicated myocardial infarction: contributing factors and prognostic significance. J Am Coll Cardiol 9: 996–1003
19. Weiss A T, Berman D S, Lew A S et al 1987 Transient ischemic dilation of the left ventricle on stress thallium-201 scintigraphy: a marker of severe and extensive coronary artery disease. J Am Coll Cardiol 9: 752–759
20. Roberti R R, Van Tosh A, Baruchin M A et al 1993 Left ventricular cavity-to-myocardial count ratio: a new parameter for detecting resting left ventricular dysfunction directly from tomographic thallium perfusion scintigraphy. J Nucl Med 34: 193–198
21. Nygaard T W, Gibson R S, Ryan J M, Gascho J A, Watson D D, Beller G A 1984 Prevalence of high-risk thallium-201 scintigraphic findings in left main coronary artery stenosis: comparison with patients with multiple- and single-vessel coronary artery disease. Am J Cardiol 53: 462–469
22. Iskandrian A S, Heo J, Lemlek J, Ogilby J D 1993 Identification of high-risk patients with left main and three-vessel coronary artery disease using stepwise discriminant analysis of clinical, exercise, and tomographic thallium data. Am Heart J 125: 221–225
23. Pollock S G, Abbott R D, Boucher C A, Watson D D, Kaul S 1991 A model to predict multivessel coronary artery disease from the exercise thallium-201 stress test. Am J Med 90: 345–352
24. Christian T F, Miller T D, Bailey K R, Gibbons R J 1992 Noninvasive identification of severe coronary artery disease using exercise tomographic thallium-201 imaging. Am J Cardiol 70: 14–20
25. Brown K A, Boucher C A, Okada R D et al 1983 Prognostic value of exercise thallium-201 imaging in patients presenting for evaluation of chest pain. J Am Coll Cardiol 1: 994–1001
26. Ladenheim M L, Pollock B H, Rozanski A et al 1986 Extent and severity of myocardial hypoperfusion as predictors of prognosis in patients with suspected coronary artery disease. J Am Coll Cardiol 7: 464–471
27. Iskandrian A S, Hakki A H, Kane-Marsch S 1985 Prognostic implications of exercise thallium-201 scintigraphy in patients with suspected or known coronary artery disease. Am Heart J 110: 135–143
28. Hilton T C, Shaw L J, Chaitman B R, Stocke K S, Goodgold H M, Miller D D 1992 Prognostic significance of exercise thallium-201 testing in patients aged greater than or equal to 70 years with known or suspected coronary artery disease. Am J Cardiol 69: 45–50
29. Kaul S, Lilly D R, Gascho J A et al 1988 Prognostic utility of the exercise thallium-201 test in ambulatory patients with chest pain: comparison with cardiac catheterization. Circulation 77: 745–758
30. Pollock S G, Abbott R D, Boucher C A, Beller G A, Kaul S 1992 Independent and incremental prognostic value of tests performed in hierarchical order to evaluate patients with suspected coronary artery disease. Validation of models based on these tests. Circulation 85: 237–248

30a. Iskandrian A S, Chae S C, Heo J et al 1993 Independent and incremental prognostic value of exercise single-photon emission computed tomographic (SPECT) thallium imaging in coronary artery disease. J Am Coll Cardiol 22: 665–670

30b. Machecourt J, Longere P, Fagret D et al 1994 Prognostic value of thallium-201 single photon emission computed tomographic myocardial perfusion imaging according to extent of myocardial defect. Study in 6926 patients with follow-up at 33 months. J Am Coll Cardiol 23: 1096–1106

31. Gill J B, Ruddy T D, Newell J B, Finkelstein D M, Strauss H W, Boucher C A 1987 Prognostic importance of thallium uptake by the lungs during exercise in coronary artery disease. N Engl J Med 317: 1486–1489
32. Kaul S, Finkelstein D M, Homma S, Leavitt M, Okada R D, Boucher C A 1988 Superiority of quantitative exercise thallium-201 variables in determining long-term prognosis in ambulatory patients with chest pain: a comparison with cardiac catheterization. J Am Coll Cardiol 12: 25–34
33. Travin M I, Boucher C A, Newell J B et al 1993 Variables associated with a poor prognosis in patients with an ischemic thallium-201 exercise test. Am Heart J 125: 335–344
34. Pamelia F X, Gibson R S, Watson D D, Craddock G B, Sirowatka J, Beller G A 1985 Prognosis with chest pain and normal thallium-201 exercise scintigrams. Am J Cardiol 55: 920–926
35. Wackers F J, Russo D J, Russo D, Clements J P 1985 Prognostic significance of normal quantitative planar thallium-201 stress scintigraphy in patients with chest pain. J Am Coll Cardiol 6: 27–30
36. Iskandrian A S, Hakki A H, Kane-Marsch S 1986 Exercise thallium-201 scintigraphy in men with nondiagnostic exercise electrocardiograms. Prognostic implications. Arch Intern Med 146: 2189–2193
37. Brown K A 1993 Critical assessment of prognostic applications of thallium-201 myocardial perfusion imaging. In: Zaret B L, Beller G A, eds. Nuclear cardiology: state of the art and future directions. Mosby Year Book, 1993, St Louis. pp 155–169
38. Gasperetti C M, Burwell L R, Beller G A 1990 Prevalence of and variables associated with silent myocardial ischemia on exercise thallium-201 stress testing. J Am Coll Cardiol 16: 115–123
39. Hilton T C, Thompson R C, Williams H, Saylors R, Fulmer H, Stowers S A 1994 Technetium-99m sestamibi myocardial perfusion imaging in the emergency room evaluation of chest pain. J Am Coll Cardiol 23: 1016–1022

39a. Brown K A, Altland E, Rowen M 1994 Prognostic value of normal technetium-99m sestamibi cardiac imaging J Nucl Med 35: 554–557

40. Gibbons R J, Fyke F E, Clements I P, Lapeyre A C, Zinsmeister A R, Brown M L 1988 Noninvasive identification of severe coronary artery disease using exercise radionuclide angiography. J Am Coll Cardiol 11: 28–34
41. Leong K, Jones R H 1982 Influence of the location of left anterior descending coronary artery stenosis on left ventricular function during exercise. Circulation 65: 109–114
42. Bonow R O, Kent K M, Rosing D R et al 1984 Exercise-induced ischemia in mildly symptomatic patients with coronary-artery disease and preserved left ventricular function. Identification of subgroups at risk of death during medical therapy. N Engl J Med 311: 1339–1345
43. Pryor D B, Harrell F E Jr, Lee K L et al 1984 Prognostic indicators from radionuclide angiography in medically treated patients with coronary artery disease. Am J Cardiol 53: 18–22
44. Lee K L, Pryor D B, Pieper K S et al 1990 Prognostic value of radionuclide angiography in medically treated patients with coronary artery disease. A comparison with clinical and catheterization variables. Circulation 82: 1705–1717
45. Jones R H, Johnson S H, Bigelow C et al 1991 Exercise radionuclide angiocardiography predicts cardiac death in patients with coronary artery disease. Circulation 84: 52–58

96. Assessment after myocardial revascularization

Matthias E. Pfisterer

With rapidly increasing numbers of coronary artery bypass graft (CABG) operations and percutaneous transluminal coronary angioplasty (PTCA) procedures performed, the number of patients presenting with clinical problems after these revascularization procedures is increasing too. The clinical questions in these patients relate to early or late complications of the procedures themselves, to new typical, or often atypical, chest pain syndromes some time after the intervention and to the prediction of outcome. In addition to their undisputed role in preoperative patient evaluation, scintigraphic methods have been used and are still used to answer these questions. The indications for scintigraphic examination of patients before and after revascularization procedures are summarized in Table 96.1. The assessment after myocardial revascularization will form the content of this chapter.

In order to appreciate the results of scintigraphic studies in these situations it is important to know the different 'modes of action' of the two revascularization procedures, the haemodynamic changes observed in the peri- and postoperative period, the coronary flow disturbance seen in the first days after angioplasty and the time course of graft closure and restenosis. In addition, one has to take into consideration whether a complete revascularization or only a revascularization of a 'culprit lesion' was attempted. Only with the understanding of these basic mechanisms can the results of scintigraphic studies be interpreted in a clinically meaningful fashion.

Table 96.1 Indications for scintigraphic evaluation of patients with revascularization procedures

A. Pre-intervention*
- > to determine myocardial function
- > to assess ischaemia/extent of myocardium at risk
- > to identify haemodynamically significant coronary artery stenoses
- > to differentiate scar from hypoperfused but viable (hibernating) myocardium

B. Post-intervention
- > to assess peri-intervention myocardial damage or recovery
- > to predict restenosis
- > to detect graft closure/restenosis (even 'silent' events)
- > to detect progression of CAD in non-revascularized vessels
- > to differentiate ischaemic from other chest pain syndromes
- > to predict long-term prognosis**

* See Chapter 4: Diagnosis of coronary artery disease and Chapter 7: Impaired ventricular function.

** See Chapter 5: Prognosis of coronary artery disease.

ASSESSMENT OF PERIOPERATIVE MYOCARDIAL DAMAGE OR RECOVERY

Background

CABG surgery and PTCA may lead to perioperative myocardial infarction which has been reported after CABG surgery at a rate ranging from 4% to over 40% depending on patient subsets studied and methods applied.[1,2] Most commonly new Q-waves in the postoperative electrocardiogram and markedly elevated myocardial enzymes are used to confirm the diagnosis, but postoperative electrocardiographic changes may be unspecific and partly due to electrical axis deviation and enzyme release is directly related to cross clamp time.[3-5] Since only a minority of patients undergo repeat angiography, there is a need for non-invasive methods to define perioperative myocardial infarction objectively.

Besides myocardial infarction as a major complication of revascularization, there is reversible deterioration of left ventricular function within the first hours after surgery[6] which has been related to cardiodepressant effects of anaesthetics, volume loading of the heart and prolonged ischaemic time. Up to hospital discharge, left ventricular ejection fraction usually rises above preoperative levels most likely due to changing loading conditions of the heart and drug effects.[7] The long-term effect of revascularization procedures on left ventricular function consists of no significant change;[8,9] however, there may be deterioration in patients with perioperative myocardial infarction or improvement in those with prior hibernating myocardial segments.[10]

Myocardial perfusion scintigraphy

Perioperative myocardial infarction has been documented scintigraphically with ^{99m}Tc pyrophosphate single-photon tomography[11] and more recently indium-111 monoclonal anti-myosin–antibody scintigraphy.[12] Whereas the first method is known to have a lower sensitivity in a setting of subendocardial necrosis,[13] the latter may be too sensitive showing some indication of myocardial injury in up to 82% of postoperative patients.[12] In contrast, newly detected persistent thallium-201 defects postoperatively not present in preoperative studies have been closely related to perioperative myocardial infarction.[14] In addition, it has been shown that persistent defects on 4 h redistribution images before surgery, which show reversibility only late[15–17] or after reinjection,[18] may markedly improve after bypass grafting indicating preoperative hibernating myocardium. Thus, it is suggested that late redistribution or reinjection imaging should be performed when non-reversible defects are observed in 4 h delayed images before revascularization.

Scintigraphic assessment of myocardial function

Based on radionuclide angiocardiography using a nuclear probe and haemodynamic measurements, Breisblatt et al[19] described an early depression in left and right ventricular function reaching a nadir at 262 ± 116 min after coronary bypass which was reversible within 24 h after surgery. Similar results have been observed by other authors.[20–22] Whereas these transient changes may be related to the method of cardioprotection, changing loading conditions or preoperative treatment with beta-blocking drugs, persistent deterioration of global or regional function usually are due to perioperative myocardial infarction. Special attention was directed to abnormal septal wall motion after CABG surgery[23,24] which has been observed repeatedly without evidence of perioperative myocardial infarction. In a recent study, Okada et al[25] could demonstrate that abnormal postoperative septal motion is usually associated with normal septal perfusion and viability. Furthermore, four recent studies showed that regional wall motion abnormalities may even improve several months after CABG surgery if it was due to hibernation as characterized by rest-redistribution or reinjection thallium-201 scintigraphy[26,27] or positron emission tomography (PET).[28,29] These results highlight the importance of preoperative scintigraphic assessment of myocardial viability to predict the functional outcome after coronary artery revascularization procedures.

ASSESSMENT OF GRAFT FUNCTION AFTER CABG SURGERY

Background

In CABG surgery, the atherosclerotic lesion is not touched as in PTCA, but bypassed except for endarterectomy of diffusedly diseased vessels. In an attempt for full revascularization of all vascular territories even vessels to scarred areas are usually grafted. Within the first 2 weeks after bypass surgery, 8–10% of bypass grafts occlude which is more than half the rate found after 1 year (12–16%).[30–33] During the following years, there is a steady deterioration of bypass grafts leading to graft occlusion in 20% after 5 and 41% after 10 years and to significant graft disease in 38% after 5 and 75% after 10 years.[33] These numbers have been somewhat improved by the use of the internal mammary artery as bypass vessel,[34] but still bypass graft occlusion due to early thrombosis or later smooth muscle cell proliferation and progression of atherosclerosis is the major limitation of this form of treatment leading to recurrent angina, infarction and death.

Myocardial perfusion scintigraphy

Scintigraphic methods have been used for many years to document improvement in myocardial perfusion after CABG surgery.[35–40] Serial thallium-201 scintigraphy has been shown to have an 80% sensitivity, 88% specificity and 86% overall accuracy in detecting or excluding graft occlusion (Fig. 96.1).[14] Occluded grafts are correctly localized only in about two thirds of cases because grafts to small areas of myocardium, multiple grafts to one vascular territory or grafts to scarred myocardium cannot be detected. In addition, postoperative reversible perfusion defects may be due to graft occlusion or progression of atherosclerosis in a non-grafted coronary artery. New graft-vessels such as the gastroepiploic artery have been evaluated by thallium-201 myocardial scintigraphy.[41] Finally, thallium-201 scintigraphy has been used to document postoperative improvement in perfusion in previously hibernating myocardium.[17,18,28] Thus, myocardial perfusion imaging is of great value in the assessment of the functional result and follow-up of CABG surgery.

Scintigraphic assessment of myocardial function

The improvement in myocardial perfusion is paralleled by an improvement in exercise left ventricular function after CABG surgery,[42–44] whereas ejection fraction at rest remains virtually unchanged in most patients.[45,46] However, it has recently been shown that regional wall motion and even global left ventricular function at rest may improve after CABG surgery in presence of ischaemic left ventricular dysfunction or hibernating myocardium before the intervention.[19–21] Furthermore, one study[48] suggested that many patients with a non-bypassable coronary artery may still benefit functionally from CABG surgery if the jeopardized myocardium is perfused by collateral vessels supplied by a stenosed artery amenable to bypass surgery.

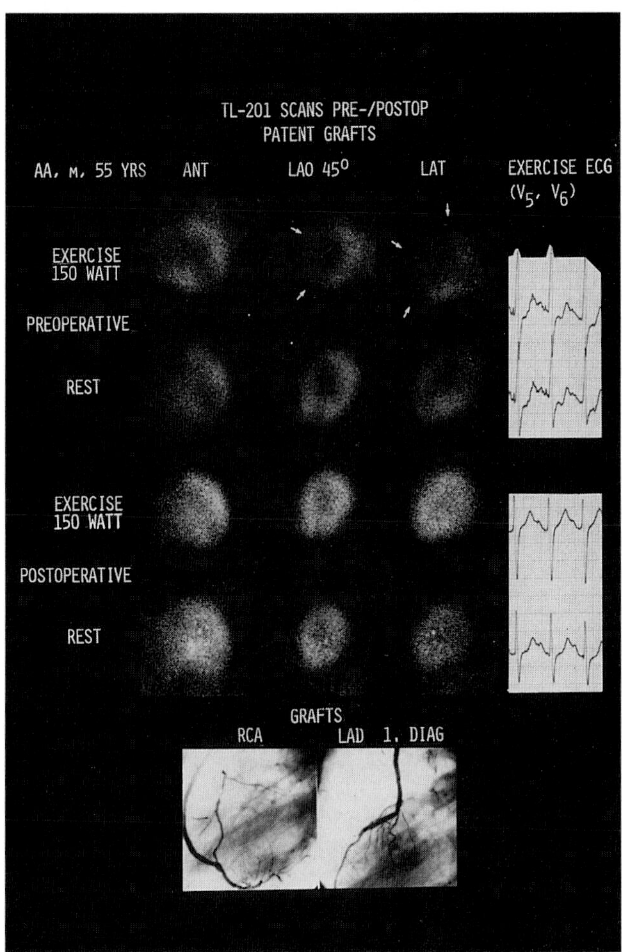

Fig. 96.1 Thallium-201 images immediately after exercise ('exercise') and 4 h later ('rest') in patient AA before and 1 year after coronary artery bypass graft surgery. Note the anteroseptal and apical ischaemia (arrows) preoperatively, which is no longer detectable after surgery in presence of open grafts to the left anterior descending (LAD) and first diagonal (1. DIAG) coronary arteries (snake graft) as well as to the right coronary artery (RCA). Maximal work levels and exercise ECG tracings are shown.[14]

PREDICTION AND DETECTION OF RESTENOSIS AFTER PTCA

Background

In contrast to CABG surgery, the coronary lesion itself is modified, compressed and ruptured by PTCA, which may lead to tears, flaps and even dissections of the intimal and medial layers of the vessel.[48] These effects, which have been visualized by angioscopy,[49] videodensitometry[50] and assessed as coronary flow reserve by quantitative angiography and Doppler measurements,[51,52] lead to early flow disturbances which may resolve or initiate either early thrombosis following platelet deposition or late restenosis due to smooth muscle cell proliferation. In serial angiographic studies it was shown that restenosis occurs mainly between 1 and 3 months after coronary angioplasty with almost no new cases after 6 months.[53,54] More recently, it has been pointed out that restenosis is no 'on–off' phenomenon, but rather a continuum from very mild to very severe obstruction.[55] The incidence of angiographically significant restenosis ranges between 20% and 50%,[56] but not all cases are associated with recurrent angina. Despite this high rate of restenosis, PTCA offers earlier, more complete relief of angina than medical therapy and is associated with better performance on the exercise test, although at higher costs and complications initially.[57] Still, prediction and detection of restenosis remains a challenge for non-invasive scintigraphic testing, since it may be silent and since the exercise electrocardiogram has repeatedly been shown to have only a low positive and negative predictive value (Table 96.2).[58–65]

Myocardial perfusion scintigraphy

Improvement in regional myocardial perfusion after successful PTCA has well been documented. With

Table 96.2 Exercise ECG to detect coronary restenosis (modified after Parisi et al [57])

First author	No. of patients	Angiographic follow-up (*n*)	Restenosis rate (%)	Sensitivity	Specificity	PPV	NPV	Timing of test
Scholl[58]	36	30	12	33 78	33 33	40 64	27 50	1 month 6 months
Rosing[59]	100	100	34	62	64	47	76	8 months
Wijns[60]	120	89	35	37	76	50	65	3–7 weeks
Ernst[61]	25	25	4	75	85	50	95	4–8 weeks
O'Keefe[63]	48	48	13	15	86	29	73	<1 month
Honan[63]	164	144	40	24	88	57	64	6 months
Bengtson[64]	209	200	25	60	69	61	84	6 months
El-Tamini[65]	31	31	45	79 93	82 100	79 100	82 94	3 days 1, 3, 6 months
Total	733	667	4 – 45	56*	73*	56*	70*	3 days–8 months

* = mean value weighted for the number in each study
PPV = positive predictive value
NPV = negative predictive value

multiple projections and single photon emission computerized tomography (SPECT), the ability to localize perfusion abnormalities and to relate them to specific vascular territories has been increased.[66,67] However, there are conflicting results of studies which were performed early after PTCA. In one study of 20 patients with successful PTCA of the left anterior descending coronary artery there was scintigraphic evidence of improved perfusion in the corresponding anteroseptal area in only 14 patients 1 week after the intervention.[68] In another investigation of 158 patients studied before and 1–2 days after successful PTCA, only 76% of perfusion abnormalities observed before the intervention improved afterwards.[69] In a semi-quantitative comparison with angiography, the correlation between the change in per cent stenosis and the improvement in thallium score was quite weak (r = 0.41). To investigate the correlation between angiographic and scintigraphic parameters of perfusion further, Powelson et al[70] studied 46 patients 1 day after PTCA with quantitative thallium-201 imaging followed by repeat angiography the next day. Thallium-201 perfusion defects were present in 13 vascular territories of 65 successfully dilated vessels, whereas significant early restenosis was present in only four of them. These findings most likely reflect the presence of early transient coronary flow abnormalities after PTCA as discussed above. Jain et al[71] reported the use of thallium-201 SPECT imaging following coronary vasodilatation with oral dipyridamole in 53 patients studied 2.9 ± 2.7 days after PTCA. Myocardial perfusion defects, present in 93% of patients before angioplasty, were reversible in 44 (83%), all of whom underwent dilatation of arteries supplying ischaemic areas. After a mean follow-up of 21.7 months, restenosis developed in 10 (71%) out of 14 patients with an ischaemic defect after angioplasty, but only in three (11.5%) of the patients without an ischaemic defect (P = 0.007).

To assess the prognostic power of thallium-201 imaging to predict angiographic restenosis, Hardoff et al[72] studied 90 consecutive patients at rest and during the stress of atrial pacing 12–24 h after angioplasty. A reversible perfusion defect in planar images was found in 38% of 104 myocardial regions supplied by the dilated coronary vessel and a subset of patients at higher risk of 6–12 months' angiographic restenosis (sensitivity 77%, specificity 67%) was identified. In contrast, late restenosis developed in only 11% of 65 vessels and in 14% of 37 patients with a non-ischaemic thallium-201 scan on day 1 (P<0.005). Multivariate logistic regression analysis selected reversible thallium-201 perfusion defect and immediate post-angioplasty residual coronary narrowing as significant independent predictors of later restenosis. Similarly, Miller et al[73] studied 50 patients 1 month after successful PTCA by rest and exercise thallium-201 scintigraphy and followed them clinically for 18 months. Delayed thallium-201 washout and a post-angioplasty pressure gradient ⩾20 mm Hg across the dilated stenosis were significantly predictive of a clinical event and 24% of patients with both abnormalities had restenosis at late follow-up. Wijns et al[60] performed planar imaging 3–7 weeks after PTCA in 120 patients, 89 of whom underwent angiographic follow-up at 6 months. The positive predictive value of an abnormal scan for restenosis was 74% and the negative predictive value was 83%. To assess the predictive accuracy of thallium-201 imaging for the diagnosis of restenosis after angioplasty, Breisblatt et al[74] evaluated 121 patients three times over a 1 year follow-up period. Four to 6 weeks after PTCA, 17 out of 121 patients complained of chest pain, nine of them had reversible scintigraphic ischaemia and all had restenosis. Of the 104 asymptomatic patients, 26 (25%) had a positive thallium-201 scan at 4–6 weeks with evidence of restenosis in 85% at 6 months and 96% at 1 year. After 3–6 months, 26 out of 28 patients with symptoms and a positive thallium-201 scan had restenosis. Ten out of 65 asymptomatic patients had a positive scan and four of them developed restenosis at 1 year. On the other hand, the 74 patients with a negative thallium-201 scan 3–6 months with or without symptoms had a low likelihood of developing restenosis. By 1 year, only five additional patients became symptomatic and four of these had previously been identified as having a positive thallium-201 study.

Although these studies suggest a relatively high predictive power of thallium-201 imaging to predict restenosis, the sensitivity of planar thallium-201 imaging performed 2.2 ± 1.2 weeks after successful PTCA in predicting restenosis in 68 patients was only 39% in a series by Stuckey et al.[75] However, the specificity of a normal study to predict continued vessel patency was 91%. In order to characterize sequential changes in myocardial perfusion after successful angioplasty and to elucidate some of these controversial findings, Manyari et al[76] studied 43 patients after 9 ± 5 days, 3.3 ± 0.6 months and 6.8 ± 1.2 months. Only patients with single vessel coronary artery disease and no evidence of prior myocardial infarction were included and all patients had angiography after 6–9 months documenting continuing patency. Serial thallium-201 studies demonstrated a progressive improvement in myocardial perfusion in the vascular territory of the dilated vessel during the follow-up period. Thus, myocardial ischaemia was diagnosed in 12 out of 43 scans recorded a few days after PTCA but in none recorded at later stages. The authors concluded that thallium-201 scans may show delayed improvement after PTCA and that therefore an abnormal thallium-201 scan soon after PTCA may not necessarily reflect residual coronary stenosis or recurrence.

To evaluate the value of myocardial perfusion scintigraphy during late follow-up of patients after coronary angioplasty, three studies reported on a total of 119 patients examined 4–8 months after the intervention

(Table 96.3).[58,59,61] The sensitivity and specificity for restenosis were 76–100% and 80–100%, respectively, with a low specificity of 46% in the study by Rosing et al,[59] most likely due to the high number of patients taking antianginal drugs during exercise testing. These values are similar to those reported for diagnostic testing with thallium-201 scintigraphy in chronic stable coronary artery disease.

Two recent studies have focused on detection of silent ischaemia after PTCA using thallium-201 imaging.[77,78] 116 patients were evaluated in a study by Hecht et al[77] to determine the ability of SPECT thallium-201 exercise and redistribution imaging to detect silent ischaemia secondary to restenosis in asymptomatic patients after PTCA and to compare it with findings in symptomatic patients. Sensitivity, specificity and accuracy for detection of restenosis by SPECT in individual patients were 96%, 75% and 88% *vs.* 91%, 77% and 85%, respectively, in the asymptomatic *vs.* symptomatic groups (P>0.05). Sensitivity and accuracy of exercise electrocardiography were significantly lower than those of SPECT imaging for patients with silent and symptomatic ischaemia (P<0.001). The authors concluded that restenosis may occur without angina despite the presence of angina before PTCA and that exercise electrocardiography is inaccurate in detecting silent ischaemia resulting from restenosis, whereas SPECT thallium-201 imaging accurately identifies restenosis in both asymptomatic and symptomatic patients. Furthermore, they pointed out that the amount of ischaemic myocardium does not differ between silent and symptomatic restenosis. These findings were confirmed in a large study of 490 consecutive patients by Pfisterer et al.[78] Six months after successful coronary angioplasty, 112 out of 405 patients (28%) had ischaemic reversible perfusion defects at planar thallium-201 scintigraphy and 60% of them were asymptomatic during the test (Fig. 96.2). Ischaemia was associated with significant coronary stenoses in 97%; in contrast, exercise electrocardiography was negative in 74% of patients with scintigraphic ischaemia and angiographic restenosis. The degree of restenosis was similar in patients with symptomatic *vs.* silent ischaemia (80 ± 16% *vs.* 81 ± 21 %). Long-term prognosis (2.2 ± 0.8 years) of

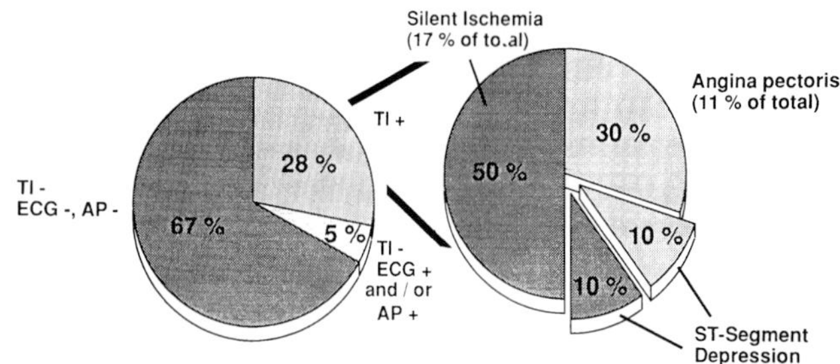

Fig. 96.2 Scintigraphic findings in 405 consecutive patients 6 months after successful PTCA. The 28% of patients (n = 112) with exercise-induced reversible perfusion defects (TL+) are shown again on the right hand side in relation to symptoms (angina pectoris or silent ischaemia) and to ST-segment depression.[78]

patients with silent ischaemia in an observational follow-up study was remarkably similar to that of symptomatic patients; a worse outcome of symptomatic patients was only found if repeat coronary angioplasty for restenosis was considered as a separate event (P<0.01). Silent and symptomatic ischaemia predicted an increased risk of recurrent ischaemic events but not of death. It was, therefore, concluded that absence of symptoms and a negative exercise electrocardiogram may not be considered indicative of a good angioplasty result. In addition, silent ischaemia due to restenosis after PTCA has a significant prognostic importance for recurrent symptomatic ischaemic events which may be reduced by repeat angioplasty.

Scintigraphic assessment of myocardial function

Improvement in myocardial perfusion after successful coronary angioplasty is associated with improvement in exercise left ventricular function as shown in several studies (Table 96.4).[61,62,79–82] In a consecutive series of 32 patients reported by Kent et al[80] left ventricular ejection fraction decreased from 55 ± 2% at rest to 51 ± 3% during exercise before angioplasty. After successful PTCA, left ventricular ejection fraction remained unchanged at rest but increased significantly during exercise to 62 ± 2% (P<0.001). The response of left ventricular ejection

Table 96.3 Radionuclide angiocardiography to detect coronary restenosis (modified after Parisi et al [57])

1st author	No. of patients	Angiographic follow-up (n)	Restenosis rate (%)	Sensitivity	Specificity	PPV	NPV	Timing of test
DePuey[82]	44	19	6	83	54	45	88	0–4 days
Rosing[59]	100	100	34	62	64	47	76	8 months
DePuey[84]	41	41	8	88	74	54	94	4–12 months
Ernst[61]	25	25	4	100	75	44	100	4–8 months
O'Keefe[62]	48	48	13	100	51	43	100	<1 month
Total	258	233	4 – 34	83*	63*	47*	88*	1 day–12 months

* = mean value weighted for the number in each study
PPV = positive predictive value
NPV = negative predictive value

fraction to exercise was abnormal in 87% of patients before *vs.* only in 19% after PTCA. Similarly, in a series of 44 patients with single vessel coronary artery disease reported by DePuey,[81] left ventricular ejection fraction at rest remained unchanged after successful PTCA (59 ± 11% *vs.* 58 ± 10% before PTCA), whereas exercise left ventricular ejection fraction increased markedly after angioplasty from 61 ± 13 % to 66 ± 12 % (P<0.001). These authors pointed out that the left ventricular ejection fraction response to exercise may only normalize in patients without prior myocardial infarction and that the improvement in exercise left ventricular ejection fraction after PTCA depends on the amount of ischaemic myocardium supplied by the dilated vessel, i.e. it is usually greater in patients with PTCA of the left anterior descending than of the right coronary artery. In addition, left ventricular function may be much more influenced by other factors such as age, sex, exercise level and anti-anginal drugs[83–87] than myocardial perfusion imaging and therefore has proven less valuable in the evaluation of patients after PTCA than perfusion imaging. In a recent study using PET imaging, Nienaber et al[88] investigated the relationship between metabolic and functional recovery of ischaemic myocardium after coronary angioplasty. They demonstrated that restoration of blood flow to ischaemic myocardium by PTCA is followed by an early improvement in perfusion but an initial persistence of abnormal metabolism and function at rest which normalized only during a late study after 68 ± 19 days.

Special aspects of left ventricular function before and after PTCA have been studied by several authors. Bonow et al[89] investigated the influence of successful PTCA on diastolic left ventricular function using high temporal resolution radionuclide angiography at rest. Before PTCA, all 25 patients had normal systolic function but 17 of them either had decreased peak filling rate or a prolonged time to peak filling rate. After successful PTCA, mean peak filling rate increased from 2.3 ± 0.6 to 2.8 ± 0.5 end-diastolic volume/s (P<0.001) and time to peak filling rate decreased from 181 ± 22 to 160 ± 18 ms (P<0.001). These results indicate that improved perfusion after successful angioplasty may normalize diastolic dysfunction at rest. Liu et al[90] measured the pulmonary blood volume ratio before and 2 weeks after successful PTCA in 31 patients with left anterior descending coronary artery stenoses. The mean pulmonary volume ratio decreased from 1.15 ± 0.10 before PTCA to 1.02 ± 0.15 afterwards. 85% of patients had an abnormal ratio of >1.06 before angioplasty *vs.* only 38% of patients after the procedure. Breisblatt et al[91] reported on their initial experience with continuous on-line monitoring of left ventricular function immediately after PTCA using a miniaturized non-imaging radionuclide detector system. Their observations suggest that this monitoring system may be particularly useful in patients with unstable lesions after coronary angioplasty. Finally, O'Keefe et al[62] tested the value of early (≤1 month) exercise radionuclide angiocardiography to predict risk of late restenosis in 48 patients. None of 17 patients with normal exercise findings had restenosis *vs.* 13 out of 31 patients with abnormal radionuclide angiographic results. Thus, by this method subgroups of patients who are at low and high risk for early restenosis after PTCA could be identified. These different findings point to multiple applications of radionuclide angiocardiography in the evaluation of patients after coronary angioplasty.

DIFFERENTIATION OF RECURRENT CHEST PAIN SYNDROMES

Background

After revascularization procedures patients may return to their treating physicians complaining of a variety of chest pain syndromes of which only a small part correspond to typical angina pectoris. Chest pain may be atypical and difficult to differentiate from true ischaemic chest pain; reasons include chest pain after thoracotomy, after resection of the internal mammary artery, due to postoperative pericarditis, neuralgy, or in many patients due to fear of

Table 96.4 Thallium-201 scintigraphy to detect coronary restenosis (modified after Parisi et al [57])

1st author	No. of patients	Angiographic follow-up (n)	Restenosis rate (%)	Sensitivity	Specificity	PPV	NPV	Timing of test
Scholl[58]	36	30	12	42	56	56	42	1 month
Rosing[59]	58	58	21	76	46	37	83	8 months
Wijns[60]	120	89	35	74	83	74	83	3 –7 weeks
Ernst[61]	25	25	4	100	80	50	100	4–8 weeks
Jain[71]	40	22	14	79	88	79	88	0–6 days
Hardoff[72]	90	71	32	77	67	53	86	12–24 hours
Total	369	295	4 – 35	75*	75*	67*	81*	12 h–8 months

* = mean value weighted for the number in each study
PPV = positive predictive value
NPV = negative predictive value

new problems. Scintigraphic tests have proven helpful in these situations to identify patients with underlying ischaemia due to graft closure or restenosis after PTCA, respectively, and to differentiate them from extracardiac chest pain syndromes.

Myocardial perfusion scintigraphy

In a study with serial thallium-201 perfusion scans after CABG surgery, Pfisterer et al[14] related postoperative symptoms and scintigraphic findings (Fig. 96.3) with angiographic results. In presence of new postoperative perfusion defects, 10 out of 12 patients (83%) with typical or atypical chest pain had at least one graft occluded. On the other hand, in the absence of new perfusion defects, only one out of 19 patients (5%) with no chest pain and one out of 11 (9%) with atypical chest pain had an occluded graft. After coronary angioplasty early symptoms (< 1 month) were usually related to incomplete revascularization or no coronary narrowing in a study reported by Joelson,[92] whereas chest pain developing between 1 and 6 months was most likely due to restenosis and later symptoms due to new significant coronary artery lesions. Quantitative exercise thallium-201 scintigraphy was used to predict recurrence of angina in 68 patients after successful PTCA by Stuckey et al.[75] The positive and negative predictive values of thallium-201 redistribution were 69% and 75% respectively, markedly higher than those of exercise electrocardiography (41% and 69%). These findings were confirmed by Hecht et al[77] who found that SPECT thallium-201 imaging was significantly more sensitive in patients with silent ischaemia (96% *vs.* 40%; $P<0.001$) and accurate (88% *vs.* 44%; $P<0.001$) than was exercise electrocardiography in detecting ischaemia with similar specificity. In patients with symptomatic ischaemia, SPECT was also more sensitive (91% *vs.* 59%; $P<0.001$) and accurate (85% *vs.* 64%; $P<0.001$) than was exercise electrocardiography, and specificity was again

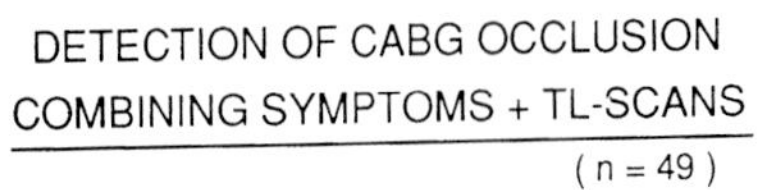

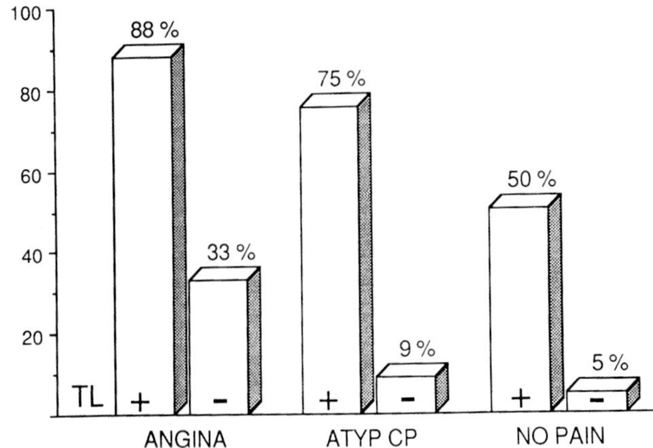

Fig. 96.3 Thallium-201 scintigraphy to detect coronary artery bypass graft occlusion in relation to symptoms 1 year after surgery. New thallium-201 perfusion defects in serial pre- and postoperative studies were considered indicative of graft occlusion.[14]

similar. SPECT was equally sensitive, specific and accurate in patients with silent or symptomatic ischaemia in contrast to the exercise electrocardiogram which was significantly more accurate in patients with symptomatic than with silent ischaemia (64% *vs.* 44%; $P<0.05$). These findings which were recently confirmed by a similar study[78] demonstrate that myocardial perfusion scintigraphy is a very useful non-invasive test to differentiate the various chest pain syndromes after coronary revascularization. It helps to identify patients with ischaemic chest pain who may profit from repeat intervention. Scintigraphic findings may also be useful in post-coronary bypass patients to identify those who will profit from PTCA as a second revascularization procedure *vs.* repeat bypass surgery.[93]

REFERENCES

1. Hultgren N H, Shettigar U R, Pfeifer J F, Angell W W 1977 Acute myocardial infarction and ischemic injury during surgery for coronary artery disease. Am Heart J 94: 146–153
2. Roberts A J 1985 Perioperative myocardial infarction in open heart surgery. In: Utley J R, ed. Perioperative cardiac dysfunction. Cardiothoracic surgery series, Vol 3. Williams & Wilkins, Baltimore, London, Los Angeles, Sydney. pp 107–121
3. du Cailar C, Maille J G, Jones W et al 1980 MB creatine kinase and the evaluation of myocardial injury following aortocoronary bypass operation. Ann Thorac Surg 29: 8–14
4. Warren S G, Wagner G S, Bethea C F, Roe C R, Newland Oldham H, Kong Y 1977 Diagnostic and prognostic significance of electrocardiographic and CPK isoenzyme changes following coronary bypass surgery: correlation with findings at one year. Am Heart J 93: 189–196
5. Schwendener R B, Pfisterer M, Skarvan K, Stulz P, Grädel E 1990 Diagnostischer Wert der C K-MB zur Beurteilung des perioperativen Infarktes der AKB-Operation. Helv chir Acta 57: 239–242
6. Mangano D T 1985 Biventricular function after myocardial revascularization in humans: deterioration and recovery patterns during the first 24 hours. Anaesthesiology 62: 571–577
7. Mahler F, Ross J Jr, O'Rourke R A, Covell JW 1975 Effect of changes in preload, afterload and inotropic state on ejection and isovolumic phase measures of contractility in the conscious dog. Am J Cardiol 35: 626–631
8. Hammermeister K E, Kennedy J W, Hamilton G W et al 1974 Aortocoronary saphenous vein bypass. Failure of successful grafting to improve resting left ventricular function in chronic angina. N Engl J Med 290: 186–192
9. Wolf N M, Kreulen T H, Bove A A et al 1978 Left ventricular function following coronary bypass surgery. Circulation 58: 63–70
10. Braunwald E, Rutherford J D 1986 Reversible ischemic left

ventricular dysfunction: evidence for the 'hibernating myocardium'. J Am Coll Cardiol 8: 1467–1470
11. Burns J B, Gladstone P J, Tremblay P C et al 1989 Myocardial infarction determined by technetium-99m pyrophosphate single-photon tomography complicating elective coronary artery bypass grafting for angina pectoris. Am J Cardiol 63: 1429–1434
12. van Vlies B, van Royen E A, Visser C A et al 1990 Frequency of myocardial indium-111 antimyosin uptake after uncomplicated coronary artery bypass grafting. Am J Cardiol 66: 1191–1195
13. Massie B M, Botvinick E H, Werner J A, Chatterjee K, Parmley W W 1979 Myocardial scintigraphy with technetium-99m stannous pyrophosphate: an insensitive test for nontransmural myocardial infarction. Am J Cardiol 43: 186–197
14. Pfisterer M, Emmenegger H, Schmitt H E et al 1982 Accuracy of serial myocardial perfusion scintigraphy with thallium-201 for prediction of graft patency early and late after coronary artery bypass surgery. A controlled prospective study. Circulation 66: 1017–1024
15. Berger B C, Watson B D, Burwell L R et al 1979 Redistribution of thallium at rest in patients with stable and unstable angina and the effect of coronary artery bypass surgery. Circulation 60: 1114–1125
16. Liu P, Kiess M C, Okada R D et al 1985 The persistent defect on exercise thallium imaging and its fate after myocardial revascularization: does it represent scar or ischemia? Am Heart J 110: 996–1001
17. Kiat H, Berman D S, Maddahi J et al 1988 Late reversibility of tomographic myocardial thallium-201 defects: an accurate marker of myocardial viability. J Am Coll Cardiol 12: 1456–1463
18. Ohtani H, Tamaki N, Yonekura Y et al 1990 Value of thallium-201 reinjection after delayed SPECT imaging for predicting reversible ischemia after coronary artery bypass grafting. Am J Cardiol 66: 394–399
19. Breisblatt W M, Stein K L, Wolfe C J et al 1990 Acute myocardial dysfunction and recovery: a common occurrence after coronary bypass surgery. J Am Coll Cardiol 15: 1261–1269
20. Gray R, Maddahi J, Berman D et al 1979 Scintigraphic and hemodynamic demonstration of transient left ventricular dysfunction immediately after uncomplicated coronary artery bypass grafting. J Thorac Cardiovasc Surg 77: 504–510
21. Reduto L A, Lawrie G M, Reid J W et al 1981 Sequential postoperative assessment of left ventricular performance with gated cardiac blood pool imaging following aortocoronary bypass surgery. Am Heart J 101: 59–66
22. Phillips H R, Carter J E, Okada R D et al 1983 Serial changes in left ventricular ejection fraction in the early hours after aortocoronary bypass grafting. Chest 83: 28–34
23. Righetti A, Crawford M H, O'Rourke R A, Schelbert H, Daily P O, Ross J Jr 1977 Interventricular septal motion and left ventricular function after coronary bypass surgery: evaluation with echocardiography and radionuclide angiography. Am J Cardiol 39: 372–377
24. Ribeiro P, Nihoyannopoulos P, Farah S et al1985 Role of transient ischemia and perioperative myocardial infarction in the genesis of new septal wall motion abnormalities after coronary bypass surgery. Br Heart J 54: 140–144
25. Okada R D, Murphy J H, Boucher C A et al 1992 Relationship between septal perfusion, viability and motion before and after coronary artery bypass surgery. Am Heart J 124: 1190–1195
26. Carrel T, Jenni R, Haubold-Reuter S, von Schulthess G, Posic M, Turina M 1992 Improvement in severely reduced left ventricular function after surgical revascularization in patients with preoperative myocardial infarction. Eur J Cardiothorac Surg 6: 479–484
27. Ragosta M, Beller G A, Wabon D D, Kaul S, Gimple L W 1993 Quantitative planar rest-redistribution TL-201 imaging in detection of myocardial viability and prediction of improvement in left ventricular function after coronary bypass surgery in patients with severely depressed left ventricular function. Circulation 87: 1630–1641
28. Takeishi Y, Tono-oka I, Kubota I et al 1991 Functional recovery of hibernating myocardium after coronary bypass surgery: does it coincide with improvement in perfusion? Am Heart J 122: 665–670
29. Marwick T H, MacIntyre W J, Lafont A, Nemes J J, Salcedo E E 1992 Metabolic responses of hibernating and infarcted myocardium to revascularization. A follow-up study of regional perfusion, function and metabolism. Circulation 85: 1347–1353
30. Chesebro J H, Clements I P, Fuster V et al 1982 A platelet inhibitor drug trial in coronary bypass operations: benefit of perioperative dipyridamole and aspirin therapy on early postoperative vein-graft patency. N Engl J Med 307: 73–78
31. Chesebro J H, Clements I P, Fuster V et al 1984 Effect of dipyridamole and aspirin on late vein-graft patency after coronary bypass operations. N Engl J Med 310: 209–214
32. Pfisterer M, Jockers G, Regenass S et al 1989 Trial of low-dose aspirin plus dipyridamole versus anticoagulants for prevention of aortocoronary vein graft occlusion. Lancet July 1: 1–7
33. Fitzgibbon G M, Leach A, Kafka H P, Leon W J 1991 Coronary bypass graft fate: long-term angiographic study. J Am Coll Cardiol 17: 1075–1080
34. Loop F D, Lytle B W, Cosgrove D M et al 1986 Influence of the internal mammary artery graft on 10 year survival and other cardiac events. N Engl J Med 314: 1–6
35. Zaret B L, Martin N D, McGowan R L, Strauss H W, Wells H P, Flamm M D 1974 Rest and exercise potassium-43 myocardial perfusion imaging for the non-invasive evaluation of aortocoronary bypass surgery. Circulation 49: 688–673
36. Lurie A J, Salel A F, Berman D S, DeNardo G L, Hurley E J, Mason D T 1976 Determination of improved myocardial perfusion after aortocoronary bypass surgery by exercise rubidium-81 scintigraphy. Circulation 54 (Suppl III): 20–23
37. Ritchie J L, Narahara K A, Trobaugh G B, Wiliams D L, Hamilton G W 1977 Thallium-201 myocardial imaging before and after coronary revascularization assessment or regional myocardial blood flow and graft patency. Circulation 56: 830–836
38. Greenberg B H, Hart R, Botvinick E H et al 1978 Thallium-201 myocardial perfusion scintigraphy to evaluate patients after bypass surgery. Am J Cardiol 42: 167–171
39. Kolibash A J, Call T D, Bush C A, Tetalman M R, Lewis R P 1980 Myocardial perfusion as an indicator of graft patency after coronary artery bypass surgery. Circulation 61: 882–887
40. Gibson R S, Watson D D, Taylor G J et al 1983 Prospective assessment of regional myocardial perfusion before and after coronary revascularization surgery by quantitative thallium-201 scintigraphy. J Am Coll Cardiol 3: 804–815
41. Kusukawa J, Hirota Y, Kawamura K et al 1989 Efficacy of coronary artery bypass surgery with gastroepiploic artery. Assessment with thallium-201 myocardial scintigraphy. Circulation (Suppl I): 135–140
42. Kent K M, Borer J S, Green M V et al 1978 Effects of coronary artery bypass on global and regional left ventricular function during exercise. N Engl J Med 298: 1434–1439
43. Carroll J D, Hess O M, Hirzel H D et al 1985 Left ventricular systolic and diastolic function in coronary artery disease: effects of revascularization on exercise-induced ischemia. Circulation 72: 119–129
44. Kawasuji M, Takemura H, Tedoriya T, Sawa S, Taki J, Iwa T 1992 Exercise response assessed by continuous monitoring of ventricular function in patients with coronary bypass operations. J Thorac Cardiovasc Surg 103: 849–854
45. Mintz L J, Ingels N B, Daughters G T, Stinson E B, Alderman E L 1980 Sequential studies of left ventricular function and wall motion after coronary arterial bypass surgery. Am J Cardiol 45: 210–216
46. Rankin J S, Newman G E, Muhlbaier L H, Behar V S, Fedor J M, Sabiston D C 1985 The effect of coronary revascularization on left ventricular function in ischemic heart disease. J Thorac Cardiovasc Surg 90: 818–832
47. Dilsizian V, Cannon III R O, Tracy C M, McIntosh C L, Clark R E, Bonow R O 1989 Enhanced regional left ventricular function after distant coronary bypass by means of improved collateral blood flow. J Am Coll Cardiol 14: 312–318
48. Block P C, Myler R K, Stertzer S, Fallon J T 1981 Morphology after transluminal angioplasty in human beings. N Engl J Med 305: 382–385
49. Ramee S R, White C J, Collins T J, Mesa J E, Murgo J P 1991 Percutaneous angioscopy during coronary angioplasty using a steerable microangioscope. J Am Coll Cardiol 17: 100–105
50. Johnson M R, Wilson R F, Skorton D J, Collins S M, White C W

1986 Coronary lumen area immediately after angioplasty does not correlate with coronary vasodilator reserve: a videodensitometric study. Circulation 74 (Suppl II): 193 (Abstract)
51. Wilson R F, Johnson M R, Marcus M L et al 1988 The effect of coronary angioplasty on coronary flow reserve. Circulation 77: 873–885
52. Zijlstra F, denn Boer A, Reiber J H C, van Es G A, Lubsen J, Serruys PW 1988 Assessment of immediate and long-term functional results of percutaneous transluminal coronary angioplasty. Circulation 78: 15–24
53. Nobuyoshi M, Kimura T, Nosak H et al 1988 Restenosis after successful percutaneous transluminal coronary angioplasty: serial angiographic follow-up of 229 patients. J Am Coll Cardiol 12: 616–623
54. Serruys P W, Luijten H E, Beatt K J et al 1988 Incidence of restenosis after successful coronary angioplasty: a time-related phenomenon. Circulation 77: 361–371
55. Beatt K J, Serruys P W, Hugenholtz P G 1990 Restenosis after coronary angioplasty: new standards for clinical studies. J Am Coll Cardiol 15: 491–498
56. Califf R M, Fortin D F, Frid D J et al 1991 Restenosis after coronary angioplasty: an overview. J Am Coll Cardiol 17: 2B–13B
57. Parisi A F, Folland E D, Hartigan P on behalf of the Veterans Affairs ACME Investigators 1992 A comparison of angioplasty with medical therapy in the treatment of single-vessel coronary artery disease. N Engl J Med 326: 10–16
58. Scholl J M, Chaitman B R, David P R et al 1982 Exercise electrocardiography and myocardial scintigraphy in the serial evaluation of the results of percutaneous transluminal coronary angioplasty. Circulation 66: 380–390
59. Rosing D R, Van Raden M J, Mincemoyer R M et al 1984 Exercise electrocardiographic and functional responses after percutaneous transluminal coronary angioplasty. Am J Cardiol 53: 36C–41C
60. Wijns W, Serruys P W, Reiber J H C et al 1985 Early detection of restenosis after successful percutaneous transluminal coronary angioplasty by exercise-redistribution thallium scintigraphy. Am J Cardiol 55: 357–361
61. Ernst S M P G, Hillebrand F A, Klein B, Ascoop C A, van Tellingen C, Plokker H W M 1985 The value of exercise tests in the follow-up of patients who underwent transluminal coronary angioplasty. Int J Cardiol 7: 267–279
62. O'Keefe J H, Lapeyre A C, Holmes D R, Gibbons RJ 1988 Usefulness of early radionuclide angiography for identifying low-risk patients for late restenosis after percutaneous transluminal coronary angioplasty. Am J Cardiol 61: 51–54
63. Honan M B, Bengtson J R, Pryor D B et al 1989 Exercise treadmill testing is a poor predictor of anatomic restenosis after angioplasty for acute myocardial infarction. Circulation 80: 1585–1594
64. Bengtson J R, Mark D B, Honan M B et al 1990 Detection of restenosis after elective percutaneous transluminal coronary angioplasty using the exercise treadmill test. Am J Cardiol 65: 28–34
65. El-Tamini H, Davies GJ, Hackett D et al 1990 Very early prediction of restenosis after successful coronary angioplasty: anatomic and functional assessment. Am Coll Cardiol 5: 259–264
66. Lim Y L, Okada R D, Chesler D A et al 1984 A new approach to quantitation of exercise thallium-201 scintigraphy before and after an intervention: application to define the impact of coronary angioplasty on regional myocardial perfusion. Am Heart J 108: 917–925
67. Mahmarian J J, Boyce T M, Goldberg R K, Cocanougher M K, Roberts R, Verani M S 1990 Quantitative exercise thallium-201 single-photon emission computed tomography for the enhanced diagnosis of ischemic heart disease. J Am Coll Cardiol 15: 318–329
68. Okada R D, Yean L L, Boucher C A, Pohost G M, Chesler D A, Block P C 1985 Clinical, angiographic, hemodynamic, perfusional and functional changes after one-vessel left anterior descending coronary angioplasty. Am J Cardiol 55: 347–356
69. DePuey E G, Roubin G S, Cloninger K G et al 1988 Correlation of transluminal coronary angioplasty parameters and quantitative thallium-201 tomography. J Invasive Cardiol 1: 40–50
70. Powelson S W, DePuey E G, Roubin G S, Berger J H, King S B III 1986 Discordance of coronary angiography and 201-thallium tomography early after transluminal coronary angioplasty. J Nucl Med 27: 6 (Abstract)
71. Jain A, Mahmarian J J, Borges-Neto S et al 1988 Clinical significance of perfusion defects by thallium-201 single photon emission tomography following oral dipyridamole early after coronary angioplasty. J Am Coll-Cardiol 11: 970–976
72. Hardoff R, Shefer A, Gips S et al 1990 Predicting late restenosis after coronary angioplasty by very early (12 to 24 h) thallium-201 scintigraphy: implications with regard to mechanisms of late coronary restenosis. J Am Coll Cardiol 15: 1486–1492
73. Miller D D, Liu P, Strauss H W, Block P C, Okada R D, Boucher C A 1987 Prognostic value of computer-quantitated exercise thallium imaging early after percutaneous transluminal coronary angioplasty. J Am Coll Cardiol 10: 275–283
74. Breisblatt W M, Weiland F L, Spaccavento L F 1988 Stress thallium-201 imaging after coronary angioplasty predicts restenosis and recurrent symptoms. J Am Coll Cardiol 12: 1199–1204
75. Stuckey T D, Burwell L R, Nygaard T W, Gibson R S, Watson D D, Beller G A 1989 Quantitative exercise thallium-201 scintigraphy for predicting angina recurrence after percutaneous transluminal coronary angioplasty. Am J Cardiol 63: 517–521
76. Manyari D E, Knudtson M, Kloiber R, Roth D 1988 Sequential thallium-201 myocardial perfusion studies after successful percutaneous transluminal coronary artery angioplasty: delayed resolution of exercise-induced scintigraphic abnormalities. Circulation 77: 86–95
77. Hecht H S, Shaw R E, Chin H L, Ryan C, Stertzer S H, Myler R K 1991 Silent ischemia after coronary angioplasty: evaluation of restenosis and extent of ischemia in asymptomatic patients by tomographic thallium-201 exercise imaging and comparison with symptomatic patients. J Am Coll Cardiol 17: 670–677
78. Pfisterer M, Rickenbacher P, Kiowski W, Müller-Brand J, Burkart F 1993 Silent ischemia after PTCA: incidence and prognostic significance. J Am Coll Cardiol 22: 1446–1454
79. Sigwart U, Grbic M, Essinger A et al 1982 Improvement of left ventricular function after percutaneous transluminal coronary angioplasty. Am J Cardiol 49: 651–657
80. Kent K M, Bonow R O, Rosing D R et al 1982 Improved myocardial function during exercise after successful percutaneous transluminal coronary angioplasty. New Engl J Med 306: 441–446
81. DePuey E G, Boskovic D, Krajcer Z et al 1983 Exercise radionuclide ventriculography in evaluating successful transluminal coronary angioplasty. Cathet Cardiovasc Diagn 9: 153–156
82. DePuey E G, Leatherman L L, Leachman R D et al 1984 Restenosis after transluminal coronary angioplasty detected with exercise-gated radionuclide ventriculography. J Am Coll Cardiol 4: 1103–1113
83. Pfisterer M, Battler A, Zaret B 1985 Range of normal values for left and right ventricular ejection fraction at rest and during exercise assessed by radionuclide angiocardiography. Eur Heart J 6: 647–655
84. Port S, Cobb F R, Coleman R E et al 1980 Effect on age on the response of the left ventricular ejection fraction to exercise. New Engl J Med 303: 1133–1137
85. Greenberg P S, Berge R D, Johnson K D et al 1983 The value and limitation of radionuclide angiocardiography with stress in women. Clin Cardiol 6: 312–317
86. Lindsay J, Nolan N G, Goldstein S A et al 1983 Effects of beta-adrenergic blocking drugs on sensitivity and specificity of radionuclide ventriculography during exercise in patients with coronary heart disease. Am Heart J 106: 271–278
87. Gibbons R J, Lee K L, Pryor D et al 1983 The use of radionuclide angiography in the diagnosis of coronary artery disease – a logistic regression analysis. Circulation 68: 740–746
88. Nienaber C A, Brunken R C, Sherman C T et al 1991 Metabolic and functional recovery of ischemic human myocardium after coronary angioplasty. J Am Coll Cardiol 18: 966–978
89. Bonow R O, Kent K M, Rosing D R et al 1982 Improved left ventricular diastolic filling in patients with coronary artery disease after percutaneous transluminal coronary angioplasty. Circulation 66: 1159–1167
90. Liu P, Kiess M C, Strauss H W et al 1986 Comparison of ejection

fraction and pulmonary blood volume ratio as markers of left ventricular function change after coronary angioplasty. J Am Coll Cardiol 8: 511–516

91. Breisblatt W M, Schulman D S, Follansbee W P 1991 Continuous on-line monitoring of left ventricular function with a new nonimaging detector: validation and clinical use in the evaluation of patients post angioplasty. Am Heart J 121: 1609–1617

92. Joelson J M, Most A S, Williams D O 1987 Angiographic findings when chest pain recurs after successful percutaneous transluminal coronary angioplasty. Am J Cardiol 60: 792–795

93. Reed D C, Beller G A, Nygaard T W, Tedesco C, Watson D D, Burwell L R 1989 The clinical efficacy and scintigraphic evaluation of post-coronary bypass patients undergoing percutaneous transluminal coronary angioplasty for recurrent angina pectoris. Am Heart J 117: 60–71

97. Radionuclides in the assessment of impaired ventricular function

Gerald G. Blackwell   Gerald M. Pohost

INTRODUCTION

The prognosis in most forms of cardiac disease is linked to ventricular function. Left ventricular (LV) volumes and ejection fraction influence prognosis in patients with coronary heart disease, the most common cause of morbidity and mortality in the Western world. These LV parameters are also important in the great number of patients afflicted with valvular heart disease and cardiac muscle disease. Assessment of right ventricular (RV) function attracts less attention yet can be of primary importance in patients with pulmonary vascular disease and congenital heart disease. Interestingly, RV function can also greatly influence the clinical status of patients with severe LV dysfunction.

Radionuclide-based techniques are well suited to assess both the RV and LV objectively. An important breakthrough in non-invasive cardiac imaging occurred with the development of nuclear cardiology techniques to assess ventricular function.[1,2] In this chapter we shall briefly review physiological and pathophysiological considerations in the assessment of myocardial performance. We shall then focus on the clinical role of nuclear cardiology in assessing impaired ventricular function.

PHYSIOLOGICAL AND PATHOPHYSIOLOGICAL CONSIDERATIONS IN THE ASSESSMENT OF VENTRICULAR FUNCTION

At the most basic level the role of the cardiovascular system is to supply adequate nutrition to living cells. The syndrome of heart failure is loosely applied when cardiac output is insufficient to meet the demands of the body as a whole or of specific organs. This term is also applied when adequate cardiac output can be accomplished only by filling pressures which cause extravasation of fluid from the systemic capillary network (right heart failure) and/or the pulmonary capillary network (left heart failure). The term 'heart failure' is entrenched in the medical literature and is often literally interpreted to implicate the heart as the only abnormally functioning organ. Radionuclide techniques can define the functional status of the heart in patients with a disordered circulation accurately. It is important to recognize, however, that maintenance of a normal circulation is dependent on the closely regulated interaction of the heart, the peripheral vasculature, and the neurohumoral system. Abnormalities in any of these subsystems can lead to absolute or relative inadequacies in the distribution of cardiac output. In recent years, the recognition and treatment of pathophysiological abnormalities extrinsic to the heart has assumed a central role in the management of many forms of clinical heart failure.

Determinants of myocardial performance

The major determinants of myocardial performance are preload, afterload, contractility, and heart rate. These parameters can be isolated and measured in the muscle mechanics laboratory but in an intact organism all four parameters act in concert to determine cardiac performance.[3] At the cellular level, 'preload' refers to the force acting to stretch the myofibre, and within physiological limits the greater the degree of end-diastolic fibre length (stretch) the greater the volume of blood ejected from the ventricle. Clinically, an increase in preload is determined by end-diastolic chamber volume, and the graphic expression of this is shown by the familiar Frank–Starling curve (Fig. 97.1). The normal cardiovascular system has a significant amount of preload reserve.[4] In other words, when contractile function is diminishing a major adaptive measure for the maintenance of an adequate cardiac output is to increase ventricular preload.

'Afterload' is defined as the force that opposes myocardial fibre shortening. The best description of afterload is given by wall stress. According to the law of Laplace:

$$\text{wall stress} \approx (\text{pressure} \times \text{radius})/\text{wall thickness}.$$

This formula incorporates a factor external to the heart

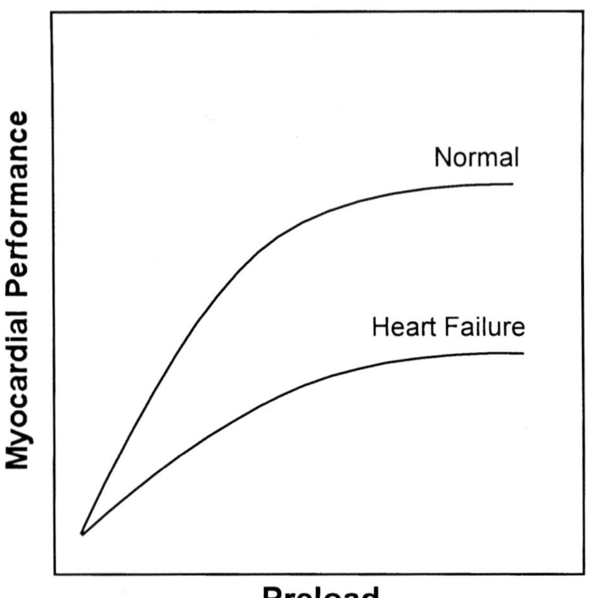

Fig. 97.1 Graphic representation of the relationship between preload and cardiac output in the normal heart and in a patient with systolic heart failure. In both curves an increase in preload results in an increase in cardiac output. In the patient with systolic heart failure the slope of the curve is flatter so that a progressive increase in proload results in a smaller incremental increase in cardiac output. High levels of preload ultimately lead to extravasation of fluid into the extravascular space.

(i.e. pressure) and the internal geometry of the heart (i.e. chamber radius and wall thickness). In addition it should be appreciated from this formula that afterload constantly changes through the cardiac cycle, as both pressure changes and geometric changes occur from diastole through systole. For this reason systolic blood pressure, though often used as a measure of afterload, is an oversimplification.

'Heart rate' influences cardiovascular performance by altering the time available for diastolic filling and the frequency with which stroke volume is delivered to the peripheral tissues. In a more complex fashion it may also directly influence the beat-to-beat inotropic state of the heart.

'Contractility' refers to the intrinsic inotropic state of the myocardium. This parameter can be very difficult to measure in the intact organism as it is intimately linked to preload, afterload and heart rate. Three categories of contractility indexes have been described: isovolumic indices, ejection phase indices, and pressure–volume loops.[3]

Isovolumic indices include the maximum rate of LV pressure rise (dP/dt), the velocity of contractile element shortening (V_{ce}), and the maximum unloaded velocity of the contractile element (V_{max}). These indices require precise pressure measurements and high temporal resolution acquisitions. Accordingly, they cannot be determined in the nuclear medicine laboratory. Ejection phase indices and pressure–volume loops are described in the following sections.

Assessment of myocardial performance: ejection phase indices

Ejection phase indices include the velocity of circumferential fibre shortening and the ejection fraction. These incorporate measurements of ventricular wall motion during the period of systolic ejection. The velocity of circumferential fibre shortening requires measurement of diastolic and systolic dimensions and is not well suited for radionuclide techniques. Ejection fraction (EF), however, is easily determined. It is defined as:

$$EF=(EDV-ESV)/EDV$$

where EDV is the end-diastolic volume and ESV is the end-systolic volume. As a dimensionless parameter it can be applied to hearts of different sizes and ejection fraction is widely used clinically in the assessment of ventricular

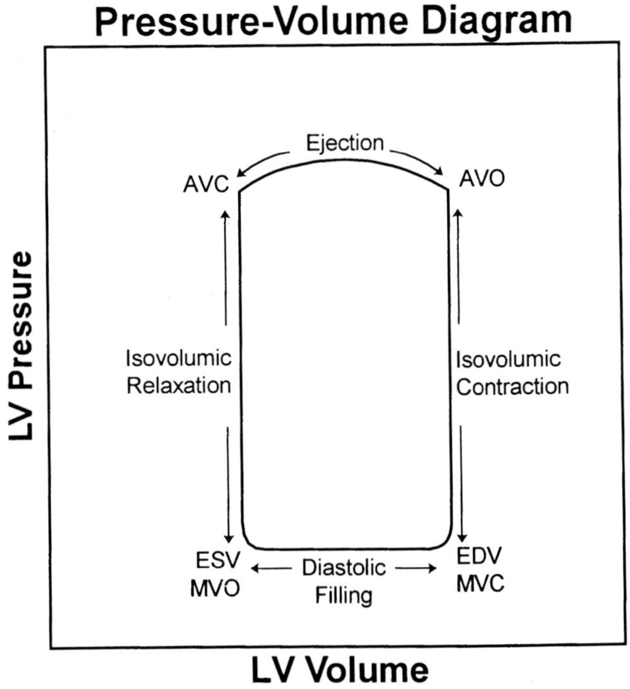

Fig. 97.2 Left ventricular (LV) pressure–volume diagram. The cardiac cycle begins with mitral valve opening (MVO). Diastolic filling proceeds until mitral valve closure (MVC) and in the normal heart end-diastolic volume (EDV) is reached with a minimal increase in LV diastolic pressure. During the period of isovolumic contraction, ventricular pressure increases with no change in ventricular volume. The ejection phase of the cardiac cycle is bounded by aortic valve opening (AVO) and closure (AVC). Completion of cardiac ejection defines ventricular end-systolic volume (ESV). During the period of isovolumic relaxation ventricular pressure falls with no change in ventricular volume. The cycle repeats with opening of the mitral valve. Pressure–volume diagrams incorporate the coupling of the ventricle to the vasculature, thereby helping to separate instrinsic abnormalities of ventricular performance from abnormalities related to altered loading conditions.

function. The major limitation of ejection fraction as a measure of contractility is that it is load dependent. Changes in either preload or afterload can cause a change in ejection fraction in the absence of a true change in contractility. This concept is perhaps best understood through ventricular pressure– volume diagrams.

Assessment of myocardial performance: pressure–volume loops

A pressure–volume loop measures the instantaneous ratio between ventricular pressure and volume, referred to as elastance.[5] This parameter varies throughout the cardiac cycle and a comprehensive, clinically useful model of both systolic and diastolic ventricular performance can be constructed (Fig. 97.2). By altering arterial pressure or LV volume, multiple loops can be constructed for an individual patient. The end-systolic points on these curves bear a direct, nearly linear relationship, the slope of which is referred to as E_{max} (Fig. 97.3).[6] This slope is insensitive to changes in loading conditions and has been touted as a load-independent index of contractility. Using this conceptual framework changes in ventricular volumes and ejection fraction can be interpreted more clearly. For example, at a constant afterload and inotropic state an increase in end-diastolic volume will produce an increase in stroke volume and ejection fraction (Fig. 97.4). Alternatively, at a constant preload and inotropic state an increase in afterload will result in a reduced stroke volume and ejection fraction (Fig. 97.5). If the inotropic state of the ventricle increases, E_{max} shifts upward and to the left. Conversely, a decrease in inotropic state, as occurs in systolic heart failure, is accompanied by a shift of E_{max} downward and to the right (Fig. 97.6). End-systolic wall stress can be subsituted for pressure to account for changes in wall thickness and ventricular size.[7] Magorien et al[8] have described a technique for defining the LV pressure–volume relation in man using equilibrium radionuclide angiography in combination with echocardiography and micromanometer pressure recordings.

RADIONUCLIDE METHODS TO ASSESS VENTRICULAR FUNCTION

The basic methods by which radiopharmaceuticals are used to assess ventricular function are covered in detail in accompanying chapters of this book. Briefly, a radiolabelled tracer, usually ^{99m}Tc, is introduced into a peripheral or central vein and radioactive emissions are

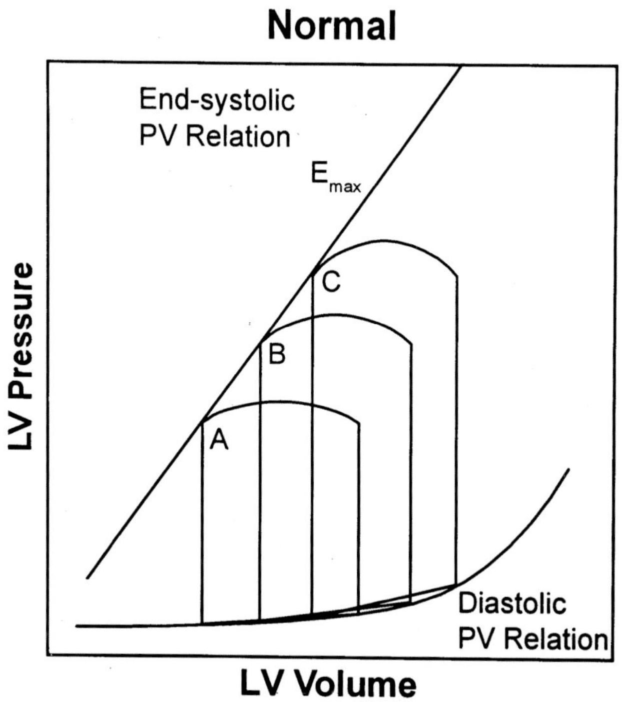

Fig. 97.3 The end-systolic pressure–volume (PV) relation and the diastolic PV relation can be defined in an individual patient by constructing PV loops at different loading conditions. Loop A is acquired at a low preload and afterload; loop B at an intermediate preload and afterload; and loop C at a high preload and afterload. If the inotropic state of the heart remains constant the end-systolic points on these curves have a nearly linear relation, the slope of which is referred to as E_{max}.

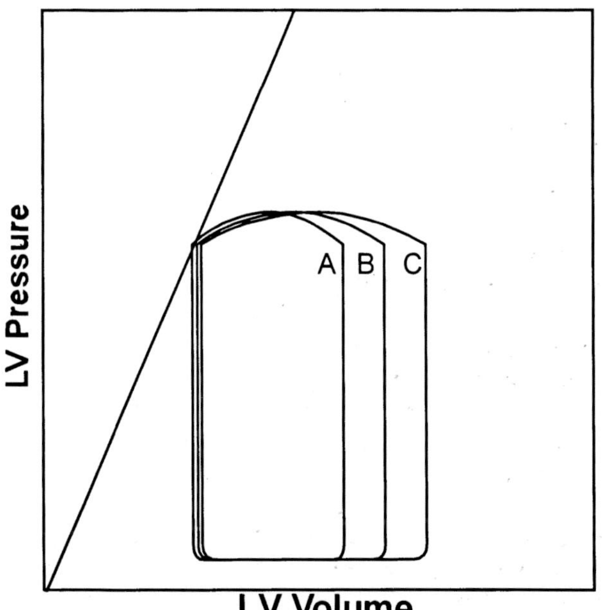

Fig. 97.4 Effect of increasing preload (LV volume) in a patient in whom afterload and inotropic state remain constant. Loop A is baseline with loop B and loop C acquired at progressively increased levels of preload. Note that stroke volume (EDV–ESV) and ejection fraction (SV/EDV) rise from loop A to loop B to loop C in the absence of a change in inotropic state. These loops underscore the influence of preload on ejection fraction. Common clinical situations associated with an increase in preload include mitral and aortic regurgitation.

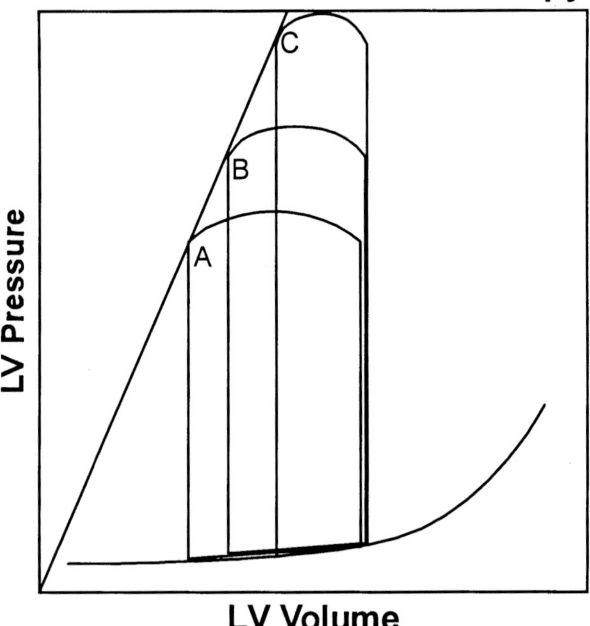

Fig. 97.5 Effect of increasing afterload (left ventricular pressure) in a patient in whom preload and inotropic state remain constant. Loop A is baseline with loop B and loop C acquired at progressively increased levels of afterload. Note that stroke volume (EDV−ESV) and ejection fraction (SV/EDV) decrease from loop A to loop B to loop C in the absence of a change in inotropic state. These loops underscore the influence of afterload on ejection fraction. Common clinical situations associated with an increased afterload include hypertension and aortic stenosis.

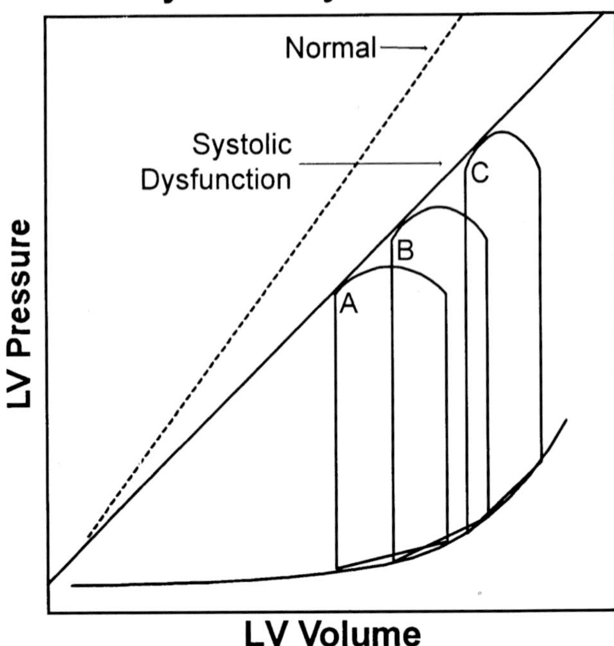

Fig. 97.6 Effect of systolic dysfunction on the pressure–volume relation. At any given level of preload and afterload a reduction in myocardial contractility (inotropy) will result in an increase in the end-systolic volume. This reduced inotropic state is demonstrated by a shift of E_{max} downward and to the right. For comparison, the dotted line represents the slope of E_{max} prior to the development of systolic dysfunction.

Table 97.1 Radionuclide techniques for assessing ventricular function

1. Gated equilibrium radionuclide angiography
2. First pass radionuclide angiography
3. Gated first pass radionuclide angiography

measured by a gamma camera appropriately positioned over the heart. The maximum number of counts will be obtained during the end-diastolic period when ventricular volume, and thus radioactive count density, is highest. The minimum number of counts will be obtained at end-systole when chamber volume and count density is at a minimum. Radioactive emissions at all other points during the cardiac cycle will fall between these two extreme values. A graphic representation of cyclic radioactive emissions from either ventricle can be displayed as a familiar time–activity curve. There are two common techniques that use these principles in assessing ventricular function; a gated equilibrium blood pool technique and a first pass technique (Table 97.1).

Gated equilibrium radionuclide angiography

The most widely applied method in clinical practice is the equilibrium gated blood pool technique, also called radionuclide angiography or multiple gated acquisition. In this method the radiopharmaceutical 'tags' red blood cells which are then allowed to equilibrate within the patient's circulation. An aliquot of blood is tagged outside the body and then reinjected (ex vivo technique), or alternatively, the tag can be made to occur exclusively within the circulation (in vivo technique). Electrocardiographic leads are attached to the patient and detection of gamma emissions synchronized (gated) to the ECG signal. With this approach each R–R interval is divided into equal time intervals (phase) and counts during each interval averaged over multiple cardiac cycles. A reconstructed image of each cardiac phase is then placed into an endless loop cine format to depict a typical cardiac contraction.

The major advantage of this method is that count density is high and resolution thereby optimized. However, accurate representation of an 'average' cardiac contraction is dependent on a stable heart rate. If R–R intervals vary widely during the acquisition, temporal misregistration occurs and image quality is severely degraded. This effect can be lessened by computer algorithms that analyse only R–R intervals falling within a specified range while rejecting all others. From a practical standpoint, the worst images are often obtained in patients with atrial fibrillation and a highly variable ventricular response.

First pass radionuclide angiography

In a first pass study the radioactive tracer is injected as a bolus into the blood stream and followed as it sequentially traverses the cardiac chambers. An advantage of this method is that excellent anatomic separation of the chambers can be achieved. This is particularly important when imaging the right ventricle. A major disadvantage of this technique is that count density is low since only several cardiac cycles can be analysed before the tracer exits the chamber of interest and equilibrates within the circulation. Specialized instrumentation is needed to record events faithfully. In addition, accurate data acquisition is dependent upon delivery of a tight bolus into the circulation. Streaming of the bolus into the right heart may adversely effect calculations of ventricular volumes and ejection fraction.

Imaging considerations for radionuclide angiography

A standard single-crystal gamma counter can be used in most circumstances but multi-crystal cameras are useful for performing first pass studies. Imaging considerations are very different for the LV and RV. For equilibrium gated blood pool scans of the LV three views are typically acquired. These are an anterior view, lateral view, and best septal separation view. The combination of these views affords an excellent method for assessing regional wall motion. The best septal separation view is usually a cranially angulated left anterior oblique view. This plane separates the LV from the RV and the LV from the LA.

Imaging the RV is considerably more difficult. In the anterior projection there is overlap of the RV and LV cavities. In the left anterior oblique projection the RA overlaps the RV cavity. Accordingly, for first pass studies a shallow right anterior oblique projection is frequently used. This view minimizes chamber overlap and is analogous to the view obtained in the cardiac catheterization laboratory.

Calculation of ventricular volumes and ejection fraction

Absolute ventricular volumes can be determined by several different techniques. Count-based, attenuation-corrected techniques have been validated but require knowledge of the equilibrium count density of aliquots of the subject's blood and careful correction for background counts and soft-tissue attenuation.[9,10] Simpler count-based methods have recently been developed which do not require either blood sampling or attenuation correction.[11,12] Ventricular volumes obtained in this fashion may be useful in following patients with several forms of chronic heart disease.

Table 97.2 Functional parameters which may be assessed by radionuclide techniques

1. Left ventricular volumes and ejection fraction
2. Right ventricular volumes and ejection fraction
3. Regional wall motion of the left and right ventricles
4. Ventricular diastolic function via time–activity curves
5. Stroke volume ratios
6. Phase mapping

Ejection fraction can also be determined from absolute volumes. More commonly, however, ejection fraction in the nuclear cardiology laboratory is obtained via:

$$EF=(EDC-ESC)/EDC$$

where EDC and ESC represent end-diastolic and end-systolic counts, respectively. Radionuclide determined ejection fractions are easy to obtain, do not require geometric assumptions and are highly reproducible assuming studies are obtained under stable haemodynamic conditions.[13–15] Accordingly, they have assumed a prominent role in the assessment of patients with normal and impaired ventricular function (Table 97.2).

Assessment of ventricular diastolic function

The importance of ventricular diastolic function has become clear in recent years. Often regarded as a passive process, it is now recognized that ventricular relaxation and chamber filling is an active, energy-requiring process which is altered early in the course of many disease states before systolic dysfunction occurs. This is especially true in patients with the two most common forms of heart disease, coronary artery disease and hypertensive heart disease. Approximately one-third of all patients with congestive heart failure have predominant diastolic dysfunction.[16] The prognosis in these patients can be poor and treatment is different from that of patients with ventricular systolic dysfunction.[17] Using radionuclides, inferences can be made regarding diastolic function by observing the filling patterns of both the RV and LV.[18–20] Alterations can occur in early diastolic filling, late diastolic filling following atrial systole, or in the peak filling rate (Fig. 97.7). In assessing diastolic ventricular properties with radionuclides strict attention must be paid to technique. For best results the patient must be in sinus rhythm with few ectopic beats and the data acquired with high temporal resolution. Age-related changes in radionuclide-derived diastolic function have also been reported.[21,22]

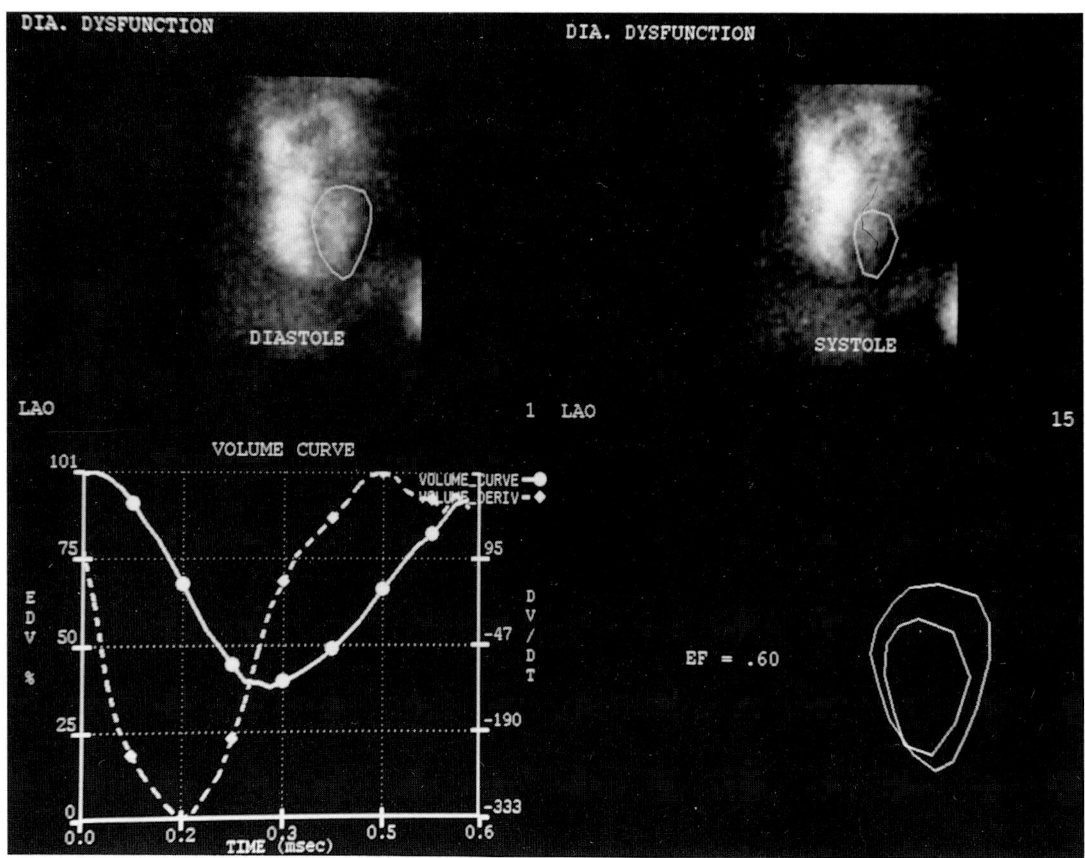

Fig. 97.7 Gated equilibrium blood pool scan in a patient with left ventricular diastolic dysfunction. Systolic function is normal as demonstrated by an ejection fraction of 60%. However, there is a prolonged diastolic filling phase consistent with diastolic dysfunction. Examination of the characteristics of activity–time curves is an accurate method of identifying diastolic dysfunction.

Continuous monitoring of ventricular performance

Attention has also been given to the continuous monitoring of ventricular function. The prototype of these devices is a detector which can be worn as a vest to provide assessment of ventricular function over the course of several hours.[15,23] Whether worn in an intensive care unit or in an ambulatory setting, these devices may provide new insight into ventricular dysfunction occurring as a result of either silent or symptomatic ischaemia.[24–26] Engineering improvements may lead to on-line monitoring of cardiac function and widespread dissemination of this technology in the future.[27]

Perfusion methods in the assessment of impaired ventricular function

Radionuclide angiography permits a direct assessment of ventricular function, but impaired ventricular function can be inferred from data acquired during myocardial perfusion imaging. Increased ventricular size and wall thickness can be appreciated qualitatively on standard ^{201}Tl images. Several studies have reported that an increase in the ratio of pulmonary to myocardial ^{201}Tl uptake is a bad prognostic sign in patients with coronary artery disease.[28–30] It must be remembered, however, that the presence of increased lung thallium is directly related to pulmonary capillary wedge pressure (PCWP) and does not distinguish between patients with systolic or diastolic heart failure.

Issues of patient care and logistical problems previously limited the use of radionuclide techniques in the face of acute ischaemic syndromes. The unique imaging characteristics of newer isonitrile compounds, however, make them more suitable for assessing patients with evolving myocardial infarction. ^{99m}Tc Sestamibi can be injected during an acute infarction yet imaged many hours later when the patient is likely to be more stable. Because there is slow washout and no significant redistribution with this compound, administration prior to an intervention such as PTCA or thrombolytic therapy provides images that depict the myocardium at risk. A second study can then be performed days later. The difference between the initial perfusion defect (myocardial area at risk) and any residual defect seen on late images can be assumed to represent myocardial salvage from interventions performed.[31]

The feasibility of this approach was originally shown by Gibbons et al[32] in patients with acute myocardial infarction. Final ^{99m}Tc sestamibi perfusion defects correlated closely with radionuclide angiography ejection fraction and regional wall motion at the time of hospital discharge. Subsequent data has extended the correlation with ejection fraction at 6 weeks and with ejection fraction, end-diastolic volume, and end-systolic volume at 1 year.[33,34]

Recently, techniques have been described which combine functional imaging with myocardial perfusion imaging using ^{99m}Tc sestamibi. Perfusion and function studies at rest and exercise have been performed in normal volunteers and patients with stable coronary artery disease.[35,36] Clinical use in patients with myocardial infarction has been demonstrated by Boucher et al[37] using first pass ejection fraction and myocardial perfusion at rest. Further work is to be expected in this exciting area.

RADIONUCLIDES IN THE ASSESSMENT OF IMPAIRED LV FUNCTION

The most common application of radionuclide angiography is in the assessment of LV function (Table 97.3).

Table 97.3 Clinical indications for resting radionuclide angiography

1. Assessment of global left and right ventricular function
2. Assessment of regional wall motion abnormalities in patients with ischaemic heart disease
3. Differentiation of systolic versus diastolic dysfunction in patients with dyspnoea
4. Serial follow-up of patients treated with doxyrubicin

Equilibrium studies acquired in different projections facilitate the evaluation of both global and regional LV systolic function (Fig. 97.8). Importantly these studies can be combined with exercise, most commonly supine bicycle ergometry, to yield insight into cardiovascular reserve. This section will focus on the identification of impaired LV function in several clinical situations.

LV function in patients with ischaemic heart disease

Data from many studies have shown that an important prognostic factor in patients with acute myocardial infarction is the status of resting LV function. Because of the accuracy, reproducibility and availability of nuclear medicine techniques most studies to date have used

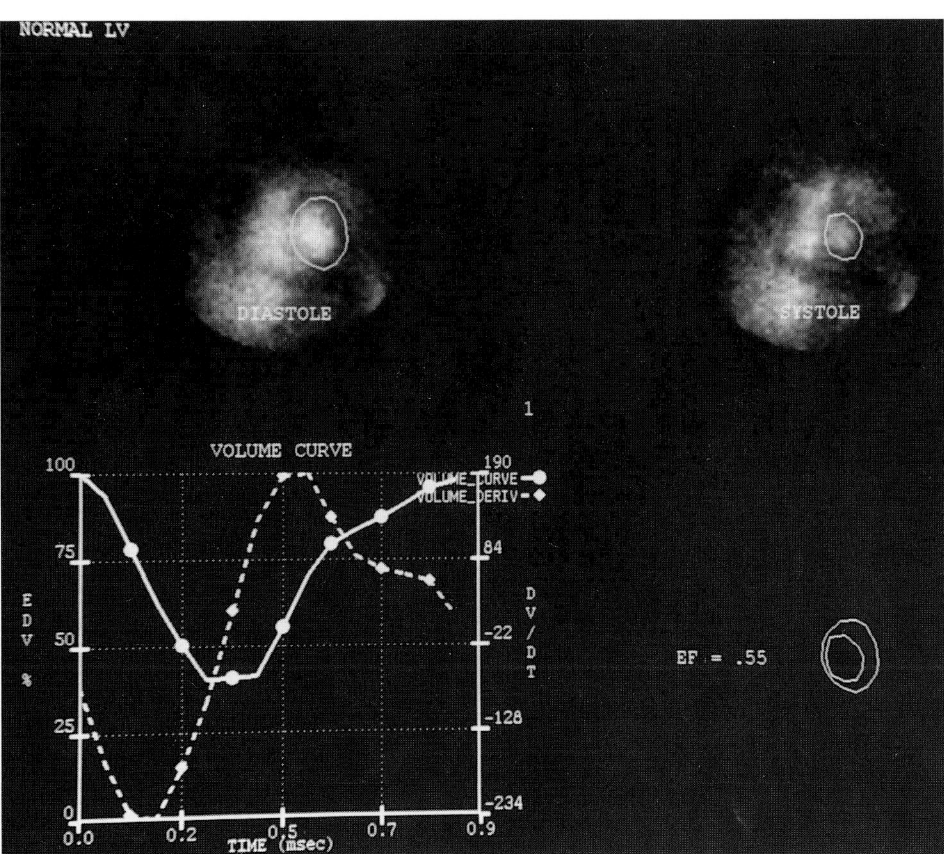

Fig. 97.8 Gated equilibrium blood pool scan in a patient with normal left ventricular systolic and diastolic performance. End-diastolic and end-systolic phases are shown in the best septal separation view. The graph displays a volume–time curve as well as the first derivative of this curve (dV/dt). Both left ventricular filling and emptying are normal.

equilibrium radionuclide angiography to measure ejection fraction.[38,39] In the widely quoted Multicenter Postinfarction Research Group study,[40] ejection fraction was the single most important determinant of prognosis, with 1 year mortality increasing exponentially in patients with an ejection fraction ≤ 40%. It should be noted that these data were acquired over 10 years ago in the pre-thrombolytic era and before widespread use of other adjunctive therapies now known to benefit post-myocardial infarction patients. Accordingly, more recent data have shown that radionuclide-determined ejection fraction remains of prognostic significance, but there has been a parallel shift downward of the survival curve. The exponential increase in mortality now occurs at an ejection fraction of approximately ≤ 30%.[41]

An area of major research and clinical importance in post-myocardial infarction patients is that of ventricular remodelling. The LV undergoes architectural changes following a myocardial infarction, particularly infarctions involving a large segment of the anterior wall. The most dramatic example of ventricular remodelling that can be recognized by radionuclide angiography is LV aneurysm formation (Fig. 97.9).[42] In most patients, however, changes in ventricular size and function occur insidiously over the course of months or longer. The segmental nature of myocardial infarction leads to a complex sequence of changes both in the infarct zone and in non-infarcted segments.[43] Ventricular volume may increase to maintain cardiac output in the face of a reduction in the number of functioning myocytes. Decreased systolic function is often accompanied by an abnormal diastolic pressure with resultant increases in both systolic and diastolic LV wall stress. Compensatory mechanisms are time dependent and influenced by the status of the infarct-related artery, the presence of critical coronary stenoses in additional territories, systemic blood pressure, and many other factors. The serial increase in ventricular volumes occurring in patients following anterior myocardial infarction can be attenuated by therapy with angiotensin converting-enzyme (ACE) inhibitors and a favourable influence of these agents on survival has been demonstrated.[44] Equilibrium radionuclide angiography is well suited for serially assessing the dynamic process of ventricular remodelling.

Radionuclide angiography in combination with exercise has also been used to assess patients with ischaemic heart

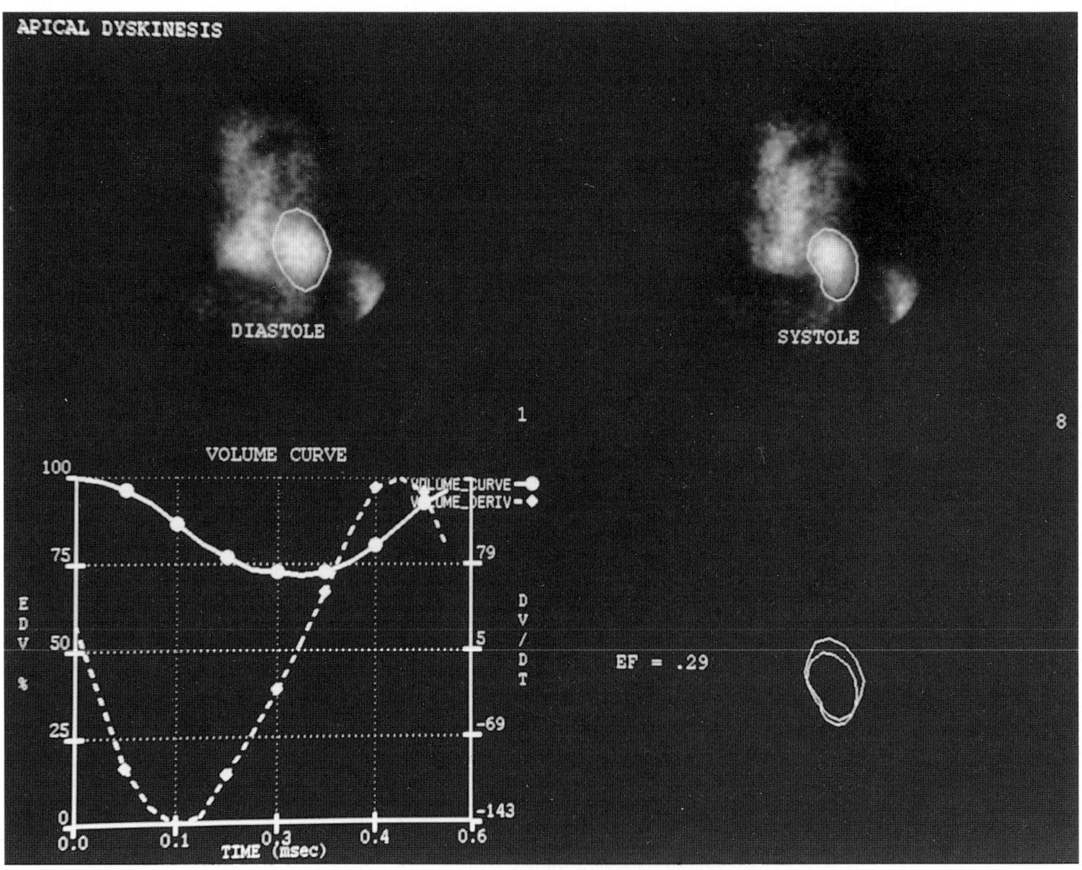

Fig. 97.9 Gated equilibrium blood pool scan in a patient with a large apical left ventricular (LV) aneurysm. There is systolic expansion of the apical segment and a markedly reduced ejection fraction. The aneurysm appears to have a wide communication with the remainder of the LV consistent with a true aneurysm.

Table 97.4 Clinical indications for exercise radionuclide angiography

1. Detection of stress-induced global and regional wall motion abnormalities for diagnosis and prognosis of patients with ischaemic heart disease
2. Assessment of right and left ventricular function in patients with chronic volume overload from valvular heart disease (i.e. aortic regurgitation and mitral regurgitation)
3. Assessment of functional capacity in patients with congestive heart failure
4. Assessment of contractile reserve of the right ventricle in patients with pulmonary heart disease and congenital heart disease

Table 97.5 Valvular lesions which may lead to an increased ejection fraction secondary to abnormal loading conditions

Lesions	*Abnormal loading conditions*
1. Mitral regurgitation	1. Decreased afterload and increased preload
2. Aortic regurgitation	2. Decreased afterload and increased preload
Valvular lesions which may lead to a decreased ejection fraction secondary to abnormal loading conditions	
Lesions	*Abnormal loading conditions*
1. Aortic stenosis	1. Increased afterload
2. Mitral stenosis	2. Decreased preload

disease (Table 97.4).[45–47] A normal exercise response is generally considered to be a rise of ≥ 5% above the resting ejection fraction level.[15] Both age- and gender-related differences have been described.[48–50] Care must be taken when analysing the many studies available because they vary in patient selection (i.e. pre/post-myocardial infarction, age, gender), number of patients, radionuclide protocol, length of follow-up and end-points analysed. In several early post-myocardial infarction studies performed with exercise, the final exercise ejection fraction was found to be a significant predictor of outcome.[51,52] Investigators have also found that the change in exercise ejection fraction from the resting value provided prognostic information in this patient population,[53,54] while other studies found no prognostic information from the change in ejection fraction with exercise.[51,55]

Several large studies have looked at exercise radionuclide angiography in patients with chronic ischaemic heart disease. Bonow et al[56] prospectively studied 117 consecutive patients with minimally symptomatic coronary artery disease and preserved resting ejection fraction (>40%). They identified a high risk group consisting of patients with three-vessel coronary disease and a decreased ejection fraction response to exercise equilibrium radionuclide angiography. In contrast, Taliercio et al[57] found no additional prognostic information from exercise radionuclide angiography after information from resting ejection fraction, age, and number of diseased coronary vessels was considered. Subtle differences in patient selection and the uninterrupted use of beta-blockers during exercise in 42% of patients in the Taliercio study versus stopping all anti-anginal therapy prior to exercise in the study by Bonow may explain these differences.[58]

More recently, Lee et al[59] reported findings from 571 consecutive medically treated patients who had upright rest and exercise radionuclide angiography performed within 3 months of cardiac catheterization. After a median follow-up period of 5.4 years the most important radionuclide predictor of survival was the exercise ejection fraction. Exercise ejection fraction was a better predictor than either rest ejection fraction or the change in ejection fraction from rest to exercise. Further, radionuclide angiography contributed additional prognostic information to data derived from clinical and catheterization variables.

Taken in total, the incorporation of an exercise protocol often yields prognostic information additional to that available from resting radionuclide angiography in patients with ischaemic heart disease.

LV function in patients with valvular heart disease

A non-invasive diagnosis of valvular heart disease can usually be made by physical examination complimented by echocardiography. Prognosis and decisions regarding surgical intervention, however, are usually based on the effect valvular lesions have on ventricular size and function.[60] Chronic valvular lesions alter ventricular loading. Accordingly, radionuclide angiography-determined ejection fractions can be either increased or decreased depending on the nature of the valvular lesion and the haemodynamics at the time of the study (Table 97.5). Despite this limitation, radionuclide angiography has been shown to be of prognostic value in patients with both chronic mitral and aortic regurgitation.[61–63] The prognostic power of radionuclide angiography may be enhanced in combination with exercise testing.

LV function in patients with cardiomyopathy

Patients with congestive heart failure unrelated to coronary artery disease, valvular disease, pericardial disease, or recognized systemic disease are classified as having cardiomyopathy. Dilated cardiomyopathy is characterized by primary systolic dysfunction and an enlarged chamber volume (Fig. 97.10). Hypertrophic and restrictive cardiomyopathies are characterized by diastolic dysfunction with small chamber volumes and typically well-preserved systolic function. As with valvular heart disease, the major role of radionuclide techniques is in serially assessing ventricular volumes and ejection fraction. Likewise, these parameters are significantly affected by the haemodynamics at the time of data acquisition.

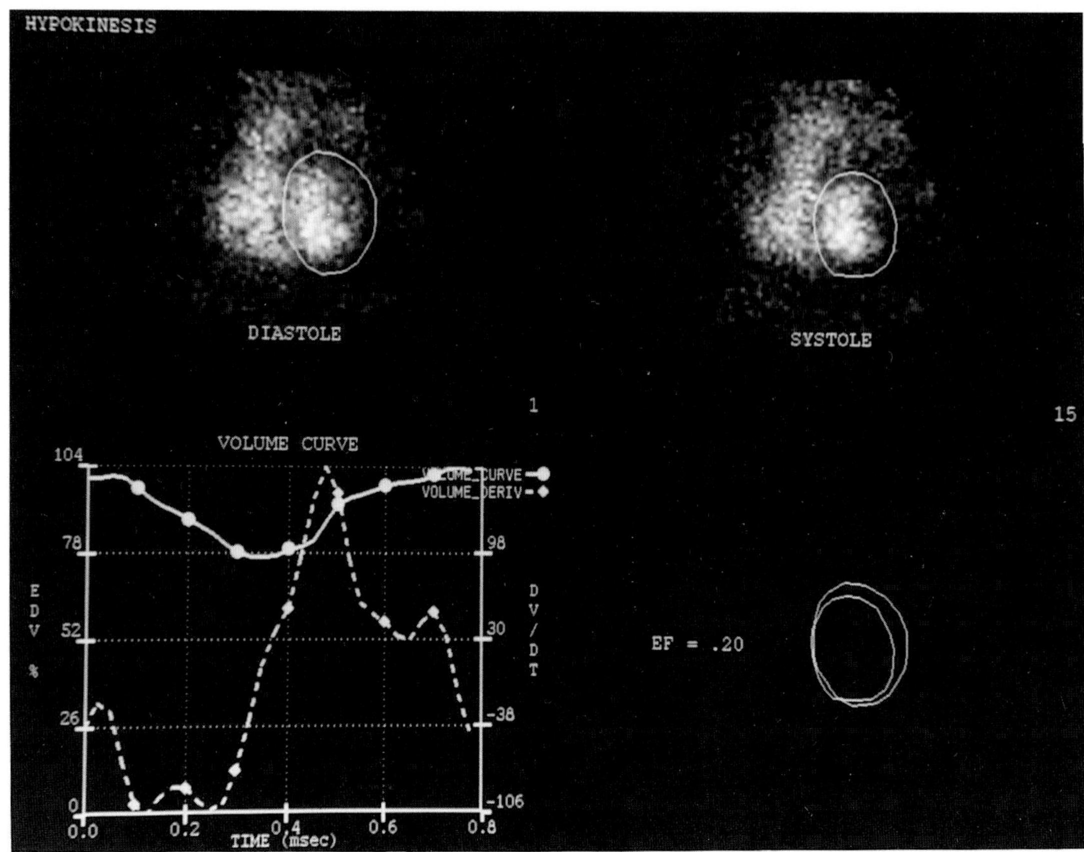

Fig. 97.10 Severe left ventricular dysfunction is demonstrated on this gated equilibrium blood pool scan from a patient with dilated cardiomyopathy. Ventricular volumes are increased and the ejection fraction is reduced. As can be appreciated on the superimposed end-diastolic and end-systolic outlines there is global hypokinesis.

It is common for dilated cardiomyopathy to produce global biventricular dysfunction and non-segmental defects on perfusion imaging. In contrast, ischaemic heart disease often produces regional wall motion and perfusion abnormalities. While large fixed defects and reversible perfusion defects favour an ischaemic aetiology, reliable non-invasive differentiation between ischaemic and non-ischaemic dilated cardiomyopathy cannot be made using radionuclide techniques alone.[64,65] Glamann et al[66] have reported their findings in 76 patients with catheter-proven non-ischaemic cardiomyopathy studied with radionuclide angiography and ^{201}Tl. In this study segmental perfusion abnormalities, regional LV dysfunction, and global RV function all failed to discriminate between those patients with ischaemic and non-ischaemic cardiomyopathy.[66] The influence of RV function in patients with LV systolic failure is discussed in a subsequent section of this chapter.

The gated blood pool findings in hypertrophic cardiomyopathy have been described by Pohost et al.[67] However, the diagnosis of hypertrophic cardiomyopathy is almost always made on the basis of a careful physical examination, ECG findings, and echocardiography. Differentiation of restrictive cardiomyopathy from constrictive pericardial disease using diastolic filling patterns from radionuclide angiography has also been reported.[68]

Doxorubicin cardiotoxicity

An established indication for radionuclide angiography is in the serial follow-up of patients treated with doxorubicin. Schwartz et al[69] studied 1487 patients treated with doxorubicin and monitored by rest radionuclide angiography in both university and community hospital settings. High risk patients were identified as having: (a) a decline of 10 ejection fraction percentage points from a normal baseline to a final level of ≤50%; (b) total doxorubicin dose of >450 mg/m^2; or (c) baseline resting ejection fraction of <50%. Based on their observations criteria have been proposed for monitoring resting radionuclide ejection fraction and discontinuing doxorubicin therapy.[69]

RADIONUCLIDES IN THE ASSESSMENT OF IMPAIRED RV FUNCTION

The location and complex geometry of the RV make it a

difficult chamber to image by any technique. The right ventricle is a thin-walled chamber which lies beneath the sternum and anterior to the dominant LV. While the shape of the normal left ventricle is approximately a prolate ellipse the shape of the normal RV varies in individuals and does not conform to a simple geometric model.[70] Ultrasound techniques are limited by poor acoustic windows and comprehensive, quantitative information about the RV can seldom be obtained by echocardiography.[71] Invasive angiography can be used to assess RV function but practical considerations and the lack of a suitable geometric model makes it impractical for routine clinical use.[72,73] Magnetic resonance imaging (MRI) assesses RV volumes and function accurately without the need for geometric assumptions.[74] Unfortunately, it requires special expertise and is not widely available.

Radionuclide methods for assessing the RV have been reported by several investigators. Acceptable images can be obtained in most patients and no geometric assumptions are required to obtain the RV ejection fraction.[73] Both first pass and gated equilibrium techniques have been applied to the RV but first pass techniques are best suited to the assessment of RV function. The shallow right anterior oblique view minimizes the effects of chamber overlap but accurate measurements depend delivery of a tight bolus of the tracer into the circulation. In non-gated first pass studies count density is low since only a limited number of cardiac cycles are available for analysis. However, RV ejection fraction using the non-gated first pass technique agrees well with contrast ventriculography.[75,76] A gated first pass technique sums the data from several cardiac cycles so that count density is increased. Multi-crystal cameras improve the ability to assess RV function using first pass techniques (Fig. 97.11). Another limitation of first pass techniques is that the long half-life of standard tracers precludes repeated studies to assess the effects of exercise or pharmacological stress on RV function.

The gated equilibrium technique provides a much higher count density for imaging the normal and abnormal RV (Figs 97.12 and 97.13). However, this technique is limited by overlap from the LV in the anterior projection and the RA in the left anterior oblique view. A shallow right anterior oblique projection seems to provide the best chamber separation for assessing the RV. Several methods for calculating RV ejection fraction using the gated equilibrium technique have been described and correlated with biplane cine-angiography and first pass techniques.[76-78] Because of the lack of a gold standard the 'true' RV ejection fraction remains unknown.[79] MRI techniques have been touted as providing a gold standard but a comparison of MRI methods and radionuclide methods has not yet been described.

A limitation of radionuclide techniques in the assessment of the RV is that they can only easily measure RV systolic and diastolic parameters. Radionuclide techniques do not allow assessment of wall thickness, pulmonary artery pressures or the position and shape of the interventricular septum. Each of these parameters can be of importance in determining the functional status of the right heart.

The following discussion will focus on the identification of impaired RV function in several clinical situations.

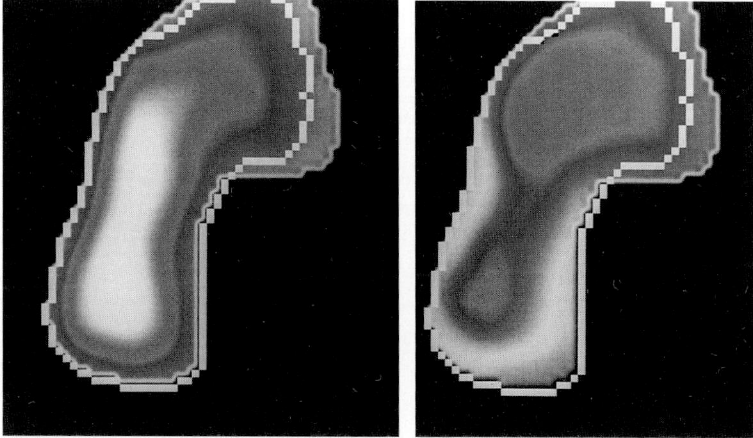

Fig. 97.11 First pass radionuclide angiogram acquired with a multi-crystal camera in a patient with well-preserved right ventricular (RV) systolic function. The left hand panel displays an outline of the RV region of interest superimposed on the RV end-diastolic image. The right hand panel displays the end-diastolic region of interest superimposed on the end-systolic image. Ejection fraction is 48%.

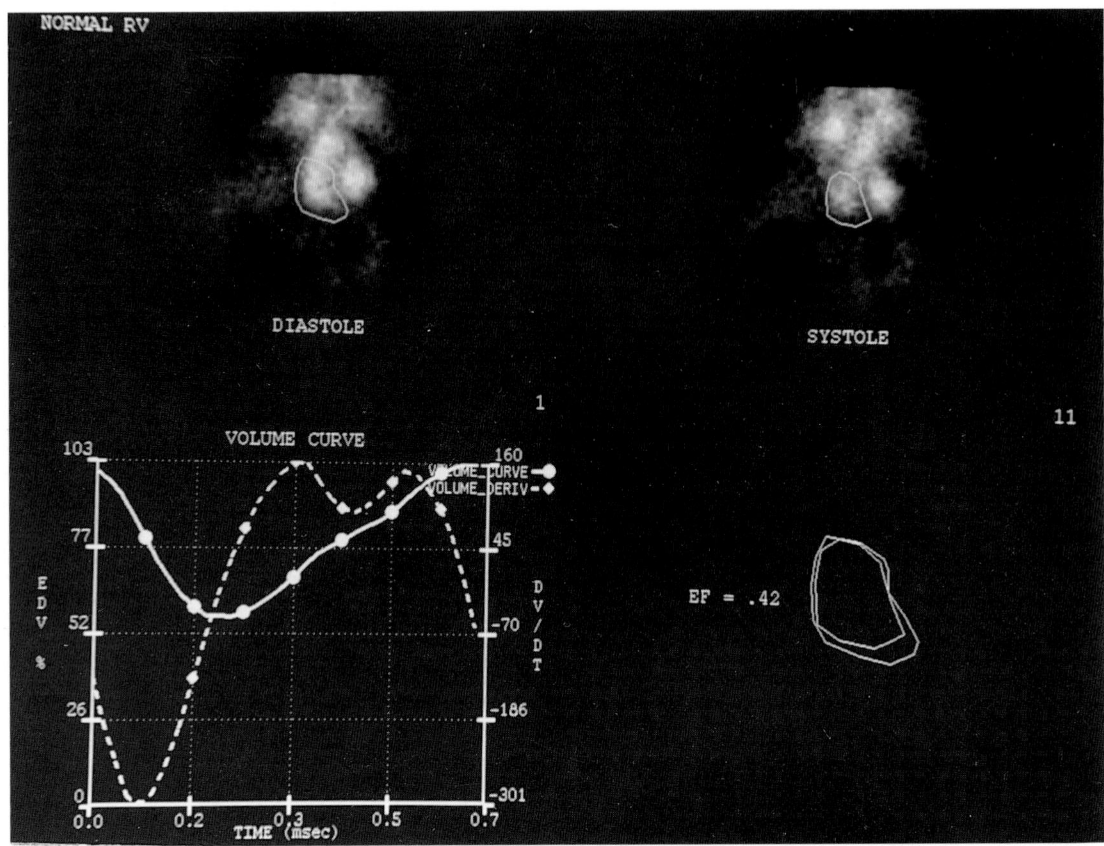

Fig. 97.12 Gated equilibrium blood pool scan in a patient with normal right ventricular (RV) systolic function. As can be appreciated from the end-diastolic and end-systolic phases in the left anterior oblique projection, it can be difficult to separate the RV from adjacent cardiac chambers.

RV function in patients with acute inferior myocardial infarction

The RV is predominantly supplied by the right coronary artery, and most patients with clinically detectable RV infarction have proximal occlusion in this vessel. Based on ECG findings, imaging studies and autopsy series, over one-third of patients with acute inferior myocardial infarction have associated RV infarction.[80] In a recent study by Zehender et al[81] patients with RV involvement, defined as ST-segment elevation in lead V_{4R}, had an in-hospital mortality of 31% versus 6% in patients without evidence of RV involvement.[81] Major complications were also increased in the group with RV involvement. Accordingly, the comprehensive radionuclide angiography evaluation of patients with acute inferior MI should include an assessment of RV as well as LV function.[82,83]

Despite the adverse prognosis of RV infarction acutely, RV systolic function may recover in the following months. Dell'Italia et al[84] used radionuclide angiography and respiratory gas exchange to study patients with RV myocardial infarction at rest and with upright exercise at least one year after their initial event. The RV ejection fraction increased significantly in these patients from 41 ± 10% to 47 ± 12% ($P<0.001$). The direction of change correlated with LV ejection fraction and the only deviations occurred in patients with abnormal pulmonary function.

RV function in patients with chronic ischaemic heart disease

The exercise response of the RV has been variable in patients with chronic coronary artery disease. Johnson et al[85] reported an increase of RV ejection fraction from 49 ± 6% to 58 ± 9% in patients with coronary disease not involving the proximal right coronary. This increase occurred despite a decrease in LV ejection fraction with exercise. In patients with disease involving the proximal right coronary artery, exercise ejection fraction may either decrease or remain unchanged.[85,86] Other investigators have reported no change in the RV ejection fraction between rest and exercise irrespective of the presence of right coronary artery disease.[87] Intuitively, determined by the RV response to exercise is a complex

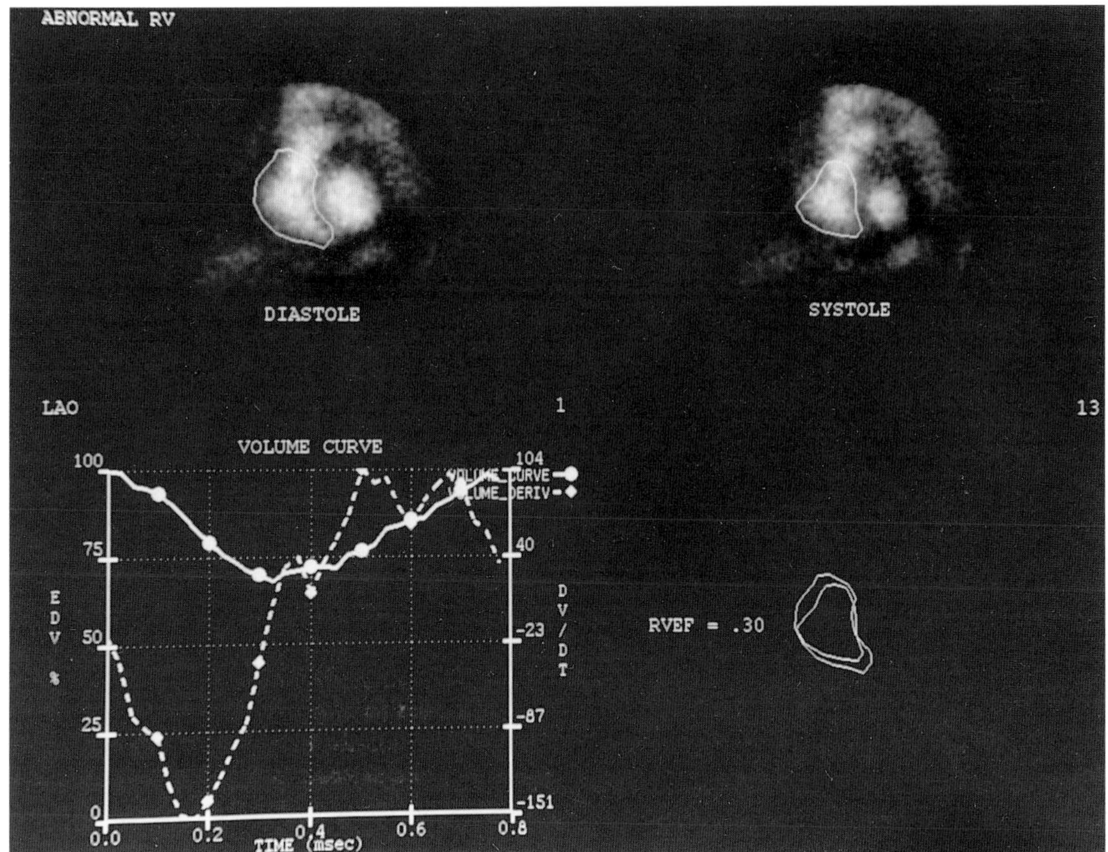

Fig. 97.13 Gated equilibrium blood pool scan in a patient with abnormal right ventricular (RV) systolic dysfunction. The RV volumes are increased and systolic function globally depressed.

interplay of systemic venous return, inducible RV ischaemia, dynamic pulmonary pressure, and changes in chamber volume mediated by ventricular interdependence.

RV function in patients with pulmonary heart disease

Radionuclide ventriculography can be used to assess RV function in patients with pulmonary heart disease.[88,89] The normally thin-walled RV chamber is accustomed to emptying into a low pressure pulmonary circulation. In patients with either primary or secondary pulmonary hypertension, RV afterload (wall stress) is increased and is inversely correlated with RV ejection fraction.[90,91] Acute afterload mismatch of the RV, as occurs with massive pulmonary embolism, can lead to RV failure and rapid death. Slowly progressive increases in pulmonary pressure permit RV adaptation by increasing wall thickness or chamber volume to preserve RV output.

In a study by Berger et al[92] RV ejection fraction was assessed in patients with chronic obstructive pulmonary disease (COPD) using a first pass technique. 19 of 36 patients had a reduced RV ejection fraction with 10 of the 19 having overt cor pulmonale. Importantly, there was a higher likelihood of developing clinical decompensation within the following year in those patients with a reduced ejection fraction.

Using a first pass technique and a multi-crystal camera, Brent et al[93] performed simultaneous measurements of RV ejection fraction and pulmonary artery pressure in 30 patients with COPD (Fig. 97.14). In their laboratory, an RV ejection fraction of <40% had a sensitivity of 75%, specificity of 100%, and positive predictive value of 100% for identifying patients with an elevated mean pulmonary artery pressure.[93]

RV function in patients with congenital heart disease

Assessment of RV function is important in many forms of congenital heart disease. In left-to-right shunt lesions pulmonary artery pressures are increased and may impair RV systolic function. In some situations (i.e. transposition of the great arteries) the morphological RV must perform as the systemic ventricle and eject blood against the high resistance of the systemic circulation. Radionuclide angiography has been validated against cine-angiography in children with a variety of congenital lesions.[94] The ability to follow these patients serially is an important

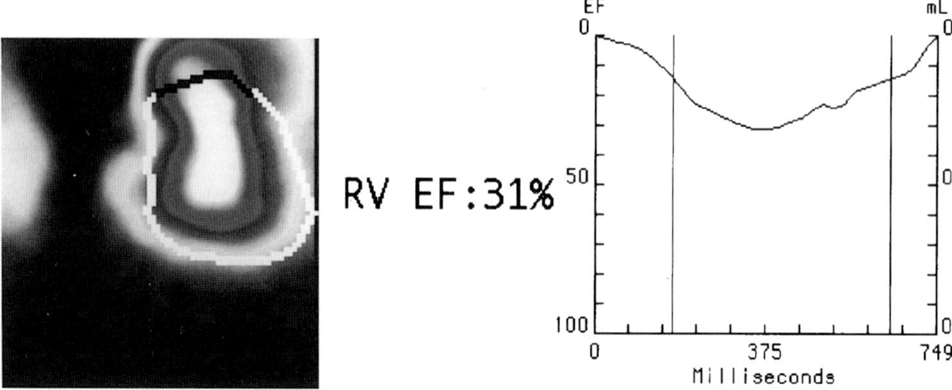

Fig. 97.14 First pass radionuclide angiography in a patient with abnormal right ventricular (RV) systolic function. The left hand panel displays the right ventricular region of interest superimposed on the RV end-systolic image. The RV ejection fraction curve demonstrates a reduced RV ejection fraction of 31%.

advantage, particularly in the increasing population of adult patients who have undergone corrective or palliative surgical procedures.

RV function in patients with LV failure

In clinical practice right heart failure is most commonly seen in association with left heart failure. Intrinsic muscle disease (cardiomyopathy) can affect both ventricles, or RV systolic dysfunction can occur as the result of passively elevated pulmonary pressures from LV dysfunction. Alternatively, LV function can be influenced by RV function through ventricular interdependence.[95] There is provocative evidence that both prognosis and exercise capacity in patients with congestive heart failure may be closely linked to RV function.[3,96,97]

Using equilibrium radionuclide angiography in combination with other invasive and non-invasive techniques, Hochreiter et al[61] studied 53 patients with chronic, severe mitral regurgitation. In this study, symptom status at entry correlated best with resting RV ejection fraction and left atrial size, while treadmill exercise performance in these patients correlated best with RV ejection fraction during exercise. RV ejection fraction was of significant prognostic value in medically treated patients with all deaths occurring in patients with an RV ejection fraction ≤30% and LV ejection fraction ≤45%. Similarly, Polack and co-workers have provided data demonstrating the prognostic value of the radionuclide-derived RV ejection fraction in patients with coronary artery disease.[98] The mechanisms responsible for these observations are unclear. However, these data underscore the important influence of RV function on determining prognosis in diseases that are often considered left heart lesions in isolation.

SUMMARY

Radionuclide-based methods have contributed greatly to our understanding of both RV and LV performance in many disease states. The development of new tracers and refinements which facilitate continuous monitoring of ventricular function should continue to make radionuclide techniques invaluable in the clinical management of patients with impaired ventricular function.

REFERENCES

1. Strauss H W, Zaret B L, Hurley P J et al 1971 A scintiphotographic method for measuring left ventricular ejection fraction in man without cardiac catheterization. Am J Cardiol 28: 575–580
2. Zaret B L, Strauss H W, Hurley P J et al 1971 A noninvasive scintiphotographic method for detecting regional ventricular dysfunction in man. N Engl J Med 284: 1165–1170
3. Dell'Italia L J, Freeman G L, Gaasch W H 1993 Cardiac function and functional capacity: Implications for the failing heart. Curr Prob Cardiol 18: 705–760
4. Ross J Jr 1976 Afterload mismatch and preload reserve: a conceptual framework for the analysis of ventricular function. Prog Cardiovasc Dis 18: 255–264
5. Sagawa K, Maughan W L, Suga H, Sunagawa K 1988 Cardiac contraction and the pressure–volume relationship. Oxford University Press, New York.
6. Kass D A, Maughan W L 1988 From 'Emax' to pressure–volume relations: a broader view. Circulation 77: 1203–1212
7. Carabello B A 1989 Ratio of end-systolic stress to end-systolic volume: is it a useful clinical tool? J Am Coll Cardiol 14: 496–498
8. Magorien D J, Shaffer P, Bush C A et al 1983 Assessment of left ventricular pressure–volume relations using gated radionuclide angiography, echocardiography and micromanometer pressure records. Circulation 67: 844–853
9. Starling M R, Dell'Italia L I, Walsh R A et al 1984 Accurate estimates of absolute left ventricular volumes in gated equilibrium radionuclide angiographic counts data using a simple geometric attenuation correction. J Am Coll Cardiol 3: 789–798
10. Links J M, Becker L C, Shindledecker J G et al 1982 Measurement of absolute left ventricular volume from gated blood pool studies. Circulation 65: 82–91
11. Massardo T, Gal R A, Grenier R P et al 1990 Left ventricular

volume calculation using a count-based ratio method applied to multigated radionuclide angiography. J Nucl Med 31: 450–456
12. Levy W C, Cerqueira M D, Matsuoka D T, Harp G D, Sheehan F H, Stratton J R 1992 Four radionuclide methods for left ventricular volume determination: comparison of a manual and an automated technique. J Nucl Med 33: 763–770
13. Upton M T, Rerych S K, Newman G E, Bounous E P, Jones R H 1980 The reproducibility of radionuclide angiographic measurements of left ventricular function in normal subjects at rest and during exercise. Circulation 62: 126–132
14. Marshall R C, Berger H J, Reduto L A, Gottschalk A, Zaret B L 1978 Variability in sequential measures of left ventricular performance assessed with radionuclide angiocardiography. Am J Cardiol 41: 531–536
15. Zaret B L, Wackers F J 1993 Nuclear cardiology (second of two parts). New Engl J Med 329: 855–863
16. Soufer R, Wohlgelernter D, Vita N A et al 1985 Intact systolic left ventricular function in clinical congestive heart failure. Am J Cardiol 55: 1032–1036
17. Setaro J F, Soufer R, Remetz M S, Perlmutter R A, Zaret B L 1992 Long-term outcome in patients with congestive heart failure and intact systolic left ventricular performance. Am J Cardiol 69: 1212–1216
18. Bonow R O, Bacharach S L, Green M V et al 1981 Impaired left ventricular diastolic filling in patients with coronary artery disease: assessment with radionuclide angiography. Circulation 64: 315–323
19. Mancini G B J, Slutsky R A, Norris S L, Bhargava V, Ashburn W L, Higgins C B 1983 Radionuclide analysis of peak filling rate, filling fraction, and time to peak filling rate. Response to supine bicycle exercise in normal subjects and patients with coronary disease. Am J Cardiol 51: 43–51
20. Inouye S. Massie B, Loge D, Topic N, Silverstein D, Simpson P et al 1984 Abnormal left ventricular filling: an early finding in mild to moderate systemic hypertension. Am J Cardiol 53: 120–126
21. Iskandrian A S, Hakki A 1986 Age-related changes in left ventricular diastolic performance. Am Heart J 112: 75–78
22. Miller T R, Grossman S J, Schectman K B et al 1986 Left ventricular diastolic filling and its association with age. Am J Cardiol 58: 531–535
23. de Yang L, Bairey C N, Berman D S, Nichols K J, Odom-Maryon T, Rozanski A 1991 Accuracy and reproducibility of left ventricular ejection fraction measurements using an ambulatory radionuclide left ventricular function monitor. J Nucl Med 32: 796–802
24. Kayden D S, Wackers F J, Zaret B L 1990 Silent left ventricular dysfunction during routine activity after thrombolytic therapy for acute myocardial infarction. J Am Coll Cardiol 15: 1500–1507
25. Tamaki N, Yasuda T, Moore R et al 1988 Continuous monitoring of left ventricular function by an ambulatory radionuclide detector in patients with coronary artery disease. J Am Coll Cardiol 12: 669–679
26. Burg M M, Jain D D, Soufer R, Kerns R D, Zaret B L 1993 Role of behavioral and psychological factors in mental stress-induced silent left ventricular dysfunction in coronary artery disease. J Am Coll Cardiol 22: 440–448
27. Broadhurst P, Cashman P, Crawley J et al 1991 Clinical validation of a miniature nuclear probe systems for continuous on-line monitoring of cardiac function and ST-segment. J Nucl Med 32: 37–43
28. Boucher C A, Zir L M, Beller G A, Okada R D, McKusick K A, Strauss H W, Pohost G M 1980 Increased lung uptake of thallium-201 during exercise myocardial imaging: clinical, hemodynamic and angiographic implications in patients with coronary artery disease. Am J Cardiol 46: 189–196
29. Kushner F G, Okada R D, Kirshenbaum H D, Boucher C A, Strauss H W, Pohost G M 1981 Lung thallium-201 uptake after stress testing in patients with coronary artery disease. Circulation 63: 341–347
30. Gill J B, Ruddy T D, Newell J B, Finkelstein D M, Strauss H W, Boucher C A 1987 Prognostic importance of thallium uptake by the lungs during exercise in coronary artery disease. N Engl J Med 317: 1485–1489
31. Gibbons R J, Holmes D R, Reeder G S, Bailey K R, Hopfenspirger M R, Gersh B J 1993 Immediate angioplasty compared with the administration of a thrombolytic agent followed by conservative treatment for myocardial infarction. N Engl J Med 328: 685–691
32. Gibbons R J, Verani M S, Behrenbeck T et al 1989 Feasibility of tomographic technetium-99m-hexakis-2-methylpropyl-isonitrile imaging for the assessment of myocardial area at risk and efficacy of thrombolytic therapy in acute myocardial infarction. Circulation 80: 1277–1286
33. Christian T F, Behrenbeck T, Pelikka P A, Huber K C, Chesebro J H, Gibbons R D 1990 Mismatch of left ventricular function and infarct size demonstrated by technetium-99m isonitrile imaging after reperfusion therapy for acute myocardial infarction: identification of myocardial stunning and hyperkinesia. J Am Coll Cardiol 16: 1632–1638
34. Christian T F, Behrenbeck T, Gersh B J, Gibbons R J 1991 Relation of left ventricular volume and function over one year after acute myocardial infarction to infarct size determined by technetium-99m sestamibi. Am J Cardiol 68: 21–26
35. Borges-Neto S, Coleman R E, Jones R H 1990 Perfusion and function at rest and treadmill exercise using technetium-99-m-sestamibi: comparison of one- and two-day protocols in normal volunteers. J Nucl Med 31: 1128–1132
36. Iskandrian A S, Heo J, Kong B, Lyons E, Marsch S 1989 Use of technetium-99m isonitrile (RP-30A) in assessing left ventricular perfusion and function at rest and during exercise in coronary artery disease, and comparison with coronary arteriography and exercise thallium-201 SPECT imaging. Am J Cardiol 64: 270–275
37. Boucher C A, Wackers F J T, Zaret B L, Mena I G 1992 Technetium-99m sestamibi myocardial imaging at rest for assessment of myocardial infarction and first-pass ejection fraction. Am J Cardiol 69: 22–27
38. Reduto L A, Berger H J, Cohen L S, Gottschalk A, Zaret B L 1978 Sequential radionuclide assessment of left and right ventricular performance following acute transmural myocardial infarction. Ann Intern Med 89: 441–447
39. Ahnve S, Gilpin E, Henning H et al 1986 Limitations and advantages of the ejection fraction for defining high risk after acute myocardial infarction. Am J Cardiol 58: 872–878 (Erratum, Am J Cardiol 1987; 59: A12)
40. The Multicenter Postinfarction Research Group 1983 Risk stratification and survival after myocardial infarction. N Engl J Med 309: 331–336
41. Zaret B L, Wackers F J, Terrin M et al 1991 Does left ventricular ejection fraction following thrombolytic therapy have the same prognostic impact described in the pre-thrombolytic era? Results of the TIMI II trial. J Am Coll Cardiol 17 (Suppl A): 214A (abstract)
42. Meizlish J L, Berger H J, Plankey M, Errico D, Levy W, Zaret B L 1984 Functional left ventricular aneurysm formation after myocardial infarction: incidence, natural history, and prognostic implications. N Engl J Med 311: 1001–1006
43. Pfeffer M A, Braunwald E 1990 Ventricular remodelling after myocardial infarction: experimental observations and clinical implications. Circulation 81: 1161–1172
44. Pfeffer M A, Braunwald E, Moye L A et al 1992 Effect of captopril on mortality and morbidity in patients with left ventricular dysfunction after myocardial infarction: results of the Survival and Ventricular Enlargement Trial. N Engl J Med 327: 669–677
45. Borer J S, Kent K M, Bacharach S L et al 1979 Sensitivity, specificity and predictive accuracy of radionuclide cineangiography during exercise in patients with coronary artery disease: comparison with exercise electrocardiography. Circulation 60: 572–580
46. Dewhurst N G, Muir A L 1983 Comparative prognostic value of radionuclide ventriculography at rest and during exercise in 100 patients after first myocardial infarction. Br Heart J 49: 111–121
47. Gibbons R J, Fyke F E III, Clements I P et al 1988 Noninvasive identification of severe coronary artery disease using exercise radionuclide angiography. J Am Coll Cardiol 11: 28–34
48. Port S, Cobb F R, Coleman R E, Jones R H 1980 The effects of age on the response of the left ventricular ejection fraction to exercise. N Engl J Med 303: 1133–1137
49. Hanley P C, Zinsmeister A R, Clements I P, Bove A A, Brown M L, Gibbons R J 1989 Gender-related differences in cardiac response to supine exercise assessed by radionuclide angiography. J Am Coll Cardiol 13: 624–629

50. Higgenbotham M B, Morris K G, Coleman E, Cobb F R 1984 Sex-related differences in normal cardiac response to upright exercise. Circulation 70: 357–366
51. Morris E G, Palmeri S T, Califf R M et al 1985 Value of radionuclide angiography in predicting specific cardiac events after acute myocardial infarction. Am J Cardiol 55: 318–324
52. Nicod P, Corbett J R, Firth B G, Lewis S E, Rude R E, Huxley R, Willerson J T 1983 Prognostic valve of resting amd submaximal exercise radionuclide ventriculography after acute myocardial infarction in high risk patients with single and multivessel disease. Am J Cardiol 52: 30–36
53. Corbett J R, Dehmer G J, Lewis S E, Woodward W, Henderson E, Parkey R W, Blomqvist C G, Willerson J T 1981 The prognostic value of submaximal exercise testing with radionuclide ventriculography before hospital discharge in patients with recent myocardial infarction. Circulation 64: 535–544
54. Hung J, Goris M L, Nash E et al 1984 Comparative value of maximal treadmill testing, exercise thallium myocardial perfusion scintigraphy and exercise radionuclide ventriculography for distinguishing high- and low-risk patients soon after acute myocardial infarction. Am J Cardiol 53: 1221–1227
55. Abraham R D, Harris P G, Rubin G S et al 1987 Usefulness of ejection fraction response to exercise one month after acute myocardial infarction in predicting coronary anatomy and prognosis. Am J Cardiol 60: 225–230
56. Bonow R O, Kent K M, Rosing D R et al 1984 Exercise-induced ischemia in mildly symptomatic patients with coronary-artery disease and preserved left ventricular function: identification of subgroups at risk of death during medical therapy. N Engl J Med 311: 1339–1345
57. Taliercio C P, Clements I P, Zinmaster A R, Gibbons R J 1988 Prognostic value and limitations of exercise radionuclide angiography in medically treated patients with coronary artery disease. Mayo Clin Proc 63: 573–582
58. Bonow R O 1988 Prognostic implications of exercise radionuclide angiography in patients with coronary artery disease. Mayo Clin Proc 63: 630–634
59. Lee K L, Pryor D B, Pieper K S et al 1990 Prognostic value of radionuclide angiography in medically treated patients with coronary artery disease: A comparison with clinical and catheterization variables. Circulation 82: 1705–1717
60. Rigo P, Alderson P O, Robertson R M et al 1979 Mesurement of aortic and mitral regurgitation by gated cardiac blood pool scans. Circulation 60: 306
61. Hochtreiter C, Niles N, Devereux R B, Kligfield P, Borer J S 1986 Mitral regurgitation: relationship of noninvasive descriptors of right and left ventricular performance to clinical and hemodynamic findings and to prognosis in medically and surgically treated patients. Circulation 73: 900–912
62. Bonow R O, Picone A L, McIntosh C L et al 1984 Reversal of left ventricular dysfunction after aortic valve replacement for chronic aortic regurgitation: Influence of duration of properative left ventricular dysfunction. Circulation 70: 570
63. Boucher C A, Wilson R A, Kanarek D J et al 1983 Exercise testing in asymptomatic or minimally symptomatic aortic regurgitation: Relationship of left ventricular ejection fraction of left ventricular pressure during exercise. Circulation 67: 1091–1100
64. O'Rourke R A, Chatterjee K, Dodge H T et al 1986 Guidelines for clinical use of cardiac radionuclide imaging: a report of the ACC/AHA task force on assessment of cardiovascular procedures. J Am Coll Cardiol 8: 1471–1483
65. Greenberg J M, Hurphy J H, Okada R D, Pohost G M, Strauss H W, Boucher C A 1985 Value and limitations of radionuclide angiography in determining the cause of reduced left ventricular ejection fraction: comparison of idiopathic dilated cardiomyopathy and coronary artery disease. Am J Cardiol 55: 541–544
66. Glamann D B, Lange R A, Corbett J R, Hillis L D 1992 Utility of various radionuclide techniques for distinguishing ischemic from nonischemic dilated cardiomyopathy. Arch Intern Med 152: 769–772
67. Pohost G M, Vignola P A, McKusik K E et al 1977 Hypertrophic cardiomyopathy: evaluation by gated blood pool scanning. Circulation 55: 92–99
68. Aroney C N, Ruddy T D, Dighero II, Fifer M A, Boucher C A, Palacious II 1989 Differentiation of restrictive cardiomyopathy from pericardial constriction: assessment of diastolic function by radionuclide angiography. J Am Coll Cardiol 13: 1007–1014
69. Schwartz R G, McKenzie W B, Alexander J et al 1987 Congestive heart failure and left ventricular dysfunction complicating doxorubicin therapy: seven-year experience using serial radionuclide angiocardiography. Am J Med 82: 1109–1118
70. Dell'Italia L J 1991 The right ventricle: anatomy, physiology, and clinical importance. Curr Prob Cardiol 16: 655–720
71. Kaul S, Tei C, Hopkins J M, Shah P M 1984 Assessment of right ventricular function using two-dimensional echocardiography. Am Heart J 107: 526–531
72. Dell'Italia L J, Starling M R, Walsh R A et al 1985 Validation of attenuation-corrected equilibrium radionuclide angiographic determinations of right ventricular volume: comparison with cast-validated biplane cineventriculography. Circulation 72: 317–326
73. Pietras R J, Kondos G T, Kaplan D, Lam W 1985 Comparative angiographic right and left ventricular volumes. Am Heart J 109: 321–326
74. Sechtem U, Pflugfelder P W, Gould R G, Cassidy M M, Higgins C B 1987 Measurement of right and left ventricular volumes in healthy individuals with cine MR imaging. Radiology 163: 697–702
75. Steele P, Kirch D, LeFree M 1976 Measurement of right and left ventricular ejection fractions by radionuclide angiography in coronary artery disease. Chest 70: 51–56
76. Morrison D A, Turgeon J, Ovitt T 1984 Right ventricular ejection fraction measurement: constrast ventriculography versus gated blood pool and gated first-pass radionuclide methods. Am J Cardiol 54: 651–653
77. Maddahi J, Berman D S, Matsuoka D T 1979 A new technique for assessing right ventricular ejection fraction using rapid multi-gated equilibrium cardiac blood pool scintigraphy. Circulation 60: 581–589
78. Holman B L, Wynne J, Zielonka J S et al 1981 A simplified technique for measuring right ventricular ejection fraction using the equilibrium radionuclide angiocardiogram and the slant-hole collimator. Radiology 138: 429–435
79. Marving J, Hoilund-Carlsen P F, Chraemmer-Jorgensen B, Gadsboll N 1985 Are right and left ventricular ejection fractions equal? Ejection fractions in normal subjects and patients with first acute myocardial infarction. Circulation 72: 502–514
80. Wellens H J J 1993 Right ventricular infarction. N Engl J Med 328: 1036–1038
81. Zehender M, Kasper W, Kauder E, Schonthaler M, Geibel A, Olschewski M, Just H 1993 Right ventricular infarction as an independent predictor of prognosis after acute inferior myocardial infarction. N Engl J Med 328: 981–988
82. Dell'Italia L J, Starling M R, Blumhardt R, Lasher J C, O'Rourke R A 1985 Comparative effects of volume loading, dobutamine, and nitroprusside in patients with predominant right ventricular infarction. Circulation 72: 1327–1335
83. Shah P K, Maddahi J, Berman D S, Pichler M, Swan H J C 1985 Scintigraphically detected predominant right ventricular dysfunction in acute myocardial infarction: clinical and hemodynamic correlates and implications for therapy and prognosis. J Am Coll Cardiol 6: 1264–1272
84. Dell'Italia L J, Lembo N J, Starling M R et al 1987 Hemodynamically important right ventricular infarction: follow-up evaluation of right ventricular systolic function at rest and during exercise with radionuclide ventriculography and respiratory gas exchange. Circulation 75: 996–1003
85. Johnson L L, McCarthy D M, Sciacca R R, Cannon P J 1979 Right ventricular ejection fraction during exercise in patients with coronary artery disease. Circulation 60: 1284–1291
86. Maddahi J, Berman D S, Matsuoka D T et al 1980 Right ventricular ejection fraction during exercise in normal subjects and in coronary artery disease patients: assessment by multiple-gated equilibrium scintigraphy. Circulation 62: 133–140
87. Berger H J, Johnstone D E, Sands J M et al 1979 Response of right ventricular ejection fraction to upright bicycle exercise in coronary artery disease. Circulation 60: 1292–1300

88. Bourge R C, Briggs D D 1991 Pulmonary heart disease. In: Pohost G M and O'Rourke R A (eds) Principles and practice of cardiovascular imaging. Little, Brown and Co., Boston, pp 773–815
89. Matthay R A, Berger H J, Davies R A, Loke J, Mahler D A, Gottschalk A, Zaret B L 1980 Right and left ventricular exercise performance in chronic obstructive pulmonary disease: Radionuclide assessment. Ann Intern Med 93: 234–239
90. Brent B N, Berger H J, Matthay R A, Mahler D, Pytlik L, Zaret B L 1982 Physiologic correlates of right ventricular ejection fraction in chronic obstructive pulmonary disease: a combined radionuclide and hemodynamic study. Am J Cardiol 50: 255–262
91. Winzelberg G G, Boucher C A, Pohost G M, McKusick K A, Bingham J B, Okada R D, Strauss H W 1981 Right ventricular function in aortic and mitral valve disease. Relation of gated first-pass radionuclide angiography to clinical and hemodynamic findings. Chest 79: 520–528
92. Berger H J, Matthay R A, Loke J, Marshall R C, Gottschalk A, Zaret B L 1978 Assessment of cardiac performance with quantitative radionuclide angiocardiography: Right ventricular ejection fraction with reference to findings in chronic obstructive pulmonary disease. Am J Cardiol 41: 897–905
93. Brent B N, Mahler D, Matthay R A, Berger H J, Zaret B L 1984 Noninvasive diagnosis of pulmonary arterial hypertension in chronic obstructive pulmonary disease: right ventricular ejection fraction at rest. Am J Cardiol 53: 1349–1353
94. Parrish M D, Graham T P Jr, Born M L 1982 Radionuclide evaluation of right and left ventricular function in children: validation of methodology. Am J Cardiol 49: 1241–1247
95. Clyne C A, Alpert J S, Benotti J R 1989 Interdependence of the left and right ventricles in health and disease. Am Heart J 117: 1366–1374
96. Baker B J, Wilen M M, Boyd C M, Dinh H, Franciosa J A 1984 Relation of right ventricular ejection fraction to exercise capacity in chronic left ventricular failure. Am J Cardiol 54: 596–599
97. Lewis J F, Webber J D, Sutton L L, Chesoni S, Curry C L 1993 Discordance in degree of right and left ventricular dilation in patients with dilated cardiomyopathy: recognition and clinical implications. J Am Coll Cardiol 21: 649–654
98. Polack J F, Holman B L, Wynne J et al 1983 Right ventricular ejection fraction: an indicator of increased mortality in patients with congestive heart failure associated with coronary artery disease. J Am Coll Cardiol 2: 217–224

98. Assessment of myocardial viability in hibernating myocardium

Robert O. Bonow

INTRODUCTION

In a proportion of patients with chronic coronary artery disease and left ventricular dysfunction, left ventricular performance is reduced as a result of regionally ischaemic or hibernating myocardium rather than irreversibly infarcted myocardium. The identification of reversibly dysfunctional myocardium is clinically relevant, as regional and global left ventricular function in such patients will improve after revascularization.[1–5] Up to one-third of patients (Fig. 98.1) with chronic coronary artery disease and left ventricular dysfunction have the potential for significant improvement in ventricular function if accurately identified and revascularized.[6] However, the ability to detect patients with such potentially reversible left ventricular dysfunction is problematic and often can be made only after revascularization. This is inadequate in many high risk patients with left ventricular dysfunction, in whom the decision to revascularize may depend upon whether the myocardium within the territory to be revascularized is viable. Hence, accurate diagnostic techniques are required that can provide this information prospectively.

A number of clinically reliable physiological markers of viability can be employed in this diagnostic process. These include indexes of regional wall motion, regional systolic wall thickening, and regional coronary blood flow. These three latter indexes are helpful in identifying viable tissue if they are normal or near-normal. However, in patients with left ventricular dysfunction arising from viable but hibernating myocardium, by definition the hibernating regions have blood flow, wall motion, and wall thickening that are severely reduced or absent.[2–5] For this reason, radionuclide tracers that reflect intact cellular metabolic processes or cell membrane integrity have intrinsic advantages over indexes of function and blood flow. For over a decade, numerous studies have shown that nuclear cardiology techniques, involving positron emission tomography (PET) and single photon methods, provide critically important viability information in patients with left

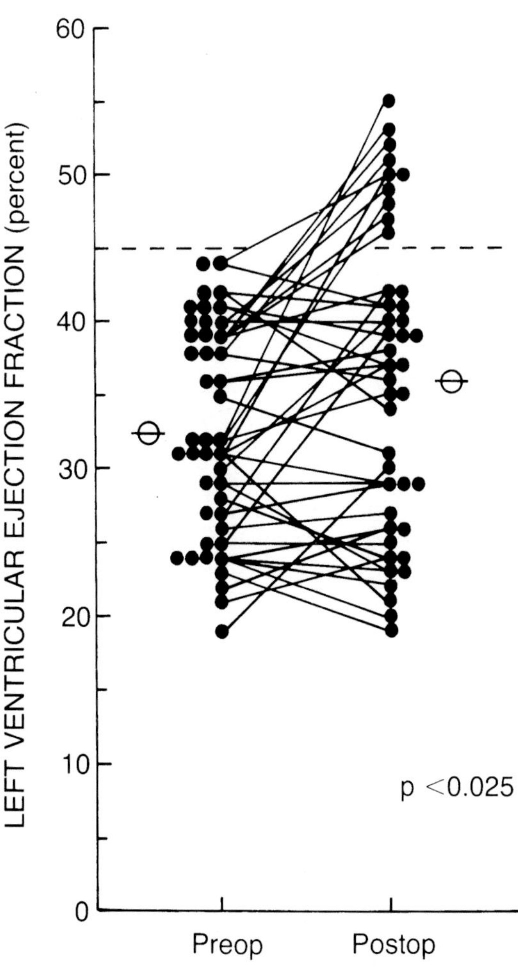

Fig. 98.1 Left ventricular ejection fraction at rest by radionuclide ventriculography before (Preop) and 6 months after (Postop) coronary artery bypass surgery in 43 patients with preoperative left ventricular dysfunction. The dashed line at 45% indicates the lower limit of normal resting ejection fraction for our laboratory. Although operation resulted in only a small increase in mean ejection fraction, substantial increases in ejection fraction were observed in 15 patients (35%), and postoperative ejection fraction was normal in 10 patients (23%). Reproduced[6] with permission of the W. B. Saunders Company.

ventricular dysfunction. This chapter will review the applications of nuclear cardiac procedures that have evolved over the past decade for the assessment of myocardial viability.

POSITRON EMISSION TOMOGRAPHY

PET has emerged as a very promising method for demonstrating viable myocardium in patients with compromised left ventricular function.[7,8] Although a number of PET methods have been developed to assess myocardial viability, the greatest experience and the greatest validation has been achieved in studies to assess whether metabolic activity is preserved in regions of severely underperfused and dysfunctional myocardium. For this purpose, ^{18}F deoxyglucose (^{18}FDG) has been employed as a marker of regional exogenous glucose utilization in such hypoperfused regions[9–15], and ^{11}C acetate has been employed as a marker of oxidative metabolism.[16] The larger cumulative patient experience thus far has been reported using ^{18}FDG. In particular, a pattern of enhanced ^{18}FDG uptake in regions with reduced perfusion (termed the ^{18}FDG–blood flow 'mismatch') indicates ischaemic or hibernating myocardium that has preferentially shifted its metabolic substrate toward glucose rather than fatty acids or lactate.[10–15] The finding of preserved metabolic activity in myocardial regions with reduced blood flow has been demonstrated in several studies to be an accurate clinical marker with which to distinguish hibernating myocardium from myocardial fibrosis, with positive and negative predictive accuracies in the range of 85% for identifying regions that will manifest improved function after revascularization.[11,16–19] The identification of viable myocardium with ^{18}FDG–blood flow mismatch has been shown in several clinical studies to be predictive of improved global left ventricular ejection fraction,[11,17,18,20] improved heart failure symptoms,[21] and improved survival after revascularization.[22–24] Thus, PET appears to yield excellent, clinically relevant viability information.

More recently, identification of preserved oxidative metabolism, using PET imaging with ^{11}C acetate, has also been shown to be an accurate marker for viable myocardium in patients with left ventricular dysfunction and for predicting recovery of regional left ventricular function after revascularization.[16] Other PET methods for assessing myocardial viability include the use of ^{15}O water to determine the amount of perfusable tissue within dysfunctional myocardial segments[25,26] and the analysis of ^{82}Rb uptake and washout kinetics in regions with impaired systolic function.[27] All three of these PET applications have thus far been employed in only small numbers of patients and will require greater clinical experience before being recommended for routine purposes.

RATIONALE FOR THALLIUM IMAGING TO ASSESS VIABILITY

The requirements for cellular viability include, among other processes, intact sarcolemmal function to maintain electrochemical gradients across the cell membrane, as well as preserved metabolic activity to generate high energy phosphates. These processes also require adequate myocardial blood flow both to deliver substrates and to wash out the metabolites of the metabolic processes. In terms of glucose utilization, lactate and hydrogen are metabolic byproducts of glycolysis which will inhibit glycolytic enzymes if they accumulate intracellularly,[28,29] leading to inability to generate high energy phosphates, cell membrane disruption, and cell death. As the retention of ^{201}Tl is an active process that is a function of cell viability and cell membrane activity, as well as blood flow, ^{201}Tl should in theory be delivered and retained by myocardial regions that also receive and retain ^{18}FDG and other metabolic tracers.

THALLIUM REDISTRIBUTION AS A MARKER OF VIABILITY

A large number of patients with coronary artery disease and dysfunctional but viable myocardium develop reversible ischaemia during exercise in regions with contractile dysfunction. Myocardial regions that are precariously balanced with reduction in flow sufficient to cause contractile dysfunction at rest are likely to become ischaemic with exercise. Hence, the majority of these regions will manifest reversible thallium perfusion defects using a standard exercise–redistribution imaging protocol (Fig. 98.2). By demonstrating ischaemic myocardium with a reversible thallium defect, an exercise–redistribution thallium study also indicates that the dysfunctional myocardium is viable, with the potential for substantial improvement in function after revascularization. However, many regions of severely ischaemic or hiber-

Exercise

Redistribution

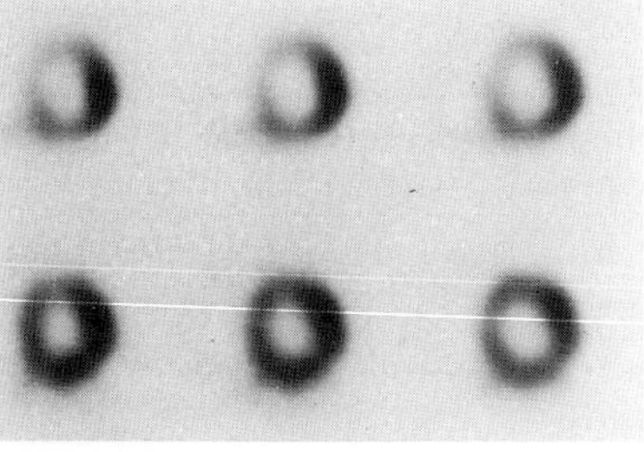

Fig. 98.2 Inducible myocardial ischaemia with reversible thallium defects in a patient with multivessel coronary artery disease, left ventricular dysfunction, and severe anteroseptal hypokinesia at rest. Exercise-induced perfusion defects in the anteroseptal and inferior regions redistribute substantially at 3–4 h. This identifies the dysfunctional anteroseptal territory as representing viable myocardium with the potential for improvement in function after revascularization.

nating myocardium appear to have irreversible thallium defects on standard exercise–redistribution imaging. It has been shown that up to 50% of regions with 'irreversible' thallium defects will improve in function after revascularization.[30–34] Thus, although the positive value of a reversible defect in predicting viable myocardium is quite high, the negative predictive value of a persistent defect is disappointingly low. It has therefore become apparent that standard thallium scintigraphy may not provide satisfactory precision in differentiating between left ventricular dysfunction arising from infarcted versus hibernating myocardium.

This has also been shown to be the case in studies directly comparing the results of regional ^{18}FDG uptake by PET and standard exercise–redistribution thallium imaging. In four initial comparative studies,[35–38] between 38% and 47% of apparently 'irreversible' thallium defects (that would have been identified as scar by standard thallium imaging) were identified as viable on the basis of ^{18}FDG uptake. Although these data suggest that metabolic imaging using PET may be superior to thallium imaging in the detection of viable myocardium, two limitations of these early studies must be emphasized. First, the severity of the reduction in thallium activity within the 'irreversible' thallium defects was not assessed. The thallium studies were interpreted as showing a defect or no defect, with no consideration for the thallium activity within the defect. This has important implications, as the magnitude of reduction in thallium activity within an irreversible defect is itself an index of viability (Fig. 98.3). In two studies comparing ^{201}Tl SPECT imaging and ^{18}FDG imaging with PET, metabolic activity indicative of viability was reported in the large majority of 'irreversible' thallium defects in which the reduction in thallium activity was only mild, but ^{18}FDG uptake was very uncommon in persistent thallium defects that were severe.[39,41] Second, the initial comparative studies of thallium scintigraphy and PET all performed post-exercise thallium imaging followed by a single redistribution study 3 to 4 h later. Recently, alternative imaging protocols have enhanced the ability of thallium imaging to detect viable myocardium.

LATE THALLIUM REDISTRIBUTION IMAGING

It has now become well established that late imaging at 8–72 h will demonstrate substantial thallium redistribution in many defects that appear to be irreversible at 3–4 h, and that this late thallium uptake is consistent with viable myocardium.[33,42–44] The number of 'irreversible' defects at 3–4 h that subsequently show reversal on late imaging (22–54%) is in some studies similar to the frequency of metabolic activity that has been demonstrated by PET studies in such apparently irreversible thallium defects. It is important to note that, although a greater number of thallium defects are shown to be reversible when late redistribution imaging is performed, the overall results of late imaging are similar to those of 3–4 h redistribution imaging. That is, the positive value of late redistribution in predicting improvement after revascularization is high (>90%),[43] but the negative predictive value of a persistent defect remains low. Roughly 50% of such defects manifest metabolic activity by PET imaging,[41] 37% improve after revascularization,[43] and 39% show enhanced relative thallium activity when thallium is reinjected at rest after completion of the 24 h study demonstrating the persistent

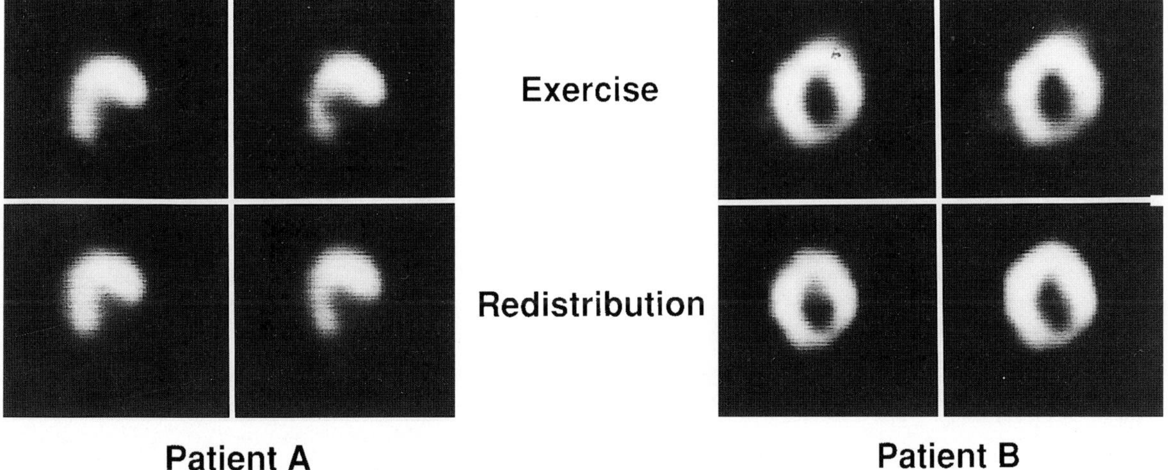

Fig. 98.3 Short axis thallium SPECT images in two patients with irreversible thallium defects involving the inferolateral region of the left ventricle. Two tomographic levels are shown for each patient. The greater severity of the persistent thallium defect in Patient A indicates a greater likelihood of irreversible myocardial damage than in Patient B, in whom the defect is only mild to moderate in severity. Thallium uptake within the defect in Patient B, reflecting adequate perfusion and intact sarcolemmal function, indicates myocardial viability.

defect.[45] Hence, it is apparent that a sizeable percentage of dysfunctional but viable myocardial segments will not demonstrate redistribution after a stress thallium study, no matter how lengthy the redistribution period.

THALLIUM REINJECTION TECHNIQUES

The reinjection of thallium at rest immediately after the standard 3–4 h redistribution image[46–48] or after a late 24 h redistribution image[45] appears to provide excellent viability information in patients with apparently irreversible thallium defects on redistribution images (Fig. 98.4). The reinjection approach surpasses the capacity of either early or late redistribution imaging for detecting viable myocardium. Thallium reinjection facilitates late uptake of thallium in viable regions with apparently irreversible defects and may be used to distinguish between viable and infarcted myocardium. Up to 49% of 'irreversible' defects on 4 h redistribution studies demonstrate improved or normal uptake after thallium reinjection.[46] Studies have also assessed whether additional redistribution of the reinjected thallium dose at 24 h provides further information. Only rarely (roughly 3% of regions) do myocardial regions without thallium uptake on images obtained immediately after reinjection show evidence of late thallium redistribution.[49] Thus, thallium reinjection at rest after 4 h redistribution provides most of the clinically relevant information pertaining to myocardial viability in regions with apparently 'irreversible' thallium defects.

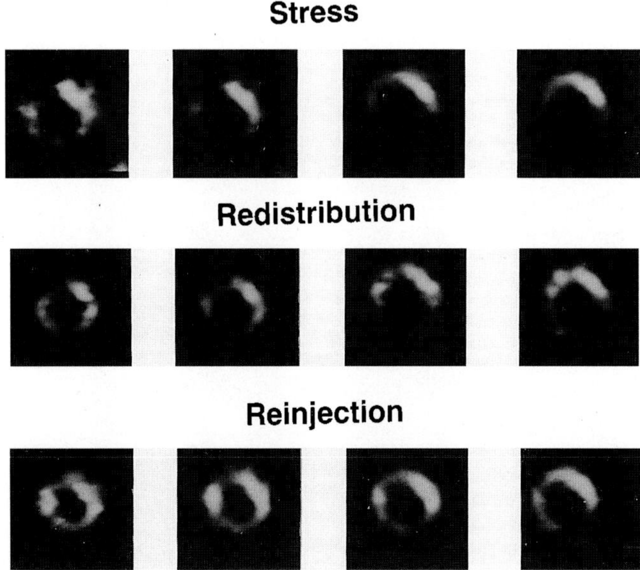

Fig. 98.4 Effects of thallium reinjection. Short axis thallium SPECT images after exercise show extensive abnormalities in anterior, septal, inferior and inferolateral perfusion. The septal defect partially reverses on 4 h redistribution images but the other defects persist. All regions improve substantially after reinjection, with the exception only of the inferolateral wall, which remains irreversible. Reproduced[6] with permission of the W. B. Saunders Company.

Thallium reinjection may be used instead of 24 h imaging in the majority of patients in whom a persistent thallium defect is observed on conventional redistribution images.

That the uptake of thallium after reinjection represents hibernating myocardium is substantiated in three subgroups of patients. First, in three studies of patients with apparently irreversible defects at 3–4 h, the positive and negative predictive accuracies of thallium reinjection for improved wall motion after revascularization has been >85%,[33,46,50] similar to those reported using metabolic PET imaging. Second, in patients with chronic coronary artery disease and left ventricular dysfunction who were also studied by PET imaging with ^{18}FDG, the majority of segments with thallium defects identified as viable by reinjection had ^{18}FDG uptake (Fig. 98.5), and hence metabolic evidence for myocardial viability.[34,39] The concordance between the thallium reinjection and ^{18}FDG uptake data is excellent, with 51% of regions with severe 'irreversible' thallium defects on 4 h redistribution studies identified as viable by both techniques.[39] Third, in patients studied by gated magnetic resonance imaging to assess regional systolic function, an excellent correlation has been observed between regional thallium activity and ^{18}FDG activity in myocardial regions with severely reduced or absent wall thickening.[40]

These latter PET data are in keeping with previous studies indicating that up to 50% of regions with 'irreversible' thallium defects have evidence of metabolic activity and thus viability by PET. This data also indicates that thallium reinjection is a convenient, clinically accurate, and relatively inexpensive method with which to identify viable myocardium in patients with chronic coronary artery disease and left ventricular dysfunction.

REST–REDISTRIBUTION THALLIUM IMAGING

The demonstration of exercise-induced ischaemia in a patient with left ventricular dysfunction has important prognostic implications that under most conditions identifies that patient as a candidate for revascularization therapy. This is especially the case in patients with left ventricular dysfunction, in whom evidence of inducible ischaemia superimposed on impaired left ventricular function at rest identifies a subgroup of patients at considerable risk of death during medical therapy. Thus, exercise–redistribution–reinjection thallium protocols are attractive, as they provide important information regarding both jeopardized myocardium and viable myocardium. However, in many patients, the sole clinical issue to be addressed may be the viability of one or more left ventricular regions with systolic dysfunction, and not whether there is also inducible ischaemia. In such patients, rest–redistribution thallium imaging is a practical approach that can yield accurate viability data. It is essential to obtain not only initial images (indicating regional

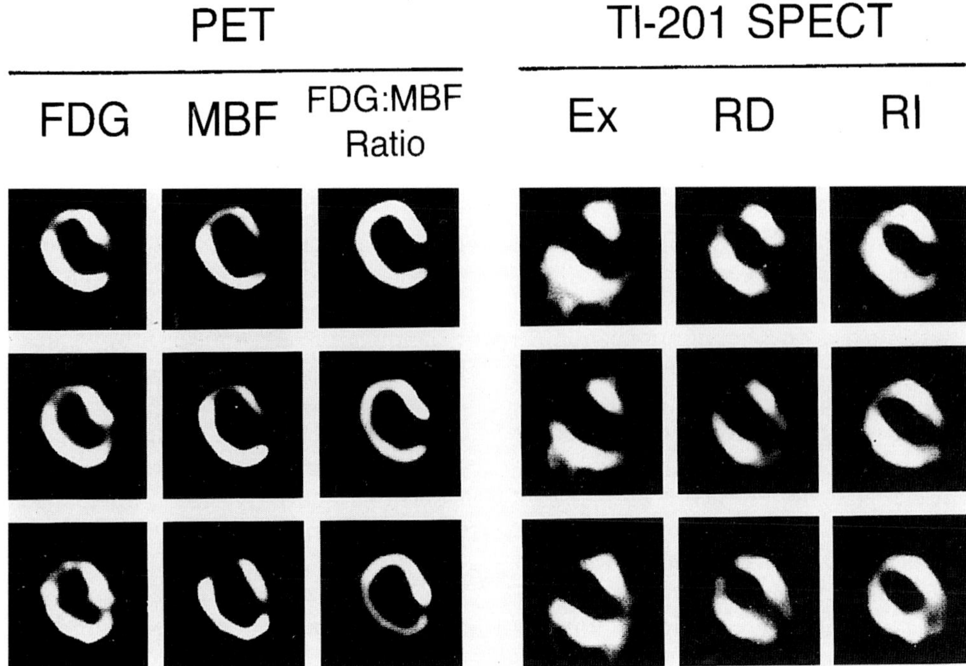

Fig. 98.5 Concordance of PET and thallium reinjection data. ^{18}F Deoxyglucose (FDG) images are shown for three tomographic levels in one patient, along with functional images of myocardial blood flow (MBF) and the FDG–blood flow ratio, generated from quantitative [^{15}O]water data with partial volume and spillover correction. The corresponding thallium data for exercise (Ex), redistribution (RD) and reinjection (RI) are shown in the right panels. The standard exercise–redistribution thallium studies demonstrate an apparently irreversible anteroapical defect. Myocardial blood flow is reduced in this region and in the septum by PET. However, the FDG images demonstrate uptake, and hence viability, in all regions, most notably the anteroapical wall. The functional images of FGD–blood flow ratio demonstrate enhanced FDG uptake relative to blood flow ('mismatch') involving the apex and septum. Thallium reinjection results in enhanced thallium uptake in the anteroapical regions, resulting in reinjection images that mirror the FDG images. Reproduced[46] with permission of the American Heart Association.

perfusion) but also subsequent redistribution images. Although the early experience with resting thallium protocols yielded mixed results regarding the predictive accuracy of rest–redistribution imaging,[51–53] recent studies indicate that a quantitative analysis of regional thallium activity in rest–redistribution studies predicts recovery of regional left ventricular function[54] and compares favourably with the results of thallium exercise–reinjection imaging and metabolic PET imaging.[55]

^{99m}TC SESTAMIBI IMAGING

^{99m}Tc sestamibi, like ^{201}Tl, requires intact cell membrane processes for retention and has been shown to be an excellent marker of cellular viability.[56–58] In experimental and clinical settings in which blood flow is restored (and hence sestamibi delivery is adequate) to previously ischaemic or damaged myocardium, uptake and retention of sestamibi parallels myocardial viability rather than perfusion alone.[57,59–61] However, unlike thallium, ^{99m}Tc sestamibi does not redistribute appreciably after its initial uptake when the tracer is injected either during exercise or at rest. Thus, sestamibi may have inherent disadvantages relative to thallium for viability assessment in clinical situations in which blood flow is severely impaired and sestamibi delivery is reduced.[62] This concept is supported by several studies suggesting that rest–exercise sestamibi imaging underestimates viable myocardium in patients with chronic coronary artery disease and left ventricular dysfunction compared to exercise–redistribution-reinjection thallium imaging.[63–65] More recently, ^{18}FDG activity indicating viability by PET imaging has been reported in a large percentage of sestamibi defects in patients with left ventricular dysfunction.[66] It should be pointed out that subsequent studies within the past year indicate that a quantitative analysis of regional sestamibi activity after an injection at rest substantially increases the accuracy for identifying viable myocardium,[67,68] and that this accuracy begins to approach that of thallium imaging and PET imaging. These latter findings are preliminary in nature and await confirmation by larger, more definitive studies.

SPECT VESUS PET FOR VIABILITY ASSESSMENT

In theory, radionuclide methods that evaluate cell membrane integrity should be as effective for assessing myocardial viability as are markers of preserved metabolic activity, as viability requires both intact membrane function and maintenance of metabolic processes. Thus, the relative efficacy of PET or SPECT to identify viable myocardium is not governed primarily by the underlying physiological processes themselves that are assessed by these techniques, but by the ability to image these processes within the existing physical limitations of the imaging devices. In this regard, there are several advantages of PET approaches. These include improved resolution and the ability to correct for photon attenuation. In addition, as noted previously, it is possible with PET to assess metabolic activity independent of perfusion. Advantages of SPECT imaging include the ability to assess inducible ischaemia along with viability as part of a routine comprehensive imaging protocol. In addition, viability can be assessed in all patients without concerns regarding the metabolic conditions of the patient, which must be standardized and controlled for ^{18}FDG PET studies. With these considerations in mind, the principal advantage of PET is the availability of attenuation correction algorithms. Each of the SPECT protocols shares the limiting feature of photon attenuation of a low energy radioisotope, in which apparently irreversible thallium or sestamibi defects suggesting fibrosis may be merely attenuation artefacts in viable tissue. Thus, it is anticipated that imaging with ^{201}Tl- or with ^{99m}Tc-based agents will never achieve the accuracy of PET imaging for viability assessment.

CLINICAL IMPLICATIONS

The identification of viable myocardium has become an area of intense interest for several reasons. Among these is the rather unique potential of nuclear cardiology techniques to distinguish viable tissue, on the basis of perfusion, cell membrane integrity, and metabolic activity, thereby providing greater precision than can be achieved by assessment of regional anatomy or function. However, there remain unresolved issues regarding the clinical applications of such techniques. First, larger scale studies comparing PET and ^{201}Tl, using reinjection techniques or resting injections, are required in patients undergoing revascularization to determine the relative efficacy of these two methods in identifying viable myocardium. There may be subgroups of patients in whom PET provides more accurate and complete data than can be accomplished using thallium imaging, but the characteristics of this subgroup are not yet fully defined. Second, further information is also required to determine the efficacy of sestamibi imaging relative to these other modalities in assessing myocardial viability. Third, the properties of the newer technetium-based perfusion tracers for viability assessment have yet to be investigated. Fourth, single photon approaches for metabolic imaging (such as ^{123}I-labelled fatty acids) appear to be promising,[69,70] and further work comparing these agents to ^{201}Tl and ^{18}FDG in the same patients are needed. Finally, although roughly 85% of dysfunctional myocardial regions identified as viable by these various imaging techniques may improve after revascularization, it is unlikely that this will actually lead to clinical benefit in 85% of patients. Whether or not a clinically relevant change in ventricular performance occurs, and whether this translates into improved lifestyle and prognosis, will depend upon a number of factors, many of which are only poorly defined at present. The amount of dysfunctional but viable myocardium certainly is one such factor. At the current time, the identification of hibernating myocardium is not by itself an indication for revascularization. As in any other patient with coronary artery disease, this decision should be based on clinical presentation, coronary anatomy, left ventricular function, and evidence of inducible ischaemia. However, the knowledge that a large region of left ventricular myocardium is hibernating rather than irreversibly damaged will greatly aid in this decision-making process.

REFERENCES

1. Rahimtoola S H 1982 Coronary bypass surgery for chronic angina – 1981: a perspective. Circulation 65: 225–241
2. Braunwald E, Rutherford J D 1986 Reversible ischemic left ventricular dysfunction: Evidence for 'hibernating' myocardium. J Am Coll Cardiol 8: 1467–1470
3. Rahimtoola S H 1989 The hibernating myocardium. Am Heart J 117: 211–213
4. Ross J Jr 1991 Myocardial perfusion–contraction matching: implications for coronay artery disease and hibernation. Circulation 83: 1076–1083
5. Dilsizian V, Bonow R O 1993 Current diagnostic techniques of assessing myocardial viability in hibernating and stunned myocardium. Circulation 87: 1–20
6. Bonow R O, Dilsizian V: Thallium-201 for assessing myocardial viability. Semin Nucl Med 21: 230–241
7. Bonow R O, Berman D S, Gibbons R J, Johnson L L, Rumberger J A, Schwaiger M, Wackers F J 1991 Cardiac positron emission tomography. A report for health professionals from the Committee on Advanced Cardiac Imaging and Technology of the Council on Clinical Cardiology, American Heart Association. Circulation 84: 447–454
8. Schelbert H R, Bonow R O, Geltman E, Maddahi J, Schwaiger M 1993 Clinical use of positron emission tomography. Position paper of the Cardiovascular Council of the Society of Nuclear Medicine. J Nucl Med 34: 1385–1388
9. Schelbert H R, Phelps M E, Hoffman E, Huang S C, Kuhl D E 1980 Regional myocardial blood flow, metabolism, and function assessed noninvasively with positron emission tomography. Am J Cardiol 80: 1269–1277
10. Marshall R C, Tillisch J H, Phelps M E, Huang S C, Carson R, Henze E, Schelbert H R 1983 Identification and differentiation of resting myocardial ischaemia and infarction in man with positron computed tomography, ^{18}F-labelled fluorodeoxyglucose and N-13 ammonia. Circulation 67: 766–778

11. Tillisch J H, Brunken R, Marshall R, Schwaiger M, Mandelkorn M, Phelps M, Schelbert H 1986 Reversibility of cardiac wall-motion abnormalities predicted by positron tomography. N Engl J Med 314: 884–888
12. Brunken R, Tillisch J, Schwaiger M, Child J S, Marshall R, Mandelkorn M, Phelps M E, Schelbert H R 1986 Regional perfusion, glucose metabolism, and wall motion in patients with chronic electrocardiographic Q wave infarctions: evidence for persistence of viable tissue in some infarct regions by positron emission tomography. Circulation 73: 951–963
13. Schelbert H R, Buxton D 1988 Insights into coronary artery disease gained from metabolic imaging. Circulation 78: 496–505
14. Fudo T, Kambara H, Hashimoto T, Hayashi M, Nohara R, Tamaki N, Yonekura Y, Senda M, Konishi J, Kawai C 1988 F-18 deoxyglucose and stress N-13 ammonia positron emission tomography in anterior wall healed myocardial infarction. Am J Cardiol 61: 1191–1197
15. Tamaki N, Yonekura Y, Yamashita K, Saji H, Magata Y, Senda M, Konishi Y, Hirata K, Ban T, Konishi J 1989 Positron emission tomography using fluorine-18 deoxyglucose in evaluation of coronary artery bypass grafting. Am J Cardiol 64: 860–865
16. Gropler R J, Geltman E M, Sampathkumaran K, Perez J E, Moerlein S M, Sobel B E, Bergmann S R, Siegel B A 1992 Functional recovery after coronary revascularization for chronic coronary artery disease is dependent on maintenance of oxidative metabolism. J Am Coll Cardiol 20: 569–577
17. Lucignani G, Paolini G, Landoni C et al 1992 Presurgical identification of hibernating myocardium by combined use of technetium-99m hexakis 2-methoxyisobutylisonitrile single photon emission tomography and fluorine-18 fluoro-2-deoxy-D-glucose positron emission tomography in patients with coronary artery disease. Eur J Nucl Med 19: 874–881
18. Carrel T, Jenni R, Haubold-Reuter S, Von Schulthess G, Pasic M, Turina M 1992 Improvement in severely reduced left ventricular function after surgical revascularization in patients with preoperative myocardial infarction. Eur J Cardiothorac Surg 6: 479–484
19. vom Dahl J, Altehoefer C, Sheehan F H, Beilin I, Uebis R, Kleinhans E, Messmer B J, Hanrath P, Buell U 1993 Recovery of myocardial function following coronary revascularization: impact of viability and long-term vessel patency as assessed by preoperative F-18 FDG PET and serial angiography (abstr). J Nucl Med 34: 23P
20. Bessozi M C, Brown M D, Hubner K F, Smith G T, Bond H W, Goodman M M, Buonocore E 1992 Retrospective post-therapy evaluation of cardiac function in 208 coronary artery disease patients evaluated by positron emission tomography (abstr). J Nucl Med 33: 885
21. DiCarli M, Khanna S, Davidson M, Harris G, Brunken R, Czernin J, Mody F, Hoh C, Stevenson L, Laks H, Hawkins R, Phelps M, Schelbert H R, Maddahi J 1993 The value of PET for predicting improvement in heart failure symptoms in patients with coronary artery disease and severe left ventricular dysfunction (abstr). J Am Coll Cardiol 21: 129A
22. Louie H W, Laks H, Milgalter E, Drinkwater D C, Hamilton M A, Brunken R C, Stevenson L W 1991 Ischemic cardiomyopathy: criteria for coronary revascularization and cardiac transplantation. Circulation 84 (Suppl III): III.290–III.295
23. Eitzman D, Al-Aouar Z, Kanter H L, vom Dahl J, Kirsh M, Deeb G M, Schwaiger M 1992: Clinical outcome of patients with advanced coronary artery disease after viability studies with positron emission tomography. J Am Coll Cardiol 20: 559–565
24. Maddahi J, DiCarli M, Davidson M, Khanna S, Rokhsar S, Tillisch J, Laks H, Schelbert H, Phelps M 1992 Prognostic significance on PET assessment of myocardial viability in patients with left ventricular dysfunction (abstr). J Am Coll Cardiol 19: 142A
25. Yamamoto Y, de Silva R, Rhodes C G, Araujo L I, Iida H, Rechavia E, Nihoyannolpoulos P, Hackett D, Galassi A R, Taylor C J V, Lammertsma A A, Jones T, Maseri A 1992 A new strategy for the assessment of viable myocardium and regional myocardial blood flow using ^{15}O-water and dynamic positron emission tomography. Circulation 86: 167–178
26. de Silva R, Yamamoto Y, Rhodes C G, Iida H, Nihoyannolpoulos P, Davies G J, Lammertsma A A, Jones T, Maseri A 1992 Preoperative prediction of the outcome of coronary revascularization using positron emission tomography. Circulation 86: 1738–1742
27. Gould K L, Haynie M, Hess M J, Yoshida K, Mullani N, Smalling R W 1991 Myocardial metabolism of fluorodeoxyglucose compared to cell membrane integrity for the potassium analogue Rb-82 for assessing infarct size in man by PET. J Nucl Med 32: 1–9
28. Opie L H 1976 Effects of regional ischaemia on metabolism of glucose and fatty acids: Relative rates of aerobic and anaerobic energy production during myocardial infarction and comparison with effects of anoxia. Circ Res 38(Suppl I): I52–74
29. Camici P, Ferrannini E, Opie L H 1989 Myocardial metabolism in ischemic heart disease: Basic principles and application to imaging by positron emission tomography. Prog Cardiovasc Dis 32: 217–238
30. Gibson R S, Watson D D, Taylor G J, Crosby I K, Wellons H L, Holt N D, Beller G A 1983 Prospective assessment of regional myocardial perfusion before and after coronary revascularization surgery by quantitative thallium-201 scintigraphy. J Am Coll Cardiol 1: 804–815
31. Liu P, Kiess M C, Okada R D, Block P C, Strauss H W, Pohost G M, Boucher C A 1985 The persistent defect on exercise thallium imaging and its fate after myocardial revascularization: Does it represent scar or ischaemia? Am Heart J 110: 996–1001
32. Manyari D E, Knudtson M, Kloiber R, Roth D 1988 Sequential thallium-201 myocardial perfusion studies after successful percutaneous transluminal coronary artery angioplasty: Delayed resolution of exercise induced scintigraphic abnormalities. Circulation 77: 86–95
33. Cloninger K G, DePuey E G, Garcia E V, Roubin G S, Robbins W L, Nody A, DePasquale E E, Berger H J 1988 Incomplete redistribution in delayed thallium-201 single photon emission computed tomographic (SPECT) images: An overestimation of myocardial scarring. J Am Coll Cardiol 12: 955–963
34. Ohtani H, Tamaki N, Yonekura Y, Mohiuddin I H, Hirata K, Ban T, Konishi J 1990 Value of thallium-201 reinjection after delayed SPECT imaging for predicting reversible ischemia after coronary artery bypass grafting. Am J Cardiol 66: 394–399
35. Brunken R, Schwaiger M, Grover-McKay M, Phelps M E, Tillisch J, Schelbert H R 1987 Positron emission tomography detects tissue metabolic activity in myocardial segments with persistent thallium perfusion defects. J Am Coll Cardiol 10: 557–567
36. Tamaki N, Yonekura Y, Yamashita K, Senda M, Saji H, Hashimoto T, Fudo T, Kambara H, Kawai C, Ban T, Konishi J 1988 Relation of left ventricular perfusion and wall motion with metabolic activity in persistent defects on thallium-201 tomography in healed myocardial infarction. Am J Cardiol 62: 202–208
37. Brunken R C, Kottou S, Nienaber C A, Schwaiger M, Ratib O M, Phelps M E, Schelbert H R 1989 PET detection of viable tissue in myocardial segments with persistent defects at Tl-201 SPECT. Radiology 65: 65–73
38. Tamaki N, Yonekura Y, Yamashita K, Mukai T, Magata Y, Hashimoto T, Fudo T, Kambara H, Kawai C, Hirata K, Ban T, Konishi J 1989 SPECT thallium-201 tomography and positron tomography using N-13 ammonia and F-18 fluorodeoxyglucose in coronary artery disease. Am J Cardiac Imaging 3: 3–9
39. Bonow R O, Dilsizian V, Cuocolo A, Bacharach S L 1991 Identification of viable myocardium in patients with chronic coronary artery disease and left ventricular dysfunction: comparison of thallium-201 with reinjection and PET imaging with ^{18}F-fluorodeoxyglucose. Circulation 83: 26–37
40. Perrone-Filardi P, Bacharach S L, Dilsizian V, Maurea S, Frank J A, Bonow R O 1992 Regional left ventricular wall thickening: relation to regional uptake of ^{18}F-fluorodeoxyglucose and thallium-201 in patients with chronic coronary artery disease and left ventricular dysfunction. Circulation 86: 1125–1137
41. Brunken R C, Mody F V, Hawkins R A, Neinaber C, Phelps M E, Schelbert H R 1992 Positron emission tomography detects metabolic activity in myocardium with persistent 24-hour single photon emission computed tomography ^{201}Tl defects. Circulation 86: 1357–1369
42. Gutman J, Berman D S, Freeman M, Rozanski A, Maddahi J,

Waxman A, Swan H J C 1983 Time to completed redistribution of thallium-201 in exercise myocardial scintigraphy: Relationship to the degree of coronary artery stenosis. Am Heart J 106: 989–995
43. Kiat H, Berman D S, Maddahi J, Yang L D, Van Train K, Rozanski A, Friedman J 1988 Late reversibility of tomographic myocardial thallium-201 defects: An accurate marker of myocardial viability. J Am Coll Cardiol 12: 1456–1463
44. Yang L D, Berman D S, Kiat H, Resser K J, Friedman J D, Rozanski A, Maddahi J 1990 The frequency of late reversibility in SPECT thallium-201 stress-redistribution studies. J Am Coll Cardiol 15: 334–340
45. Kayden D S, Sigal S, Soufer R, Mattera J, Zaret B L, Wackers F Th J 1991 Thallium-201 for assessment of myocardial viability: Quantitative comparison of 24-hour redistribution imaging with imaging after reinjection at rest. J Am Coll Cardiol 18: 1480–1486
46. Dilsizian V, Rocco T P, Freedman N M T, Leon M B, Bonow R O 1990 Enhanced detection of ischemic but viable myocardium by the reinjection of thallium after stress-redistribution imaging. N Engl J Med 323: 141–146
47. Rocco T P, Dilsizian V, McKusick K A, Fischman A J, Boucher C A, Strauss H W 1990 Comparison of thallium redistribution with rest 'reinjection' imaging for detection of viable myocardium. Am J Cardiol 66: 158–163
48. Tamaki N, Ohtani H, Yonekura Y, Nohara R, Kambara H, Kawai C, Hirata K, Ban T, Konishi J 1990 Significance of fill-in after thallium-201 reinjection following delayed imaging: Comparison with regional wall motion and angiographic findings. J Nucl Med 31: 1617–1623
49. Dilsizian V, Smeltzer W R, Freedman N M T, Dextras R, Bacharach S L, Bonow R O 1991 Thallium reinjection after stress-redistribution imaging: does 24 hour delayed imaging following reinjection enhance detection of viable myocardium? Circulation 83: 1247–1255
50. Nienaber C A, de la Roche J, Camarius H, Montz R 1993 Impact of ^{201}thallium reinjection imaging to identify myocardial viability after vasodilation-redistribution SPECT. J Am Coll Cardiol 21: 283A (abstr)
51. Berger B C, Watson D D, Burwell L R, Crosby I K, Wellons H A, Teates C D, Beller G A 1979 Redistribution of thallium at rest in patients with stable and unstable angina and the effect of coronary artery bypass surgery Circulation 60: 1114–1125
52. Iskandrian A S, Hakki A, Kane S A, Goel I P, Mundth E D, Hakki A, Segal B L 1983 Rest and redistribution thallium-201 myocardial scintigraphy to predict improvement in left ventricular function after coronary artery bypass grafting. Am J Cardiol 51: 1312–1316
53. Mori T, Minamiji K, Kurogane H, Ogawa K, Yoshida Y 1991 Rest-injected thallium-201 imaging for assessing viability of severe asynergic regions. J Nucl Med 32: 1718–1724
54. Ragosta M, Beller G A, Watson D D, Kaul S, Gimple L W 1993 Quantitative planar rest-redistribution 201Tl imaging in detection of myocardial viability and prediction of improvement in left ventricular function after coronary bypass surgery in patients with severely depressed left ventricular function. Circulation 87: 1630–1641
55. Dilsizian V, Perrone-Filardi P, Arrighi J A, Bacharach S L, Quyyumi A A, Freedman N M T, Bonow R O 1993 Concordance and discordance between stress-redistribution-reinjection and rest-redistribution thallium imaging for assessing viable myocardium. Circulation 88: 941–952
56. Freeman I, Grunwald A M, Hoory S, Bodenheimer M M 1991 Effect of coronary occlusion and myocardial viability on myocardial activity of technetium-99m-sestamibi. J Nucl Med 32: 292–298
57. Sinusas A J, Watson D D, Cannon J M, Beller G A 1989 Effect of ischemia and postischemic dysfunction on myocardial uptake of technetium-99m-labelled methoxyisobutyl isonitrile and thallium-201. J Am Coll Cardiol 14: 1785–1793
58. Beanlands R S B, Dawood F, Wen W H, McLaughlin P R, Butany J, D'Amati G, Liu P P 1990 Are the kinetics of technetium-99m methoxyisobutyl isonitrile affected by cell metabolism and viability? Circulation 82: 1802–1814
59. Edwards N C, Ruiz M, Watson D D, Beller G A 1990 Does Tc-99m sestamibi given immediately after coronary reperfusion reflect viability? Circulation 82: III–542 (abstr)
60. Li Q S, Matsumura K, Dannals R, Becker L C 1990 Radionuclide markers of viability in reperfused myocardium: comparison between ^{18}F-2-deoxyglucose, ^{201}Tl, and ^{99m}Tc-sestamibi. Circulation 82: III–542 (abstr)
61. Christian T F, Behrenbeck T, Pellikka P A et al 1990 Mismatches of left ventricular function and perfusion with Tc-99m-isonitrile following reperfusion therapy for acute myocardial infarctions: identification of myocardial stunning and hyperkinesia. J Am Coll Cardiol 16: 1632–1638
62. Bonow R O, Dilsizian V 1992 Thallium-201 and technetium-99m-sestamibi for assessing viable myocardium. J Nucl Med 33: 815–818
63. Cuocolo A, Pace L, Ricciardelli B, Chiariello M, Trimarco B, Salvatore M 1992 Identification of viable myocardium in patients with chronic coronary artery disease: comparison of thallium-201 scintigraphy with reinjection and technetium-99m methoxyisobutyl isonitrile. J Nucl Med 33: 505–511
64. Marzullo P, Sambuceti G, Parodi O 1992 The role of sestamibi scintigraphy in the radioisotopic assessment of myocardial viability. J Nucl Med 33: 1925–1930
65. Marzullo P, Parodi O, Reisenhofer B, Sambeceti G, Picano E, Distante A, Gimelli A, L'Abbate A 1993 Value of rest thallium-201/technetium-99m sestamibi scans and dobutamine echocardiography for detecting myocardial viability. Am J Cardiol 71: 166–172
66. Sawada S G, Allman K C, Muzik O, Beanlands R S B, Wolfe E R Jr, Gross M, Fig L, Schwaiger M 1994 Positron emission tomography detects evidence of viability in rest technetium-99m sestamibi defects. J Am Coll Cardiol 23: 92–98
67. Dilsizian V, Arrighi J A, Diodati J G, Quyyumi A A, Bacharach S L, Marin-Neto J A, Uddin S, Bonow R O 1994 Myocardial viability in patients with chronic ischemic left ventricular dysfunction: comparison of ^{99m}Tc-sestamibi, ^{201}thallium, and ^{18}F-fluorodeoxyglucose. Circulation 89: 578–587
68. Udelson J E, Coleman P S, Matherall J A, Pandian N G, Gomes A R, Griffith J L, Shea N L, Oates E, Konstam M A 1994 Predicting recovery of severe regional ventricular dysfunction: comparison of resting scintigraphy with thallium-201 and technetium-99m sestamibi. Circulation 89: (in press)
69. Tamaki N, Kawamoto M, Yonekura Y, Fujibayashi Y, Takahashi N, Konishi J, Nohara R, Kambara H, Kawai C, Ikekubo K, Kato H 1992 Regional metabolic abnormality in relation to perfusion and wall motion in patients with myocardial infarction: assessment with emission tomography using an iodinated branched fatty acid analog. J Nucl Med 33: 659–667
70. Murray G, Schad N, Ladd W et al 1992 Metabolic cardiac imaging in coronary artery disease with severe left ventricular dysfunction: assessment of myocardial viability with ^{123}I-iodophenylpentadecanoic acid imaged by a multicrystal camera and correlation with transmural myocardial biopsy. J Nucl Med 33: 1269–1277

99. Infarct-avid imaging in acute myocardial infarction

Jamshid Maddahi

INTRODUCTION

Despite significant progress in the non-invasive detection and treatment of coronary artery disease, acute myocardial infarction (MI) still represents one of its major complications. In the United States approximately 1.5 million people suffer an MI each year. In management of patients with suspected or known MI, important clinical steps are to confirm the diagnosis, to assess the size of the patient's infarction, and to determine prognosis, in order to optimize care.

The diagnosis of myocardial necrosis in patients suspected of having acute MI may be difficult despite the number of diagnostic procedures available. Although electrocardiographic (ECG) abnormalities can be identified in most patients with acute MI, correlation of serial ECG changes with pathological findings indicates that the accuracy of diagnosis by this method is <80%.[1,2] Limitations include the size and specific location of infarction, previous infarction, conduction defects, acute pericarditis, electrolyte abnormalities, and cardioactive drugs.[1,3,4] Diagnosis of transmural lateral and posterior infarction is less accurate than diagnosis of either transmural anterior or inferior infarction.[4] Non-specific ST-segment depression and/or T-wave inversion are ECG features associated with non-transmural (subendocardial, non-Q-wave) MI that may also appear in other conditions in patients presenting with chest pain, including stable and unstable angina pectoris.[4]

Elevated serum enzyme levels provide a sensitive means of diagnosing acute MI, but there are drawbacks.[5] An elevated CK-MB fraction is highly specific, but CK-MB levels peak in the first day after infarction. Optimal performance requires frequent serial measurements within the first 24 h after infarction. If only single measurements are available, the sensitivity of CK-MB determination is between 34% and 57%.[6] Total CK levels remain elevated longer than CK-MB, but elevation in total CK is less specific for MI.[7] Even if serial measurements are obtained in the appropriate time frame, the specific diagnosis of acute MI depends upon the observation of a classic rise and fall of serum enzyme levels. Elevated CK and CK-MB fraction serum levels may be missed in late presenting patients. Non-definitive enzymatic findings occur in 10–20% of patients including those who present with disparity of CK and CK-MB levels, minimal elevations of CK-MB or total CK, or sustained elevations without independent verification of diagnosis.[8,9] Traditional CK-MB enzyme studies are less reliable in assessing the extent of infarction, especially in patients following thrombolysis. Successful reperfusion causes rapid, profound enzymes release even from quite small infarcts. When MI is the result of intermittent coronary occlusion, enzyme release is erratic and routine protocols for obtaining blood samples for enzyme determination do not allow reliable analysis of CK-MB release.

In patients suspected of having MI, the concurrent appearance of new Q-waves and elevated CK-MB fraction provides specific evidence of acute MI. However, at least 18% of patients with cardiac enzyme patterns suggesting acute MI have non-diagnostic ECGs, and as many as 30% of patients with ECG evidence of acute MI have normal enzyme measurements.[2,10]

Two-dimensional echocardiography or radionuclide ventriculography may be used to demonstrate the presence and size of MI by the presence and extent of regional wall motion abnormalities. However, ventricular function, especially in the early post-infarction state, is often artificially depressed in the presence of stunned or hibernating myocardium. In these circumstances, ventricular function may not improve for days or even months despite the presence of viable myocardium, making the early use of these measurements a less precise prognostic indicator for the assessment of long term outcome.

Myocardial perfusion imaging with ^{201}Tl and ^{99m}Tc-labelled sestamibi demonstrates the presence, extent and location of a perfusion abnormality but a non-reversible defect does not establish the absence of viable myocardium; this makes it difficult to differentiate stunned myocardium from myocardial infarction. Furthermore, myocardial perfusion imaging with these agents does not distinguish acute from old MI.

Infarct avid imaging provides a direct means of identifying an acute MI. ^{99m}Tc-labelled pyrophosphate (^{99m}Tc PYP) and ^{111}In-labelled antimyosin monoclonal antibody (^{111}In antimyosin) are two currently available infarct avid imaging agents. In this chapter, [^{111}In]antimyosin imaging will be discussed first and its characteristics will then be compared with those of ^{99m}Tc PYP.

INFARCT AVID IMAGING WITH [^{111}IN]ANTIMYOSIN MONOCLONAL ANTIBODY

Antimyosin monoclonal antibody (Myoscint, Centocor) is an Fab fragment of murine monoclonal antibody which binds specifically to an antigenic site on the heavy chain of human myosin. Myosin is an intracellular protein found in myocytes and is not exposed when the cell membrane is intact. Destruction of cell membrane during myocardial necrosis exposes myosin and allows its binding with antimyosin monoclonal antibody.

Specificity of antimyosin for myocardial necrosis

Several studies have demonstrated the specificity of antimyosin antibodies for binding to necrotic myocardium and specifically to myofibrils. In 1976, Khaw et al[11] showed, in dogs, that uptake of ^{125}I-labelled F(ab′)$_2$ fragments of polyclonal rabbit antibody was six times greater in the endocardial myocardium of the infarcted zone than in normal myocardium, and 3.3 times greater in the epicardial myocardium. Another study[12] showed a close correlation between the zone of infarction, defined by absence of TTC staining and macro-autoradiographically determined antimyosin antibody uptake. Micro-autoradiography also indicated that the antibody concentrated only in myocardium shown to be necrotic by haematoxylin–eosin staining. In 1987 Khaw et al[13] demonstrated a close correlation between the area of infarction, as determined by TTC staining, and uptake of i.v. ^{99m}Tc-labelled Fab fragments of monoclonal antimyosin antibody. It has been further demonstrated that ^{111}In antimyosin Fab is not taken up by severely ischaemic but viable myocardium.[14] In an in vitro study, polyclonal rabbit antimyosin antibody against mouse myosin was bound to fluorescent microspheres.[15] Damaged and undamaged culture-grown cells were exposed to the antimyosin microspheres. The study demonstrated substantial adsorption of the antimyosin microspheres to necrotic myocytes. Non-necrotic myocytes showed low levels of non-specific binding (Fig. 99.1).

Jain et al[16] studied a patient who died of ventricular rupture 1 day after ^{111}In antimyosin imaging and 6 days after acute MI. There was good agreement between the area of antimyosin uptake on post-mortem autoradiography and infarcted tissue determined by TTC staining and histopathological examination. The infarction demonstrated intense focal uptake on ante-mortem images (Fig. 99.2). These investigators also reported another patient who died 12 h after antimyosin injection; at 48 h post-infarction there was also correlation of histopathological evidence of infarction and antimyosin uptake, although no ante-mortem imaging was performed.[17]

Estimating the size of myocardial infarction

The extent of antimyosin antibody uptake is related to the size of the MI. Khaw et al[18] studied reperfused myocardial infarctions in dogs, and showed a good agreement between TTC staining and imaging performed after i.v. injection of antimyosin antibody, although ^{99m}Tc PYP imaging tended to overestimate infarct size. Another animal study[19] found a close correlation between infarct size measured by antimyosin single photon emission computerized tomography (SPECT) and TTC staining. This type of analysis may be important in view of the

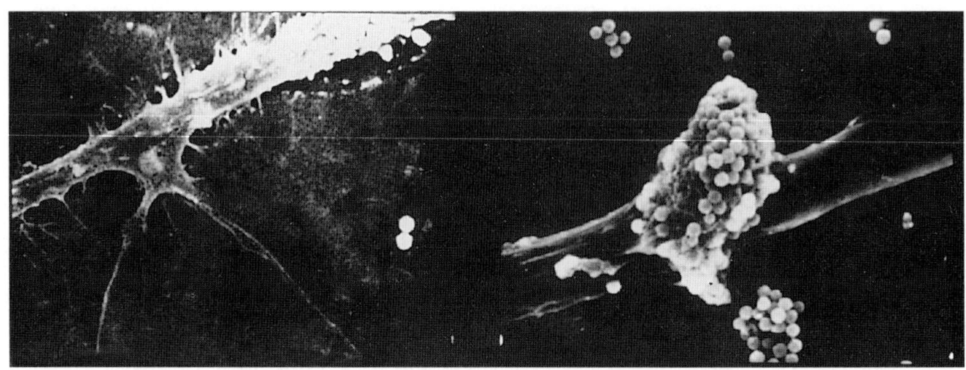

Fig. 99.1 In vivo binding of antibody coated microspheres to necrotic myocardium.

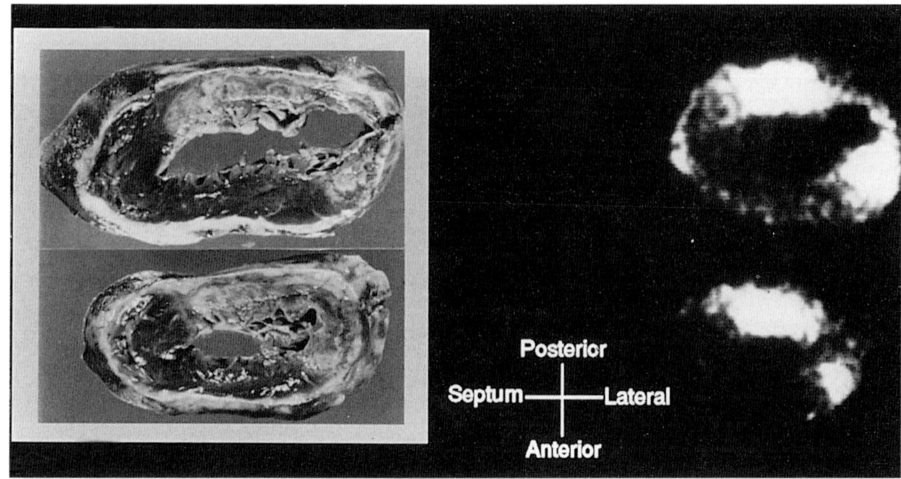

Fig. 99.2 Comparison of post-mortem necrosis and [^{111}In]antimyosin uptake in man.

increasing clinical use of thrombolysis and angioplasty in acute infarction.

SPECT imaging with ^{99m}Tc antimyosin was used by Khaw et al[20] to evaluate infarct size (in grams) and was compared with angiography and CK blood levels. There was a linear correlation between SPECT determination of infarct size and the length of the hypokinetic myocardial segment on angiography. ^{99m}Tc PYP SPECT images measured an infarct size almost twice that of antimyosin antibody imaging. The extent of antimyosin uptake also correlated with peak CK levels.[20] Johnson et al[19] reported significant correlation between infarct size measured by SPECT imaging of ^{111}In antimyosin uptake and ejection fraction. SPECT antimyosin infarct size also correlated with peak CK levels in those patients who did not have reperfusion.

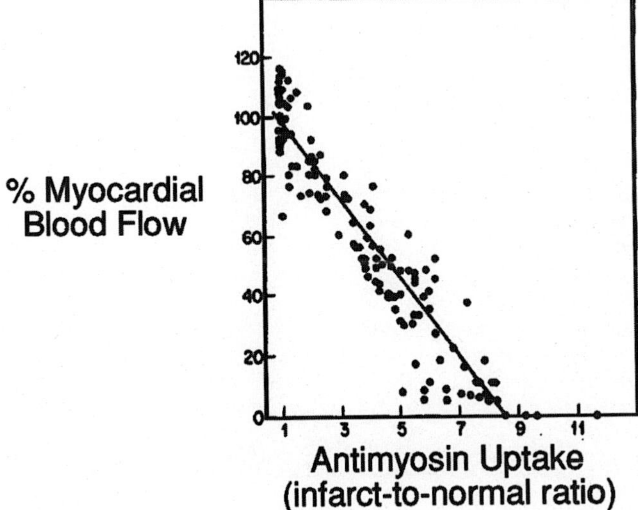

Fig. 99.3 Correlation between blood flow and ^{111}In antimyosin uptake in a permanent occlusion experiment.

Khaw et al have demonstrated that antimyosin monoclonal antibody is taken up by the necrotic tissue in proportion to the amount of necrosis, with maximal uptake in areas with severely reduced myocardial blood flow (Fig. 99.3). It appears that even in the presence of a totally occluded vessel, antimyosin monoclonal antibody reaches the infarcted tissue by diffusion. These features make ^{111}In antimyosin monoclonal antibody a suitable tracer for the detection of myocardial necrosis in humans.

Clinical safety

^{111}In Antimyosin antibody has been intensively tested for its safety in humans. A major concern was the possibility of immunological reactions caused either by the antibody reacting against human tissues or by human antimouse antibody (HAMA) response to the murine antibody molecule. HAMA can interfere with the diagnostic or therapeutic use of murine monoclonal antibodies.

In Phase I, II and III multicentre clinical trials, 1742 serum samples were obtained from over 600 patients who had received ^{111}In antimyosin murine antibody Fab.[21] Serum samples were obtained before antimyosin injection, at the time of hospital discharge, and at 3–8 weeks after injection and there was no evidence of antimyosin-induced HAMA. None of the patients developed allergy or anaphylaxis, and there was no serum sickness. All symptoms were attributed to acute MI, co-existent medical conditions, or other medications. Thirty patients in this group died, all because of the severity of their coronary artery disease.

A clinical trial was performed to evaluate the immune response to single and multiple i.v. administrations of ^{111}In antimyosin antibody Fab.[21] 182 patients with recent MI were given a total of 254 injections, with patients receiving from one to five doses of antibody over a 1 year period. There was no increase in HAMA levels.

Two patients had HAMA detected in preinjection serum samples but developed no increases in HAMA levels after injection. The very low antigenic potential of the antibody may be related in part to the use of the Fab fragment rather than the whole antibody molelcule, as well as the 0.5 mg dose.

Dosimetry

After i.v. injection, ^{111}In antimyosin clears from the blood exponentially and blood activity is reduced to 20% within 24 h, providing a good target-to-background ratio. Blood activity drops to 10% at 48 h. Since most of the circulating antimyosin is excreted in the urine, the kidney is the critical organ. The dose to the kidney is 9.53 rads per 2 mCi of ^{111}In DTPA. The total body dose is 0.86 rads per 2 mCi.

Clinical detection of MI

^{111}In antimyosin antibody is useful in patients presenting with ischaemic chest pain for determining whether infarction occurred, where infarction is located, and how extensive it is. These issues were evaluated in the antimyosin phase III clinical trial,[22] conducted in 25 sites, 16 in the USA and nine in Europe. 497 patients with chest pain that was thought to be due to an MI were studied. 2 mCi of ^{111}In antimyosin was injected within 72 h of chest pain and planar images were obtained 24 and 48 h after injection. CK-MB was measured every 6 h for 36 h and ECGs were obtained every 12–24 h for 5 days. These data were used to categorize patients into four groups:

- acute Q-wave MI
- acute non Q-wave MI
- unstable angina pectoris
- chest pain without myocardial necrosis or resting ischaemia.

^{111}In Antimyosin images were evaluated by a blinded panel of nuclear cardiologists.

The sensitivity of [^{111}In]antimyosin for the detection of myocardial necrosis was 87.5% in 257 patients with MI based on clinical, ECG or enzymatic criteria. The sensitivity for the detection of Q-wave infarction was 91% and for the detection of non Q-wave infarction it was 76%. The specificity of antimyosin was 95% in 40 patients with chest pain but without MI or ischaemia. No significant differences in sensitivity were seen when results were examined using consecutive 6 h intervals (0–6 h up to >48 h). Positive ^{111}In antimyosin images were obtained in all eight patients with definitive MI injected within 6 h of the onset of chest pain (including one injected 2.6 h after onset).

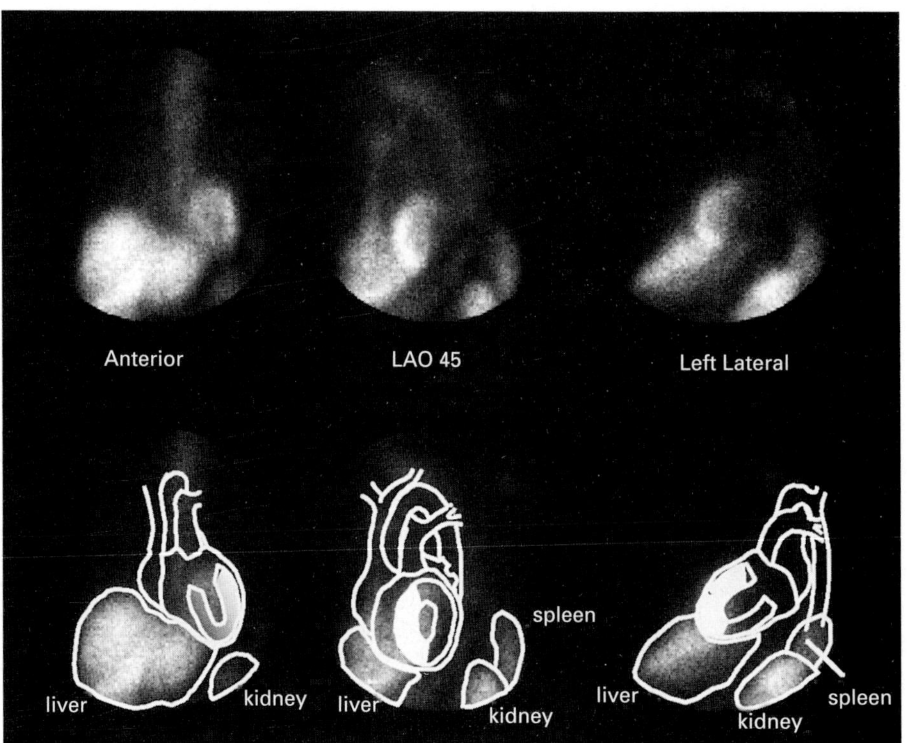

Fig. 99.4 ^{111}In antimyosin antibody images obtained at approximately 24 h after injection demonstrating abnormal focal myocardial uptake in the anterior, septal and apical regions of the left ventricle corresponding to an anteroseptal myocardial infarction. Uptake by the liver and kidneys may also be noted.

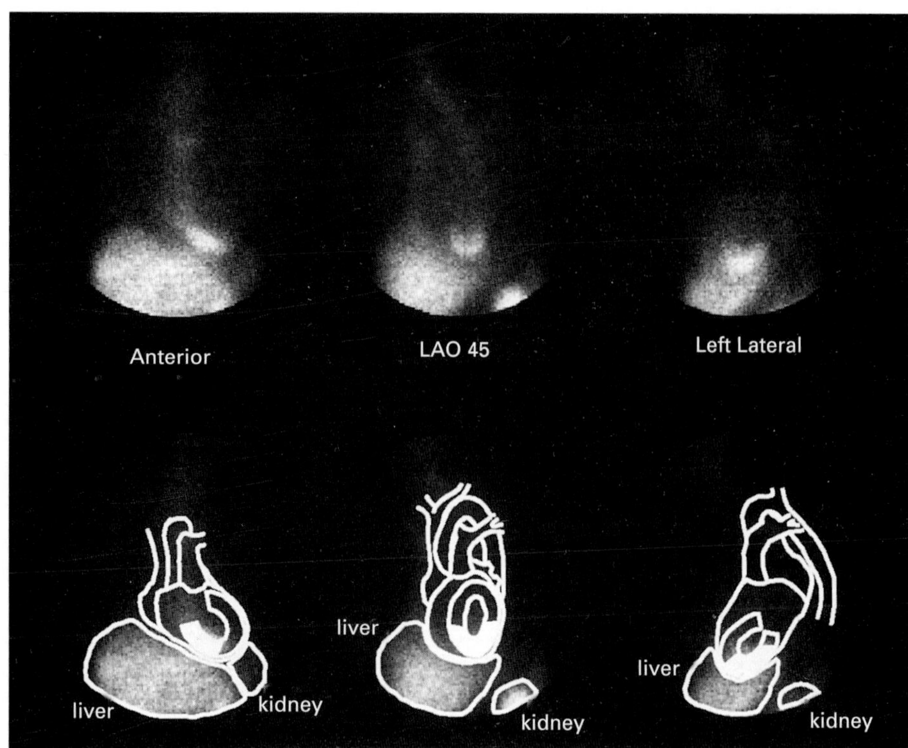

Fig. 99.5 ^{111}In antimyosin antibody images obtained at approximately 24 h after injection in a patient with a small inferior myocardial infarction.

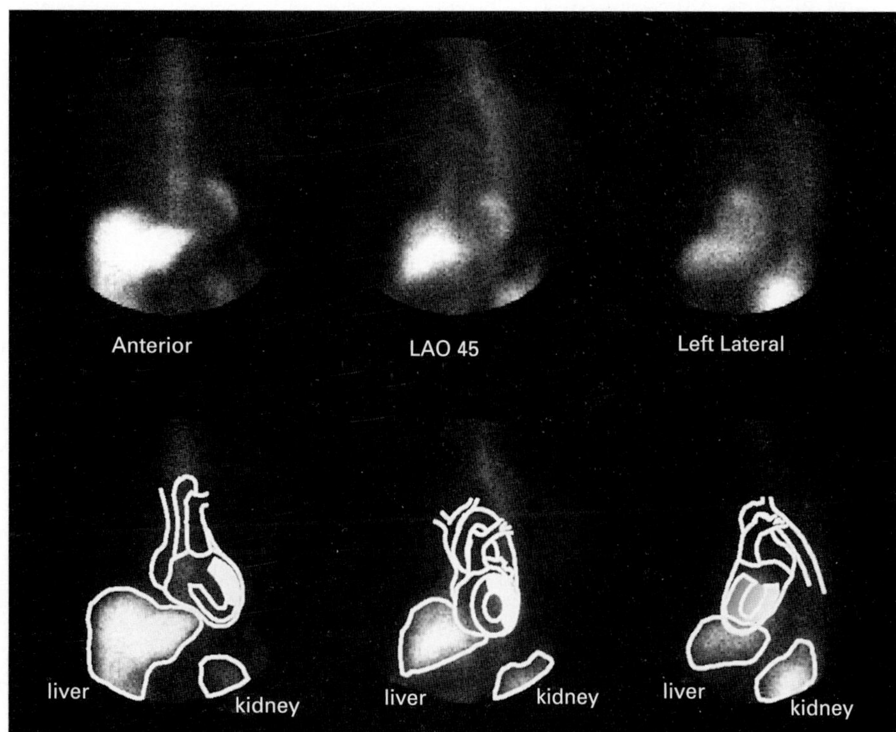

Fig. 99.6 Positive ^{111}In antimyosin antibody images obtained in a patient with acute lateral wall myocardial infarction.

182 patients with acute Q-wave MI and positive ^{111}In antimyosin images had Q-wave infarcts localized by ECG. The concordance of ^{111}In antimyosin with ECG was 91% in these patients (Figs 99.5–99.7). There was also a high degree of localization concordance in patients with definitive findings even when non-Q-wave infarcts were considered.

Utility for diagnosis of MI in equivocal cases

Patients not infrequently present with equivocal or conflicting ECG or enzymatic findings that make the diagnosis of MI uncertain. Examples are patients who have conduction disturbances, those who might have suffered infarction during bypass surgery or coronary angioplasty, and those following thrombolysis therapy or with non-Q-wave infarction. Patients who present late after developing symptoms suspicious of an ischaemic event also pose a diagnostic problem.

In the multicentre trial,[23] equivocal or conflicting ECG or enzyme results were seen frequently. Almost one-third of these patients could not be classified definitively as having acute MI, unstable angina, or chest pain of non-ischaemic origin based on ECG findings, clinical presentation and CK. In order to assess the value of antimyosin imaging all data were used to classify the patients into those with and without MI. This 'best guess' classification for the presence of MI was then correlated with the results of antimyosin images, with uptake of antimyosin interpreted as evidence of necrosis. In 73% of these patients there was agreement between the two classifications.

Bayes' Theorem may also be used to address the question whether patients with a non-definitive diagnosis of myocardial necrosis may benefit from antimyosin study. Bayes' Theorem states that the probability of disease after a given test depends on the pre-test likelihood of the disease, as well as the sensitivity and specificity of the test. Using the sensitivity and specificity of ^{111}In antimyosin study determined from the multicentre trial, we observe that the greatest discrimination between positive test responders and those with a negative study is achieved in patients who have an intermediate likelihood of necrosis. In such patients the presence of a positive study indicates a high likelihood of myocardial necrosis, while a negative study essentially rules out the presence of myocardial necrosis.

^{111}In Antimyosin uptake in unstable angina

^{111}In Antimyosin imaging can show uptake in some patients with unstable angina. This suggests that myocardial necrosis can occur in some patients with unstable angina. Phase III clinical trials indicated a 37% incidence of ^{111}In antimyosin uptake in patients with unstable angina, a pattern that could not be distinguished from that seen in patients with acute MI. The extent of uptake was positively correlated with the risk of further cardiac events in patients with infarction and with unstable angina. The uptake of ^{111}In antimyosin in patients with unstable angina and its high specificity for necrotic myocardium suggests that some myocardial necrosis is present in many patients with unstable angina, in spite of the absence of traditional indicators of myocardial necrosis. This finding is supported by post-mortem studies in patients with unstable angina.[24,25]

Persistent positive uptake of ^{111}In antimyosin in older MI

The uptake of ^{111}In antimyosin Fab by infarcted myocardium may persist after the acute period, although the intensity of uptake appears to diminish. In one investigation, infarcted myocardium demonstrated focal antimyosin uptake as long as 9 months after the acute infarction.[26] All 17 patients studied less than <1 month after acute infarction had focal uptake. Of seven patients studied 1–9 months after infarction, two had negative scans at 1 and 2 months. Five had focal uptake. In two of the patients with uptake in more recent infarcts, older infarcts were not visualized at 8 months and 8.5 years after those events. Patients with infarcts <1 week old generally had more intense uptake than those with older infarcts.

In a multicentre study of 182 patients receiving ^{111}In antimyosin Fab between 1 day and 68 weeks after acute MI, a steadily diminishing frequency of uptake was seen with increasing age of the infarct.[27] 68% of those patients studied <2 months after acute infarction had positive scans, decreasing to 50% at 4–6 months after infarction and 23% at 8–10 months. There was persistent uptake with both transmural and non-transmural infarctions. In a subset of the previous study, 40 patients were examined 3 days to 9 months after infarction.[28] 36 of 40 patients had ^{111}In antimyosin uptake. These patients were compared with a group of 50 imaged within 2 days of acute infarction. The ratio of heart-to-lung activity was significantly higher in the early post-infarction group. There was an inverse correlation between the ratio and the age of the infarct.

The uptake of ^{111}In antimyosin Fab by infarcted myocardium, occurring after the acute event, may affect its use in differentiating between acute and old myocardial injury occurring within 1 year. Therefore, in patients who may have had prior MI, a positive Fab scan should be interpreted using all available clinical information.

Application of ^{111}In antimyosin imaging for prognosis of MI

Patient prognosis following acute MI is related to the amount of necrotic myocardium and the amount that is at risk. In acute ischaemic syndromes (acute MI and unstable angina) and following thrombolysis, the amount of necrotic myocardium and the amount of jeopardized myocardium is unpredictable and may not be accurately assessed by clinical, enzyme and ECG findings. ^{111}In Antimyosin images may be used in several ways to assess prognosis.

Semiquantitative method

^{111}In Antimyosin images may be analysed semiquantitatively to assess the extent of myocardial necrosis on either planar or SPECT images. In the multicentre trial the extent of myocardial necrosis was evaluated from the three view planar images by a method shown in Fig. 99.5. Each view of the left ventricle was divided into six segments and each segment was visually scored for the presence of ^{111}In antimyosin uptake as mild, moderate or intense. It is important to note that summing the number of involved segments from all three views may overestimate the extent of necrosis since regions of the left ventricle are seen in more than one view. Furthermore, apparent uptake in one region may be caused by 'shine-through' of ^{111}In antimyosin from another. Localization is therefore best accomplished by confirming uptake in at least two views. In order to assess the location and the extent of myocardial necrosis more accurately, the three planar images were translated into a composite image of the entire left ventricle using the polar map method that has been described for ^{201}Tl SPECT imaging. The polar map display not only demonstrated the location of ^{111}In antimyosin uptake but also allowed assessment of the percentage of the entire left ventricular myocardium with ^{111}In antimyosin uptake expressed as the number of positive segments divided by the total number of evaluable segments, which is 18.

A linear relationship was noted between the number of segments with ^{111}In antimyosin uptake and the incidence of cardiac death, non-fatal MI, and either of these two events during the 5 month follow-up period.[29] The cumulative cardiac death rate during the follow-up period ranged from 4% in patients with a negative study to over 30% in patients with extensive uptake. Receiver–operating curve (ROC) analysis demonstrated that $\geqslant$ 10 segments of uptake best discriminated patients with a low risk (5%) from those with a high risk (25%). In patients who could not be classified as having definite MI (because of conflicting or equivocal clinical findings, ECG, or cardiac enzyme results), the incidence of major cardiac events was 36% in those with extensive uptake compared with 4% in those without extensive uptake (relative risk of 9:1) (Fig. 99.7). The presence of extensive uptake had superior and independent prognostic value compared with all of the other variables that were included in multivariate analysis such as Killip Class, age, presence of Q-wave, ischaemia, peak CK, and prior MI. Therefore, it appears that the information gained from antimyosin uptake was independent of all other clinical variables evaluated, alone or in combination, and added new prognostic information. However, ejection fraction and extent of perfusion abnormality were not measured hence and the relative role of ^{111}In antimyosin imaging is unknown.

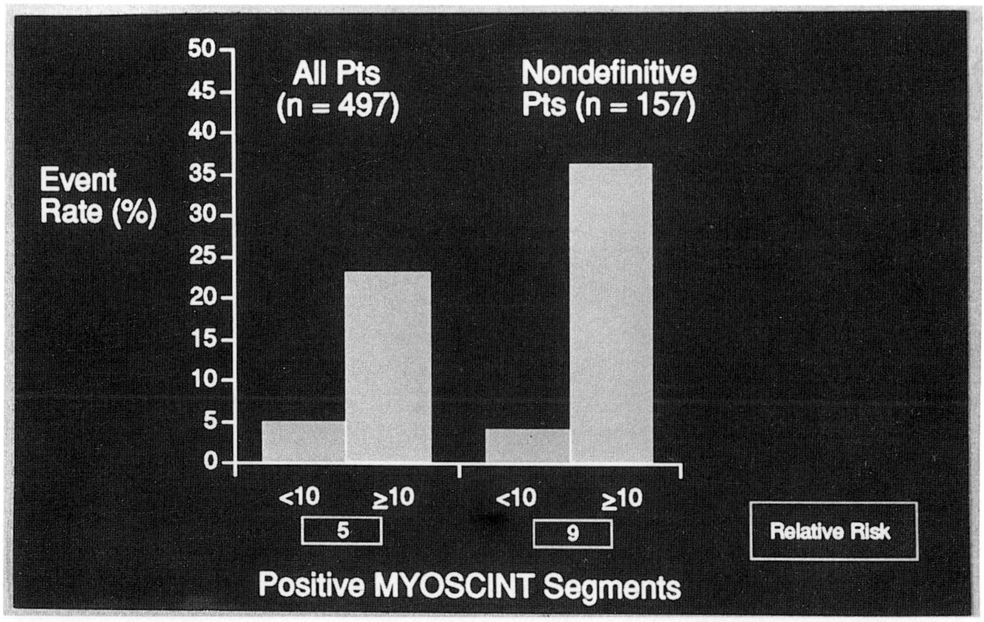

Fig. 99.7 Risk of cardiac death or non-fatal myocardial infarction, predicted by the extent of ^{111}In antimyosin uptake in all patients and a subgroup of patients with non-definitive evidence of myocardial infarction. (Also shown in colour on Plate 30.)

Intensity of myocardial uptake of [^{111}In]antimyosin

In quantifying the extent of myocardial necrosis, it is important to determine whether the necrosis involves the full thickness of the myocardium, or whether it is interspersed with viable myocardium. One approach may be to measure the intensity of regional ^{111}In antimyosin uptake. Van Vlies et al[30] described a count density index (CDI), which is the ratio of count densities in the myocardium and the left lung. The lower the ratio, the less the volume of necrosis in a given region and the smaller likelihood that it is transmural. Van Vlies et al demonstrated that in the subgroup of 21 patients with their first MI who were treated with thrombolytic therapy, CDI correlated with two-dimensional echocardiographic estimates of regional wall motion 5–9 days after admission. In patients with mild asynergy in at least one segment, CDI was significantly lower than in those with severe asynergy (1.6 *vs.* 2.5).

Another indication that CDI reflects the density of infarction was provided by Van Vlies et al[31] in a study of 55 patients with first uncomplicated acute MI, defined as Killip Class I or II, no severe heart failure and no significant arrhythmias. There was 18 events within 6 months, eleven occurring within 6 weeks of the infarction. Events recorded were cardiac death, further infarction, unstable angina, the need for bypass surgery or PTCA, and recurrent ischaemia. In patients with an event, the mean CDI was 1.82 but in patients without an event, it was 2.2 ($P < 0.01$). The positive predictive value of a CDI of 2.0 was 57% but the negative predictive value was 93%, suggesting that CDI identifies a subgroup of patients with a low chance of recurrent ischaemic events.

Dual-isotope imaging

Another approach to determining the extent of necrosis and of viable but jeopardized myocardium is dual isotope imaging, using ^{201}Tl and ^{111}In antimyosin in conjunction. Several patterns may be observed (Fig. 99.8):

- normal uptake of ^{201}Tl without antimyosin uptake indicating normal myocardium
- reduced ^{201}Tl uptake without ^{111}In antimyosin uptake suggesting resting ischemia (if defect is reversible) or prior infarction (if ^{201}Tl defect is non-reversible)
- absence of ^{201}Tl uptake in areas with antimyosin uptake suggesting transmural necrosis
- presence of some ^{201}Tl uptake in an area of antimyosin uptake indicating non-transmural infarction.

In a given patient, different extent of one or more of these regional patterns may be observed.

A study of 42 patients performed by Johnson et al[32] has substantiated the concept that these patterns may have prognostic implications. In patients with matching areas of abnormality consistent with transmural infarction, there were no ischaemic events. However, among the 23 patients with a mismatch pattern, i.e. areas of ^{201}Tl reduction without ^{111}In antimyosin uptake (suggesting the presence of ischaemia), there were further ischaemic

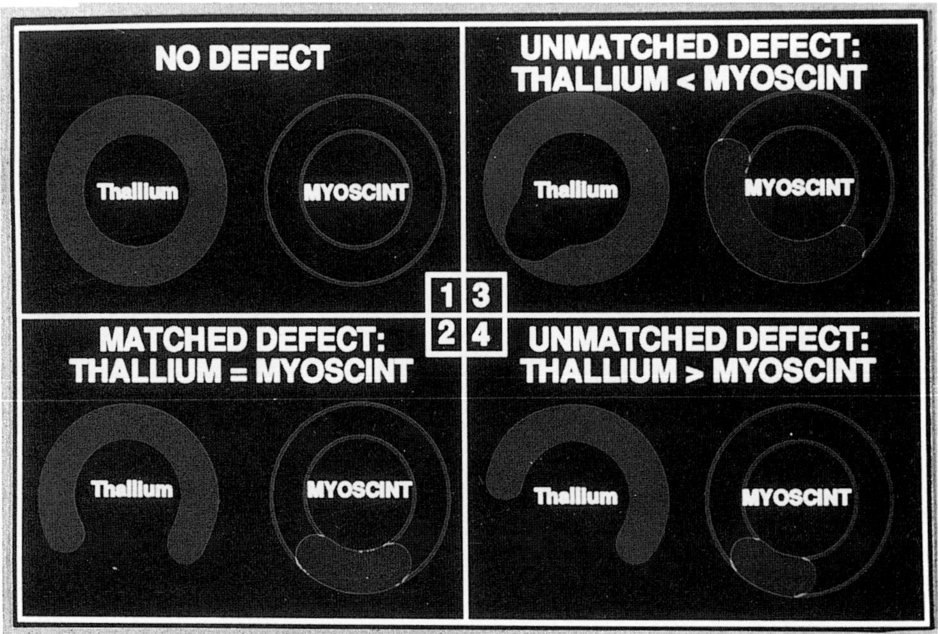

Fig. 99.8 Diagrammatic representation of dual isotope (^{201}Tl and ^{111}In antimyosin) image patterns. (Also shown in colour on Plate 30.)

events in 16 patients. Furthermore, of five patients who showed ^{111}In antimyosin and ^{201}Tl overlap in the same areas, four had evidence of ischaemia. Thus, dual isotope imaging early after thrombolysis may help to identify patients at risk of further ischaemic events.

^{111}In ANTIMYOSIN ANTIBODY VS. ^{99m}Tc PYROPHOSPHATE (PYP)

Infarct avid scintigraphy may provide unique and valuable information unavailable from other diagnostic imaging modalities. ^{99m}Tc PYP has received only limited acceptability due, in part, to practical limitations restricting its usefulness in clinical settings. ^{111}In Antimyosin overcomes many of the limitations that have prevented wider acceptance of ^{99m}Tc PYP, and offers distinct and practical advantages in the detection of the presence, location and extent of MI.

Time window for detection of MI

^{99m}Tc PYP has a restrictive time window for successful detection of an acute MI, with an acceptable level of sensitivity both delayed in onset and limited in duration. The optimal time for imaging with ^{99m}Tc PYP depends upon residual blood flow or redevelopment of blood flow to the region of infarction; this optimal sensitivity often does not occur until 48 to 72 h following infarction.[33–41] This delay often necessitates serial ^{99m}Tc PYP injections and imaging because some patients develop a positive image later than usual.[42] Such a delay has also limited the usefulness of ^{99m}Tc PYP in guiding acute interventions designed to reduce infarct size.[43] After 48 to 72 h, the sensitivity then declines over the next week and ^{99m}Tc PYP scintigrams may be normal by 5 days after acute infarction.[35] This variable temporal sensitivity often excludes patients otherwise most likely to benefit from infarct-avid scintigraphy, i.e. patients with an equivocal diagnosis or presenting late after a suspicious episode of chest pain. In contrast, there appears to be no significant variation in ^{111}In antimyosin sensitivity during this period. Studies to date indicate that the high sensitivity of ^{111}In antimyosin is constant for 2 weeks after acute infarction.[26] The Phase III trial confirmed that it also provides successful early detection even when injected within hours of an episode of chest pain. Thus, patients outside the time window available for detection with ^{99m}Tc PYP may be successfully evaluated using ^{111}In antimyosin.

Specificity for detection of MI

The specificity of ^{99m}Tc PYP for acute MI has been estimated at 50–60% in several studies comprising planar imaging with ECG or enzymes.[35] In a large multicentre trial, which was part of the Multicentre Investigation of the Limitation of Infarct Size (MILIS), the specificity of ^{99m}Tc PYP was 64%.[44] The explanation for this relatively low figure was the common occurrence of mildly increased diffuse uptake. This pattern of uptake adds substantially to the difficulty in interpretation of ^{99m}Tc PYP images, and occurs in approximately one-third of all patients imaged and in approximately 50% of patients with non-Q-wave infarctions.[38,45] In contrast, cardiac images obtained with ^{111}In antimyosin could be interpreted as positive or negative in all but a few patients in the Phase III trial, (with acute infarcts generally appearing as distinct focal abnormalities), giving a specificity of 95%. Cardiac uptake of ^{99m}Tc PYP can also occur in a variety of disease states not associated with acute MI such as pericarditis, cardiac metastases, valvular calcification, and secondary hyperparathyroidism or other causes of dystrophic cardiac calcification.[41] In contrast, cardiac uptake of ^{111}In antimyosin is specific for necrotic myocardium.

Non-cardiac thoracic uptake

Non-cardiac thoracic uptake of ^{99m}Tc PYP can interfere or be confused with cardiac activity on planar images. Approximately 50% accumulates in the skeleton;[46] sternal and costal activity is significant and is present in every image of the thorax. Additional overlapping activity can also arise from calcified costal cartilage, normal or diseased breast, and from skin and chest wall following cardioversion, surgery or other trauma.[41] In contrast, overlying thoracic structures demonstrate minimal-to-mild ^{111}In antimyosin activity, which does not significantly obscure or interfere with cardiac planar images. Liver uptake of ^{111}In antimyosin, however, may interfere with visualization of small areas of inferior wall uptake.

Estimation of infarct size

Current clinical interest in risk assessment and in interventional therapy to reduce or limit infarction has placed considerable emphasis on the estimation of infarct size. Although ^{99m}Tc PYP, like ^{111}In antimyosin, is taken up only by irreversibly injured necrotic cells, its accumulation in the myocardium is not proportional to the degree of myocardial necrosis.[41,47] Maximal concentration of ^{99m}Tc PYP occurs in regions of 20–40% decreased blood flow, which typically occur at the periphery of the infarction, while the infarct centre receives very little activity.[47,49] When employing in-vivo imaging techniques the non-uniform distribution produces intensive uptake at the infarct periphery. This 'doughnut ring' effect results in an overestimate of infarct size. Although this effect can be lessened using sophisticated algorithms, quantification of infarct size using ^{99m}Tc PYP is difficult.[19,20] In contrast, animal experiments have demonstrated that ^{111}In antimyosin distributes throughout infarcted tissue. In dogs, infarct size in ^{111}In antimyosin images agrees closely with tissue size.[13,19] In direct comparisons of both agents, ^{99m}Tc PYP overestimates infarct size.[13] Similarly, in man, ^{111}In antimyosin images agrees closely with post-mortem infarct size.[16,17,50,51] As a result of the more central localization of ^{111}In antimyosin within an infarct, visual images obtained with this agent properly convey a sense of total damaged tissue, while quantitation may be accomplished by straightforward approaches (e.g. bull's-eye display methods applied to planar images in the Phase III trial and to tomographic images employed by other investigators.[19,20,52]

ACKNOWLEDGEMENTS

The author wishes to thank Mercedes Bocanegra for typing and preparation of the manuscript and Diane Martin for preparation of the figures.

REFERENCES

1. Levine H D, Phillips E 1951 Appraisal of the newer electrocardiography correlations in one hundred and fifty consecutive cases. N Engl J Med 245: 833
2. Rude R E, Poole W K, Muller J E et al 1983 Electrocardiographic and clinical criteria for recognition of acute myocardial infarction based on analysis of 3,697 patients. Am J Cardiol. 52: 936–942
3. Savage R M, Wagner G S, Ideker R E et al 1977 Correlation of postmortem anatomic findings with electrocardiographic changes in patients with myocardial infarction. Retrospective study of patients with typical anterior and posterior infarcts. Circulation 55: 279
4. Cooksey J D, Dunn M, Massie E 1977 Clinical vectorcardiography and electrocardiography, 2nd edn. Year Book Medical Publishers, Chicago, p 361
5. Lee T H, Goldman L 1986 Serum enzyme assays in the diagnosis of acute myocardial infarction. Recommendations based on quantitative analysis. Ann Intern Med. 105: 221
6. Lee T H, Weisberg M, Cook E F et al 1986 Clinical impact of creatine kinase-MB for diagnosis of myocardial infarction in the emergency room. Arch Intern Med
7. Sobel B E, Shell W E 1972 Serum enzyme determinations in the diagnosis and assessment of myocardial infarction. Circulation 45: 471
8. Dillon M C, Calbreath D F, Dixon A M et al 1982 Diagnostic problems in acute myocardial infarction: CK-MB in the absence of abnormally elevated total creatine kinase levels. Arch Intern Med 142: 33
9. White R D, Grande P, Califf L et al 1985 Diagnostic and prognostic significance of minimally elevated creatine kinase-MB in suspected acute myocardial infarction. Am J Cardiol 55(13 pt 1): 1478
10. Zarling E J, Sexton H, Milnor P Jr 1983 Failure to diagnose acute myocardial infarction; the clinicopathologic experience at a large community hospital. JAMA 250: 1177–1181
11. Khaw B A, Beller G A, Haber E, Smith T W 1976 Localization of cardiac myosin-specific antibody in myocardial infarction. J Clin Invest 58: 439–446
12. Khaw B, Fallon J, Beller G et al 1979 Specificity of localization of myosin-specific antibody fragments in experimental myocardial infarction. Circulation 60: 1527–1531
13. Khaw B A, Strauss H W, Moore R et al 1987 Myocardial damage delineated by indium-111 antimyosin Fab and technetium-99m pyrophosphate. J Nucl Med 28: 76–82
14. Nedelman M A, Schaible T F, Manspeaker H F et al 1990 Evaluation of antimyosin uptake in reversibly injured ("stunned") myocardium. J Nucl Med 31: 795
15. Khaw B A, Scott J, Fallon J T et al 1982 Myocardial injury: quantitation by cell sorting initiated with antimyosin fluorescent spheres. Science 217: 1050–1053
16. Jain D, Crawley J C, Lahiri A et al 1990 Indium-111-antimyosin images compared with triphenyl tetrazolium chloride staining in a patient six days after myocardial infarction. J Nucl Med 31: 231–233
17. Jain D, Lahiri A, Crawley J C W et al 1988 ^{111}In-antimyosin imaging in a patient with acute myocardial infarction: post-mortem correlation between histopathologic and autoradiographic extent of myocardial necrosis. Am J Cardiac Imaging 2: 158–161
18. Khaw B A, Beller G A, Haber E 1978 Experimental myocardial infarction imaging following intravenous administration of iodine-131 labeled antibody (Fab') fragments specific for cardiac myosin. Circulation 57: 743–750
19. Johnson L L, Lerrick K S, Coromilas J et al 1987 Measurement of infarct size and percentage myocardium infarcted in a dog preparation with single photon-emission computed tomography, thallium-201, and indium-111-monoclonal antimyosin Fab. Circulation 76: 181–190
20. Khaw B A, Gold H K, Yasuda T et al 1986 Scintigraphic quantification of myocardial necrosis in patients after intravenous injection of myosin-specific antibody. Circulation 74(3): 501–508
21. Data on file. Centocor, Inc., Malvern, PA 19355, USA
22. Berger H, Lahiri A, Leppo J, Makler T, Maddahi J, Mintz G, Strauss H W and Antimyosin Multicenter Trial Group, Centocor, Inco, Malvern, PA 1988 Antimyosin imaging in patients with ischemic chest pain: initial results of phase III multicenter trial. J Nucl Med 29(5): 805
23. Berger H J and the Antimyosin Multicenter Trial Group, Centocor, Inc., Malvern, PA 1988 Antimyosin imaging in patients with chest pain but without a definitive diagnosis of myocardial infarction or unstable angina. Circulation 78(4): II-493
24. Donsky S S, Curry G C, Parkey R W et al 1976 Unstable angina pectoris: clinical angiographic, and myocardial scintigraphic observations. Br Heart J 38: 257–263
25. Buja L M, Poliner L R, Parkey R W et al 1977 Clinicopathologic study of persistently positive technetium-99m stannous pyrophosphate myocardial scintigrams and myocytolytic degeneration after myocardial infarction. Circulation 56: 1016–1023
26. Tamaki N, Yamada T, Matsumori A, Yoshida A, Fujita T, Ohtani H, Watanabe Y, Yonekura Y, Endo K, Konishi J, Kawai C 1990 Indium-111-antimyosin antibody imaging for detecting different stages of myocardial infarction: comparison with technetium-99m-pyrophosphate imaging. J Nucl Med 31: 136–142
27. Gewirtz H, Leppo J, Makler P T et al The safety and diagnostic accuracy of delayed and repeated injections of indium-111 labeled antimyosin in ischemic heart disease. Centocor Clinical Study C04I-005
28. Liu X J, Jain D, Senior R et al 1990 A quantitative method for assessing age of myocardial infarction from antimyosin images. J Nucl Med 31: 782
29. Berger H J and the Antimyosin Multicenter Trial Group, Centocor, Inc., Malvern, PA 1988 Prognostic significance of the extent of antimyosin uptake in unstable ischemic heart disease: Early risk stratification. Circulation 78(4): II-131
30. Van Vlies B, Baas J, Visser C 1989 Predictive value of indium-111 antimyosin uptake for improvement of left ventricular wall motion after thrombolysis in acute myocardial infarction. Am J Cardiol 64: 176–181
31. Van Vlies B, von Royen E A, Fioretti P et al 1990 Predictive value of early indium-111 antimyosin scintigraphy for ischemic events after first myocardial infarction. J Nucl Med 31: 782
32. Johnson L L, Seldin D W, Keller A M, Wall R M, Bhatia K, Bingham C O, Tresgallo M E 1990 Dual isotope thallium and indium antimyosin SPECT imaging to identify acute infarct patients at further ischemic risk. Circulation 81: 37–45
33. Willerson J T, Parkey R W, Bonte F J et al 1975 Acute subendocardial myocardial infarcts detected by technetium-99m

stannous pyrophosphate myocardial scintigrams. Circulation 51: 436–441
34. Willerson J T, Parkey R W, Bonte F J et al 1975 Technetium stannous pyrophosphate myocardial scintigrams in patients with chest pain of varying etiology. Circulation 51: 1046–1052
35. Willerson J T, Buja M L, Parker R W et al 1987 Infarct-avid myocardial scintigraphy to detect acute myocardial infarction. Cardiac Nucl Med 251–261
36. Berman D S, Amsterdam E A, Hines H H et al 1977 Problem of diffuse cardiac uptake of Tc-pyrophosphate in the diagnosis of acute myocardial infarction: Enhanced scintigraphic accuracy by computerized selective blood pool subtraction. Am J Cardiol 40: 768–774
37. Marcus M L, Kerber R E 1977 Present status of the technetium-99m pyrophosphate scintigram. Circulation 56: 335–339
38. Massie B M, Botvinick E H, Werner J A et al 1979 Myocardial scintigraphy with technetium-99m stannous pyrophosphate: an insensitive test for nontransmural myocardial infarction. Am J Cardiol 43: 186–192
39. Holman B L, Goldhaber S Z, Kirsch C M et al 1982 Measurement of infarct size using single photon emission computed tomography and technetium-99m pyrophosphate: a description of method and comparison with patient prognosis. Am J Cardiol 50: 503–511
40. Jansen D E, Corbett J R, Wolfe C L et al 1985 Quantification of myocardial infarction: a comparison of single photon-emission computed tomography with pyrophosphate to serial plasma MB-creatine kinase measurements. Circulation 72: 327–333
41. Lewis S E, Parker R W, Bonte F J et al 1988 Infarct-avid imaging in acute myocardial infarction. Diagn Nucl Med. 1: 399–413. 2nd edn. Gottschalk A, Hoffer P B, Potchen E J (eds). Williams & Wilkins, Baltimore M D
42. Malin F R, Rollo D, Gertz E W 1978 Sequential myocardial scintigraphy with technetium-99m stannous pyrophosphate following myocardial infarction. J Nucl Med 19: 1111–1115
43. Toltzis R J, Gershen M C 1987 Non-invasive test selection in the coronary care unit. In: McGershon (ed), Cardiac nuclear medicine. McGraw-Hill, New York, pp 263–296
44. Turi Z G, Rutherford J D, Roberts R, Muller J E, Jaffe A S, Rude R E, Parker C, Raabe D S, Stone P H, Hartwell T D, Lewis S E, Parkey R W, Gold H K, Robertson T L, Sobel B E, Willerson J T, Braunwald E, Cooperating Investigators from MILIS Study Group 1985 Electrocardiographic, enzymatic and scintigraphic criteria of acute myocardial infarction as determined from study of 726 patients (a MILIS study). Am J Cardiol 55: 1463–1468
45. Berman D S, Amsterdam E A, Hines H H et al 1977 New approach to interpretation of technetium-99m pyrophosphate scintigraphy in detection of acute myocardial infraction. Am J Cardiol 39: 341–346
46. Holman B L 1984 Infarct-avid scintigraphy. In: Freeman L M (ed) Freeman and Johnson's clinical radionuclide imaging, vol 1, 3rd edn. W B Saunders, Philadelphia pp 537–562
47. Buja L M, Tofe A J, Kulkarni P V et al 1977 Sites and mechanisms of localization of technetium-99m phosphorous radiopharmaceuticals in acute myocardial infarcts and other tissues. J Clin Invest 60: 724–740
48. Zaret B L, DiCola V C, Donabedian R K et al 1976 Dual radionuclide study of myocardial infarction. Relationships between myocardial uptake of potassium-43, technetium-99m stannous pyrophosphate, regional myocardial blood flow and creatine phosphokinase depletion. Circulation 53: 422–428
49. Rude R, Parkey R W, Bonte F J et al 1977 Clinical implication of the "doughnut" pattern of uptake in myocardial imaging with technetium-99m stannous pyrophosphate. Circulation 56: m-561
50. Hendel R C, McSherry B A, Leppo J A 1990 Myocardial uptake of indium-111 labeled antimyosin in acute subendocardial infarction: clinical, histochemical, and autoradiographic correlation of myocardial necrosis. J Nucl Med 31: 1851–1853
51. Nakata T, Sakukibara T, Noto T et al 1991 Myocardial distribution of indium-111-antimyosin Fab in acute inferior and right ventricular infarction: comparison with technetium-99m-pyrophosphate imaging and histologic examination. J Nucl Med 32: 865–867
52. Antunes, M L, Seldin D W et al 1989 Measurement of acute Q-wave myocardial infarct size with single photon emission computed tomography imaging of indium-111 antimyosin. Am J Cardiol 777–783

100. Myocardial infarction: the assessment of thrombolysis

John J. Mahmarian   Mario S. Verani

The treatment of acute myocardial infarction has had its greatest advancement over the last decade, particularly with the development of new thrombolytic agents and mechanical interventions to restore coronary flow. Numerous studies have shown a survival benefit in patients treated acutely with thrombolytic agents[1–5] which persists over at least a year of follow-up.[6] The presumed mechanism by which lytic agents reduce mortality is through myocardial salvage. Determining the degree of myocardial salvage after infarction would therefore seem advantageous when evaluating individual patients, and could be used as a surrogate end point for mortality in future clinical trials evaluating new forms of therapy. Quantifying myocardial salvage has been attempted by assessing changes in regional[7–11] and global left ventricular function,[8–22] and by myocardial perfusion imaging using quantitative planar and tomographic techniques.[21–28] These methods have met with variable success due to a variety of technical considerations, and patient differences in the extent of myocardium at risk for infarction during coronary occlusion.

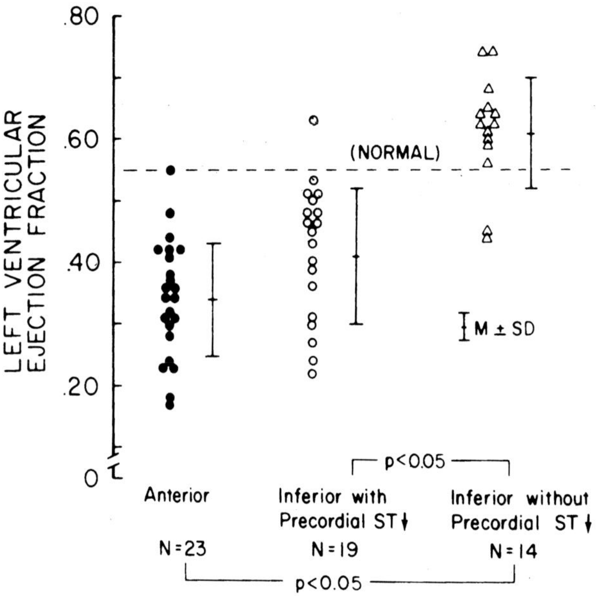

Fig. 100.1 Left ventricular ejection function related to the electrocardiographic location of acute myocardial infarction. Note the significant heterogeneity in ejection fraction in patients with anterior and inferior infarction. The horizontal dashed line denotes the lower limit of normal for left ventricular ejection fraction. (Reproduced with permission from Shah et al[29].)

DETERMINING MYOCARDIUM AT RISK AND INFARCT SIZE

The left ventricular ejection fraction is commonly used as an indirect measure of infarct size, although it has long been appreciated that the final ejection fraction after acute infarction varies widely in individual patients and is only partially related to infarct location.[29,30] Shaw et al[29] demonstrated in the pre-thrombolytic era that patients admitted with their first Q-wave infarction had ejection fractions ranging from below 20% to well over 60% as measured by gated radionuclide angiography. Patients with anterior infarction had a significantly lower mean ejection fraction compared to those with inferior infarction, but there was substantial individual overlap (Fig. 100.1). This has also been observed using myocardial perfusion imaging, which allows a more accurate quantitative assessment of infarct size than the ejection fraction.[26,31–32] Thus, infarct size cannot be predicted a priori based on infarct location.

The extent of myocardium at risk is also highly variable following occlusion of a specific coronary artery as observed both in animal models[33] and clinical trials.[34–36] In a recent study using first-pass radionuclide angiography, the left ventricular ejection fraction was determined immediately before and during transient coronary artery occlusion in patients undergoing angioplasty.[36] During occlusion of the left anterior descending artery, the left ventricular ejection fraction significantly decreased compared to baseline (55 ± 13% to 32 ± 11%, p=0.0001) whereas right coronary artery occlusion had minimal effects (49 ± 12% to 46 ± 13%). However, in individual patients, the amount of myocardium at risk from a given

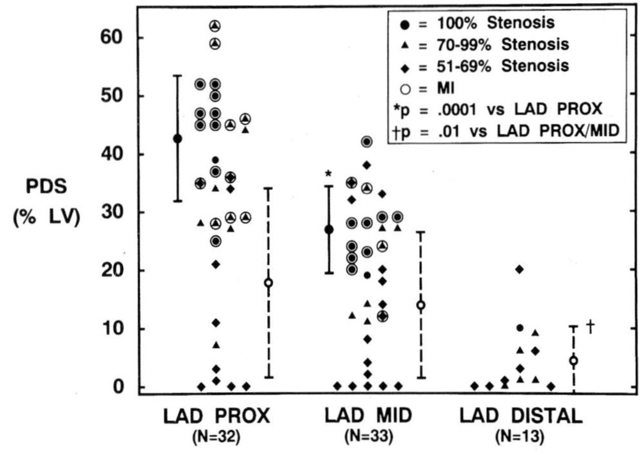

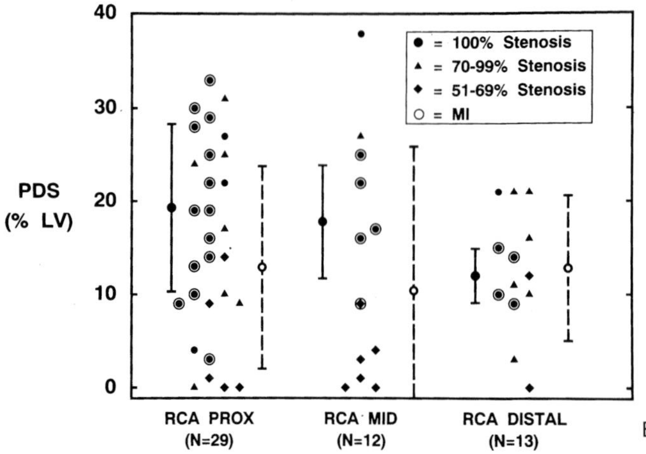

Fig. 100.2 Mean left ventricular perfusion defect size (PDS) in patients with (solid bar) and without (broken bar) myocardial infarction (MI) for the left anterior descending (LAD) (A) and right (RCA) (B) coronary arteries with proximal (prox) MID or distal stenosis. Although proximal LAD stenosis (A) generally led to a larger perfusion defect size than did MID or distal stenosis, there was significant individual vessel heterogeneity. This was also observed for the right coronary artery. The anatomic information was imprecise at predicting the extent of jeopardized myocardium. (Reproduced with permission from Mahmarian et al[39].)

coronary occlusion varied considerably. Twenty-three per cent of patients during right or circumflex occlusions had a >10% drop in ejection fraction whereas 18% of patients during left anterior descending occlusion had a <10% decrease. Similar results have been reported using exercise thallium-201(^{201}Tl) perfusion scintigraphy.[37–39] Although proximal left anterior descending artery stenosis produces perfusion defects approximately twice as large as proximal right or circumflex stenosis, the size of the risk zone varies widely even at similar stenosis locations within a specific coronary artery[39] (Fig. 100.2).

The impact of coronary occlusion on infarct size as assessed by perfusion imaging or the left ventricular ejection fraction is not definable from knowing the coronary anatomy. Furthermore, there are no clinical patient characteristics which can predict the extent of myocardium at risk. Thus, in placebo controlled trials assessing benefit with thrombolytic agents, unless the size of the risk zone is known, the extent of myocardial salvage cannot be determined because the final infarct size is inseparably linked to the initial size of the area at risk.

LEFT VENTRICULAR EJECTION FRACTION

Although the left ventricular ejection fraction is known to impart important prognostic information,[40–42] it is imprecise for detecting coronary reperfusion or measuring therapeutic benefit following thrombolysis. Since the ejection fraction is affected by cardiac loading conditions, heart rate, intrinsic regional contractility, the duration of the ischaemic insult, the location of infarction, the initial size of the risk zone, as well as the actual infarct size, it is impossible to sort out to what extent each of these parameters contributes to the final ejection fraction value.[27,43,44] Thus, a single resting ejection fraction obtained prior to hospital discharge in patients enrolled in a randomized trial of thrombolytic therapy *vs.* placebo might demonstrate variable results, not based on the therapy per se, but rather due to unrecognized differences in the above parameters in an otherwise seemingly closely matched population. This dilemma is apparent from many of the large, randomized placebo-controlled trials assessing the efficacy of thrombolytic therapy with the ejection fraction.[13–16,19,21,22]

In order to control for the known wide disparity in myocardium at risk during acute infarction, several studies have assessed the left ventricular ejection fraction prior to administering a thrombolytic agent and again several weeks later.[7–12,17,18,20] By using each patient as his/her own control, the sequential change in ejection fraction might prove to be a more meaningful expression of myocardial salvage than a single measurement after infarction. Most of these studies have shown a significant improvement in group mean left ventricular function with early recanalization of the infarct-related artery. However, assessing benefit in individual patients remains difficult since cardiac loading conditions and heart rate will invariably differ from the time of initial infarction to several weeks later. Furthermore, regional myocardial stunning within the reperfused area and reversible hypercontractility of non-infarct regions add yet greater complexity.[27,43] Thus, although the left ventricular ejection fraction is useful for assessing sequential group changes in clinical trials this is clearly not an optimal measure of thrombolytic success in individual patients.

MYOCARDIAL PERFUSION SCINTIGRAPHY

Myocardial perfusion scintigraphy is an attractive method for assessing the extent of infarction since the uptake of

Table 100.1 Myocardial perfusion agents

	^{201}Tl	^{99m} sestamibi	^{99m}Tc-teboroxime
Energy	80 keV	140 keV	140 keV
Dose	3 mCi	25–30 mCi	25–30 mCi
Physical $t_{1/2}$	72 h	6 h	6 h
Cardiac uptake	linear	linear	linear
Extraction	0.75	0.65	0.90
Cardiac clearance		5–6 h	2 min (68%) 78 min (32%)
Redistribution	+++	+/o	+/o
Hepatic clearance		30 min	90 min
Imaging post-injection	5–10 min	up to 6 h	1–2 min

^{201}Tl and more recently developed technetium-based radiopharmaceuticals is not affected by cardiac loading conditions, heart rate, myocardial stunning, or regional differences in left ventricular contractility as noted with the ejection fraction. The myocardial uptake of ^{201}Tl, technetium-99m (^{99m}Tc) sestamibi and teboroxime is directly related to blood flow,[45–49] allowing accurate quantification of the area at risk during coronary occlusion. There are some important differences, however, between these radioisotopes (Table 100.1). ^{201}Tl is actively transported into myocardial cells whereas ^{99m}Tc sestamibi (Cardiolite) and teboroxime passively cross intact cell membranes. ^{201}Tl then redistributes substantially from normal regions to hypoperfused areas[45,50] whereas sestamibi redistributes only minimally[47,51,52] and so can define the myocardial area at risk during coronary occlusion, even when imaging is performed several hours after the initial injection. Teboroxime is rapidly taken up by the myocardium but unlike sestamibi washes out within minutes[53] so that rapid imaging is required.

EXPERIMENTAL STUDIES WITH THALLIUM-201

Although ^{201}Tl has been used extensively in cardiac imaging for the detection of coronary disease and myocardial ischaemia, its utility in the setting of acute infarction may be somewhat limited.

In animals with sustained coronary occlusion, the final infarct size is synonymous with the area at risk. In this model of permanent occlusion, initial ^{201}Tl activity within the infarct zone correlates very well with coronary blood flow as measured by radiolabelled microspheres.[50] However, the relative gradient in thallium activity between the normal myocardium and the infarct zone decreases over time due to isotope washout from the normal regions (Fig. 100.3). Due to the kinetics of ^{201}Tl, the count activity within the infarct zone might appear to improve over time relative to the normally perfused myocardium, with an artifactual reduction in scintigraphic infarct size.

This phenomenon is exaggerated following reperfusion[50] where myocardial thallium concentrations not only

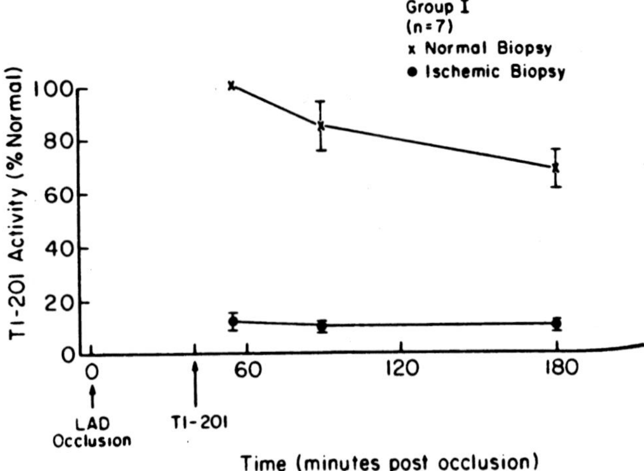

Fig. 100.3 Myocardial thallium ^{201}Tl time–activity curves in dogs after 3 hours of sustained coronary artery occlusion. Note the constancy of low counts in the area of the infarct zone (ischaemic biopsy) *vs.* the decrease in counts from the normal myocardium over time. (Reproduced with permission from Granato et al[50].)

decrease in normal regions but steadily increase within the ischaemic zone resulting in a far greater reduction in the thallium gradient than observed during sustained coronary artery occlusion. Furthermore, when ^{201}Tl is administered immediately after reperfusion, excessive activity is found within the reperfused area due to vascular reactive hyperaemia which leads to an underestimation of infarct size.

Based on these observations, in order to accurately determine the myocardial area at risk (and hence the degree of salvage) cardiac imaging with ^{201}Tl should be performed shortly after isotope administration and preferably prior to giving thrombolytic agents. Since infarct size is directly related to the duration of coronary occlusion, withholding thrombolytic therapy for up to an additional hour in order to perform a baseline perfusion scan would seem both impractical and unethical.

EXPERIMENTAL STUDIES WITH TECHNETIUM-99m SESTAMIBI

The feasibility of using ^{99m}Tc sestamibi perfusion scintigraphy for quantifying infarct size and the degree of myocardial salvage following coronary reperfusion has been recently investigated in our animal laboratory.[54] In a model of sustained coronary occlusion, a close correlation was found between the quantified tomographic and pathologic infarct sizes (Fig. 100.4). This observation has been confirmed by others.[52,55] Furthermore, there is a close correlation between initial sestamibi uptake and occluded flows by microspheres,[52,55] but unlike ^{201}Tl, the relative gradient in sestamibi activity between normally perfused and infarcted zones does not decrease substantially over time.[52,55] Thus, the risk zone quantified by sestamibi

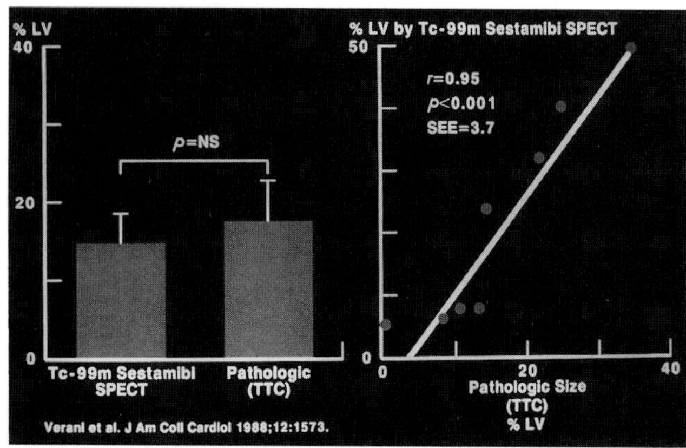

Fig. 100.4 Comparison of tomographic (SPECT) and pathologic infarct sizes in 13 dogs with permanent coronary occlusion. LV = left ventricle; TTC = triphenyltetrazolium chloride. (Reproduced with permission from Verani et al[54].)

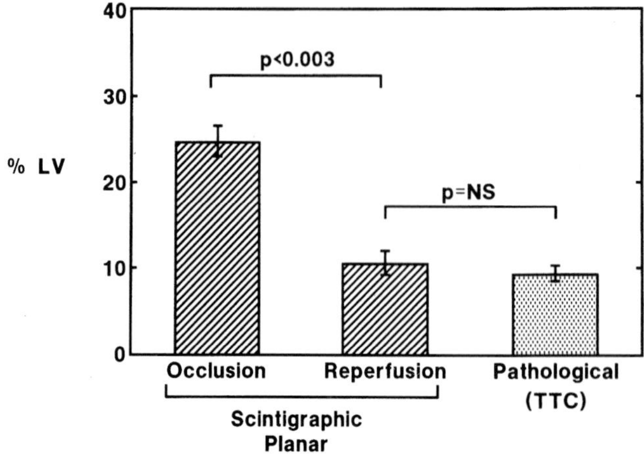

Fig. 100.5 Comparison of planar scintigraphic defect size during occlusion and following reperfusion with pathologic infarct size in 12 dogs. Note the final scintigraphic infarct size after reperfusion is similar to the pathologic infarct size. The difference between the initial defect during occlusion and the final infarct size after reperfusion is the extent of myocardial salvage. Abbreviations as in Figure 100.4. (Reproduced with permission from Verani et al[54].)

scintigraphy is comparable to that defined by pathology independent of temporal constraints.

In an animal model of occlusion followed by coronary reperfusion, the scintigraphic and anatomic risk zones during occlusion were comparable in size, and both were significantly larger than the perfusion defect quantified after coronary reperfusion (Fig. 100.5).[54] Importantly, however, the scintigraphic perfusion defect size after reperfusion was similar to the pathologic infarct size. Other investigators have likewise demonstrated a close correlation in animals between scintigraphic and pathologic infarct sizes which is not influenced by the early reactive hyperaemia observed following rapid reperfusion.[52,55] These series of experiments support the concept that serial sestamibi imaging during acute infarction can delineate the area at risk during occlusion and subsequently provide a quantitative assessment of the degree of myocardial salvage after reperfusion.

CLINICAL TRIALS USING THALLIUM-201 SCINTIGRAPHY

The largest reported placebo-controlled study evaluating myocardial salvage after thrombolytic therapy has been published by the Western Washington Study Group using intracoronary[21] and intravenous[22] streptokinase. In the intracoronary trial, patients were randomized within 12 h of acute infarction (mean 276 min) to either streptokinase or placebo. Of the 232 survivors, 207 had assessment of left ventricular perfusion at a mean time of 62 ± 35 days. As shown in Table 100.2, no significant reduction in infarct size was observed as reflected indirectly by the left ventricular ejection fraction or the quantified ^{201}Tl perfusion defect size, despite a significant survival benefit with thrombolytic therapy.

In the intravenous streptokinase trial, patients were treated within 6 h of symptoms (mean time 209 min) and had gated radionuclide angiography and tomographic imaging performed several (8.2 ± 7.5) weeks later. Although the total perfusion defect size was significantly smaller in patients treated with streptokinase (15 ± 13%) *vs.* placebo (19 ± 13%, p=0.03), the left ventricular ejection fraction did not significantly improve.

The lack of a more substantial benefit with streptokinase in these trials probably reflects study design rather

Table 100.2 Western Washington Trial results

	Placebo	Intracoronary SK		Placebo	Intravenous SK	
Ejection fraction						
Total	46 ± 14% (*N*=92)	46 ± 14% (*N*=115)	NS	47 ± 15% (*N*=95)	51 ± 15% (*N*=110)	0.08
ANT MI	41 ± 15% (*N*=38)	37 ± 14% (*N*=51)	NS	37 ± 15% (*N*=33)	43 ± 19% (*N*=31)	NS
INF MI	49 ± 13% (*N*=54)	53 ± 10% (*N*=64)	NS	52 ± 12% (*N*=62)	54 ± 12% (*N*=79)	NS
<3 h to therapy	49 ± 15% (*N*=20)	46 ± 14% (*N*=25)	NS	49 ± 15% (*N*=51)	51 ± 14% (*N*=55)	NS
Perfusion defect size						
Total	20 ± 12% (*N*=48)	19 ± 13% (*N*=52)	NS	19 ± 13% (*N*=97)	15 ± 13% (*N*=110)	0.03
ANT MI	23 ± 13% (*N*=16)	28 ± 12% (*N*=24)	NS	27 ± 13% (*N*=34)	23 ± 15% (*N*=31)	NS
INF MI	18 ± 11% (*N*=32)	12 ± 13% (*N*=28)	NS	14 ± 12% (*N*=63)	12 ± 11% (*N*=79)	NS
<3 h to therapy	19 ± 10% (*N*=9)	19 ± 11% (*N*=10)	NS	18 ± 13% (*N*=51)	13 ± 12% (*N*=55)	0.05

Abbreviations: ANT = anterior; INF = inferior; MI = myocardial infarction; SK = streptokinase

than drug efficacy. First, most patients (78%) in the first trial and 48% of those in the second study were treated >3 h after infarction, which may have limited the extent of myocardium that was salvageable. Second, the left ventricular ejection fraction and the tomographic studies were not performed in all patients due to subsequent deaths after hospital discharge. The higher mortality rate in the placebo group may be reflective of patients with larger infarcts and lower ejection fractions. By eliminating these patients, the mean placebo ejection fraction might have been spuriously raised and the perfusion defect size decreased. Third, although baseline characteristics were similar between those receiving placebo and active therapy, unrecognized differences in the initial area at risk between the groups might have precluded detecting a significant benefit as assessed by the ejection fraction or scintigraphic infarct size. Several smaller clinical trials, however, performing sequential ^{201}Tl imaging before and after thrombolytic therapy[23–25] have demonstrated myocardial salvage with coronary reperfusion. Nonetheless, the practicality of this approach is questioned due to the need for rapid acute imaging prior to administering thrombolytic therapy.

CLINICAL TRIALS USING TECHNETIUM-99m SESTAMIBI

The physical properties and kinetics of ^{99m}Tc sestamibi are ideal for assessing the area at risk during acute infarction and the final infarct size several days later (Fig. 100.6). The effects of thrombolysis and angioplasty on reducing infarct size have recently been reported using this method.

Patients with anterior infarction have a significantly larger scintigraphic risk zone (53 ± 17%) than those with inferior or lateral infarcts (24 ± 18%), despite considerable individual patient variability.[26] This may explain why in large clinical trials most of the survival benefit with thrombolytic agents has been observed in patients with anterior rather than inferior infarction, since the former generally have more severe left ventricular dysfunction and a higher mortality. However, there is clearly a subset of patients with inferior infarction who have a large extent of myocardium at risk, where early coronary reperfusion would be desirable.

If one considers a clinically important infarct as one which involves ≥20% of the left ventricle,[56] this is observed in virtually all patients with anterior infarction but also in approximately 1/2 of those with inferior/lateral infarcts.[26,57] As previously pointed out, there are no clinical or angiographic variables which can predict the size of the myocardial risk zone, emphasizing the clinical utility of sestamibi perfusion imaging in the acute infarction setting when contemplating therapeutic options.

Imaging with ^{99m}Tc sestamibi also allows an accurate estimate of myocardial salvage following a given therapeutic intervention. As in animal models of occlusion/reperfusion, clinical studies using sequential planar or tomographic perfusion imaging have likewise demonstrated reductions in infarct size with thrombolytic compared to conventional therapy when each patient is used as his/her own control.[26–28,57–59] In a recent multicentre pilot study, 10 out of 11 (91%) patients treated with thrombolytics achieved myocardial salvage compared to only 1 out of 4 patients treated conventionally (Fig. 100.7).[26] The mean extent of myocardial salvage was 13% (range 0–33%, p<0.003) for those receiving thrombolytics *vs.* −4% (range 4–11%) for the placebo group. These results are qualitatively similar to those reported using planar scintigraphy.[28] Furthermore, patients who achieve early reperfusion with thrombolytic

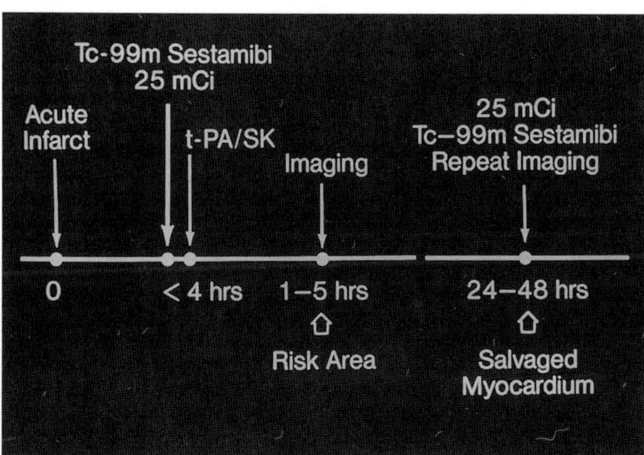

Fig. 100.6 Protocol sequence for assessing area at risk and extent of myocardial salvage using ^{99m}Tc sestamibi. SK = streptokinase; tPA = tissue plasminogen activator.

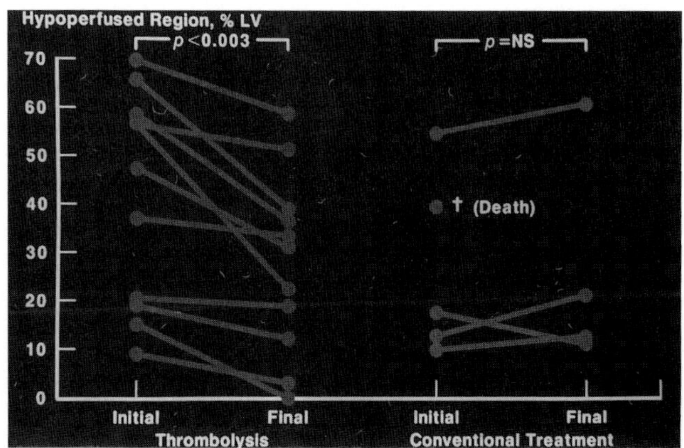

Fig. 100.7 Initial hypoperfused region (myocardium at risk) and final hypoperfused zone (infarct size) for patients treated with thrombolysis and conventional therapy. In patients receiving thrombolysis there was a significant decrease in defect size consistent with myocardial salvage. (Reproduced with permission from Gibbons et al[26].)

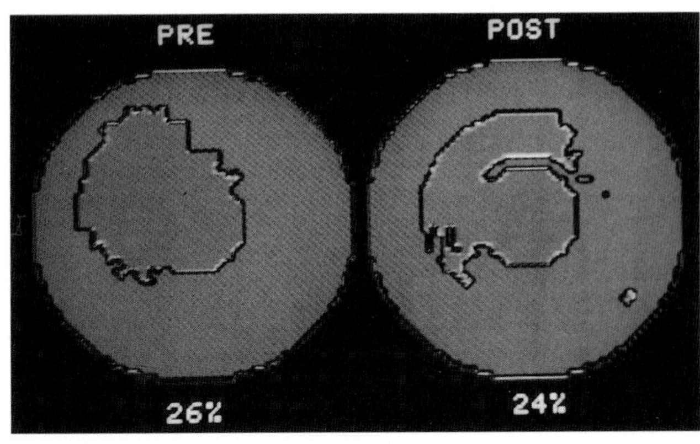

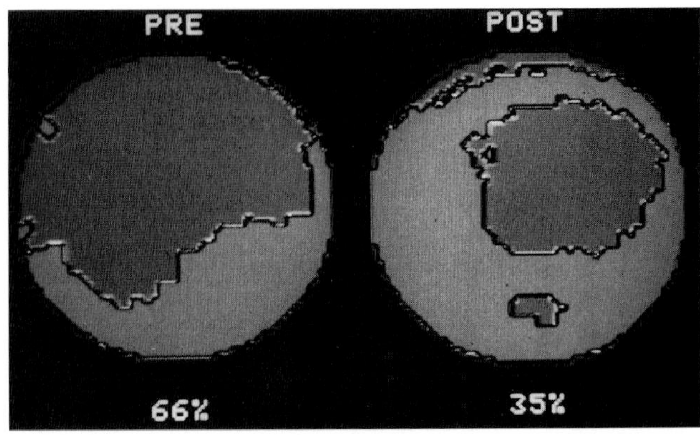

Fig. 100.8 Quantified perfusion defects displayed as polar maps for patients pre- and post-thrombolytic therapy with r-TPA. The patient in A had an initial risk zone quantified as 26% of the left ventricle and involving the apex and anterior septum (left). No improvement was observed following thrombolytic therapy (right). This patient at cardiac catheterization had an occluded MID left anterior descending coronary artery. The patient in B had an acute anterior wall infarction with the initial risk zone quantified as 66% of the left ventricle and involving the anterior, apical, septal, lateral and inferoapical regions (left). The scan 48 h later shows a residual infarct size of 35% indicating 47% myocardial salvage (right). On cardiac catheterization this patient had a residual 50% stenosis involving the proximal LAD coronary artery. Abbreviations as in Figure 100.2.

therapy have the greatest extent of myocardial salvage in contrast with those who have a persistently occluded artery.[28] Figure 100.8 illustrates the scintigraphic results in two patients studied with sequential sestamibi imaging.

Although achieving early vessel patency is important for reducing infarct size, several other variables contribute toward myocardial salvage. Christian et al[59] recently studied 89 patients who had early coronary reperfusion with either thrombolytic therapy (*N*=32) or acute angioplasty (*N*=57). All patients had sestamibi perfusion imaging pre- and post-reperfusion and coronary angiography prior to hospital discharge. In a multivariate analysis, the initial extent of myocardium at risk contributed most to the final absolute infarct size, although the per cent of myocardium salvaged was similar whether patients had large or small initial defects. The presence of collateral flow to the infarct-related artery and the time from occlusion to reperfusion also significantly contributed to the model for predicting final infarct size (r^2=0.70). These results are consistent with studies reporting an enhanced survival benefit when thrombolytic therapy is given to patients who have anterior infarction,[1] and particularly within several hours of chest pain.[1] Furthermore, patients who do not achieve reperfusion but have collaterals to the infarct-related artery have a smaller enzymatic infarct size than those who have no collaterals.[60]

The assessment of therapeutic benefit with perfusion scintigraphy has recently been compared to the resting left ventricular ejection fraction. A close inverse correlation is observed between the final infarct size assessed by perfusion scintigraphy and the resting global and regional left ventricular ejection fraction. However, in the study by Christian et al, over 1/3 of patients achieving successful reperfusion had either a significant increase or decrease in global left ventricular function from discharge to 4–6 weeks later.[43] Other studies have likewise shown that patients with significant myocardial salvage by scintigraphy may still have dyssynergy within the region of infarction at hospital discharge.[27] In the study by Santoro et al,[27] six out of seven patients with significant myocardial salvage by perfusion scintigraphy showed no improvement in regional wall motion by echocardiography until several weeks after infarction. Conversely, patients without scintigraphic improvement following thrombolytic therapy had no improvement in their serial echocardiograms. These

MYOCARDIAL SALVAGE DURING ACUTE INFARCTION
Tc-99M SESTAMIBI

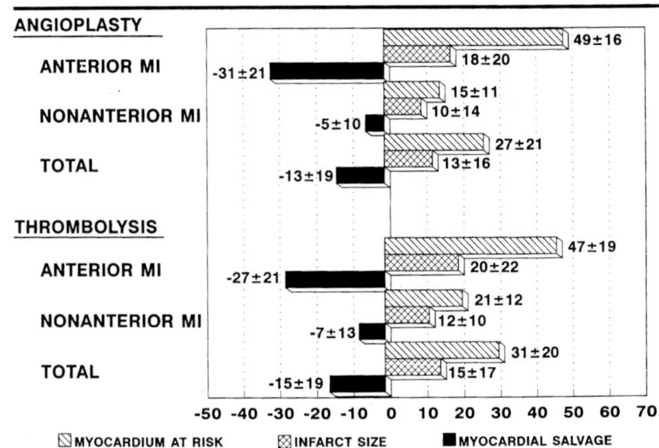

Fig. 100.9 The results of acute angioplasty of the infarct-related artery versus thrombolytic therapy with r-TPA for reducing infarct size.[63] Note that patients with anterior infarction had an initial myocardium at risk 2–3 fold larger than those with non-anterior infarction, although the standard deviations were large. Angioplasty and thrombolytic therapy were comparable for salvaging myocardium. MI = myocardial infarction.

results stress the importance of perfusion scintigraphy for assessing myocardial salvage since left ventricular stunning within the infarct zone or hyperkinesis in non-infarct regions early post-infarction can be misleading.

Sequential perfusion scintigraphy with sestamibi may also be used to evaluate the benefits of coronary angioplasty in patients with evolving myocardial infarction. In a recent study reported by Gibbons et al,[61] 180 patients with acute infarction were randomized to either initial therapy with tissue plasminogen activator or immediate angioplasty. Randomization was stratified according to the onset of chest pain and the site of infarction. The baseline characteristics of the two patient groups were similar. As shown in Figure 100.9, patients with anterior infarction had a significantly greater extent of myocardium at risk than patients with non-anterior infarcts, but the degree of myocardial salvage with either treatment was comparable. The ejection fraction at discharge, not surprisingly, was very similar between those who were randomized to thrombolytic therapy ($50 \pm 10\%$) *vs.* angioplasty ($53 \pm 11\%$). Thus, it would appear from these initial data that even when facilities are readily available to perform angioplasty within the first several hours after infarction, the benefit achieved appears to be no better than that obtained by the simple administration of an intravenous thrombolytic agent.

FUTURE DIRECTIONS

The technology to quantify the extent of myocardial salvage following acute infarction has allowed assessment of various therapeutic modalities. Unfortunately, ^{99m}Tc sestamibi scintigraphy requires repeat imaging over a several day interval so that failure to reperfuse is recognized at a time when restoring flow may have no beneficial effect. A major future advance would be to serially assess changes in myocardial perfusion over relatively short (1/2 to 1 h) time intervals in order to determine whether reperfusion had occurred, and so allow time to further intervene in patients who did not respond to initial therapies. An ideal perfusion agent for this task would have flow characteristics similar to thallium-201, a very short myocardial half-life to allow rapid sequential imaging, and a favourable energy profile. In many respects ^{99m}Tc teboroxime is well-suited for this kind of evaluation (Table 100.2), but due to its very fast myocardial washout and slow clearance from the liver, acute imaging is feasible but very difficult with this agent.

REFERENCES

1. Gruppo Italiano per lo Studio della Streptochinase nell' Infarto Miocardico (GISSI) 1986 Effectiveness of intravenous thrombolytic treatment in acute myocardial infarction. Lancet 1: 397–402
2. ISAM Study Group 1986 A prospective trial of intravenous streptokinase in acute myocardial infarction (ISAM): mortality, morbidity, and infarct size at 21 days. N Engl J Med 314: 1465–1471
3. ISIS-2 (Second International Study of Infarct Survival) Collaborative Group 1988 Randomised trial of intravenous streptokinase, oral aspirin, both, or neither among 17,187 cases of suspected acute myocardial infarction: ISIS-2. Lancet 2: 349–360
4. AIMS Trial Study Group 1988 Effect of intravenous APSAC on mortality after acute myocardial infarction: preliminary report of a placebo-controlled clinical trial. Lancet 1: 545–559
5. Anglo-Scandinavian Study of Early Thrombolysis Study Group 1988 Trial of tissue plasminogen activator for mortality reduction in acute myocardial infarction. Anglo-Scandinavian Study of Early Thrombolysis (ASSET). Lancet 2: 525–530
6. Rovelli F, deVita C, Feruglio G A, Lotto A, Selvini A, Tognoni G, GISSI investigators 1987 GISSI Trial: early results and late follow-up. J Am Coll Cardiol 10: 33B–39B
7. Touchstone D A, Beller G A, Nygaard T W, Tedesco C, Kaul S 1989 Effects of successful intravenous reperfusion therapy on regional myocardial function and geometry in humans: a tomographic assessment using two-dimensional echocardiography. J Am Coll Cardiol 13: 1506–1513
8. Sheehan F H, Braunwald E, Canner P et al 1987 The effect of intravenous thrombolytic therapy on left ventricular function: a report of tissue-type plasminogen activator and streptokinase from the Thrombolysis in Myocardial Infarction (TIMI Phase I) Trial. Circulation 75: 817–829
9. Sheehan F H, Mathey D G, Schofer J, Krebber H J, Dodge H T 1983 Effect of interventions in salvaging left ventricular function in acute myocardial infarction: a study of intracoronary streptokinase. Am J Cardiol 52: 431–438
10. Anderson J L, Marshall H W, Bray B E et al 1983 A randomized trial of intracoronary streptokinase in the treatment of acute myocardial infarction. N Engl J Med 308: 1321–1328
11. Raizner A E, Tortoledo F A, Verani M S et al 1985 Intracoronary thrombolytic therapy in acute myocardial infarction: a prospective, randomized, controlled trial. Am J Cardiol 55: 301–308
12. Smalling R W, Fuentes F, Matthews M W et al 1983 Sustained improvement in left ventricular function and mortality by intracoronary streptokinase administration during evolving myocardial infarction. Circulation 68: 131–138
13. White H D, Norris R M, Brown M A et al 1987 Effect of intravenous streptokinase on left ventricular function and early survival after acute myocardial infarction. N Engl J Med 317: 850–855
14. DeFeyter P J, VanEenige M J, VanDerWall E E et al 1983 Effects of spontaneous and streptokinase-induced recanalization on left ventricular function after myocardial infarction. Circulation 67: 1039–1044
15. Kennedy J W, Martin G V, David K B et al 1988 The Western Washington intravenous streptokinase in acute myocardial infarction randomized trial. Circulation 77: 345–352
16. O'Rourke M, Baron D, Keogh A et al 1988 Limitation of myocardial infarction by early infusion of recombinant tissue-type plasminogen activator. Circulation 77: 1311–1315
17. Rentrop K P, Feit F, Blanke H et al 1984 Effects of intracoronary streptokinase and intracoronary nitroglycerin infusion on coronary angiographic patterns and mortality in patients with acute myocardial infarction. N Engl J Med 311: 1457–1463
18. Khaja F, Walton J A, Brymer J F et al 1983 Intracoronary fibrinolytic therapy in acute myocardial infarction. N Engl J Med 308: 1305–1311
19. Simoons M L, Serruys P W, van den Brand M et al 1986 Early thrombolysis in acute myocardial infarction: limitation of infarct size and improved survival. J Am Coll Cardiol 7: 717–728
20. Guerci A D, Gerstenblith G, Brinker J A et al 1987 A randomized trial of intravenous tissue plasminogen activator for acute myocardial infarction with subsequent randomization to elective coronary angioplasty. N Engl J Med 317: 1613–1618

21. Ritchie J L, Davis K B, Williams D L, Caldwell J, Kennedy J W 1984 Global and regional left ventricular function and tomographic radionuclide perfusion: The Western Washington intracoronary streptokinase in myocardial infarction trial. Circulation 70: 867–875
22. Ritchie J L, Cerqueira M, Maynard C, Davis K, Kennedy J W 1988 Ventricular function and infarction size: the Western Washington intravenous streptokinase in myocardial infarction trial. J Am Coll Cardiol 11: 689–697
23. DeCoster P M, Melvin J A, Detry J-MR, Brasseur L A, Beckers C, Col J 1985 Coronary artery reperfusion in acute myocardial infarction: assessment by pre- and postintervention thallium-201 myocardial perfusion imaging. Am J Cardiol 55: 889–895
24. Schuler G, Schwarz F, Hofmann M et al 1982 Thrombolysis in acute myocardial infarction using intracoronary streptokinase: assessment by thallium-201 scintigraphy. Circulation 66: 658–664
25. Markis J E, Malagold M, Parker J A et al 1981 Myocardial salvage after intracoronary thrombolysis with streptokinase in acute myocardial infarction. N Engl J Med 305: 777–782
26. Gibbons R J, Verani M S, Behrenbeck T et al 1989 Feasibility of tomographic 99mTc-hexakis-2-methoxy-2-methylpropyl- isonitrile imaging for the assessment of myocardial area at risk and the effect of treatment in acute myocardial infarction. Circulation 80: 1277–1286
27. Santoro G M, Bisi G, Sciagra R, Leoncini M, Fazzini P F, Meldolesi U 1990 Single photon emission computed tomography with technetium-99m hexakis 2-methoxyisobutyl isonitrile in acute myocardial infarction before and after thrombolytic treatment: assessment of salvaged myocardium and prediction of late functional recovery. J Am Coll Cardiol 15: 301–314
28. Wackers F J, Gibbons R J, Verani M S et al 1989 Serial quantitative planar technetium-99m isonitrile imaging in acute myocardial infarction: efficacy for noninvasive assessment of thrombolytic therapy. J Am Coll Cardiol 14: 861–873
29. Shah P K, Pichler M, Berman D S, Singh B N, Swan H J C 1980 Left ventricular ejection fraction determined by radionuclide ventriculography in early stages of first transmural myocardial infarction. Relation to short-term prognosis. Am J Cardiol 45: 542–546
30. Kumpuris A G, Quiñones M A, Kanon D, Miller R R 1980 Isolated stenosis of left anterior descending or right coronary artery: relation between site of stenosis and ventricular dysfunction and therapeutic implications. Am J Cardiol 46: 13–20
31. Mahmarian J J, Pratt C M, Borges-Neto S, Cashion W R, Roberts R, Verani M S 1988 Quantification of infarct size by thallium-201 single-photon emission computed tomography during acute myocardial infarction in man: comparison with enzymatic estimates. Circulation 78: 831–839
32. Mahmarian J J, Pratt C M, Nishimura S, Abreu A, Verani MS 1993 Quantitative adenosine 201-Tl single-photon emission computed tomography for the early assessment of patients surviving acute myocardial infarction. Circulation 87: 1197–1210
33. Reimer K A, Ideker R E, Jennings R B 1981 Effect of coronary occlusion site on ischemic bed size and collateral blood flow in dogs. Cardiovasc Res 15: 668–674
34. Feiring A J, Johnson M R, Kioschos J M, Kirchner P T, Marcus M L, White C W 1987 The importance of the determination of the myocardial area at risk in the evaluation of the outcome of acute myocardial infarction in patients. Circulation 75: 980–987
35. Bertrand M E, Lablanche J M, Fourrier J L, Traisnel G, Mirsky I 1988 Left ventricular systolic and diastolic function during acute coronary artery balloon occlusion in humans. J Am Coll Cardiol 12: 341–347
36. Verani M S, Lacy J L, Guidry G W et al 1992 Quantification of left ventricular performance during transient coronary occlusion at various anatomic sites in humans: a study using tantalum-178 and a multiwire gamma camera. J Am Coll Cardiol 19: 297–306
37. Iskandrian A S, Lichtenberg R, Segal B L et al 1982 Assessment of jeopardized myocardium in patients with one-vessel disease. Circulation 65: 242–247
38. DePace N L, Iskandrian A S, Nadell R, Colby J, Hakki A-H 1983 Variation in the size of jeopardized myocardium in patients with isolated left anterior descending coronary artery disease. Circulation 67: 988–994
39. Mahmarian J J, Pratt C M, Boyce T M, Verani M S 1991 The variable extent of jeopardized myocardium in patients with single vessel coronary artery disease: quantification by thallium-201 single photon emission computed tomography. J Am Coll Cardiol 17: 355–362
40. Bigger J T Jr, Fleiss J L, Kleiger R, Miller J P, Rolnitzky L M, for the Multicenter Post-Infarction Research Group 1984 The relationships among ventricular arrhythmias, left ventricular dysfunction and mortality in the 2 years after myocardial infarction. Circulation 69: 250–258
41. Becker L C, Silverman K J, Bulkley B H, Kallman C H, Mellits E D, Weisfeldt M 1983 Comparison of early 201-Tl scintigraphy and gated blood pool imaging for predicting mortality in patients with acute myocardial infarction. Circulation 67: 1272–1282
42. Sanz G, Castaner A, Betriu A et al 1987 Determinants of prognosis in survivors of myocardial infarction: a prospective clinical angiographic study. N Engl J Med 306: 1065–1070
43. Christian T F, Behrenbeck T, Pellikka P A, Huber K C, Chesebro J H, Gibbons R J 1990 Mismatch of left ventricular function and infarct size demonstrated by technetium-99m isonitrile imaging after reperfusion therapy for acute myocardial infarction: identification of myocardial stunning and hyperkinesia. J Am Coll Cardiol 16: 1632–1638
44. Wackers F J, Berger H J, Weinberg M A, Zaret B L 1982 Spontaneous changes in left ventricular function over the first 24 hours of acute myocardial infarction: implications for evaluating early therapeutic interventions. Circulation 66: 748–754
45. Nishiyama H, Adolph R J, Gabel M, Lukes S J, Franklin D, Williams C C 1982 Effect of coronary blood flow on thallium-201 uptake and washout. Circulation 65: 534–542
46. Leppo J A, Meerdink D A 1989 Comparison of the myocardial uptake of a technetium-labeled isonitrile analogue and thallium. Circ Res 65: 632–639
47. Okada R D, Glover D, Gaffney T, Williams S 1988 Myocardial kinetics of technetium-99m-hexakis-2-methoxy-2-methylpropyl-isonitrile. Circulation 77: 491–498
48. Marshall R C, Leidholdt E M Jr, Zhang D Y, Barnett C A 1990 Technetium-99m hexakis 2-methoxy-2-isobutyl isonitrile and thallium-201 extraction, washout, and retention at varying coronary flow rates in rabbit heart. Circulation 82: 998–1007
49. Leppo J A, Meerdink D J 1990 Comparative myocardial extraction of two technetium-labeled BATO derivatives (SQ30217, SQ32014) and thallium. J Nucl Med 31: 67–74
50. Granato J E, Watson D D, Flanagan T L, Gascho J A, Beller G A 1986 Myocardial thallium-201 kinetics during coronary occlusion and reperfusion: influence of method of reflow and timing of thallium-201 administration. Circulation 73: 150–160
51. Liu P, Houle S, Mills L, Dawood F 1987 Kinetics of Tc-99m MIBI in clearance in ischemia-reperfusion: comparison with Tl-201 Circulation 76 (Suppl IV): IV–216 (Abstract)
52. Sinusas A J, Trautman K A, Bergin J D et al 1990 Quantification of area at risk during coronary occlusion and degree of myocardial salvage after reperfusion with technetium-99m methoxyisobutyl isonitrile. Circulation 82: 1424–1437
53. Narra R K, Nunn A D, Kuczynski B L, Feld T, Wedeking P, Eckelman W C 1989 A neutral technetium-99m complex for myocardial imaging. J Nucl Med 30: 1830–1837
54. Verani M S, Jeroudi M O, Mahmarian J J et al 1988 Quantification of myocardial infarction during coronary occlusion and myocardial salvage after reperfusion using cardiac imaging with technetium-99m hexakis 2-methoxyisobutyl isonitrile. J Am Coll Cardiol 12: 1573–1581
55. DeCoster P M, Wijns W, Cauwe F, Robert A, Beckers C, Melin J A 1990 Area-at-risk determination by technetium-99m-hexakis-2-methoxyisobutyl isonitrile in experimental reperfused myocardial infarction. Circulation 82: 2152–2162
56. Mahmarian J J, Cochran A J, Marks G F, Verani M S 1993 Models for predicting long-term outcome after acute myocardial infarction

by quantitative adenosine tomography. J Nucl Med 34: 54P (Abstract)

57. Christian T F, Gibbons R J, Gersh B J 1991 Effect of infarct location on myocardial salvage assessed by technetium-99m isonitrile. J Am Coll Cardiol 17: 1303–1308
58. Pellikka P A, Behrenbeck T, Verani M S, Mahmarian J J, Wackers F J Th, Gibbons R J 1990 Serial changes in myocardial perfusion using tomographic technetium-99m-hexakis-2-methoxy-2-methylpropyl-isonitrile imaging following reperfusion therapy of myocardial infarction. J Nucl Med 31: 1269-1275
59. Christian T F, Schwartz R S, Gibbons R J 1992 Determinants of infarct size in reperfusion therapy for acute myocardial infarction. Circulation 86: 81–90
60. Habib G B, Heibig J, Forman S A et al 1991 Influence of coronary collateral vessels on myocardial infarct size in humans: results of phase I thrombolysis in myocardial infarction (TIMI) Trial. Circulation 83: 739–746
61. Gibbons R J, Holmes D R, Reeder G S, Bailey K R, Hopfenspirger M R, Gersh B J 1993 Immediate angioplasty compared with the administration of a thrombolytic agent followed by conservative treatment for myocardial infarction. N Engl J Med 328: 685–691

101. Congenital heart disease

Edward J. Baker

INTRODUCTION

Congenital malformations of the heart affect about eight newborn infants in a thousand. They usually present clinically within the first year of life. The most serious malformations present within a few hours of birth. An important difference between congenital heart defects and acquired heart disease is the presence of intracardiac communications between the left and right sides of the heart, so-called shunts. Shunts in which the flow of blood is exclusively from the left side of the heart to the right lead to an increased blood flow to the lungs. Shunts in which the blood flows in both directions, or predominantly from the right side of the heart to the left, cause desaturated blood to enter the systemic arterial circulation. Defects with such bidirectional shunting present clinically with arterial hypoxia or central cyanosis. There are no cardiac defects in which shunting only occurs from the right side of the heart to the left. Not all congenital malformations of the heart involve shunts. Some solely involve the cardiac valves or the arterial trunks.

Congenital heart disease is commonly divided into cyanotic and non-cyanotic types. This is not a very valuable physiological differentiation. A better classification is: defects with simple left-to-right shunts (Table 101.1); cyanotic defects with bidirectional shunts (Table 101.1); cyanotic defects that have complete mixing (Table 101.2); and defects with no shunts (Table 101.3).

Complete mixing (Table 101.2) occurs where there is an absence of a pathway, usually an atrioventricular valve, on one side of the heart. This means that all the blood within the heart, systemic venous and pulmonary venous, has to pass through a common pathway. Therefore, all blood leaving the heart, whether it goes to the systemic circulation or the lungs, has a uniform oxygen content.

The malformations listed in Table 101.3 do not necessarily have an intracardiac shunt, but they can, and often do, coexist with a lesion that does have a shunt. Thus combinations such as coarctation with a ventricular septal defect and pulmonary stenosis with an atrial septal defect are frequently found.

Some cardiac malformations are complex and cannot be described in these simple terms. In order to simplify the description of these complex hearts the method of sequential segmental analysis has been developed[1]. The heart is divided into four segments; the great veins, the atria, the ventricles, and the arterial trunks. Abnormalities are described in each of these segments and in the connec-

Table 101.1 Relative incidence of defects with left-to-right shunts and bidirectional shunts

	Relative incidence
Defects with simple left-to-right shunts	
Ventricular septal defect	28%
Persistent ductus arteriosus	10%
Atrial septal defect	7%
Defects with bidirectional shunts	
Transposition of the great arteries (complete transposition)	6%
Tetralogy of Fallot	5%
Double outlet right ventricle	1%
Truncus arteriosus	1%

Table 101.2 Relative incidence of defects with complete mixing

Defects with complete mixing	Relative incidence
Pulmonary atresia	2%
Mitral atresia	1%
Tricuspid atresia	1%
Total anomalous pulmonary venous drainage	1%

Table 101.3 Relative incidence of defects which usually have no shunts

Defects which usually have no shunts	Relative incidence
Aortic stenosis	5%
Pulmonary stenosis	5%
Coarctation of the aorta	5%

Table 101.4 Sequential segmental analysis of the heart

Segment	Examples
Atrial situs	Solitus Inversus Left isomerism Right isomerism
Venous connections of the atria	Total or partial anomalous pulmonary venous connection Anomalous systemic venous connection
Atrioventricular connection	Concordant Discordant Absent left connection (mitral atresia) Absent right connection (tricuspid atresia) Double inlet left ventricle
Ventriculoarterial connection	Concordant Discordant (transposition) Double outlet right ventricle
Associated anomalies	Ventricular septal defect Atrial septal defect Pulmonary or aortic stenosis Coarctation of the aorta

tions between them (Table 101.4). A concordant connection is one that would be expected from the morphology (e.g. the right atrium connected to the right ventricle), while a discordant connection is the reverse of the expected (e.g. left ventricle connected to pulmonary trunk).

RADIONUCLIDE IMAGING

When radionuclide imaging of congenital heart defects was first performed there was a tendency to concentrate on the anatomy of defects. In reality, congenital heart defects are too complex and the resolution of radionuclide techniques too low for them to have such a clinical role. Selective cineangiography, cross-sectional echocardiography and, most recently, magnetic resonance imaging provide excellent high resolution images of cardiac anatomy and are widely available. Radionuclide scans should not be performed unless cardiac anatomy has already been established and it is the assessment of function that is the major role of radionuclide techniques.

LEFT-TO-RIGHT SHUNTS

If a first-pass radionuclide angiogram is acquired in the anterior projection in a patient without a shunt, the bolus will pass through the right heart, the lungs, the left heart and into the systemic circulation (Fig. 101.1). Time–activity curves acquired from either of the lung fields show a single peak of activity. This peak falls rapidly and is followed by a second broad peak as the radionuclide returns to the heart from the systemic veins. A time–activity curve from the systemic circulation shows no activity until after the lung peak (Fig. 101.2).

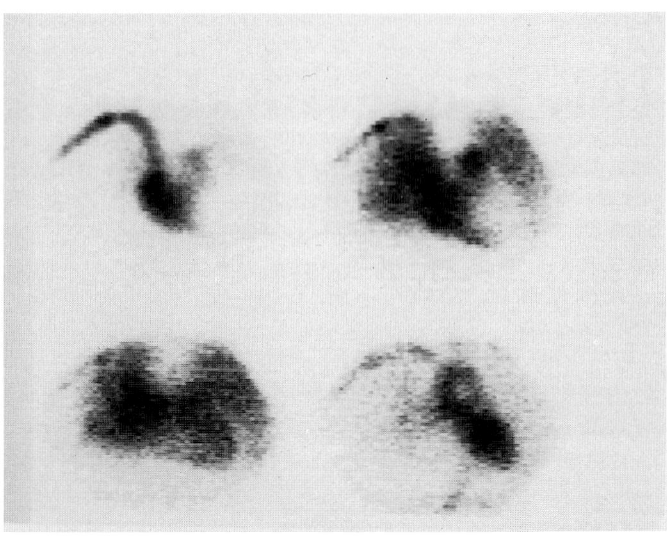

Fig. 101.1 Four frames from a first-pass radionuclide angiogram acquired in the anterior projection. The bolus passes through the right side of the heart, the lungs, the left side of the heart and into the systemic circulation. At the end of the angiogram the left heart phase of the study is seen clearly and the lung fields have virtually cleared.

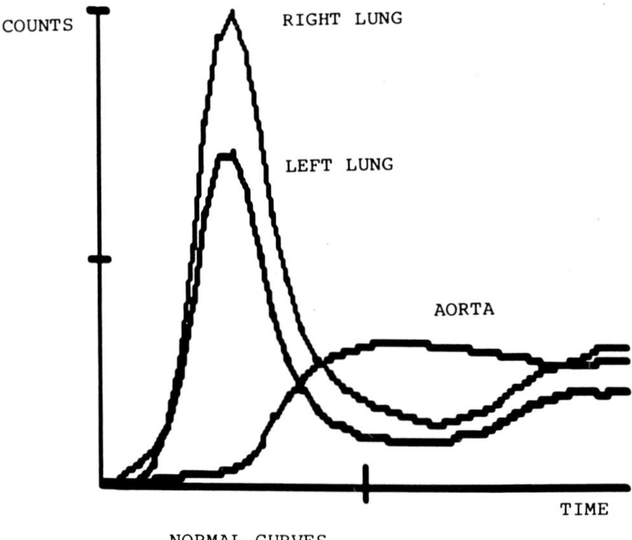

Fig. 101.2 Normal first-pass time–activity curves from regions of interest over the right lung, the left lung and the aorta beneath the diaphragm. The pulmonary time–activity curves have a single initial peak and the aorta only begins to fill after the pulmonary phase.

If there is a left-to-right shunt, some of the radionuclide returning to the left heart from the lungs crosses through the shunt and returns to the lungs and this early recirculation is characteristic. On viewing the angiogram it shows as persistence of activity in the lung fields with poor

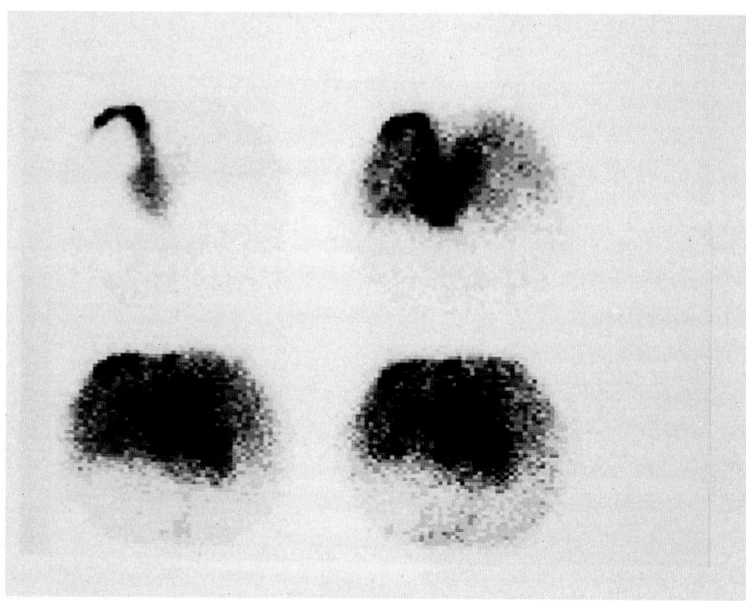

Fig. 101.3 Four frames from a first-pass angiogram in a patient with a ventricular septal defect. The left heart phase of the study is indistinct (c.f. Fig. 101.1). There is persistence of activity in the lungs at the end of the study.

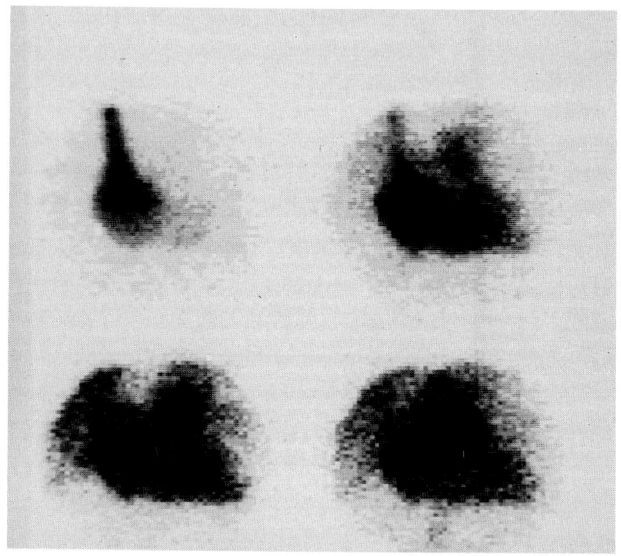

Fig. 101.4 A first-pass angiogram in a patient with an atrial septal defect. The right ventricle is dilated. The lung fields do not clear at the end of the study because of recirculation through the left-to-right shunt.

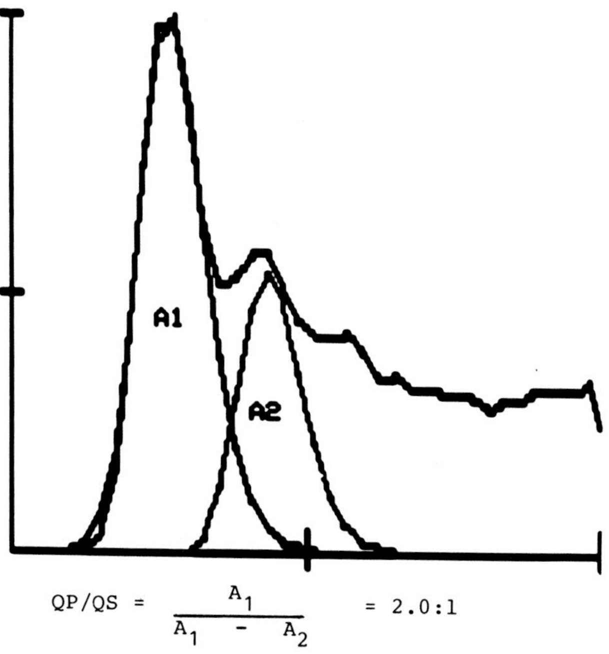

Fig. 101.5 A pulmonary time–activity curve in a patient with a left-to-right shunt. Recirculation through the shunt means that the first-pass peak is closely followed by repeated peaks of activity that merge together leaving a high level of residual activity in the lungs as the study ends.

definition of the left heart phase of the study (Fig. 101.3 and 101.4). The pulmonary time–activity curve is also characteristic. The first peak in activity in the lung fields begins to diminish, but this is interrupted by an early recirculation peak from the left-to-right shunt. Further recirculation peaks follow merging into one another, so that there is a persistently high level of activity in the lung fields (Fig. 101.5).

The accurate measurement of left-to-right shunts is essential in the management of many patients with congenital heart defects. In clinical practice the most common method was, until recently, to make the measurement during diagnostic cardiac catheterization using oximetry. This method has major drawbacks.[2,3] With the development of accurate non-invasive methods of demonstrating cardiac anatomy the frequency of diagnostic catheterization has fallen. It would now be unusual to perform catheterization simply to measure the size of a left-to-right shunt. One relic of oximetric measurement remains, however: the size of left-to-right shunt is usually expressed as the ratio of pulmonary and systemic flow (Q_p/Q_s). In the normal circulation pulmonary and systemic flows are equal. When there is a left-to-right shunt the pulmonary flow increases relative to the systemic flow and Q_p/Q_s is greater than 1. A Q_p/Q_s of 2.0 indicates a moderate left-to-right shunt; anything less than this is small. A Q_p/Q_s of 3.0 or greater indicates a large left-to-right shunt.

Several non-invasive methods of measuring left-to-right shunts have been described.[4] First-pass radionuclide angiography and Doppler echocardiography are the most commonly used. The Doppler technique is operator dependent and most regard it as being only semi-quantitative. The radionuclide technique is well established and validated.

Radionuclide measurement of left-to-right shunts

A first-pass radionuclide angiogram is acquired in the anterior projection using a compact and rapid bolus of technetium-99m. Images are acquired at two frames per s over a period of 20 s in a young child, 30 s in an older child or adult. The radionuclide should be administered through an in-dwelling cannula. The largest cannula possible should be used and it is best sited at the right antecubital fossa. In small children the largest and most proximal vein possible should be used. Great care has to be taken to ensure that the radionuclide reaches the heart as a compact bolus. This is best done by loading the radionuclide, in as small a volume as possible, into a short piece of intravenous tubing connected to the cannula. When the angiogram is acquired, the radionuclide should be flushed in rapidly with 10 ml of saline in a small baby, 20 ml in a larger child or adult. If possible the patient should fully abduct their shoulder so that the veins of the axilla are straightened. If care is taken, a technically satisfactory bolus can be administered in the majority of patients. This method can be used in an uncooperative child, if the child is restrained, but it is better to use sedation if necessary.

The quality of the bolus should be checked by creating a time–activity curve over the superior vena cava (Fig. 101.6). The bolus should be no more than 2 s in width. If the bolus is unsatisfactory, either too wide or split, the study should not be analysed further. The images should be inspected in a cine loop to look for evidence of intracardiac shunting. Time–activity curves are created over the lung fields and beneath the diaphragm over the systemic circulation.

Two methods have been described for the analysis of the pulmonary time–activity curve. In the first, the peak activity of the first-pass curve is measured (C_1). The level of activity at a time equal to twice that to the first peak is then measured (C_2). The ratio of C_1/C_2 is proportional to the Q_p/Q_s. A regression equation can be derived by comparing the C_1/C_2 ratio with the Q_p/Q_s measured oximetrically.[4]

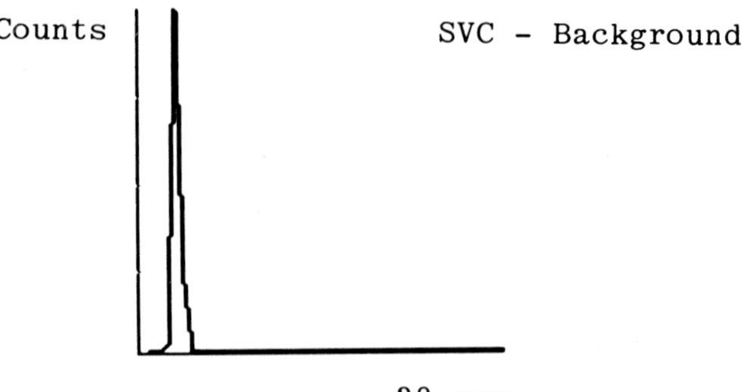

Fig. 101.6 A time–activity curve from a region of interest drawn over the superior vena cava. Background counts have been subtracted. This good quality bolus is a single peak less than 2 s wide.

The second and preferred method is the gamma variate technique.[5,6] The area under the first peak is measured by computer fit of a gamma variate function to the time–activity curve. This area (A_1) is proportional to the pulmonary blood flow. Then the area under the first recirculation peak is estimated by fitting a second gamma variate function. This second area (A_2) is proportional to the flow through the left-to-right shunt, which is equal to the difference between the systemic and pulmonary blood flows (Fig. 101.7). The systemic blood flow is therefore proportional to A_1–A_2. Provided there is no right-to-left shunt, Q_p/Q_s can be calculated as:

$$\frac{Q_p}{Q_s} = \frac{A_1}{A_1 - A_2}$$

This method requires some operator experience with

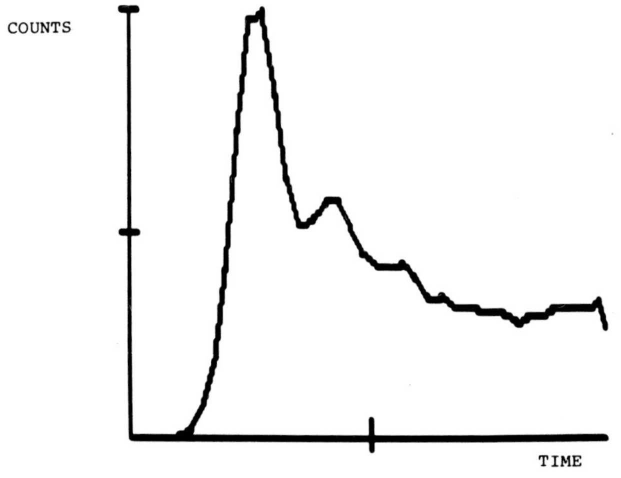

Fig. 101.7 Computer gamma variate curve fitting to a pulmonary time–activity curve from a first-pass angiogram to calculate the pulmonary to systemic flow ratio (Q_p/Q_s).

computer curve fitting. It has been found to be reproducible and, for patients with simple left-to-right shunts, it correlates well with measurement of the left-to-right shunt oximetrically (Fig. 101.8).[7,8] The agreement with oximetric measurements is much stronger for the gamma variate technique than for the C_1/C_2 method. The gamma variate analysis should be able to detect and measure left-to-right shunts (reliably) down to a Q_p/Q_s of 1.2. It is certainly as sensitive as oximetric measurement and for patients with simple anatomy and it is probably more accurate.[8]

There are significant limitations to the radionuclide method. The measurement of Q_p/Q_s is only valid in patients with simple left-to-right shunts (ventricular septal defects and atrial septal defects), and it is not valid where there is bidirectional shunting or multiple sources of pulmonary blood flow (e.g. persistent ductus arteriosus).[8] This is an important shortcoming, but suitable cases make up about 40% of congenital heart defects, so it is widely applicable. When cardiac function is poor or when there is severe valvular regurgitation the pulmonary transit time is prolonged and this may lead to an overestimation of the size of a left-to-right shunt. Results in these circumstances must be interpreted with care.

Despite these limitations, the radionuclide technique is a valuable technique in patients with congenital heart defects. It is valid at all ages and can be used in outpatients or inpatients who are critically ill. Clinically, non-invasive measurement of left-to-right shunts is indicated in two main groups of patients. Preoperatively it is used to determine the need for surgery. Postoperatively it is used to assess the results of surgery demonstrating the presence of residual shunts and measuring their size.

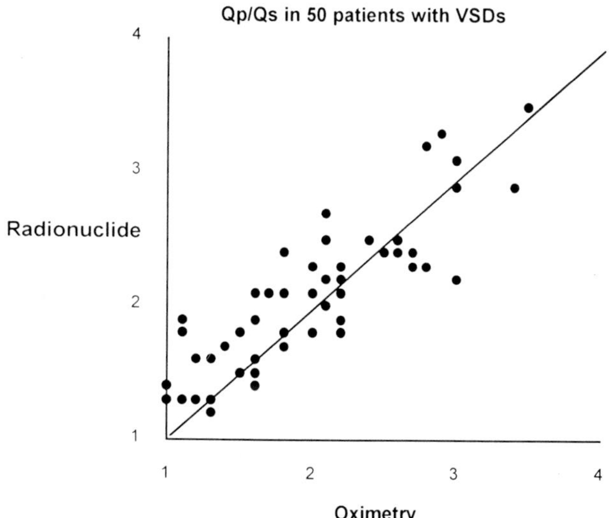

Fig. 101.8 A comparison of the pulmonary to systemic flow ratio measured in 50 patients with ventricular septal defects both by oximetry during cardiac catheterization and by first-pass radionuclide angiography, using the gamma variate method. (Redrawn with permission from Baker et al 1985[8])

RIGHT-TO-LEFT SHUNTS

There are many ways of detecting intracardiac shunts from right-to-left.[9] Colour Doppler echocardiography is very sensitive and it is the most useful. Measurement of the rise in arterial pO_2 in oxygen is also a sensitive and valuable technique. Radionuclide techniques have a limited role. Right-to-left shunts can be detected in first-pass radionuclide angiograms by the early appearance of activity in the left side of the heart or aorta (Fig. 101.9). In a normal first-pass angiogram activity should not be detected in the aorta until after the pulmonary phase of the study.

Analysis of the time–activity curve of the aorta can be used to estimate the size of a right-to-left shunt.[10] The method of analysis is derived from that originally described for the analysis of dye dilution curves. Right-to-left shunts can also be detected and measured by the injection into a peripheral vein of radionuclide-labelled particles that are trapped in the pulmonary and systemic capillaries.[11] Either human albumin microspheres or macro-aggregated albumin may be given safely in the presence of a right-to-left shunt. ^{99m}Tc-labelled microspheres are preferred. They can be given in a dose of 3×10^4 microspheres per square metre of body surface area.[12]

Isolated measurements of right-to-left shunts are of little clinical value. Pure right-to-left shunting is rare. It is seen in pulmonary arteriovenous fistulae. In cardiac malformations with systemic hypoxia there is either bidirectional shunting (Table 101.1) or complete mixing (Table 101.2). Where there is a bidirectional shunt the pulmonary to systemic blood flow cannot be calculated from the right-to-left shunt alone. If there is complete mixing, the distribution of microspheres between the systemic and pulmonary circulations is proportional to the pulmonary to systemic flow ratio.

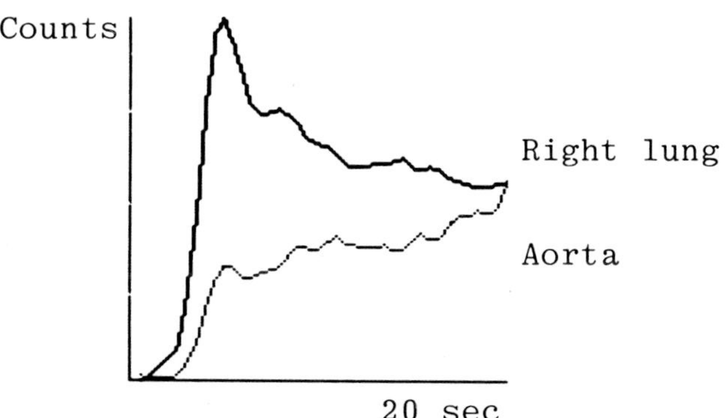

Fig. 101.9 Pulmonary and aortic time–activity curves from a first-pass angiogram in a patient with the tetralogy of Fallot. There is bidirectional shunting. The pulmonary curve is characteristic of a left-to-right shunt, with a persistently high level of activity at the end of the study. The aortic curve shows early appearance of activity, simultaneously with the first lung peak. This indicates that a right-to-left shunt is present.

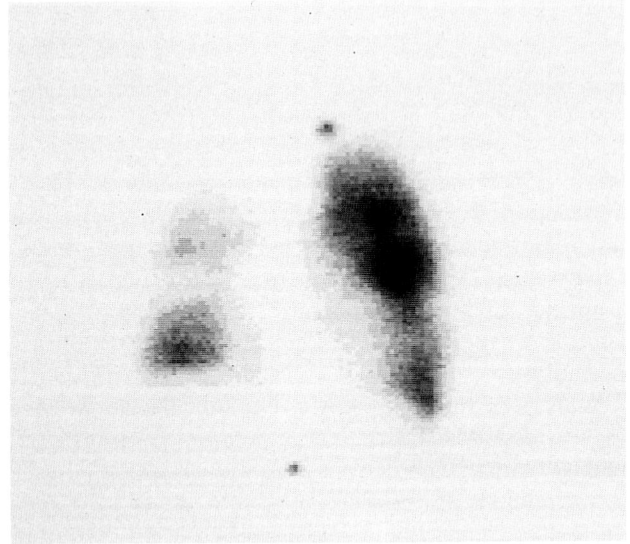

Fig. 101.10 An anterior lung perfusion scan in a patient with a complex form of pulmonary atresia. There are multiple perfusion defects, reflecting abnormalities in the pulmonary arteries that are typical of this condition.

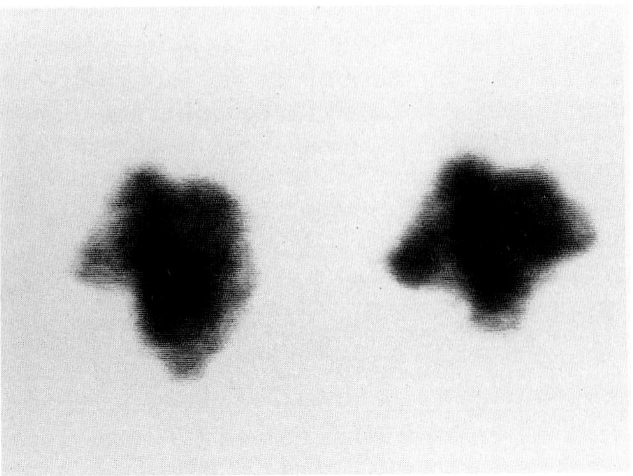

Fig. 101.11 Diastolic and systolic frames from an electrocardiogram gated equilibrium blood pool scan in a patient with tricuspid atresia. A 30 degree left anterior oblique projection with 25 degrees of craniocaudal tilt has been used. The left ventricle is dilated, but contracts well. The right ventricle is severely hypoplastic and cannot be identified in these views.

PULMONARY PERFUSION STUDIES

Radionuclide imaging has been used to study lung perfusion after corrective surgery for congenital heart defects[13] and to assess the patency and function of surgically created systemic to pulmonary artery shunts.[14] Pulmonary perfusion defects may be present in patients with congenital abnormalities of the pulmonary arteries or may occur following surgery (Fig. 101.10).[15] Balloon angioplasty and stent implantation are now established techniques for pulmonary arterial stenosos.[16] Pulmonary perfusion studies both before and after these procedures are essential to assess the success of these interventions.

MEASUREMENT OF LEFT VENTRICULAR FUNCTION

The left ventricular ejection fraction can be measured from either the first-pass angiogram or from an equilibrium gated blood pool angiogram. In congenital heart disease both have been validated against cineangiographic measurements of ventricular volume,[17–19] but the equilibrium method is generally preferred.

The first-pass method can only be used when there are no intracardiac shunts. The presence of either left-to-right or right-to-left shunts means that there is no discrete left heart phase to the study. Left ventricular counts cannot be distinguished from counts coming from the lungs or right atrium and ventricle. In patients with no shunts first-pass analysis is possible, but in small children the count rate from first-pass angiograms may be inadequate.[17]

The blood pool study does not suffer from these problems and should be used in most cases. Nevertheless there are problems in patients with congenital heart disease, mainly because of the abnormal anatomy. Equilibrium imaging requires an oblique plane which separates the left ventricular blood pool from the other chambers of the heart and great arteries. With normal anatomy this can be achieved with a modified left anterior oblique projection, but the projection may need to be modified in patients with congenital heart disease and knowledge of the cardiac anatomy is essential (Fig. 101.11). For instance in patients with a dilated right ventricle, an atrial septal defect, or transposition of the great arteries, a more lateral projection is usually needed. If the left ventricle is dilated, or the right hypoplastic, a more anterior projection may be best. In most cases craniocaudal angulation is essential in order to separate atrial counts from the left ventricle. In individual cases various imaging planes should be tried until the best is found. In rare cases, particularly those with cardiac malposition, a satisfactory imaging plane may not be achieved.

A disadvantage of the equilibrium method is the length of time taken to acquire sufficient counts. In small children the imaging time is likely to be longer than in adults and the child must be either cooperative or sedated.

RIGHT VENTRICULAR FUNCTION

Right ventricular function can be assessed from equilibrium blood pool studies, but measurement of the ejection fraction is difficult.[18] Satisfactory separation of right ventricular counts from the remainder of the heart is not possible with normal anatomy and when the cardiac anatomy is distorted the situation is usually worse. First-pass analysis of right ventricular function is more helpful, but it cannot be used if there is a right-to-left shunt, because there is no discrete right heart phase to the angiogram. An electrocardiogram gated first-pass angiogram enables the maximum number of counts to be obtained, but even then the count rate is not ideal.[20]

While radionuclide imaging does have drawbacks for the measurement of right ventricular function, so do all other clinical methods. In patients with congenital heart defects the right ventricular function may be especially important. This is the case in patients with tetralogy of Fallot after surgery, and following the Mustard or Senning operations for transposition. Despite its problems, radionuclide imaging is valuable in following up these patients.

MYOCARDIAL PERFUSION

Abnormal myocardial perfusion is frequently found in patients with congenital heart disease, but its significance is poorly understood. It is not appropriate to use criteria developed in adults for the interpretation of myocardial perfusion studies in congenital heart disease.

Abnormal myocardial perfusion has been described using thallium-201 in transient myocardial ischaemia of the newborn,[21] cardiomyopathies,[22] and congenital coronary artery abnormalities,[23] but the resolution of thallium images is low and interpretation in small children is difficult. Because of these problems, there is little clinical experience of thallium-201 imaging in congenital heart disease. The development of ^{99m}Tc-labelled myocardial perfusion imaging agents may lead to a better understanding of myocardial perfusion in these patients. Certainly, with ^{99m}Tc-labelled methoxy isobutyl isonitrile, perfusion defects have been demonstrated in various groups of patients after surgery.[24] The clinical significance of these defects is, as yet, uncertain.

CLINICAL ROLE OF RADIONUCLIDE IMAGING

There are many different techniques for imaging and studying patients with congenital heart defects. For these to be used appropriately the strengths and weaknesses of each must be understood. The mainstay of diagnosis is echocardiography. This is capable of giving a precise anatomical diagnosis and, with Doppler and colour flow imaging, it can also provide functional information. Because a full understanding of the anatomy is essential in order to plan and analyse radionuclide studies, the cardiologist and nuclear medicine physician must collaborate both in deciding whether a radionuclide study is appropriate and in interpreting the results.

Radionuclide imaging is a practical and well validated

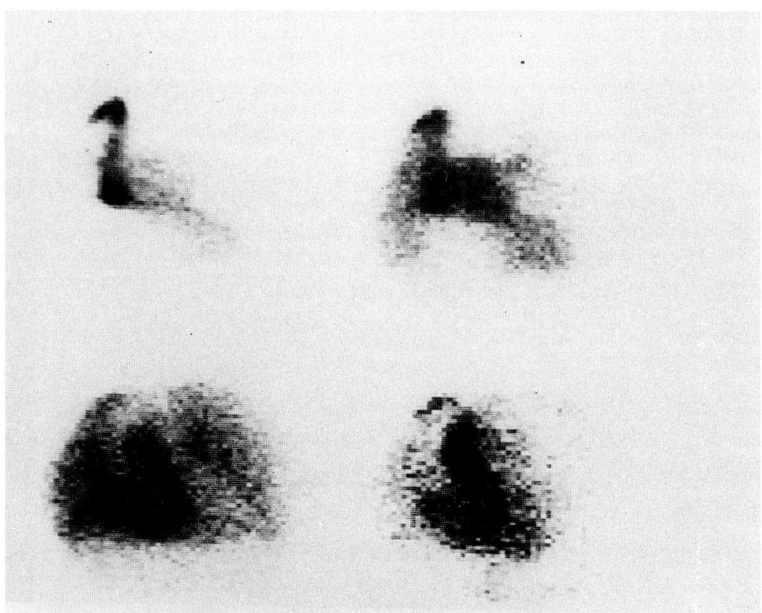

Fig. 101.12 Four frames from a first-pass angiogram in a patient with transposition of the great arteries who has had a Senning operation. A baffle has been created across the atria to redirect the flow of blood. The activity flows from the superior vena cava diagonally across the atria into the left ventricle and from there to the lungs. Returning from the lungs the activity flows across the atria into a dilated tight ventricle and then into the aorta. At the end of the study there is still a little activity in the lungs, indicating a small left-to-right shunt. Electrocardiogram gating of this study can be used to analyse right ventricular (i.e. the systemic ventricle) function.

technique to measure simple left-to-right shunts and measure ventricular function. It can therefore provide important clinical information in preoperative assessment and, probably most importantly, the long-term postoperative follow-up of patients with congenital heart disease (Fig. 101.12). Studies of pulmonary perfusion are important in the assessment of operations and interventions affecting the pulmonary arteries. Imaging myocardial perfusion is poorly understood, but may have an important role in the expanding group of postoperative patients.

REFERENCES

1. Anderson R H, MacCartney F J, Shinebourne E A, Tynan M 1987 Paediatric cardiology. Churchill Livingstone, London
2. Miller H C, Brown D J, Miller G A H 1974 Comparison of formulae used to estimate oxygen saturation of mixed venous blood from cava samples. Br Heart J 36: 446–451
3. Barratt-Boyes R G, Wood E H 1957 Oxygen saturation of blood in the vena cava, right heart chambers and pulmonary vessels of healthy subjects. J Lab Clin Med 50: 93–106
4. Boehrer J D, Lange R A, Willard J E, Grayburn P A, Hills L D 1992 Advantages and limitations of methods to detect, localize, and quantitate intracardiac left-to-right shunting. Am Heart J 124: 448–455
5. Askenazi J, Ahnberg D S, Korngold E, LaFarge C G, Maltz D L, Treves S 1976 Quantitative radionuclide angiocardiography: detection and quantitation of left to right shunts. Am J Cardiol 37: 382–387
6. Alserson P O, Jost R G, Strauss A W, Boonvisut S, Markham J 1975 Radionuclide angiocardiography: improved diagnosis and quantitation of left to right shunts using area ratio techniques in children. Circulation 51: 1136–1143
7. McIlveen B M, Murray I P C, Giles R W, Molk G H, Scarf C M, McCredie R M 1981 Clinical application of radionuclide quantitation of left to right shunts in children. Am J Cardiol 47: 1273–1278
8. Baker E J, Ellam S V, Lorber A, Jones O D H, Tynan M J, Maisey M N 1985 The superiority of radionuclide over oximetric measurement of left to right shunts. Br Heart J 53: 535–540
9. Boehrer J D, Lange R A, Willard J E, Grayburn P A, Hills L D, Boehrer 1993 Advantages and limitations of methods to detect, localize, and quantitate intracardiac right-to-left and bidirectional shunting. Am Heart J 125: 215–220
10. Peter C A, Armstrong B E, Jones R H 1981 Radionuclide quantitation of right to left shunts in children. Circulation 64: 572–577
11. Gates G F, Orme H W, Dore E K 1971 Measurement of cardiac shunting with technetium labelled albumin aggregates. J Nucl Med 12: 746–749
12. Baker E J, Malamitsi J, Jones O D H, Maisey M N, Tynan M J 1984 Use of radionuclide labelled microspheres to show the distribution of the pulmonary perfusion with multifocal pulmonary blood supply. Br Heart J 52: 72–76
13. Alderson P O, Boonvisut S, McKnight R C, Hartman A F, 1976 Pulmunary perfusion and ventilation imbalance in children after total repair of tetralogy of Fallot. Circulation 53: 332–337
14. Friedman W F, Braunwald E, Morrow A G 1968 Alterations in regional blood flow in patients with congenital heart disease studied by radioisotope scanning. Circulation 37: 747–758
15. Haroutunian L M, Neill C A, Wagner H N 1969 Radioisotope scanning of the lung in cyanotic congenital heart disease. Am J Cardiol 23: 387–395
16. Tynan M, Qureshi S 1993 Interventional catheterization in congenital heart disease. Curr Opinion Cardiol 8: 114–118
17. Baker E J, Ellam S V, Tynan M J, Maisey M N 1985 First pass measurement of left ventricular function in infants and children. Eur J Nucl Med 10: 422–425
18. Parrish M D, Graham T P, Bender H W, Jones J P, Patton J, Partain C L 1982 Radionuclide angiographic evaluation of right and left ventricular function in children: validation of methodology. Am J Cardiol 49: 1241–1247
19. Baker E J, Ellam S V, Maisey M N, Tynan M J 1984 Radionuclide measurement of left ventricular ejection fraction in infants and children. Br Heart J 51: 275–279
20. Baker E J, Shaobu C, Clarke S E M, Fogelman I, Maisey M N, Tynan M 1986 Radionuclide measurement of right ventricular function in atrial septal defects, ventricular septal defects and complete transposition of the great arteries. Am J Cardiol 57: 1142–1146
21. Gilday D L 1981 Radionuclides in paediatric cardiology. In: Freeman L M, Weissman H S, eds. Nuclear medicine annual. Raven Press, New York. pp 251–273
22. Dunn R F, Uren R F, Sadich N et al 1982 Comparison of thallium 201 scanning in idiopathic dilated cardiomyopathy and severe coronary artery disease. Circulation 66: 804–810
23. Finley J P, Howman-Giles R, Gilday D L, Olley P M, Rowe R D 1978 Thallium-201 myocardial imaging in anomalous left coronary artery arising from the pulmonary artery: applications before and after medical and surgical treatment. Am J Cardiol 42: 675–680
24. Hayes A M, Kakadekar A, Parsons J M et al 1992 Anatomical correction for transposition of the great arteries: myocardial perfusion with Tc99m MIBI. J Amer Coll Cardiol 19: 2

PART D

Developing areas

102. Single photon imaging of myocardial metabolism: the role of ^{123}I-labelled fatty acids and ^{18}F deoxyglucose

F. C. Visser J. J. Bax F. F. Knapp

INTRODUCTION

Metabolism is a basic process of the heart, because it produces the high energy phosphates needed for cardiac contraction and maintenance of cell integrity. The first alteration during ischaemia is a change in cardiac metabolism, even before changes in cardiac function occur or ECG changes appear. These considerations stress the importance of the study of myocardial metabolism in cardiac disease.

Under physiological conditions most of the energy requirements of the heart are derived from oxidation of free fatty acids. In contrast, during ischaemia oxidation of fatty acids is reduced or stopped and energy is derived from anaerobic glycolysis. Therefore, radiolabelled fatty acid and glucose analogues may be used to study these aspects of cardiac metabolism. In this chapter the scintigraphic characteristics of the ^{123}I-labelled fatty acids and ^{18}F deoxyglucose (^{18}FDG) are discussed along with the results of clinical studies.

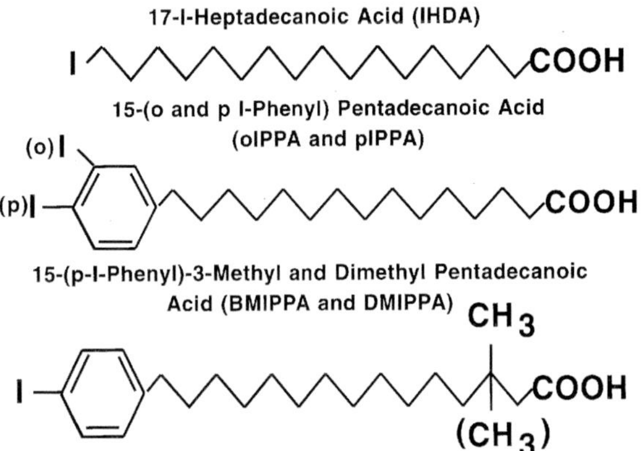

Fig. 102.1 Structural formula of the three classes of radioiodinated fatty acids. *Top*: iodoalkyl fatty acids. *Middle*: terminal iodophenyl fatty acids. The labeling site of radioiodide is different between oIPPA and pIPPA. *Bottom*: methyl-branched fatty acids. The addition of a second methylgroup (–CH3) to BMIPPA results in DMIPPA.

^{123}I-LABELLED FREE FATTY ACIDS

For patient studies, a variety of free fatty acids radiolabelled with ^{11}C and ^{123}I have been developed. One of their advantages in comparison with the positron emitters is that radioiodide can be traced with conventional gamma-cameras, and is therefore potentially applicable in routine nuclear medicine. ^{123}I has an energy of 159 KeV, which is almost optimal when using sodium iodide detectors. The disadvantage of limited in-depth resolution in planar fatty acid imaging can be overcome using single photon emission computerized tomographic (SPECT) imaging.

Scintigraphic characteristics

Although a large number of ^{123}I-labelled fatty acid analogues have been developed, a limited number have been used in patient studies and include the following (Fig. 102.1):

- iodoalkyl fatty acids: 17-I-heptadecanoic acid (IHDA) and 17-I-hexadecanoic acid (IHA)
- terminal iodophenyl fatty acids: 15-(*p*-I-phenyl)pentadecanoic acid (pIPPA) and 15-(*o*-I-phenyl)pentadecanoic acid (oIPPA)
- methyl-branched fatty acids: 15-(*p*-I-phenyl)-3-R,S-methylpentadecanoic acid (3-BMIPPA), 15-(*p*-I-phenyl)-9-R,S-methylpentadecanoic acid (9-BMIPPA) and 14-(*p*-I-phenyl)-3-R,S-methyltetradecanoic acid (IPBMTA).

IHDA and IHA

After uptake, a major part of the fatty acid is immediately oxidized, splitting off the radioiodide, which leaves the cell and enters the circulation, giving rise to background activity. A minor part is stored in lipids, mainly phospholipids (Fig. 102.2). Scintigraphy is performed by acquisition of serial planar images of the myocardium, followed

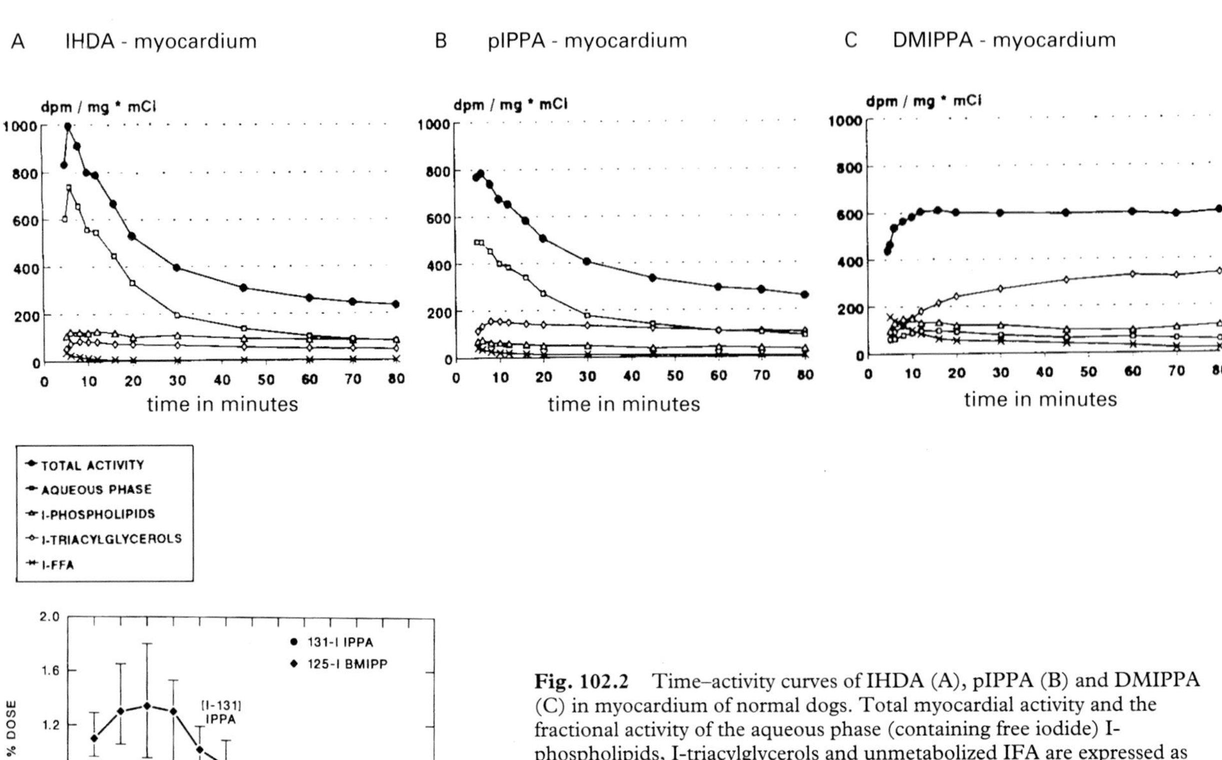

Fig. 102.2 Time–activity curves of IHDA (A), pIPPA (B) and DMIPPA (C) in myocardium of normal dogs. Total myocardial activity and the fractional activity of the aqueous phase (containing free iodide) I-phospholipids, I-triacylglycerols and unmetabolized IFA are expressed as disintegrations per minute per milligram myocardium per injected dose (dpm/mg/mCi). (Reprinted with permission of the Journal of Nuclear Medicine.) D Comparison of washout rates of pIPPA and BMIPPA activity in the outflow tract of Langendorff perfused rat hearts. Higher values for pIPPA represent greater washout. (Reprinted with permission of the Annals of Nuclear Medicine.)

by the generation of time–activity curves of defined regions of interest.

With IHDA the three parameters of uptake, % oxidation and washout or clearance of radioactivity can be obtained from the time–activity curves.[1] The time–activity curve can be described as either a bi-exponential or as mono-exponential plus constant. Correction for free iodide has been used but the need for this background subtraction is debatable. Although the structures of the IHA and IHDA fatty acid analogues are slightly different, the time–activity curves are similar. Due to the relatively rapid disappearance of the tracer under normal conditions (elimination half-time ($T\frac{1}{2}$) in patients varies between 18 and 33 min) SPECT imaging is not possible. However, exercise[2,3] or lactate loading[4] results in delayed washout, thus permitting SPECT acquisition.

pIPPA and oIPPA

Because of the high background activity of IHDA and IHA, Machulla et al[5] proposed stabilization of radioiodine by attachment to a terminal phenyl group of fatty acids and developed pIPPA. The pIPPA analogue is catabolized to *p*-iodobenzoic acid (pIBA) which is either directly excreted or transformed in the liver to *p*-iodohippuric acid and then excreted by the kidneys.[6] Rapid excretion would lower levels of radioactivity in the blood, resulting in more favourable heart-to-blood ratios. Uptake of pIPPA and global turnover is similar to that of IHDA[7] and most of it, although less than IHDA, is oxidized (Fig. 102.2). The pIPPA isomer is incorporated to a greater degree than IHDA into triacylglycerols, and to lesser degree into phospholipids. In addition, pIPPA clearance from the myocardium is slightly slower ($T\frac{1}{2}$ higher) than that of IHDA. From the scintigraphic data the uptake, clearance and fatty acid extraction can be obtained. The fatty acid extraction can be measured when the ^{123}I-labelled fatty acid is administered simultaneously with ^{201}Tl.[8] Although the position of the radiolabel in the phenyl ring is the only difference between oIPPA and pIPPA, their metabolism is quite different in humans. In animal experiments oIPPA is rapidly oxidized, accompanied by a very low rate of incorporation into triacylglycerols.[9] In contrast, in humans oIPPA is well retained with $T\frac{1}{2}$ >200 min,[10] allowing measurement of uptake differences between normal and diseased myocardium.

Methyl-branched iodinated fatty acids

These have been designed to overcome the problem of

rapid clearance of radioactivity of the 'straight-chain' fatty acids, due to oxidation. Although the position of the methyl group differs in the three ^{123}I-labelled fatty acid analogues discussed here, which have been used in clinical studies, the global effect is that oxidation is apparently prevented or changed by the introduction of the methyl group. This results in prolonged myocardial retention. In animal experiments it was demonstrated that 3-BMIPPA and DMIPPA was mainly incorporated into triacylglycerols and to a lesser extent into diacylglycerols and phospholipids[11,12] (Fig. 102.2). The long myocardial retention allows determination of uptake differences between normal and diseased myocardium. It was demonstrated that there was a relation between the uptake of BMIPPA and ATP concentration of the myocardium.[13]

Clinical applications

The following clinical topics have been studied with ^{123}I-labelled free fatty acids:

- diagnosis of coronary artery disease (CAD)
- changes in fatty acid metabolism in CAD
- detection of myocardial infarction and tissue viability
- bypass surgery/PTCA
- dilated and hypertrophic cardiomyopathy
- valvular disease.

Changes in fatty acid metabolism during ischaemia and diagnosis of CAD

Uptake and oxidation of natural fatty acids is diminished during ischaemia and a greater fraction of the extracted fatty acids is stored in lipids. In ischaemic animal studies the altered oxidation/storage pattern has been demonstrated for ^{123}I-labelled fatty acids.[14–16] A number of studies with patients at rest with radioiodinated fatty acids have demonstrated that the normal scintigraphic pattern is disturbed in patients with CAD. In ischaemic regions, decreased uptake and extraction,[17–19] reduced clearance of radioactivity of the straight-chain radioiodinated fatty acids,[6,18–22] and a decrease in the relative oxidation size[20] or component ratio[23] is observed. Reduced uptake is also observed with the methyl-branched fatty acids.[12,24] Possibly, the altered metabolic handling at rest can be regarded as a metabolic variety of silent ischaemia. However, the clinical relevance of this finding has yet to be resolved.

Detection of CAD by exercise fatty acid scintigraphy has been the subject of a number of studies. Metabolic imaging may be more sensitive than other modalities to detect CAD, because fatty acid oxidation strongly depends on oxygen supply. Thus, even in conditions where a relative lack in aerobic oxidation is completely compensated by anaerobic glycolysis, fatty acid metabolism may be 'visibly' disturbed. Both oIPPA,[25]

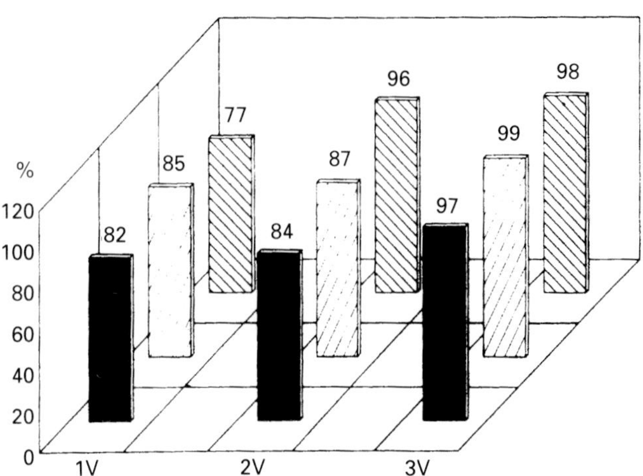

Fig. 102.3 Diagnostic value of exercise pIPPA scintigraphy to detect coronary artery disease. Sens: sensitivity; spec: specificity; ppv: positive predictive value; 1V: one vessel disease; 2V: two vessel disease; 3V: three vessel disease. (Reprinted with permission of the Annals of Nuclear Medicine.)

pIPPA[8,26–28] and 9-BMIPPA[29] have demonstrated a high sensitivity to detect CAD (Fig. 102.3). Hansen et al[26] and Chouraqui et al[29] concluded that fatty acid imaging is at least as sensitive as ^{201}Tl perfusion scintigraphy for the detection of CAD. With IHDA more conflicting results have been published[30–32] and these contrasting results are probably due to methodological problems. These problems are related with the short acquisition period and the curve-fitting and background correction procedures.[33–35]

Detection of myocardial infarction and tissue viability

Myocardial infarction is easily identified by reduced tracer uptake with the straight-chain as well as with the methyl-branched fatty acids.[36–38] However, infarct detection and localization can be performed with other clinical tools such as ECG, cardiac enzyme determination and echocardiography. Thus, ^{123}I-labelled fatty acids do not represent a cost-effective tool for this application.

Myocardial viability is very important and clinically much less easy to ascertain. The only diagnostic tools which currently recognize tissue viability are positron emission tomography (PET) imaging with ^{18}FDG and ^{201}Tl imaging. However, PET imaging is costly, complex and time-consuming and would not be expected to be routinely available in the near future. An important study has been published by Murray et al[39] using IPPA in combination with a multicrystal gamma-camera. They assessed tissue viability by myocardial biopsies and by comparison of ventricular function before and after revascularization. Compared to biopsy, IPPA sensitivity for viability was 92% and specificity 86%. 80% of the IPPA

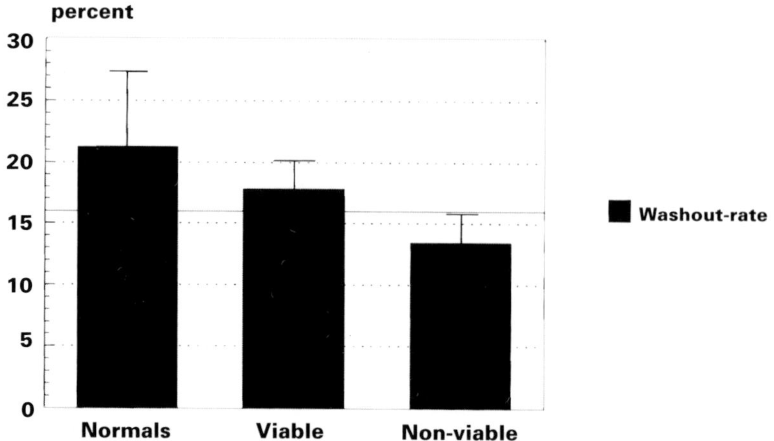

Fig. 102.4 Washout rates (mean and SD) of pIPPA in normal, viable and non-viable myocardium (biopsy proven). The solid horizontal line represents the threshold for viability.

viable segments showed improvement after revascularization (Fig. 102.4). Henrich et al[40] published a comparison between SPECT oIPPA uptake and PET FDG uptake in myocardial infarction patients with persistent ^{201}Tl defects. Twenty-two percent of the patients had both normal oIPPA and FDG uptake in the ^{201}Tl defects. Also, a significant correlation of oIPPA and FDG uptake was found in the ^{201}Tl defects.[40] Tamaki et al[41] compared BMIPPA with FDG uptake and found that the sensitivity of BMIPPA imaging to detect increased FDG uptake was 88% with a specificity of 80%.

Studies with IHDA related the clearance rate of radioactivity with tissue viability. Increased elimination of radioactivity compared to controls was associated with infarcted tissue and decreased elimination with ischaemia.[42,43] However, increase in elimination is also

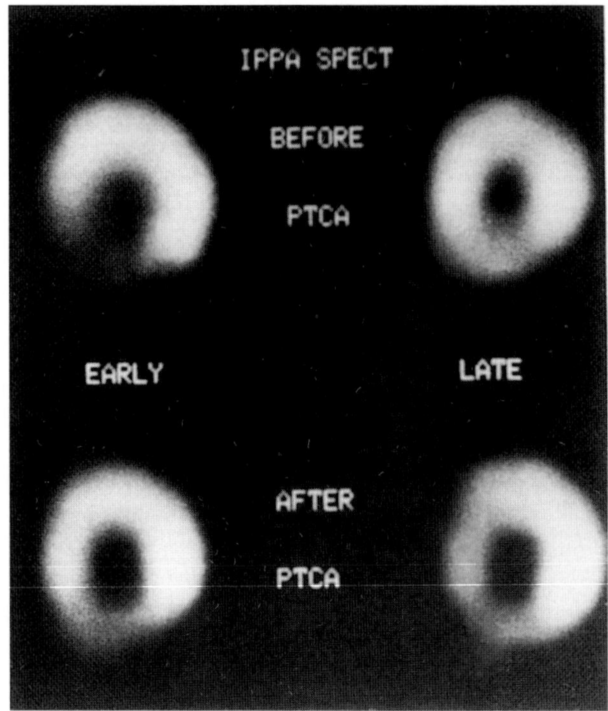

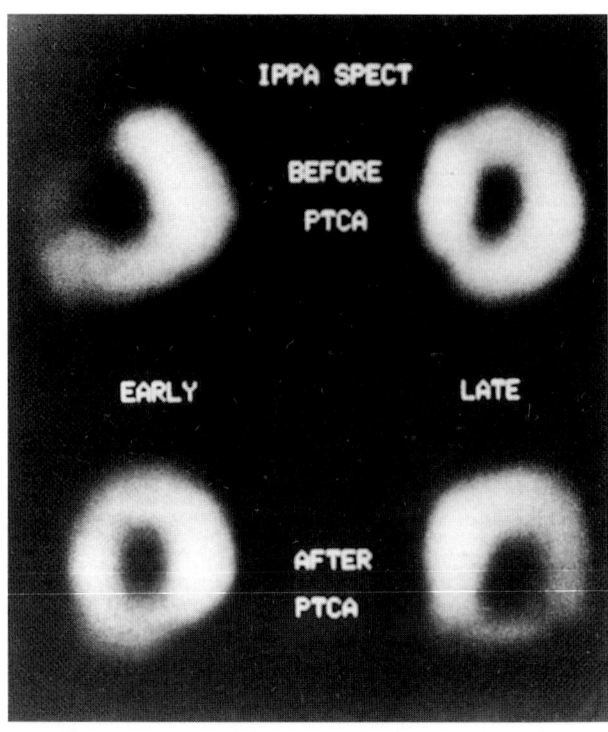

Fig. 102.5 A Early (exercise) and late (rest) pIPPA tomograms of a patient with a 90% RCA stenosis and without an infarction prior to (*top*) and after(*bottom*) PTCA. *Top left*: diminished tracer uptake is observed in the septal and inferior wall. *Top right*: at the late image relative normalization of uptake is observed in these segments. This indicates slow pIPPA turnover in these segments. This pattern is normal after PTCA (*bottom*).
B Early and late pIPPA tomogram of a patient with an 80% stenosis of the LAD without infarction. A relatively increased uptake of pIPPA is seen at the late tomogram in the anteroseptal region, indicating slow pIPPA turnover. This slow turnover is persistent after PTCA. (Reprinted with permission of the Annals of Nuclear Medicine.)

found in patients without infarction.[44] Stoddart et al[45] and Roessler et al[46,47] found a weak relation between clearance rates and improvement in ventricular function. On the other hand, Chappuis et al[48] showed in a canine occlusion–reperfusion model that heptadecanoic acid uptake was found to be the single most important predictor of viability, whereas ^{201}Tl was only of limited importance. These observations suggest that viability may well be demonstrated with radioiodinated fatty acids.

Bypass surgery/PTCA

Interestingly, there seems to be a dissociation between restoration of flow and metabolism after revascularization, since the uptake and turnover of iodinated fatty acids normalizes only in some of the patients.[32,49–51] The significance of this finding is not clear, but may indicate restenosis, incomplete revascularization, cellular ischaemia or focal necrosis. Alternatively it may indicate a delay in restoration of some aspects of fatty acid transport and metabolism, which is very sensitive to ischaemia (Fig. 102.5). Similar studies with ^{201}Tl after bypass surgery indicate that reversible defects may not completely disappear.[52]

Dilated and hypertrophic cardiomyopathy

Studies in patients with congestive cardiomyopathy indicate that regional uptake/extraction of fatty acids is inhomogeneously reduced and that clearance of the radioactivity from the myocardium is altered (Fig 102.6).[19,21,23,37,53–56] In contrast, the study of Rabinovitch et al[57] showed abnormal uptake and turnover in only two out of 16 patients with cardiomyopathy of different aetiology. In patients with hypertrophy and hypertrophic cardiomyopathy,[54,58–61] a heterogeneous decrease in uptake and extraction was noted and the latter was related with degree of hypertrophy (Fig. 102.7).[62] These studies indicate that discrimination between the different aetiologies of the dilated cardiomyopathies cannot be expected from metabolic studies. Possibly metabolic imaging can better discriminate between ischaemic and idiopathic congestive cardiomyopathy than other non-invasive tools. Also, metabolic imaging can possibly discriminate between physiological and pathological hypertrophy and the

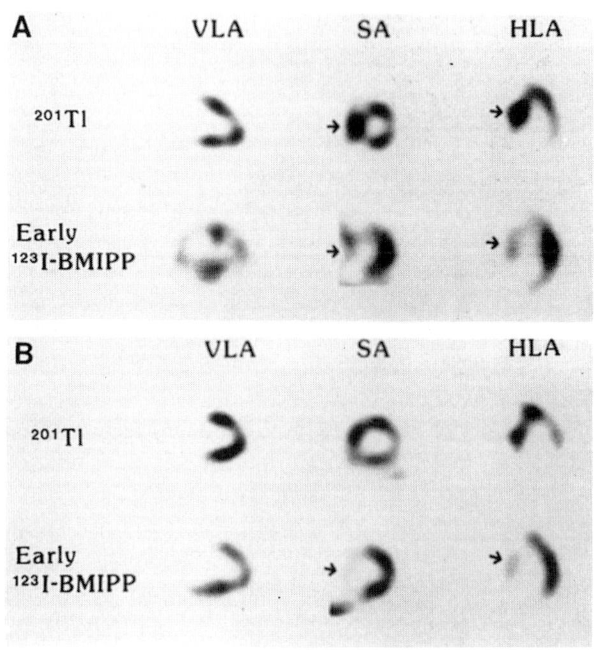

Fig. 102.7 BMIPPA tomograms of 2 patients with septal hypertrophy. The uptake of BMIPPA uptake in the septum is lower compared to the thallium-201 uptake. (Reprinted with permission of the Annals of Nuclear Medicine.)

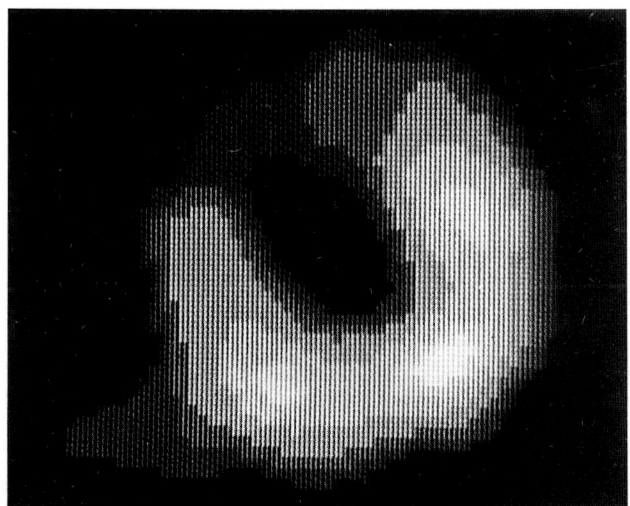

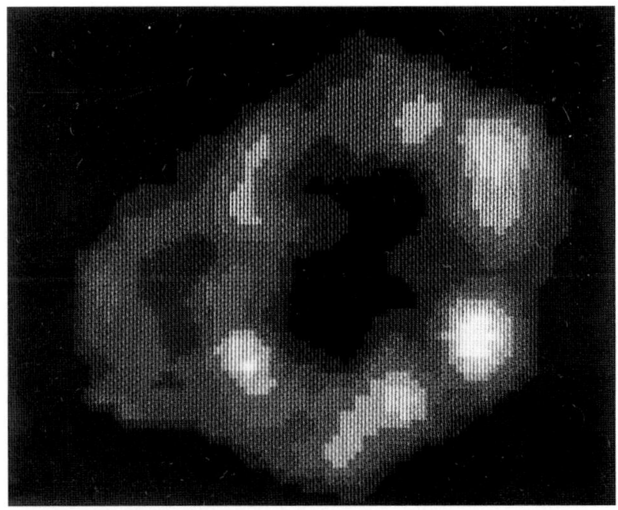

Fig. 102.6 A Homogeneous uptake of IHDA in a normal subject. B Inhomogeneous uptake of IHDA in a patient with congestive cardiomyopathy. (Reprinted with permission of the Journal of Nuclear Medicine.)

influence of therapy may be assessed by metabolic studies.[63]

Valvular heart disease

The diagnosis and assessment of the severity of valvular heart disease can routinely be determined with non-invasive techniques such as Doppler echocardiography. The timing of valvular replacement can still represent a problem because premature replacement exposes patients to the risks inherent in surgery, reoperation and long-life anticoagulants. In contrast, replacement too late may lead to persistent damage of the ventricle. In this respect metabolic studies may play a role, on the hypothesis that functional changes of the myocardium may be preceded by metabolic changes. Notohamiprodjo et al[64] studied patients with IPPA before and after valve replacement because of severe aortic stenosis. They found that fatty acid transport was impaired in these patients before surgery and that severely impaired fatty acid transport did not recover after valve replacement in contrast to patients with moderately reduced fatty acid transport. Thus, fatty acid imaging may have a unique role in the timing decision of valve replacement.

In summary, a variety of radioiodinated fatty acids with specific metabolic behaviour have been developed and have been applied in different cardiac diseases. Because metabolism is essential for maintaining cellular integrity and cardiac contraction, the major advantage of using radioiodinated fatty acids is that they provide a specific insight into metabolic abnormalities, obtainable with widely available gamma-cameras. Although metabolic studies are not yet established diagnostic tools like the perfusion agents, the potential is such that in the future radioiodinated fatty acids will have their clinical application.

^{18}F DEOXYGLUCOSE

The clinical use of 18FDG with PET has been discussed earlier, and discussion here will therefore be brief. Studies show that ^{18}FDG uptake is increased after exercise in ischaemic regions of patients with stable angina pectoris,[65] and in unstable angina patients at rest.[66] More importantly, increased ^{18}FDG uptake (relative to a flow tracer) following myocardial infarction has been demonstrated in a substantial number of patients, indicating the presence of viable myocardium.[67,68] Schwaiger et al[69] demonstrated that maintenance of glucose uptake in the area of infarction could result in improvement of regional left ventricular function, whereas in areas with a consistent decrease of flow and ^{18}FDG uptake, improvement of ventricular function did not occur. Assessment of the presence of viable myocardium in areas of contractile dysfunction is important, because patients with depressed ventricular function may benefit from a revascularization procedure (bypass surgery or PTCA). This has been demonstrated by Tillisch et al[70] and Tamaki et al.[71] The positive and negative values for predicting the presence or absence of ventricular function improvement in these two studies were 78–85% and 78–92%, respectively. These values indicate that improvement of function can be predicted quite accurately using ^{18}FDG imaging by PET.

Also, in a preliminary study of the prognostic information from increased ^{18}FDG uptake Eitzman et al[72] suggested that patients with impaired left ventricular function and metabolic evidence of myocardial ischaemia appear to have the most clinical benefit from a revascularization procedure. Thus PET has proved to be an important clinical tool for specific cardiological questions. However, the costs and complexity of the PET devices and the long acquisition periods for assessing ^{18}FDG uptake in patients has limited the widespread clinical use of these diagnostic tools.

Recently, it has been demonstrated that ^{18}FDG uptake can be visualized with conventional gamma-cameras equipped with a 511 keV collimator.[73,74] The great advantage of this approach is that conventional gamma-cameras are widely available, which would allow viability assessment in routine clinical practice. This is also possible because the relatively long half-life of ^{18}F enables the commercial production of ^{18}FDG, transportation and off-site use of the tracer. In this section the initial study results will be discussed for both planar and SPECT ^{18}FDG imaging.

Planar ^{18}FDG imaging

In a recent study we assessed the feasibility of planar ^{18}FDG imaging in 51 patients after myocardial infarction. Patients were studied 5 $\pm$2 days after infarction and underwent rest ^{18}FDG imaging in the three standard projections after oral glucose loading. Also, in the same imaging projections rest ^{201}Tl images were obtained shortly after tracer injection. Early ^{201}Tl imaging has been shown to be a reliable marker of myocardial flow distribution.[75]

To evaluate ^{18}FDG image quality, the images were interpreted by two observers and judged as good, moderate or poor. 27 patient studies were judged as good, 17 as moderate and five as poor. Also, heart/lung and heart/liver ratios were calculated by drawing ROIs over normal heart areas and over lung and liver regions. ^{18}FDG heart/lung and heart/liver were 2.5$\pm$0.4 and 1.8$\pm$0.3, respectively compared to 2.4$\pm$0.4 and 1.1$\pm$0.2 respectively for ^{201}Tl images. Thus planar ^{18}FDG scintigraphy is feasible, yielding adequate image quality for analysis (Fig. 102.8).

To determine the relation between ^{18}FDG and ^{201}Tl

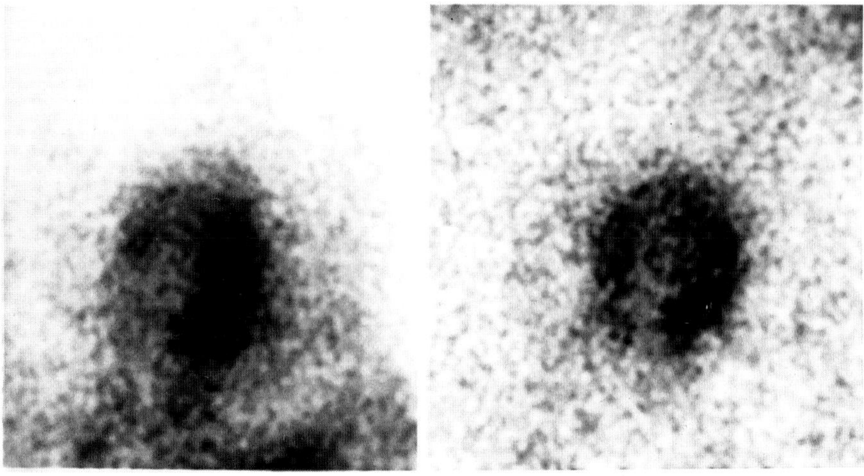

Fig. 102.8 LAO 45° view of ^{201}Tl (*left*) and of FDG uptake in a patient with a recent anteroseptal infarction. FDG uptake in the septal region is relatively increased compared to the ^{201}Tl uptake.

uptake and to see if increased ^{18}FDG uptake could be demonstrated in these infarct patients, images were semi-quantitatively analysed using circumferential profiles after

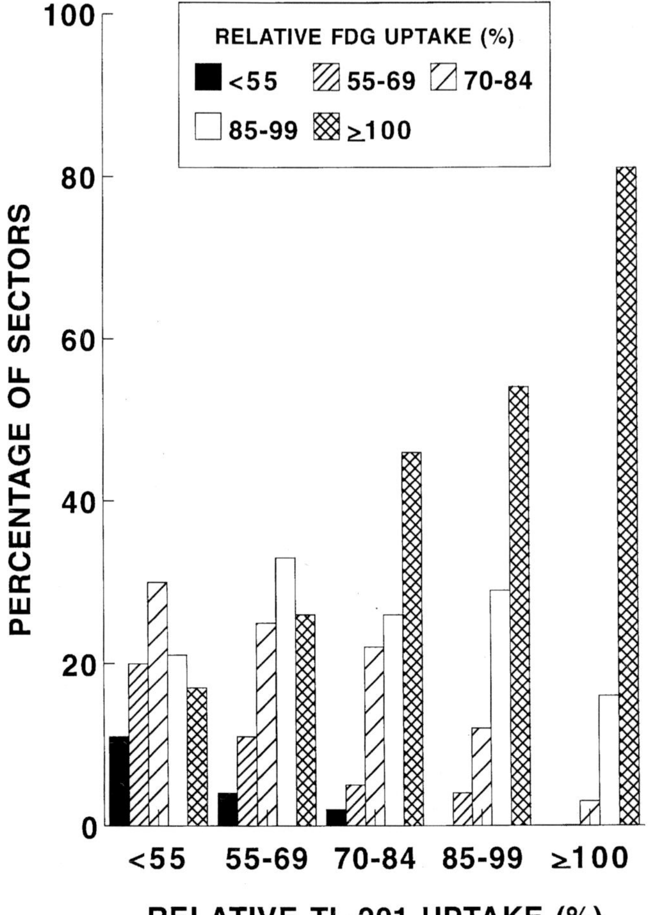

Fig. 102.9 Bar graph showing the relative FDG uptake in 15% quartiles in relation to the relative ^{201}Tl uptake. FDG and ^{201}Tl uptake is expressed as a percentage of the lower limit of normal (>100% uptake is normal uptake). Especially in the moderately reduced ^{201}Tl tracer defects, FDG uptake is preserved.

background subtraction. Segmental ^{201}Tl and ^{18}FDG activities were expressed as a percentage of the lower limit of normal (relative ^{201}Tl and ^{18}FDG activities). These lower limits of normal for ^{201}Tl and ^{18}FDG activities were determined in 31 and 12 subjects respectively. Figure 102.9 shows the distribution of relative ^{18}FDG activity in myocardial segments with normal and abnormal ^{201}Tl uptake after dividing segments into 15% quartiles. These results demonstrate that, especially in the moderately reduced ^{201}Tl segments, ^{18}FDG uptake was higher than ^{201}Tl uptake (51% of segments with a relative ^{201}Tl uptake >70% showed a normal ^{18}FDG uptake). Applying the criteria of Marshall et al[67] for infarction and ischaemia (modified for planar images), we demonstrated that 41% of patients had signs of ischaemia in the area of infarction, which indicates the presence of viable tissue.

The data clearly demonstrate that increased ^{18}FDG uptake can be observed with planar ^{18}FDG imaging. From the data of Williams et al,[76] it can be inferred that increased ^{18}FDG uptake as obtained by planar imaging is, in the same manner as PET, related to improvement of ventricular function. They observed in their study that 83% of the segments with improvement in regional ventricular function and/or improvement of ^{201}Tl uptake in previously fixed defects had increased ^{18}FDG uptake prior to surgery.

SPECT ^{18}FDG imaging

Recently, SPECT ^{18}FDG imaging has also been performed in the same manner as described for planar imaging, with the exception that ^{18}FDG studies were performed after a hyperinsulinaemic euglycaemic glucose clamp.[77] This technique is used instead of oral glucose loading, and its purpose is to increase blood insulin levels to promote glucose and ^{18}FDG uptake. Nine patients and nine normals were studied. The tomographic slices of

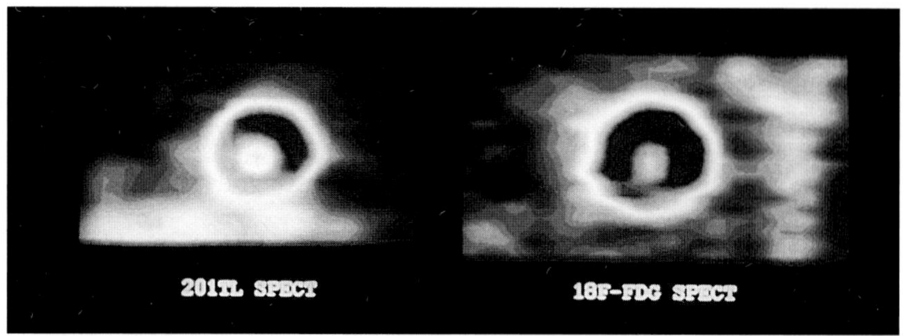

Fig. 102.10 ^{201}Tl and FDG uptake in a SPECT study of a patient with a previous inferoseptal infarction. Especially in the septal area, FDG uptake is preserved. (Also shown in colour on Plate 30.)

patients showed an adequate to good image quality with heart/lung ratios for ^{18}FDG of 6.6 ±2.1 and for ^{201}Tl of 2.6 ±0.6. Of the nine infarct patients four showed increased ^{18}FDG uptake in the area of infarction, indicating the presence of viable myocardium. An example of a patient with increased ^{18}FDG uptake is shown in Figure 102.10.

These data are consistent with those from Stoll et al[78] who studied 30 patients with ^{18}FDG SPECT after oral glucose loading combined with sestamibi SPECT. 87% of mild hypokinetic segments had normal ^{18}FDG uptake, 8% showed mismatches and 5% showed matches. In contrast, 44% of akinetic segments had matched defects, 27% mismatched defects and 29% were normal. Their data confirm that ^{18}FDG SPECT is feasible in routine clinical practice.

Thus, the available data suggest that myocardial viability can be determined using ^{18}FDG and conventional gamma-cameras. Although this approach will not meet the PET standards in terms of resolution and quantitation, the application seems justified as Tillisch et al[70] found that only large myocardial areas with flow/metabolism mismatch improved after surgical revascularization.

Using planar scintigraphy, overlap of myocardial activity from normal myocardium may mask areas with ischaemia or infarction. Despite this, the data of Williams et al[76] suggest that viability can be demonstrated in this manner. Furthermore, SPECT ^{18}FDG imaging reduces the problem of overlap. However, the relative value of planar and SPECT ^{18}FDG scintigraphy compared to PET and compared to ^{201}Tl reinjection and rest-redistribution studies needs to be established.

Finally, as gamma-cameras are operational in community hospitals and because the physical half-life of ^{18}F enables off-site use of ^{18}FDG, application in routine clinical practice may be possible for viability assessment, risk-stratification and for prediction of functional recovery after myocardial infarction.

REFERENCES

1. Van Eenige M J, Visser F C, Duwel C M B, Karreman A J P, Van Lingen A, Roos J P 1988 Comparison of 17-iodine-131 heptadecanoic acid kinetics from externally measured time–activity curves and from serial myocardial biopsies in an open-chest canine model. J Nucl Med 29: 1934–1942
2. Visser F C, Van Eenige M J, Duwel C M B, Van Lingen A, Roos J P 1990 radioiodinated fatty acid scintigraphy of the normal human myocardium during exercise testing: A new interpretation. Nuc Compact 21: 236–240
3. Kuikka J T, Mustonen J N, Uusitupa M I J, Rautio P, Vanninen E, Laakso M, Lansimies E, Pyorala K 1991 Demonstration of disturbed free fatty acid metabolism of myocardium in patients with non-insulin-dependent diabetes mellitus with iodine-123-heptadecanoic acid. Eur J Nucl Med 18: 475–481
4. Duwel C M B, Visser F C, Van Eenige M J, Den Hollander W, Roos J P 1990 The fate of (131)I-1-7-iodoheptadecanoic acid during lactate loading: Its oxidation is strongly inhibited in favor to its esterification. A radiochemical study in the canine heart. Nuklearmedizin 29: 30–33
5. Machulla H J, Marsmann M, Dutchka K 1980 Biochemical concept and synthesis of a radioiodinated phenyl fatty acid for in vivo metabolic studies of the myocardium. Eur J Nucl Med 5: 171–173
6. Dudczak R, Schmolinger R, Kletter K, Frischauf H, Angelberger P 1983 Clinical evaluation of 123I-labeled p-phenylpentadecanoic acid for myocardial scintigraphy. J Nucl Med All Sci 27: 267–279
7. Sloof G W, Visser F C, van Eenige M J, Comans E F I, Teerlink T, Herscheid J D M, van der Vusse G J, Knapp F F 1993 Comparison of uptake, oxidation and lipid distribution of 17-iodoheptadecanoic acid, 15-(p-iodophenyl)pentadecanoic acid and 15-(p-iodophenyl)-3,3-dimethylpentadecanoic acid in normal canine myocardium. J Nucl Med 34: 649–657
8. Vyska K, Machulla H J, Stremmel W, Faßbender D, Knapp W H, Notohamiprodjo G, Gleichmann U, Meyer H, Knust E J, Körfer R 1988 Regional myocardial free fatty acid extraction in normal and ischemic myocardium. Circulation 78: 1218–1233
9. Beckurts T E, Shreeve W W, Schieren R, Feinendegen L E 1985 Kinetics of different (123)I- and (14)C-labelled fatty acids in normal and diabetic rat myocardium in vivo. Nucl Med Commun 6: 415–424
10. Antar M A, Spohr G, Herzog H H, Kaiser K P, Notohamiprodjo G, Vester E, Schwartzkopf B, Lösse B, Machulla H J, Shreeve W W, Feinendegen L E 1986 15-(ortho-123I-phenyl)-pentadecanoic acid, a new myocardial imaging agent for clinical use. Nucl Med Commun 7: 683–696
11. Ambrose K R, Rice D E, Goodman M M, Knapp F F 1987 Effect

of 3-methyl-branching on the metabolism in rat hearts of radioiodinated iodovinyl long chain fatty acids. Eur J Nucl Med 13: 374–379

12. Knapp F F, Goodman M M, Ambrose K R, Som P, Brill A B, Yamamoto K, Kubota K, Yonekura Y, Dudczak R, Angelberger P, Schmolinger R 1987 The development of radioiodinated 3-methylbranched fatty acids for evaluation of myocardial disease by single photon techniques. In: van der Wall E E (ed) Non-invasive imaging of cardiac metabolism. Martinus Nyhoff, Dordrecht, pp 159–201
13. Fujibayashi Y, Yonekura Y, Takemura Y, Wada K, Matsumoto K, Tamaki N, Yamamoto K, Konishi J, Yokoyama A 1990 Myocardial accumulation of iodinated beta-methyl-branched fatty acid analogue, iodine-125-15-(p-iodophenyl)-3-R, S-methylpentadecanoic acid (BMIPP), in relation to ATP concentration. J Nucl Med 31: 1818–1822
14. Hudon M P J, Lyster D M, Jamieson W R E, Qayumi A K, Sartori C 1990 The metabolism of 15-p-[123I]-iodophenylpentadecanoic acid in a surgically induced canine model of regional ischemia. Eur J Nucl Med 16: 199–204
15. Visser F C, Sloof G W, Comans E, Eenige van M J, Knapp F F 1990 Metabolism of radioiodinated heptadecanoic acid in the normal and ischemic dog heart. Eur Heart J Suppl 137 (abstract)
16. Rellas J R, Corbett J R, Kulkarni P V, Morgan C, Devous M D, Buja L M, Bush L, Parkey R W, Willerson J T, Lewis S E 1983 Iodine-123 phenylpentadecanoic acid: detection of acute myocardial infarction and injury in dogs using an iodinated fatty acid and single-photon emission tomography. Am J Cardiol 52: 1326–1332
17. Reske S N 123I-phenylpentadecanoic acid as a tracer of cardiac free fatty acid metabolism. Experimental and clinical results. Eur Heart J 6 (Suppl B): 39–47
18. Reske S N, Koischwitz D, Reichmann K, Machulla H J, Simon H, Knopp R, Winkler C 1984 Cardiac metabolism of 15 (p-I-123 phenyl)pentadecanoic acid after intracoronary tracer application. Eur J Radiol 4: 144–149
19. Railton R, Rodger J C, Small D R, Harrower A D B 1987 Myocardial scintigraphy with I-123 heptadecanoic acid as a test for coronary heart disease. Eur J Nucl Med 13: 63–66
20. Eenige van M J, Visser F C, Duwel C M B, Roos J P 1990 Clinical value of studies with radioiodinated heptadecanoic acid in patients with coronary artery disease. Eur Heart J 11: 258–268
21. Freundlieb C, Hoeck A, Vyska K, Feinendegen L E, Machulla H J, Stoeklin G 1980 Myocardial imaging and metabolic studies with [17-123I]iodoheptadecanoic acid. J Nucl Med 21: 1043–1050
22. Visser F C, Eenige van M J, Van der Wall E E, Westera G, van Engelen C J, van Lingen A, de Cock C C, den Hollander W, Heidendal G A K, Roos J P 1985 The elimination rate of 123I-heptadecanoic acid after intracoronary and intravenous administration. Eur J Nucl Med 11: 114–119
23. Fridrich L, Pichler M, Gassner A, Vagner M, Mostbeck G, Eghbalian F 1985 Tracer elimination in I-123-heptadecanoic acid: half-life, component ratio and circumferential profiles in patients with cardiac disease. Eur Heart J 6 (Suppl B): 61–70
24. Dudczak R, Schmollinger R, Angelberger P, Knapp F F, Goodman M M 1986 Structurally modified fatty acids: clinical potential as tracers of metabolism. Eur J Nucl Med 12: S45–S48
25. Kaiser K P, Vester E, Grossmann K, Geuting B, Loesse B, Feinendegen L E 1990 15-(ortho-I-123-phenyl)pentadecanoic acid (OPPA) in the human myocardium: clinical applications. Nuc Compact 5: 213–215
26. Hansen C L, Corbett J R, Pippin J J, Jansen D E, Kulkarni P V, Ugolini V, Henderson E, Akers M, Buja L M, Parkey R W, Willerson J T 1988 Iodine-123 phenylpentadecanoic acid and single photon emission computed tomography in identifying left ventricular regional metabolic abnormalities in patients with coronary heart disease: comparison with thallium-201 myocardial tomography. J Am Coll Cardiol 12: 78–87
27. Kennedy P L, Corbett J R, Kulkarni P V, Wolfe C L, Jansen D E, Hansen C L, Buja L M, Parkey R W, Willerson J T 1986 Iodine 123-phenylpentadecanoic acid myocardial scintigraphy: usefulness in the identification of myocardial ischaemia. Circulation 74: 1007–1015
28. Schad N, Wagner R K, Hallermeier J, Daus H J, Vattimo A, Bertelli P 1990 Regional rates of myocardial fatty acid metabolism: comparison with coronary angiography and ventriculography. Eur J Nucl Med 16: 205–212
29. Chouraqui P, Maddahi J, Henkin R, Karesh S M, Galie E, Berman D S 1991 Comparison of myocardial imaging with Iodine-123-iodophenyl-9-methyl pentadecanoic acid and Thallium-201-Chloride for assessment of patients with exercise-induced myocardial ischaemia. J Nucl Med 32: 447–452
30. Van der Wall E E, Heidendal G A K, den Hollander W, Westera G, Roos J P 1981 Metabolic myocardial imaging with I-123 labeled heptadecanoic acid in patients with angina pectoris. Eur J Nucl Med 6: 391–396
31. Hoeck A, Freundlieb C, Vyska K, Feinendegen L E, Rost R, Schuerch P M, Hollmann W The influence of rehabilitation training on fatty acid metabolism in patients after myocardial infarction. In: Faivre G, Bertrand A, Cherrier F, Amor M, Neiman J L (eds) Non invasive methods in ischaemic heart disease. Specia, Nancy, pp 300–303
32. Stoddart P G P, Papouchado M, Vann Jones J, Wilde P 1990 Practical and technical problems of myocardial imaging with 17-(123-iodo)-heptadecanoic acid. Nuc Compact 5: 244–247
33. Eenige van M J, Visser F C, Duwel C M B, Bezemer P D, Karreman A J P, Roos J P 1987 Analysis of myocardial time–activity curves of 123I-heptadecanoic acid I. Curve fitting. Nucl Med 26: 241–247
34. Eenige van M J, Visser F C, Karreman A J P, Duwel C M B, Bezemer P D, Roos J P 1987 Analysis of myocardial time–activity curves of 123I-heptadecanoic acid II. The acquisition time. Nucl Med 26: 248–252
35. Eenige van M J, Visser F C, Karreman A J P, Bezemer P D, Westera G, Lingen van A, Roos J P 1991 Analysis of time–activity curves related to myocardial metabolism. The case of ^{123}I-heptadecanoic acid. Nucl Med Commun 12: 115–125
36. Fischman A J, Saito T, Dilsizian V, Rocco T P, Yasuda T, Gonzalez E, Elmaleh D, Strauss H W 1989 Myocardial fatty acid imaging: Rationale, comparison of (11)C- and (123)I-labeled fatty acids, and potential clinical utility. Am J Card Imag 3: 288–296
37. Abdullah A Z, Hawkins L A, Britton K E, Elliot A T, Stephens J D 1981 I-123-labeled heptadecanoic acid as myocardial imaging agent: comparison with thallium-201 and first pass nuclear ventriculography. Nucl Med Comm 2: 268–277
38. Van der Wall E E, Heidendal G A K, den Hollander W, Westera G, Roos J P 1980 I-123 labeled hexadecenoic acid in comparison with Thallium-201 for myocardial imaging in coronary heart disease. Eur J Nucl Med 5: 401–405
39. Murray G, Schad N, Ladd W, Allie D, Vander Zwag R, Avet P, Rocket J 1991 Metabolic cardiac imaging in severe coronary disease: assessment of viablity with iodine-123-iodophenylpentadecanoic acid and multicrystal gamma camera, and correlation with biopsy. J Nucl Med 33: 1269–1277
40. Henrich M M, Vester E, Lohe von der E, Herzog H, Simon H, Kuikka J T, Feinedegen L E The comparison of 2-F18-deoxyglycose and 15-(ortho-131-phenyl) pentadecanoic acid uptake in persisting defects of Thallium-201 tomography in myocardial infarction. J Nucl Med 32: 1353–1357
41. Tamaki N, Kawamoto M, Yonekura Y, Fujibayashi Y, Magata Y, Torizuka T, Tadamura E, Nohara R, Sasayama S, Konishi J Assessment of fatty acid metabolism using I-123 branched fatty acid: comparison with positron emission tomography. Ann Nucl Med (in press)
42. Van der Wall E E, den Hollander W, Heidendal G A K, Westera G, Majid P A, Roos J P 1981 Dynamic myocardial scintigraphy with 123I-labeled free fatty acids in patients with myocardial infarction. Eur J Nucl Med 6: 383–389
43. Visser F C, Westera G, Eenige van M J, Van der Wall E E, Heidendal G A K, Roos J P 1985 Free fatty acid scintigraphy in patients with successful thrombolysis after acute myocardial infarction. Clin Nucl Med 10: 35–39
44. Reske S N 1987 Cardiac metabolism of I-123 phenylpentadecanoic acid. In: van der Wall E E (ed) Non-invasive imaging of cardiac metabolism. Martinus Nyhoff, Dordrecht, pp 139–158
45. Stoddart P G P, Papouchado M, Wilde P 1987 Prognostic value of 123-iodo-heptadecanoic acid imaging in patients with acute myocardial infarction. Eur J Nucl Med 12: 525–528

46. Roessler H, Hess T, Weiss M, Noelpp U, Mueller G, Hoeflin F, Kinser J 1983 Tomographic assessment of myocardial metabolic heterogeneity. J Nucl Med 24: 285–296
47. Roessler H, Noelpp U, Toth T, Schubiger P A, Hunziker H R On the prognostic potential of the sequential 123-I-HDA-tomoscintigram after the first MI. Eur Heart J 6(Suppl B): 49–55
48. Chappuis F, Meier B, Belenger J, Blauenstein P, Lerch R 1990 Early assessment of tissue viability with radioiodinated heptadecanoic acid in reperfused canine myocardium: comparison with thallium-201. Am Heart J 119: 833–841
49. Fridrich L, Gassner A, Sommer G, Kneussl M, Kassal H, Klicpera M, Salomonowitz E 1986 Dynamic 123I-HDA myocardial scintigraphy after aortocoronary bypass grafting. Eur J Nucl Med 12: S24–S26
50. Stoddart P G P, Papouchado M, Jones J V, Wilde P 1987 Assessment of percutaneous transluminal coronary angioplasty with ^{123}IODO-heptadecanoic acid. Eur J Nucl Med 12: 605–608
51. Kropp J, Likungu J, Kirchhoff P G, Knapp F F, Reichmann K, Reske S N, Biersack H J 1991 Single photon emission tomography imaging of myocardial oxidative metabolism with 15-p-123Iiodophenyl pentadecanoic acid in patients with coronary artery disease and aorto-coronary bypass grafting. Eur J Nucl Med 18: 467–474
52. Fioretti P, Reijs A E M, Neumann D, Taams M, Kooij P P M, Bos E, Reiber J H C 1988 Improvement in transient and persistent perfusion defects on early and late post-exercise thallium-201 tomograms after coronary artery bypass grafting. Eur Heart J 9: 1332–1338
53. Hoeck A, Freundlieb C, Vyska K, Loesse B, Erbel R, Feinendegen L E 1983 Myocardial imaging and metabolic studies with [17-123I]iodoheptadecanoic acid in patients with idiopathic congestive cardiomyopathy. J Nucl Med 24: 22–28
54. Knapp W H, Vyska K, Machulla H J, Notohamiprodjo G, Schmidt U, Knust E J, Gleichmann U 1988 Double-nuclide study of the myocardium using 201Tl and 123I labeled fatty acids in non-ischemic myocardial diseases. J Nucl Med 27: 72–78
55. Schad N, Daus H J, Ciavolella M, Maccio A 1987 Non-invasive functional imaging of regional rate of myocardial fatty acid metabolism. Cardiologia 32: 239–247
56. Ugolini V, Hansen C L, Kulkarni P V, Jansen D E, Akers M S, Corbett J R 1988 Abnormal myocardial fatty acid metabolism in dilated cardiomyopathy detected by I-123 phenylpentadecanoic acid and tomographic imaging. Am J Cardiol 62: 923–928
57. Rabinovitch M A, Kalff V, Allen A, Rosenthal A, Albers J, Das S K, Pitt B, Swanson D P, Manger T, Rogers W L, Thrall J H, Beierwaltes W H 1985 123I-hexadecanoic acid metabolic probe of cardiomyopathy. Eur J Nucl Med 10: 222–227
58. Livni E, Elmaleh D R, Barlai-Kovach M M, Goodman M M, Knapp F F, Strauss H W 1985 radioiodinated beta-methyl phenyl fatty acids as potential tracers for myocardial imaging and metabolism. Eur Heart J 6(Suppl B): 85–89
59. Notohamiprodjo G, Vyska K, Knapp W H, Brauns N, Gleichmann U, Machulla H J, Knust E J 1990 Fatty acid extraction in hypertrophied myocardium in hypertensive heart disease. Nuc Compact 5: 241–243
60. Kurata C, Tawarahara K, Taguchi T, Aoshima S, Kobayashi A, Yamazaki N, Kawai H, Kaneko M 1992 Myocardial emission computed tomography with iodine-123-labeled beta-methyl-branched fatty acids in patients with hypertrophic cardiomyopathy. J Nucl Med 33: 6–13
61. Heterogeneous myocardial distribution of iodine-123 15-(p-iodophenyl)-3-R,S-methylpentadecanoic acid (BMIPP) in patients with hypertrophic cardiomyopathy. Eur J Nucl Med 19: 775–782
62. Wolfe C L, Kennedy P L, Kulkarni P V, Jansen D E, Gabliani G I, Corbett J R 1990 Iodine-123 phenylpentadecanoic acid myocardial scintigraphy in patients with left ventricular hypertrophy: alterations in left ventricular distribution and utilization. Am Heart J 119: 1338–1347
63. Som P, Oster Z H, Kubota K, Goodman M M, Knapp F F Jr, Sacker D F, Weber D A 1989 Studies of a new fatty acid analog (DMIVN) in hypertensive rats and the effect of verapamil using ARG microimaging. Nucl Med Biol, Int J Radiat Appl Instrum part B 16: 483–490
64. Notohamiprodjo G, Minami K, Korfer R 1993 Non-invasive assessment of the myocardial fatty acid transport in patients with severe aortic stenosis for the evaluation of patient prognosis and of timing for surgical treatment. In: Abstractbook of the First International Congress of Nuclear Cardiology, Cannes, France, 1993, p 504 (abstract).
65. Camici P, Araujo L, Spinks T et al 1986 Increased uptake of 18F-fluordeoxyglucose in postischemic myocardium of patients with exercise-induced angina. Circulation 74: 81–88
66. Araujo, L I, Camici P, Spinks T J, Jones T, Maseri A 1988 Abnormalities in myocardial metabolism in patients with unstable angina as assessed by positron emission tomography. Cardiovasc Drug Ther 2: 41–46
67. Marshall R C, Tillisch J H, Phelps M E et al 1983 Identification and differentiation of resting myocardial ischemia and infarction in man with positron computed tomography, 18F-labeled fluorodeoxyglucose and N-13 ammonia. Circulation 67: 766–777
68. Brunken R, Tillish J, Schwaiger M et al 1986 Regional perfusion, glucose metabolism, and wall motion in patients with chronic electrocardiographic Q wave infarctions: evidence for persistence of viable tissue in some infarct regions by positron emission tomography. Circulation 73: 951–963
69. Schwaiger M, Brunken R, Grover-McKay M et al 1986 Regional myocardial metabolism in patients with acute myocardial infarction assessed by positron emission tomography. J Am Coll Cardiol 8: 800–808
70. Tillisch J R, Marshall R et al 1986 Reversibility of cardiac wall motion abnormalities predicted by positron tomography. N Engl J Med 314: 884–888
71. Tamaki N, Yonekura Y, Yamashita K et al 1989 Positron emission tomography using fluorine-18 deoxyglucose in evaluation of coronory artery bypass grafting. Am J Cardiol 64: 860–865
72. Eitzman D, Al-Aouar Z, Kanter H L et al 1992 Clinical outcome of patients with advanced coronary artery disease after viability studies with positron emission tomography. J Am Coll Cardiol 20: 559–565
73. Hoeflin F, Ledermann H, Noelpp U, Weinreich R, Roesler H 1989 Routine 18F-deoxy-2-fluoro-d-glucose (18FDG) myocardial tomography using a normal large field of view gamma camera. Angiology 140: 1058–1064
74. Van Lingen A, Huijgens P C, Visser F C et al 1992 Performance characteristics of a 511-keV collimator for imaging positron emitters with a standard gamma camera. Eur J Nucl Med 19: 315–321
75. Maddahi J, Garcia E V, Berman D S, Waxman A, Swan H J C, Forrester J S 1981 Improved noninvasive assessment of coronary artery disease by quantitative analysis of regional stress myocardial distribution and washout of thallium-201. Circulation 64: 924–931
76. Williams K A, Taillon L A, Stark V J 1992 Quantitative planar imaging of glucose metabolic activity in myocardial segments with exercise thallium-201 perfusion defects in patients with myocardial infarction: comparison with late (24-hour) redistribution thallium imaging for detection of reversible ischaemia. Am Heart J 124: 294–304
77. Knuuti M J, Nuutila P, Ruotsalainen U, Saraste M, Härkönen R, Ahonen A, Teräs M, Haaparanta M, Weggelius U, Haapanen A, Hartiala J, Voipio-Puekki L 1992 Euglycemic hyperinsulinemic clamp and oral glucose load in stimulating myocardial glucose utilization during positron emission tomography. J Nucl Med 33: 1255–1262.
78. Stoll H P, Hellwig N, Ozbek C, Oberhausen E, Schieffer 1993. Myocardial viability detected by F-18-deoxyglucose–Tc-99m-sestamibi dual isotope single photon emission tomography (SPECT). J Am Coll Cardiol 21: 250A

103. Clinical applications of positron emission tomography

Heinrich R. Schelbert

INTRODUCTION

Positron emission tomography (PET) expands the research and clinical capabilities of nuclear medicine for several reasons:

- PET yields tomographic images that reflect quantitatively the regional tracer activity concentrations in organs
- it employs a vast array of tracer substances labelled with positron-emitting isotopes, e.g. ^{15}O, ^{13}N, ^{11}C and ^{18}F, i.e. radioactive isotopes of elements that constitute major portions of living matter
- its high temporal resolution capability permits the delineation of the tissue kinetics of radiotracers in tissue
- if combined with appropriate tracer compartment models, it affords the in vivo application of tracer kinetic principles for the non-invasive quantification of regional functional processes, e.g. blood flow and substrate metabolism.

This chapter reviews technical aspects of PET as they relate to clinical studies, describes quantitative approaches to the study of the human heart, and then focuses on the contributions of PET to the diagnosis and management of patients with cardiovascular disease. Foremost among its clinical applications in cardiac disease are the detection of coronary artery disease and of its consequences on regional substrate metabolism.

* The author is affiliated to the Laboratory of Structural Biology and Molecular Medicine, University of California, operated for the U.S. Department of Energy by the University of California under Contract #DE-AC03-76-SF00012. This work was supported in part by the Director of the Office of Energy Research, Office of Health and Environmental Research, Washington D.C., by Research Grants #HL 29845 and #HL 33177, National Institutes of Health, Bethesda, MD and by an Investigative Group Award by the Greater Los Angeles Affiliate of the American Heart Association, Los Angeles, CA.

METHODOLOGIC ASPECTS

Image acquisition and analysis

Current PET scanners have an internal opening of about 50–60 cm and an axial field of view of 16–17 cm. The intrinsic axial and in-plane resolution approaches 4–5 mm in the centre of the field of view. In order to reduce the statistical noise of the images, reconstruction filters are used which lower the effective spatial resolution to about 7–10 mm.

Acquisition of images of the uptake of radiotracers in myocardium is preceded by acquisition of transmission images for about 15–20 min. Transmission images display the heterogeneous attenuation of photons throughout the thorax. During image reconstruction, they correct for photon attenuation of the emission images. After tracer injection, it is critical to record the emission images in exactly the same position in order to avoid image artefacts. More recently, software algorithms have been developed and validated for correction of body motion between the transmission and the emission images.[1] The relatively short axial field of view of only about 10 cm with older and of about 15–16 cm with newer tomographs requires careful patient positioning. Therefore, many tomographs permit acquisition of a 'rectilinear scan' of the chest which depicts the cardiac silhouette. With the aid of on screen 'cursors', the patient is then moved automatically into the most appropriate position within the tomograph.

Acquisition of emission images depends on the type of information sought with PET. Characteristically, static images depict the relative distribution of tracer concentrations in organs, and thus provides qualitative information on regional functional processes. Depending on the specific type of tracer, 1–40 min are allowed for tracer clearance from blood or for metabolic trapping of the tracer in the myocardium (e.g. 5 min for ^{13}N ammonia or 40 min for ^{18}F deoxyglucose); images are then acquired for 15–20 minutes. Quantification of regional functional processes such as blood flow and glucose utilization rates requires rapid acquisition of serial images, e.g. of 1–12 s frames. Typically, after serial images have been recorded, a final static image is taken for accurate assignment of regions of interest for determining the regional tracer tissue kinetics.

Because PET images are recorded in a transaxial orientation, most laboratories now employ reorientation software routines in order to display the tracer activity concentrations in the form of short axis and vertical and horizontal long axis cross sections of the left ventricular myocardium.[2–4] Reorientation also minimizes effects of regional partial volume and, thus, artefactual reductions in observed regional tracer tissue concentrations. The short axis cuts can be assembled into polar maps; similar to cartographic approaches, this particular format displays the three-dimensional distribution of functional processes in the form of a two-dimensional map.[2,3,5] Alternatives include the three-dimensional topographic display[6] or true three-dimensional representations of the left ventricular myocardium with colour coding of blood flow or metabolic abnormalities.[7] The 'geographic display methods' depict the location and the extent of abnormalities of blood flow and metabolism, and are suitable for quantifying the extent and severity of functional abnormalities.[6,8,9]

Radiotracers of blood flow and metabolism

While the number of positron-emitting tracers for probing and quantifying functional processes of the human myocardium is virtually unlimited, clinically most useful have been tracers of myocardial blood flow, glucose utilization, fatty acid and oxidative metabolism.

Tracers of myocardial blood flow

Used most widely are ^{13}N ammonia, ^{82}Rb and ^{15}O water. Each tracer offers specific advantages as well as disadvantages. The cyclotron-produced ^{13}N ammonia and the generator-available ^{82}Rb are retained in myocardium in proportion to flow and therefore offer static images of the relative distribution of myocardial blood flow.[10–13] The physical half-life of ^{82}Rb (only 75 s) can result in low count images but affords serial evaluations of myocardial blood flow in rapid succession. The 10 min physical half-life of ^{13}N ammonia requires 30–40 min time intervals between serial studies, yet gives high count density images of better diagnostic quality. It should be emphasized that the net extraction (the product of the first pass extraction fraction and of blood flow) increases non-linearly with blood flow because of a progressive flow-dependent decline in the first pass extraction fraction. In contrast, the net extraction of ^{15}O water increases with flow linearly, one of several reasons why it meets more closely the criteria of an ideal tracer of blood flow.[14–16] However, ^{15}O water exchanges rapidly between blood and surrounding tissues, so that blood pool subtraction techniques are needed to delineate its uptake in the myocardium. Also, the tracer clears rapidly from myocardium so that static images are generally of low count density. This tracer is therefore used mostly for quantitative flow measurements.

Tracers of substrate metabolism

Several radiotracers permit the evaluation and quantification of specific aspects of myocardial substrate metabolism. Given the notion of free fatty acid as the heart's preferred fuel substrate, early studies focused on ^{11}C palmitate.[17] This labelled long chain fatty acid provides largely qualitative information on the myocardium's fatty acid metabolism. Its bi-exponential clearance from the myocardium implies a distribution of the tracer label between at least two functional pools of different sizes and turnover rates.[18,19] It is now clear that the rapid clearance curve component reflects the fraction of fatty acid that immediately undergoes oxidation (both β-oxidation and oxidation via the TCA cycle); the clearance rate corresponds to the flux of substrate through the oxidative pathway.[20–22] In contrast, the slow clearance curve component corresponds to the fraction of labelled palmitate that enters the endogenous lipid pool consisting mainly of triglycerides and phospholipids.[23] While quantitative measurements of total fatty acid metabolism have not become available with PET, the clearance curve morphology nevertheless offers useful information (Fig. 103.1). For example, during preferential fatty acid oxidation, the relative size of the rapid clearance curve component is large and its slope is steep.[20] Increases in cardiac work and, consequently, in oxygen consumption, enhance the relative size of the rapid clearance curve component and accelerate the clearance rate (Fig. 103.1).[24] Conversely, if myocardium shifts to glucose as its major oxidative substrate, the rapid clearance curve component declines and its slope becomes less steep.[20] Acute myocardial ischaemia produces similar changes as a reflection of impaired fatty acid oxidation and increased fatty acid deposition in the endogenous lipid pool.[19,23,25]

Animal experimental and clinical investigations with PET have emphasized the myocardium's ability to shift between substrates. Such shifts in substrate utilization and oxidation can be demonstrated also with ^{18}F 2-fluoro-2-deoxyglucose (^{18}FDG).[26–28] This glucose analogue exchanges across the capillary and sarcolemmal membranes in proportion to glucose as its tracer; it then competes with glucose for hexokinase for phosphorylation to ^{18}FDG-6-phosphate.[26,29] Unlike glucose-6-phosphate, the phosphorylated glucose analogue is a poor substrate for glycogen synthesis, the fructose phosphate shunt and glycolysis, and thus becomes virtually trapped in the myocardium. Regional ^{18}F activity concentrations in

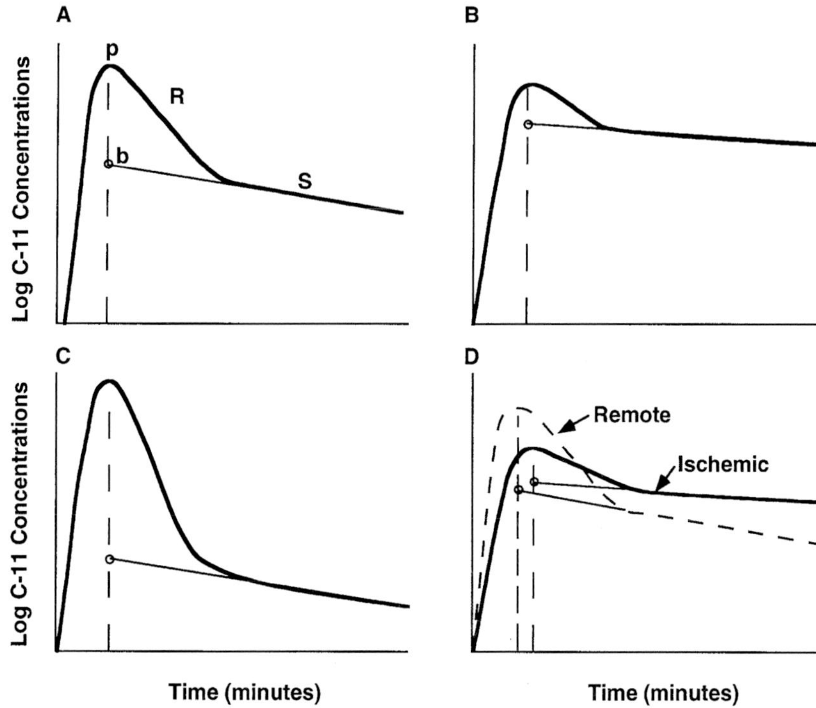

Fig. 103.1 Clearance pattern of ^{11}C palmitate from myocardium. A depicts the characteristic bi-exponential clearance pattern where the relative size $(p-b)/P$ and slope (R) of the rapid clearance phase correspond to the fraction of tracer undergoing oxidation immediately and where the relative size (b/p) and slope (S) of the slow clearance phase correspond to the fraction of tracer that is incorporated into the endogenous lipid pool and its turnover rate. This clearance curve is seen in the fasted state where the major fraction of tracer is oxidized immediately. B demonstrates the changes in the clearance kinetics of ^{11}C palmitate as induced by a shift in myocardial substrate metabolism from free fatty acids to carbohydrates. While myocardial oxygen consumption remains constant, the increase in oxidation of glucose is paralleled by a decrease in fatty acid oxidation as reflected by decline in the relative size and slope of the rapid clearance curve component. C depicts the change in the clearance curve morphology as induced by an increase in cardiac work. The increased oxygen consumption is reflected on the time–activity curve by an increase in the relative size and slope of the rapid clearance curve component as a reflection of greater fatty acid oxidation. D depicts a similar pattern, though regional, in acutely ischaemic myocardium where fatty acid oxidation is impaired (curve designated 'ischemic') as compared to normal fatty acid oxidation in remote myocardium (curve designated as 'remote').

myocardium as depicted on static images therefore reflect the relative distribution of regional rates of exogenous glucose utilization. Under conditions of preferred fatty acid oxidation, ^{18}FDG clears only slowly from blood with little if any uptake in myocardium.[30,31] Similar findings occur in patients with diabetes mellitus. Conversely, if myocardium preferentially oxidizes glucose, uptake of ^{18}FDG by myocardium is high and its clearance from blood is rapid. Animal and human investigations have demonstrated a similar regional augmentation of ^{18}FDG uptake as an expression of increased glycolysis in acute ischaemic situations;[32,33] in this case, the uptake is confined to a region with reduced myocardial blood flow and impaired contractile function (see below).

Myocardial oxygen consumption can be quantified with ^{11}C-labelled acetate[34,35] or, as proposed more recently, with molecular ^{15}O.[36] The ^{11}C acetate approach has been extensively explored and validated;[34,35,37–39] ^{11}C acetate readily exchanges across the cellular and mitochondrial membranes, becomes esterified to acetyl-CoA, is metabolized through the TCA cycle and then released from the myocardium in the form of ^{11}C-labelled CO_2. The rate of release of label from myocardium correlates linearly with the myocardial oxygen consumption. It is important to point out that the tissue clearance rate reflects only a rate constant and not (unlike the glucose measurements) an estimate of true substrate or mass flux. Recent biochemical studies have indicated that the clearance rate constant largely depends on the turnover rate of the glutamate pool.[40] Accordingly, changes in the size of this pool or of pools of other metabolites of the TCA cycle will alter the clearance rate constant independently of an actual change of the flux rate of the TCA cycle. Studies are currently underway to establish and validate a true tracer compartment model that will yield estimates of true substrate (mass) flux rather than only flux rates.[41]

Detection of coronary artery disease

In conventional radionuclide imaging, treadmill exercise is the preferred method for inducing flow defects in the stenosis-dependent myocardial territory. For detection of coronary artery disease with PET most laboratories employ pharmacological stress, because the patient needs to remain in exactly the same position during the rest and stress imaging sessions. In order to avoid reconstruction artefacts, the emission images must remain aligned exactly with the transmission images. Either ^{13}N ammonia or ^{82}Rb serve as tracers of myocardial blood flow. Dipyridamole or adenosine are administered i.v. for the induction of coronary vasodilation.

The rationale for pharmacological stress is that significant coronary stenoses attenuate the flow reserve in the dependent myocardium.[42] As initially demonstrated in animal experiments, myocardial blood flow at rest may be maintained normal even in the presence of severe coronary stenosis (approximately up to 85–90% luminal diameter narrowing).[12,42,43] However, less severe stenoses attenuate responses in myocardial flow to coronary vasodilation.

The blood flow images are analysed by visual inspection or, more recently, by comparison to laboratory-specific databases of normal. Semiquantitative image analysis, e.g. normalization of tracer concentrations to the injected tracer dose, are believed to enhance the accuracy of disease detection especially in instances of balanced lesions or left main stenosis.[44] If myocardial tissue activity concentrations do not increase from the rest to the hyperaemic study then pharmacological stress might have been inadequate, or alternatively, coronary artery disease may be severe and extensive.

The diagnostic accuracy of PET exceeds that reported for ^{201}Tl SPECT imaging. As listed in Table 103.1, sensitivities range from 84% to 98% and specificities from 78% to 100%.[43,45–47] Studies comparing both approaches in the same patient populations offer even more support for the higher diagnostic performance of PET (Table 103.2).[48–50] One study reported similar sensitivities and specificities for both approaches while another study in 201 patients observed a higher sensitivity with PET than with SPECT. A third study in 81 patients found a higher specificity for PET than for SPECT but similar sensitivities. Several reasons might account for these results. The Tamaki study[48] employed first generation PET scanners with low spatial resolution capabilities. The higher sensitivity versus the higher specificity in the two more recent studies[49,50] may be related to interpretative differences, e.g. image analysis at different points on the receiver–operator characteristics (ROC) curve.

Table 103.1 Detection of coronary artery disease by PET: summary of all reported studies

Study	No. of patients	Sensitivity (%)	Specificity (%)	Accuracy (%)
Schelbert et al[43]	45	97	100	98
Yonekura et al[46]	50	93	100	94
Demer et al[45]	156	94	95	94
Williams et al[47]	146	98	93	94
Stewart et al[49]	81	84	88	85
Go et al[50]	202	93	78	90
Mean ±		93±5	92±8	91±5

Table 103.2 Detection of coronary artery disease by PET and by SPECT

Study	No. of Patients	Sensitivity (%)		Specificity (%)		Accuracy (%)	
		SPECT	PET	SPECT	PET	SPECT	PET
Stewart et al[49]	81	84	84	53	88*	79	85*
Go et al[50]	202	76	93*	80	78	77	90
Tamaki et al[48]	48	96	98	–	–	–	–

* Stastically significant differences between SPECT and PET.
The study by Tamaki et al does not include patients without coronary artery disease; therefore no values for specificity are available.

While these initial studies have relied largely on visual or semiquantitative analysis, more recent developments suggest that region-specific thresholds for abnormal tracer uptakes may yield even higher diagnostic accuracies.[7,51] Despite the discordant results of these initial intra-patient comparisons, it is important to point out that the overall diagnostic accuracy of the PET approach exceeded that of SPECT, even though the diagnostic gain has been relatively modest. The diagnostic gain may be due to several factors. One is the appropriate correction for measured (rather than assumed) photon attenuation which minimizes effective image artefacts. This correction accounts for the absence of gender-related differences in the relative distributions of myocardial tracer concentrations as observed frequently with SPECT. Additional reasons are the higher spatial and contrast resolution capabilities of PET, so that even small or subtle flow reductions are identified.

On the other hand, the high diagnostic accuracy of PET does not negate the value of conventional SPECT or planar approaches with ^{201}Tl- or ^{99m}Tc-labelled flow tracers for the detection of coronary artery disease. In laboratories equipped with both SPECT and PET, one might submit those patients to PET in whom SPECT is likely to yield equivocal or falsely positive findings. Such patients include those in whom coronary artery disease is expected to be only mild or who have a low pre-test probability of the disease. One might equally assign to PET those patients with a high likelihood of attenuation artefacts on SPECT, e.g. women or obese patients.

QUANTIFICATION OF MYOCARDIAL BLOOD FLOW

The ^{13}N ammonia and ^{15}O water approaches have been widely employed for measurements of regional myocardial blood flow in the human. Estimates of flow at rest appear to be somewhat higher with the ^{15}O water than with the ^{13}N ammonia approach,[15,16,52–54] presumably because of different approaches for the correction of partial volume and spillover of activity between myocardium and blood. Furthermore, blood flow values in normal volunteers exhibit considerable interindividual variations, which may be due to method-related factors but also, more importantly, because of interindividual variations in cardiac work and oxygen demand.[55] Therefore most laboratories relate individual flow estimates to the rate pressure product as a readily available though incomplete index of cardiac work. Other studies have demonstrated proportionate increases in blood flow and cardiac work during supine bicycle exercise[56] or inotropic stimulation with dobutamine.[57]

The myocardial flow reserve of the normal human myocardium has been extensively explored with pharmacological vasodilation using either i.v. dipyridamole[52] or adenosine.[58] There is evidence that the myocardial flow reserve declines with age;[55,59] one study has demonstrated an age-dependent decline in hyperaemic blood flows, but a second and more extensive investigation failed to demonstrate such a decline in the maximum hyperaemic flow. However, it has been shown that resting blood flow progressively rises with age as a function of increasing rate pressure product, so that myocardial flow reserve as the ratio of hyperaemic to resting blood flow significantly falls with age.[55] This information may be important; for example, a somewhat lower flow reserve in myocardium supplied by normal coronary arteries in chronic coronary artery disease patients might imply angiographically non-detectable disease when compared to younger normal volunteers, but would prove to be normal when compared to an age matched control population.

The availability of quantitative flow measurements has prompted an intensive search for possible abnormalities in patients with syndrome X.[58,60–62] Observations in this particular disorder have thus far however remained inconclusive. Some investigators have noted normal myocardial flow reserves; some have reported subgroups with increased resting and attenuated hyperaemic blood flows; others have pointed to heterogeneities in blood flow at rest and during dipyridamole-induced hyperaemia.

Similarly, hypertrophic cardiomyopathy has been the subject of several investigations.[63] Measurements of myocardial blood flow unequivocally demonstrated a markedly attenuated flow reserve that was not confined to the hypertrophied interventricular septum but involved also the lateral wall, conventionally thought to be normal. In a small group of patients with hypertrophic cardiomyopathy, supine bicycle exercise failed to produce an increase in blood flow, presumably because of excessive extravascular resistive forces.[64] On the other hand this finding might account for the ischaemia-like clinical symptomatology in such patients.

There are numerous investigations that have examined the resting and hyperaemic blood flows in cardiac transplants.[65–68] Generally, baseline blood flow was observed to be increased in proportion to the increase in the rate pressure product, while hyperaemic blood flow was found to be normal. A more recent study demonstrated a marked reduction in blood flow reserve during acute transplant rejection.[68] This was because of an increase in resting blood flows in excess of cardiac work as well as a marked reduction in hyperaemic blood flow. These observations provide a rationale for clinical restriction of physical activity during rejection in order to minimize injury from rejection and, at the same time, suggest a possible role for monitoring immunosuppressive treatment in rejecting cardiac allografts.

Other studies have explored the effects of coronary artery stenosis on resting and hyperaemic blood flow. As expected, maximum hyperaemic blood flow is markedly attenuated in stenosis-dependent myocardium. Successful angioplasty fully restored hyperaemic blood flow and thus myocardial flow reserve, even though more recent studies indicate that such normalization does not occur immediately after angioplasty.[69] The flow reserve was found to be attenuated at 7 days after angioplasty but normal at 4 months.[70] Several laboratories currently correlate the angiographic stenosis severity with flow reserve at maximum hyperaemic flow.[71–73] While these studies are currently in progress, initial results indicate considerable flow variations for the same angiographic stenosis severity. These initial findings raise questions as to the true 'gold standard' of stenosis severity, i.e. quantitative arteriography as compared to functional flow measurements. It might imply that functional rather than anatomic information would characterize disease severity more accurately, and would allow the monitoring of its progression or the effects of mechanical or pharmacological interventions.

ASSESSMENT OF MYOCARDIAL VIABILITY

The widespread use of interventional revascularization and the increased availability of cardiac transplantation underscore the need for diagnostic approaches that identify accurately viable myocardium and its extent. To be clear, myocardial viability is an issue only when regional or global left ventricular function is impaired. Diagnostic approaches seek to determine whether an impairment of contractile function is reversible if blood flow is restored. Thus, regional contractile function must be taken into account. In other words, regardless of any scintigraphic findings (for example on the conventional stress–rest redistribution imaging with ^{201}Tl) viability is not an issue if regional or global left ventricular wall motion is normal at rest. The issue is to distinguish a potentially reversible from an irreversible impairment of contractile function. For the same reason it is important to determine how well any 'viability test' predicts the outcome in contractile function after blood flow has been restored. Additional criteria are important. For example, can viability assessment predict whether global rather than merely regional left ventricular function improves? Can it predict a potential improvement in the symptoms related to congestive heart failure, and can it be used to stratify patients to a specific therapeutic approach? Can it identify those patients who are likely to benefit from revascularization? Conversely, can it provide additional evidence that cardiac transplantation is in fact the most appropriate therapeutic option in a given patient, or does it support the decision to assign a patient to conservative management?

Given the large number of tracers and possibilities, PET offers several avenues for the assessment of myocardial viability. These avenues are based on the evaluation and quantification of myocardial blood flow, transmembranous ion exchange and substrate metabolism. Foremost at present are

- blood flow-metabolism imaging
- the water perfusable tissue index
- the ^{82}Rb uptake and retention approach
- the determination of oxidative metabolism with ^{11}C acetate.

Imaging of myocardial blood flow and glucose metabolism

This approach, which has now been accepted by many laboratories, entails two steps. First, the relative distribution of myocardial blood flow is evaluated with a positron-emitting tracer of blood flow, e.g. ^{13}N ammonia or ^{82}Rb. Second, ^{18}FDG is used for the evaluation of regional rates of exogenous glucose utilization; preserved or even enhanced ^{18}FDG uptake in dysfunctional myocardial regions is the hallmark of myocardial viability. The approach is based on early observations in experimental animals with acutely induced myocardial ischaemia.[32,74] While the explanations of the underlying mechanisms have been extrapolated from the acute ischaemic situation to chronic conditions, it remains uncertain whether they in fact do apply to more chronic reductions in blood flow as frequently noted in chronic coronary artery disease patients. It is possible, as Opie suggests,[75] that membrane-related, glycolytically derived ATP is essential for cell survival (i.e. maintenance of transmembranous ion concentration gradients) which may indeed account for the enhanced ^{18}FDG uptake.

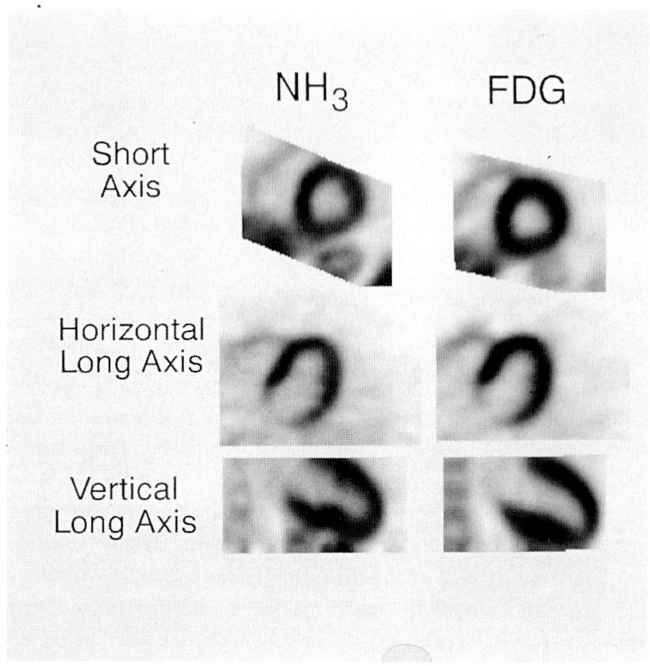

Fig. 103.2 Reoriented short axis (**top**) and vertical and horizontal long axis cuts (**middle, bottom**) of myocardial blood flow with N-13 ammonia (**left**) and of ^{18}FDG uptake (**right**) in a patient with moderate hypokinesis of the anterior wall. Note the homogeneous distribution of blood flow and glucose metabolism.

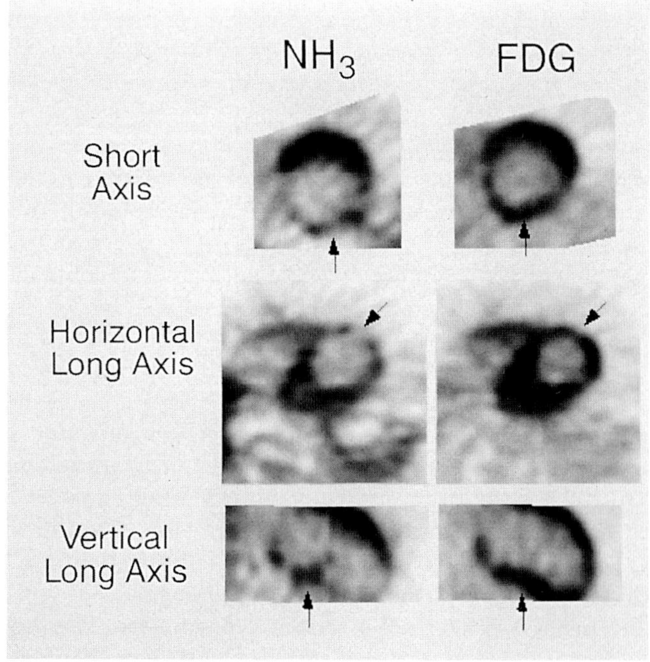

Fig. 103.3 Blood flow–metabolism mismatch pattern in a patient with akinesis of the inferior wall. The display is the same as in Fig. 103.2. Note the decreased blood flow in the inferior wall on the ^{13}N ammonia images and the preserved or even modestly enhanced ^{18}FDG uptake in the same region.

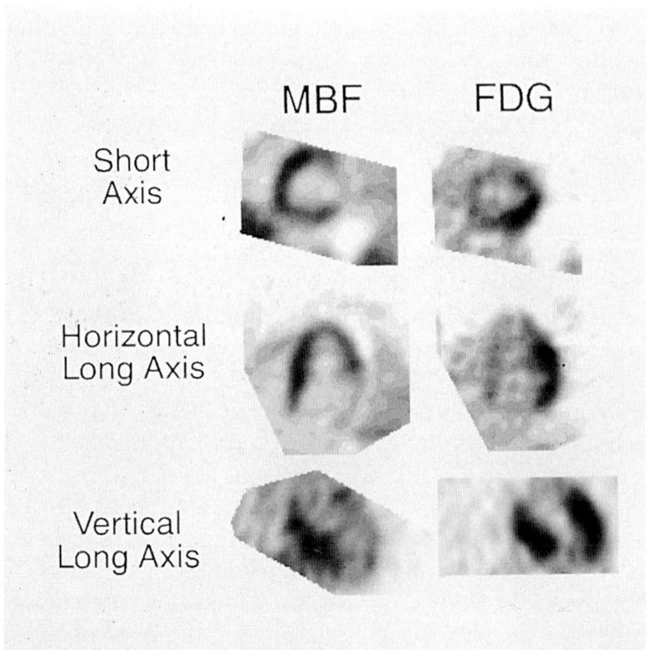

Fig. 103.4 Blood flow metabolism mismatch pattern in a patient with severe hypokinesis of the lateral wall. The display is identical to that in Fig. 103.2. Note the decreased blood flow in the lateral and posterolateral wall on the ^{13}N ammonia images. The ^{18}FDG images reveal only modest tracer uptake in normally perfused myocardium but a striking increase in the hypoperfused lateral wall. Unlike the patient shown in Fig. 103.3 who was examined after oral administration of 75 g of glucose, the patient in this study was examined after a 5 h fasting period. Because normal myocardium preferentially utilizes free fatty acid in this condition, glucose utilization, and consequently ^{18}FDG uptake, is low (although increased in the reversibly injured lateral wall).

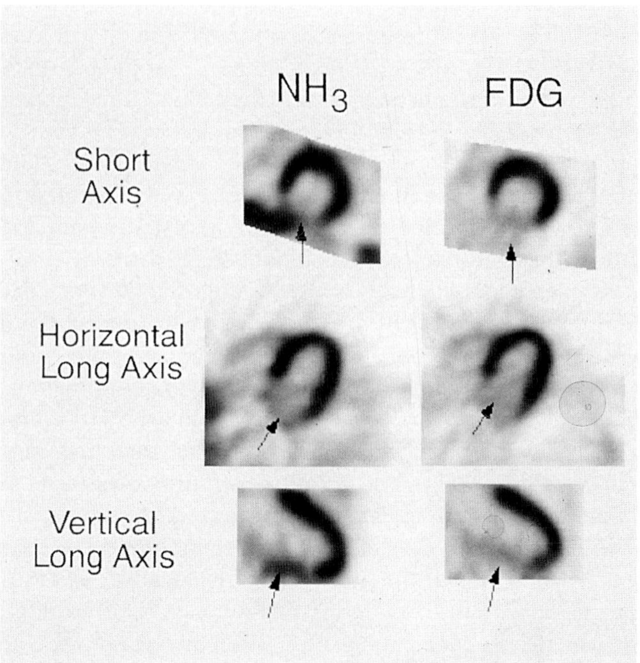

Fig. 103.5 Blood flow metabolism match in a patient with akinesis of the inferior wall. The display is identical to that in Fig. 103.2. Note the decreased ^{13}N ammonia uptake in the inferior wall indicating reduced myocardial blood flow. This is associated with a concordant reduction in ^{18}FDG uptake.

Segments with impaired contractile function exhibit on blood flow metabolism imaging three distinctly different patterns:

1. Blood flow and ^{18}FDG uptake are normal (Fig. 103.2).
2. Blood flow is reduced but glucose utilization is increased relative to blood flow or is even enhanced relative to normal and remote myocardium, known as 'blood flow–metabolism mismatch pattern' (Figs 103.3 and 103.4).
3. Blood flow and ^{18}FDG are concordantly reduced, known as 'blood flow–metabolism match' (Fig. 103.5).

The severity of regional flow reduction and their extent as well as the magnitude of the relative or absolute increases in ^{18}FDG uptake are readily established on visual analysis. Semiquantitative image analysis may also be used for circumferential activity profile techniques or polar mapping in comparison to laboratory-specific data bases of normal.

Some laboratories have developed modifications to the original technique: one is a 'hybrid' approach in which blood flow is evaluated with ^{99m}Tc sestamibi and SPECT;[76] another is the study of the relative distribution of blood flow with ^{11}C acetate[4] whose uptake parallels myocardial blood flow;[77] lastly, the relative myocardial uptake of only ^{18}FDG is examined. Regional uptake thresholds may thus distinguish between viable and non-viable myocardium.[78,79]

It should be emphasized that the term 'match' does not imply the complete absence of 'viable' or 'normal' myocardium. For example, subendocardial scar tissue may coexist with normal myocardium in the more epicardial layers. Conversely, the term 'mismatch' does not imply that contractile function will fully recover after successful restoration of blood flow. Rather, scar tissue, normal myocytes and functionally compromised cells coexist frequently. The amount of functional improvement attainable through revascularization depends on the fractional distribution of these three general types of cell populations in a given myocardial region. It is also thought that normal blood flow and normal or enhanced glucose utilization in dysfunctional myocardial regions primarily reflect 'stunning', while reduced blood flow may signify 'hibernation'. In view of the well-known transmural gradients in the severity of an ischaemic injury, it is also possible that the latter condition represents an admixture of scar tissue and stunned myocardium or even coexistence of all three types of functionally compromised tissues.

Preliminary studies noted an almost complete loss of myocardial flow reserve in match and mismatch segments.[80] Observations in collateral dependent human myocardium with normally maintained blood flow implied that contractile dysfunction can be associated with a severely impaired myocardial flow reserve.[81,82] The impaired contractile function in this case was attributed to 'repetitive' stunning – an alternative explanation for the chronic but reversible dysfunctional state. Such dysfunctional segments contain a substantial fraction of 'dedifferentiated myocytes', which characteristically exhibit a loss of contractile filaments, glycogen granules and multiple small though ultrastructurally normal mitochondria.[81,83] While these cells may represent the structural correlate of the enhanced glucose uptake, they may also represent the 'lower end' of the entire spectrum of functionally though reversibly compromised myocytes.

Several clinical investigations have established the high predictive accuracies of the blood flow–glucose metabolism patterns (see Table 103.3) as a measure of viability, by using post-revascularization outcome of contractile improvement.[4,78,84–91] Positive predictive accuracies as reported in these investigations in a cumulative total of 274 patients range from 52% to 95% and negative predictive accuracies from 78% to 100%.

Most of the investigations listed above compared the relative distribution of ^{18}FDG uptake to that of regional myocardial blood flow assessed with either ^{13}N ammonia or ^{82}Rb and PET. Two studies employed a 'hybrid' approach in which ^{99m}Tc sestamibi and SPECT gave no significant loss in predictive accuracies.[88,91] Of further note is that the study by Knuuti et al[78] employed only ^{18}FDG imaging with PET. The relative ^{18}FDG uptake in dysfunctional segments served as a predictor of the post-revascularization outcome in regional contractile function. In this particular study, the optimum threshold for discriminating viable from non-viable myocardium, determined retrospectively, was found to be a relative tracer uptake of 85–90%.

There are a number of factors that might account for the interstudy differences in predictive accuracies. While most studies administer ^{18}FDG 1 h after an oral glucose load, some laboratories prefer the use of tracer in the fasted state.[85,86] This approach, as recently demonstrated in our laboratory,[92] might uncover even small amounts of reversibly compromised myocardium. Yet, such small amounts of compromised tissue may be of little consequence for a post-revascularization improvement in regional contractile function, and thus lower the specificity of the blood flow–metabolism imaging approach. Another reason for the reported variability in predictive accuracies, as for example in the study by Gropler et al,[4] may be differences in the analyses of the blood flow–metabolism pattern. These investigators normalized the relative uptake of both the tracer of blood flow and of ^{18}FDG to their respective highest tracer activity concentrations, and employed ratios of ^{18}FDG to flow tracer concentrations as criteria for 'matches' and 'mismatches'. This differs from the original technique which normalized the myocardial ^{18}FDG uptake to the myocardial region with the highest uptake of flow tracer (upper 10% of activity concentrations) and defined matches and mismatches by tracer differences rather than ratios.[74] Ratios of tracer concentrations may be more sensitive to statistical noise than differences, especially when regional count densities are low. Moreover, the normalization of both tracer distributions to

Table 103.3 Detection of hibernation in dysfunctional myocardium by ^{18}FDG uptake, using the gold standard of improvement in function by revascularization

Study	No. of patients	No. of segments	^{18}FDG present (%)	^{18}FDG absent (%)
Tillisch et al[84]	17	67	85	8
Tamaki et al[85]	22	46	78	22
Tamaki et al[86]	11	56	80	0
Marwick et al[89]	16	85	68	21
vom Dahl et al[90]	40	not given	75	14
Lucignani et al[88]	14	54	95	20
Carrel et al[87]	21	53	79	17
Gropler et al[100]	34	116	52	19
Knuuti et al[78]	48	90	85	16
vom Dahl et al[91]	51	153	77	12
Mean ±			77±7	15±11

[^{18}F]DG present indicates a blood flow–metabolism mismatch or enhanced or preserved FDG uptake in dysfunctional myocardial regions as compared to ^{18}FDG absent, which indicates a match or absent glucose utilization. Segments refers to the numbers of dysfunctional segments in each study. In the studies by Lucignani et al[88] and by vom Dahl et al,[91] myocardial blood flow was evaluated with ^{99m}Tc sestamibi and SPECT while glucose utilization was examined with ^{18}FDG PET. The data presented by Knuuti et al[78] are derived from ^{18}FDG PET images only using a threshold for the relative tracer uptake of 85–90%. Gropler et al[100] report a relatively low positive predictive value. This value improved to 72% when only akinetic and dyskinetic segments were analysed (see text for details). For the study by vom Dahl et al[90] the positive predictive accuracy is listed only for segments with marked and not for mild mismatches.

different maxima may lower the accuracy of distinguishing matches from mismatches, and thus adversely affect the predictive accuracies. It is of interest that in the Gropler study, the predictive accuracy improved when only severely dysfunctional segments were analysed. Presumably, such segments exhibited more severe flow defects and thus were correctly identified by this modified approach.

The reported interstudy differences in predictive accuracies underscore the need for standardization of study protocols. Most laboratories now employ oral glucose loading (75–100 g glucose) about 1 h prior to the ^{18}FDG injection. This stimulates insulin secretion and thus improves the myocardial uptake of the tracer.[30,74] More challenging are patients with diabetes mellitus in whom regular i.v. administration of small amounts of insulin usually succeeds in adequate uptake of tracer in myocardium and tracer clearance from blood. The hyperinsulinaemic euglycaemic clamp may serve as another alternative for obtaining high quality images in diabetic patients,[93,94] although this approach may render clinical studies more cumbersome and impractical.

The water-perfusable tissue index

Determination of this index requires several steps. The routinely recorded transmission images reflect the overall tissue density or volume. They are corrected for blood volume after labelling of red blood cells with ^{15}O carbon monoxide. An image of the extravascular tissue density or volume is obtained and is then analysed for the fraction that rapidly exchanges ^{15}O water.[95] The approach is predicated on the assumption that viable myocardium exchanges free water rapidly, whereas necrotic myocytes or scar tissue do not. Initial observations in early post-infarction and in chronic coronary artery disease patients have been encouraging. A perfusable tissue index > 0.7 consistently predicted post-revascularization improvements in segmental contractile function. In contrast, wall motion remained unchanged if the perfusable tissue index was less than 0.7.[96,97] Although this method shortens considerably PET determinations of myocardial viability, it awaits validation in animal experimental studies. Given its complexities, it will be essential to examine the utility of this index in patients with reduced left ventricular ejection fractions. Lastly, it remains uncertain whether it adequately distinguishes between functionally compromised but viable and normal myocardium.

^{82}Rb uptake and retention

Fundamental to this approach is that only viable myocardium retains actively the cation Rb^+ (substituting for K^+ on the sodium–potassium pump). Thus, loss of tracer from myocardium between the initial uptake and the subsequent retention image signifies loss of viability, whereas retention of tracer indicates viable myocardium. An initial comparison with the now widely employed ^{18}FDG method has been encouraging.[6,98] Further, a recent report described a 3 year follow-up of 35 patients studied with the ^{82}Rb uptake and retention method. The authors concluded that the absence of viable myocardium was the single most powerful predictor of mortality. Yet, of the 25 patients (or 71% of all patients in this study) with viability diagnosed using ^{82}Rb, 20 patients (or 80%) underwent revascularization, which may force a re-evaluation. It also remains unknown whether revascularization in these patients produced an improvement in left ventricular function and in congestive heart failure symptoms.

Measurement of oxidative metabolism with ^{11}C acetate

This is based on the idea that glycolytically derived ATP is inadequate for cell survival. Accordingly, oxidative metabolism must be sustained. Studies in both early post-infarction patients and chronic coronary artery disease patients have demonstrated that ^{11}C acetate clearance rates in reversibly compromised myocardium do not differ significantly from those in remote myocardium but are significantly reduced in irreversibly dysfunctional segments.[99,100] Based on these initial findings the same group of investigators defined two standard deviations below the mean of

Table 103.4 Effect of revascularization on left ventricular ejection fraction (LVEF)

Author	No. of patients	Extensive mismatch region				Small or no mismatch region			
		n*	Pre-LVEF	Post-LVEF	*P*	*n**	Pre-LVEF	Post-LVEF	*P*
Tillisch et al[84]	17	11	30±11	45±14	<0.05	6	30±11	31±12	NS
Marwick et al[89]	24	9	37±11	40±9	NS	15	38±13	38±13	NS
Carrel et al[87]	23	21	34±14	52±11	<0.01	–	–	–	–
Lucignani et al[88]	14	13	38±5	48±4	<.001	–	–	–	–
Depré et al[102]	23	†	43±18	52±15	†		35±9	24±8	†
Besozzi et al[101]	56	49	29±12	41±11	†	7	43±10	39±16	†

* *n* = number of patients with or without mismatches.
† Values not given.

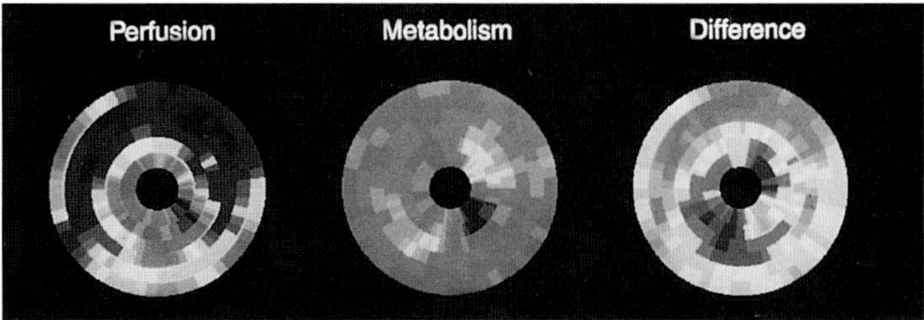

Fig. 103.6 Polar map displays of perfusion metabolism in a patient with reduced blood flow in the inferior wall (blue). Note the homogeneous ^{18}FDG uptake as seen on the polar map of metabolism. The difference polar map (**left**) reveals a blood flow–glucose metabolism mismatch (red). (Also shown in colour on Plate 30.)

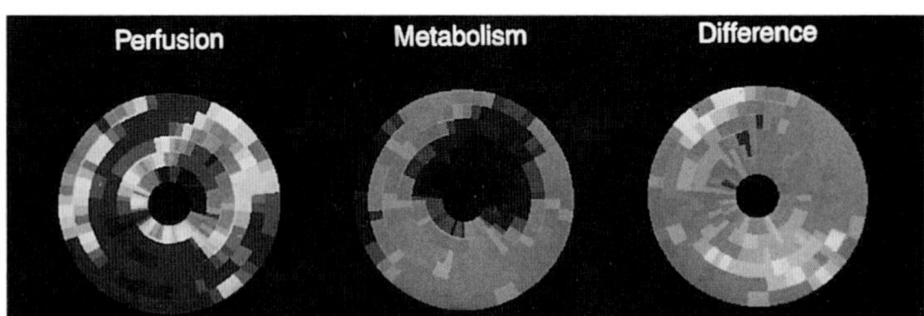

Fig. 103.7 Polar map displays of perfusion and metabolism in a patient with LAD disease. Note the extensive perfusion abnormality affecting the anterior wall. The metabolism polar map indicates a concordant zone of decreased ^{18}FDG uptake (dark blue). Accordingly, the difference polar map fails to reveal a blood flow–metabolism mismatch. The polar maps at the bottom depict a blood flow–metabolism match. As noted on the polar map of myocardial perfusion, blood flow is decreased in the inferior wall. This is associated with a concordant reduction in ^{18}FDG uptake. Accordingly, the difference polar map as shown on the right does not reveal any regional increases in the difference in the uptake of ^{18}FDG and ^{13}N ammonia. (Also shown in colour on Plate 30.)

normal of ^{11}C acetate clearance rates as the lower threshold for 'viability'. In a series of 34 chronic coronary artery disease patients with regional wall motion abnormalities, the investigators reported a 67% positive and an 89% negative predictive accuracy for the post-revascularization outcome in regional contractile function.[4] While these results are highly promising and while the use of a single tracer such as acetate would facilitate PET viability studies, it will be important to test these findings in patients with severely depressed left ventricular function, and in other laboratories.

BLOOD FLOW–METABOLISM IMAGING AND GLOBAL LEFT VENTRICULAR FUNCTION

An early study demonstrated a correlation between the geographic extent of a blood flow–metabolism mismatch and the post-revascularization improvement in left ventricular function.[84] For example, the left ventricular ejection fraction remained unchanged when only one or no myocardial segments exhibited a blood flow–metabolism mismatch (Table 103.4). Conversely, in patients with two or more myocardial regions with mismatches, the left ventricular ejection fraction improved from 30±11 to 45±14% ($P<0.05$) when re-examined 12–18 weeks after surgical revascularization. More recent studies have confirmed these earlier observations.[81,87,88,101,102] A post-revascularization improvement in the exercise capacity[89] or an increase in the left ventricular ejection fraction with exercise after surgical revascularization as compared to no significant change at baseline[87] have also been reported. It is anticipated that newer, more quantitative methods for determining the extent and severity of such 'mismatches'[5] will predict more accurately the gain in left ventricular function following revascularization.

BLOOD FLOW–METABOLISM IMAGING AND RISK STRATIFICATION

Imaging of myocardial blood flow and of glucose utilization with PET can also provide information on the long term morbidity and mortality of patients with ischaemic heart disease. For example, Tamaki et al[103] observed in 84 coronary artery disease patients that a segmental increase in ^{18}FDG uptake over a 23 month follow-up period was the single most accurate predictor of a subsequent cardiac event, e.g. death, non-fatal myocardial infarction, unstable angina or late revascularization. On logistic regression analysis, ^{18}FDG uptake in a single myocardial region offered a higher predictive power than the number of stenosed vessels, findings on ^{201}Tl redistribution scintigraphy or left ventricular ejection fraction. It should be emphasized, however, that the patients in this study had relatively well-preserved left ventricular ejection fractions compared to patients with severely impaired left ventricular functions in other retrospective studies.[101,104,105]

During average follow-up periods of 12–13 months, survival of patients with severely depressed left ventricular ejection fractions (generally $< 35\%$) and blood flow–metabolism mismatches was significantly lower than for those with matches only.[104,105] Similarly, patients with mismatches revealed a higher incidence of cardiac events such as myocardial infarction or revascularization than patients with only blood flow metabolism matches. The same investigations suggested that interventional revascularization in patients with mismatches significantly lowered cardiac morbidity and improved patient survival. For example, surveying 82 and 93 patients each, the 12 or 13 month mortality was 4% and 12% in patients with matches. This compared to mortality rates of 33% and 41% in patients with mismatches when treated conservatively. Conversely, patients with mismatches undergoing either angioplasty or coronary artery bypass grafting had mortalities of only 4% and 12%.[104,105]

These follow-up studies also imply a correlation between blood flow–metabolism patterns on PET and a change in the functional state of patients. For example, only about a quarter of patients with or without mismatches treated conservatively or with matches but submitted to revascularization reported a significant improvement in congestive heart failure symptoms or a change from New York Heart Association functional class III or IV to class I or II. This was different in patients with mismatches who had been submitted to coronary revascularization. In the latter group, 80% of patients initially in functional class III or IV had only mild or no symptoms of congestive heart failure at the time of follow-up.[104] Expressed somewhat differently in the second study[105] the average chance of improvement in functional class was significantly greater in patients with mismatches and revascularization as compared to patients with matches only, treated either conservatively or with revascularization, or patients with mismatches treated conservatively. In aggregate, these studies suggest that a mismatch identifies a patient with reduced left ventricular function to be at high risk. Conversely, this risk can be reduced by interventional revascularization.

CONCLUSIONS

Clinical investigations performed to date have demonstrated the high diagnostic accuracy of PET for the detection of coronary artery disease as well as for the identification of myocardial viability. It would seem that the latter approach is especially important for stratifying patients with endstage cardiac disease to the most appropriate and cost-effective treatment. The observations to date suggest further that PET can be cost-effective. If used appropriately, e.g. in patients with severely depressed left ventricular function, it is more likely than alternative diagnostic approaches to yield unequivocal results. It can therefore reduce the need for more expensive invasive diagnostic techniques and thus shorten the diagnostic process. Furthermore, PET findings might become useful for assigning potential transplant candidates to interventional revascularization. Initial diagnostic and therapeutic algorithms have been proposed for such patients.[106]

More generally, it is likely that the increased use of already existing or currently emerging tracer techniques with PET and the ability to quantify regional functional processes will expand the scope of clinical applications of PET to other aspects of cardiovascular disease, to the characterization and early diagnosis of non-coronary-related diseases, as well as to define and monitor new pharmacological treatments.

ACKNOWLEDGEMENTS

The author wishes to thank Diane Martin for preparing the illustrations and Eileen Rosenfeld for her skilful assistance in preparing this manuscript. The author is also grateful to Dr J. vom Dahl for additional information on findings published thus far in only preliminary form.

REFERENCES

1. Hoh C, Dahlbom M, Harris G et al 1993 Automated iterative three-dimensional registration of Positron Emission Tomography images. J Nucl Med 34: 2009–2018
2. Hicks K, Ganti G, Mullani N, Gould K L 1989 Automated quantitation of three-dimensional cardiac positron emission tomography for routine clinical use. J Nucl Med 30: 1787–1797
3. Kuhle W, Porenta G, Huang S-C, Phelps M, Schelbert H 1992 Issues in the quantitation of reoriented cardiac PET images. J Nucl Med 33: 1235–1242
4. Gropler R J, Geltman E M, Sampathkumaran K et al 1993 Comparison of carbon-11-acetate with fluorine-18-fluorodeoxyglucose for delineating viable myocardium by positron emission tomography. J Am Coll Cardiol 22: 1587–1597
5. Porenta G, Kuhle W, Czernin J et al 1992 Semiquantitative assessment of myocardial viability and perfusion utilizing polar map displays of cardiac PET images. J Nucl Med 33: 1623–1631
6. Yoshida K, Gould K 1993 Quantitative relation of myocardial infarct size and myocardial viability by positron emission tomography to left ventricular ejection fraction and 3-year mortality with and without revascularization. J Am Coll Cardiol 22: 984–997
7. Laubenbacher C, Rothley J, Sitomer J et al 1993 An automated analysis program for the evaluation of cardiac PET studies: Initial results in the detection and localization of coronary artery disease using nitrogen-13-ammonia. J Nucl Med 34: 968–978
8. Sun K, De Groof M, Hansen H, Selin C, Schelbert H 1993 Quantification of the extent and severity of perfusion defects in

canine myocardium by PET polar mapping. J Am Coll Cardiol 21: 461A
9. Czernin J, Porenta G, Müller P et al 1991 Perfusion defect extent determines LV function in patients with PET ischemia. Circulation 84: II–474
10. Schelbert H R, Phelps M E, Hoffman E J, Huang S C, Selin C E, Kuhl D E 1979 Regional myocardial perfusion assessed with N-13 labeled ammonia and positron emission computerized axial tomography. Am J Cardiol 43: 209–218
11. Schelbert H R, Phelps M E, Huang S C et al 1981 N-13 ammonia as an indicator of myocardial blood flow. Circulation 63: 1259–1272
12. Gould K L, Schelbert H R, Phelps M E, Hoffman E J 1979 Noninvasive assessment of coronary stenoses with myocardial perfusion imaging during pharmacologic coronary vasodilation. V. Detection of 47 percent diameter coronary stenosis with intravenous nitrogen-13 ammonia and emission-computed transaxial tomography in intact dogs. Am J Cardiol 43: 200–208
13. Mullani N A, Goldstein R A, Gould K L et al 1983 Perfusion imaging with rubidium-82: I. Measurement of extraction and flow with external detectors. J Nucl Med 24: 898–906
14. Bergmann S R, Fox K A A, Rand A L et al 1984 Quantification of regional myocardial blood flow in vivo with $H_2\,^{15}O$. Circulation 70: 724–733
15. Bergmann S R, Herrero P, Markham J, Weinheimer C J, Walsh M N 1989 Noninvasive quantitation of myocardial blood flow in human subjects with oxygen-15-labeled water and positron emission tomography. J Am Coll Cardiol 14: 639–652
16. Araujo L, Lammertsma A, Rhodes C et al 1991 Noninvasive quantification of regional myocardial blood flow in coronary artery disease with oxygen-15-labeled carbon dioxide inhalation and positron emission tomography. Circulation 83: 875–885
17. Weiss E S, Hoffman E J, Phelps M E et al 1976 External detection and visualization of myocardial ischemia with 11C-substrates in vitro and in vivo. Circ Res 39: 24–32
18. Schön H R, Schelbert H R, Najafi A et al 1982 C-11 labeled palmitic acid for the noninvasive evaluation of regional myocardial fatty acid metabolism with positron computed tomography. I. Kinetics of C-11 palmitic acid in normal myocardium. Am Heart J 103: 532–547
19. Schön H R, Schelbert H R, Najafi A et al 1982 C-11 labeled palmitic acid for the noninvasive evaluation of regional myocardial fatty acid metabolism with positron computed tomography. II. Kinetics of C-11 palmitic acid in acutely ischemic myocardium. Am Heart J 103: 548–561
20. Schelbert H R, Henze E, Schön H R et al 1983 C-11 palmitate for the noninvasive evaluation of regional myocardial fatty acid metabolism with positron computed tomography. III. In vivo demonstration of the effects of substrate availability on myocardial metabolism. Am Heart J 105: 492–504
21. Schelbert H R, Henze E, Sochor H et al 1986 Effects of substrate availability on myocardial C-11 palmitate kinetics by positron emission tomography in normal subjects and patients with ventricular dysfunction. Am Heart J 111: 1055–1064
22. Fox K A A, Abendschein D R, Ambos H D, Sobel B E, Bergmann S R 1985 Efflux of metabolized and nonmetabolized fatty acid from canine myocardium. Implications for quantifying myocardial metabolism tomographically. Circ Res 57: 232–243
23. Rosamond T L, Abendschein D R, Sobel B E, Bergmann S R, Fox K A A 1987 Metabolic fate of radiolabeled palmitate in ischemic canine myocardium: Implications for positron emission tomography. J Nucl Med 28: 1322–1329
24. Grover-McKay M, Schelbert H R, Schwaiger M et al 1986 Identification of impaired metabolic reserve by atrial pacing in patients with significant coronary artery stenosis. Circulation 74: 281–292
25. Schelbert H R, Henze E, Schön H R et al 1983 C-11 palmitic acid for the noninvasive evaluation of regional myocardial fatty acid metabolism with positron computed tomography. IV. In vivo demonstration of impaired fatty acid oxidation in acute myocardial ischemia. Am Heart J 106: 736–750
26. Phelps M E, Hoffman E J, Selin C E et al 1978 Investigation of $[^{18}F]$ 2-fluoro-2-deoxyglucose for the measurement of myocardial glucose metabolism. J Nucl Med 19: 1311–1319
27. Ratib O, Phelps M E, Huang S C, Henze E, Selin C E, Schelbert H R 1982 Positron tomography with deoxyglucose for estimating local myocardial glucose metabolism. J Nucl Med 23: 577–586
28. Choi Y, Bruinken R C, Hawkins R A et al 1993 Factors affecting myocardial 2-[F-18]fluoro-2-deoxy-D-glucose uptake in positron emission tomography studies of normal humans. Eur J Nucl Med 20: 308–318
29. Sokoloff L, Reivich M, Kennedy C et al 1977 The [14C]-deoxyglucose method for the measurement of local cerebral glucose utilization: theory, procedure and normal values in the conscious and anesthetized albino rat. J Neurochem 28: 897–916
30. Berry J, Baker J, Pieper K, Hanson M, Hoffman J, Coleman R 1991 The effect of metabolic milieu on cardiac PET imaging using fluorine-18-deoxyglucose and nitrogen-13-ammonia in normal volunteers. J Nucl Med 32: 1518–1525
31. Choi Y, Brunken R, Hawkins R et al 1993 Factors affecting myocardial 2-[F-18]fluoro-2-deoxy-D-glucose uptake in positron emission tomography studies of normal humans. Eur J Nucl Med 20: 308–318
32. Schelbert H R, Phelps M E, Selin C, Marshall R C, Hoffman E J, Kuhl D E 1980 In: Advances in clinical cardiology: quantification of myocardial ischemia. Gehard Witzstrock, New York. pp 437–447
33. Camici P, Araujo L I, Spinks T et al 1986 Increased uptake of 18F-fluorodeoxyglucose in postischemic myocardium of patients with exercise-induced angina. Circulation 74: 81–88
34. Buxton D B, Nienaber C A, Luxen A et al 1989 Noninvasive quantitation of regional myocardial oxygen consumption in vivo with [1-11C] acetate and dynamic positron emission tomography. Circulation 79: 134–142
35. Brown M, Marshall D R, Burton B S, Sobel B E, Bergmann S R 1987 Delineation of myocardial oxygen utilization with carbon-11-labeled acetate. Circulation 76: 687–696
36. Bol A, Melin J, Essamri B et al 1991 Assessment of myocardial oxidative reserve with PET: comparison with Fick oxygen consumption. Circulation 84: II–425
37. Armbrecht J J, Buxton D B, Schelbert H R. Validation of [1-11C] acetate as a tracer for noninvasive assessment of oxidative metabolism with positron emission tomography in normal, ischemic, post-ischemic and hyperemic canine myocardium. Circulation 81: 1594–1605
38. Armbrecht J J, Buxton D B, Brunken R C, Phelps M E, Schelbert H R 1989 Regional myocardial oxygen consumption determined noninvasively in humans with [1-11C] acetate and dynamic positron tomography. Circulation 80: 863–872
39. Henes C G, S.R. B, Walsh M N, Sobel B E, Geltman E M 1989 Assessment of myocardial oxidative metabolic reserve with positron emission tomography and carbon-11 acetate. J Nucl Med 30: 1489–1499
40. Ng C, Huang S, Schelbert H, Buxton D 1991 Tracer kinetic modeling for delineating C-11 acetate as a tracer for myocardial oxidative metabolism. J Nucl Med 32: 910
41. Sun K, Cyhen K, Huang S et al 1993 A workable compartmental model for simultaneous measurement of myocardial blood flow and oxygen consumption using C-11 acetate. J Nucl Med 34:
42. Gould K L, Lipscomb K, Hamilton G W 1974 Physiologic basis for assessing critical coronary stenosis. Instantaneous flow response and regional distribution during coronary hyperemia as measures of coronary flow reserve. Am J Cardiol 33: 87–94
43. Schelbert H R, Wisenberg G, Phelps M E et al 1982 Noninvasive assessment of coronary stenoses by myocardial imaging during pharmacologic coronary vasodilation. VI. Detection of coronary artery disease in man with intravenous N-13 ammonia and positron computed tomography. Am J Cardiol 49: 1197–1207
44. Gould K L, Goldstein R A, Mullani N A et al 1986 Noninvasive assessment of coronary stenoses by myocardial perfusion imaging during pharmacologic coronary vasodilation. VIII. Clinical feasibility of positron cardiac imaging without a cyclotron using generator-produced rubidium-82. J Am Coll Cardiol 7: 775–789
45. Demer L L, Gould K L, Goldstein R A et al 1989 Assessment of coronary artery disease severity by positron emission tomography.

Comparison with quantitative arteriography in 193 patients. Circulation 79: 825–835
46. Yonekura Y, Tamaki N, Senda M et al 1987 Detection of coronary artery disease with 13N-ammonia and high-resolution positron-emission computed tomography. Am Heart J 113: 645–654
47. Williams B R, Jansen D E, Wong L F, Fiedotin A F, Knopf W D, Toporoff S J 1989 Positron emission tomography for the diagnosis of coronary artery disease: A non-university experience and correlation with coronary angiography. J Nucl Med 30: 845
48. Tamaki N, Yonekura Y, Senda M et al 1988 Value and limitation of stress thallium-201 single photon emission computed tomography: comparison with nitrogen-13 ammonia positron tomography. J Nucl Med 29: 1181–1188
49. Stewart R, Schwaiger M, Molina E et al 1991 Comparison of rubidium-82 positron emission tomography and thallium-201 SPECT imaging for detection of coronary artery disease. Am J Cardiol 67: 1303–1310
50. Go R, Marwick T, MacIntyre W et al 1990 A prospective comparison of rubidium-82 PET and thallium-201 SPECT myocardial perfusion imaging utilizing a single dipyridamole stress in the diagnosis of coronary artery disease. J Nucl Med 31: 1899–1905
51. Khanna S, DeGroof M, Maddahi J et al 1992 Quantitative analysis of adenosine stress N-13 ammonia myocardial perfusion PET images: definition of normal limits and criteria for detection and localization of coronary artery disease. J Nucl Med 33: 825
52. Chan S, Brunken R, Czernin J et al 1992 Comparison of maximal myocardial blood flow during adenosine infusion with that of intravenous dipyridamole in normal men. J Am Coll Cardiol 20: 979–985
53. Hutchins G, Schwaiger M, Rosenspire K, Krivokapich J, Schelbert H, Kuhl D 1990 Noninvasive quantification of regional blood flow in the human heart using N-13 ammonia and dynamic positron emission tomographic imaging. J Am Coll Cardiol 15: 1032–1042
54. Bellina C, Parodi O, Camici P et al 1990 Simultaneous in vitro and in vivo validation of nitrogen-13-ammonia for the assessment of regional myocardial blood flow. J Nucl Med 31: 1335–1343
55. Czernin J, Müller P, Chan S et al 1993 Influence of age and hemodynamics on myocardial blood flow and flow reserve. Circulation 88: 62–69
56. Krivokapich J, Smith G T, Huang S C et al 1989 13N ammonia myocardial imaging at rest and with exercise in normal volunteers. Quantification of absolute myocardial perfusion with dynamic positron emission tomography. Circulation 80: 1328–1337
57. Krivokapich J, Huang S-C, Schelbert H 1993 Assessment of the effects of dobutamine on myocardial blood flow and oxidative metabolism in normal human subjects using nitrogen-13 ammonia and carbon-11 acetate. Am J Cardiol 71: 1351–1356
58. Shelton M E, Senneff M J, Ludbrook P A, Sobel B E, Bergmann S R 1993 Concordance of nutritive myocardial perfusion reserve and flow velocity reserve in conductance vessels in patients with chest pain with angiographically normal coronary arteries. J Nucl Med 34: 717–722
59. Senneff M, Geltman E, Bergmann S, Hartman J 1991 Noninvasive delineation of the effects of moderate aging on myocardial perfusion. J Nucl Med 32: 2037–2042
60. Geltman E, Henes C, Senneff M, Sobel B, Bergmann S 1990 Increased myocardial perfusion at rest and diminished perfusion reserve in patients with angina and angiographically normal coronary arteries. J Am Coll Cardiol 16: 586–595
61. Camici P G, Gistri R, Lorenzoni R et al 1992 Coronary reserve and exercise ECG in patients with chest pain and normal coronary angiograms. Circulation 86: 179–186
62. Galassi A, Crea F, Araujo L et al 1993 Comparison of regional myocardial blood flow in syndrome x and one-vessel coronary artery disease. Am J Cardiol 72: 134–139
63. Camici P, Chiriatti G, Oorenzoni R et al 1991 Coronary vasodilation is impaired in both hypertrophied and nonhypertrophied myocardium of patients with hypertrophic cardiomyopathy: a study with nitrogen-13 ammonia and positron emission tomography. J Am Coll Cardiol 17: 879–886
64. Nienaber C, Gambhir S, Vaghaiwalla Mody F et al 1993 Regional myocardial blood flow and glucose utilization in symptomatic patients with hypertrophic cardiomyopathy. Circulation 87: 1580–1590
65. Krivokapich J, Stevenson L, Kobashigawa J, Huang S-C, Schelbert H 1991 Quantification of absolute myocardial perfusion at rest and during exercise with positron emission tomography after human cardiac transplantation. J Am Coll Cardiol 18: 512–517
66. Rechavia E, Araujo L, De Silva R et al 1992 Dipyridamole vasodilator response after human orthotopic heart transplantation: Quantification by oxygen-15-labeled water and positron emission tomography. J Am Coll Cardiol 19: 100–106
67. Senneff M J, Hartman J, Sobel B E, Geltman E M, Bergmann S R 1993 Persistence of coronary vasodilator responsivity after cardiac transplantation. Am J Cardiol 71: 333–338
68. Chan S, Kobashigawa J, Stevenson L et al 1991 Basal myocardial blood flow is increased but maximal flow is decreased during acute cardiac transplant rejection: A non-invasive quantitative study. J Am Coll Cardiol 17: 58A
69. Walsh M N, Geltman E M, Steele R L et al 1990 Augmented myocardial perfusion reserve after coronary angioplasty quantified by positron emission tomography with H215O. J Am Coll Cardiol 15: 119–127
70. Uren N G, Crake T, Lefroy D C, DeSilva R, Davies G J, Maseri A 1993 Delayed recovery of coronary resistive vessel function after coronary angioplasty. J Am Coll Cardiol 21: 612–621
71. Beanlands R, Muzik O, Sutor R et al 1992 Noninvasive determination of regional perfusion reserve in coronary artery disease using N-13 ammonia PET. J Nucl Med 33: 826
72. Uren N, Melin J, De Bruyne B et al 1993 Maximal myocardial flow as a function of stenosis severity in man. Circulation 88: 1–274
73. Di Carli M, Czernin J, Sherman T et al 1993 Relationship between stenosis severity, hyperemic blood flow, flow reserve and coronary resistance in CAD patients. Circulation 88: I-647
74. Marshall R C, Tillisch J H, Phelps M E et al 1983 Identification and differentiation of resting myocardial ischemia and infarction in man with positron computed tomography 18F-labeled fluorodeoxyglucose and N-13 ammonia. Circulation 67: 766–778
75. Opie L H 1990 Myocardial ischemia – metabolic pathways and implications of increased glycolysis. Cardio Drugs and Ther 4: 777–790
76. Altehoefer C, Kaiser H-J, Dörr R et al 1992 Fluorine-18 deoxyglucose PET for assessment of viable myocardium in perfusion defects in 99mTc-MIBI SPET: a comparative study in patients with coronary artery disease. Eur J Nucl Med 19: 334–342
77. Chan S, Brunken R, Phelps M, Schelbert H 1991 Use of the metabolic tracer C-11 acetate for evaluation of regional myocardial perfusion. J Nucl Med 32: 665–672
78. Knuuti M, Nuutila P, Ruotsalainen U et al 1993 The value of quantitative analysis of glucose utilization in detection of myocardial viability by PET. J Nucl Med 34: 2068–2075
79. Bonow R, Dilsizian V, Cuocolo A, Bacharach S 1991 Identification of viable myocardium in patients with chronic coronary artery disease and left ventricular dysfunction: Comparison of thallium scintigraphy with reinjection and PET imaging with F-18-fluorodeoxyglucose. Circulation 83: 26–37
80. Czernin J, Porenta G, Rosenquist G et al 1991 Loss of coronary perfusion reserve in PET ischemia. Circulation 84: II-47
81. Vanoverschelde J-L, Wijns W, Depre C et al 1993 Mechanisms of chronic regional postischemic dysfunction in humans: New insights from the study of noninfarcted collateral-dependent myocardium. Circulation 87: 1513–1523
82. Sambuceti G, Parodi O, Marzullo P et al 1993 Regional myocardial blood flow in stable angina pectoris associated with isolated significant narrowing of either the left anterior descending or left circumflex coronary artery. Am J Cardiol 72: 990–994
83. Flameng W, Suy R, Schwarz F et al 1981 Ultrastructural correlates of left ventricular contraction abnormalities in patients with chronic ischemic heart disease: determinants of reversible

segmental asynergy post-revascularization surgery. Am Heart J 102: 846
84. Tillisch J, Brunken R, Marshall R et al 1986 Reversibility of cardiac wall motion abnormalities predicted by positron tomography. New Engl J Med 314: 884–888
85. Tamaki N, Yonekura Y, Yamashita K et al 1989 Positron emission tomography using fluorine-18 deoxyglucose in evaluation of coronary artery bypass grafting. Am J Cardiol 64: 860–865
86. Tamaki N, Ohtani H, Yamashita K et al 1991 Metabolic activity in the areas of new fill-in after thallium-201 reinjection: comparison with positron emission tomography using fluorine-18-deoxyglucose. J Nucl Med 32: 673–678
87. Carrel T, Jenni R, Haubold-Reuter S, Von Schulthess G, Pasic M, Turina M 1992 Improvement of severely reduced left ventricular function after surgical revascularization in patients with preoperative myocardial infarction. Eur J Cardiothorac Surg 6: 479–484
88. Lucignani G, Paolini G, Landoni C et al 1992 Presurgical identification of hibernating myocardium by combined use of technetium-99m hexakis 2-methoxyisobutylisonitrile single photon emission tomography and fluorine-18 fluoro-2-deoxy-D-glucose positron emission tomography in patients with coronary artery disease. Eur J Nucl Med 19: 874–881
89. Marwick T, MacIntyre W, Lafont A, Nemec J, Salcedo E 1992 Metabolic responses of hibernating and infarcted myocardium to revascularization: a follow-up study of regional perfusion, function, and metabolism. Circulation 85: 1347–1353
90. vom Dahl J, Eitzman J, Al-Auoar Z, Hicks R, Schwaihger M 1992 Myokardial Perfusion und Glukosestoffwechsel als prädiktive Parameter der segmentellen Wandbewegung nach Koronarrevaskularization. Z Kardiol 81: 165
91. vom Dahl J, Altehoefer C, Sheehan F H et al 1994 Myocardial viability assessed by combined nuclear imaging using myocardial scintigraphy and positron emission tomography: Impact on treatment and functional outcome following revascularization. J Am Coll Cardiol
92. Chan A, Czernin J, Brunken R, Choi Y, Krivokapich J, Schelbert H R 1993 Effects of fasting on the incidence of blood flow metabolism mismatches in chronic CAD patients. J Am Coll Cardiol 21: 129A
93. Knuuti M, Nuutila P, Ruotsalainen U et al 1992 Euglycemic hyperinsulinemic clamp and oral glucose load in stimulating myocardial glucose utilization during positron emission tomography. J Nucl Med 33: 1255–1262
94. vom Dahl J, Herman W, Hicks R et al 1993 Myocardial glucose uptake in patients with insulin-dependent diabetes mellitus assessed quantitatively by dynamic positron emission tomography. Circulation 88: 395–404
95. Iida H, Rhodes C, de Silva R et al 1991 Myocardial tissue fraction – correction for partial volume effects and measure of tissue viability. J Nucl Med 32: 2169–2175
96. Yamamoto Y, De Silva R, Rhodes C et al 1992 A new strategy for the assessment of viable myocardium and regional myocardial blood flow using ^{15}O-water and dynamic positron emission tomography. Circulation 86: 167–178
97. de Silva R, Yamamoto Y, Rhodes C G et al 1992 Preoperative prediction of the outcome of coronary revascularization using positron emission tomography. Circulation 86: 1738–1742
98. Gould L, Yoshida K, Hess M, Haynie M, Mullani N, Smalling R 1991 Myocardial metabolism of fluorodeoxyglucose compared to cell membrane integrity for the potassium analogue rubidium-82 for assessing infarct size in many by PET. J Nucl Med 32: 1–9
99. Gropler R, Siegel B, Sampathkumaran K et al 1992 Dependence of recovery of contractile function on maintenance of oxidative metabolism after myocardial infarction. J Am Coll Cardiol 19: 989–997
100. Gropler R, Geltman E, Sampathkumaran K et al 1992 Functional recovery after coronary revascularization for chronic coronary artery disease is dependent on maintenance of oxidative metabolism. J Am Coll Cardiol 20: 569–577
101. Besozzi M C, Brown M D, Hubner K F et al 1992 Retrospective post therapy evaluation of cardiac function in 208 coronary artery disease patients evaluated by positron emission tomography. J Nucl Med 33: 885
102. Depre C, Melin J, Vanoverschelde J, Borgers M, Wijns W 1993 Assessment of myocardial viability after bypass surgery by pre-operative PET flow-metabolism measurements and ultrastructural analysis of myocardial biopsies. Circulation 88: I-99
103. Tamaki N, Kawamoto M, Takahashi N et al 1993 Prognostic value of an increase in fluorine-18 deoxyglucose uptake in patients with myocardial infarction: Comparison with stress thallium imaging. J Am Coll Cardiol 22: 1621–1627
104. Di Carli M, Davidson M, Little R et al 1994 Prognosis in patients with coronary artery disease and left ventricular dysfunction; the value of myocardial perfusion and metabolism imaging by positron emission tomography. Am J Cardiol
105. Eitzman D, Al-Aouar Z, Kanter H et al. Clinical outcome of patients with advanced coronary artery disease after viability studies with positron emission tomography. J Am Coll Cardiol 20: 559–565
106. Louie H, Laks H, Milgalter E et al 1991 Ischemic cardiomyopathy: criteria for coronary revascularization and cardiac transplantation. Circulation 84: III-290–III-295

104. Nuclear techniques in the assessment of myocardial innervation

André Syrota   Héric Valette

INTRODUCTION

Cardiac innervation plays a key role in the genesis and evolution of heart disease and is a target of many drugs. It involves several steps: the synthesis of the neurotransmitter by the nerves, its release in the synaptic cleft, the binding to the receptor inducing the physiological response of the effector, and the metabolism or the re-uptake of the neurotransmitter. Presynaptic function, i.e. re-uptake and release of the neurotransmitter, can be assessed using positron emission tomography (PET) and 'false adrenergic neurotransmitters', but single photon emission tomography (SPET) or planar imaging with ^{123}I- or ^{131}Imetaiodobenzylguanidine (MIBG) are more widely used. Receptors form a class of intrinsic membrane proteins defined by the high affinity and specificity with which they bind ligands. Receptors are associated directly or indirectly with membrane ion channels which open or close after a conformational change of the receptor induced by the binding of the neurotransmitter. In heart disease, anatomical or functional modifications of cardiac innervation have been extensively reported. Alterations in receptors have been demonstrated from samples collected by endomyocardial biopsy, either during surgery or autopsy. SPET and PET using appropriate ligands and quantitative methods have opened a large field for clinical investigation in patients suffering from heart disease. The methodology is based on the synthesis of a radioligand, usually a selective receptor antagonist. Mathematical compartmental models applied to concentration *vs.* time curves obtained during saturation or displacement experiments are able to provide the value of the receptor concentration and of the rate constants of the ligand–receptor interaction. Therefore, nuclear medicine has a great potential for the investigation of cardiac innervation in different physiological situations and in heart disease.

PATHOPHYSIOLOGICAL ASPECTS OF CARDIAC INNERVATION IN HEART: ANIMAL AND HUMAN STUDIES IN VITRO

Presynaptic adrenergic neuronal function

Elevated circulating norepinephrine or increased myocardial norepinephrine release may induce hypertrophy, myocyte calcium overload, arrhythmias or desensitization of beta-adrenergic receptor pathways. The neuronal uptake-1 function is the principal means for terminating the action of norepinephrine. An impairment of this process induces an overexposure of the myocytes to norepinephrine, which is released from the adrenergic nerve terminal or delivered by the coronary circulation.

Congestive heart failure

Heart failure is associated with an increase in circulating norepinephrine level related to the severity of the disease. Various alterations of intramyocardial adrenergic innervation occur, including decrease in catecholamine content, impairment of norepinephrine uptake–release, and lesions of nerve terminals.[1,2] Evidence for depression of the uptake-1 function in heart failure has been reported in animals as well as in humans.[1] An increased norepinephrine release has been reported[3,4,5] while opposite findings have also been described.[2] These conflicting results may be due to methodological differences or to different patient populations.

Ischaemic heart disease

Extensive myocardial catecholamine depletion and adrenergic denervation are observed in the infarcted area. Myocardial neuronal injury is a two-step process induced by energy deficiency. As a first step, norepinephrine is lost from the storage vesicles; the second step is the rate-limited transport of intracellular norepinephrine through the cellular membrane by the uptake-1 carrier. After a prolonged period of ischaemia, the carrier reverses its normal net transport direction.

Hypertrophic cardiomyopathy

Abnormalities of the cardiac adrenergic function mainly include changes in catecholamine synthesis or turnover, alterations of norepinephrine neuronal release–uptake, and decreased myocardial catecholamine content.[6] The pathophysiological importance and the nature of the adrenergic disorders in primary hypertrophic cardiomyopathy are controversial. A decreased norepinephrine uptake function has been found using in vivo pharmacological techniques.[7]

Cardiac adrenergic receptors

The relationship between the biochemical changes in the beta-adrenergic receptor/adenylate system and the pathophysiological state has created the potential for the development of new interventional strategies.

Denervation supersensitivity

Surgical denervation of dog heart results in beta-adrenergic receptor up-regulation and supersensitivity.[8] The mechanism of supersensitivity is due in part to up-regulation of beta-adrenergic receptors, but is mainly related to the lack of norepinephrine re-uptake caused by the absence of sympathetic nerve endings.[9]

Desensitization

One potential mechanism for the changes in the beta-adrenergic receptor–G protein–adenylyl cyclase complex involves desensitization, secondary to the chronic exposure to high levels of norepinephrine at the receptor sites.[10]

Myocardial ischaemia

Experimental ischaemia has been shown to produce an increase in beta-receptor density. This is probably due to the externalization of intracellular receptors at the cell surface.[11]

Hypertension and myocardial hypertrophy

In rodents with renovascular hypertension or spontaneously hypertensive rats, beta-adrenergic receptor density is either normal[12] or depressed.[13] In rats and dogs with aortic banding, beta-adrenergic receptor number has been found increased[14] or unchanged.[15] In patients with primary hypertrophic cardiomyopathy, no change in beta-adrenergic receptor density has been found.[16]

Congestive heart failure

Sympathetic nervous system stimulation is one of the main compensatory mechanisms supporting the failing heart. As failure progresses, cardiac stores of norepinephrine are depleted. Circulating norepinephrine concentration is elevated and is directly related to the degree of ventricular dysfunction and the risk of death. Even though the plasma levels of norepinephrine are elevated, inotropic response to exogenous catecholamines is abnormal.[17,18] Alpha-receptor density is unchanged or slightly increased. This alpha-1-receptor pathway may play a key role in the stimulation of cardiac hypertrophy. Heart failure induces a loss of beta-1-receptors, while beta-2-receptor density remains constant.[19] Beta-receptor density begins to decrease in mild heart failure and becomes further reduced as heart failure progresses.[20]

Cardiac acetylcholine receptors

Much less information is available on these, probably because the parasympathetic neurotransmission plays a lesser role than that of sympathetic neurotransmission in the diseased myocardium. However, since muscarinic agonists antagonize the stimulating effect of adrenergic hyperactivity in the heart, changes in their function, parallel to the observed alteration of adrenergic neurotransmission, would be expected to occur. Indeed, in a dog model, cardiac failure has been associated with slight dysfunction of the cardiac muscarinic receptors.[21] However, no significant abnormalities have been found by in vitro binding techniques in myocardium from end-stage heart failure patients.[22]

EVALUATION OF PRESYNAPTIC NEURONAL FUNCTION

MIBG imaging

Complex and invasive pharmacological studies requiring both arterial and venous samplings are the only means to determine in humans the kinetics of tissue uptake and release of norepinephrine. Scintigraphic imaging using metaiodobenzylguanidine (MIBG; a structural analogue of norepinephrine) as a tracer allows us to assess non-invasively the adrenergic neuronal function. MIBG shares the same uptake and storage mechanisms as norepinephrine.[23] MIBG is unmetabolizable by catechol-*O*-methyl transferase or monoamine oxidase. Two types of uptake system for MIBG have been identified. The uptake-1 system, that dominates at low concentrations, is sodium and ATP dependent and is inhibited by tricyclic antidepressants. It has been shown recently that the norepinephrine transporter is responsible for the specific uptake of MIBG in man.[24] Pharmacological behaviour of MIBG has been extensively studied.[25–32]

^{123}IMIBG was first used in humans to localize pheochromocytoma;[33] in the same year, its use for imaging the myocardium in normal volunteers was reported.[33] In patients with pheochromocytoma, MIBG cardiac accumulation was inversely related to plasma concentrations and urinary excretion rate of catecholamine.[35] A faster clearance of ^{131}IMIBG from the heart of patients with adrenergic dysfunction was reported.[17] In vivo quantification of myocardial MIBG activity has technical limitations. Tomographic imaging provides an opportunity to study the regional distribution of MIBG.[18] However, the severe decrease in MIBG uptake which may be observed in heart disease hinders the use of SPET imaging in routine examination. To overcome this limitation, higher doses of MIBG (10 mCi ^{123}I) have been used for SPET imaging while a 3–4 mCi ^{123}I dose is suitable for planar imaging.[18,36] However, since absolute quantification is not available in SPET, this technique does not provide information accurate enough to compare the absolute MIBG uptake in different subjects.

Planar imaging represents an alternative solution, but shares technical limitations of SPET imaging and has limitations of its own. Ideally the cardiac region of interest should include myocardial wall radioactivity and should exclude adjacent lung and liver activities. Ventricular enlargement may induce an underestimation of the myocardial radioactivity. Pulmonary and liver 'cross-talk' in the cardiac region of interest may induce an overestimation of the myocardial activity. Hence, the activity measured over a left ventricular region may represent only a crude estimate. The upper mediastinum, a non-target area for MIBG, can therefore be used for normalization, and cardiac MIBG uptake may be evaluated as the heart-to-mediastinum activity ratio.[36,37] Such an index may permit evaluation of a large number of patients with a simple and reproducible technique (Fig. 104.1).

The actual neuronal uptake of the amount of MIBG taken by the myocardium is probably the most important question to be addressed when estimating the clinical value of MIBG imaging. MIBG uptake measured 3–4 h after injection appears to be the best index of neuronal accumulation of the tracer. In humans, the uptake-2 pathway is probably much less important than in other animal species, as shown by heart transplanted patients in whom a tenfold decrease in cardiac MIBG uptake was found.[38,39] This suggests that MIBG uptake through the uptake-2 pathway is low in the human heart.

Decreased MIBG uptake in the failing heart

Accumulation and retention of the tracer were reduced in patients with idiopathic cardiomyopathy.[35] Scintigraphically determined ^{123}IMIBG activity correlated with MIBG radioactivity measured from endomyocardial biopsy samples.[37] Furthermore, myocardial ^{123}IMIBG uptake correlated with myocardial endogenous norepinephrine concentration. ^{123}IMIBG uptake also correlated with left ventricular ejection fraction,[37] with right and left catheterization parameters such as cardiac index,

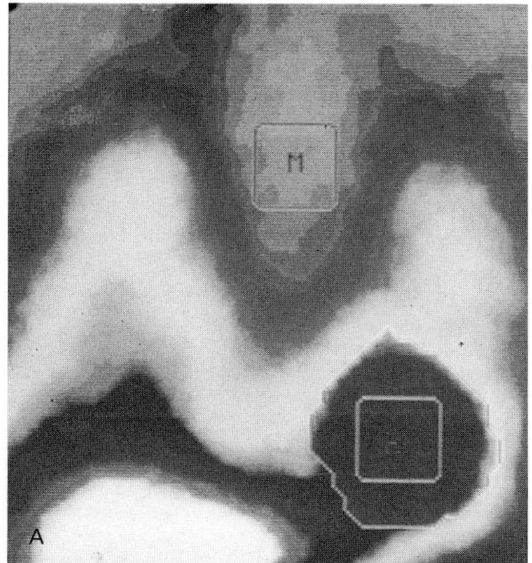

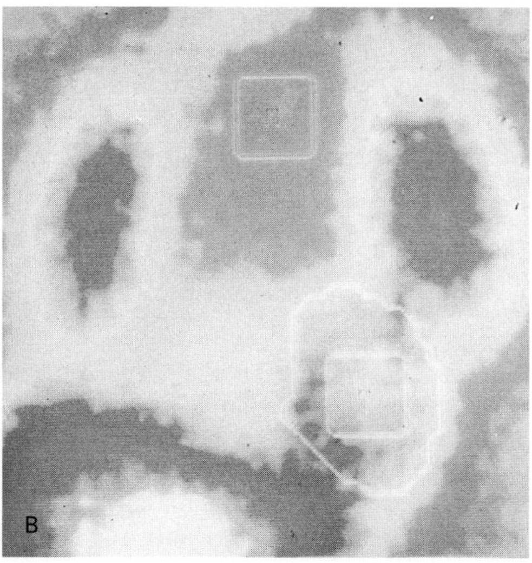

Fig. 104.1 Scintigraphic images obtained 4 h after injection of 3–4 mCi of ^{123}IMIBG (anterior view of the chest). Cardiac MIBG uptake is quantified as the ratio of heart (H) activity to mediastinal activity (M).
A Control subject. B Patient with moderate congestive heart failure: a decrease in myocardial MIBG uptake is clearly seen. (Also shown in colour on Plate 31.)

and with left ventricular end-diastolic pressure.[40] A similar relationship between markers of left ventricular dysfunction and adrenergic disorders has been reported.[18] In particular, elevated circulating norepinephrine concentration has been shown to be a potent prognostic marker in a large population of patients with heart failure. Therefore, the relationship repeatedly found between decreased MIBG uptake and altered indices of left ventricular function suggests that MIBG imaging may be a good prognostic marker. Results of a study of 90 patients with congestive heart failure have already supported this idea.[36] A multivariate stepwise regression discriminant analysis showed that cardiac MIBG uptake was the most potent predictor of survival. Moreover, multivariate life table analysis showed that the best predictor for life duration was also cardiac MIBG uptake.[36] These abnormalities are partially reversible under therapy known to act on sympathetic system hyperactivation. In patients with moderate heart failure, a significant increase in cardiac ^{123}I MIBG uptake was found after a 6-month therapy with captopril, while circulating norepinephrine level measured at rest remained unchanged.[41] Therefore, increased circulating concentration of norepinephrine is not the only factor involved in the decrease of cardiac MIBG uptake. In patients with moderate heart failure, a significant decrease in cardiac MIBG uptake may coexist with normal circulating concentrations of norepinephrine.[41] Thus, MIBG imaging may be helpful in deciding on transplantation for those patients with heart failure, and to evaluate the timing of this.

Ischaemic heart disease

Sympathetic nerve endings appeared to be more sensitive to ischaemia than the myocytes. Denervated myocardium with absent MIBG uptake was shown to be supersensitive to adrenergic stimulation. In a normal heart, tomographic images of the left ventricle showed a similar and parallel distribution of MIBG and thallium activity.[32] In patients with myocardial infarction related to a single vessel disease, the same pattern was observed. The MIBG uptake, after the initial acute global depression, recovered partially after approximately 2 months.[32] The chronic ischaemic situation has also been extensively studied.[42] Prognosis after myocardial infarction is related to the degree of left ventricular dysfunction and to the presence of ventricular arrhythmias. Abnormalities in cardiac adrenergic function have been implicated as a contributing factor to arrhythmogenesis.[43] In patients recovering from acute myocardial infarction, the neuronal damage was more extensive than the perfusion defect and was correlated to left ventricular regional wall motion abnormalities and to the occurrence of ventricular arrhythmias. In this way, new insights on the pathophysiology of numerous cardiac disorders can be offered. The extent of the MIBG defect size is larger than the thallium defect size 2 weeks after infarction.[38] In patients studied 1–3 months after a myocardial infarction with a dual isotope tomographic imaging protocol (^{201}Tl dipyridamole and ^{123}I MIBG), a significant difference was found between the uptake of the tracers in the necrotic, ischaemic and normal areas (Fig. 104.2).[44] The defect sizes were significantly different for ^{201}Tl and for the ^{123}I MIBG images. In a few patients, ^{123}I MIBG uptake was higher than ^{201}Tl uptake in the border zone of the necrotic area and in the ischaemic areas. This higher uptake was not correlated with the presence of a ^{201}Tl redistribution.[44] The difference in the defect size was smaller than in other studies, suggesting a partial reinnervation as observed in dogs.[43] A mismatch between thallium uptake and MIBG uptake was also found in patients with a remote myocardial infarction and ventricular tachycardia.[42]

Primary hypertrophic cardiomyopathy

MIBG scintigraphy studies show a significant decrease in the tracer uptake (Fig. 104.3). Tomographic quantitative analysis of ^{123}I MIBG uptake combined with ^{201}Tl tomographic imaging has suggested that this decrease predominates in the most hypertrophic myocardial areas.[45] These findings have confirmed previous data obtained using in vivo invasive methods[46] and have suggested that impaired adrenergic nerve function is

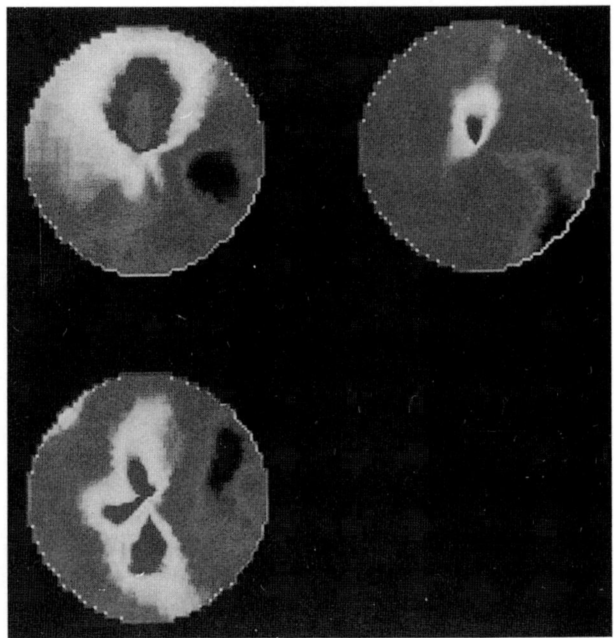

Fig. 104.2 ^{201}Tl and ^{123}IMIBG 'bull's eye' images of a patient with a left anterior descending coronary artery stenosis. Post-exercise ^{201}Tl image (upper left) shows a large anterior defect which 'fills-in' on 3 h delayed images (upper right). On the ^{123}I MIBG image, acquired 5 h after exercise, the defect is much larger than on the delayed perfusion bull's eye. (Also shown in colour on Plate 31.)

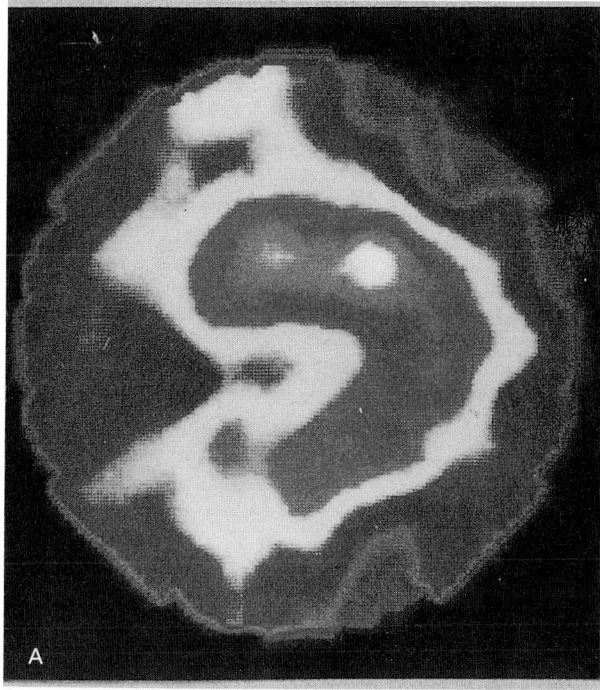

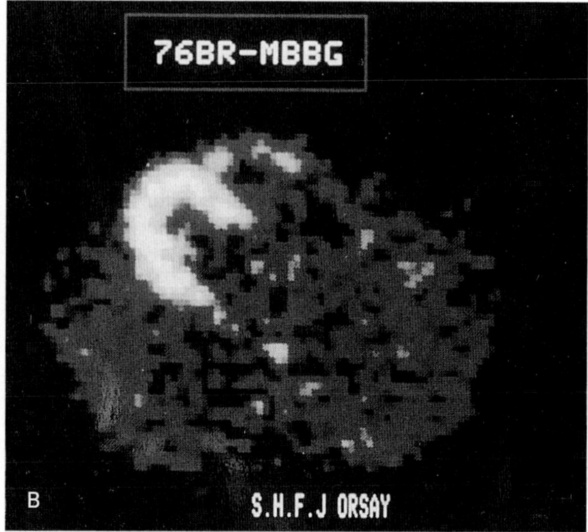

Fig. 104.3 SPET image obtained after injection of 3–4 mCi of ^{123}I MIBG (A) in a patient with a primary hypertrophic cardiomyopathy (mainly septal hypertrophy). Single static PET image obtained after injection of 1 mCi of [^{76}Br]MBBG (B) in a control subject. Acquisition duration was 60 min. (Also shown in colour on Plate 32.)

involved in mechanisms of primary hypertrophic cardiomyopathy. Moreover, a link between the severity of the disease and the decrease in MIBG uptake has been suggested.[47] Thus, MIBG scintigraphy could provide helpful clinical and pathophysiological information.

PET imaging of sympathetic nerve terminal

Poor quantification in SPET imaging restrains the neuronal adrenergic function study of the heart with MIBG. Development of new PET ligands may overcome these limitations.

6-^{18}F Fluorometaraminol[48–51] was the first 'false neurotransmitter' to be used as a tracer for PET studies. Metaraminol is a good index of uptake-1, but the relatively low specific activity of the ^{18}F-labelled compound suggested that the doses of both labelled and unlabelled 6-fluorometaraminol necessary to obtain high count rate images would be too high to allow its clinical use.

^{11}C Hydroxyephedrine, a methyl derivative of metaraminol, has been synthesized at a high specific activity;[52] it showed a high neuronal selectivity in rat heart as indicated by the 93% decrease in uptake in animals pre-treated with desipramine. Similarly, after epicardial phenol application, the dog heart showed a 77% reduction of ^{11}C hydroxyephedrine uptake.[53] Hydroxyephedrine is a better index of the uptake-1 function than MIBG. Human studies in healthy volunteers and in heart-transplanted patients demonstrated the lack of haemodynamic effects of the compound:[54] in transplanted patients, uptake was found to be reduced by 76%.[55] Combined studies of perfusion and neuronal function using ^{11}C hydroxyephedrine in patients with acute myocardial infarction showed neuronal dysfunction in the ischaemic area.[56] In patients with heart failure, a decrease of tracer retention was also observed.[57] The degree of abnormality varied regionally, indicating a heterogeneous pattern of adrenergic nerve dysfunction. Cardiac diabetic neuropathy was also evidenced with this tracer: retention of ^{11}C-hydroxyephedrine was more markedly reduced at the apex than at the base of the left ventricle. The extent of defective uptake of ^{11}C-hydroxyephedrine correlated with the severity of postural hypotension.[58]

In vivo behaviour of (+)-6-^{18}F fluoronorepinephrine and 6-^{18}F fluorodopamine[59,60] has been compared in baboons. (+)-6-^{18}F Fluoronorepinephrine demonstrated a higher myocardial uptake than 6-^{18}F Fluorodopamine and a longer biological half-life. 6-^{18}F Fluorodopamine was also metabolized faster. Further characterization of the in vivo behaviour is needed for this compound, the published data being discrepant.[61,62]

A bromo-analogue of MIBG has been recently studied in rats and dogs;[63,64] in vitro and in vivo behaviour of this compound was closer to that of norepinephrine than that of MIBG. Preliminary results in humans showed a prolonged myocardial retention, a rapid clearance from blood and a high heart-to-lung ratio.

Due to the rapid sequestration of all these compounds by the amine pump, the uptake of these tracers is directly linked to myocardial blood flow. Therefore, for a clinical purpose, their use should be associated with the study of coronary blood flow using $^{15}OH_2O$ or $^{13}N\text{-}NH_3$.

PET imaging of the presynaptic parasympathetic innervation

Several attempts have been made to select a specific inhibitor of intravesicular storage of acetylcholine. Eighty compounds including succinylcholine, phenylcyclidine, quinacrine and AH 5183 (vesamicol) have been tested in vitro,[65] only the last of which demonstrated an inhibition concentration inducing a 50% decrease in the response in the nanomolar range.[65] Therefore several vesamicol derivatives have been recently labelled and evaluated for SPET and PET imaging,[66,67] the published results showing that the compounds are either quickly metabolized or too lipophilic. In isolated working rat hearts, (−)^{18}F fluoroethoxybenzovesamicol shows promise to probe cholinergic neuron of the heart.[68]

EVALUATION OF MYOCARDIAL RECEPTOR DENSITY

The main problem of in vivo cardiac receptor studies is to reduce data from receptor binding experiments to parameters such as receptor density, affinity constants and rate constants.[69,70] The in vivo analysis uses PET, which is a quantitative technique. This methodology is much more complicated than the in vitro analysis on tissue homogenates or on autoradiographic slices, although the basic principles are similar. A mathematical model is necessary to calculate receptor density.

Beta-adrenergic receptors

Several antagonists such as propranolol,[71] practolol,[72] pindolol,[73] atenolol,[74] CGP 12177,[75,76] carazolol[77] and metoprolol[78] have been labelled with ^{11}C or ^{18}F. They differ in affinity, liposolubility and subtype selectivity.

Both ^{11}C pindolol and ^{11}C CGP 12177 have a high affinity and a low lipophilicity. ^{11}C CGP 12177 presents strong advantages. It is a potent hydrophilic beta-blocker, usually considered to have no beta-adrenoceptor subtype selectivity, although a low beta-1 selectivity has been demonstrated on rat ventricular microsomes.[79] It has low non-specific binding on membranes and low intracellular uptake,[80,81] and does not bind to receptors that are removed from the plasma membrane and internalized during short-term desensitization.[82] As a ligand that is not taken up by cells, it is therefore an ideal probe to specifically measure in vivo the cell surface receptors, which are the 'functionally active' beta-receptors. Until now, only CGP 12177 has been used successfully for the in vivo quantification of beta adrenergic receptors.[83]

Beta adrenergic receptor density (Fig. 104.4) has been measured in the dog ventricular myocardium by PET;[83] the concentration of available binding sites was 31±4 pmol/ml of tissue. The use of ^{11}C CGP 12177 for clinical investigation has been also validated.[84] Left ventricular beta-receptor density was evaluated in 10 patients with an idiopathic dilated cardiomyopathy and eight control subjects. The clinical tolerance of the coinjection protocol was good. Left ventricular concentration of beta-receptors (Fig. 104.5) was decreased by 53% in patients, which agreed with previous in vitro data. The PET beta-receptor concentration was compared to the beta-receptor density determined on left ventricle endomyocardial biopsy samples of the same patients using ^{3}H CGP 12177. Results obtained with the two techniques were strongly correlated. Moreover, decreased beta-receptor concentration was well correlated with the contractile responsiveness to intracoronary dobutamine infusion, indicating a direct link between level of down-

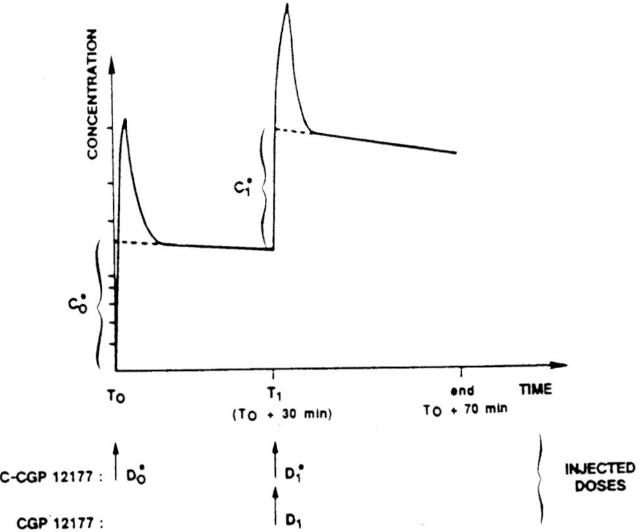

Fig. 104.4 The graphical method is based on a specific experimental protocol and justified by the properties of the CGP 12177 kinetics. In particular, a few minutes after the injection of the labelled ligand, the myocardial time–concentration curve takes the shape of a plateau with a slight slope. The receptor concentration is estimated by using two experimental myocardial concentration values calculated from the PET time–concentration curve. C_0* represents the intercept on the concentration axis of the straight line (logarithmic scale) extrapolated back from the plateau following the first injection. C_1* represents the difference between the concentration at 30 min, extrapolated back from the straight line obtained after the second injection, and the concentration measured just before this second injection. The proposed graphical method estimates the receptor concentration using five values: the two measured concentrations C_0* and C_1*, and the three doses D_0*, D_1* and D_1 that are the known masses of labelled (*) and unlabelled CGP 12177 injected.

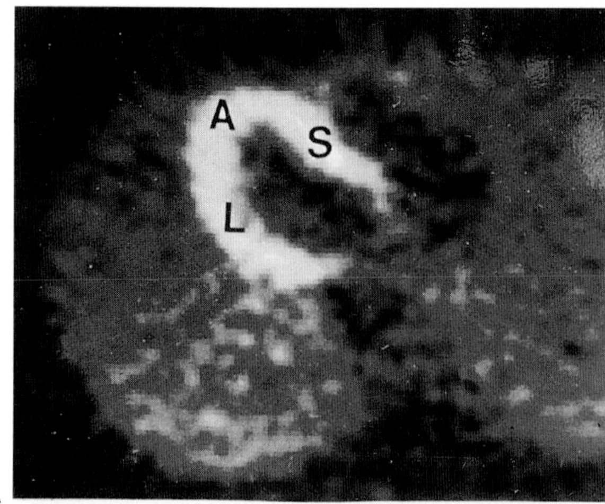

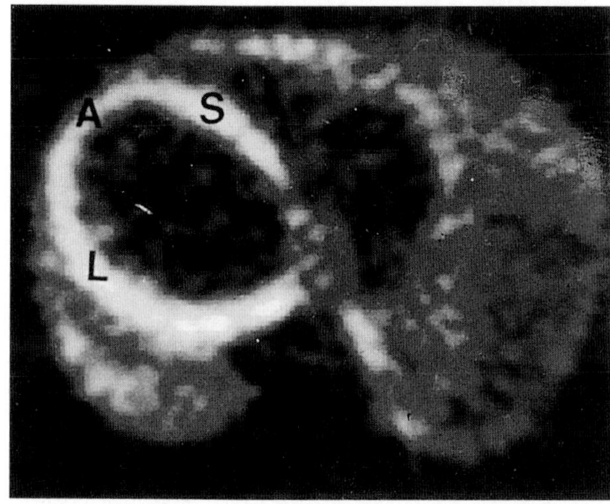

Fig. 104.5 PET slices showing the myocardial distribution of ^{11}C CGP 12177 in a control subject (A) and in a patient with congestive heart failure (B). The images are scaled to their own maximum, therefore they do not show the two-fold decrease in beta-adrenergic receptor density calculated from the dynamic series. (Also shown in colour on Plate 32.)

regulation process assessed by PET and the corresponding impaired biological effect. A relationship between the decrease in beta receptor density and the neuronal norepinephrine function has been evidenced using PET with CGP 12177 and MIBG planar scintigraphy.[85] This finding supports the hypothesis of beta-receptor down-regulation due to adrenergic presynaptic nerve dysfunction.

Alpha-adrenergic receptors

^{11}C Prazosin, a selective alpha-1-adrenergic blocker with K_d value in 100–200 pM range,[86] was evaluated in dogs.[87] PET scans showed a high and homogeneous myocardial uptake. However, the validation of criteria needed for the characterization of receptors could not be achieved, probably because of excessive non-specific binding.

Muscarinic acetylcholine receptors

^{11}C methylquinuclidinyl benzylate (MQNB) has been used to study the muscarinic acetylcholine receptor in vivo by PET.[88] MQNB is a hydrophilic antagonist which is not trapped in the cells.[89,90] It is not extracted by the lungs and it displays a high affinity for the cholinergic receptors in rat heart homogenates.[91,92] All the criteria needed to characterize the muscarinic receptor have been validated in dogs and baboons.[93]

The receptor density measured in dogs, using ^{11}C MQNB and a multi-injection protocol (Fig. 104.6), was found to be 42 ± 11 pmol/ml tissue.[94] This value is similar to that obtained in rat heart homogenates with ^{3}H MQNB.[93] A simplified protocol was validated in human volunteers[95] and applied to a group of six patients who underwent heart transplantation 4.7±2.3 months earlier. No difference in the concentration of muscarinic receptor was found in transplanted patients compared to control subjects.

CONCLUSION

Neuroimaging techniques have begun to be applied to the study of cardiac physiology and disease. They represent a potent means to investigate in vivo the neurotransmission. These techniques can contribute to a better understanding of the regulation of cardiac function by the autonomic nervous system. Preliminary investigations of neurotransmission abnormalities in patients with heart disease have already suggested that this kind of approach can be clinically relevant. In particular, the use of the detection of

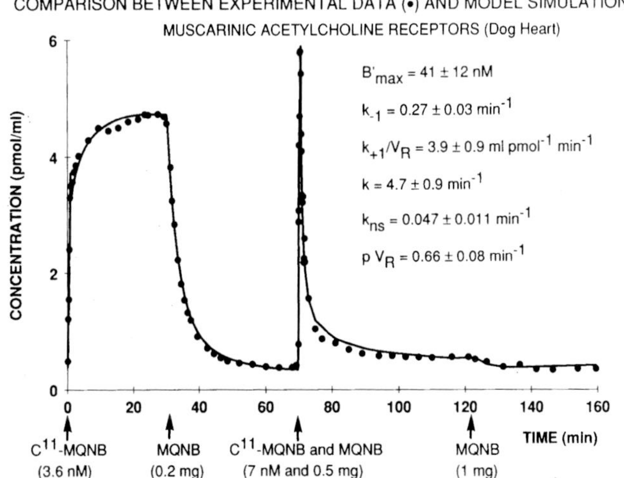

Fig. 104.6 The non-equilibrium non-linear model is based on a specific experimental protocol and justified by the properties of the MQNB kinetics. A few minutes after the injection of ^{11}C MQNB, the myocardial time–concentration curve takes the shape of a plateau. The injection of a large amount of unlabelled MQNB resulted in rapid decrease in myocardial content of ^{11}C MQNB. The coinjection of ^{11}C MQNB and unlabelled MQNB produced a peak of radioactivity in the myocardium.

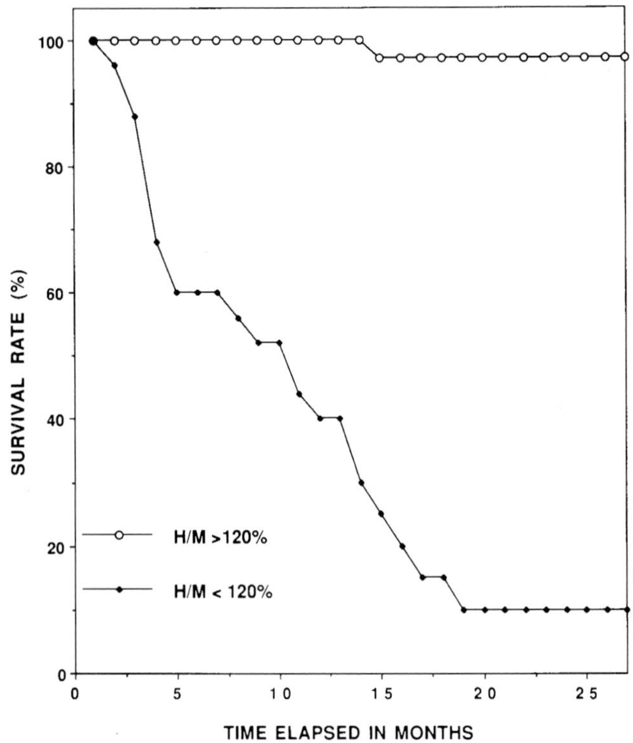

presynaptic abnormalities by MIBG imaging may represent a potent tool to make a decision for heart transplantation (Fig. 104.7). Moreover, the combined use of PET with ^{11}C CGP 12177 and ^{123}I MIBG planar scintigraphy in patients with an idiopathic dilated cardiomyopathy, showing a relationship between the altered adrenergic neuronal function and the beta-adrenergic down-regulation, has suggested that alterations at the presynaptic level could participate in the myocardial overexposure to norepinephrine. The demonstration of partial reinnervation after heart transplantation has provided new insights concerning the function of the human transplanted heart. Therapeutic agents such as angiotensin-converting-enzyme inhibitors, which have been shown on improve cardiac function and survival, have also improved the adrenergic presynaptic function. These findings suggest that neuroimaging techniques have the potential to help physicians in patient management and evaluation of therapy.

Fig. 104.7 The survival curve (life table analysis) shows the good prognostic value of the myocardial ^{123}IMIBG uptake in patients with congestive heart failure. A threshold value of 120% (this value being 196±33% in normal subjects) made a clear-cut difference between the life duration of the two groups of patients.

REFERENCES

1. Petch M C, Nayler W G 1979 Uptake of catecholamines by human cardiac muscle in vitro. Br Heart J 41: 336–339
2. Rose C, Burgess J H, Cousineau D 1985 Tracer norepinephrine kinetics in coronary circulation of patients with heart failure secondary to chronic pressure and volume overload. J Clin Invest 76: 740–747
3. Swedberg K, Viquerat C, Rouleau J L et al 1984 Comparison of myocardial catecholamine balance in chronic congestive heart failure and in angina pectoris without failure. Am J Cardiol 54: 783–786
4. Hasking G J, Esler M D, Jenning G L, Burton D, Johns J A, Korner P I 1986 Norepinephrine spillover to plasma in patients with congestive heart failure: evidence of increased overall and cardiorenal sympathetic nervous activity. Circulation 73: 615–621
5. Meredith I T, Eisenhofer G, Lambert G W, Dewar E M, Jennigs G L, Esler M D 1993 Cardiac sympathetic nervous activity in congestive heart failure. Evidence for increased neuronal norepinephrine release and preserved neuronal uptake. Circulation 88: 136–145
6. Ganguly P K, Lee S L, Beamish R E, Dhalla N S 1989 Altered sympathetic system and adrenoreceptors during the development of cardiac hypertrophy. Am Heart J 18: 520–525
7. Brush J E, Eisenhofer G, Garty M et al 1989 Norepinephrine kinetics in hypertrophic cardiomyopathy. Circulation 79: 836–844
8. Vatner D E, Lavallee M, Amano J, Finizola A, Homcy C J, Vatner S F 1985 Mechanisms of supersensitivity to sympathetic amines in the chronically denervated heart of the conscious dog. Circ Res 57: 55–64
9. Gilbert E M, Eiswirth C C, Mealey P C, Larrabee P, Herrick C M, Bristow M R 1989 β-Adrenergic supersensitivity of the transplanted human heart is presynaptic in origin. Circulation 79: 344–349
10. Sibley D R, Lefkowitz R J 1987 Beta-adrenergic receptor-coupled adenylate cyclase. Biochemical mechanisms of regulation. Mol Neurobiol 1: 121–154
11. Maisel A S, Motulsky H J, Insel P A 1985 Externalisation of beta-adrenergic receptors promoted by myocardial ischemia. Science 230: 183–186
12. Giachetti A, Clark T L, Berti F 1982 Subsensitivity of cardiac beta-adrenoceptors in renal hypertensive rats. J Cardiovasc Pharmacol 1: 467–471
13. Hammond H K, Roth D A, Insel P A et al 1992 Myocardial β-adrenergic receptor expression and signal transduction after chronic volume-overload hypertrophy and circulatory congestion. Circulation 85: 269–280
14. Vatner De, Homcy C J, Sit S P, Manders W T, Vatner S F 1984 Effects of pressure overload left ventricular hypertrophy on β-adrenergic receptors, and responsiveness to catecholamines. J Clin Invest 73: 1473–1482
15. Cervoni P, Herzlinger H, Lai F M, Tanikella T 1981 A comparison of cardiac reactivity and beta-adrenoceptor number and affinity between aorta-coarcted hypertensive and normotensive rat. Br J Pharmacol 74: 517–523
16. Wagner J A, Sax F L, Weisman H F et al 1989 Calcium-antagonist receptors in the atrial tissue of patients with hypertrophic cardiomyopathy. N Engl J Med 320: 755–761
17. Nakajo M, Shimabukuro K, Miyaji N et al 1985 Rapid clearance of iodine-131 MIBG from the heart and liver of patients with adrenergic dysfunction and pheochromocytoma. J Nucl Med 26: 357–365
18. Henderson E B, Kahn J K, Corbett J R et al 1988 Abnormal 123-I Myocardial washout and distribution may reflect myocardial adrenergic derangement in patients with congestive heart cardiomyopathy. Circulation 78: 1192–1199
19. Bristow M R, Ginsburg R, Umans V et al 1986 Beta-1 and beta-2 adrenergic receptor subpopulations in nonfailing and failing human ventricular myocardium: coupling of both receptor subtypes to muscle contraction and selective beta-1 receptor down-regulation in heart failure. Circ Res 59: 297–309
20. Fowler M B, Laser J A, Hopkins D L, Minobe W, Bristow M R 1986 Assessment of the beta-adrenergic receptor pathway in the

intact failing human heart: progressive receptor down-regulation and subsensitivity to agonist response. Circulation 74: 1290–1294
21. Vatner D E, Lee D L, Schwarz K R et al 1988 Impaired cardiac muscarinic receptor function in dogs with heart failure. J Clin Invest 81: 1836–1842
22. Böhm M, Gierschik P, Jakobs K H, Pieske B, Schnabel P, Ungerer M, Erdmann E 1990 Increase of Gi alpha in human hearts with dilated but not ischemic cardiomyopathy. Circulation 82: 1249–1265
23. Wieland D M, Brown L E, Les Roger W et al 1981 Myocardial imaging with a radioiodinated norepinephrine storage analog. J Nucl Med 22: 22–31
24. Glowniak J V, Kilty J E, Amara S G, Hoffman B J, Turner F E 1993 Evaluation of metaiodobenzylguanidine uptake by the norepinephrine, dopamine and serotonine transporters. J Nucl Med 34: 1140–1146
25. Jacques S, Jr, Tobes M C, Sisson J C 1984 Comparison of the sodium dependency of uptake of metaiodobenzylguanidine and norepinephrine into cultured bovine adrenomedullary cells. Mol Pharmacol 26: 539–546
26. Tobes M C, Jacques S, Wieland D M, Sisson J C 1985 Effect of uptake on inhibitors on the uptake of norepinephrine and metaiodobenzylguanidine. J Nucl Med 26: 897–907
27. Sisson J C, Wieland D M, Sherman P, Mangner T J, Tobes M C, Jacques S 1987 Metaiodobenzylguanidine as an index of the adrenergic nervous system integrity and function. J Nucl Med 28: 1620–1624
28. Gasnier B, Roisin M P, Scherman D, Coornaert S, Desplanches G, Henry J P 1986 Uptake of meta-iodobenzylguanidine by bovine chromaffin granule membranes. Molec Pharmacol 29: 275–280
29. Sisson J C, Shapiro B, Meyers L et al 1987 Metaiodobenzylguanidine to map the adrenergic nervous system in man. J Nucl Med 28: 1624–1636
30. Sisson J C, Lynch J J, Johnson J et al 1988 Scintigraphic detection of regional disruption of adrenergic neurons in the heart. Am Heart J 116: 67–76
31. Dae M W, O'Connel J W, Botvinick E H et al 1989 Scintigraphic assessment of regional cardiac adrenergic innervation. Circulation 79: 634–644
32. Rabinovitch M A, Rose C P, Rouleau J L et al 1987 Metaiodobenzylguanidine (131I) scintigraphy detects impaired myocardial sympathetic neuronal transport function of canine mechanical-overload heart failure. Circ Res 61: 797–804
33. Sisson J C, Frager M S, Valk T W et al 1981 Scintigraphic localisation of pheochromocytoma. J Nucl Med 305: 12–17
34. Kline R C, Swanson D P, Wieland D M, Thrall J H, Milton D G, Pitt B, Beierwaltes W H 1981 Myocardial imaging in man with 123-I metaiodobenzyl-guanidine. J Nucl Med 21: 129–132
35. Nakajo M, Shapiro B, Glowniak J, Sisson J C, Beierwaltes W H 1983 Inverse relationship between cardiac accumulation of meta-131-iodobenzylguanidine (I-131 MIBG) and circulating catecholamines in suspected pheochromocytoma. J Nucl Med 24: 1127–1134
36. Merlet P, Valette H, Dubois Randé J L et al 1992 Prognostic value of cardiac MIBG imaging in patients with congestive heart failure. J Nucl Med 33: 471–477
37. Schofer J, Spielmann R, Schubert A, Weber K, Schlüter M 1988 Iodine-123 metaiodobenzylguanidine scintigraphy: a non invasive method to demonstrate myocardial adrenergic system disintegrity in patients with idiopathic dilated cardiomyopathy. J Am Coll Cardiol 12: 1252–1258
38. Glowniak J V, Turner F E, Palac R T, Lagunas-Solar M C, Woodward W R 1989 Iodine-123 metaiodobenzylguanidine imaging of the heart in idiopathic congestive cardiomyopathy and cardiac transplants. J Nucl Med 30: 1182–1191
39. Dae M W, De Marco T, Botvinick E H et al 1992 Scintigraphic assessment of MIBG uptake in globally denervated human and canine hearts. Implications for clinical studies. J Nucl Med 33: 1444 –1450
40. Merlet P, Dubois Randé J L, Adnot S et al 1992 Myocardial beta adrenergic desensitization and neuronal norepinephrine uptake function in idiopathic cardiomyopathy. J Cardiovasc Pharmacol 19: 10–16
41. Merlet P, Attlan G, Agostini D et al 1992 Improvement of cardiac uptake-1 function induced by captopril in patients with idiopathic cardiomyopathy (abstract). Eur Heart J 13: 169
42. Stanton M S, Tuli M M, Radtke N L et al 1989 Regional sympathetic denervation after myocardial infarction in human detected noninvasively using 123-I-metaiodobenzylguanidine. J Am Coll Cardiol 14: 1519–1526
43. Inoue H, Zipes D P 1987 Results of sympathetic denervation in the canine heart: supersensitivity that may be arrhythmogenic. Circulation 75: 877–887
44. Valette H, Merlet P, Bourguignon M et al 1990 Dual isotope tomographic imaging: a Thallium 201–I123 metaiodobenzylguanidine comparative study in coronary artery disease (abstract). Eur J Nucl Med 16: 405
45. Nakajima K, Bunko H, Taki J, Shimizu M, Muramori A, Hisada K 1990 Quantitative analysis of 123I-metaiodobenzylguanidine (MIBG) uptake in hypertrophic cardiomyopathy. Am Heart 119: 1329–1337
46. Kawai C, Yui Y, Sasayama S, Matsumori A 1983 Myocardial catecholamines in hypertrophic and dilated (congestive) cardiomyopathy. J Am Coll Cardiol 2: 834–840
47. Bourguignon M, Valette H, Merlet P et al 1989 123-I Metaiodobenzylguanidine (MIBG) cardiac imaging as an index of the severity of cardiomyopathies. In: Schmidt H A E, Buraggi G L (eds) Nuclear medicine trends and possibilities in nuclear medicine. Schattauer, Stuttgort. pp 281–283
48. Mislankar S G, Gildersleeve D L, Wieland D M, Massin G C, Mulholland G K, Toorongian S A 1988 6-[18F]Fluorometaraminol: a radiotracer for in vivo mapping of adrenergic nerves of the heart. J Med Chem 31: 362–366
49. Wieland D M, Rosenpire K C, Hutchkins G D et al 1990 Neuronal mapping of the heart with 6-18F fluorometaraminol. J Med Chem 33: 956–964
50. Goldstein D S, Brush J E, Eisendorfer G, Stull R, Esler H 1988 In vivo measurement of neuronal uptake of norepinephrine in the human heart. Circulation 78: 41–48
51. Goldstein D S, Chang P C, Eisenhofer G et al 1990 Positron emission tomographic imaging of cardiac sympathetic innervation and function. Circulation 81: 1606–1621
52. Rosenpire K, Haka M S, Van Dort M E, Jewett D M, Gildersleeve D L, Schwaiger M, Wieland D M 1990 Synthesis and preliminary evaluation of carbon-11-meta-hydroxyephedrine: a false transmitter agent for neuronal imaging. J Nucl Med 31: 1328–1334
53. Wieland D M, Hutchins G D, Rosenspire K C, Haka M S, Sherman P S, Pisani T L, Nguyen N T B, Schwaiger M 1989 (C 11)Hydroxyephedrine: a high specific activity alternative to 6-(F18)fluorometaraminol for heart neuronal imaging (abstract). J Nucl Med 30(5): 767
54. Schwaiger M, Kalff V, Rosenpire K et al 1990 Noninvasive evaluation of sympathetic nervous system in human heart by positron emission tomography. Circulation 82: 457–464
55. Schwaiger M, Hutchkins G D, Kalff et al 1991 Evidence for regional catecholamine uptake and storage sites in the transplanted human heart by positron emission tomography. J Clin Invest 87: 1681–1690
56. Allman K C, Wolfe E, Sitomer J, Hutchkins G, Wieland D, Schwaiger M 1991 C-11 Hydroxyephedrine assessment of regional myocardial sympathetic neuronal function following acute myocardial infarction in man (abstract). J Nucl Med 32: 1040
57. Schwaiger M, Hutchins G, Rosenpire K, Haka M S, Wieland D 1990 Quantitative evaluation of the sympathetic nervous system in patients with cardiomyopathy. J Nucl Med 31: 792–798
58. Allman K C, Stevens M J, Wieland D M, Hutchkins G D, deGradp T R, Schwaiger M 1992 Neuronal imaging with PET for the quantitative characterization of cardiac diabetic neuropathy (abstract). Circulation 86(4): 246
59. Ding Y-S, Fowler J S, Gatley S J, Dewey S L, Wolf A P 1991 Synthesis of high specific activity (+)- and (–)-6-(18F)fluoronorepinephrine via the nucleophilic aromatic substitution reaction. J Med Chem 34: 767–771
60. Ding Y-S, Fowler J S, Gatley S J, Dewey S L, Wolf A P, Schlyer D J 1991 Synthesis of high specific activity of 6-(18F)fluorodopamine

for positron emission tomography studies of sympathetic nervous tissue. J Med Chem 34: 861–863
61. Ding Y S, Fowler J S, Dewey S L, Logan J, Schyler D J, Gatley S J, Volkow N D, King P T, Wolf A P 1993 Comparison of high specific activity (–) and (+)-6-(^{18}F)fluoronorepinephrine and 6-(^{18}F)fluorodopamine in baboons: heart uptake, metabolism and the effect of desipramine. J Nucl Med 34: 619–629
62. Goldstein S, Eisenhofer G, Dunn B B et al 1992 PET imaging of cardiac sympathetic innervation using 6-(^{18}F)fluorodopamine: initial findings in humans (abstract). Ciculation 86(4): I247
63. Loc'h C, Mardon K, Valette H, Brutesco C, Merlet P, Syrota A, Mazière B 1993 Preparation and pharmacological characterization of ^{76}Br-metabromobenzylguanidine. J Nucl Med 34: 1739–1744
64. Valette H, Loc'h C, Mardon K et al 1993 ^{76}Br-Metabromobenzyl-guanidine: a PET radiotracer for mapping of sympathetic nerves of the heart. J Nucl Med 34: 1739–1744
65. Anderson D C, King S C, Parsons S M 1983 Pharmacological characterization of the acetylcholine transport system in purified Torpedo electric organ synaptic vesicles. Mol Pharmacol 24: 48–54
66. Widén L, Erikson L, Ingvar M, Parsons, Rogers G A, Stone-Elender S 1993 Positron emission tomography studies of central cholinergic nerve terminals (abstract). J Nucl Med 33(5): 1011
67. Kuhl D E, Koeppe R A, Fessler J A, Minoshima S, Ackermann R J, Carey J E, Frey K A, Wieland D M 1993 In vivo mapping of cholinergic neurons in the human brain using SPECT and (–)-5-(I-123) iodobenzovesamicol (abstract). J Nucl Med 34(5): 25
68. DeGrado T R, Mullholland G K, Melon P G, Nguyen N, Wieland D M, Schwaiger M 1992 Evaluation of F-18(-)flouroethoxybenzovesamicol (FEOBV) as a new PET tracer of cholinergic neuron of the heart (abstract). Circulation 86(4): 246
69. Delforge J, Syrota A, Mazoyer B: Experimental design optimization: theory and application to estimation of receptor model parameters using dynamic positron emission tomography. Phys Med Biol 34: 419–435
70. Syrota A 1991 Positron emission tomography: evaluation of cardiac receptors. In: Marcus M L, Skorton D J, Schelbert H R, Wolf G L, Braunwald E (eds) Cardiac imaging – principles and practice: a companion of Braunwald's heart disease. W B Saunders, Philadelphia, pp 1256–1270
71. Berger G, Mazière M, Prenant C, Sastre J, Syrota A, Comar D 1982 Synthesis of 11C propranolol. J Radioanal Chem 74: 301–306
72. Berger G, Prenant C, Sastre J, Syrota A, Comar D 1983 Synthesis of a beta-blocker for heart visualization. [11C]Practolol. Int J Appl Radiat Isot 34: 1556–1557
73. Prenant C, Sastre J, Crouzel C, Syrota A 1987 Synthesis of 11C-Pindolol. J Label Compds Radiopharm 24: 227–232
74. Antoni G, Ulin J, Långström B 1989 Synthesis of the 11-C-labelled β-adrenergic ligands atenolol, metoprolol and propranolol. Appl Radiat Isot 40: 561–572
75. Boullais C, Crouzel C, Syrota A 1986 Synthesis of 4-(3-t-butylamino-2-hydroxypropoxy)-benzimidazol-2(11C)-one (CGP 12177). J Label Compds Radiopharm 23: 565–567
76. Hammadi A, Crouzel C 1991 Asymetric synthesis of (2S) and (2R)-4-(butylamino-2-hydroxypropoxy-benzamidazol-2-C-11)one (S) and (R) (C-11 CGP 12177) from optically active precursors. J Lab Compds Radiopharm 29: 681–690
77. Berridge M S, Terris H A, Vesselle J M 1992 Preparation and in vivo binding of 11-C-carazolol, a radiotracer for the beta-adrenergic receptor. Nucl Med Biol 19: 563–567
78. de Groote T J, van Warde A, Elsinga P H, Visser G M, Brodde O E, Vaalburg W 1993 Synthesis and evaluation of 1'-(18-F)fluorometoprolol as a potential tracer for the visualization of β-adrenoceptors with PET. Nucl Med Biol 20(5): 637–642
79. Nanoff C, Freissmuth M, Schütz W 1989 The role of a low beta-1 adrenoceptor selectivity of [3H]CGP-12177 for resolving subtype-selectivity of competitive ligands. Naunyn-Schmiedebergs Arch Pharmacol 336: 519–525
80. Staehelin M, Hertel C 1983 [3H]CGP-12 177, a beta-adrenergic ligand suitable for measuring cell surface receptors. J Receptor Res 3: 35–43
81. Staehelin M, Simons P, Jaeggik, Wigger N 1983 CGP-12 177. A hydrophilic beta-adrenergic receptor radioligand reveals high affinity binding of agonists to intact cells. J Biol Chem 258: 3496–3502
82. Hertel C, Muller P, Portenier H, Staehelin M 1983 Determination of the desensitization of beta-adrenergic receptors by [3H]CGP-12 177. Biochemistry 216: 669–674
83. Delforge J, Syrota A, Lancon J P et al 1991 Cardiac beta-adrenergic receptor density measured in vivo using PET, CGP 12177 and a new graphical method. J Nucl Med 32: 739–748
84. Merlet P, Delforge J, Syrota A et al 1993 Positron emission tomography with 11-C-CGP 12177 to assess β-adrenergic receptor concentration in idiopathic dilated cardiomyopathy. Circulation 87: 1169–1178
85. Merlet P, Delforge J, Dubois Randé J L et al 1992 In vivo evaluation of mechanisms of down regulation in idiopathic dilated cardiomyopathy using positron emission tomography (PET) and MIBG imaging (abstract). J Nucl Med 33: 896
86. Skomedal T, Aass H, Osnes J B 1984 Specific binding of ^{3}H-prazosin to myocardial cells isolated from adult rats. Biochem Pharmacol 33: 1897–1906
87. Ehrin E, Luthra S K, Crouzel C, Pike V W 1988 Preparation of carbon-11 labelled prazosin, a potent and selective alpha-1 adrenoceptor antagonist. J Label Compds Radiopharm 25: 177–183
88. Mazière M, Comar D, Godot J M, Collard P, Cepeda P, Nacquet R 1981 In vivo characterization of myocardium muscarinic receptors by positron emission tomography. Life Sci 29: 2391–2397
89. Gossuin A, Maloteaux J M, Trouet, Laduron P 1984 Differentiation between ligand trapping into intact cells and binding on muscarinic receptors. Biochim Biophys Acta 804: 100–106
90. Watson M, Yamamura H I, Roeske W R 1986 [^{3}H]Pirenzepine and (–)-[^{3}H]quinuclidinyl benzilate binding to rat cerebral cortical and cardiac muscarinic cholinergic sites. I. Characterization and regulation of agonist binding to putative muscarinic subtypes. J Pharmacol Exp Ther 237: 411–418
91. Chaumet-Riffaud Ph, Girault M, Syrota A 1984 Characterization of muscarinic cholinergic receptors in the isolated perfused rat heart. J Physiol (London) 348: 11–15
92. Syrota A, Paillotin G, Davy J M, Aumont M C 1984 Kinetics of in vivo binding of antagonist to muscarinic cholinergic receptor in the human heart studied by positron emission tomography. Life Sci 35: 937–945
93. Syrota A, Comar D, Paillotin G, Davy J M, Aumont M C, Stulzaft O, Mazière B 1985 Muscarinic cholinergic receptor in the human heart evidenced under physiological conditions by positron emission tomography. Proc Natl Acad Sci (USA) 82: 584–588
94. Delforge J, Janier M, Syrota A et al 1990 Noninvasive quantification of muscarinic receptors in vivo with positron emission tomography in the dog heart. Circulation 82: 1494–1504
95. Delforge J, Le Guludec D, Syrota A, Bendriem B, Crouzel C, Salma M, Merlet P 1993 Quantification of myocardial muscarinic receptors with PET in humans. J Nucl Med 34: 981–991

105. Nuclear techniques in the assessment of thrombosis and atheroma

Helmut Sinzinger Juan Flores

INTRODUCTION

Arterial lesions may start in the fetus (stage I atherogenesis). While the vascular system apparently has the capacity to remove these lesions, at least some of them may undergo stepwise progression, the cause and severity being dependent on life-style risk factors (smoking, hyperlipidaemic mother, etc.). A stepwise, but silent progression (stage II) of the disease after decades may result in acute clinical manifestation (stage III) which, with regard to the coronary arteries, is associated with sudden death in about one-third.

One of the key mechanisms of human atherogenesis is the formation of thrombus on the intimal wall, at the site of vascular injury.[1] The thrombus is composed of platelets and fibrin which may be dissolved subsequently by the eicosanoid system or fibrinolysis. However, it may become incorporated, leading to a localized thickening of the wall and an eccentric thickening. Cellular mechanisms are also involved with the migration and proliferation of smooth muscle cells[2] as well as an adhesion and invasion of mononuclear cells which become macrophages that undergo transformation to foam cells after extensive lipid uptake.[3] Together with the smooth muscle, foam cells and the trapping of lipids by arterial glycosaminoglycans, the disturbed arterial lipid metabolism is another key event occurring in early disease. The onset of the disease is in part genetically determined, while the three main risk factors for developing atherosclerosis, i.e. elevated LDL-cholesterol (>130 mg/dl), cigarette smoking and hypertension, are relevant factors in determining the spontaneous course as well as the onset of the disease.

Clinicians' attention has been focused mainly on manifest arterial disease, where the application of radioisotopic techniques has an established role. However, nuclear medicine techniques are still only of limited value for contributing to the presymptomatic diagnosis of atherosclerosis. Attempts to prevent rather than to repair existing lesions in the various vascular segments, as well as considerable improvements in technical equipment and new methodologies, suggest that nuclear techniques could have a place among other non-invasive diagnostic techniques in the detection of early atherosclerosis. In particular, the approach to image the functional importance of atheroma may gain importance and become a useful indication for the use of radioisotopic techniques at a rather early stage (stages I and II) of the disease.

DETECTION OF INTIMAL THROMBUS FORMATION

Fibrinogen

Shortly after coronary artery thrombus was detected in vivo by [^{131}I]fibrinogen injection,[4] [^{123}I]fibrinogen was claimed to detect atherosclerotic plaques.[5] The authors found a significantly increased tracer uptake 20 h after tracer application. In none of the three major vascular beds, however, did this methodology achieve clinical acceptance. Neither morphological control (in experimental animals and anecdotal in humans) nor clinical follow-up data were promising, because of a high rate of false positive and false negative results.

Antibodies

Monoclonal antibodies (GC4 and T2G1) reacting either with purified high molecular weight digest products of fibrinogen, fibrin or cross-linked fibrin, or with thrombin cleavage site-specific epitope of des-FPA des-FPB-fibrin and other antibodies, have not been used sufficiently often in human arterial disease to allow meaningful conclusions.

Although promising data have been reported in 20 patients suffering from acute peripheral arterial thrombus using specific monoclonal ^{111}In-labelled antibody (P 256 Fab′), their use to detect atheromatous lesions is still remote.

Platelet labelling

The deposition of platelets occurs only in thrombogenic arterial segments. Sensitivity testing in the carotid region indicates that the lesion has to contain at least 0.1% of the total injected dose in order to allow scintigraphic detection. Furthermore, platelet accumulation can be imaged only if the plaque-to-blood ratio exceeds 4.0–5.0.[6] The dynamic process of platelet contact, residence, deposition and incorporation into the vascular wall as well as embolization needs more frequent imaging. The kinetics over human lesions may vary considerably. Morphological control reveals that part of the radiotracer is found in the platelets on the vascular surface (intimal thrombus, ulcerative lesion) or incorporated into the vascular wall along with mononuclear elements. While experimental lesions do show severe platelet deposition after vascular damage, the extent of platelet deposition during spontaneous atherosclerosis in humans is dramatically lower, probably reflecting the difference in the activity of the disease (Table 105.1). Very active human lesions may appear within 1 h, but the majority require between 12 and 24 h.

The prevalence of spontaneously positive lesions in healthy adults in their twenties and thirties is below 10%. In patients with manifest vascular disease above the age of 60 the prevalence of positive lesions in the carotid arteries is about 50%, while in the coronary arteries and the peripheral arteries it is again much lower, about 10%. The decrease in the prevalence of positive lesions in asymptomatic patients indicates a higher activity of the atherosclerotic disease at a younger age. Interestingly enough, in young patients with cerebrovascular disease below the age of 40 this percentage exceeds 80%, indicating that the platelet uptake correlates with the activity of atherosclerotic lesions rather than their severity or their extent. Isaka et al,[7] however, detected a correlation between enhanced platelet uptake and the extent of angiographically proven lesions ($P<0.001$). Platelet deposition was recorded in 41% of angiographically verified lesions compared with 13% of angiographically unaffected areas.

Table 105.1 Imaging of spontaneous human atherosclerosis after ^{111}In-oxine platelet labelling

Reference	Vessel
14 Davis et al (1980)	Carotid
15 Goldman et al (1982)	Carotid
16 Heyns et al (1982)	Aneurysms
17 Kessler and Trabant (1982)	Carotid
18 Powers et al (1982)	Carotid
19 Kimura et al (1982)	Carotid
7 Isaka et al (1984)	Carotid
20 Sinzinger et al (1984)	Aneurysms
21 Sinzinger and Fitscha (1984)	Femoral

While an acute occlusion of the femoral artery can be imaged in more than 90% of patients by ^{111}In-oxine-labelled platelets, only 25% of those with myocardial infarction investigated within 24 h of the onset of chest pain show an area of increased platelet uptake corresponding to an occluded coronary artery in the angiogram. The high blood background as well as problems with gating heart and respiratory function interfere with the sensitivity of the technique.

False positive images may be obtained in the carotid artery region by tortous vessels (for review see ref. 8). Furthermore, platelet accumulation at the site of a haematoma in varicose veins, at inflammatory sites and around malignant tumours, may also lead to false positive results.

Follow-up monitoring

Regular follow-up of scintigraphically positive lesions revealed that the majority remain unchanged over some months, the scans may therefore be used to monitor the efficacy of drugs in experimental animals (for review see ref. 8) and in humans (Table 105.2).

As the target–background ratio is extremely variable, the timing of the subtraction of the blood background is a problem. The most promising approach has been to determine the blood background from ^{113}In-oxine-labelled platelets still circulating, but this has not been performed widely enough to allow definite conclusions.

Table 105.2 Monitoring of antiplatelet therapy in human arteries (and implanted grafts)

Reference	Vessel	Lesion	Drug
22 Huang and Harper (1981)	Graft/ aneurysm	–	ASA, DIP, SP
23 Pumphrey et al (1982)	Aorto-femoral	Dacron	ASA/DIP
24 Ritchie et al (1982)	Shunt	–	SP
25 Stratton and Ritchie (1982)	Graft	Dacron	SP
26 Stratton et al (1983)	Graft	Dacron	Ticlopidine
21 Sinzinger and Fitscha (1984)	Femoral	Lesion	PGI_2
27 Fitscha et al (1985)	Femoral	Lesion	Taprostene
28 Kessler et al (1985)	Femoral	Lesion	ASA
29 Fitscha (1986)	Femoral	Lesion	Iloprost
30 Sinzinger et al (1987)	Femoral	Lesion	ASA
31 Sinzinger et al (1990)	Femoral	Lesion	ISDN, PGE_1

Vascular graft

Arterial grafts show extensive uptake of platelets even years after implantation. Its extent has been claimed to be a parameter of the reocclusion rate. There are contradictory results regarding angioplasty, and it remains unclear whether enhanced platelet deposition correlates with later reocclusion. The role of drugs for decreasing or delaying reocclusion has not been clearly assessed.

Positron emission tomography

^{68}Ga-oxine (tropolone and MPO) has been used successfully in a small number of patients. Although the platelet accumulation at certain lesion sites takes time, a 3.5-fold accumulation of ^{68}Ga-labelled platelets has been found in a scraped aorta as compared to the normal segment. The short half-life, the radiation dose (spleen) and the possibility that the ^{68}Ga-labelled platelets might reflect a circulating rather than an adhering population might be limiting factors.

IMAGING OF LIPID METABOLISM IN ATHEROSCLEROTIC PLAQUES

Low density lipoprotein (LDL) imaging in patients has been introduced by Lees et al.[9] Arterial wall metabolism has been studied using lipoproteins obtained by ultracentrifugation according to density, or immunoaffinity chromatography. ^{99m}Tc, ^{111}In, ^{123}I, ^{125}I and ^{131}I have been used as tracers. In human and rabbit arterial tissue the LDL entry kinetics exhibit characteristic behaviour reflecting the qualitative endothelial surface lining, i.e. normal, denuded or repaired (Fig. 105.1), while the quantitative uptake of the lesions correlates with the vascular cholesterol ester content.[10] The prevalence of positive lesions and the extent of LDL entry is the highest in the carotid arteries. LDL lesion imaging in the coronary arteries is very difficult. In hyperlipoproteinaemic patients the prevalence of visible positive lesions is higher than in normolipidaemics. Follow-up studies after various time intervals show stable behaviour of the lesions, by quantitative uptake and kinetic criteria.

To assess the kinetics of LDL entry requires repeated imaging, which makes it difficult to perform repeated blood background subtraction. Autologous LDLs have the advantage reflecting physiological behaviour, while (unphysiological) cholesteryl ester analogues might be better to image the process of accumulation because of resistance to the action of intracellular cholesteryl ester hydrolysis.[11]

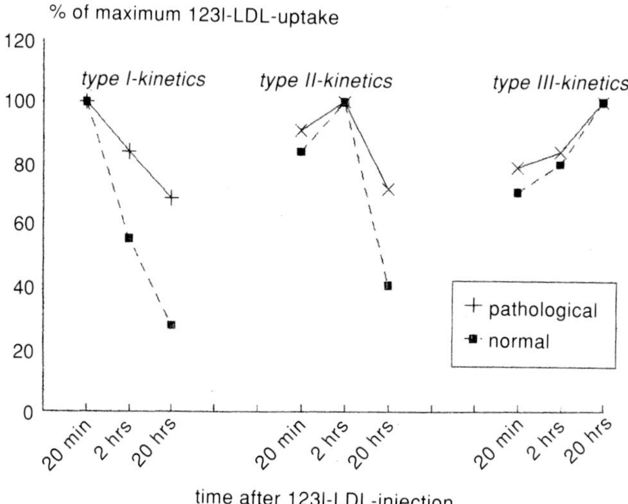

Fig. 105.1

IMAGING OF CELLULAR ASPECTS OF ATHEROSCLEROSIS

Once in the arterial wall monocytes show phagocytosis and start to accumulate (mainly oxidized) LDL,[12] finally becoming lipid-laden foam cells. Injection of radiolabelled autologous monocytes (purity >90%) allows visualization of atherosclerotic lesions after 1–4 h.[13] In contrast to platelet LDL uptake, the monocyte entry rate in positive lesions is quite low. There is no correlation at all to ^{111}In-oxine platelet positive lesions, while 40–60% of the LDL positive areas coincide.

OTHER APPROACHES

Non-specific polyclonal immunoglobulin G

Foam cells are predominantly macrophage-derived and bear abundant Fc receptors to bind non-specific polyclonal Ig and Fc fragments. ^{111}In-labelled polyclonal IgG may therefore be used to image experimental atherosclerosis in rabbits after balloon-catheter injury of the abdominal aorta. Although data on positive imaging do exist, almost no controlled information is available concerning human arteries.

Porphyrins

Several haematoporphyrins have been used to image experimental lesions in rabbits, the optimal uptake being found between 24 and 48 h. Human data, however, are again not yet available.

CONCLUSION

Functional imaging of atheroma may become clinically useful in the future using specific (coagulation, lipoproteins, mononuclear cells) and unspecific radiolabelling agents. None of the techniques used so far has achieved widespread clinical application. For some techniques, such as platelet labelling and LDL labelling, considerable experience exists, while most of the other approaches are still only occasionally performed and thus lack proof of clinical value. Imaging has been mainly performed in the carotid and peripheral vessels, while coronary arteries remain difficult by any of the existing methods.

REFERENCES

1. Rokitansky C V 1852 Über einige der wichtigsten Krankheiten. K.u.K. Hof- und Staatsdruckerei, Vienna
2. Virchow R 1856 Phlogose und Thrombose im Gefä §-system. Gesammelte Abhandlungen zur wissenschaftlichen Medizin. Hirsch, Berlin
3. Anitschkow N N 1933 Experimental arteriosclerosis in animals. In: Cowdry E C (ed) Arteriosclerosis. A survey of the problem. Macmillan, New York, pp 271–322
4. Moschus C B, Oldewurtel H A, Lahivi K 1974 Incorporation of ^{131}I-fibrinogen in a coronary artery thrombus detected in vivo with a scintillation camera. Cardiovasc Res 8: 715–720
5. Mettinger K I, Larsson S, Ericson K et al 1978 Detection of atherosclerotic plaques in arteries by the use of ^{123}I-fibrinogen. Lancet i: 242–244
6. Dewanjee M K 1990 Radiolabelled platelets in monitoring of drug efficacy in animal models. Thromb Haemorrh Dis 1: 37–51
7. Isaka Y, Kimura K, Yoneda S et al 1984 Platelet accumulation in carotid atherosclerotic lesions: semiquantitative analysis with ^{111}Indium platelets and ^{99m}technetium human serum albumin. J Nucl Med 25: 556–563
8. Sinzinger H, Virgolini I 1990 Nuclear medicine and atherosclerosis. Eur J Nucl Med 17: 160–178
9. Lees R S, Lees A M, Strauss H W 1983 External imaging of human atherosclerosis. J Nucl Med 24: 154–161
10. Virgolini I, Rauscha F, Lupattelli G et al 1991 Autologous low-density lipoprotein labelling allows characterization of human atherosclerotic lesions in vivo as to presence of foam cells and endothelial coverage. Eur J Nucl Med 18: 948–951
11. DeGalan M R, Schwendner S W, Skinner W S et al 1988 ^{125}Iodine cholesteryl iopanoate for measuring extent of atherosclerosis in rabbits. J Nucl Med 29: 503–508
12. Gerrity R G 1981 The role of the monocyte in atherosclerosis. I. Transition of blood-borne monocytes into foam cells in fatty lesions. Am J Pathol 103: 181–190
13. Sinzinger H, Virgolini I, Rauscha F et al 1990 Autologous ^{111}In-oxine monocyte scintigraphy in atherosclerosis. Eur J Nucl Med 16: 503
14. Davis H H, Siegel B A, Welch M J 1980 Scintigraphic detection of an arterial thrombus with ^{111}In-labelled autologous platelets. J Nucl Med 21: 548–549
15. Goldman M, Leung J C Y, Chandler S T et al 1982 Imaging carotid artery disease with ^{111}In-labelled platelets: a combined clinical and theoretical study. In: Raynaud C (ed) Nuclear medicine and biology. Pergamon, Paris, pp 887–890
16. Heyns A du P, Lotter M G, Badenhorst P N et al 1982 Kinetics and fate of ^{111}indium-labelled platelets in patients with aortic aneurysms. Arch of Surg 117: 1170–1174
17. Kessler C, Trabant R 1982 Thrombozytenszintigraphie mit ^{111}Indium. Arch Psychiatr Nervenkr 231: 449
18. Powers W J, Siegel B A, David H H et al 1982 ^{111}Indium platelet scintigraphy in cerebrovascular disease. Neurology 32: 938–943
19. Kimura K, Isaka Y, Etani H et al 1982 In-^{111} labelled autologous platelet scintigraphy for the detection of vascular thrombi in ischemic cerebrovascular disease. In: Raynaud C (ed) Nuclear medicine and biology. Pergamon, Paris, pp 1750–1761
20. Sinzinger H, Fitscha P, O'Grady J 1984 Detection of aneurysms by gamma-camera imaging after injection of autologous labelled platelets. Lancet ii: 1365–1367
21. Sinzinger H, Fitscha P 1984 Epoprostenol and platelet deposition in atherosclerosis. Lancet i: 905–906
22. Huang T W, Harker L A 1981 ^{111}In-platelet imaging for detection of platelet deposition in abdominal aneurysms and prosthetic arterial grafts. Am J Cardiol 47: 882–889
23. Pumphrey C W, Dewanjee M K, Chesebro J H et al 1982 A new method for quantifying human platelet vascular graft interaction and the effect of platelet-inhibitor therapy. In: Raynaud C (ed) Nuclear medicine and biology. Pergamon, Paris, pp 895–897
24. Ritchie J L, Lindner A, Hamilton G W et al 1982 ^{111}In-oxine platelet imaging in hemodialysis patients: detection of platelet deposition at vascular access sites. Nephrology 39: 334–339
25. Stratton J R, Ritchie J L 1982 Sulfinpyrazone fails to inhibit platelet deposition on Dacron prosthetic grafts in man. Circulation 66: 55
26. Stratton J R, Thiele B L, Ritchie J L 1983 Natural history of platelet deposition on Dacron aortic bifurcation grafts in the first years after implantation. Am J Cardiol 52: 371–374
27. Fitscha P, Kaliman J, Sinzinger H 1985 Gamma-camera imaging after autologous human platelet labelling with ^{111}In-oxine-sulfate: a key for assessing the efficacy of prostacyclin treatment in active atherosclerosis? In: Schrör K (ed) Prostaglandins and other eicosanoids in the cardiovascular system. Karger, Basel, pp 352–361
28. Kessler C, Henningsen H, Reuther R et al 1985 Szintigraphie mit ^{111}In-markierten Thrombozyten: Therapiekontrolle bei Acetylsalicylsäure (ASS) – behandelten Schlaganfallpatienten. Nuc Compact 16: 30–31
29. Fitscha P 1986 Prostaglandine in Pathogenese und Therapie der peripheren arteriellen Verschlu§krankheit (PVK). In: Kraupp O, Sinzinger H, Widhalm K (eds) Atherogenesis VII. Wilhelm Maudrich, Vienna, pp 124
30. Sinzinger H, O'Grady J, Fitscha P et al 1987 Diminished platelet residence time on active human atherosclerotic lesion in vivo – evidence for an optimal dose of aspirin? Prostagl Leukotr Essent Fatty Acids 34: 89–93
31. Sinzinger H, Fitscha P, O'Grady J et al 1990 Synergistic effect of prostaglandin E1 and isosorbide dinitrate in peripheral vascular disease. Lancet i: 627–628

SECTION 8

Basic sciences

106. Basic physics of nuclear medicine

Brenda Walker Peter Jarritt

THE ORIGIN OF RADIATION

● What is the relationship between the structure of the atom and the production of radiation?

▲ To understand the principle of radioactive decay it is necessary to consider the structure of the atom. In the simplest model, suggested by Bohr, an atom consists of a central nucleus of protons and neutrons with electrons orbiting about the nucleus in discrete energy levels or 'shells'. The shells are denoted by the letters K, L, M, etc., K referring to the innermost shell (shell number n=1), L being the next shell (n=2), etc. The maximum number of electrons in any one shell = $2n^2$ (Fig. 106.1A).

In the neutral atom the number of electrons is exactly equal to the number of protons in the nucleus. In a stable atom the electrons remain in their discrete orbits. Electrons may be moved to higher shells (**excitation**) or be completely removed from the atom (**ionization**), but this requires energy to be given to the electron, e.g. from a particle or photon. The energy required to remove an electron from a shell is called the **binding energy** and it is greatest for the shells closest to the nucleus. When an electron is removed from an inner shell of an atom, an electron from an outer shell fills the vacancy and energy is then released (Fig. 106.1B). This energy is equal to the difference in binding energy of the two shells. These emissions are known as **characteristic X-rays** as they have different values for different elements. An alternative to characteristic X-ray emission is **Auger electron emission**. In this process the energy released by the outer shell electron is given to another electron, which then leaves the atom (Fig. 106.1C). In this example the energy of the Auger electron is equal to the binding energy of the K shell minus the sum of the binding energies of the shells having the two vacancies, i.e. the L shell. Because two vacancies exist further characteristic X-rays can result.

● What do the numbers in the names of the routine nuclear medicine radionuclides refer to, e.g. gallium-67, thallium-201, iodine-131?

▲ The atomic nucleus is composed of protons and neutrons and is characterized by the number of each it contains. The number of protons determines the **atomic number *Z*** of the atom. The total number of protons and neutrons, known as the nucleons, determines the **mass number *A*** of the nucleus and ***N*, the neutron number**, is equal to A minus Z. The notation now used is

$${}^{A}_{Z}\mathbf{X}_{N}$$

where X represents the chemical element to which the atom belongs. For example, ${}^{131}{}_{53}\mathrm{I}_{78}$ represents one of the radioactive nuclides of the element iodine. All iodine atoms have atomic number 53, therefore it can be omitted from the notation. The neutron number (N) can be calculated and therefore may also be omitted. The simpler, yet still correct notation, then becomes ${}^{131}\mathrm{I}$. Some radionuclides of iodine are ${}^{123}\mathrm{I}$, ${}^{125}\mathrm{I}$, ${}^{131}\mathrm{I}$. The changing numbers indicate that the neutron number is changing.

The term **nuclide** is used to describe a particular nuclear composition. Nuclides that have the same number of protons (i.e. atomic number Z) are called **isotopes**. Isotopes of an element have the same chemical properties but differ physically. Nuclides that have the same number of neutrons (i.e. neutron number N) are called **isotones**, and nuclides that have the same total number of neutrons and protons (i.e. mass number A) are called **isobars**.

● Why are some nuclides radioactive?

▲ There are combinations of protons and neutrons which produce stable nuclei and others which produce unstable nuclei. The most stable state of a nucleus is

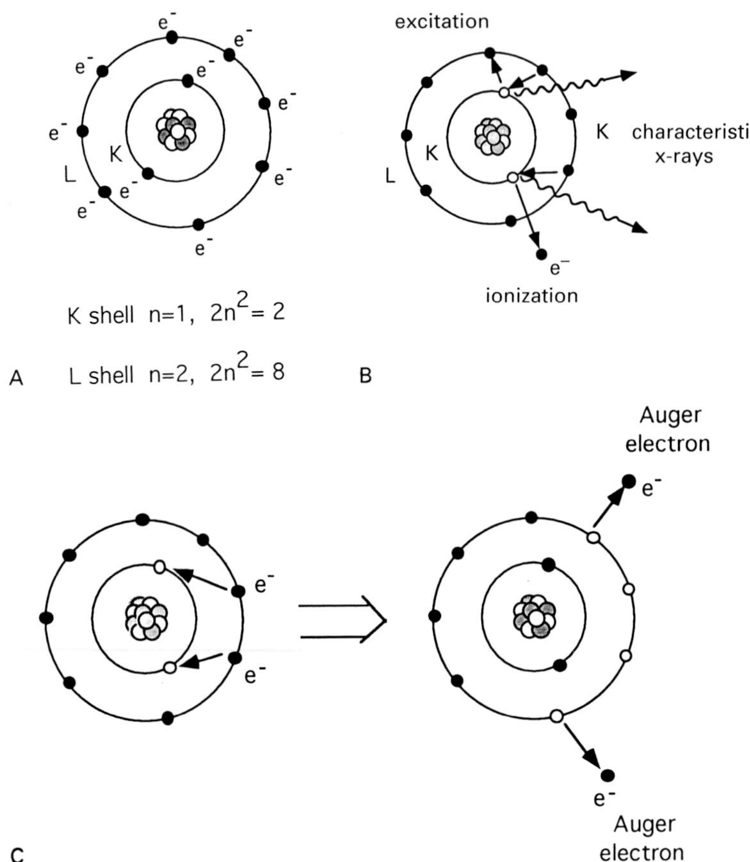

Fig. 106.1 (A) The Bohr model of the atom, showing only the K and L shell configurations. (B) Characteristic X-ray emission. (C) Auger electron emission.

called the '**ground**' state. In an unstable nucleus the nucleons are in an '**excited**' state and must release energy to reach the ground state. This usually happens more or less instantaneously. The nucleus may, however, remain in an excited state for a measurable time; this is called a **metastable state,** and it may then be considered as a separate nuclide. Two nuclides with the same Z, A and N but differing only in their energy states are called **isomers**. The process of de-excitation is called **isomeric transition.**

The neutron-to-proton ratio in the nucleus determines its stability. Figure 106.2 shows a plot of N *vs.* Z for stable nuclei and also shows a plot of $N = Z$ for comparison. The imaginary line identifying the stable nuclei is known as the '**line of stability**'. It can be seen that the N/Z ratio for stability increases as Z increases, i.e. as the elements become heavier. All elements with $A > 209$ are unstable, e.g. uranium-235 and uranium-238. In the transformation of an unstable nucleus to a more stable nucleus, energy is emitted in the form of particles such as alpha- and beta-particles, and in some cases photons (gamma-rays). This is the process of **radioactive decay**.

An unstable or radioactive nucleus is called the **parent** nucleus, and the more stable product nucleus is called the

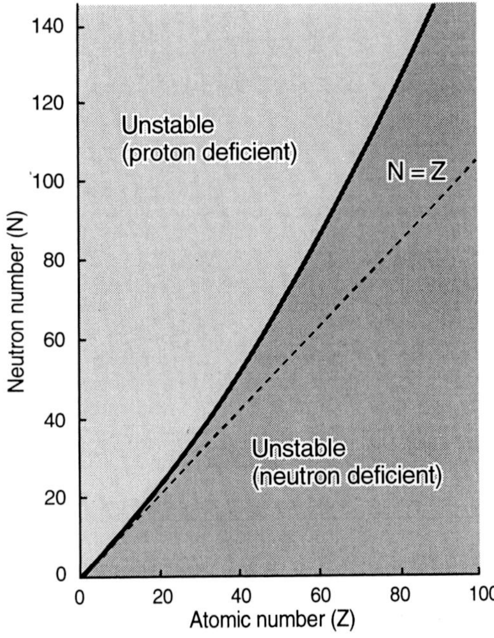

Fig. 106.2 Schematic of the 'line of stability', showing that as Z increases the N/Z ratio for stability increases. The $N=Z$ line is shown for comparison. Unstable nuclides with N/Z above the 'line of stability' are 'proton deficient' and decay by β^-; those below the line are 'neutron deficient' and decay by β^+, electron capture and alpha emission.

daughter nucleus. We then refer to **parent–daughter** relationships.

Unstable or radioactive nuclides each have a set of characteristic properties, e.g. the mode of decay, energy and half-life of the emission. Because these basic properties are characteristic of the nuclide it is referred to as a **radionuclide**. The term **radioisotope** is sometimes used but is not strictly correct and should only be used when identifying a particular radioactive isotope of a family, e.g. ^{123}I, ^{131}I. The term **radionucleotide** is occasionally used in the literature but is incorrect.

● **How can information about each nuclide be readily obtained?**

▲ A source of information about all stable and unstable nuclides is the **Chart of the Nuclides**. This shows the nuclides of all known elements in increasing mass number, atomic number and neutron number. The decay data of the unstable nuclides are provided within their appropriate 'box', and patterns of decay can be traced using this chart. An example of a portion of a typical chart is shown in Figure 106.3.

THE MECHANISMS OF RADIOACTIVE DECAY

● **What are the modes of decay?**

▲ There are several forms of radioactive decay depending on the original state of the unstable nucleus, i.e. whether it is neutron deficient or proton deficient (Fig. 106.2).

Alpha decay

This occurs in very heavy elements, i.e. $Z > 83$. The unstable nucleus ejects an alpha-particle which consists of two neutrons and two protons (a helium nucleus).

The decay may be represented as

$${}^{A}_{Z}X \rightarrow {}^{A\text{-}4}_{Z\text{-}2}Y \quad \text{e.g. } {}^{238}_{92}\text{U} \rightarrow {}^{234}_{90}\text{Th}$$

Radionuclides which decay by alpha emission are not used in nuclear medicine imaging as alpha-particles are very highly ionizing and have only a very short range in tissue.

Beta minus decay

This occurs when a nucleus has too many neutrons, i.e. it is proton deficient (Fig. 106.2), and it transforms a neutron into a proton plus an electron, known as a beta minus particle (β^-), and a neutrino (ν). The total energy released is shared between the electron and the neutrino. The neutrino has no mass or charge and will not be considered further as it plays no role in nuclear medicine. The mass number remains unchanged. The decay may be described as

$$\text{n} \rightarrow \text{p} + \text{e}^- + \nu$$

This may also be represented as

$${}^{A}_{Z}X \rightarrow {}^{A}_{Z+1}Y \quad \text{e.g. } {}^{90}_{39}\text{Y} \rightarrow {}^{90}_{40}\text{Zr}$$

The daughter product is a different element to the parent, as it has an atomic number increased by 1. Beta-particles are emitted with a continuous energy spectrum ranging from zero to a maximum value depending on the radionuclide. The average energy of the beta particles is $E \sim E_{max}/3$. Beta particles have only a very short range in

54 Xe	^{124}Xe	^{125}Xe	^{126}Xe	^{127}Xe	^{128}Xe (stable)	^{129}Xe (stable)	^{130}Xe	^{131}Xe (stable)	^{132}Xe
53 I	**^{123}I** 13.2 h EC γ 159.0 ↘	**^{124}I** 4.18 d EC β^+ 2.14,1.53 ↘	**^{125}I** 60.1 d EC γ 35.5 ↘	**^{126}I**	**^{127}I** (stable)	**^{128}I**	↖ **^{129}I** 1.57×10^7 y β^- .15 γ 39.6	**^{130}I**	↖ **^{131}I** 8.04 d β^- .606,... γ 364.5,...
52 Te	^{122}Te	**^{123}Te**	**^{124}Te** (stable)	**^{125}Te**	^{126}Te (stable)	^{127}Te	^{128}Te	^{129}Te	^{130}Te

Z ↑ N →

[shaded box] stable nuclides
EC electron capture
γ gamma rays (in keV)
β^-, β^+ electron,positron decay (in MeV)

isotopes →
isotones ↑
isobars ↘

Fig. 106.3 The Chart of the Nuclides. A small section illustrating the nuclides of iodine and the decay paths of the most common iodine radioisotopes.

tissue before being absorbed and are therefore unsuitable for imaging.

Some beta-emitting radionuclides may leave the daughter nucleus in an excited energy state, and the stable state is reached by the immediate emission of one or more gamma-rays, e.g. ^{131}I. These radionuclides may be used for imaging but are not ideal because of the high radiation dose from the β^- emission.

Beta plus or positron decay

This occurs when a nucleus has too many protons, i.e it is neutron deficient (Fig. 106.2) and it transforms a proton into a neutron plus a positron (β^+), and a neutrino. The mass number A remains unchanged:

$$p \rightarrow n + e^+ + \nu$$

This may also be represented as

$$^A_Z X \rightarrow {}^A_{Z-1} Y \quad \text{e.g. } {}^{11}_{6}C \rightarrow {}^{11}_{5}B$$

Like beta-particles, positrons are emitted in a continuous spectrum up to a maximum energy. The important and recognizable feature of positron decay is **annihilation radiation**. A positron cannot exist at rest, and therefore when it has expended all its kinetic energy it combines with an electron and their mass is converted into energy in the form of two 0.511 MeV gamma-rays 180° apart. For this form of decay to occur a minimum energy of 1.022 MeV is required, any excess energy being given to the positron. As with β^- decay the daughter nucleus may have excess energy and therefore other gamma emissions, as well as the 0.511 MeV gamma-rays, may accompany positron emission. With the advent of positron emission tomography (PET) cameras the use of positron emitters in nuclear medicine has increased dramatically. The utilization of the 180° gamma-rays in coincidence counting is the backbone of the instrumentation (see Ch. 110).

Electron capture

If the nucleus does not have sufficient energy to decay by positron emission, the excess protons may be reduced by electron capture. In this case an orbital electron is 'captured' by the nucleus and a proton transforms into a neutron plus a neutrino:

$$p^+ + e^- \rightarrow n + \nu$$

This may also be represented, like the positron equation, as

$$^A_Z X \rightarrow {}^A_{Z-1} Y \quad \text{e.g. } {}^{51}_{24}Cr \rightarrow {}^{51}_{23}V$$

This leaves a vacancy in an orbital electron shell, most probably the K shell, and so characteristic X-rays will be emitted. Thus electron capture decay will be accompanied by a characteristic X-ray of the daughter radionuclide and in some cases, when excess energy is remaining, also a gamma-ray. Many radionuclides used in nuclear medicine decay by electron capture (Table 106.1). The characteristic X-ray energies increase with the mass number A of the nuclide, e.g. the X-rays characteristic of vanadium resulting from the decay of ^{51}Cr are only 5 keV and are undetectable, whereas those characteristic of mercury resulting from the decay of ^{201}Tl range from 68 to 80 keV and are used in gamma-camera imaging. The 27 keV characteristic X-ray produced in the decay of ^{125}I is used for 'in vitro' counting.

Table 106.1 Radionuclides used in nuclear medicine which decay by electron capture

Radionuclide	Principal gamma emissions (keV) and useable characteristic X-rays ( )
^{51}Cr	320
^{57}Co	122, 136
^{67}Ga	93, 185, 300
^{111}In	171, 245
^{123}I	159
^{125}I	35.5 (27)
^{201}Tl	167 (68–80)

Internal conversion

This form of decay occurs when a radionuclide, rather than emitting a gamma-ray, transfers its energy to an orbital electron which is ejected instead of the gamma-ray. Characteristic X-rays or Auger electrons follow internal conversion. Unlike β^- decay, conversion electrons have discrete energies. This decay process is important in radiation dosimetry calculations.

● **What is the meaning of the 'm' in the symbol ^{99m}Tc?**

▲ Technetium-99m decays by **isomeric transition**. When a nucleus decays by beta emission the daughter nucleus is often left in an excited state with the immediate emission of a gamma-ray. The excited state may, however, exist for a measurable time, and the decay process is then considered as two separate events, the excited daughter nucleus decaying by isomeric transition from a metastable state. This metastable state is indicated by adding an m to the mass number. The great advantage of this form of decay for nuclear medicine imaging studies is the availability of a gamma-emitting radionuclide which emits only gamma-rays, thus reducing the radiation dose to the patient.

^{99m}Tc, with a half-life of 6 hours, is produced in a generator (see Ch. 110) from the parent ^{99}Mo, a beta-emitter

Table 106.2 Metastable radionuclides which have been used in nuclear medicine

Parent	$t_{1/2}$	Daughter	$t_{1/2}$
^{113}Sn	120 d	^{113m}In	100 min
^{81}Rb	4.6 h	^{81m}Kr	13.3 s
^{87}Y	80 h	^{87m}Sr	2.8 h
^{195m}Hg	40 h	^{195m}Ag	30.6 s
^{191}Os	15 d	^{191m}Ir	4.96 s

with a 66 hour half-life. There are other clinically useful metastable radionuclides (Table 106.2).

● What are radionuclide decay schemes?

▲ It is helpful to illustrate the decay of a radionuclide diagramatically. This is called a decay scheme. The rules for drawing a decay scheme are:

- The parent and daughter nuclei are identified as broad horizontal lines.
- β^- decay is shown by a diagonal line going from left to right, i.e. $Z+1$.
  β^+, electron capture and alpha decay are shown by a diagonal line going from right to left, i.e. $Z-1$, $Z-2$.
- Excited energy states are represented by horizontal lines.
- Vertical lines between the energy levels indicate the gamma-rays emitted.

Simplified decay schemes for some routine nuclear medicine radionuclides are shown in Figure 106.4. Everything a physician needs to know for clinical use is highlighted in these diagrams, and the useable characteristic X-rays have also been added. Complete information on the decay of a wide range of radionuclides used in nuclear medicine are provided in the MIRD data.[1]

● What are the differences between X-rays and gamma-rays?

▲ X-rays and gamma-rays have exactly the same properties; they differ only in their origin. X-rays come from the atomic structure outside the nucleus and are produced by excitation and ionization of electrons in the atom, whereas gamma-rays are produced from excess energy in the nucleus of the atom. Gamma-rays are emitted from the excited nucleus with discrete energies from well-defined energy levels and are characteristic of the particular radionuclide decaying. In many cases a series of gamma-rays are emitted. X-rays are emitted in a continuous spectrum which may have characteristic X-rays superimposed, with discrete energy states (from K, L, M shells) for different elements.

● How is radioactive decay determined and quantified?

▲ The decay of a radioactive nuclide is a random process. The radioactive atoms decay spontaneously and it is not possible to predict precisely the time when a radioactive nucleus will transform into a more stable nucleus. Only the probability of disintegration in a particular time can be stated. The probable rate of decay at any time is proportional to the number of atoms present at that time. The decay process can therefore be characterized by a decay constant λ, which is the fractional loss per unit time.

If there are N radioactive atoms present it can be stated that the rate of decay is dN/dt, where dN radioactive atoms are decaying in a small time interval dt. This is known as the radioactivity A.

$$A = dN/dt = -\lambda N$$

The minus sign indicates that N is decreasing.

Rearranging this equation

$$dN/N = -\lambda dt$$

Integrating from $_0$ t$_0$ t

$$\ln N_t - \ln N_0 = -\lambda t \quad (1)$$

Taking exponentials

$$N_t = N_0 e^{-\lambda t}$$

Since $A_0 = -\lambda N_0$ and $A_t = -\lambda N_t$ then

$$A_t = A_0 e^{-\lambda t} \quad (2)$$

Remembering that decay is a random process, radioactivity is actually an average decay rate.

● What is meant by the SI units of radioactivity?

▲ SI units are the units of radioactivity now used in most countries. They replace the Curie system. The SI unit of **radioactivity** is the **becquerel (Bq)**:

1 Bq = 1 disintegration per second

(1 curie = 3.7×10^{10} Bq)

Radioactivity administered for diagnostic nuclear medicine is in the **MBq** (10^6 Bq) range, and for therapy in the **GBq** (10^9 Bq) range.

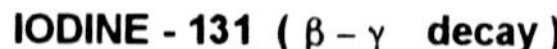

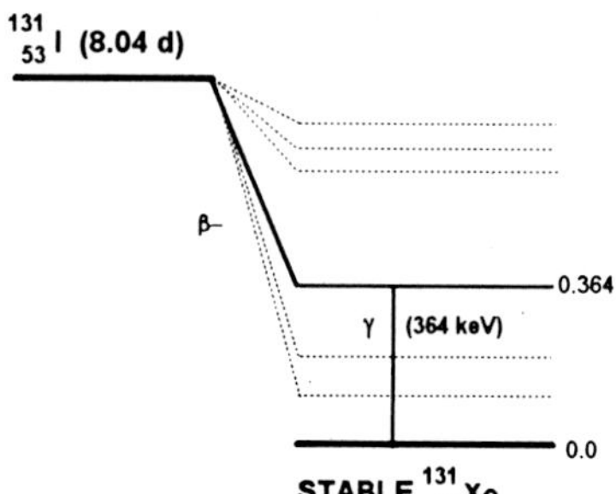

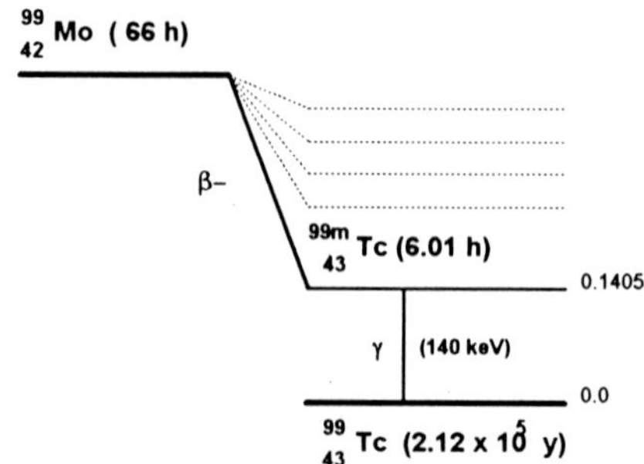

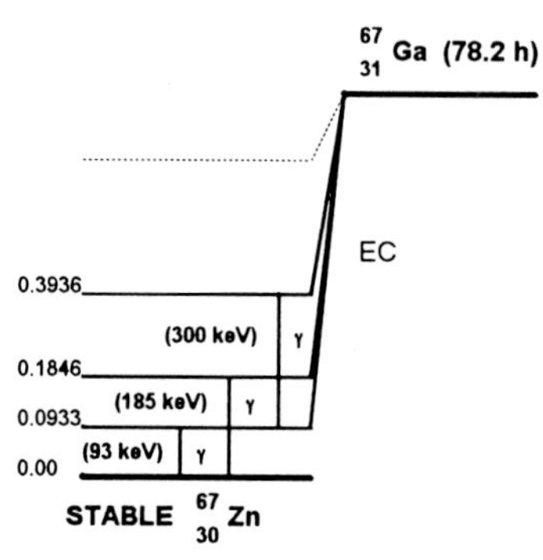

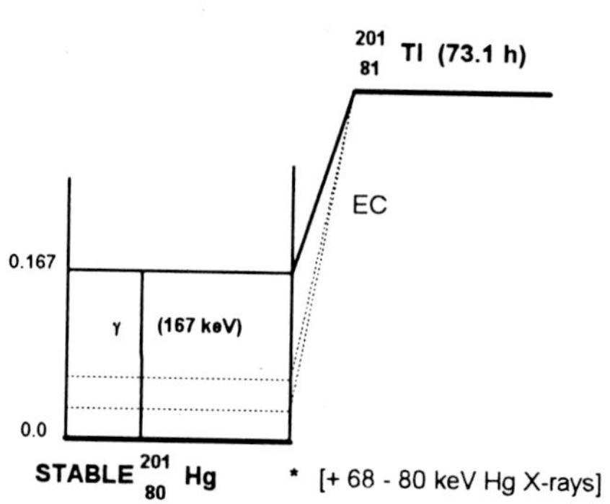

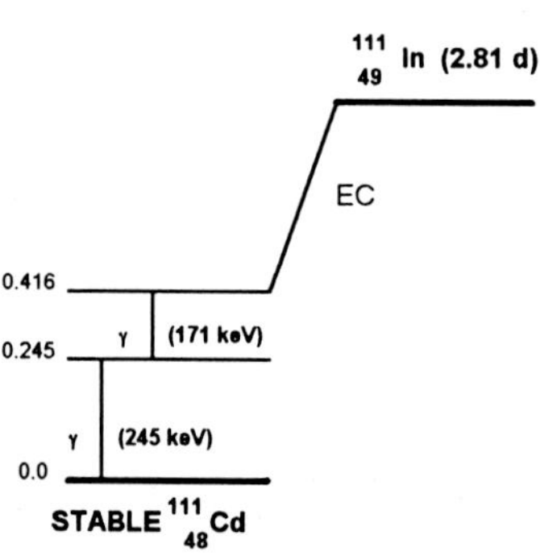

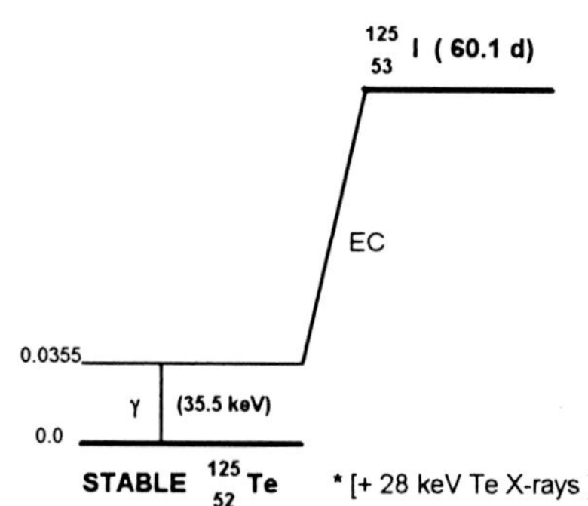

Fig. 106.4 Decay schemes of common nuclear medicine radionuclides. Only the most important and useful decay paths are shown. The clinically useful characteristic X-rays have been added to the schema.

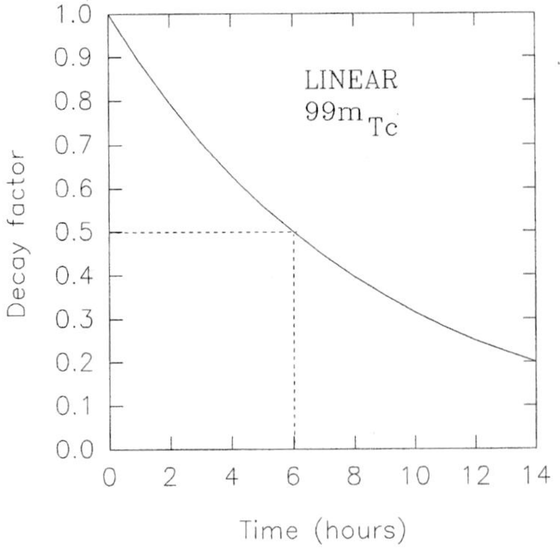

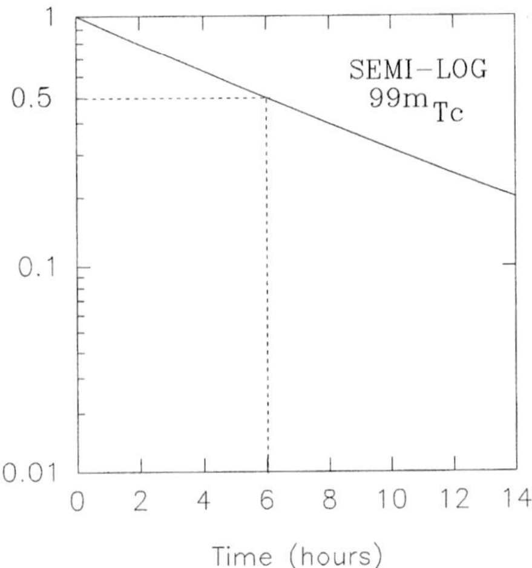

Fig. 106.5 Graphical measurement of the physical half-life of ^{99m}Tc showing linear and semilogarithmic plots.

● What is meant by 'half-life' and how is it determined?

▲ The half-life of a radionuclide is the period over which half the atoms will disintegrate. It is unique for each radionuclide. Using the decay equation (eqn 2)

$$A_o/2 = A_o\, e^{-\lambda t_{1/2}}$$
$$1/2 = e^{-\lambda t_{1/2}}$$
$$\ln(1/2) = -\ln(2) = -\lambda t_{1/2}$$
$$\text{or } 0.693 = \lambda t_{1/2}$$
$$\lambda = 0.693/t_{1/2} \quad (3)$$

This can be drawn graphically either by using a linear x–y scale, which produces an exponential curve, or by converting the y-axis to a logarithmic scale, which produces a straight line (Fig. 106.5). This is explained by studying the decay equation (eqn 1), which can be written as

$$\ln A_t = -\lambda t + \ln A_o$$

which takes the form of the straight line equation $y = mx + c$, where λ equals the slope m and A_o the y-axis intercept c. This is the quickest and simplest way to determine the fraction of decay over a time period provided the half-life is known. If the original activity is known then the amount present at any time may be determined.

● Is a correction for radioactive decay necessary in clinical studies?

▲ When performing quantitative analysis on a patient study over a period of time, it may be necessary to correct for the physical decay of the radionuclide so that the values obtained only represent the physiological changes present. The importance of decay correction depends on the half-life of the radionuclide being used and the duration of the study. When short acquisition times are involved, such as first-pass studies with ^{99m}Tc radionuclides, then decay correction is unnecessary. However with quantitative studies taking several hours using ^{99m}Tc, decay correction is essential. Quantitative studies taking several days and involving radionuclides such as ^{67}Ga, ^{201}Tl and ^{131}I require decay correction.

This may be done by using the decay equation (eqn 2) and substituting for λ (eqn 3):

$$A_t = A_o e^{-0.693t/t_{\frac{1}{2}}}$$

The counts A_t at a known time t post injection must be determined (this could be from an area of interest on a camera image, or blood samples counted in an autogamma-counter). Because A_t, $t_{1/2}$ and t are known, A_o may be calculated. The changing counts A_t would be corrected for each time period t since the start of the study.

● What is specific activity and why is it relevant?

▲ Specific activity is the ratio of radionuclide activity to total **mass** of the element or compound present. Examples of the units used are: kBq/μg, MBq/mg, GBq/g.

The highest possible specific activity is the 'carrier-free' specific activity, when all the atoms or molecules present are radioactive, i.e. there is no stable tracer present. Most radionuclides used in nuclear medicine are in this category because a high specific activity is desirable so that the mass of element or compound present does not cause any physiological change to the system – the essential requirement of a 'tracer' study.

Specific activity should not be confused with specific concentration, which is the ratio of radionuclide activity to total **volume** of the compound, e.g. MBq/ml.

Knowledge of the exact amount of a particular chemical or drug given to the patient is essential as the toxicity of the drug is dependent on the amount administered. The distribution of a radiochemical in a biological system may also depend on the amount of carrier present. Specific activity is calculated for a given radioactivity are as follows.

Calculation of specific activity of ^{99m}Tc

Radioactivity is defined by the decay equation:

$$A = dN/dt = -\lambda N$$

where A is the activity in disintegrations per second (becquerels), N is the number of atoms present and λ is the decay constant.

One gram of an element contains $6.02 \times 10^{23}/W$ atoms (6.02×10^{23} = Avogadro's number, W = atomic weight of the element in grams). The number of becquerels in 1 g of a pure radionuclide is

$$\lambda(6.02 \times 10^{23})/W$$

$$= (0.693/t_{1/2})(6.02 \times 10^{23})/W$$

$$= 4.17 \times 10^{23}/t_{1/2} W \text{ Bq/g}$$

For a typical patient administered radioactivity of 370 MBq of ^{99m}Tc ($W = 99$; $t_{1/2} = 6$ h $= 2.16 \times 10^4$s), the amount of carrier-free ^{99m}Tc is therefore

$$\frac{(370 \times 10^6) \times (2.16 \times 10^4) \times 99}{4.17 \times 10^{23}} = \sim 2 \text{ ng}$$

Thus, the specific activity is 185 MBq/ng or 185 GBq/μg.

THE MECHANISMS FOR THE DETECTION OF RADIATION IN NUCLEAR MEDICINE

● How does radiation interact with matter?

▲ The interaction of different radiations with matter, such as particulate radiation, i.e alpha- and beta-particles, and non-particulate radiation, i.e. photons or gamma-rays, plays a vital role in the detection and measurement of radiation in nuclear medicine. These interactions determine the design of all instrumentation for patient use, patient safety and laboratory procedures, and they determine the need for radiation protection procedures as they are the means by which radiation dose is delivered to tissue. Ionizing radiation is so named because interaction with matter results in electrons being ejected from atoms causing ion pairs.

The two types of interaction must be considered separately as the particulate radiation causes primary ionization only, whereas the high-energy electrons, resulting from gamma-ray interactions, cause indirect or secondary ionization.

● What are the important interactions of particulate radiation with matter?

▲ **Alpha-particles** lose energy by ionizing the matter through which they travel. They lose energy rapidly because of their high mass, therefore their range is very small, e.g. a 5 MeV alpha particle has a range of ~ 4.0 cm in air and ~ 0.05 mm in tissue. They are highly ionizing owing to their double charge. The number of ion pairs produced per millimetre is defined as the **specific ionization**. Because alpha-particles have high specific ionization, thus causing high radiation dose if ingested, they play no role in nuclear medicine imaging. They may, however, have a role in therapy.

Beta-particles interact with matter in a similar way to alpha-particles, but because they are much lighter and have only a single charge they can penetrate further before absorption, e.g. a 1 MeV beta-particle has a range in air of ~ 300 cm and in tissue of ~ 0.4 cm. The specific ionization of beta-particles is in the order of 100 times less than alpha-particles.

Bremsstrahlung electromagnetic radiation is caused by high-energy beta-particles passing through the electric field of a nucleus. The electron is deflected and loses energy by radiation, giving a continuous X-ray spectrum. The intensity of bremsstrahlung radiation (braking radiation) is proportional to the square of the atomic number of the absorber. This is why high atomic number (Z) materials such as tungsten are used in X-ray tubes, to produce a high X-ray yield. Also low-Z materials such as plastic and glass are used to shield beta-emitting radionuclides to minimize the bremsstrahlung radiation.

● Why are beta-emitters such as phosphorus-32 and yttrium-90 unsuitable for nuclear medicine imaging studies?

▲ Phosphorus-32 and yttrium-90 decay by pure beta emission. This means that they have very short penetrating power of only millimetres in tissue before depositing all their energy and causing ionization. The patient will receive a high radiation dose and external detection can only be achieved by measuring the bremsstrahlung radiation produced, which has a wide energy range, and therefore only a blurred very low resolution image is achieved on a gamma-camera. It is important to note however that ^{32}P and ^{90}Y are used for therapeutic purposes, as the radiation dose from the absorption of the beta-particles has a high probability of killing cancer cells. ^{90}Y is also used for radionuclide synovectomy (see Ch. 88). ^{131}I is also used therapeutically (see Ch. 72) because it is a beta-emitter and also has the added advantage of producing gamma-rays, which can be detected externally. ^{131}I has been used for nuclear medicine imaging in the past, mainly for thyroid and renal imaging, but has now been replaced by technetium-labelled products in order to reduce the radiation dose to the patient. Unfortunately, many radionuclides of biological interest are pure beta-emitters, e.g. ^{3}H, ^{14}C, and cannot be used for imaging because of their high absorption. They are used, however, for 'in vitro' studies using liquid scintillation counting.

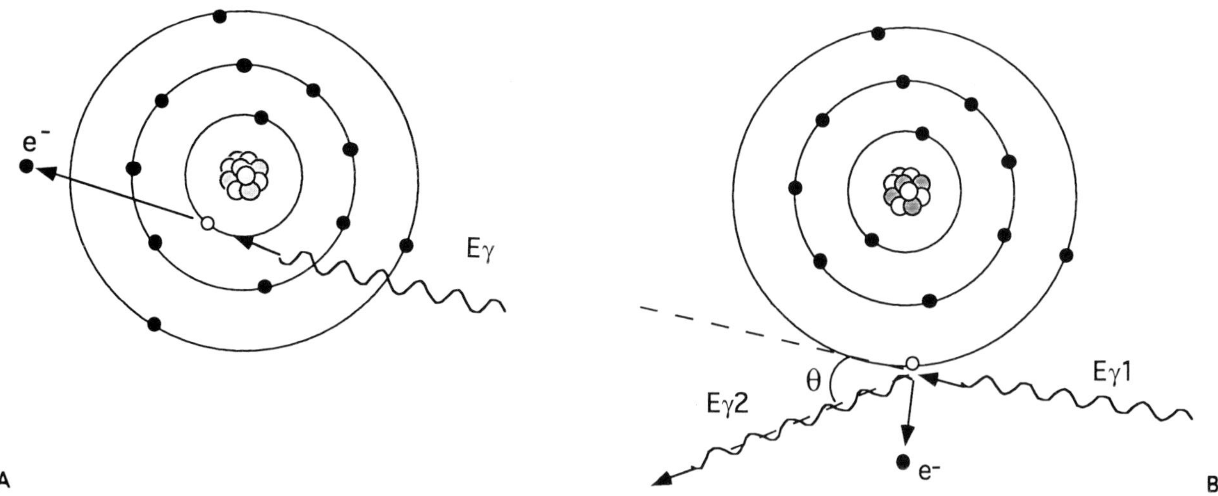

Fig. 106.6 Interaction of gamma rays with matter. (A) Photoelectric effect. (B) Compton scattering.

● **What are the important interactions of gamma-rays with matter?**

▲ The two most important interactions of gamma-rays with matter, in the energy range associated with nuclear medicine, are the **photoelectric effect** and **Compton scattering**. As the physical principles of imaging are progressively described it will become evident that these two interactions play key roles. The photoelectric effect predominates in the design of the instrumentation, and at the gamma-ray energies used in nuclear medicine Compton scattering is the predominant interaction in tissue. Compton scattering is a source of error in the absolute quantification of SPECT, and much research is being carried out in this field.

Photoelectric effect

In this interaction the atom absorbs all of the gamma-ray energy and the energy is then used to eject an electron from the atom. This electron, from an inner shell and called a photoelectron, has an energy equal to the gamma-ray energy minus the binding energy of the electron shell (Fig. 106.6A). The number of photoelectrons produced is related to the atomic number (Z) of the absorbing material and the energy (E) of the incident gamma-ray ($\alpha\ Z^3/E^3$). This is one of the reasons why sodium iodide ($Z = 53$) is used as the detector in nuclear medicine instrumentation. It also explains why radionuclides with very low-energy gamma-rays may not be used for external detection as the gamma-rays will be stopped in tissue primarily by the photoelectric effect, causing unnecessary radiation dose to the patient. As the energy of the gamma-ray increases the role of the photoelectric effect decreases.

Compton scattering

Compton scattering occurs when the incident gamma-ray collides with an outer shell electron of the atom. Only a portion of the incident gamma-ray energy ($E_{\gamma 1}$) is given to the electron, called the recoil electron, and a reduced energy gamma-ray ($E_{\gamma 2}$) is scattered at an angle θ (Fig. 106.6B). The energy of the scattered gamma-ray is given by the equation

$$E_{\gamma 2} = E_{\gamma 1}/[1 + (E_{\gamma 1}/0.511)(1-\cos\theta)]\ \text{MeV}$$

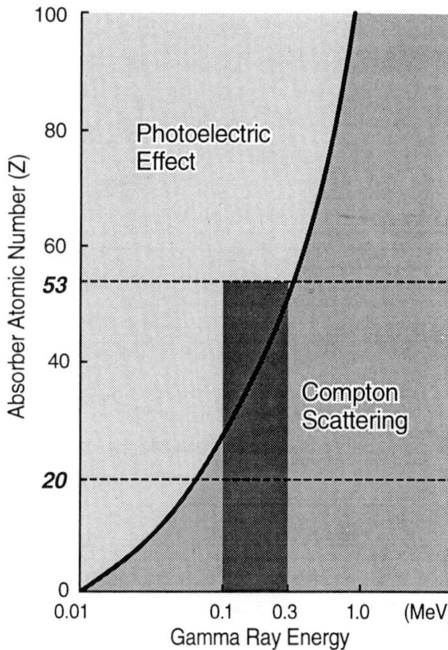

Fig. 106.7 Absorber atomic number (Z) versus gamma-ray energy, showing the most probable interactions in the nuclear medicine imaging energy range ~ 100–300 keV. Tissue ($Z \leq 20$) and sodium iodide (Z=53) atomic numbers are highlighted, showing Compton scatter to be the predominant interaction in tissue and the photoelectric effect in the sodium iodide detector.

The energy of the recoil electron, E_{e1}, is given by

$$E_{e1} = E_{\gamma 1} - E_{\gamma 2}$$

The maximum recoil electron energy occurs when the gamma-ray is scattered at 180°, i.e. backscattered. The minimum recoil electron energy is at a scattering angle of near zero. At low gamma-ray energies the energy received by the recoil electron is very small regardless of scattering angle, but this recoil energy increases as the incident gamma-ray energy increases. The varying scattered gamma-ray energies play an important role in the elimination of Compton-scattered gamma-rays in nuclear medicine imaging, e.g. ^{99m}Tc, with an incident energy of 140 keV, has a maximum recoil electron energy of 49.0 keV and minimum scattered gamma-ray energy of 91.0 keV. It is important to remember that multiple Compton scattering may occur as a gamma-ray passes through matter and as the scattered gamma-ray loses its energy it may eventually be absorbed by the photoelectric effect. This is an important consideration in the design of imaging instrumentation, as the inclusion of Compton-scattered gamma-rays in the detection process reduces the resolution of the final image.

● How are gamma-rays attenuated in different materials?

▲ The attenuation of gamma-rays in tissue and in detector material is one of the determining factors for the selection of particular radionuclides for nuclear medicine imaging. If the gamma-ray has a very low energy it will not penetrate tissue and will be totally absorbed by the photoelectric effect. This means that the patient will receive a high radiation dose and no gamma-rays will be transmitted through the patient in order to produce an image. As the energy of a gamma-ray increases, Compton scattering will become the predominant interaction in tissue. Gamma-rays will be detected externally, but because of the Compton process they will have lost energy and will have been deflected from their original path, introducing an uncertainty in the detection of the original event's location. As the energy increases further some of the gamma-rays of a particular energy will penetrate the tissue without absorption or scatter, and it is these gamma-rays which are optimal for imaging.

In the detector, however, high absorption is required, and therefore the photoelectric effect is the most desirable interaction, hence the use of sodium iodide. As the energy of the incident gamma-ray striking the detector increases, Compton scatter may occur and these gamma-rays of reduced energy may not be detected, unless the gamma-ray is eventually totally absorbed by the photoelectric effect. More gamma-rays may be absorbed by increasing the detector thickness, but loss of resolution will then occur. In summary, the photoelectric interaction is unacceptable in the patient but essential in the detector. Compton scatter in the patient and detector causes loss of sensitivity and resolution. However, it cannot be avoided at the energies used in nuclear medicine imaging. Figure 106.7 illustrates the relative frequency with which the photoelectric effect and Compton scatter occur with increasing absorber atomic number *Z* and increasing gamma-ray energy.

● Why is a radionuclide with a photon energy less than 70 keV unsuitable for gamma-camera imaging?

▲ The low keV means that the predominant interaction of the gamma-rays in tissue will be the photoelectric effect. A very high percentage of the gamma-rays will be absorbed in the tissue or Compton scattered, and therefore few unscattered gamma-rays will be available for external detection. This is not a problem in 'in vitro' small-sample gamma counting, and much lower energy radionuclides, such as ^{125}I with a 35 keV gamma-ray, are used routinely for radioimmunoassay work.

● Why are radionuclides with energies in the range 100–200 keV considered the most suitable for gamma-camera imaging?

▲ The energy range 100–200 keV is deemed the most suitable for imaging a patient with a gamma-camera for two reasons. Firstly, the energy is high enough that a large percentage of the gamma-rays can penetrate the tissue without being absorbed by the photoelectric effect or be Compton scattered (the intensity of a beam of 140 keV gamma-rays is reduced by half by approximately 5 cm of tissue). Figure 106.7 highlights that if an interaction with tissue does take place the predominant interaction in this energy range is Compton scatter. Secondly, in this energy range the unscattered gamma-rays that leave the patient and reach the sodium iodide detector of the gamma-camera are stopped predominantly by the photoelectric effect or by multiple Compton scattering followed by photoelectric absorption.

● Why is technetium-99m used for the majority of nuclear medicine imaging studies?

▲ Technetium-99m is considered an ideal radionuclide for nuclear medicine because:

- It is a **pure gamma emitter**. The radiation dose to the patient is therefore reduced compared with particulate emissions.
- It has a short physical **half-life of 6 h**. The majority of nuclear medicine studies are performed in less than 4 h. The use of radionuclides with half-lives much greater than the required scanning time

increases the radiation dose to the patient unnecessarily.

- It has a gamma-ray **energy of 140 keV**. Gamma-cameras perform most efficiently with gamma-ray energies between 100 and 200 keV.
- It is **carrier free**, i.e. there is no stable isotope of the element present. 37 GBq of ^{99m}Tc weighs less than 1 μg. Most patient doses are less than 1 GBq, therefore the amount injected is in the nanogram range.
- It can be **produced cheaply** in large volume from a generator in a nuclear medicine department.
- It can exist in various **valency states**, thus allowing the preparation of a wide range of radiopharmaceuticals.

● How is radioactivity accurately measured before administration to a patient?

▲ Gamma-radiation may be detected either by the conversion of energy to light, as in the sodium iodide crystal or by ionization which produces positive and negative ion pairs. Ionization is used in the design of most **dose calibrators**, the instruments used to ensure that the correct amount of radioactivity is administered to the patient. The dose calibrator comprises an ionization chamber to measure the radiation by virtue of the number of ion pairs produced. An electrometer measures the electric current produced which, for a particular energy of radiation, is directly proportional to the radioactivity being measured. Detector efficiency varies with the energy and number of gamma-rays emitted. Unlike a sodium iodide detector, there is no energy discrimination in an ionization chamber and therefore the dose calibrator must be calibrated for all the radionuclides to be measured. The radioactivity in the vial or syringe is then provided directly on a digital readout in units of becquerels or curies.

FURTHER READING

There are a variety of textbooks dedicated to the basic physics of nuclear medicine and, in particular, the interested reader may find more detailed information in Sorenson & Phelps.[2]

REFERENCES

1. Weber D A, Eckerman K F, Dillman L T, Ryman J C 1989 MIRD: radionuclide data and decay schemes. The Society of Nuclear Medicine, New York
2. Sorenson J A, Phelps M E 1987 Physics in nuclear medicine, 2nd edn. Grune & Stratton, Orlando

107. Nuclear medicine imaging instrumentation

Stefan Eberl   Robert E. Zimmerman

THE GAMMA-CAMERA

● What is a gamma-camera?

▲ The gamma-camera was first developed by Anger in 1958[1] and is now almost exclusively used for all single photon nuclear medicine imaging. While the size and shape of the detector and electronic processing of signals have altered since its inception, the basic components and principles of the gamma-camera have changed little over that time. It consists of a detector mounted on a gantry for easy positioning close to the patient and an electronic processing console. The gamma-camera is now usually either connected to or incorporates a computer for further image processing and display.

It is important to note that, unlike X-ray machines, gamma-cameras do not emit any ionizing radiation, but merely detect radiation emitted from the patient or other sources. An introduction to the gamma-camera is given in this section. For further reading, references 2 and 3 or other textbooks on nuclear medicine instrumentation are recommended.

● How does a gamma-camera work?

▲ The gamma-camera consists of two main functional units, the detector and the processing electronics. The detector is responsible for the primary detection of the gamma-rays and contains the scintillation crystal, photomultiplier (PM) tubes and preamplifiers. The detector is well shielded from stray radiation and is mounted on a stand for optimum positioning with respect to the organ being imaged. Shielding of the detector is usually fabricated from lead or tungsten, which means that all movements must be either motor driven or counterbalanced because of the weight involved. The processing electronics may be located within the detector or in an associated console and consists of signal-processing circuits, pulse height analysis circuitry and the display system. It is now common to include digital image processing in the console, allowing much of the operations and settings of the gamma-camera to be controlled from a single keyboard.

The simplified block diagram of a gamma-camera (Fig. 107.1) demonstrates its basic components and

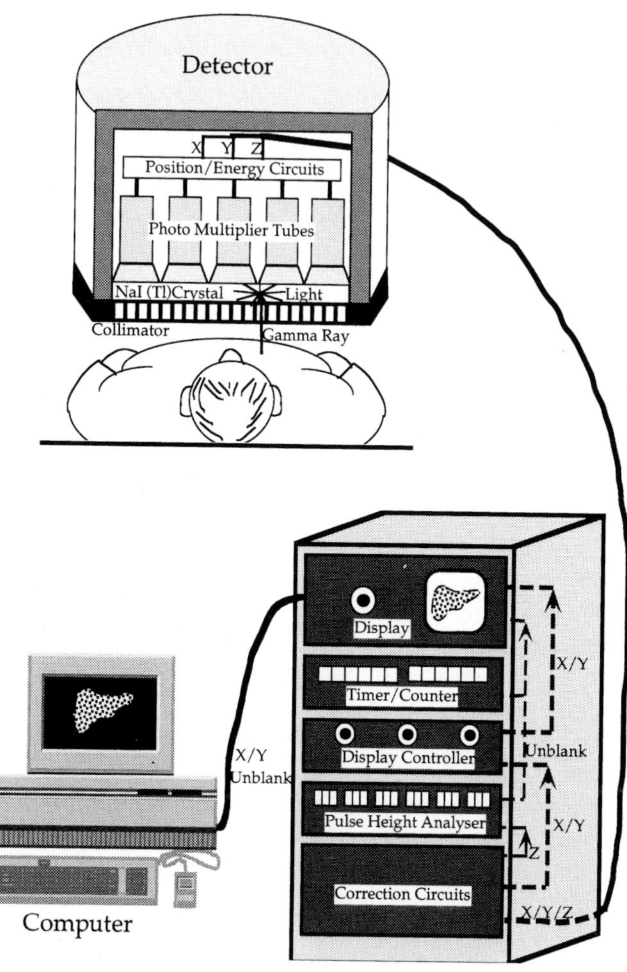

Fig. 107.1 Block diagram showing the main components of a gamma-camera for detecting, processing and imaging gamma-rays emanating from the patient. In this diagram, the imaging computer is shown as an add-on to the basic gamma-camera. However, the computer is now frequently integrated directly into the gamma-camera.

principle of operation. A detailed description of the various components is given below. However, overall the detection of gamma-rays and their display proceeds as follows: gamma-rays emitted by the patient and which pass through the collimator are converted into light by the NaI(Tl) crystal. The **photomultiplier (PM) tubes** convert the light into electrical signals which are fed into the position/energy circuitry which produce the X and Y position signals and the Z (energy) signal. The X and Y signals give the coordinate position of the gamma-ray interaction in the crystal, while the size of the Z or energy signal is proportional to the energy of the gamma-ray. These signals are further processed by the correction circuits to remove inherent, systematic distortions. The **pulse height analyser (PHA)** analyses the height of the Z signal to generate the unblank signal whenever the detected gamma-ray energy is within a selected range. Image rotation, magnification, etc. can be selected by the display controller and its X/Y outputs are fed together with the unblank pulse from the PHA to the cathode ray tube (CRT), which displays the detected gamma-ray at the appropriate position on its screen. The X, Y and unblank signals are also usually connected to a built-in or, as shown in Figure 107.1, an external digital computer for further processing and display.

Collimator

Gamma-rays are difficult to control. They have no electrical charge and thus cannot be deflected using electric or magnetic fields. While they are in the electromagnetic spectrum, their energy is too high to be reflected or focused like visible light. However, they can be attenuated through absorption or scatter, and this process is utilized in the collimator. The collimator consists of channels through which gamma-rays can pass and which are separated by lead septa. Only gamma-rays travelling within the narrow solid angle of acceptance of the collimator holes can pass unhindered through the channels to the detector. Other photons will be attenuated (absorbed/scattered) by the collimator septa. Thus the gamma-rays reaching the crystal will form a planar projection of the isotope distribution within the organ being imaged. Note, however, that gamma-photons scattered either within the patient or the collimator can still reach the crystal. These scattered photons can blur and degrade the image. As energy is lost through scattering, contributions of scattered radiation to the image can be reduced by discriminating against lower energy photons with the pulse height analyser.

Collimators play a very important part in the final image quality achieved. They are very inefficient devices, with only a small fraction (typically around 0.02%) of the gamma-rays emitted from the patient reaching the detector crystal. Collimator design is a compromise between **efficiency (sensitivity)** and the accuracy with which the spatial origin of the gamma-ray can be determined, i.e. the **resolution** of the collimator. The solid angle of acceptance increases with increasing channel diameter or decreasing channel length, and hence the collimator's sensitivity will increase. However, at the same time its resolution will worsen. Conversely, improvements in resolution are usually gained at the expense of sensitivity.

While the sensitivity of the collimator as a function of distance is fairly constant, its resolution degrades with increasing distance. It is thus important to have the organ being imaged as close as possible to the collimator. The thickness of the lead septum is governed by the maximum gamma-ray energy to be used with the collimator. Thicker septa are required to adequately attenuate higher energy gamma-rays. However, the efficiency and/or the resolution degrade with thicker septa.

The parallel-hole collimator shown in Figure 107.2 provides a direct projection of the organ activity distribution onto the crystal without any magnification or reduction in size. However, other collimator constructions are possible which can magnify or reduce the image to allow better visualization of small organs or to allow large organs to be imaged with a relatively small detector. Some of these collimators are illustrated in Figure 107.3, including the converging, diverging and pinhole collimators.

Collimators are not adaptable to different energy ranges and resolution/sensitivity compromises, thus it is necessary to acquire several different types to suit a range of applications. Parallel-hole collimators are currently used for most nuclear medicine studies. Parallel-hole collimators available include a range of low-energy collimators such as high-resolution, general-purpose, high-sensitivity, ultra-

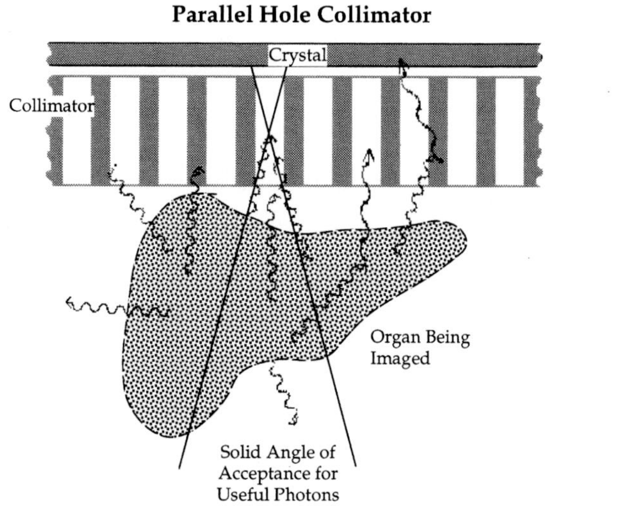

Parallel Hole Collimator

Crystal

Collimator

Organ Being Imaged

Solid Angle of Acceptance for Useful Photons

Fig. 107.2 Image formation with a parallel-hole collimator. The solid angle of acceptance determines which gamma-rays can reach the detector and hence determines the resolution and sensitivity of the collimator. Smaller angles of acceptance provide improved resolution, but at the expense of sensitivity. Note that unwanted gamma-rays scattered in either the patient or collimator can reach the detection crystal in addition to the desirable primary photons.

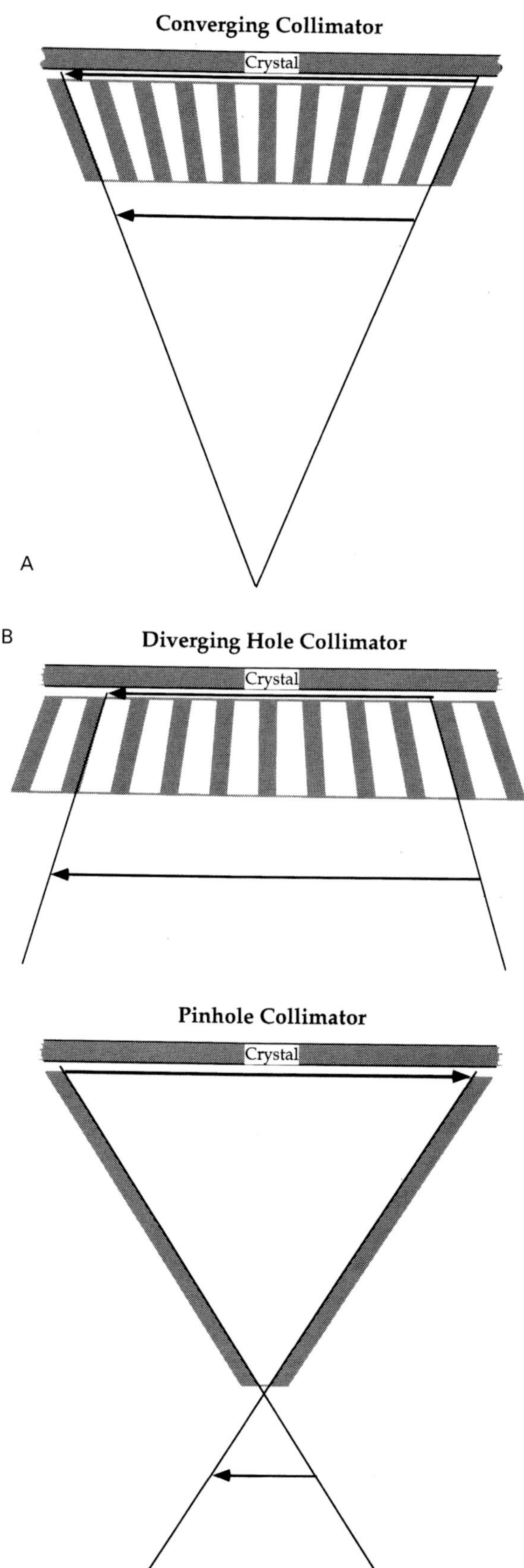

high-resolution collimators as well as medium- and high-energy collimators. With the widespread availability of large field of view (≥ 40 cm) gamma-cameras, diverging collimators are now only used in special cases. Pinhole collimators can provide the best resolution and image definition for small organs. However, their sensitivity is typically rather poor. Further, magnification changes with distance from the collimator, which can result in distortion for organs with appreciable thickness. There are also other types of specialized collimators available such as fan and cone beam collimators. These are specifically designed for brain and heart tomographic studies.

NaI(Tl) detector crystal

The object of the scintillation crystal is to convert the gamma-photons into light. A single sodium iodide crystal (NaI) is almost exclusively used in all gamma-cameras. The sodium iodide crystal is normally doped with a small amount of thallium (Tl) to increase the light production at room temperature. It has a high atomic weight (Z=53) and is relatively dense, therefore it has good stopping power for the gamma-ray energies used in nuclear medicine. The energy of the gamma-rays is converted to light in the blue to ultraviolet range of the spectrum. The number of light photons produced is directly proportional to the energy of the gamma-ray, with typically 30 photons being produced per keV of incident gamma-rays. Thus, for the 140 keV gamma rays from ^{99m}Tc, the most frequently used isotope for nuclear medicine studies, approximately 4200 light photons are produced.

The size of the crystal determines the field of view of the gamma-camera. Crystals range in diameter from about 25 cm to 50 cm. Rectangular crystals up to a size of about 60 cm by 38 cm are also available. The thickness of the crystal ranges from about 6 mm to 13 mm, with the most popular thickness being about 9.5 mm. Sensitivity tends to increase with increasing crystal thickness, particularly for the higher energy gamma-photons. However, as with the collimators, increasing thickness tends to degrade resolution, thus again a compromise is taken. The crystal is hygroscopic and thus has to be hermetically sealed against moisture, which would otherwise destroy the properties of the crystal. This is achieved by enclosing the crystal in a thin aluminium case with an optical window between the crystal and PM tubes. The crystal is very fragile and

Fig. 107.3 (left) Non-parallel-hole collimator configurations. (A) The converging collimator can be used to magnify a small organ to use more of the available detector area and hence improve resolution. (B) The diverging hole collimator allows large organs to be completely imaged with relatively small detectors. (C) The pinhole collimator has only a single hole and again provides magnification of small organs. The best resolution can be achieved with this collimator, but at the expense of sensitivity. Note that with these three collimators, image size changes as a function of distance, which can introduce distortions when imaging large organs.

should not be subjected to either thermal or mechanical shock.

Photomultiplier tubes

The purpose of the photomultiplier tube is to detect the light generated in the crystal and convert it into an amplified electrical signal. It consists of a photocathode, a string of dynodes and an anode all encased in an evacuated glass envelope. When the light photons from the crystal hit the photocathode, electrons are emitted through the photoelectric effect. The number of electrons emitted is proportional to the number of light photons reaching the photocathode. The dynodes are at positive potentials with respect to the photocathode, and thus the negatively charged photoelectrons will be accelerated towards the first dynode, releasing a larger number of secondary electrons. These are then accelerated through the other dynode stages, with an increasing number of electrons being released at each stage until about 1 million times as many electrons appear at the anode as started at the cathode. These electrons can be detected as a flow of current and can be converted into a time-varying voltage that is proportional to the energy of the absorbed gamma-ray.

Position/energy circuits

The light photons produced by a single gamma-ray interaction in the crystal are detected by several PM tubes in the vicinity of the interaction. The amount of light reaching a particular PM tube, and hence its electrical output signal, is determined by its distance from the gamma-ray interaction point in the crystal. From the relative output of the PM tubes and their position, the location of the gamma-ray interaction in the crystal can be estimated with an accuracy much greater than the physical size of the PM tubes. This estimation of positions is usually performed with a position-weighted network of resistors or capacitors connected to the PM tube outputs. The value of the resistors or capacitors is related to the position of the corresponding PM tube on the surface of the crystal. The position network produces X and Y position signals which are proportional to the X and Y position coordinate, respectively, of the gamma-ray interaction in the crystal.

The summation of the PM tube outputs provides an energy or Z signal which is proportional to the total light produced and hence the energy of the gamma-ray. To increase the accuracy of both the position and energy signals, only PM tubes in the vicinity of the gamma-ray interaction are allowed to contribute to its position and energy signals. This avoids noise from PM tubes at a large distance adversely affecting the accuracy of the signal.

Correction circuits

There are a number of factors which affect the efficiency of the light detection. PM tubes have a rather non-uniform response to light as a function of position across their entry windows. The efficiency of converting light to electrical signals can also vary between PM tubes, despite careful matching and adjustment. Light production and collection in the crystal can vary as a function of position. These and other factors can all introduce systematic errors in the position and energy signals. A correction map of these errors is generated and stored in the correction module by imaging sources at known locations and intensities. These corrections are then subsequently applied to all position and energy signals to produce an undistorted image. This is illustrated in Figure 107.4, which demonstrates the severe non-uniformities being introduced by positioning errors which are successfully eliminated by the position correction circuits.

Pulse height analyser

As mentioned previously, scatter as well as primary gamma-photons can reach the crystal and are detected. Inclusion of scattered photons causes a loss of resolution and contrast in the image, and it is thus desirable to exclude them as much as possible from the image. When gamma-rays are scattered, they lose some of their energy, with the exact amount of energy lost being a function of the scatter angle. The larger the angle through which gamma-rays are scattered, the larger the energy loss. Thus it is possible to exclude at least some of the scattered photons by only accepting gamma-rays above a certain energy threshold. This task is performed by the pulse height analyser, which only produces an output signal if the Z or energy signal from the detector, and hence the gamma-ray energy, is within specified lower and upper limits. The region between these limits is called the **energy window**.

Some radionuclides, such as ^{67}Ga, ^{111}In, ^{201}Tl and ^{75}Se, emit gamma-rays at more than one energy. Multiple windows in the pulse height analyser allow use of all the gamma-photon energies from these radionuclides, while still keeping scatter to a minimum. Alternatively, multiple windows may be used to simultaneously acquire images from different isotopes administered to the patient. Most current gamma-cameras include at least three windows in their pulse height analyser.

Display controller

The display controller is used to select the final orientation of the image on the CRT and film. It can rotate, mirror or invert the image to provide a consistent display of the image irrespective of the orientation of the patient in front

UNIFORMITY 7/ 1/93

UNIFORMITY IMAGES

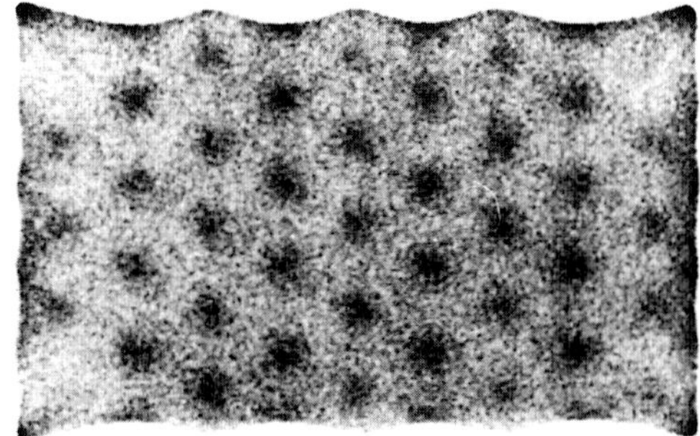

Without Linearity Correction

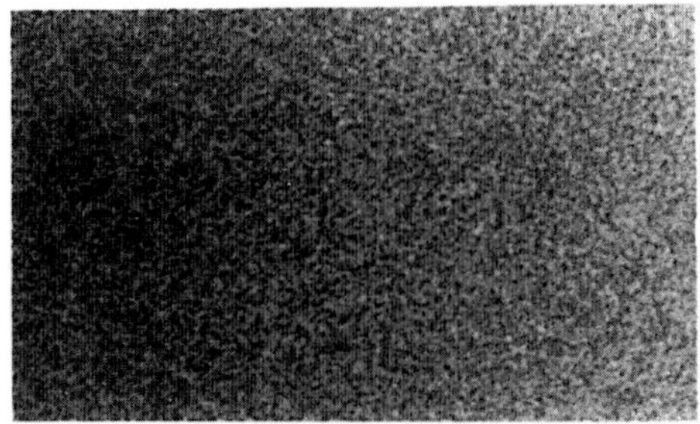

With Linearity Correction

Fig. 107.4 Gross non-uniformities introduced by systematic mispositioning of detected gamma-rays towards the centre of the PM tubes. Linearity correction eliminates these misplacements and yields the expected uniform image.

of the detector. Most display controllers also include an ability to electronically magnify or shift the image for easier visualization. Note, however, that unlike magnification with the pinhole or converging collimators, electronic magnification does not improve resolution.

Timer/counter

The counter records the number of gamma-rays detected in the PHA windows. Together with the timer it can be used to accumulate a certain number of detected gamma-rays (counts) on the film or expose the film for a predetermined time to provide consistent images. Typically 500 000 to 1 million counts are collected for a fairly standard image, although the number of counts per image may be considerably lower in dynamic studies.

Display

The cathode ray tube (CRT) displays each valid gamma-ray detected as a single dot on the screen. The final *X* and *Y* position signals are applied to the horizontal and vertical deflection plates of the CRT respectively, while the unblank signal from the PHA is used to turn on the electron beam of the CRT. The electron beam is deflected in proportion to the applied position signals before it strikes the phosphor of the screen and produces a single dot of light. Thus the position of the light dot on the screen has a direct correspondence to the position of the gamma-ray interaction in the crystal. Since the CRT can only display one dot at a time, the light generated on the screen is integrated photographically, typically on special *X*-ray film, to form the final image for viewing by the physician.

● **What is the difference between digital and analogue cameras?**

▲ There are three 'styles' of cameras currently available:

1. analogue, with or without, an attached computer;
2. integrated camera and computer; and
3. a truly digital camera.

An **analogue camera** is one that permits integration of the image directly onto film. There may be an attached computer as in the configuration shown in Figure 107.1. The computer is functionally separate from the main gamma-camera, with image integration occurring on film and simultaneously being collected on the computer, if desired. Since in this type of gamma-camera the final position signals and display are in analogue form, it is referred to as an analogue gamma-camera. However, even in these types of cameras, the position and energy corrections are carried out using digital circuitry.

It is now increasingly common for manufacturers to integrate a computer system directly into the gamma-camera console. In this case most processing from the correction circuits onwards is carried out in digital form. In these systems, integration of the image information no longer occurs on photographic film, but in computer memory. The images can then be stored on disk and displayed on standard computer displays. This allows much greater flexibility in selecting appropriate image contrast and brightness, removing the necessity for repeat scans in some instances. While various dials and controls on the console are used for selecting appropriate imaging settings such as PHA windows on analogue gamma-cameras, these settings can be controlled directly from a single computer keyboard.

A **truly digital** camera digitizes the output of each PMT and performs the position calculation using a digital algorithm. Of course, correction for linearity, energy and uniformity can be performed within this digital camera. PHA selection, display and other functions occur totally within the digital realm.

● What are the different gamma-camera configurations?

▲ A large variety of different gamma-camera configurations are offered by manufacturers. They can be roughly classified according to the size and number of detectors. Typical large field of view (FOV) gamma-cameras have a detector diameter ranging from about 35 cm to 40 cm, which are large enough to cover most organs without having to resort to a diverging collimator. However, for total body scans, detectors up to 53 cm diameter or rectangular detectors up to 60 cm × 38 cm provide advantages over the standard large FOV detectors. Smaller detectors in the range 25–30 cm are typically employed in mobile gamma-cameras. These gamma-cameras are usually motor driven and allow studies to be obtained in ward areas on patients too sick to travel to the department. As the weight of these systems has to be kept to a minimum, only enough shielding for the lower energy isotopes such as ^{99m}Tc and ^{201}Tl is usually incorporated into the detector.

Multidetector systems have recently gained increasing popularity. Dual detector systems with large opposing detectors provide for optimal total body scanning, allowing both anterior and posterior total body images to be obtained in a single pass. They also offer significant sensitivity advantages for some SPECT studies. Three heads arranged in a triangular configuration can offer a threefold improvement in sensitivity for brain tomographic studies. This improved sensitivity can be used to advantage to reduce the study time, increase the total counts collected or provide high-resolution images by trading sensitivity against resolution in the collimator design. Other multidetector configurations include dual head, right angle and four-head systems as well as ring-type systems specifically designed for brain SPECT.

The exact configuration of the gamma-camera selected will depend on the types of studies to be performed on the system, other gamma-cameras already installed in the department and, of course, budgetary constraints, as multidetector systems tend to be substantially more expensive than single detector systems.

● What influences nuclear medicine image quality?

▲ Compared with radiographs, nuclear medicine images have rather poor resolution, and the number of photons making up an image are several orders of magnitude lower than those of a typical radiograph. Radiography can provide high-resolution anatomical detail. However, despite the poorer resolution, through suitable tracers, nuclear medicine can provide an indication of regional functional differences, highlighting pathology before anatomical changes are necessarily apparent. Thus some of the inherent shortcomings of the imaging technique are overcome by the inherently high contrast between normal and abnormal tissue in nuclear medicine imaging.

The final quality of the nuclear medicine image is determined by a number of factors, including the resolution, the amount of scatter included, the total number of photons contributing to the image and the uniformity of response across the detector, and these will be discussed in detail below.

Resolution

Resolution of an imaging system is the degree with which the representation of an object is blurred in the final image. This concept is illustrated in Figure 107.5. A very well-defined, narrow source when imaged with imperfect resolution results in a blurred image of the source spread over a larger area of the image. The resolution is defined as the amount of spread introduced to a narrow point source by measuring the **full-width at half-maximum (FWHM)** in the image. Occasionally the full-width at tenth maximum (FWTM) is also quoted to define further the characteristics of the imaging system.

The intrinsic resolution of gamma-cameras ranges from about 3 mm to 4.5 mm FWHM. However, the addition of a parallel-hole collimator degrades the resolution to 6–12 mm at a distance of 10 cm from the collimator. Resolution worsens with increasing distance from colli-

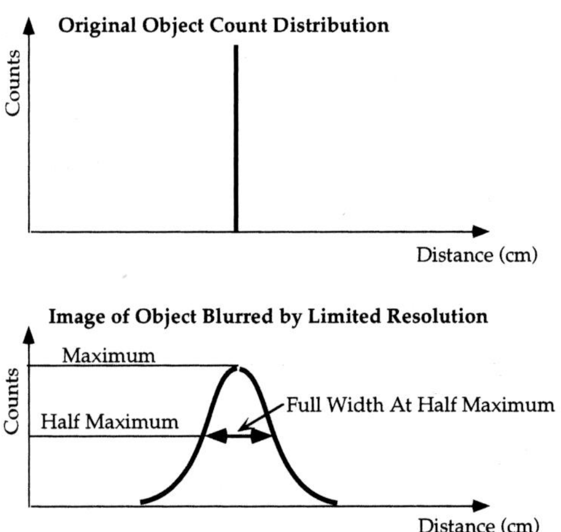

Fig. 107.5 Blurring of an ideal point source count profile by the limited resolution of the gamma-camera. Rather than being focused on a single spot, the counts from the point source are spread over a large area. The resolution in terms of full-width at half-maximum (FWHM) can be measured directly from the point spread function as shown.

mator, degrading further to 12–20 mm at a distance of 20 cm. Thus, the choice and design of collimator has a very strong bearing on the final image quality achieved.

Lack of resolution causes loss of contrast for small lesions, particularly those smaller than 1–2 times the FWHM. The resolution also determines the minimum distance between two objects in order to differentiate them as two distinct entities on the final image. Typically the distance between objects needs to be at least one FWHM to be easily distinguishable, however bars with separation down to about 0.75 times FWHM should be distinguishable.

Scatter

It is a basic assumption of nuclear medicine imaging that a gamma-ray detected in the crystal originated from a radioactive decay somewhere along a straight line drawn from the crystal at an angle defined by the collimator. This basic assumption certainly holds for unscattered gamma-rays which do travel in a straight line. However, once scattered, the origin of the gamma-ray can no longer be determined because the scatter angle and its point of origin are not known. The only way to distinguish scattered from primary, unscattered gamma-rays is by their energy. A typical energy spectrum for ^{99m}Tc obtained from a gamma-camera is shown in Figure 107.6. Just like the spatial resolution, the **energy resolution** of the gamma-camera is quite poor, being typically 10–12% FWHM. Thus, to ensure good sensitivity by including most primary photons, a rather large PHA window of typically 20% is used. For ^{99m}Tc gamma-ray emissions at 140 keV, a 20% window translates into energies of 126–154 keV being accepted in the PHA window. With such a large window, a significant number of scattered events also contribute to the image. Techniques to reduce the scatter contribution include using an asymmetric window around the photopeak, shifted towards the high-energy range. Various

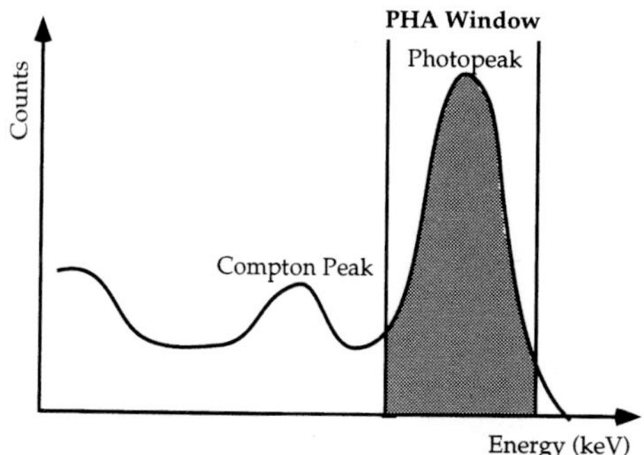

Fig. 107.6 Typical energy spectrum obtained from a gamma-camera with the pulse height analyser (PHA) window also shown. While some scattered as well as primary gamma-rays fall within the PHA energy window, all the scattered gamma-rays with detected energies below the lower window level are eliminated from the image.

image-processing techniques have also been developed to provide an estimate of scatter, which can then be subtracted from the image to reduce the effect of scatter. However, at this stage scatter cannot be entirely eliminated, and these correction schemes tend to increase the noise in the image.

Number of photons contributing to the image

Nuclear medicine images are photon limited. The number of gamma-photons contributing to the image is several orders of magnitude lower than the number of photons contributing to an X-ray film or photographic image. Radioactive decay is a random process, i.e. there is a random fluctuation in the number of photons contributing to any area in the image. This random fluctuation is referred to as image noise. The exact amount of noise is a function of the number of photons contributing to the image, with the standard deviation of the noise being given by the square root of the number of photons collected. The higher the number of photons, the better the signal-to-noise ratio and the better the image quality.

There are a number of ways to increase the number of photons contributing to the image. The image could be acquired for a longer time, but this can increase patient discomfort and loss of resolution owing to patient motion as well as reduce patient throughput. Further, when trying to follow fast changes in activity distribution, the image collection time is dictated by the rate of change in the tracer concentration, restricting the collection time for each image. The amount of radioactive tracer injected into the patient could be increased. However, this results in a higher radiation dose to the patient. Further, as radiotracer activity is increased, more and more gamma-rays are lost because of gamma-camera processing speed limitations until a point is reached at which increasing activity will provide little gain or even loss of the number of photons contributing to the image. As mentioned previously, high-sensitivity collimators could be used, but this causes a loss in resolution. Thus the number of photons contributing to an image is again a compromise.

Uniformity of detector response

Ideally, if the gamma-camera is exposed to a uniform source of activity, the resultant image should also be perfectly uniform. However, because of imperfections in the detection system, the correction circuits and collimator, some non-uniformity in sensitivity can be observed across the detector. It is important to keep this non-uniformity as small as possible to reduce the likelihood of artefactual lesions appearing in the image. In modern gamma-cameras, non-uniformities of $<5\%$ over the whole detector area and $<3\%$ over small areas can be readily achieved.

● **What types of image collections can be performed with a gamma-camera?**

▲ Gamma-cameras support both static and dynamic collection, and with suitable accessories whole-body studies, gated cardiac studies and tomographic studies can also be performed.

Static images are acquired when the radioactive distribution is essentially constant during the time required to acquire the images. Static imaging usually entails acquiring several views of an organ including anterior, posterior and lateral views for typically about 500 000 to 1 million counts.

Much physiological information can be obtained observing tracer uptake and clearance from organs. Dynamic studies are a series of sequential images, each collected for a predetermined amount of time. The image rate depends on the rate of change of the tracer and can range from several images per second to one image every tens of minutes or even longer. Particularly for high image rates, the images are very count limited and the main benefit is gained from the functional aspect of the image sequence.

A single, contiguous image of the skeletal system can be obtained even with a limited detector size by scanning the detector across the patient through either bed or detector motion. This is termed a **whole-body** or **area scan** and is particularly useful for bone scanning, but also for localizing metastases or tumours in the body.

Synchronizing the collection of a set of images to the ECG allows images of the beating heart to be formed and hence its function can be determined. This synchronization is termed gating, hence these studies are called gated studies. The exact mechanisms of collecting these studies are dealt with in another section.

By rotating the gamma-camera around the patient and acquiring images at multiple angles, tomographic slices can be reconstructed. Single photon emission computerized tomography (SPECT) is dealt with in detail in Chapter 109.

REFERENCES

1. Anger H O 1958 Scintillation camera. Rev Scient Inst 29, 27–33
2. Williams L E 1987 Nuclear medical physics. CRC Press, Boca Raton
3. Davies E R, Thomas W E G 1988 Nuclear medicine: application to surgery. Castle House Publications, Tunbridge Wells

108. The computer and its application in nuclear medicine

Roger R. Fulton Brian F. Hutton

DIGITAL ACQUISITION AND DISPLAY

● How is a nuclear medicine image formed?

▲ In nuclear medicine, a digital image consists of a rectangular matrix of pixels, each of which contains a value representing the number of counts recorded in the portion of the gamma-camera field of view to which it corresponds.

For normal monochrome display, pixels containing the highest counts are displayed at maximum brightness (white), and those with the lowest counts at minimum brightness (black). Pixels containing counts between these limits are displayed in intermediate shades of grey (Fig. 108.1). Modern computer displays are capable of displaying in both colour and monochrome. Both modes of display are achieved by mixing red, green and blue (RGB) signals in particular proportions. Each different colour is a unique mix of RGB signals. Displays differ in the number of different colours they can display. For the interpretation of nuclear medicine images, displays with 256 different grey scales/colours have gained wide acceptance.

The way in which the available colours are used to display the image has an important bearing on its appearance, and hence may influence the diagnosis. The process of mapping the range of counts contained in the image to the available colours is called **scaling**. In its simplest form, scaling involves assigning an appropriate display level to each pixel, such that its displayed brightness is proportional to the counts it contains. This entails dividing the range of counts in the image, say 0–2047, by the number of display levels, say 256. Each display level then corresponds to a range of counts of size 2048/256, or eight counts. Thus pixels having counts in the range 0–7 will be displayed in the first display level, pixels with counts in the range 8–15 in the second display level, and so on.

This scheme is 'fair' in that it does not 'favour' any particular range of counts. However, it is often not the most appropriate scaling. It may well be that most of the pixels of diagnostic interest occupy a much narrower range

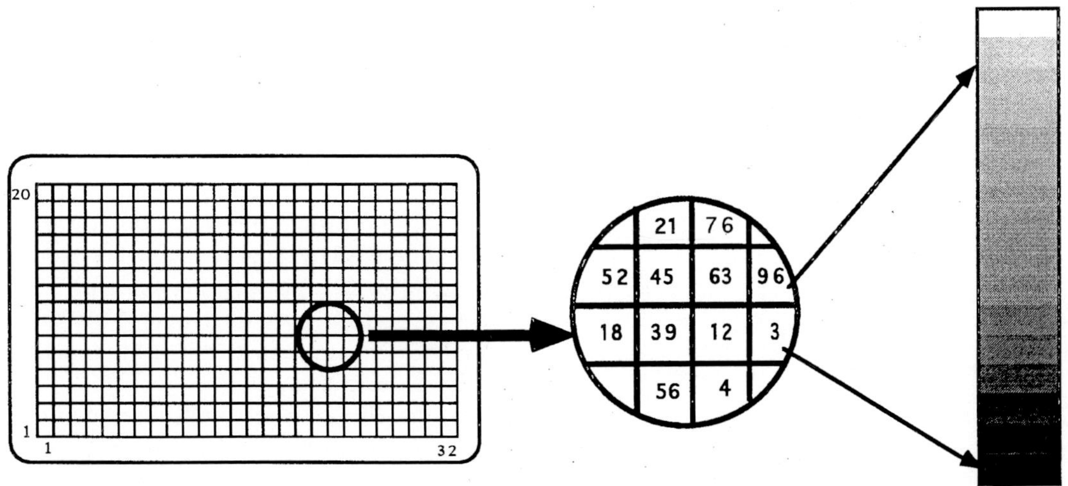

Fig. 108.1 Digital image display. Each pixel accumulates a certain number of counts. When the image is displayed, the brightness of the pixel is proportional to the counts.

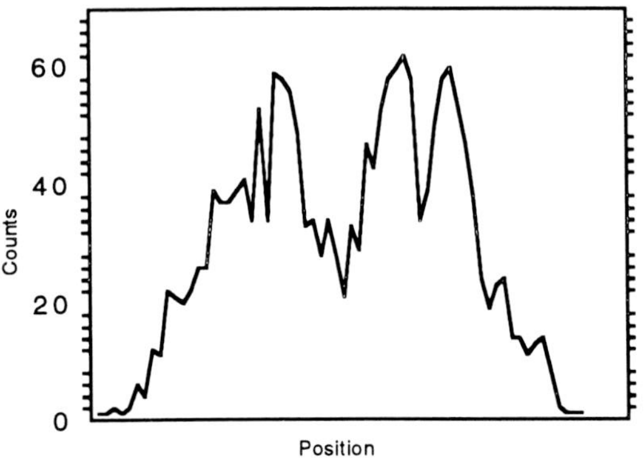

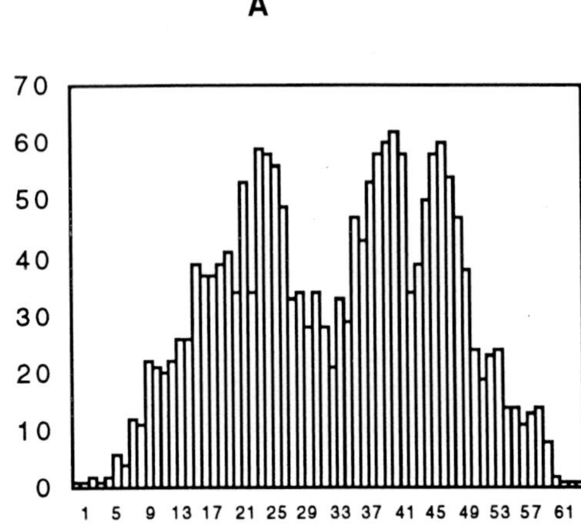

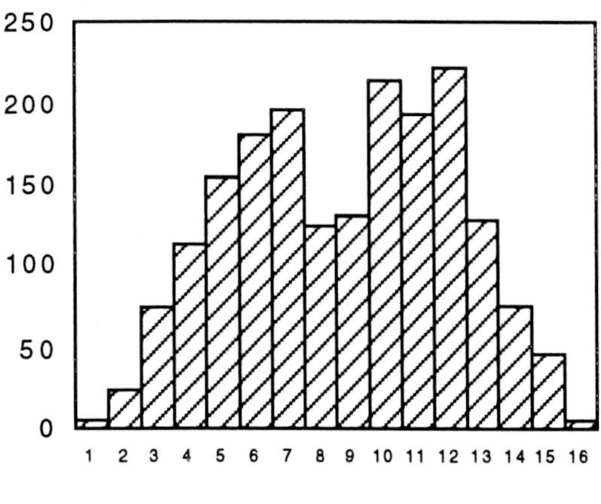

Fig. 108.2A A profile through a 64 × 64 thallium myocardial radioactivity distribution. The profile is sampled at 64 (B), and 16 positions (C).

of counts than the image as a whole. In an extreme situation, for example, if certain pixels contain exceptionally high counts, the pixels of interest may cover a substantial range of counts, but be forced into a small number of display levels. A better use of the available display levels is to scale between the minimum and maximum counts in the pixels of interest, excluding other pixels from the scaling procedure. This is accomplished by **thresholding**, i.e. defining a count range to which all the available display levels will be allocated. Pixels outside this range are displayed in a display level identical to that of the minimum or maximum of the range. The limits of the range are usually expressed as a percentage of the maximum pixel in the image.

● How can we best choose the matrix size?

▲ A 64 × 64 image consists of 4096 pixels. If we assume that each pixel requires one byte for storage, the image will occupy 4096, or 4K, bytes of storage. On the other hand, a 256 × 256 image occupies 64K bytes. A disk can therefore store 16 times as many 64 × 64 images as 256 × 256. Clearly, in order to conserve disk space, we should not use an acquisition matrix that is any larger than necessary.

When a digital image is acquired, the radioactivity distribution in the gamma-camera's field of view is 'sampled' at equally spaced points on a grid. Let us consider a profile through the radioactivity distribution (Fig. 108.2A). This profile is a continuous function. As we shall see later, any continuous function is equivalent to a sum of pure sine functions of different frequencies and amplitudes. When we acquire a digital image of the radioactivity distribution, the sampling points should be sufficiently close together to identify the full detail of the profile. In Figure 108.2B, the profile has been sampled at 64 positions which, visually, appears to faithfully reproduce most of the detail in the original profile. Figure 108.2C shows the profile sampled at 16 rather than 64 positions, illustrating the loss of detail that occurs when the sampling is too coarse. Since the finest detail in the profile is contained in the highest frequency components, we therefore need to sample in such a way that these high-frequency components are detected.

Knowledge of the spatial resolution of the camera tells us the highest frequency which the camera can contribute to the profile. Gamma-camera spatial resolution is normally quoted as the full-width at half-maximum (FWHM) of a profile through a point source. Two point sources one FWHM apart can just be resolved as separate sources. Hence the gamma-camera is incapable of detecting frequencies higher than 1/FWHM, and we can reasonably asssume that this is the highest frequency present in the image.

The **sampling theorem** tells us that in order to recover $f(x)$ exactly, it must be sampled at a rate greater than twice its highest frequency.[1] Hence we must sample the image at intervals less than FWHM/2. Let us take a concrete example by assuming that the gamma-camera's spatial resolution (with the collimator) is 7.2 mm (FWHM). From the sampling theorem we must take samples at intervals less than FWHM/2, i.e. less than 3.6 mm. If the width of the camera detector to which the image matrix corresponds is 400 mm, then the required number of samples is greater than 400/3.6, i.e. >111. In this case, therefore, a 128 × 128 acquisition would be sufficient to realize the full resolution of the camera.

It should be noted that in certain instances it may not be necessary to obtain images with the highest possible resolution, for example in certain dynamic studies where it is only desired to obtain a time–activity curve for an entire organ. In such cases, it may be sufficient, and save disk space, to collect the study in a coarser matrix.

● What is interpolation?

▲ Interpolation is a technique that is used in several areas of image processing and/or display. It typically involves determining the best estimate of the value of a point lying between two samples (pixels). It is a technique used, for example, in image rotation to determine values for a rotated image in which the rotated image pixels do not correspond exactly to the original pixel geometry.

There are several interpolation methods. One of the simplest, **linear interpolation**, makes the assumption that values between any pair of adjacent sample points are given by the straight line connecting them. A less precise method, **nearest neighbour interpolation**, on the other hand, simply involves taking the value of the nearest sample.

Another example of interpolation is the display of an image using a matrix size greater than that used for acquisition. Acquiring a nuclear medicine image with a particular matrix size is equivalent to sampling the count density at a number of equally spaced points on a rectangular grid. Interpolation is used to increase the number of pixels for display purposes, for example from 64 × 64 to 128 × 128. Interpolating coarse matrices sometimes makes them more pleasing to the eye. However, it is important to remember that this does *not* improve resolution, which is controlled by the sampling used to acquire the original image.

Figure 108.3 shows the interpolation of an image to double the matrix dimensions. Each new pixel receives a value based on itself and its nearest neighbours,[2] for example

$$e_1 = \frac{3e + b + d + a/\sqrt{2}}{S} \quad (1)$$

where

$$S = \frac{1}{e}\left[12e + 2b + 2f + 2h + 2d + \frac{a + c + g + i}{\sqrt{2}}\right] \quad (2)$$

This procedure preserves the counts in any given area.

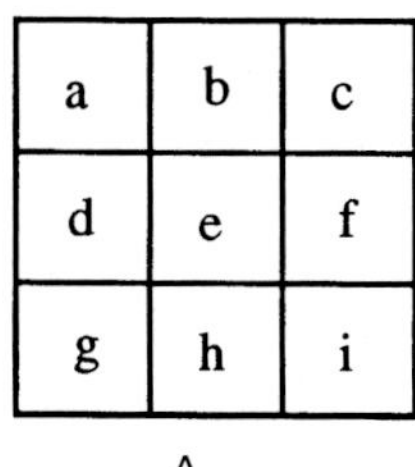

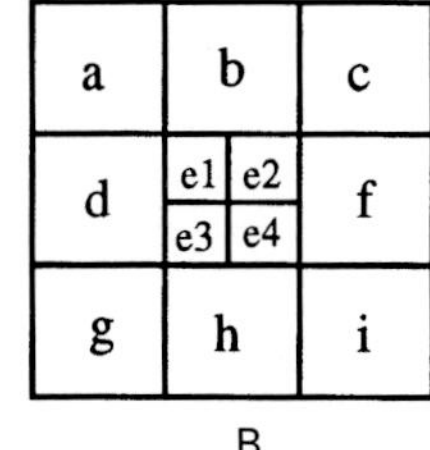

Fig. 108.3 Interpolation of a digital image. Each pixel in the original image is subdivided into four new pixels, each of which receives a value derived from its nearest neighbours.

● What does data compression involve?

▲ Digital images consume large quantities of disk storage. The size, in bytes, of an image is given by the product of its dimensions and the number of bytes occupied by each pixel. The latter is called 'pixel depth'. If the dimensions are doubled, the size of the image increases by a factor of 4. Table 108.1 lists some typical image sizes, assuming square matrices and a pixel depth of 2. Note that image size increases as the square of the matrix dimension.

Image sizes have an impact on nuclear medicine in several ways. Firstly, image size limits the number of images that a computer system can accommodate at one time. Secondly, when images are copied to an archival medium such as magnetic tape or optical disk, the image sizes dictate how many images the archival device can store. The third effect arises when computers transfer images over a network. The larger the image, the longer the transfer takes, and the more load is placed on the network. An increased load is undesirable because it degrades network performance for other users.

It is therefore desirable to keep the size of images to a minimum by ensuring that image dimensions are no larger than required for adequate sampling. An additional way to reduce image size is to compress the data, using a **data compression** technique. Data compression involves encoding the data into a more compact form, using a computer algorithm. The compressed data set can then be archived, or transmitted over a network. Before the data set can be used, however, it must be decoded, or 'uncompressed'. The compression and uncompression steps

Table 108.1 The number of bytes required to store images of typical dimensions, given that two bytes are used to represent the value of each pixel

Matrix size	Size (bytes)
32 × 32	2 048
64 × 64	8 192
128 × 128	32 768
256 × 256	131 072
512 × 512	524 288
1024 × 1024	2 097 152

involve some computational effort (and time), and this must be balanced against the gains obtained.

A simple, and commonly used, data compression algorithm is **run-length encoding**. This technique compresses sequences of repeated bytes. For example, consider a segment of an image file within which, say, 100 consecutive bytes contain the value 0. Run-length encoding compresses the sequence into two bytes, the first containing the repeated value (0) and the second the number of repetitions (100).

● Three-dimensional (3-D) display – what techniques are available?

▲ The conventional way of viewing reconstructed slice data from tomographic studies is as multiple slices. With this form of presentation the interpretation of spatial inter-relationships can be difficult, particularly for the inexperienced. Three-dimensional (3-D) displays provide an overview of multiple slices in a single image, and enhance the perception of spatial inter-relationships.

Three-dimensional displays are necessarily 2-D pictures (more than two dimensions cannot be displayed at one time on a conventional computer screen). The 3-D effect is produced by depth cues, such as illumination and shading. There are four basic methods[3] of displaying 3-D data – multislice display, 2-D mapping, surface rendering and volume rendering. An example of 2-D mapping is the familiar 'bull's-eye' display, which displays profiles of adjacent short-axis myocardial slices as concentric annuli.

Surface rendering is a method of displaying the surface of an object. The first task in surface rendering is to delineate the surface. This is usually done by some automated binary operation, such as setting a cut-off threshold. Each voxel in the volume is classified as to whether it is within the object or not. The surface is then rendered, using illumination and shading to convey depth information.

Surface rendering has some major disadvantages in nuclear medicine. Firstly, it provides no information about the interior of the object. While the interior of the object may be of limited importance in many studies performed with structural imaging modalities, it is of major importance in functional imaging. Secondly, accurate delineation of the surface is difficult in nuclear medicine due to the relatively poor resolution of the imaging techniques, and the fact that patterns of radiotracer uptake do not necessarily conform to anatomical boundaries. Surface rendering appears to be best suited to the display of data derived from the structural imaging modalities, such as computed X-ray tomography (CT) and magnetic resonance imaging (MRI). However, surface-rendered images are not entirely without use in nuclear medicine. They can be used to good effect in graphical displays to indicate where in an organ selected slices come from. The 3-D surface display aids the physician's interpretation of the spatial inter-relationships of the displayed slices. Colour-coded functional information can be overlaid on a surface display, permitting an appreciation of the spatial variation of a functional parameter from a single, easily interpreted image.

Volume rendering[4] on the other hand, as its name implies, presents information from the entire volume imaged. Volume rendering begins with a cube of data, e.g. a stack of reconstructed slices. The data are forward projected along parallel ray paths at a number of equally spaced angles encompassing 360°. If voxel values along the rays are summed, the result will be planar images similar to the original projections. Alternatively, maximum voxel images can be produced by finding the maximum voxel along each ray, and placing its value in the appropriate pixel of the rendered image. This improves contrast and emphasizes the most intense objects, which are of greatest interest in hotspot scanning. Depth cues come from a weighting using simulated exponential attenuation that is applied before finding the maximum voxel. Displaying these so-called depth-weighted maximum voxel images in rotating cine format considerably enhances depth perception.

FOURIER THEORY AND FILTERING

● What is the purpose of filtering?

▲ Possibly the least understood, yet one of the most important, aspects of image processing is that of filtering. The purpose of this section is to discuss filtering with few mathematical terms so as to provide an intuitive understanding. By 'exposing' this 'black art' the reader may be encouraged to explore further with less of a phobia! A good starting point for further reading is Parker.[5]

In a strict sense filtering is any operation which is applied sequentially within a neighbourhood of each point of an image (or curve). Examples are image or curve smoothing, edge enhancement or restoration. In nuclear medicine filtering has wide application not only in general image processing but also in specialized areas such as image reconstruction (SPECT and PET) and tracer kinetic analysis.

● How does filtering apply to a nuclear medicine image?

▲ The gamma-camera is used to image the distribution of activity in the body. Consider the gamma-camera to be a 'black box' in which emitted gamma-rays are converted to an image of the activity distribution (Fig. 108.4). The final image is a blurred representation of the activity distribution; in fact, each point of activity is blurred. In essence the gamma-camera acts as a filter and produces an output (image) that is directly related to the input (object) in a predictable way for each element of the input [defined by the point response function of the system, $h(x,y)$].

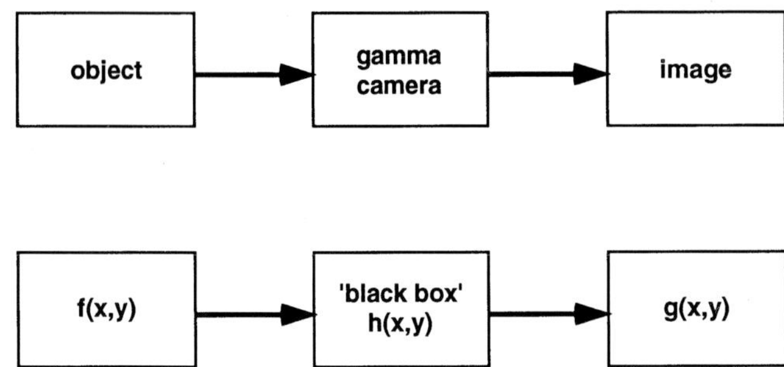

Fig. 108.4 Diagrammatic representation of image formation. The gamma-camera can be considered as a device which filters acquired data to form a final image.

A similar process can be performed on a computer by replacing the 'black box' with a filter function. By defining the appropriate function, a similar **smoothing** effect can be achieved (e.g. nine-point smooth). Alternatively, the opposite effect can be achieved, termed **restoration** or resolution recovery. With appropriate definition the filter can be defined so as to attempt to reverse the smoothing action of the gamma-camera.

● How does filtering apply to time–activity curves?

▲ The passage of a radioactive tracer through an organ system (e.g. the kidneys) can be considered in a similar way (Fig. 108.5). The tracer exiting from the organ will bear some relationship to the administered tracer, however it will be affected by the tracer passage through the organ. The measured activity in the organ will be defined similarly to the gamma-camera image provided that two conditions are met:

1. The response to the sum of small inputs is the same as the sum of the responses to each input (linearity).
2. A time shift to the input produces the same time shift in the output (stationarity).

In this example the kidneys act as a filter, in a temporal (time) sense rather than spatial sense, as in the case of the gamma-camera.

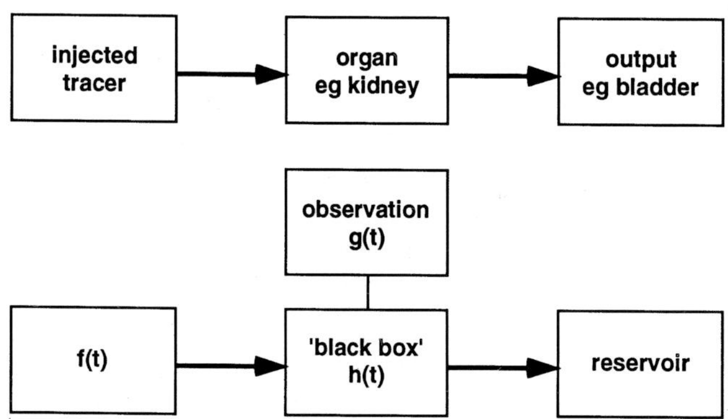

Fig. 108.5 Tracer passage through a biological system. A linear system can be used to describe the behaviour of an organ in the way it influences the passage of a tracer.

● What is meant by the terms convolution, deconvolution and mean transit time?

▲ As a tracer passes through an organ, the counts recorded by an external detector depend on the input of tracer to the organ (or input function) and the response of the organ to that input. The result for the special case of an impulse (or perfect bolus) is defined as the **impulse response function**. Similarly for a gamma-camera, this will be the system's response to a single input (a single point of activity). In general, for any input, the observed result is determined by a **convolution** of the input function with the impulse response function. Convolution is denoted by an asterisk (⋆), i. e.

$$g(x,y) = f(x,y) \star h(x,y) \quad (3)$$

or

$$g(t) = f(t) \star h(t) \quad (4)$$

These equations simply state that the detected counts (or final image) can be described by the sum of responses to a set of impulses, each of which undergoes an identical process defined by the impulse response function (h).

Convolution can be best understood by considering the following three-point curve smoothing operation. (A similar example could be the nine-point smooth applied to a 2-D image.) If the filter function (corresponding to the impulse response function) is 0.2, 0.6, 0.2; for each element, the output will be given by

$$g(t-1) = 0.2\,f(t)$$
$$g(t) = 0.6\,f(t)$$
$$g(t+1) = 0.2\,f(t)$$

The final output will be the sum of all input responses:

		$t-1$	t	$t+1$	$t+2$
$f(t)$	→	$0.2f(t)$	$0.6f(t)$	$0.2f(t)$	
			+	+	
$f(t+1)$	→		$0.2f(t+1)$	$0.6f(t+1)$	$0.2f(t+1)$
				+	+
$f(t+2)$	→			$0.2f(t+2)$	$0.6f(t+2)$
					+
$f(t+3)$	→				$0.2f(t+3)$
		↓	↓	↓	↓
		$g(t-1)$	$g(t)$	$g(t+1)$	$g(t+2)$

In the case of an organ system the impulse response function will more normally have a form as illustrated in Figure 108.6, in which there is a minimum residence time or transit time but overall a range of times for transit of the tracer through the organ. It is clear that the output must occur at some time after the input has arrived! The response (measured over the organ rather than output) is shown as a sum of the individual impulse responses.

In the case of time–activity curves, it is difficult, given a measurement of the organ itself, to determine the response or function of the organ independent of the input function

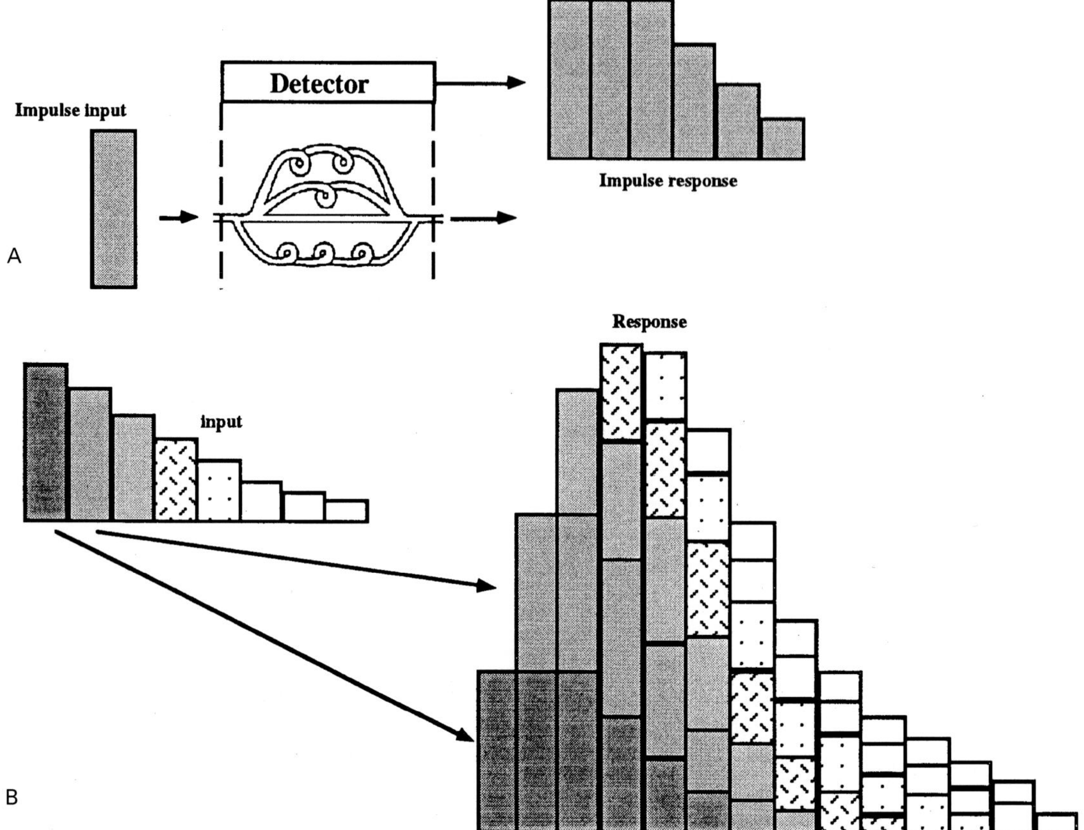

Fig. 108.6 Concept of convolution and impulse response function: when a perfect bolus of activity is injected (A), the observed activity in the kidney, for a tracer which is 100% extracted and excreted, will be as shown. The tracer remains in the kidney for a short time prior to excretion. For the more general case of an input of tracer as shown (B), each element of the tracer can be considered a perfect bolus whose transfer through the kidneys will be identical to that in A. The observed activity over the kidneys will simply reflect a sum of overlapping impulse response functions.

shape. In contrast, knowledge of the response to a perfect impulse defines exactly how the organ responds and has more direct physiological interpretation. The problem therefore is to deduce the impulse response function from the measured response and input function (determined from a region placed over the heart or a large blood vessel, or measurement of blood samples). This is obtained by determining that function (h) which satisfies $g(t) = f(t) \star h(t)$. The process needed is **deconvolution,** the opposite of convolution. Generally, deconvolution is performed either using matrix inversion or using Fourier or Laplace transforms.

The **mean transit time** is frequently measured as a single index of function, being the mean time that an element takes to pass through the system under examination. This can be measured directly from the impulse response function (IRF) as the area under the IRF divided by the height at time $t = 0$. Mean transit times are used in renal studies (Ch. 25), gastric studies (Section III) and elsewhere in nuclear medicine.[6]

For filters defined over a small neighbourhood a direct convolution or deconvolution may be efficient. However, if the filter function (kernel) is large, direct calculation can be time-consuming. Also, in defining appropriate filters, alternative approaches can offer advantages in certain circumstances. In particular, Fourier transforms have widespread application, permitting filters to be tailored for specific purposes.

● What is the Fourier transform?

▲ A sine wave can be fully described by its frequency and amplitude (and phase). Thus, a single sine wave can be represented as a single point when plotted on amplitude versus frequency axes. Although hard to intuitively accept, it can be proven mathematically that any curve (Fig. 108.7A), no matter what its shape, can be broken into a sum of sine waves of various frequencies and amplitudes (Fig. 108.7B). These can be plotted on the amplitude versus frequency axes (Fig. 108.7C). This plot has identical meaning to the original curve provided one recognizes that the original curve is the sum of sine waves of various frequencies weighted by the amplitudes as represented on the Fourier plot.

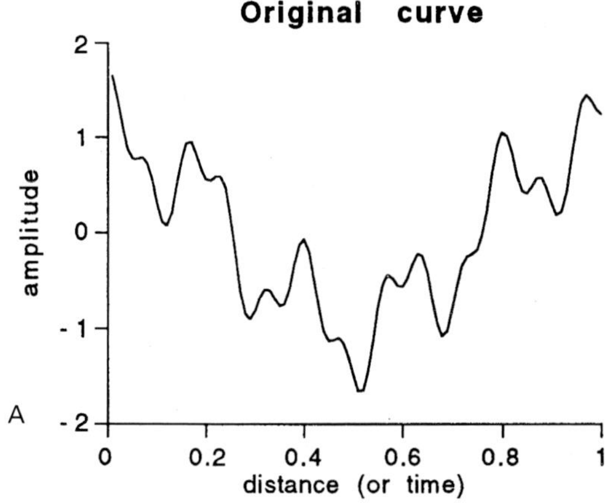

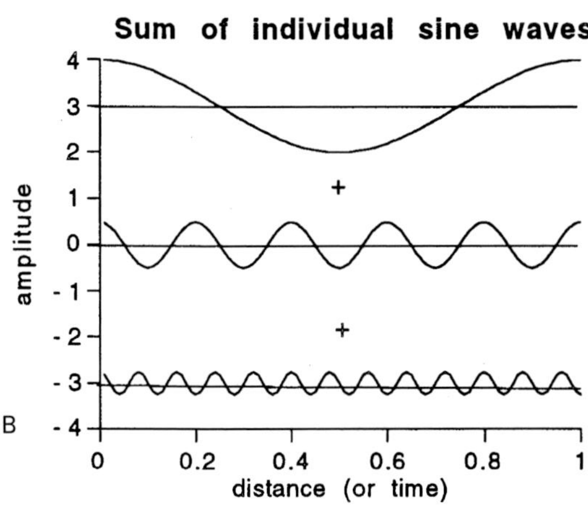

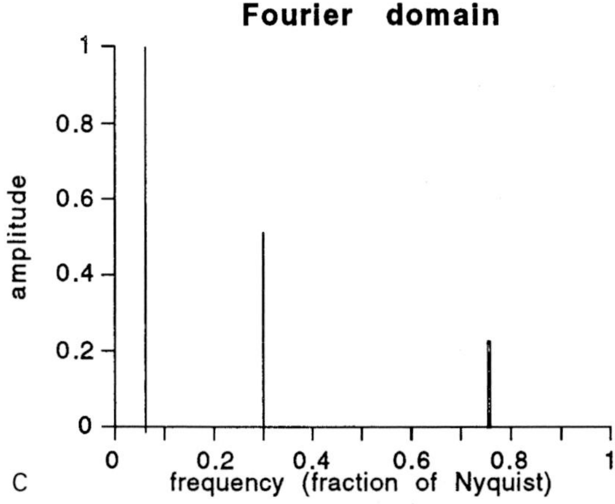

Fig. 108.7 The Fourier transform: the function represented in A consists of the sum of three sine waves each having different frequency and amplitude (B). They can be plotted on an alternative set of axes: amplitude versus frequency (C). This plot, which is the Fourier transform of the original curve, simply illustrates those frequencies which, weighted by the respective amplitudes, sum to provide the original curve.

In practice, the function required to transform data for this alternative set of axes is the **Fourier transform** (FT). The FT simply provides an alternative means of describing the data. Note that the FT of a 2-D image also has two dimensions. Typically the FT of a continuous curve has a continuum of frequencies represented, rather than discrete frequencies (Fig. 108.8) The frequency can be 1/time in the case of a time–activity curve or may involve units 1/distance (spatial frequency) in the case of an image.

The inverse FT provides an exact reverse process which simply transforms the data back to the normal activity–time (or distance) axes.

● What happens when you take the Fourier transform of a function?

▲ A useful analogy is to consider travelling by air from London to Sydney, moving into a different environment where it may be more convenient to undertake certain operations, e.g. Sydney has a warmer climate. One can easily take the inverse transform (the return flight to London), back to the 'real' world; however, the effects of the 'operation' in Sydney are still visible – the suntan, the loss in weight due to a healthy diet, exercise, etc. Similarly, the FT allows one to move to an alternative 'domain' (location) where it is more convenient to perform certain operations. The effect is still visible when returning to the 'real domain', and, indeed, an equivalent operation could be performed, albeit less conveniently, in that original location e.g. use of a sun lamp instead of the actual sun!.

It is useful to consider the transform of a delta function (i.e. a perfect point source). This particular transform (Fig. 108.8A), surprisingly, has *all* frequencies represented at unit amplitude. A perfect imaging system (which has no loss in resolution) would therefore be one which preserves amplitude at all frequencies. What happens in reality is that a point source will be imaged with loss of resolution (e.g. as a Gaussian function whose FT is also Gaussian). The poorer the resolution, the more the amplitude is decreased at higher frequencies. In the Fourier domain, high spatial frequencies represent fine detail and high resolution. Use of a lower resolution collimator will degrade resolution, further decreasing amplitude at high frequencies (Fig. 108.8B). Therefore we can interpret a reduction in high frequencies as a smoothing operation and, conversely, enhancement of high frequencies as a restoring or sharpening operation.

An extremely important property of Fourier space is that the implementation of the convolution operation becomes a simple multiplication, performed at each frequency. Thus

$g = f \star h$ is equivalent to (5)

$$g = \mathrm{FT}^{-1}\ [\mathrm{FT}(f) \times \mathrm{FT}\ (h)] \qquad (6)$$

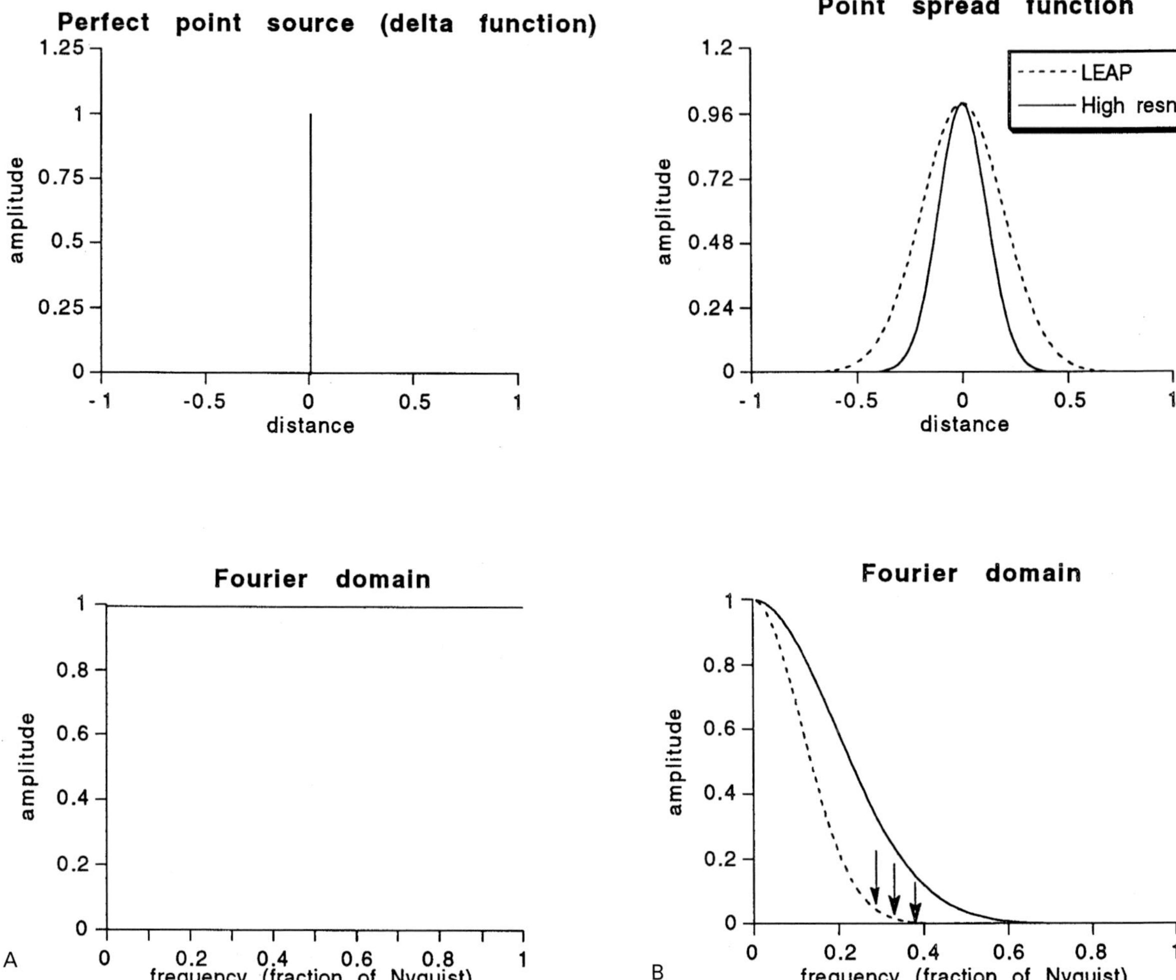

Fig. 108.8 Fourier transforms and filtering: the Fourier transform of a perfect point source has all frequencies present at unit amplitude (A). In the case of an image of a point source the profile, which is typically bell shaped (Gaussian), has a Fourier transform, which illustrates that high frequencies are represented with lower amplitude (B). Use of a lower resolution collimator results in further reduction of amplitude at high frequency.

Although appearing to be more complex than direct convolution (eqn 5), use of the FT can be computationally faster, particularly if the filter kernel is large.

Furthermore, a filter function that achieves exact restoration can be theoretically defined in terms of the FT of the impulse response function [modulation transfer function (MTF)]. It is that function [$X(f)$] such that

$$X(f) \times \text{MTF} = 1 \text{ at all frequencies} \qquad (7)$$

(which we know is the FT of a perfect point source). Unfortunately, perfect restoration is never possible because of the presence of noise (normally considered white noise in nuclear medicine, present at low amplitude at all frequencies). Restoration, multiplying by the inverse of the MTF, leads to high-amplitude noise at high frequencies, requiring some compromise to be made. This involves reduction of amplitude at high frequency, with restoration consequently limited to lower frequencies. A similar strategy is used in reconstruction filtering (see Ch. 109).

● What is the Nyquist frequency?

▲ In order to adequately preserve a particular frequency in a digital image (or curve) the data must have sufficient sampling. The sampling theorem states that there must be more than two digital samples (measured values or pixels) per cycle of that particular frequency otherwise the frequency will not be accurately preserved. The **Nyquist frequency** (f_N) is defined as the maximum frequency which could be recovered with a particular matrix size [f_N=1/(2 × pixel size)]. Given this definition, provided the image is adequately sampled, the Nyquist frequency will be larger than any frequency present in the image.

Aliasing may occur when the number of samples is too small. This is a result of introducing false information at lower frequencies owing to misrepresentation of frequencies that are too high to measure. One well-known example occurs when imaging a bar phantom with an inappropriate matrix size. Even though visual identification of this pattern may not be expected, sometimes a bar pattern, not necessarily in the correct orientation, can be visualized.

● What is meant by cut-off frequency or critical frequency and filter order?

▲ Nuclear medicine most commonly utilizes low-pass filters (reconstruction is an exception), which involves maintaining low-frequency amplitudes while reducing amplitude at higher frequencies. The **cut-off** or **critical frequency** (f_c) defines the point at which the filter produces significant high-frequency suppression. This parameter, therefore, largely defines the filter shape. Filter **order** determines the rate at which filter amplitude falls off [as illustrated for the Butterworth filter (Fig. 108.9), a widely used low-pass smoothing filter]. In the case of the Metz filter,[7] a restoration filter, the point at which high-frequency suppression occurs is determined by the filter **power**.

● What is a Hanning filter?

▲ A filter that is widely available, particularly for use in combination with SPECT reconstruction, is the Hanning filter. The fact that no such filter exists may therefore come as some surprise! At some stage in the development of image processing there has been confusion regarding two similar, but different, filters attributed to Hann and Hamming. In fact, the Hann filter (frequently mistakenly called the Hanning filter) is a special case of the generalized Hamming filter. The subtle difference can be seen in the two equations for these filters:

Generalized Hamming:

$$h(t) = a + (1-a)\cos(\pi f/f_c) \text{ if } |f| \leq f_c, 0 \text{ otherwise} \quad (8)$$

where $a<1$ and f_c is critical frequency.

Hann

$$h(t) = 0.5 + 0.5\cos(\pi f/f_c) \text{ if } |f| \leq f_c, 0 \text{ otherwise} \quad (9)$$

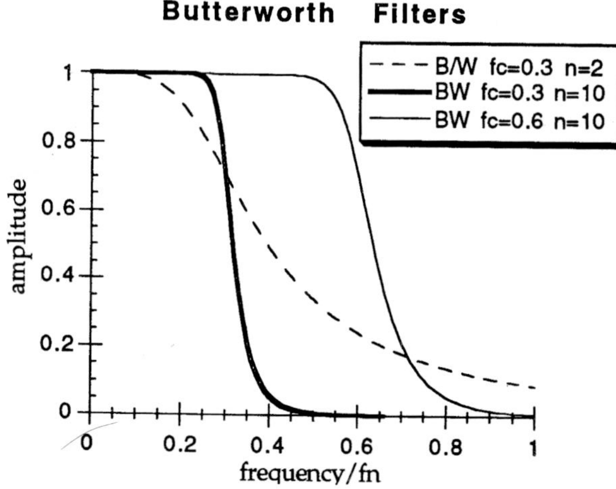

Fig. 108.9 Butterworth filter. The Butterworth filter is defined by two parameters: the critical (or cut-off) frequency defines the point at which the curve drops significantly (0.7 max), whereas the order defines the slope of the filter curve, with low order corresponding to low gradient.

● How do you compare filters from one system with those from another?

▲ Several manufacturers use alternative units for frequency such that f_c for 'equivalent' filters may be defined differently dependent on matrix size or zoom factor. The possible frequency units are illustrated in Figure 108.10. Lack of standardization can lead to considerable confusion. Provided frequency is defined in 'absolute' units (cm^{-1}), then the same filter will apply independent of matrix size. Failure to recognize this can lead to serious problems if matrix size is changed, as illustrated in Figure 108.11. When matrix size is changed from a 64 × 64 to a 128 × 128 matrix, pixel size, and consequently the Nyquist frequency, changes. Obviously the absolute frequencies present in the image are unaltered provided there is adequate sampling. However a filter with f_c defined relative to the Nyquist frequency will have totally different effects on the two images.

Other differences exist in the implementation of certain filters by manufacturers. The end-user cannot be confident of duplicating results in a different laboratory unless identical equipment is used or the differences in implementation are perfectly understood and appropriate compensation applied.

● What filter to use when?

▲ A common question, particularly in SPECT, is 'What is the best filter to use for a particular application?'. Although we can benefit from the experience of others, strictly speaking 'best' should be defined as the filter that best satisfies the criteria defined on a particular site, for a particular application. This should include the degree of smoothness required, likely count level and practicality of implementation.

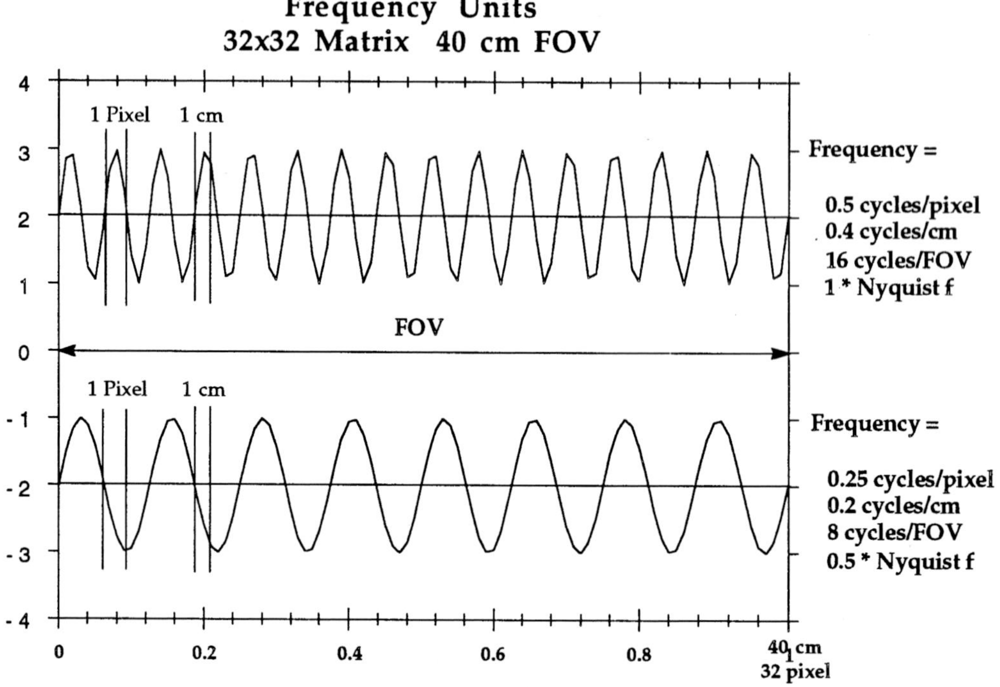

Fig. 108.10 Frequency units: several alternative units can be used to describe frequency. For a 32 × 32 matrix and 40 cm field size, the Nyquist frequency can be defined as 16 cycles per field of view (FOV), or 0.5 cycles/pixel or 0.4 cycles/cm.

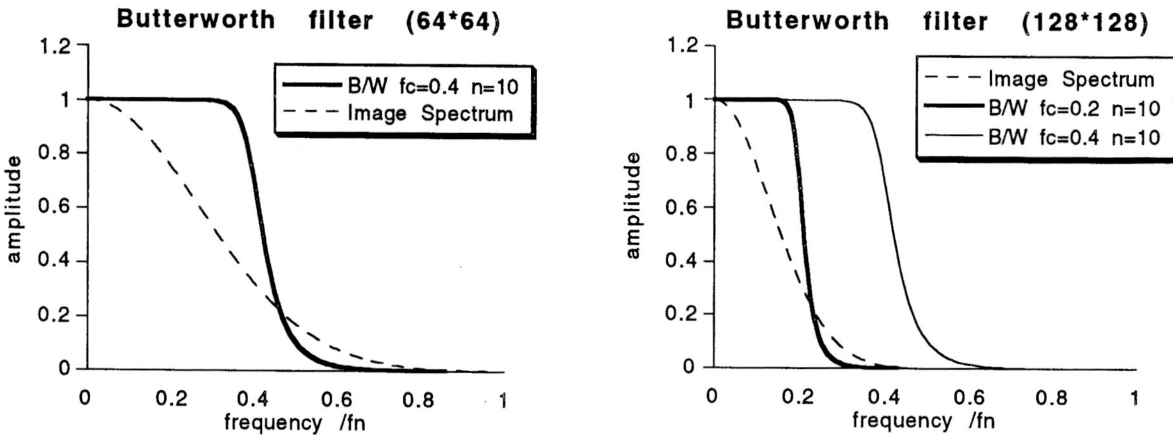

Fig. 108.11 Change in matrix size. The Fourier transforms of an image obtained using 64 × 64 and 128 × 128 matrices are illustrated. The Nyquist frequency ($f_N = 1/2a$ where a = pixel size) is different for the two matrix sizes. Therefore a filter defined in terms of f_N may look identical in shape but will have a dramatically different effect on the two images. If the filter is defined in absolute units (cycles/cm) then the filter will have the same effect, independent of matrix size.

The objective in most nuclear medicine studies should be to use as high a critical frequency as possible within the constraints of the noise present. The better the counting statistics the higher the critical frequency that can be used. If the image looks too noisy, use a reduced critical frequency. Simple experimentation can be used for any particular image with the selected range of possible f_c values based on previous experience.

In the case of restoration filters, these are based on the Fourier transform of the measured resolution for the system (MTF). It is possible to introduce false information if the defined MTF does not match the system MTF. For example, use of an inappropriate MTF could result in an attempt to restore more than was originally lost, with unreliable results. Given the variation of resolution with distance from a gamma-camera, these restoration filters can, at best, provide 'average' compensation as they assume constant resolution.

Rigorous demonstration of the optimal filter to use for a particular class of images, at a particular count level and using a particular instrument and protocol requires a full receiver operating curve (ROC) analysis. This is beyond the scope of most departments, who must rely on more subjective methods. Remember that 'beauty is in the eye of the beholder', and so the reporting physician may have a preference for a particular image appearance. Provided the basis for filter definition is sufficiently well understood, practitioners should be able to determine their own preference.

IN VIVO QUANTIFICATION OF RADIOACTIVITY

● What is background correction?

▲ Background correction is designed to remove counts due to activity in structures overlying and underlying the organ of interest. One way to estimate the counts due to background is to define a region of interest (ROI) adjacent to, but not overlapping, the organ. The average counts per pixel recorded in the background ROI are assumed to represent the background contribution to the counts recorded in each pixel of the organ. The background-corrected count in the organ ROI is then given by

$$C_{net} = C_{orig} - C_{bkg} \frac{Npix_{organ}}{Npix_{bkg}} \tag{10}$$

where C_{orig} and C_{net} are the original and background-corrected counts in the organ ROI respectively, C_{bkg} is the number of counts in the background ROI, and $Npix_{organ}$ and $Npix_{bkg}$ are the numbers of pixels in the organ and background ROIs respectively.

This technique assumes a uniform background distribution. However, background may be markedly non-uniform in certain cases. Overestimation of background may also occur, because the full depth of the patient contributes to the background ROI, while, over the organ itself, background only comes from that part of the patient's depth not occupied by the organ. A strategy used to counter both of these effects, as is used in thallium planar myocardial studies, is to estimate the background at each pixel based upon the background at points on a boundary circumscribing the heart.[8,9] This method is usually referred to as **interpolative background subtraction**.

A rectangular boundary region (Fig. 108.12) is defined which encloses the heart. The background B at point P within the boundary is then calculated as

$$B = \frac{w_a a + w_b b + w_c c + w_d d}{w_a + w_b + w_c + w_d} \tag{11}$$

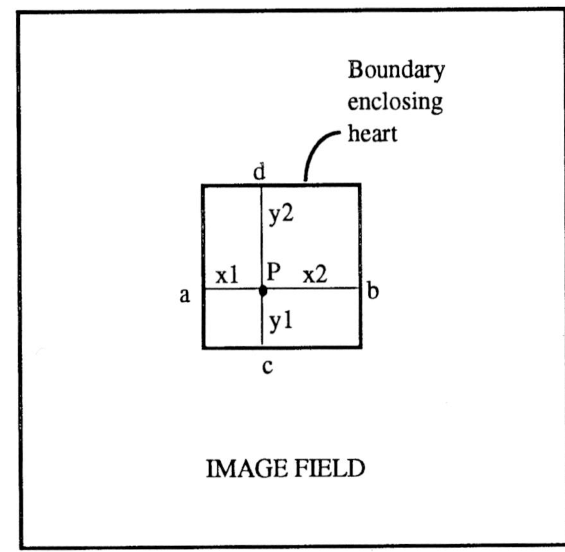

Fig. 108.12 Interpolative background subtraction. A rectangular boundary surrounds the organ of interest. The background at the point *P* is calculated as the weighted sum of the boundary pixels *a*, *b*, *c* and *d*.

where *a*, *b*, *c* and *d* are the image counts at the boundary positions shown, which are at distances x_1, x_2, y_1 and y_2 from the point *P* respectively, and

$$w_a = \frac{x_2}{x_1} + k$$

$$w_b = \frac{x_1}{x_2} + k$$

$$w_c = \frac{y_2}{y_1} + k$$

$$w_d = \frac{y_1}{y_2} + k \tag{12}$$

The constant *k* is normally set to 2 to produce a fall-of of background from extracardiac activity approximating that which would be encountered at the borders of an isolated organ. For a fuller description the reader is referred to the paper by Watson et al.[9]

● How is in vivo activity measured?

▲ It is frequently desirable to quantify the activity in a particular organ or lesion. Methods exist whereby an accurate estimate of the radioactivity in an organ or lesion can be obtained with a conventional gamma-camera. The activity can be calculated from the counts recorded within a region of interest (ROI) placed over the object, after corrections for background, scatter, attenuation and gamma-camera sensitivity have been applied.

Attenuation of gamma-rays as they traverse the body to the gamma-camera will lead to a false underestimate of the radioactivity in the organ. If the depth of the organ and the attenuation coefficients of the tissues traversed are known, an attenuation correction factor can be calculated. The attenuation-corrected count C_{corr} can be obtained from

$$C_{corr} = C_0 e^{\mu d} \tag{13}$$

where C_0 is the measured count, and $e^{\mu d}$ represents the effective attenuation factor for a point source at depth d. Typically, however, the distribution of attenuation and the depth of the organ are unknown, and an alternative method of correcting for attenuation is required. One approach frequently taken, referred to as the **conjugate view method**, is to use the **geometric mean** of opposing views of the organ.[10,11] The geometric mean of two quantities is defined as the square root of their product.

With reference to Figure 108.13, we have

$$\begin{aligned} I_1 &= \text{measured counts from detector 1} \\ &= I_0 e^{-\mu a} \\ I_2 &= \text{measured counts from detector 2} \\ &= I_0 e^{-\mu b} \end{aligned} \tag{14}$$

where $b = D - a$.

$$\begin{aligned} \text{The geometric mean counts} &= \sqrt{I_1 \cdot I_2} \\ &= I_0 e^{\frac{-\mu D}{2}} \end{aligned} \tag{15}$$

Note that the geometric mean count is independent of a and b, i.e. it is independent of the depth of the source in the attenuating medium. To calculate the activity contained in the organ from opposing views, the first step is to calculate the geometric mean image. Then the activity, A, in the organ can be obtained as

$$A = \sqrt{\frac{I_1 \cdot I_2}{e^{-\mu D}}} \cdot \frac{f_i}{c} \text{ MBq} \tag{16}$$

where c represents the system calibration factor (counts/min/MBq), and f_i is a correction factor for source attenuation and source thickness, i.e.

$$f_i = \frac{\left(\frac{\mu_s \cdot t_s}{2}\right)}{\sinh\left(\frac{\mu_s \cdot t_s}{2}\right)} \tag{17}$$

where t_s is the source thickness, and μ_s is the effective total linear attenuation coefficient across the source. Note that

$$\sinh x = \frac{e^x - e^{-x}}{2} \tag{18}$$

The above approach assumes that photon attenuation is a monoexponential phenomenon. This is not strictly true in practice due to the presence of scattered photons in the photopeak. The effect of these photons is to give a falsely high measure of the emissions from a source, an effect which increases with depth for a source in a uniform scattering medium. Hence the assumption of monoexponential attenuation is imperfect. To correct for scatter, Wu & Siegel[12] introduced the build-up factor $B(d)$. It is defined as

$$B(d) = \frac{C}{C_0 e^{\mu d}} \tag{19}$$

where C_0 is the count rate measured in air, C is the count rate at depth d cm and μ is the narrow-beam linear attenuation coefficient for soft tissue (0.15 cm for ^{99m}Tc).

The build-up factor is dependent on the radionuclide used, the source depth, source size, source thickness and

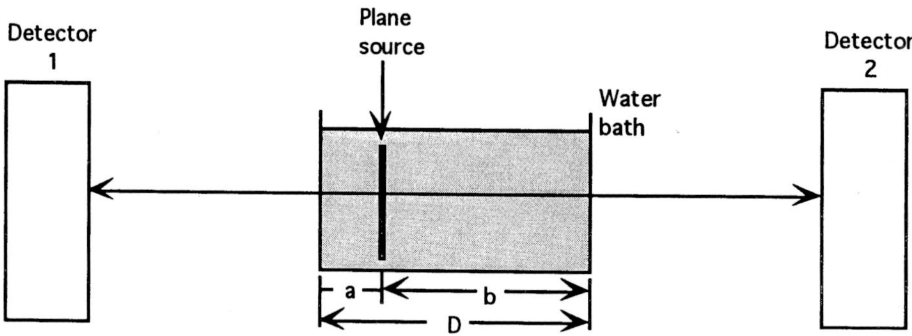

Figure 108.13 The conjugate view method of correcting for attenuation for point, line and plane sources of activity.

camera parameters (collimator, window). For ^{99m}Tc it has a value 1.0 at zero depth, increasing to approximately 1.3 at 15 cm.

DYNAMIC PROCESSING

● How are quantitative physiological parameters calculated for an organ?

▲ The images constituting a dynamic study can be viewed as a cine, which allows easy interpretation of changes in regional radioactivity distribution within the camera field of view over the duration of the study. However, the information obtained from viewing a cine, while often useful diagnostically, is qualitative. As a result, classification of organ function as normal or abnormal, other than in relatively extreme cases, is difficult from the cine alone. An unbiased quantitative parameter of organ function is preferable, since it permits comparison with a range of normal values.

To obtain quantitative parameters,[13] the first step is to plot a graph of the activity *vs.* time in a region of interest (ROI) defined over the organ. This graph is called a **a time–activity curve** (TAC). If there is a significant amount of radioactivity in the tissues overlying or underlying the organ, the organ TAC should be background corrected before any further processing is done.

Following background correction, the organ TAC depicts the changes in the amount of tracer in the organ with time. A multitude of approaches exist whereby numeric parameters can be obtained from an organ TAC. In many cases it is sufficient to determine a parameter which differentiates between disease states but which itself may not be precisely interpreted in a physiological sense. A simple example of a numeric parameter is the frame-number of the images in which the TAC attains its maximum value, T_{max}. This will always be a number in the range 1–N, where N is the number of images in the dynamic study. Another example which can be easily derived from the organ TAC is the maximum rate of increase or decrease in count rate.

Alternatively, direct physiologically based parameters can be estimated provided that an appropriate model of the tracer kinetics can be defined.[14] The most commonly applied model defines the system under consideration as a set of compartments between which the tracer exchanges (Fig. 108.14). Each compartment (which can be either a physical space or biochemical species) is considered as an instantaneously well-mixed, homogeneous entity. The amount of detectable tracer which is added must be small enough that the system is unperturbed, and the overall system must be in a steady state. The amount of tracer leaving a compartment is assumed to be proportional to the amount of tracer (Q_i) in the compartment at a point in time. The rate constants (k_i) determine the rate of transfer

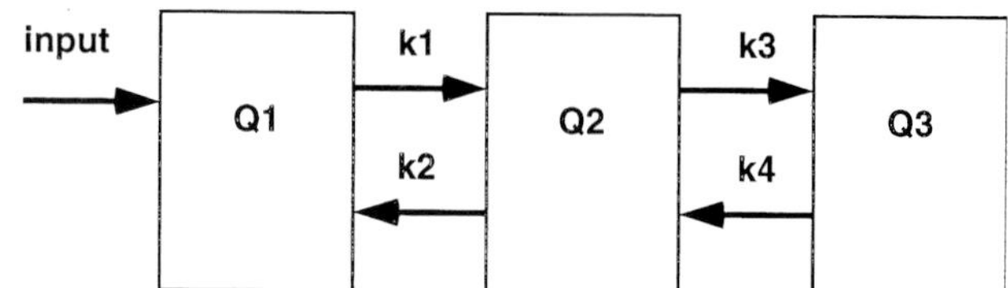

Fig. 108.14 Diagrammatic representation of a compartmental model. The rate constants relate to tracer exchange between compartments. An example of the three compartments could be (i) blood or plasma, (ii) intracellular concentration of non-metabolized tracer and (iii) metabolized tracer. The compartments represent either different physical spaces or different chemical species.

of the tracer from one compartment to its neighbouring compartments(s).

The tracer kinetics can be described by a set of differential equations whose solution typically involves multiple exponentials. Determination of parameters (k_1–k_4) involves curve fitting of observed data using the appropriate equation. The delivery of tracer, or input function, must also be taken into consideration. Compartmental models have particularly widespread application in positron emission tomography (PET), as discussed in a separate section (Ch. 110).

● What are functional (or parametric) images?

▲ The creation of a **functional image** does not require the definition of regions of interest. Instead, every pixel in the image is treated as a distinct ROI, from which a TAC is derived. Every TAC is analysed to derive a particular parameter of interest, e.g. T_{max}. Each calculated parameter value is then stored in the corresponding pixel of the functional image. Taking T_{max} as an example, each pixel of the functional image will receive a value between 1 and N. When displayed, the functional image will depict the regional variation in T_{max}. In greyscale display, bright areas will represent relatively high T_{max} (e.g. late arrival of tracer).

Functional images provide a particularly useful means of presenting dynamic data in a compressed form. The image essentially presents a dynamic sequence of images as a single image. There are many useful examples of functional images. Notable examples are the Fourier or '**phase and amplitude**' images derived from gated blood pool image sequences (see Ch. 90). These are derived by fitting a cosine-shaped curve to each pixel's TAC to determine the phase and amplitude of that pixel, i.e.

$$c(t) = A \cdot \cos(\omega t + \phi) \qquad (20)$$

where $c(t)$ is the counts for a pixel at time t, A denotes amplitude, ϕ denotes phase and ω is the frequency of the cosine function.

Phase images very graphically demonstrate regions of wall motion abnormality that may not be clearly identifiable in cine display. In particular, abnormalities can be detected in surfaces normal to the viewing angle, where no edge is visible.

Care should be taken when interpreting functional images since they assume that the model being applied is valid for each pixel. In planar dynamic imaging, the time–activity curve is not necessarily an accurate representation of the physiological behaviour of the tissue of interest, because it may also, to some degree, reflect the function of other overlapping structures. The observed time–activity curve may need to be treated as a weighted sum of separate curves corresponding to these overlapping structures.

● **What is factor analysis?**

▲ Factor analysis[15] provides a means of identifying the predominant kinetic patterns present in a dynamic study. This essentially involves classifying the pixel time–activity curves into a preselected number of classes, each of which represents a fundamental pattern of kinetic behaviour. For example, in gated heart blood pool (GHBP) studies, factor analysis might be expected to identify two classes of curves corresponding to the atria and ventricles. Each of these classes represents a basic physiological component, or factor.

Factor analysis calculates the extent to which each pixel's time–activity curve corresponds to each factor curve. Pixels are assigned a coefficient for each factor. A coefficient close to 1 for a given factor means that the pixel exhibits the typical kinetic pattern for that factor, whereas a coefficient close to 0 means that the pixel exhibits very little of the typical kinetic behaviour.

A factor image is a functional image produced by storing the value of the coefficient in each pixel. When displayed, the colour scale will depict the extent to which each pixel exhibits the factor's typical kinetic pattern. If pixels overlap structures with dissimilar kinetic behaviour, their time–activity curves may exhibit a mixture of the dominant kinetic patterns, and be assigned relatively high coefficients for more than one factor.

Care must be taken when interpreting factor curves as these do not necessarily have a direct physiological meaning. Their main use is in classification which may aid in disease discrimination.

NETWORKS AND IMAGE TRANSFER

● **What options are there for transferring data?**

▲ In recent years most vendors of nuclear medicine imaging equipment have moved away from proprietary computer designs towards general-purpose computer platforms such as the IBM PC, the Macintosh and various desktop workstations running the Unix operating system. By adopting these relatively highly developed and widely used computer systems, for which numerous hardware and software options are available, the vendors are now able to offer support for industry standards in several important areas, including networking.

Networks are groups of interconnected computer systems. A network which extends over a limited geographical area, e.g. a single hospital department, is called a **local area network** (LAN). By far the most common means of connecting computers in LANs is **ethernet.** Ethernet is a standard which defines how data are transferred (the protocol), and the physical medium (cable). It uses a method called carrier-sense multiple access with collision detect (CSMA/CD) to share a common cable among several computers. CSMA/CD operates as follows. When a computer wishes to transmit data to another computer on the network, it first listens to ensure that the cable is not in use. If the cable is in use, it waits for a random period of time before listening again. If the cable is not in use, the computer transmits, and at the same time listens to ensure that another computer did not commence transmitting at the same time. When two or more computers attempt to transmit at the same time, a 'collision' is said to occur. The collision is detected by all the computers involved, and each waits for a random period of time before trying again. Data are transmitted at a rate of 10 Mbits/s on ethernet.

Obviously, the heavier the traffic on the network, the higher the probability of collisions becomes. All transmissions on ethernet are broadcasts, i.e. every transmission is seen by every computer on the LAN. The data are encapsulated in packets. Each packet contains the unique ethernet address of the destination computer. A packet is only accepted by the computer for which it is intended. All other computers on the network ignore it.

Another important networking standard which, like ethernet, is available for all commonly used computer platforms is **TCP/IP** (transmission control protocol/internet protocol). TCP/IP is a set of protocols which were designed to allow the interconnection of dissimilar computer systems. It makes no assumptions about the nature of the connection between the computers.

Two important programs which come with TCP/IP and rely upon it for their operation are **TELNET** and **FTP** (file transfer protocol). TELNET allows you to log into another computer on the network and use it as if you were sitting at the remote computer's keyboard. In this mode of operation your local computer is acting as a 'virtual terminal' to the remote computer.

FTP facilitates file transfer between computers and, like TELNET, it is used in the same way whether the remote computer is in another country or in the same room. The user invokes FTP, specifying the Internet (see below) address of the remote computer, and logs in with a user name and password. Once logged in, the user can use the standard file-oriented FTP commands GET and PUT to move files in either direction between the local and remote computers. Any two computers on a network can exchange files with FTP provided they have TCP/IP software installed.

TCP/IP is available for all the non-proprietary computer systems supplied with nuclear medicine imaging equipment today. Therefore if all the computer systems in a department are connected to a LAN, the physical transfer of clinical data files between the systems can be achieved with FTP, even if the equipment is supplied by different vendors.

Because TCP/IP can operate over links of many different kinds, it has been possible to use it to create a worldwide virtual network, called the **Internet**, which links thousands of institutions, and millions of users, in scores of countries. The Internet is a network of networks, linked by many different kinds of physical links, including modems, leased lines, ethernet, satellites and optical fibres. All of this complexity is hidden from the Internet user. In order to connect to a computer on the Internet, the user just invokes TELNET, specifying the unique Internet address of the desired computer. The distance to the remote computer is of no consequence. It is just as easy to connect to a computer on the other side of the world as another computer on a LAN. The Internet is called a virtual network, because the user gains the impression that all the computers on Internet are attached to his/her LAN. The only effect of distance is that the speed of communication is limited to that of the slowest link in the chain. For international connections, a speed of 64 kbits/s is common.

The **network file system** (NFS) is another networking standard which facilitates the sharing of data by multiple computers on a LAN. With NFS, it is possible to access files stored on remote computers as if they were stored on the local computer. NFS access to files is actually achieved over a network, but this detail is hidden from the user. It provides greater convenience than FTP, because files do not have to be physically transferred to the local system before they can be operated upon. NFS is, like TCP/IP, available for all commonly used computer systems.

● **How are networking advances impacting nuclear medicine?**

▲ Modern networking standards such as NFS and TCP/IP have effectively solved the once perplexing problem of physically moving clinical data files between different vendors' computer systems. Once transferred however, the files cannot be used until they have been converted into the clinical data format of the destination system. All vendors have different proprietary clinical data formats. To counter this a standard file format called **Interfile**[16] has been defined for exchange purposes. The idea is that each vendor develops software to convert its proprietary format to Interfile, and vice versa. Files in Interfile format may then be freely interchanged between different vendors' systems. Interfile supports a wide range of nuclear medicine data, including static, dynamic, gated and SPECT studies, as well as regions of interest and curves.

Another standard with, to some degree, similar aims, but with an initial brief extending beyond nuclear medicine to encompass several medical imaging modalities, is ACR/NEMA 2.0, or as it is now known, **DICOM**. The objectives of ACR/NEMA are to define a complete communication protocol for medical imaging applications going beyond Interfile, which simply defines a standard file format.

REFERENCES AND FURTHER READING

DIGITAL ACQUISITION AND DISPLAY

1. Stearns S D 1983 Digital signal analysis. Hayden, Rochelle Park
2. Goris M L, Briandet P A 1983 A clinical and mathematical introduction to computer processing of scintigraphic images. Raven Press, New York.
3. Wallis J W, Miller T R 1991 Three-dimensional display in nuclear medicine and radiology. J Nucl Med 32: 534–546
4. Wallis J W, Miller T R 1990 Volume rendering in three-dimensional display of SPECT images. J Nucl Med 31: 1421–1430

FOURIER THEORY AND FILTERING

5. Parker J A 1991 Image reconstruction in radiology. CRC Press, Boca Raton
6. Peters A M 1993 A unified approach to quantification by kinetic analysis in nuclear medicine. J Nucl Med 34: 706–713
7. King M A, Penny B C, Glick S J 1988 An image dependent Metz filter for nuclear medicine images. J Nucl Med 29: 1980–1989

IN VIVO QUANTIFICATION OF RADIOACTIVITY

8. Goris M L, Daspit S G, McLaughlin P et al 1976 Interpolative background subtraction. J Nucl Med 17: 744–747
9. Watson D D, Campbell N P, Read E K et al 1981 Spatial and temporal quantitation of plane thallium myocardial images. J Nucl Med 22: 577–584
10. Macey D J, Marshall R 1982 Absolute quantitation of radiotracer uptake in the lungs using a gamma camera. J Nucl Med 23: 731
11. Thomas S R, Gelfand M J, Burns G S et al 1983 Radiation absorbed-dose estimates for the liver, spleen, and metaphyseal growth complexes in children undergoing gallium-67 citrate scanning, Radiology 146: 817
12. Wu R K, Siegal J A 1984 Absolute quantitation of radioactivity using the buildup factor. Med Phys 11: 189

DYNAMIC PROCESSING

13. Gelfand M J, Thomas S R 1988 Effective use of computers in nuclear medicine. McGraw-Hill, New York

14. Kuikka J T, Bassingthwaighte J B, Henrich M M, Feinendegen L E 1991 Mathematical modelling in nuclear medicine. Eur J Nucl Med 18: 351–352
15. Samal M 1993 Factor analysis revisited – a potential key for clinicians. Eur J Nucl Med 20: 562–564

NETWORKING AND IMAGE TRANSFER

16. Cradduck T D, Bailey D L, Hutton B F, Deconninck F, Busemann-Sokole E, Bergmann H, Noelpp U 1989 A standard protocol for the exchange of nuclear medicine image files, Nucl Med Commun 10: 703–713

109. Single photon emission computerized tomography

Dale L. Bailey J. Anthony Parker

INTRODUCTION

● What is SPECT?

▲ SPECT stands for single photon emission computerized tomography. It is a technique for producing cross-sectional images of radiotracer distribution in the body. It is called *single* photon tomography to distinguish it from another form of radionuclide emission tomography known as positron emission tomography (PET), which records dual photons arising from positron emissions from radioactive nuclei. In truth, many of the radionuclides that are imaged in nuclear medicine with SPECT emit a number of photons as they decay, but it is still a single photon counting technique. SPECT has found many applications in conventional nuclear medicine because, as a tomographic technique, it has the ability to remove overlying structures which may obscure an abnormality; in this sense it greatly improves the contrast. The data in SPECT are acquired in a similar manner to other nuclear medicine procedures except that views are usually acquired over 180° or 360° in small angular steps (e.g. 3°). The resolution in SPECT is governed by the same mechanisms as in planar images: the collimator, the photon energy, the distance from the source to the detector and the duration of the acquisition primarily determine the quality of the final result. An overview of the SPECT process is shown in Figure 109.1.

ACQUISITION

● How many angles should be used to acquire the data?

▲ The number of angles sufficient to reconstruct faithfully the organ (or area) of interest is determined by the spatial resolution of the gamma-camera. This will vary for different combinations of radionuclide, collimator, count rate, etc. In general, the following relationship is a guide to the number of projection angles N_p to acquire (over 180°):[1]

$$N_p \geq \pi M/2$$

where M is the number of sample elements in the projection (e.g. 64, 128). This is only an indication and it assumes that the proper number of sample elements has been used for the projection, but it gives a reasonable approximation.

● Is it better to acquire twice as many angles for half the time, or spend a longer time at fewer angles?

▲ Once the number of projections is sufficient to match the spatial resolution of the study, there is little benefit in increasing the number of projections acquired. In general, twice the number of projections for half the time per projection should give an identical result to the fewer angles for twice as long. However, if the projection is more finely sampled (e.g. 128 instead of 64), then the number of projections needs to be increased. Increasing the number of angles will lead to slightly increased acquisition time in step-and-shoot mode (owing to more rotations and settling time at each projection) and increased disk space, processing and reconstruction time (e.g. double the number of angles at which to back-project).

● What methods can be used in the acquisition to optimize the reconstructed resolution?

▲ The following steps can be taken at acquisition time and will contribute to better resolution in the final result:

• *Counts count!* Increasing the acquisition time or the administered dose, or using a physiological manipulation to increase the amount of tracer available to the organ of interest (e.g. fasting) will permit the use of a reconstruction window with a higher cut-off, thereby giving higher resolution reconstructions.

• *Apply planar acquisition principles.* Optimize the subject–detector distance (no aerial scanning). In brain

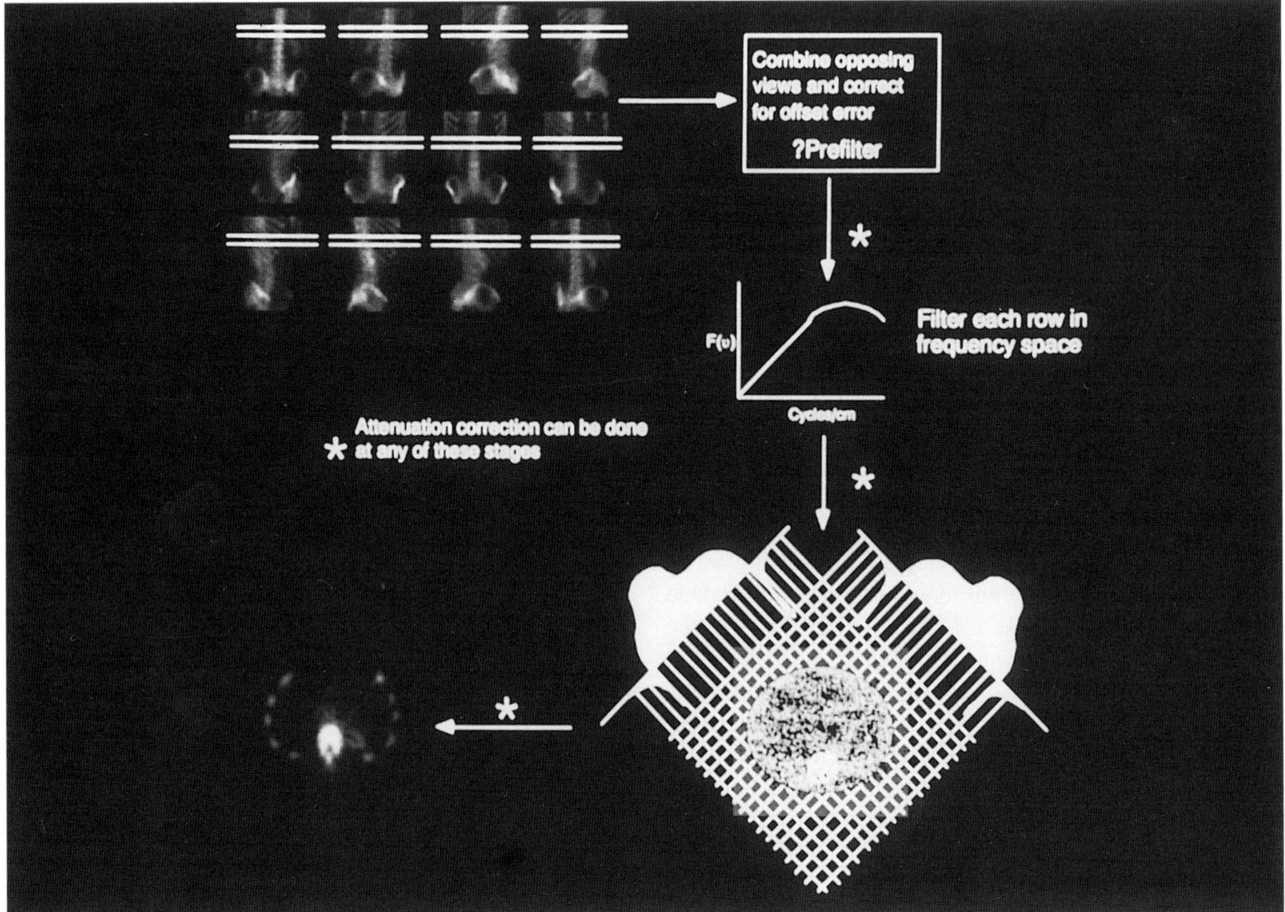

Fig. 109.1 An overview of the SPECT image formation process is shown. The data acquired on the gamma-camera are firstly corrected for image offset errors and opposing views are combined (for 360° acquisitions) and optionally prefiltered to achieve noise suppression and/or resolution recovery. Then each row is filtered with the reconstruction filter and rows from the same slice are back-projected to form the reconstructed image. Attenuation correction can be applied before, in the process of or after back-projection.

scanning, for example, using a gamma-camera that is cut away on one side or a slant-hole collimator that can be angled to avoid the shoulder but still maintain close proximity to the head gives a decided advantage over a conventional parallel-hole collimator at a greater radius of rotation.

• *Avoid moving targets.* Restrict acquisitions in which the radionuclide distribution is not static, but redistributing. If this cannot be avoided, a shorter acquisition may be an acceptable compromise.

• *Limit patient movement.* Patient motion can result in dramatic artefacts. Restraints are often useful. More cooperative subjects may be helped by the use of external cues, such as lining up an object with a spot on the ceiling or similar. A pillow under the knees to ease the strain on the back is surprisingly effective.

• *Choose the right collimator.* As a general rule, to achieve a twofold increase in the reconstructed resolution requires eight times the counts (resolution is a function of sensitivity to the third power).[2] The signal-to-noise ratio in the acquisition data will be much poorer when a collimator with low sensitivity is used.

• *Think about the situation.* If the target organ or structure is located peripherally on one side of the body, an optimized 180° acquisition will probably lead to a better result than a 360° one. An example is in the case of SPECT of the lumbosacral spine: here the patient can be positioned prone and the data acquired over 180° posteriorly. This results in higher resolution reconstructions. Similarly, ^{201}Tl myocardial perfusion studies have been shown to have better contrast using a 180° acquisition as the resolution is better.

● **Is it better to use a high-resolution collimator, and hence acquire fewer counts, or a general-purpose collimator, which trades resolution for sensitivity?**

▲ As in all aspects of nuclear medicine, a balance must

always be struck between resolution and sensitivity, and this is no less true in SPECT. However, it has been clearly shown that higher resolution imaging, which leads to improved contrast, needs fewer counts for a given signal-to-noise ratio (SNR) than imaging with a lower resolution device if the window on the reconstruction filter is adjusted appropriately.[3] This principle is known as the signal amplification technique (SAT).[4] For equivalent SNR, the contrast in the reconstruction is inversely proportional to the square root of the number of acquired counts; this suggests that a decrease in sensitivity can be tolerated as spatial resolution is improved.

This trade-off between counts and resolution can be shifted with multihead cameras. Using a multihead camera the same number of counts can be acquired at the same resolution in a shorter time, or increased counts at higher resolution in the same time as for a single headed camera. To a lesser extent the same effect occurs with fan beam collimators.

- **How is the bladder filling artifact minimized in pelvic bone SPECT?**

▲ Some of the worst reconstruction artifacts are produced by changes between adjacent projections (Fig. 109.2). Bladder filling is a slow process, so that there is relatively little change between the sequential images except for the first and last images. The artifact from this difference is projected back in the direction of this projection. Starting and ending the projection in the posterior projection will minimize the bladder filling artifact and will position it away from the hip region.

- **What are the limitations of 180° acquisitions?**

▲ Images from the two different sides of the body are often strikingly different, primarily because of the differential attenuation of the radiotracer at different angles. It is amazing that 180° aquisitions have been so useful in

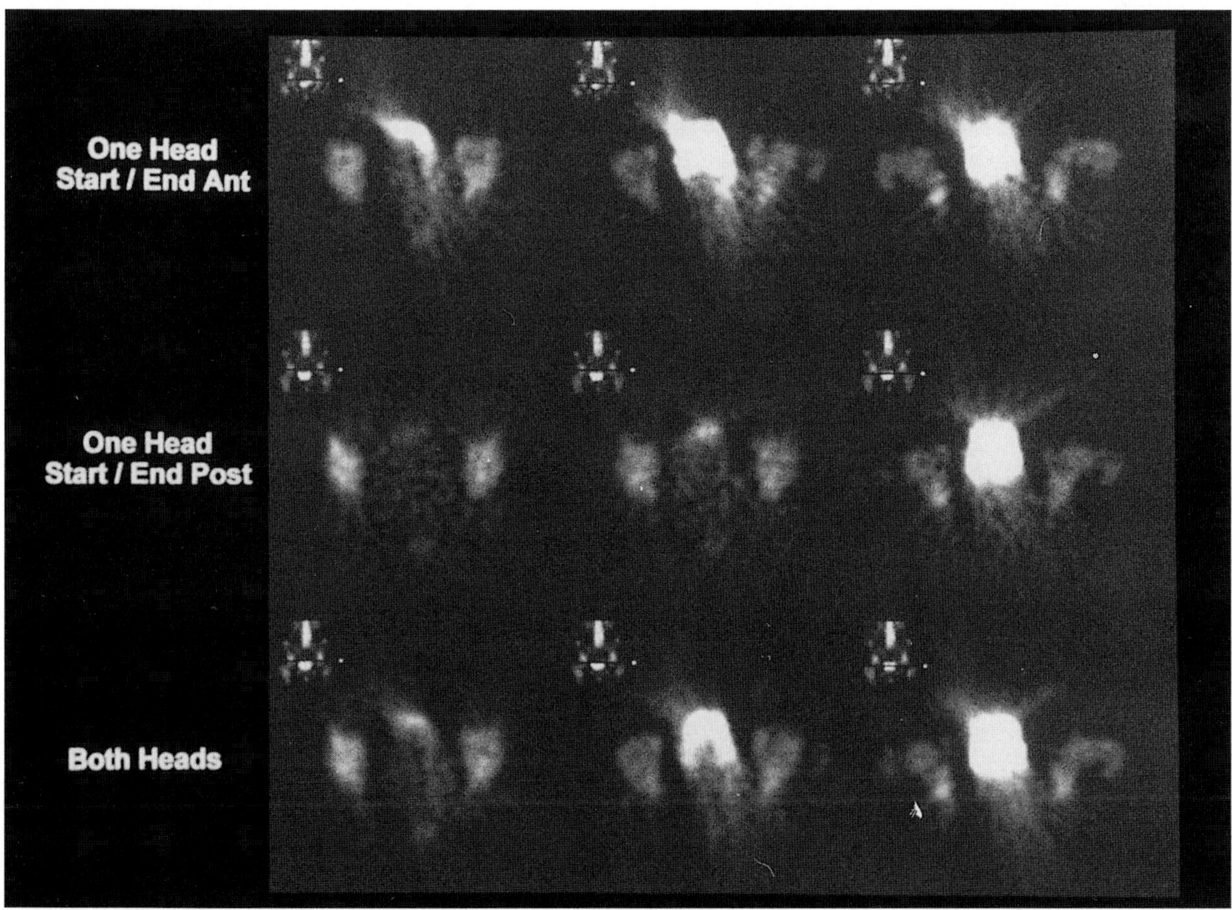

Fig. 109.2 This figure shows reconstructed SPECT images at three different levels in the pelvis. The data were collected using a 360° rotation with a two-headed camera. The top row shows reconstructed images using data from only the head which began and ended in the anterior projection. The second row shows reconstructed images using data from only the head which began and ended in the posterior projection. The third row shows reconstructed images using the data from both heads. The top row of images (start/end in the anterior projection) shows the most artifact, and the middle row of images (start/end in the posterior projection) shows the least artifact and the artifact is symmetrical. The bottom row of images (both heads) is intermediate between these two. Furthermore, the bladder artifact affects all of the slices in the top and bottom rows, but has little effect on the more cephalic slices in the middle row.

specialized situations.[5] However, 180° aquisitions can produce considerably more artifacts than 360° aquisitions, so one needs to select their use carefully.[6] With a 360° acquisition the data from opposing angles are combined, and this evens out the variation in resolution and attenuation with depth to some extent. This is not the case for 180° acquisitions. Mathematically, the last image is followed by the first image, so 180° acquisitions work best when the starting and ending images are bland and the general activity distribution appears relatively similar. Also, attenuation and scatter corrections for 180° studies are less straightforward to implement.

RECONSTRUCTION THEORY

● **How can the computer work out the internal distribution of a tracer from the planar projections?**

▲ The planar views are simply the summation of the count rates at each point along the projection through the body (complicated by attenuation, but this problem will be dealt with later). Each point is seen at every projection angle. At different angles different points are summed together. This process is like a gigantic number of simultaneous equations. The unknowns are the individual count rates at each location. Solving these equations allows the reconstruction of the radiotracer distribution that gave rise to the acquired projections.

The computer could go about solving the simultaneous equations by eliminating variables, but that method does not work very well with noisy data. There are methods known as iterative reconstructions which are similar to solving simultaneous equations. The iterative reconstruction methods do not afford as much insight about the reconstruction process as do the methods which are based on a process called back-projection.

The principle which underpins the backprojection method is known as the projection slice theorem. It states that the one-dimensional Fourier transform of the projection of an object at an angle θ is equal to a slice through the two-dimensional Fourier transform of the object at the angle θ. This is illustrated in Figure 109.3. Thus, a transform performed on the raw data is equivalent to a 'spoke' through the transform of the reconstructed image. If many spokes from different angles are combined a representation of the originating radiotracer distribution can be formed.

Back-projection involves projecting the acquired data back across the reconstruction matrix. At each angle the counts from each ray sum are evenly distributed between each element on the ray. After doing this from a large number of angles the elements with the highest count rate have the most counts, but unfortunately elements without any activity also get some counts. In order to understand these complicated processes, we always start with simple objects, and the simplest of these is a point source. The back-projected image of a point source is a star. The distance between the lines of the star increase with increasing distance from the point source. If the distance from the point source is r, then the value of the final back-projected value is $1/r$. If there are a lot of projection angles, then it makes sense to say that the density of the lines in a region is proportional to $1/r$ (Fig. 109.4). All of these extra lines lead to a very blurred reconstruction. We consider that each point in the image acts independently of those around it, and so each behaves like a star. The combined effect of all of these star artefacts is to produce a very blurred image of little use. However, this can be corrected by filtering the data, either before or after reconstruction.

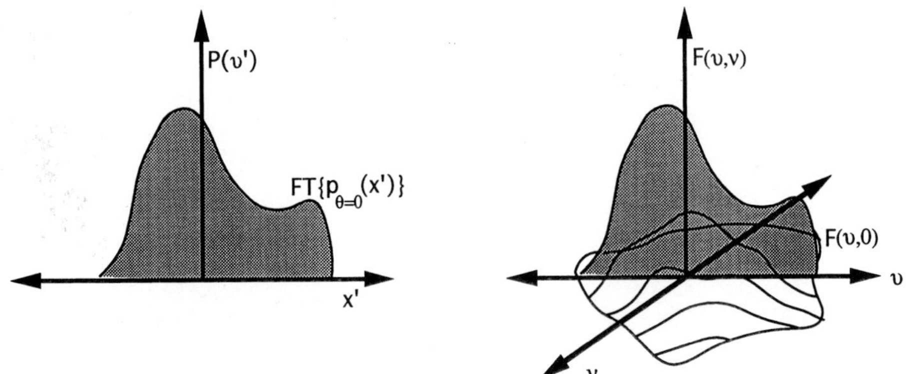

Fig. 109.3 The projection slice theorem states that the one-dimensional Fourier transform of the projection of an object at an angle θ (left) is equal to a slice through the two-dimensional Fourier transform of the object at the angle θ (right). Many projections at different angles will look like a number of spokes, and this can be transformed to give the reconstructed image.

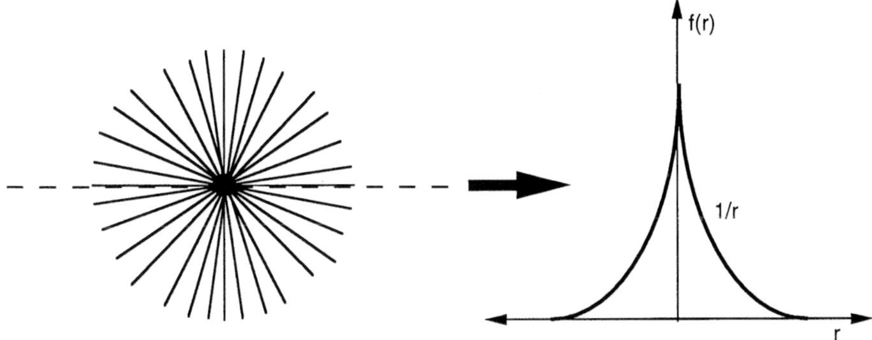

Fig. 109.4 The reconstruction of a point source by simple back-projection gives a star-like pattern. A profile through the reconstruction shows that it behaves as a $1/r$ function with increasing distance from the point. This is true for every point in the reconstruction. It is this star artefact that the filtering step removes.

● **Why is the reconstruction called *filtered* back-projection?**

▲ A method was described in 1971 that overcame the $1/r$ problem by the use of a filtering step[7] before back-projection. Correcting for the $1/r$ effect before back-projection removes the blurring, and is implemented as a convolution operation. Why does this work? A feature of the correcting function (which because of its shape is referred to as the ramp function) is that it contains negative side-lobes about the peak in the spatial domain (see Fig. 109.5). These negative components serve to cancel out the unwanted contributions outside the point and eventually lead to the desired result, a mathematically exact reconstruction (in the absence of any noise in the projection data).

● **Why is there a 'window' applied to the ramp filter, and what is its effect?**

▲ An unwanted characteristic of the ramp filter is that it is perfectly designed to amplify the noise in the data. It enhances the higher spatial frequencies in the data (the fine detail), of which noise is a constant component. A simple example shows that projection data in which each pixel contains noise at a 5% level will lead to a reconstruction with almost 50% standard deviation for all pixels in the object if a simple ramp filter is used.[8] This can be limited to some extent by the operation of windowing the ramp filter.

Windowing means that the ramp filter is altered to prevent it greatly amplifying the noise component of the image. Thus we allow the ramp filter to behave like a ramp filter in that part of the frequency spectrum where we require its 'deblurring' attributes but, at a point above which we know that the data contains very little information (fine detail) and noise predominates, the ramp filter is modified to behave more like a 'noise-suppression' filter. There are a great number of filters used to window the ramp, for example Shepp–Logan, Parzen, Hann, Hamming, Butterworth, etc. All have the same basic effect – they modify the ramp at higher spatial frequencies to restrict noise amplification. Figure 109.6 shows a bone scan (top row) and gallium scan (bottom), both roughly at the level of the liver with different windows applied to the ramp filter. The images on the left are reconstructed using

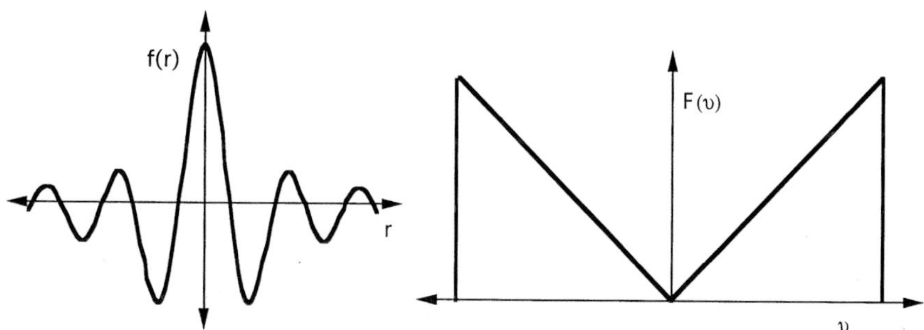

Fig. 109.5 The ramp filter's form in the spatial (left) and frequency (or Fourier, right) domain is shown. The negative side-lobes in the spatial domain serve to cancel out the unwanted contributions that would have given rise to the $1/r$ blurring in the reconstructed image.

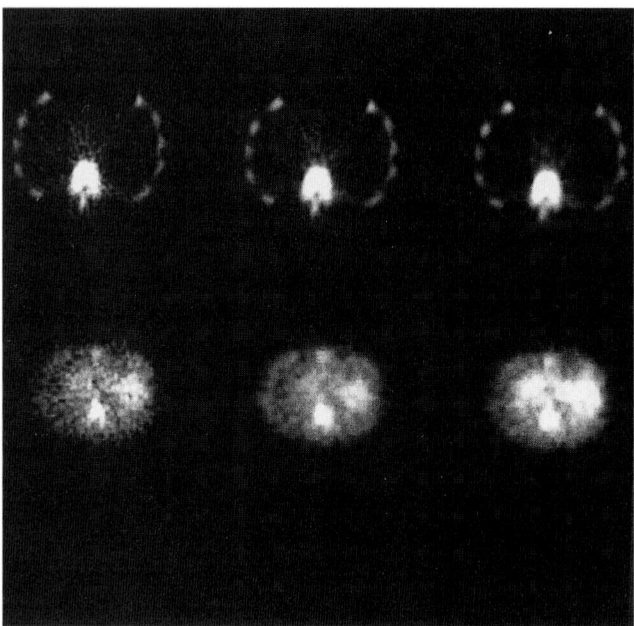

Fig. 109.6 Examples of bone (top row) and gallium (bottom row) scans at approximately the level of the liver. The reconstruction windows were: left, unwindowed ramp; centre, Hamming window cut off at 1.5 times the Nyquist frequency; and right, Hamming windowed ramp with cut-off equal to the Nyquist frequency.

an unwindowed ramp filter, the central images using a Hamming window cut off at at 1.5 times the Nyquist frequency (see Ch. 108), and the reconstructions on the right used a Hamming window cut off at the Nyquist frequency. The images show the change in the nature of the noise, and the loss of resolution, with changes in the window. The fine detail of the bone scan is best visualized with a 'sharper' image on the left, whereas the low-frequency structures seen in the gallium scan are best appreciated with a 'softer' reconstruction window.

● What is the effect of prefiltering on filtered back-projection and should the reconstruction window be modified in any way?

▲ Prefiltering refers to processing of the data before any attempt at reconstruction is made. It allows relatively straightforward two-dimensional filtering to be implemented and is often implemented simply to suppress noise by averaging with neighbouring pixels. More complicated operations include resolution recovery (i.e. image sharpening). Two common approaches that do combine these are the (so-called) Weiner and Metz filters. Both filters seek to restore resolution in the image, but include a term to suppress noise as well. It is generally assumed that the output of these operations is a projection set with better resolution and less noise. If only noise suppression is required, a filter such as a 2-D Butterworth can be used, which is essentially a low-pass filter (i.e. high frequencies including noise are suppressed).

Usually the reconstruction window is modified, compared with the unfiltered case, after these operations as noise has been largely removed. It is common to use an unwindowed ramp filter in the reconstruction, based on the premise that the projection data have little noise after the prefiltering step. Prefiltering, if used with care, affords great opportunities to improve reconstructed quality as it can improve resolution in the projection data as well as suppress noise. For further information, see some of the papers by King et al[9] and Miller & Sampathkumaran.[10]

● How do fan and cone beam reconstructions differ from those acquired with a parallel-hole collimator?

▲ A fan beam collimator is one that is focused in one direction only, so that its focus is a line. The data still come from one transaxial plane, but with some magnification. Magnification of the image means that more of the detector is being used to view the area of interest, and this implies an increase in sensitivity. There is also an improvement in resolution in much the same way as a pinhole collimator improves resolution, by using a larger detector area to view a smaller object. The data from a fan beam acquisition can be reformatted, knowing the angulation on the collimator, to a parallel-beam geometry and reconstructed with a conventional 2-D filtered back-projection algorithm.

A cone beam collimator focuses to a point. By doing so it affords the greatest sensitivity improvement possible with conventional collimation, as it is maximizing the area of detector irradiated by the object. A cone beam acquisition requires a fully 3-D reconstruction algorithm, however, and these are computationally demanding. Some algorithms to do this have recently become available.[11]

● What is a statistical or iterative reconstruction, and how do they work? What do they offer? Why are they seldom used?

▲ The methods based on spatial frequencies (i.e. back-projection) give us a very efficient method of reconstruction, but they assume that the data are simple projection ray sums. When other effects such as attenuation, scatter and statistical noise are present, these methods are susceptible to creating artefacts. A more general method is iterative reconstruction. The key to iterative reconstruction is a good understanding of the data collection process so that it can be modelled on the computer. The iterative methods are based on a set of sequential approximations.

The iterative methods start with some guess about the reconstructed image. Then the computer determines what the aquired data would be if that guess was correct. The difference between that guess and the acquired data is the error. Some types of reconstructions are based on modifications suggested by the errors. The reconstructed errors can be used to correct the guess of the image. This process is then repeated a number of times. There are a large number of variations on this process, but the basic idea is one of successive approximations. The iterative methods have a great advantage in that many different types of effects can be included – attenuation, scatter, collimator resolution as a function of depth, etc. The key to the iterative methods is a good model of the data collection process. The disadvantage of the iterative methods is that reconstruction takes more time. As computer power continues to improve, more widespread use of iterative reconstruction methods in nuclear medicine is likely.

● **What is the difference between axial resolution and slice spacing? Are the slices not just 1 pixel thick?**

▲ The slices may be 1 pixel thick, but what does that 1 pixel mean? Axial resolution is a term that describes the blurring in the axial direction in SPECT, which is just the resolution in the axis of rotation of the gamma-camera. SPECT does nothing magical to alter this. Slice spacing, though, refers to the distance between the centres of the adjacent reconstructed slices. This clearly depends on the acquisition matrix size selected, and is independent of the physical parameter 'resolution'. Axial resolution changes with collimator, radionuclide, radius of rotation of the detector, the prefiltering employed and other parameters. Slice spacing depends only on the matrix size. In the final images there are a large number (e.g. 64) of overlapping slices that are spaced 1 pixel apart. There is a great overlap in SPECT in adjacent slices.

ATTENUATION CORRECTION

● **Why correct for attenuation?**

▲ In SPECT there are two unknowns in the projection data; the first is the unknown internal distribution of the radiotracer, and the second is the unknown distribution of tissue densities. The latter, of course, is the basis of X-ray imaging and CT in particular. Attenuation has a large effect on the data. In a typical head, the photons emitted from the centre of the head will be reduced by 4–5 times compared with the edge of the head simply because of attenuation; in the abdomen it can be up to a factor of 10 (for 140 keV photons). Neglecting this effect will lead to an underestimate of the true radiotracer concentration, which will be most pronounced at the centre of the body. Furthermore, variations in attenuation can create artefacts in the reconstruction, because the successive projections are not consistent with each other.

The size of the object and the density of the tissues contained determines the attenuation. There is less attenuation in the chest than the abdomen because of the lungs. The bones have slightly more attenuation than the soft tissues, although this effect is smaller at 140 keV than in routine radiographs.

● **What types of corrections are available, and what are their merits and demerits?**

▲ Attenuation correction techniques fall into three categories depending on whether they are applied before, during or after the back-projection process. The easiest to implement are the prereconstruction corrections,[12,13] which are simple geometric calculations based on an assumed body shape and constant density. The attenuation correction during the back-projection merely applies an exponential weighting term to the data as it is distributed across the reconstruction matrix.[14,15] Again this is fairly simple to implement. The post-reconstruction corrections, the best-known example of which is the Chang method,[16] calculate the average attenuation to each point in the reconstructed image from a large number of angles. These methods have the attraction of being able to incorporate actual body density, or CT, measurements to improve accuracy. However, even using body density measurements in a post-reconstruction correction does not guarantee an accurate reconstruction.

● **Is it possible to correct for attenuation exactly?**

▲ None of these methods gives an exact correction, although some may come very close. Iterative attenuation correction techniques following back-projection that incorporate measured body density data offer great promise[17–19] and are being implemented by an increasing number of manufacturers. These methods will quite likely achieve better than 95% accuracy in a variety of situations. The iterative reconstruction techniques are also of great interest in this area as they can accurately incorporate the attenuation into their knowledge of the object as it is reconstructed. Given a good model of the object and the imaging system, the most accurate method is probably with an iterative reconstruction approach.

SCATTER CORRECTION

● **What is the difference between scatter and attenuation correction?**

▲ Interaction of photons with matter via the Compton effect gives rise to both attenuation and scatter. (The photoelectric effect also causes attenuation, but it is less important for tissue at 140 keV.) By attenuation we generally mean photons removed from the photon beam altogether, whereas scatter refers to photons which are deflected into the line of sight of the detector by a Compton interaction. When it comes to correcting for these effects, the two are inextricably linked. It is usual, though, to apply corrections for them separately.

● **What is the magnitude of the degradation due to scatter alone?**

▲ Scatter accounts for between 30% and 50% of the total counts acquired in a SPECT study with ^{99m}Tc. An illustration of the geometry of scattered events is shown in Figure 109.7. These will be back-projected and attributed to origins that are different from their true ones. This will lead to a decrease in contrast and an increased background over the image. Also, it makes the projections inconsistent with each other and back-projection does not work well under these circumstances.

● **Many methods of scatter correction have been described, but which is best?**

▲ A number of approaches to scatter correction have been proposed and fall into two main categories:

1. **energy window manipulations** such as asymmetric windows about the photopeak,[20] dual windows over the photopeak and a lower ('scatter') window,[21] splitting the photopeak with a pair of windows,[22,23] multiple windows[24] or energy-weighted acquisition;[25]
2. **pre or post-processing** operations such as Metz or Weiner filtering,[9] and deconvolution or convolution–subtraction.[26,27]

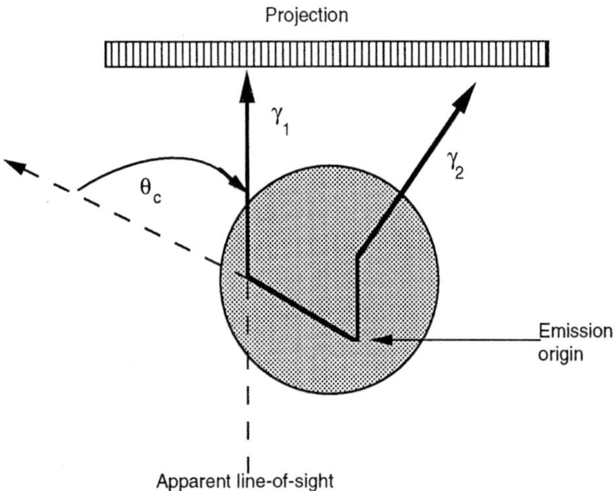

Fig. 109.7 Photon scattering via the Compton effect is shown. The deflection of the photon after the interaction is known as the Compton angle. In this example γ_1, which originally was emitted in a direction that would not have been detected at the projection angle shown, is scattered into the line of sight of the detector. Its position will be attributed to somewhere along the apparent line of response and it will therefore be misallocated. The net effect of photons like this will be to increase the background, thereby reducing contrast. The photon γ_2 on the other hand should have been recorded, but because of the scattering is deflected out of the line of response (it could of course be recorded if the detector was at a different angle, but it would also be misallocated in that example).

The answer as to which method to use depends on the reason for correcting for scatter. If it is merely to improve contrast, then the **dual window** scatter correction method would be perfectly adequate and is simple to implement. If accurate quantification of uptake is required, a more sophisticated method such as the **convolution–subtraction** method could be used (with care!). This requires a little more knowledge about the imaging environment and some experimental work beforehand usually to determine extra parameters to get the best answer. Some of the recent developments with photopeak splitting and multiple energy windows look very promising.

ERRORS DUE TO LIMITED RESOLUTION AND MOTION

● **What do the terms partial volume effect, spillover and recovery coefficient mean?**

▲ All measurement devices have some limit to their resolution, whether it is a ruler or an electron microscope, and the gamma-camera is no different. This means that at some point there exists a limit beyond which small structures become indistiguishable from each other if they are juxtaposed. Similarly, a small object appears larger than it actually is if it is less than the resolution of the system. This means that the signal is smeared over a larger area than it actually occupies signal diluted when it is reconstructed. What does remain faithfully preserved, however, are the total counts reconstructed. Thus the object appears to be larger and to have a lower radioactive concentration than it actually has. The partial volume refers to that portion of the resolution volume of the imaging system occupied by the object.

Spillover is another phenomenon which is caused by the limited resolution of the system. It represents the activity in one area of radiotracer accumulation (e.g. the heart wall in a myocardial perfusion study, or grey matter in a cerebral blood flow or metabolism study) that is 'spilled into' an adjacent area with a different radiotracer concentration (the chamber of the heart or the white matter in these examples) because of the limited resolution. This causes incorrect reconstructed concentrations in *both* of these areas.

The recovery coefficient is the ratio of the reconstructed count density to the true count density for objects less than the resolution volume, and therefore diluted by the partial volume effect. The simplest experimental way to determine it is to reconstruct different-sized objects containing the same solution of radionuclide and examine

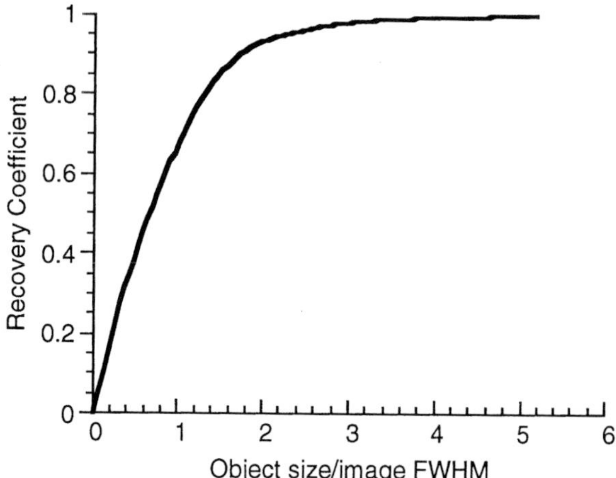

Fig. 109.8 The recovery coefficient of a rectangular object measured by a system with an isotropic Gaussian line spread function is plotted in terms of the system resolution. This curve can be implemented if the system FWHM is known. (After Hoffman & Phelps et al[2].)

the count density of the result. The recovery coefficient can give a correction factor, which is just a numerical multiplier, based on some knowledge of the real size and shape of the object of interest (e.g. a tumour) that corrects for the partial volume effect (see Fig. 109.8). It is usually determined by experimenting with different-sized objects under identical conditions to that encountered in the clinical situation; clearly, this is often hard to emulate. It does not correct for the dilution or blurring in a spatial sense but attempts to quantify accurately the uptake concentration. Anatomical modalities such as X-ray CT, MRI and ultrasound can be used to get a better assessment of the size of the object, and this information can be used to select the appropriate recovery factor.

- **What effect does physiological motion, such as diaphragmatic movement, have on reconstructed SPECT data?**

▲ There are many types of physiological motion – the beating of the heart, respiration, gastrointestinal peristalsis, bladder filling. Motion which is rapid and repetitive, such as beating of the heart, will tend to affect each of the projection images in a similar fashion. This type of motion will result in loss of resolution, but otherwise will not produce artefacts during reconstruction. Motion that affects the projection images differently will tend to produce artefacts. In cardiac imaging, the change in depth of respiration after exercise will change the position of the heart from the beginning to the end of data collection, resulting in upward creep of the heart. The change in diaphragm position changes the attenuation of the inferior wall. Therefore, in this example the most noticeable artefacts occur in the inferior wall. Some examples of the artefacts produced by patient motion are shown in Figure 109.9.

- **What can be done to limit the effect of physiological motion?**

▲ There is no simple answer to this question. In some circumstances the data collection can be modified. Starting and ending collection in the posterior projection can limit the bladder filling artefact as described previously. If possible, data collection can be timed to minimize physiological motion. For example, if data collection is delayed after exercise, then the effect of changing depth of respiration can be minimized. However, this is not always possible. In the case of ^{201}Tl imaging, delaying collection to minimize respiratory artefact must be weighed against the effects of early tracer redistribution.

- **Can the computer correct for the artefacts due to motion?**

▲ It is important to emphasize that it is always better to limit motion during collection than to correct for it during reconstruction. The largest amount of work on motion correction has dealt with myocardial imaging. There are two broad categories of motion – motion of the whole patient and motion within the patient. Motion of the whole patient may produce large effects, but motion of the heart due to respiration can also produce measurable effects. The most difficult problem is measuring the motion. After measuring the motion, the projection images can be digitally shifted to correct for the motion. Motion can be tracked either by using a fiducial marker such as a point source of activity, or by trying to track an object within the body. Tracking the object of interest, such as the myocardium, has the advantage that both whole-patient motion and motion of the heart with respect to the body can be taken into account. However, tracking an object within the body can be difficult, since in general the image of the object changes as the projection angle changes. In special circumstances this method has, however, been made to work.

NOISE

- **Why are SPECT reconstructions so noisy when, really, the acquisition time is quite lengthy?**

▲ Reconstruction by filtered back-projection is inherently a noise amplification process as the ramp filter multiplies the high frequencies in the image (of which noise is a component) by a greater amount than the lower frequencies. The noise level that might be expected intuitively based on, for example, the total acquired counts is wide of the mark because of this filtering process. The reconstructed signal-to-noise ratio (SNR) can be approximated when using a ramp filter by the equation:[28]

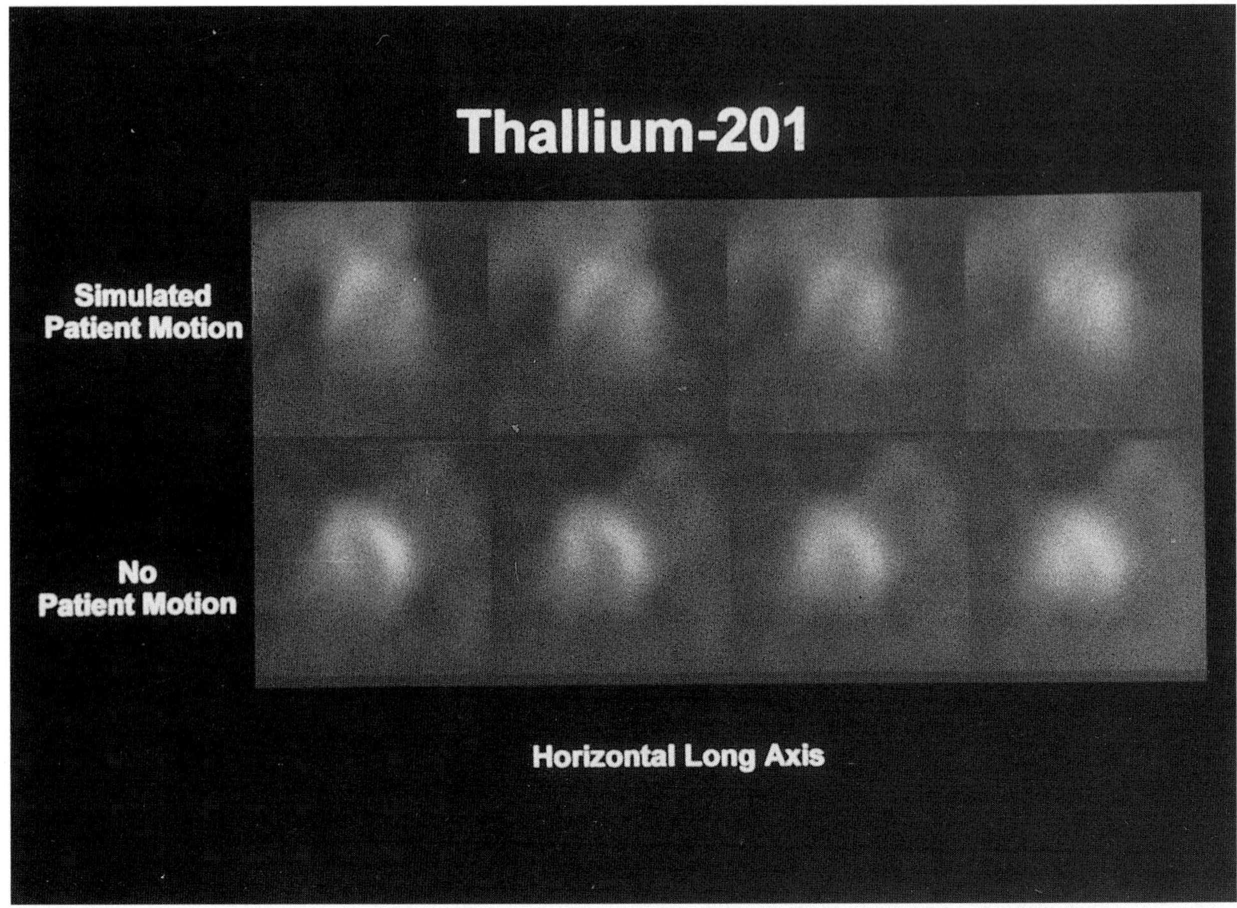

Fig. 109.9 This figure shows reconstructed SPECT images of a normal myocardial perfusion scan performed with ^{201}Tl. In the top row, 16 of 60 projections were translated to simulate patient motion. Although only a relatively small number of projections were affected, the images are totally uninterpretable. The bottom row shows the images reconstructed from the data with no patient motion. These images show a normal distribution of ^{201}Tl. Note, however, the decreased activity in the background outside the heart. This decreased activity is an artifact due to uncorrected breast attenuation.

$$SNR = \sqrt{N_r}/\sqrt[4]{R}$$

where N_r is the reconstructed count per pixel and R is the number of resolution elements containing activity. The intuitive noise level from Poisson statistics is just $\sqrt{N_r}$

Using this equation with a count density in the reconstruction of 400 counts/pixel with roughly 2000 resolution elements (≈64×642) the SNR for a reconstruction will be

$$\begin{aligned} SNR &= \sqrt{N_r}/\sqrt[4]{R} \\ &= \sqrt{400}/\sqrt[4]{2000} \\ &\approx 20/6.7 \\ &\approx 3.0 \end{aligned}$$

Intuitively assuming Poisson statistics would suggest that $400/\sqrt{400} = 20$ would be the SNR – clearly there is a big difference.

● Is noise the same at each point in the reconstructed object?

▲ Factors such as attenuation and sampling (accentuated towards the centre of the field of view) make this a complicated issue. In general reconstruction theory however, the absolute value of the noise is constant across the object independent of the underlying value.[29] In SPECT, when the corrections for attenuation are applied the effect is to magnify the centre values, and hence the noise, more than at the outer portion of the object. This leads to varying noise across the object.

● Why is a 'blob'-like pattern frequently seen in areas of constant count density?

▲ The noise in a reconstructed image is very different to the noise in a planar image. In a planar image the noise at each point is independent of the noise at any other point – this type of noise is called white noise. The noise in the projection images is white noise, but this noise is filtered during reconstruction. In the reconstructed image there is reduced low-frequency noise and increased high-frequency noise. This type of noise has a blob-like structure when reconstructed. The 'grain' of the reconstructions will change with the window selected for modifying the ramp filter. The noise structure is important in visual detection tasks as human observers do less well detecting objects in structured noise.

QUANTIFICATION

● **What is meant by 'quantification' in SPECT?**

▲ The term quantification has two potential meanings in SPECT: firstly it means to reconstruct radioactivity distributions and calibrate them in absolute activity terms [e.g. total activity (MBq) in an organ or concentration (kBq/cm^3)], and secondly it implies taking this process one step further and converting this absolute activity measure to a biological measure (e.g. blood flow in ml/min). For this, extra information about the nature of the tracer in vivo is usually required, such as the arterial blood concentration of the tracer in the period of time after injection, and analysis using models that 'compartmentalize' the tracer's distribution throughout the body (see Ch. 108).

Sometimes the term quantification is used in conjunction with the determination of organ volumes, but we prefer to use the term in relation to a measure of radioactivity (a functional measure) rather than volume (a structural measure), which anatomical modalities are better equipped to estimate.

● **What problems are likely to be encountered in calculating uptake in a tumour for the purposes of radiation therapy planning? Is a simple relative uptake estimation sufficient?**

▲ Treatment planning would appear to be an excellent application for quantitative SPECT. The aspects that would be needed to achieve this would be:

1. an accurate attenuation correction;
2. an accurate scatter correction;
3. ability to calibrate the SPECT system to convert count density to radioactivity concentration;
4. knowledge of the size of the tumour to allow for partial volume corrections;
5. knowledge of the kinetics of the tracer/treatment radionuclide to assess total integrated uptake and hence the dose to be delivered;
6. spillover from surrounding regions which might have high concentrations of the radioactive compound (e.g. blood pool or often the liver).

The problems that might be encountered are obvious in points (1), (2) and (4) above. A relative measure might be achieved by calibration against a small vial of the same radiotracer, or placing a mock tumour in a body phantom, but it is unlikely that either of these situations will encounter the same distribution, attenuation, and background problems as in the patient. These methods will give an indication of uptake, but accurate dose estimates will be prone to large errors.

It is obvious that these six requirements are very demanding. Because there are so many factors to consider, it is important that the methods be carefully checked with realistic phantoms or, when possible, biopsy material. Meticulous attention to detail and good-quality control are essential. It might seem simpler to obtain a relative measure by calibration against a small vial of the same radiotracer, or by placing a mock tumour in a body phantom. However, neither of these methods replicates the actual distribution exactly. These methods are better used for quality control than for primary quantification in a patient.

FURTHER READING

For a more in-depth discussion of many of the aspects discussed in this section the reader is referred to the following, which we have found to be useful: for acquisition and reconstruction in general see Sorenson & Phelps,[28] Mueller et al,[30] Brooks & Di Chiro,[31] Vardi et al[32] and Parker;[33] in attenuation correction there have been a number of papers comparing different approaches, such as Moore[34], Webb et al,[35] and Murase et al;[36] likewise, in scatter correction see Gilardi et al;[37] little exists in the literature about errors due to partial volume effects and motion (or more correctly) how to compensate for them), but the editorial by Parker[38] summarizes the issues; in a similar vein noise is summarized in Sorenson & Phelps;[28] quantification in SPECT is still in the realm of the 'under development', but for some interesting studies see Osborne et al,[39] and Rowell et al.[40]

REFERENCES

1. Bracewell R N, Riddle A C 1967 Inversion of fan-beam scans in radio-astronomy. Astrophys J 150: 427
2. Hoffman E J, Phelps M E 1986 Positron emission tomography: principles and quantitation. In: Phelps M, Mazziotta J, Schelbert H (eds) Positron emission tomography and autoradiography: principles and applications for the brain and the heart. Raven Press, New York, pp 273–276
3. Muehllehner G 1985 Effect of resolution improvement on required count density in ECT imaging: a computer simulation. Phys Med Biol 30: 163–173
4. Phelps M E, Huang S-C, Hoffman E J, Plummer D, Carson R 1982 An analysis of signal amplification using small detectors in positron emission tomography. J Comput Assist Tomogr 3: 551–565
5. Eisner R K, Nowak D J, Pettigrew R, Fajman W 1986 Fundamentals of 180° acquisition and reconstruction in SPECT imaging. J Nucl Med 27: 1717–1728

6. Knesaurek K, King M A, Glick S J, Penney B C 1989 Investigation of causes of geometric distortion in 180° and 360° angular sampling in SPECT. J Nucl Med 30: 1666–1675
7. Ramachandran G N, Lakshminarayanan A V 1971 Three-dimensional reconstruction from radiographs and electron micrographs: applications of convolutions instead of Fourier transforms. Proc Natl Acad Sci USA 68: 2236–2240
8. Budinger T F, Derenzo S E, Greenberg W L, Gullberg G T, Huesman R H 1978 Quantitative potentials of dynamic emission computed tomography. J Nucl Med 19: 309–315
9. King M A, Schwinger R B, Doherty P W, Penney B C 1984 Two-dimensional filtering of SPECT images using the Metz and Weiner filters. J Nucl Med 25: 1234–1240
10. Miller T R, Sampathkumaran K S 1982 Design and application of finite impulse response digital filters. Eur J Nucl Med 7: 22–27
11. Gullberg G T, Zeng G L, Datz F L, Christian P E, Tung C-H, Morgan H T 1992 Review of convergent beam tomography in single photon emission computed tomography. Phys Med Biol 7: 507–534
12. Budinger T F, Gullberg G T 1974 Three-dimensional reconstruction in nuclear medicine emission imaging. IEEE Trans Nucl Sci NS-21: 2–20
13. Kay D B, Keyes Jr J W 1975 First order corrections for absorption and resolution compensation in radionuclide Fourier tomography. J Nucl Med 16: 540–541
14. Gullberg G T, Budinger T F 1981 The use of filtering methods to compensate for constant attenuation in single-photon emission computed tomography. IEEE Trans Biomed Eng BME-28: 142–157
15. Tretiak O J, Metz C 1980 The exponential radon transform. SIAM J Appl Math 39: 341–354
16. Chang L T 1978 A method for attenuation correction in radionuclide computed tomography. IEEE Trans Nucl Sci NS-25: 638–643
17. Morozumi T, Nakajima M, Ogawa K, Yuta S 1984 Attenuation correction methods using the information of attenuation distribution for single photon emission CT. Med Imag Tech 2: 20–28
18. Malko J A, Van Heertum R L, Gullberg G T, Kowalsky W P 1986 SPECT liver imaging using an iterative attenuation correction algorithm and an external flood source. J Nucl Med 27: 701–705
19. Bailey D L, Hutton B F, Walker P J 1987 Improved SPECT using simultaneous emission and transmission tomography. J Nucl Med 28: 844–851
20. Koral K F, Clinthorne N H, Rogers W L 1986 Improving emission-computed tomography quantification by compton-scatter rejection throughout offset windows. Nucl Instr Meth Phys Res A242: 610–614
21. Jaszczak R, Greer K L, Floyd C E, Harris C C, Coleman R E 1983 Improved SPECT quantification using compensation for scattered photons. J Nucl Med 25: 893–900
22. King M A, Hademenos G, Glick S J 1992 A dual photopeak window method for scatter correction. J Nucl Med 33: 605–612
23. Pretorius P H, van Rensburg A J, van Aswegen A, Lötter M G, Serfontein D E, Herbst C P 1993 The channel ratio method of scatter correction for radionuclide image quantitation. J Nucl Med 34: 330–335
24. Gagnon D, Todd-Pokropek A, Arsneault A, Dupras G 1989 Introduction to holospectral imaging in nuclear medicine for scatter subtraction. IEEE Trans Med Imag TMI-8: 245–250
25. DeVito R P, Hamill J J, Trefert J D, Stoub E W 1989 Energy-weighted acquisition of scintigraphic images by analysis of energy spectra. J Nucl Med 30: 2029–2035
26. Axelsson B, Msaki P, Israelsson A 1984 Subtraction of compton-scattered photons in single photon emission computerized tomography. J Nucl Med 25: 490–494
27. Msaki P, Axelsson B, Dahl C M, Larsson S A 1987 Generalised scatter correction method in SPECT using point scatter distribution functions. J Nucl Med 28: 1861–1869
28. Sorenson J A, Phelps M E 1987 Physics in nuclear medicine. Grune & Stratton, Orlando, FL, pp 419–423
29. Rutherford R A, Pullen B R, Goddard J, Isherwood I 1975 Quantitative information from the EMI scanner. In: Todd-Pokropek A and Raynaud C (eds), Information processing in scintigraphy. CEA, Orsay, pp 353–376
30. Mueller S P, Polak J F, Kijewski M F, Holman B L 1986 Collimator selection for SPECT brain imaging: the advantage of high resolution. J Nucl Med 27: 1729–1738
31. Brooks R A, Di Chiro G 1975 Theory of image reconstruction in computed tomography. Radiology 117: 561–572
32. Vardi Y, Shepp L A, Kaufmann L 1985 A statistical model for positron emission tomography. J Am Stat Assoc 80: 8–37
33. Parker J A 1990 Image reconstruction in radiology. CRC Press, Boca Raton
34. Moore S C 1982 Attenuation compensation. In: Ell P J and Holman B L (eds), Computed Emission Tomography. Oxford University Press, New York, pp 339–360
35. Webb S, Flower M A, Ott R J, Leach M O 1983 A comparison of attenuation correction methods for quantitative single photon emission computed tomography. Phys Med Biol 28: 1045–1056
36. Murase K, Itoh H, Mogami H, Ishine M, Kawamura M, Iio A, Hamamoto K 1987 A comparitive study of attenuation correction algorithms in single photon emission computed tomography (SPECT). Eur J Nucl Med 13: 55–62
37. Gilardi M-C, Bettinardi V, Todd-Pokropek A, Milanesi L, Fazio F 1988 Assessment and Comparison of Three Scatter Correction Techniques in Single Photon Emission Computed Tomography. J Nucl Med 29: 1971–1979
38. Parker J A 1993 Effect of motion on cardiac SPECT imaging. J Nucl Med 34: 1355–1356
39. Osborne D, Jaszczak R J, Greer K, Lischko M, Coleman R E 1985 SPECT quantification of Technetium-99m microspheres within the canine lung. J Comput Assist Tomogr 9: 73–77
40. Rowell N P, Flower M A, Cronin B, McCready V R 1993 Quantitative single-photon emission tomography for tumour blood flow measurement in bronchial carcinoma. Eur J Nucl Med 20: 591–599

110. Positron emission tomography

Steven R. Meikle Magnus Dahlbom

PRINCIPLES OF POSITRON EMISSION TOMOGRAPHY (PET)

● How does a PET scanner detect and localize positrons?

▲ The PET scanner does not detect positrons directly, but uses important features of **positron annihilation** to determine their spatial location. A positron is an anti-particle of an electron with the same mass but opposite charge. When emitted from the unstable nucleus (see p. 106.6), the positron has some initial kinetic energy that is lost through collisions with neighbouring electrons in surrounding tissue. When the positron loses all or most of its energy it eventually recombines with an electron to form a positronium. The lifetime of the positronium is very short. It annihilates, converting all its mass into energy in the form of two photons. The energy of each of these photons is always 511 keV (equal to the resting energy of the electron and the positron) and they are always emitted in opposite directions, to conserve energy and momentum (Fig. 110.1).

The fact that the annihilation photons are emitted simultaneously and in opposite directions is the fundamental basis for detection and localization of the positron emitter. A technique known as **coincidence detection** is used.[1–3] Scintillation detectors composed of inorganic crystals, such as bismuth germanate (BGO), and photomultiplier tubes are placed on opposite sides of the radiation source. The signals from the two detectors are fed into separate amplifier and energy discrimination circuits. If these circuits both produce a signal within a very narrow time interval (in the nanosecond range), a coincidence event has been detected.

Since annihilation photons are emitted in opposite directions, the detection of a coincidence event localizes the positron annihilation to a point lying somewhere on the line that joins the two detectors. This line is referred to as a coincidence line. A typical PET scanner consists of hundreds of such detectors forming a ring that surrounds the patient or, alternatively, opposing detector banks.

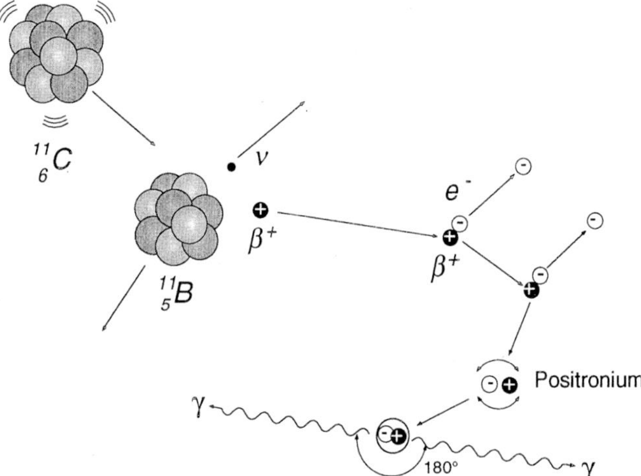

Fig. 110.1 An example of radioactive decay by positron emission. The unstable ^{11}C nucleus emits a positron (β^+) and a neutrino (υ) and, in the process, decays to stable ^{11}B. The positron travels a short distance in tissue, colliding with surrounding electrons and gradually losing energy, before forming a positronium. Almost instantaneously, the positronium annihilates, forming two gamma-rays (γ) with equal energy (511 keV) emitted at 180° to each other. It is these gamma-rays that are detected by the PET scanner and used to localize the positron emitter.

During a PET scan, several million coincidence events are recorded, forming a large number of intersecting coincidence lines and providing information about the quantity and spatial location of positron emitters within the body.

● How is a PET image formed?

▲ The following discussion refers to ring-type PET scanners, although the principles of image formation are similar for other detector configurations. Each detector in a circular array can form a coincidence line with any one of a number of opposing detectors. The location and direction of any given coincidence line is unique, and the collection of a large number of these coincidence lines forms the data set from which the cross-sectional image

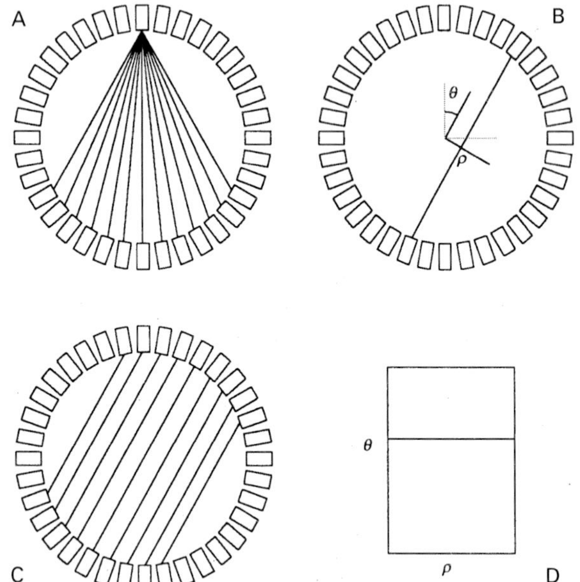

Fig. 110.2 A detector can be in coincidence with any of a number of opposing detectors, forming a fan of coincidence lines (A), each of which has a unique offset (ρ) and angle (θ) with respect to the scanner axis (B). The coincidence lines can be separated into sets that are parallel with each other (C) and rearranged into a two-dimensional sinogram (D), in which each row represents a view of the object at a particular angle. The sinogram is a convenient format in which to store the data prior to reconstruction.

can be reconstructed. Acquired coincidences are stored as two-dimensional matrices, in which the horizontal direction describes the offset (ρ) from the centre of the field of view and the vertical direction describes the projection angle (θ). This two-dimensional matrix is referred to as a **sinogram,** and provides a convenient means of storing the projection data prior to the image reconstruction step (Fig. 110.2).

Before reconstructing the image, the sinogram data must be corrected for **detector non-uniformity** of response and attenuation of photons within the body. In an ideal PET system with a large number of detectors, the efficiency of each coincidence line will be identical. However, owing to geometrical variations, differences in energy discrimination, detector gains, etc. there may be significant variation in detection efficiency between detector elements in the system. To avoid introduction of artefacts in the final image it is, therefore, necessary to equalize these variations in detection efficiency. The variations can be measured using a source that exposes all detectors with uniform photon flux. The correction is analogous to the uniformity correction procedure that is used in SPECT. Attenuation correction is performed to compensate for the reduction in measured coincidences due to absorption of one or both of the annihilation photons within the body. This procedure is discussed in detail below.

Once these corrections have been performed, the value in a given sinogram element represents the summation of all coincidence events occurring along the corresponding coincidence line. This is similar to X-ray CT, except that the sum of photons emitted from within the body is recorded rather than the sum of photons transmitted through the body (from an external source). Images can then be reconstructed from the sinogram data, most commonly using the filtered back-projection algorithm (see Ch. 109). A series of parallel two-dimensional trans-axial images is obtained, typically spaced 3 mm apart and covering an axial field of view of 10–15 cm.

● Does a PET scanner only detect valid coincidences?

▲ Ideally, the only coincidence events recorded by a positron tomograph are those which arise from a unique positron annihilation that occurred along the line between two activated detectors. These are referred to as **true coincidences**, or 'trues', and they carry useful information about the location of the positron emitter. However, other types of coincidence events occur which degrade the measurement, including **accidental, scatter and multiple coincidences**[4] (Fig. 110.3).

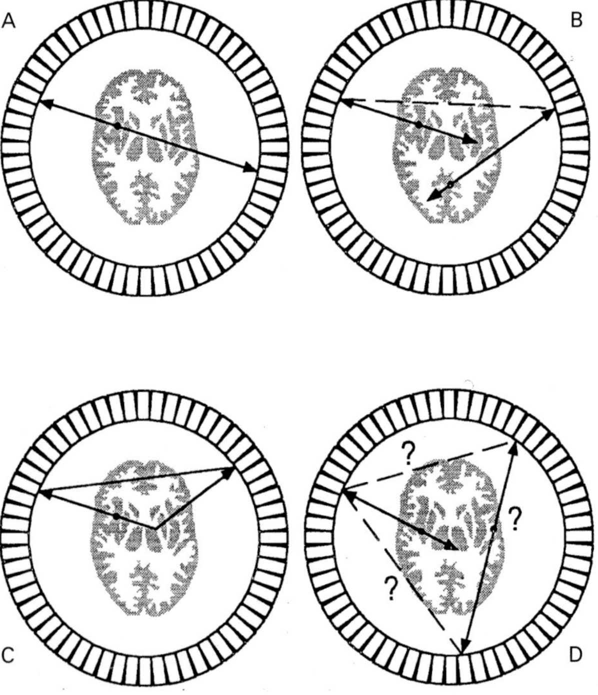

Fig. 110.3 Not all coincidence events detected by a PET scanner contain useful information. Those that arise from unique positron annihilations without deviation of the emitted photons are referred to as trues (A). True coincidences carry information about the spatial location of the positron source. Accidental coincidences are those that arise from unrelated isotope decays (B) and, therefore, do not help to locate a unique positron emission. Spatial information may also be lost if one or both of the annihilation photons undergo Compton scattering in the body (C), or if multiple photons (more than two) are in coincidence with each other as a result of two or more positron annihilations (D), creating ambiguity about positioning.

Accidental coincidences

When positron annihilation occurs, two 511 keV photons are emitted simultaneously. Therefore, the detectors should ideally produce the logic signals simultaneously. However, because of limitations in the scintillation detectors and the processing electronics, there is uncertainty in the exact timing of the logic pulses. Because of this uncertainty, coincidence events have to be accepted within a certain finite time interval, typically 12 ns. Because of the finite width of the coincidence time window there is a possibility that two unrelated photons will be detected and registered as a coincidence. These unrelated events are referred to as accidental or random events. Since accidental events are produced by photons emitted from unrelated isotope decays, they do not carry any spatial information about the activity distribution. It is therefore necessary to correct for these events that would otherwise produce an undesired background in the final images.[5] The accidental coincidence rate can be measured. However, the measurement may add significantly to the noise in the final image, particularly at high count rates.

Scatter coincidences

Scattered events are those in which one or both of the annihilation photons are diverted from their original path before reaching the detector as a result of Compton interactions with electrons in surrounding tissue. The coincidence detection technique assumes that events recorded by a detector pair originate from an annihilation located on a line connecting the two detectors. For a scattered event this is not true and, as a result, the coincidence event is mispositioned. The number of scatter coincidences as a proportion of those measured is typically 15%, and the effect is to add an almost structureless background to the image, resulting in loss of contrast. Photons lose energy through scattering collisions and therefore, in theory, can be distinguished from unscattered events on the basis of energy. However, the energy resolution of PET detectors is poor, and only large-angle scatter events in which appreciable energy is lost can be discriminated. Scatter can be more efficiently removed by lead or tungsten collimation placed between each imaging slice.[6] The **interplane septa**, typically 1 mm thick and 12–16 cm long, eliminate scattered events originating from regions outside a given slice.

Multiple coincidences

Although only two detectors are required to be activated within the coincidence time window to register a valid coincidence, at high count rates it is possible that three or more detectors are involved. This occurs if more than one positron annihilates during the coincidence time window. In this case it becomes ambiguous how the event should be positioned. To resolve the ambiguity, these multiple coincidences, which are easily distinguished from unique coincidences, are normally discarded. However, since they contain information about the quantity and spatial location of positron emissions, albeit ambiguous information, discarding them causes count rate loss in the system.

● How is attenuation correction performed?

▲ Recall that a valid coincidence event requires the simultaneous detection of both photons arising from a positron annihilation. If either photon is absorbed within the body, a coincidence will not take place. The probability of detection, therefore, depends on the combined path of both photons. Since this is the same for all sources lying on the line that joins the two detectors, the probability of attenuation is the same for all such sources, independent of position.

This can be understood by considering a point source located x cm inside the boundary of a cylinder of diameter D (Fig. 110.4). If the linear attenuation coefficient of the material in the cylinder is μ, then the proportion of

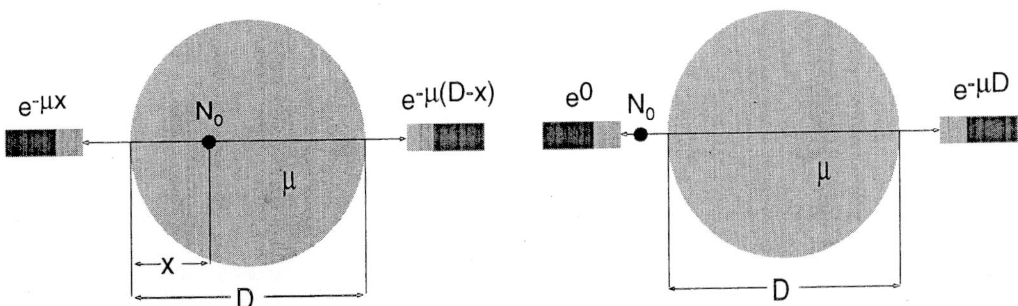

Fig. 110.4 One of the unique features of PET is that, for a given coincidence line, the probability of photon absorption (attenuation) is the same for any source, independent of its location along the line. This is true even if the source is external to the object. This makes it relatively straightforward to correct for attenuation using an external (transmission) source. As a result, PET images can be calibrated in terms of absolute tracer concentration.

emitted photons that reach the near detector is $e^{-\mu x}$ and the proportion of photons that reach the far detector is $e^{-\mu(D-x)}$. Then, the number of detected coincidences, N, given an initial count rate, N_0, is determined by combining these two probability terms:

$$N = N_0[e^{-\mu x} \times e^{-\mu(D-x)}] = N_0 e^{-\mu D} \quad (1)$$

Thus, the probability of coincidence detection is independent of source depth, x. This is true, even if the source is positioned outside the body. In this case, the probability terms are e^0 and $e^{-\mu D}$ for the nearest and farthest detectors respectively, and the number of detected coincidences is:

$$N = N_0(e^0 \times e^{-\mu D}) = N_0 e^{-\mu D} \quad (2)$$

which is the same as that obtained for the internal source. Therefore, the probability of attenuation for all sources along a given line of response can be determined by comparing the count rate from an external, or transmission, source with the unattenuated count rate from the same source when the patient is not in the tomograph, referred to as a **blank scan**.

A transmission scan typically takes 20 min to acquire and is normally performed before the PET tracer is administered. The transmission count rate is measured for all possible lines of response using one or more rod sources that rotate around the patient or, alternatively, a stationary ring source. The transmission sources contain a long-lived positron emitter, for example ^{68}Ge ($t_{1/2}$= 275 days), which is retracted behind lead shielding when not in use. It is interesting that, despite the higher energy of annihilation photons (511 keV) compared with single photon emitters (e.g. ^{99m}Tc, 140 keV), the magnitude of attenuation is typically higher in PET than in SPECT. For example, annihilation photons passing through the centre of the thorax are typically reduced by a factor of 50 compared with less than 10 in SPECT. This is because in PET the combined photon path passes through the entire body rather than just the distance from the source to the detector.

ALTERNATIVE PET MODALITIES

● What is time-of-flight PET?

▲ There is a difference in arrival times of the annihilation photons unless the annihilation occurs exactly midway between the detectors. Since these photons have velocity equal to the speed of light, the time difference is extremely small. For example, an annihilation that occurs 10 cm closer to one detector than the other results in a time difference of 0.67 ns. The difference in arrival times is ignored in conventional PET systems but is used to improve the quality of image reconstructions in time-of-flight systems. Current technology is unable to detect a difference in arrival times less than about 0.3 ns, resulting in time-of-flight resolution of about 5 cm. This is clearly insufficient to obviate image reconstruction using conventional methods. However, the additional information that time of flight provides can be used to constrain back-projection to the general region where the event is assumed to have originated (e.g. a circle of radius 5 cm). This results in less noise amplification during image reconstruction, providing better signal-to-noise ratio in the reconstructed image.[7]

There are practical problems with time-of-flight PET that have limited its widespread application. Firstly, with currently achievable time-of-flight resolution, the improvement in signal-to-noise ratio is only observed in reasonably uniform regions of the image, whereas it is normally the more detailed structures that are of interest. Secondly, detectors such as BaF_2 and CsF, which are suitable for time of flight because of their rapid scintillation decay, have lower density than non-time-of-flight detectors such as BGO. This causes a loss of counting efficiency owing to poor absorption of 511 keV photons. Thus, the signal-to-noise gains of time-of-flight reconstruction are somewhat offset by the lower efficiency of these detectors. The discovery and development of a fast, high-density detector for time-of-flight PET may result in its more widespread use in the future.

● What is total-body PET imaging?

▲ PET has in the past focused on imaging of single organ systems, such as the brain and the heart. The main reason for this is the somewhat limited axial field of view on most PET systems. A technique for extending the axial field of view of the PET scanner has recently been developed, whereby the patient bed is moved slowly through the tomograph under computer control as data are acquired.[8,9] This technique allows imaging of larger sections of the body, which has been particularly useful in oncological imaging, when there may be many sites of interest throughout the body (Fig. 110.5). The technique has been

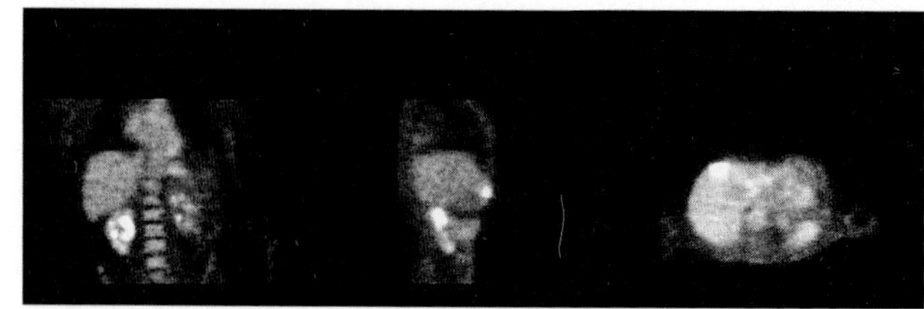

Fig. 110.5 Representative coronal, sagittal and transaxial sections from a total-body PET scan using [^{18}F]2-fluoro-2-deoxy-D-glucose (FDG). These images show the normal accumulation of FDG in liver, spleen, kidneys and skeletal muscle, as well as a focal abnormality in the right lobe of the liver corresponding to a metastatic lesion.

used with [^{18}F]2-fluoro-2-deoxy-D-glucose (FDG) for detection and localization of disease, as well as staging and assessment of response to therapy, particularly in colon carcinoma and tumours of the head and neck region.[10]

The requirement to image the whole body during the limited time that the patient can remain motionless in the scanner raises some difficult methodological issues. For example, conventional methods for performing attenuation correction are inadequate to handle the relatively noisy data acquired by total-body scanning.[11] To obtain quantitative measurements from total-body scanning requires alternative approaches to attenuation correction and the ability to simultaneously acquire emission and transmission data.[12] However, these requirements are not beyond the capabilities of current PET technology.

● What is three-dimensional (3-D) PET?

▲ Lead or tungsten septa are normally used to separate adjacent imaging planes and prevent photons that are detected in one imaging plane from being in coincidence with photons detected in other imaging planes (2-D mode). Although these are perfectly valid events and would result in up to a 10-fold increase in efficiency of the PET scanner, they are not normally permitted because this requires a special image reconstruction algorithm capable of reconstructing data acquired at all angles in three dimensions. Such a three-dimensional (3-D) algorithm had not been exploited in PET until recently.[13–15] The development of 3-D image reconstruction algorithms has resulted in current-generation PET scanners having the capability to remove the interplane septa and acquire and reconstruct data in three dimensions, resulting in significant gains in counting efficiency.[16,17] The increased efficiency in 3-D acquisition mode can be used to improve image quality in low-count studies, reduce the administered radiation dose or reduce scan time in clinical studies (Fig. 110.6).

There are, however, some drawbacks to 3-D PET, the main one being the significant increase in scatter coincidences recorded. Scattered events may account for up to 45% of measured coincidences in 3-D (similar to SPECT) compared with approximately 15% in 2-D. Therefore, some of the increase in efficiency provided by 3-D acquisition is the result of unwanted events. The increase in scatter is due to the removal of interplane septa. Correction for the presence of scatter in the measurements is required to obtain quantitative values from 3-D PET studies.[18,19] Despite the drawbacks, 3-D PET offers great potential for improving the quality and/or throughput of PET studies.

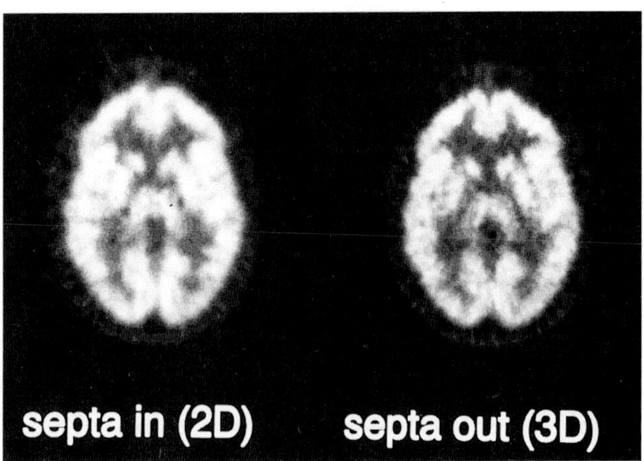

Fig. 110.6 Transaxial 2-D and 3-D [^{18}F]FDG images of the brain performed on the same patient. The image on the left was acquired for 30 min with the interplane lead septa in place (2-D mode). The image on the right was acquired for just 5 min with the interplane septa removed (3-D mode). Image quality is similar for both studies demonstrating that the improved efficiency of 3-D PET can be used to increase patient throughput.

PET PERFORMANCE CHARACTERISTICS

● What factors affect spatial resolution in PET?

▲ There are three main factors that affect the spatial resolution of PET images. These are the size of the individual detectors, **non-collinearity** of annihilation photons and **positron range**, which is the finite distance a positron travels before annihilating.

Detector size

The PET scanner consists of several hundred discrete detectors that form a ring surrounding the patient. Each pair of opposing detectors forms a channel of finite width, determined by the width of the individual detectors (typically 6 mm). Any coincidence pair that falls inside this channel will be detected by the same pair of detectors and assigned the same spatial location. Reducing the size of the detectors reduces the variation in spatial positioning within this channel. Therefore, the accuracy of spatial positioning of coincidence events is primarily limited by the size of the individual detectors. The major gains in spatial resolution of PET scanners in recent years have resulted from reducing the size of the detectors (Fig. 110.7).

Non-collinearity

One of the fundamental assumptions made in PET is that when a positron annihilates with an electron the resulting annihilation photons travel in exactly opposite directions. However, this is not always true. Unless the

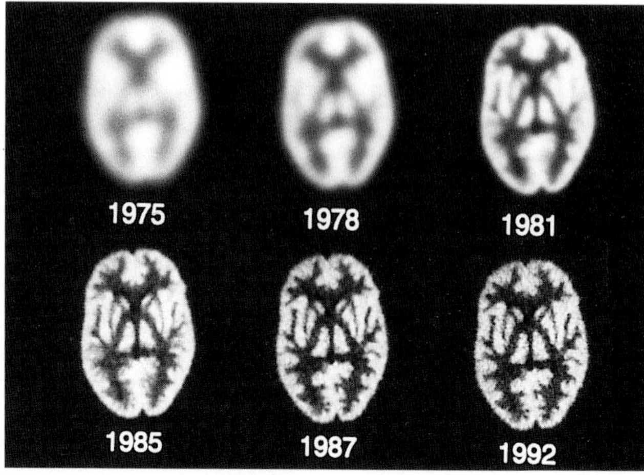

Fig. 110.7 Improvements in spatial resolution of PET scanners have occurred primarily as a result of reducing the size of individual detectors. Here, these improvements are shown by simulation for the period from 1975, when the first PET scanner for human studies was introduced, up to 1992. Current-generation PET scanners can resolve structures down to approximately 5 mm in size.

positron–electron pair comes to a complete rest, the particle will have some residual momentum when it annihilates. Since momentum must be conserved, the annihilation photons which result have some net directional component rather than emitting exactly 180° apart. This introduces a small error (typically <0.5°) in positioning the annihilation event. The impact of this error on overall image resolution depends on the diameter of the detector ring and is independent of positron energy. Non-collinearity degrades the spatial resolution of a whole-body PET scanner with 100 cm ring diameter by approximately 2 mm.

Positron range

Another assumption of PET is that the point of positron annihilation corresponds to the exact location of the radioactive atom from which it originated. However, positrons are emitted from the unstable nucleus with a continuous range of energies and, therefore, travel a finite distance, gradually losing energy, before annihilating. For example, the positrons emitted from a ^{18}F nucleus have energy up to 0.63 MeV and may travel 2–3 mm in tissue before annihilating.[20] Although this distance seems large, the error introduced in spatial localization depends on the direction of travel. If, for example, the direction of positron travel is towards one of the coincidence detectors, there is no error introduced. If, on the other hand, the positron travels in a direction orthogonal to the line between the two detectors, the error is maximized. On average, the positron range results in approximately a 0.2 mm mispositioning error for ^{18}F and 1.2 mm for the more energetic ^{15}O (see Table 110.1).[21,22]

These physical processes impose a fundamental limitation on the spatial resolution that can be achieved in PET of 2–3 mm (current commercial PET scanners have spatial resolution of approximately 5 mm). There is no such limitation in SPECT and, therefore, superior resolution compared with PET is theoretically achievable.

Table 110.1 Maximum energies, ranges and spatial resolution contribution for positron emitters commonly used in PET[20–22]

Isotope	E_{max} (keV)	Max range (mm)	FWHM (mm)
^{18}F	0.63	2.6	0.22
^{11}C	0.96	4.2	0.28
^{13}N	1.20	5.4	0.35
^{15}O	1.74	8.4	1.22
^{82}Rb	3.15	17.1	2.60

- **How does the physical performance of a PET scanner compare with that of a SPECT camera?**

▲ The parameters that describe the physical performance of SPECT and PET instruments include counting efficiency, spatial resolution, energy resolution and count rate performance. The relative importance of these parameters depends on the type of study being performed.

Counting efficiency

This refers to the proportion of emitted photons that are detected and contribute to the final image. The higher the counting efficiency, the better the instrument makes use of the available photon flux and the lower the noise level in the images. This is particularly important in low-count studies such as receptor–ligand studies. The counting efficiency of PET scanners is typically about 0.5% in 2-D mode. This compares with approximately 0.02% in SPECT using a single head system, a factor of 25 lower. These figures increase to approximately 3% for PET scanners operated without the interplane septa (3-D mode) and nearly 0.1% for a triple head camera using fan-beam collimation. Thus, PET maintains a 30-fold advantage in efficiency over SPECT.

Spatial resolution

This refers to the precision with which emissions can be localized. In PET this is determined by both scanner design and the physical processes of positron annihilation, as outlined above. In SPECT, spatial resolution is determined only by camera design, including collimator geometry. The variation in spatial resolution within the field of view differs for SPECT and PET systems. In PET, resolution is nearly uniform within the imaging plane, but is not necessarily the same in the axial (body axis) direction as it is in-plane. This is because of differences in

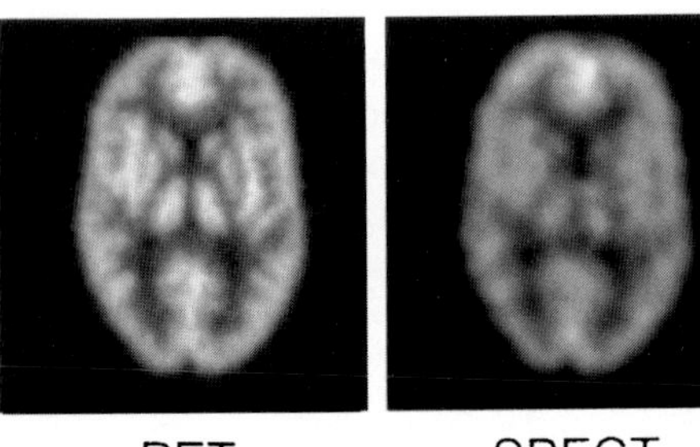

Fig. 110.8 Transaxial images of a realistic brain phantom using current-generation SPECT and PET instrumentation. Activity in the phantom and acquisition times were varied to achieve approximately the same number of acquired counts in both studies. These images demonstrate the similarity in spatial resolution between the two modalities, given sufficient counting statistics. SPECT images were performed on a Trionix Triad triple head camera (Trionix Research Laboratories, Twinsburg, OH, USA) with fan beam collimation. PET images were acquired on an ECAT 951 whole-body tomograph (CTI/Siemens, Knoxville, TN, USA) operated in 2-D mode.

detector size and spacing in each direction. However, in most current scanners spatial resolution is essentially isotropic. Also, spatial resolution is largely unaffected by operating in 3-D mode. In SPECT, spatial resolution is the same axially as it is across the imaging plane. However, there is a significant loss of spatial resolution within the imaging plane as depth in the object increases. Despite these differences, the gap between SPECT and PET in terms of absolute spatial resolution has become almost negligible in recent years and is 5–7 mm in both cases given ideal imaging conditions (Fig. 110.8).

Energy resolution

Energy resolution is the precision with which the detection system can determine the energy of detected photons. This, in turn, determines the ability of the system to discriminate between valid, unscattered photons and those that have lost their spatial information through scattering within the body or the detector itself. The result is loss of accuracy of spatial localization and poor image contrast. In both PET and SPECT this is primarily determined by the light output characteristics of the scintillator. Specifically, more light produced for each photon deposited in the crystal results in more information about photon energy being transferred to the detection system. The light output of BGO used in PET is much poorer (approximately 12% by comparison) than that of sodium iodide (NaI) used in SPECT. The error in energy discrimination is approximately 20% for 511 keV photons on a current generation PET scanner, compared with less than 11% for 140 keV photons on a current-generation SPECT camera. Despite this, the fraction of accepted events that undergo scattering is lower in PET because of the presence of interplane septa, typically 15% compared with up to 40% in SPECT.

Count rate performance

This parameter describes the response of the imaging system to inreasing the amount of radioactivity within the field of view. Ideally, the detected count rate increases linearly with increasing activity. However, in any counting system, a point is reached where the circuit is unable to process all incoming events as they arrive too rapidly. The count rate response then becomes non-linear. It is important to maintain a linear count rate response in high-count studies such as cerebral blood flow studies using the short-lived [^{15}O]water. A measure of count rate performance is the count rate at which a 20% loss is observed. This is similar for current-generation PET and SPECT systems; approximately 75 000 counts/s. Count rate performance is similar for PET operated in 2-D and 3-D modes. However, in 3-D, the 20% count rate loss is achieved at much lower radioactivity concentrations (typically 7–10 times lower) because of the increase in efficiency. In both modalities, count rate performance is adversely affected by the channelling of electronic signals through common circuitry, or multiplexing.[23,24] Unique to PET, the count rate performance is further limited by the necessity to process unwanted random coincidences, which form a large fraction of detected events at high count rates.

PET QUANTIFICATION

● Why is PET said to be quantitative?

▲ Three unique features of PET enable physiological variables, such as blood flow, metabolic rates and receptor density, to be measured in vivo. Firstly, the ability to perform accurate attenuation correction makes it possible to relate measured count rates to absolute tracer concentrations. Secondly, since all projections are acquired simultaneously, without any detector motion, rapid sequential images can be acquired, enabling the change in tracer concentration with time to be studied. The third and most important feature of PET is that positron emitters such as ^{11}C, ^{15}O and ^{18}F are readily incorporated into important biological compounds such as carbon monoxide, water and the glucose analogue, FDG. This, combined with the ability to measure the change in absolute tracer concentrations with time, enables their fate in vivo to be modelled using well-established tracer kinetic models.[25]

● How are physiological variables measured?

▲ The quantitative nature of PET lends itself to the application of tracer kinetic models for determining physiological variables of interest. The most common type of models employed are linear compartmental models, in which rate constants describe the rate of exchange of tracer between discrete compartments (see p. 108.13).

To estimate the rate constants for a particular compartmental model, it is necessary to know both the model input function (e.g. the blood activity versus time curve) and the model output (e.g. the tissue activity versus time curve). The input function can be obtained by taking serial blood samples from a radial artery and counting them in a calibrated gamma well counter. The tissue curve can be obtained by plotting counts versus time for defined regions of interest on the reconstructed PET images. The tissue and blood curves are supplied to a curve-fitting procedure, along with initial estimates of the rate constants, which attempts to find the optimal values of the rate constants, given the chosen compartmental model. Once the values of the rate constants are determined, relevant physiological variables can be derived. In general, the errors in parameter estimation increase with the complexity of the tracer model employed. For this reason, compartmental models used in PET are normally simplified to contain two or three compartments at most.

The most common tracer kinetic model used in PET is the three-compartment model for FDG[26,27] (Fig. 110.9). The compartments represent FDG in plasma, FDG in tissue and phosphorylated FDG in tissue (FDG-6-P). Phosphorylation of FDG is mediated by the hexokinase enzyme and, unlike glucose, is the terminal reaction step. The fact that FDG does not continue to be metabolized through the glycolytic pathway is an advantage for modelling purposes, as this means that the number of compartments and, therefore, the number of rate constants that need to be determined is manageable. The rate constants, k_1–k_4, represent the following processes:

k_1 = rate of transport of FDG from plasma to the tissue space
k_2 = rate of transport of FDG from tissue back to the vascular space
k_3 = rate of phosphorylation of FDG to form FDG-6-P
k_4 = rate of dephosphorylation of FDG-6-P to form FDG.

After estimating the values of k_1-k_4 by curve fitting, the metabolic rate of glucose utilization (MRGlc) is calculated as:

$$\mathrm{MRGlc} = \frac{C_\mathrm{p}}{\mathrm{LC}}\left(\frac{k_1 k_3}{k_2 + k_3}\right) \tag{3}$$

where C_p is the glucose concentration in the blood during the PET scan and LC is the lumped constant which accounts for differences in transport and phosphorylation between FDG and glucose.

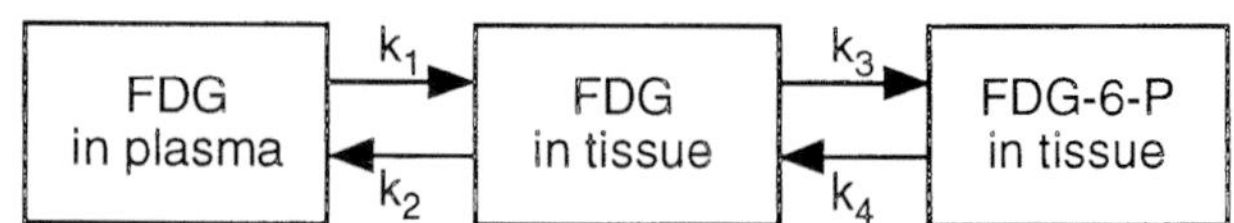

Fig. 110.9 A three-compartment model describing the kinetics of FDG in vivo. The compartments represent FDG in plasma, FDG in tissue and phosphorylated FDG in tissue (FDG-6-P) produced via the hexokinase reaction. For each dynamic FDG PET study, the values of the rate constants, k_1–k_4, for a given region of interest are determined by curve fitting and used to derive the metabolic rate of glucose utilization (MRGlc).

● How are parametric images generated in PET?

▲ If a given tracer model is sufficiently insensitive to noise, a stable solution may be found for an individual pixel rather than groups of pixels enclosed in a region of interest. If this is the case, the tracer model can be applied to every pixel in the image and a parametric image can be generated. In a parametric image, each pixel contains the parameter value of best fit determined by the model-fitting procedure. An example is [^{15}O]water, which can be represented by a two-compartment model, allowing generation of parametric images of either blood flow or volume of distribution. In most cases, three-compartment models, such as the FDG model, are too unstable to allow parametric images to be created.

An alternative approach for generating parametric images is the so-called **Patlak graphical technique**.[28,29] The method applies to any tracer that is irreversibly trapped in the tissue space within the measurement time interval. In other words, the tracer must have unidirectional uptake. If this condition is satisfied, the ratio of tissue to blood activity over time can be expressed as a straight-line plot. The fraction of blood activity taken up by tissue per unit time, or uptake constant, is given by the slope of the straight line and can be used to derive physiological variables.

Using FDG as an example, with the assumption that the rate of dephosphorylation of FDG in tissue is negligible, the myocardial tissue activity, C_t, at any point in time comprises a fraction, F, of the blood activity, C_b, and the amount of tracer delivered to the tissue up to that point in time:

$$C_t(t) = FC_\mathrm{b}(t) + K\int_0^t C_\mathrm{b}(s)\,\mathrm{d}s \tag{4}$$

K is the tissue uptake constant, which is equivalent to the combined rate constant term in equation 3, $\frac{k_1 k_3}{k_2+k_3}$. By plotting $C_t(t)/C_\mathrm{b}(t)$ versus $\int_0^t C_\mathrm{b}(s)\mathrm{d}s/C_\mathrm{b}(t)$, a straight-line plot is obtained with K given by the slope and F given by the y-intercept. Linear regression is performed on each pixel to determine K. These values are converted to metabolic rates as in equation 3, producing an image calibrated in units of μmol/min/g (Fig. 110.10).

The graphical technique is relatively insensitive to

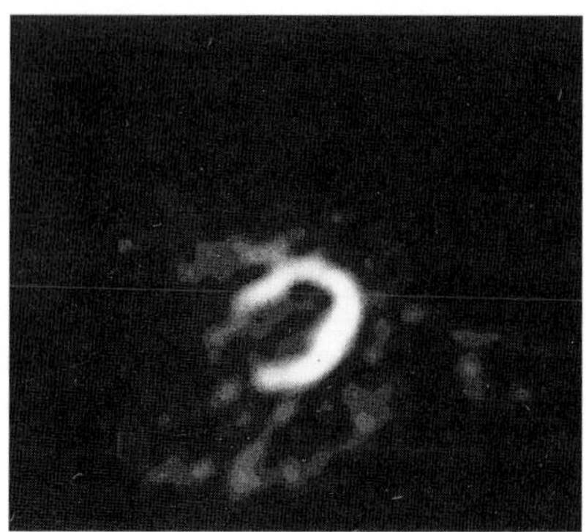

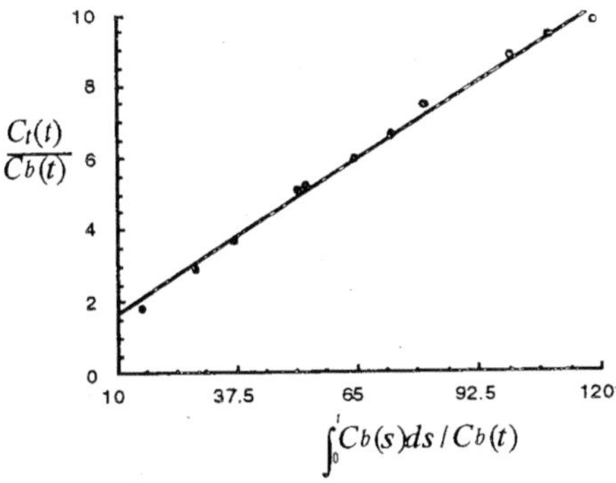

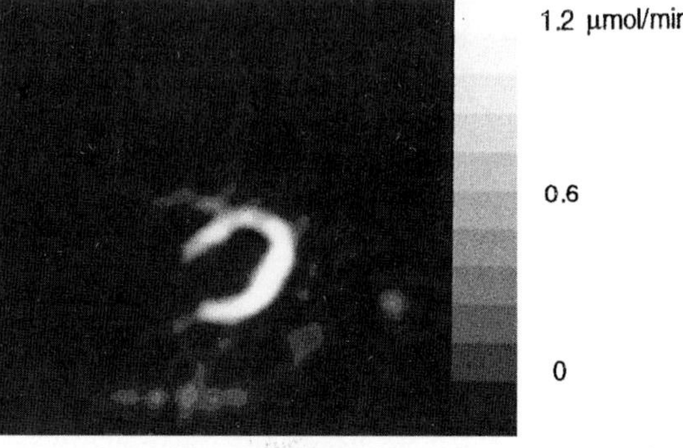

Fig. 110.10 The top image is taken from a dynamic sequence of transaxial [^{18}F]FDG images of the heart. The Patlak plot in the middle was generated from the activity versus time curves for a left ventricular blood pool region of interest and a myocardial tissue region of interest. The myocardial metabolic rate of glucose utilization (MMGlc) can be derived from the slope of the straight-line plot. If this is calculated for every pixel in the image, the parametric image of MMGlc values shown at the bottom can be generated.

noise and has the advantage that it can be easily automated for practical use in a range of tracer studies, including non-PET studies such as determination of glomerular filtration rate using ^{99m}Tc-labelled DTPA[30]

- **When is arterial blood sampling required?**

▲ Tracer kinetic models require measurements of the change in tissue and arterial plasma activity concentrations over time. The tissue measurements are provided by the PET scanner, while plasma measurements are normally obtained by withdrawing arterial blood samples during the imaging procedure. Obtaining arterial blood samples is the most invasive aspect of PET, but it is not always performed. For example, most PET centres do not perform this level of quantification in clinical studies, relying only on visual assessment of the images. Also, there are alternatives to direct arterial sampling for obtaining the model input function.

One alternative is to use arterialized venous blood sampling.[27] This involves heating the hand to approximately 45°C using a water bath or electric blanket, causing arterial blood in the terminal arterioles to be shunted to the venous circulation. Arterialized venous blood samples are then withdrawn, usually from a cubital fossa vein. Alternatively, if a pool of arterial blood is within the field of view of the PET scanner during imaging, the input function can be obtained directly from the images. An example of this is cardiac PET, in which the arterial activity can be estimated from the left ventricular chamber, which is always in the field of view.[31]

RADIATION DOSIMETRY

- **How does radiation dosimetry in PET compare with SPECT?**

▲ The radiation exposure to a patient from a PET study is primarily due to the positron itself rather than the 511 keV annihilation photons that result.[32] Recall that a positron is a charged particle with the same mass as an electron but opposite charge. Such particles cause more ionizing damage for a given distance travelled in tissue compared with a photon of similar energy. Also, positrons are relatively energetic particles with energies ranging up to 0.63 MeV for ^{18}F and up to 3.15 MeV for ^{82m}Rb. A large fraction of this energy is deposited within a few millimetres of the point of origin. By comparison, most commonly used tracers used in SPECT are pure single photon emitters of relatively low energy (e.g. ^{99m}Tc, 140 keV), with minor local energy deposition from internal conversion electrons. Offsetting this, positron emitters are generally quite short-lived compared with single photon emitters (e.g. 110 min for ^{18}F compared with 6.02 h for ^{99m}Tc).

The effective dose to the patient from an administered activity of 370 MBq of [^{18}F]FDG for a cerebral metabolic study is approximately 7.4 mSv. This compares with 6.8 mSv for a 740 MBq administered activity of ^{99m}Tc for a ^{99m}Tc-labelled HMPAO cerebral perfusion study. The three most highly exposed organs for [^{18}F]FDG are the bladder, heart and brain. Other PET tracers with shorter half-lives, such as ^{15}O ($t_{1/2}$ = 120 s), deliver a much smaller radiation dose, allowing larger activities to be employed.

As a consequence, however, a large fraction of the radiation dose is delivered to tissues and organs on the routes of administration (e.g. upper airways from inhaled activity).

The main hazard to technologists working in PET is from handling unshielded sources, for example when dispensing, calibrating and administering patient doses, and when withdrawing venous and arterial blood samples. In these cases, as for the patient, the positron causes most of the radiation damage and the main dose is to the skin of the fingers. A few millimetres of Perspex, aluminium or glass provides effective shielding for positrons from small sources. When not being directly handled, all positron-emitting sources are shielded with lead typically 3 cm thick to shield staff from the 511 keV photons. Other precautions include wearing protective eye glasses when handling liquid sources to protect the cornea and lens of the eye from both radiation and biological hazards. Rooms in which radioactive gases are used should have adequate exhaust systems and be under negative pressure with respect to adjoining areas. Apart from these precautions, the usual measures apply, including maintaining distance and minimizing time spent near radioactive sources. Radiation exposure is generally higher for technologists working in PET than for those working with single photon emitters. In a busy PET centre, annual whole-body and extremity doses may be up to 5 mSv and 30 mSv respectively, depending on the type of studies performed.[33] This is approximately double the corresponding values for the non-PET nuclear medicine technologist.

REFERENCES

1. Nicholson P W 1974 Nuclear electronics. Wiley, New York
2. Phelps M E, Hoffman E J, Mullani N A, Ter-Pogossian M M 1975 Application of annihilation coincidence detection to transaxial reconstruction tomography. J Nucl Med 16: 210–224
3. Phelps M E, Hoffman E J, Mullani N A, Ter-Pogossian M M 1975 Transaxial emission reconstruction tomography: coincidence detection of positron-emitting radionuclides.In: DeBlanc H, Sorenson J A (eds) Non-invasive brain imaging, radionuclides and computed tomography. Society of Nuclear Medicine, New York, pp 87–109
4. Hoffman E J, Phelps M E 1986 Positron emission tomography: principles and quantitation. In: Phelps M E, Mazziotta J C, Schelbert H R (eds) Positron emission tomography and autoradiography. Principles and applications for the brain and heart. Raven Press, New York: pp 237–286
5. Hoffman E J, Huang S C, Phelps M E, Kuhl D E 1981 Quantitation in positron emission tomography: 4. Effect of accidental coincidences. J Comput Assist Tomogr 5: 391–400
6. Hoffman E J, Phelps M E, Huang S C et al 1981 A new tomograph for quantitative positron emission computed tomography of the brain. IEEE Trans Nucl Sci 28: 99–103
7. Mullani N A, Markham J, Ter-Pogossian M M 1980 Feasibility of time of flight reconstruction in positron tomography. J Nucl Med 21: 1095–1097
8. Guerrero T M, Hoffman E J, Dahlbom M, Cutler P D, Hawkins R A, Phelps M E 1990 Characterization of a whole body imaging technique for PET. IEEE Trans Nucl Sci 37: 676–680
9. Dahlbom M, Hoffman E J, Hoh C K et al 1992 Whole-body positron emission tomography: Part I. Methods and performance characteristics. J Nucl Med 33: 1191–1199
10. Hawkins R A, Hoh C, Dahlbom M et al 1991 PET cancer evaluations with FDG (editorial). J Nucl Med 32: 1555–1558
11. Meikle S R, Dahlbom M, Cherry S R 1993 Attenuation correction using count-limited transmission data in positron emission tomography. J Nucl Med 34: 143–150
12. Thompson C J, Ranger N T, Evans A C 1989 Simultaneous transmission and emission scans in positron emission tomography. IEEE Trans Nucl Sci 36: 1011–1016
13. Kinahan P E, Rogers J G 1989 Analytic 3-D image reconstruction using all detected events. IEEE Trans Nucl Sci NS-36: 964–968
14. Townsend D W, Spinks T, Jones T et al 1985 Three dimensional reconstruction of PET data from a multi-ring camera. IEEE Trans Nucl Sci 36: 1056–1065
15. Defrise M, Townsend D W, Geissbuhler A 1990 Implementation of three-dimensional image reconstruction for multi-ring tomographs. Phys Med Biol 35: 1361–1372
16. Cherry S R, Dahlbom M, Hoffman E J 1991 3-D positron emission tomography using a conventional multi-slice tomograph without septa. J Comput Assist Tomogr 15: 655–668
17. Bailey D L, Jones T, Spinks T J, Gilardi M C, Townsend D W 1991 Noise equivalent count measurements in a neuro-PET scanner with retractable septa. IEEE Trans Med Imag 10: 256–260
18. Grootoonk S, Spinks T J, Jones T, Michel C, Bol A 1991 Correction for scatter using a dual energy window technique with a tomograph operated without septa. Conference Record of the 1991 IEEE Medical Imaging Conference, Santa Fe. IEEE, Piscataway, NJ, pp 1569–1573
19. Cherry S R, Meikle S R, Hoffman E J 1993 Correction and characterization of scattered events in three-dimensional PET using scanners with retractable septa. J Nucl Med 34: 671–678
20. Cho Z H, Chan J K, Eriksson L et al 1975 Positron ranges obtained from biomedically important positron-emitting radionuclides. J Nucl Med 16: 1174–1176
21. Phelps M E, Hoffman E J, Huang S C, Ter-Pogossian M M 1975 Effect of positron range on spatial resolution. J Nucl Med 16: 649–652
22. Derenzo S E 1979 Precision measurement of annihilation point spread distributions for medically important positron emitters. 5th International Conference on Positron Annihilation. The Japan Institute of Metals, Sendai, Japan, pp 819–824
23. Sorenson J A 1975 Deadtime characteristics of Anger cameras. J Nucl Med 16: 284–288
24. Germano G, Hoffman E J 1988 Investigation of count rate and deadtime characteristics of a high resolution PET system. J Comput Assist Tomogr 12: 836–846
25. Huang S-C, Phelps M E 1986 Principles of tracer kinetic modelling in positron emission tomography and autoradiography. In: Phelps M E, Mazziotta J C, Schelbert H R (eds) Positron emission tomography and autoradiography. Principles and applications for the brain and heart. Raven Press, New York, pp 287–346
26. Sokoloff L, Reivich M, Kennedy C et al 1977 The (^{14}C)-deoxyglucose method for the measurement of local cerebral glucose utilization: theory, procedure and normal values in the conscious and anesthetized albino rat. J Neurochem 28: 897–916
27. Phelps M E, Huang S-C, Hoffman E J, Selin C, Sokoloff L, Kuhl D E 1979 Tomographic measurement of local cerebral glucose metabolic rate in humans with (F-18)2-fluoro-2-deoxy-D-glucose: validation of method. Ann Neurol 6: 371–388
28. Rutland M D 1979 A single injection technique for subtraction of blood background in ^{131}I-hippuran renograms. Br J Radiol 52: 134–137
29. Patlak C S, Blasberg R G, Fenstermacher J D 1983 Graphical evaluation of blood-to-brain transfer constants from multiple-time uptake data. J Cereb Blood Flow Metab 3: 1–7
30. Rutland M R 1985 A comprehensive analysis of renal DTPA studies. I. Theory and normal values. Nucl Med Commun 6: 11–20

31. Weinberg I N, Huang S-C, Hoffman E J et al 1988 Validation of PET-acquired input functions for cardiac studies. J Nucl Med 29: 241–247
32. Harper P V, Lathrop K A 1992 Special aspects of positron dosimetry. In: Watson E E, Schlafke-Stelson A T (eds) 5th International Radiopharmaceutical Dosimetry Symposium, Oak Ridge, TN. Oak Ridge Associated Universities, pp 366–370
33. McCormick V A, Miklos J A 1993 Radiation dose to positron emission tomography technologists during quantitative versus qualitative studies. J Nucl Med 34: 769–772

111. Radioisotope production

R. E. Boyd D. J. Silvester

● **What is the historical basis for the production of radionuclides?**

▲ The single step signalling the start of radioisotope production occurred in 1898, when **Marie** and her husband **Pierre Curie** ground up a 100 g sample of pitchblende and began the search for a hitherto unknown new element. This investigation resulted from Marie's belief, based on evidence of unusual radiation intensity, that the uranium ore, pitchblende, might contain another more active substance than uranium. Within a few months the Curies succeeded in showing that pitchblende contained not just one but in fact two new elements, for which Marie coined the description **radioactive**. The first of the new elements resembled bismuth in its chemical behaviour and was named **polonium** after the country of Marie's birth. The second was found to be very like barium but its radioactivity was of such intensity that the Curies decided to call this element **radium**.

While these discoveries were corroborated by spectroscopy, much bigger samples were needed to facilitate the measurement of atomic weights before their existences could be considered as unequivocally proven. To achieve this, Marie Curie embarked on what may be regarded as the first large-scale operation in radioisotope production which yielded, after 4 years' labour on 100 kg of pitchblende residues, a mere 100 mg of radium.

The radioactive transformation process was very puzzling to the many scientists who studied it in the first decade of this century. Radioactivity was recognized as an atomic property, yet as more naturally occurring radioactive species were discovered it became impossible to allocate a place for all of them in the periodic table of elements. They could not all be new elements. Measurement of the chemical properties of these radioactive substances indicated that while some exhibited properties similar to those of known chemical elements, others showed properties which were identical to existing substances.

It was the chemist **Frederick Soddy** who, in 1913, first proposed a theory of **isotopes**, recognizing that these new substances were actually radioactive forms of existing elements, and that more than one atomic species could occupy the same place in the periodic table. Even in those early days, low levels of radiation could be detected with a fair degree of sensitivity, and hence a trace of a radioactive isotope of a particular element could serve to identify the presence of that element in a system. Almost immediately many important practical implications were demonstrated by **George de Hevesy** and **Fritz Paneth**, and their experiments clearly identified the potential for radioactive tracers in chemical and biological studies. In 1919, **Ernest Rutherford** was successful in achieving a feat that had been the goal of alchemists in bygone days, that is transmutation of the elements. By irradiating the gas nitrogen with alpha-particles, he found that a different element, oxygen, was formed. In 1924 the first clinical study with a radioactive tracer was carried out by **Blumgart** and **Weiss**. By injecting a decay product of radium into one arm and detecting its arrival in the other arm they measured blood circulation time. They showed that the time taken was increased in patients with heart disease.

The early work was performed with the few naturally occurring radioactive substances, which limited the scope for their use as tracers. This situation changed dramatically when radioisotopes were produced artificially.

In 1933, **Irene Curie** and **Frederic Joliot** discovered that some light elements themselves became radioactive after being bombarded with radiation from a polonium source.

By 1934, **Ernest Lawrence** had conceived and built an electrical apparatus, called a cyclotron, to produce fast-moving charged particles. When he used this device to irradiate a carbon target with deuterons accelerated to about 3 million electron volts (MeV), he found the target was radioactive with a half-life of about 10 min after the beam was switched off. Following this experiment, the path was opened to the discovery and production of many more radioisotopes from the cyclotron.

In the same year, 1934, **Enrico Fermi** commenced a programme of systematically irradiating all the elements in the periodic table with neutrons. While success was not apparent for the elements from hydrogen to oxygen, in the next 60 elements from fluorine onwards Fermi discovered some 40 new radioactive species as a result of neutron bombardment. Fermi's group was the first to expose uranium to neutrons and record the production of several radioactive entities; however, it took a further 4 years of research before these observations could be explained. In 1938 **Otto Hahn** and **Fritz Strassman**, having taken the utmost pains over their experimental analyses, concluded that neutron bombarded uranium atoms split into two radioactive fragments. From this concept was developed the theory of **nuclear fission**.

Neutrons used in these experiments were then only available from certain radioactive substances, such as radon or polonium, mixed with the element beryllium. When the principle of nuclear fission was enunciated, Fermi suggested that the fission process might also produce free neutrons and that these could be capable of inducing further fission events, leading to a **chain reaction**. (Fig. 111.1).

In 1942, Fermi was able to prove correct his prediction when the first atomic pile was assembled at the University of Chicago. Subsequently more atomic piles (reactors) were constructed in the USA, initially as part of the military programme to develop nuclear weapons, later for the production of tracers for more peaceful applications.

● What are the desirable properties of radionuclides used in nuclear medicine?

▲ The radionuclides used in **diagnostic** nuclear medicine are selected on the basis of their ability to provide useful clinical information while exposing the patient to only minimal radiation. The **selection criteria** to guarantee this stipulation include the conditions that the radionuclide should:

- possess a relatively short half-life which is commensurate with the duration of the investigative procedure.
- not emit particulate radiation (that is no alpha- and beta-radiation)
- emit gamma-radiation of energy high enough to be detectable even if emitted from deep seated tissues.
- not emit gamma-radiation of energy so high as to make detection inefficient or spatial discrimination ineffective
- be available in the highest possible **specific activity** (the measure of the mass of that particular element that is associated with unit radioactivity; units Becquerels per gram) to avoid invoking a toxic response or affecting the biochemistry of the patient.

In **therapeutic** nuclear medicine a different set of selection criteria apply. In this case the aim is to locate the radionuclide precisely within the tissues to be treated such that the lesion is subjected to effective short range destructive radiation. To achieve this the preferred radionuclide should:

- be of sufficiently short half-life to minimize the period

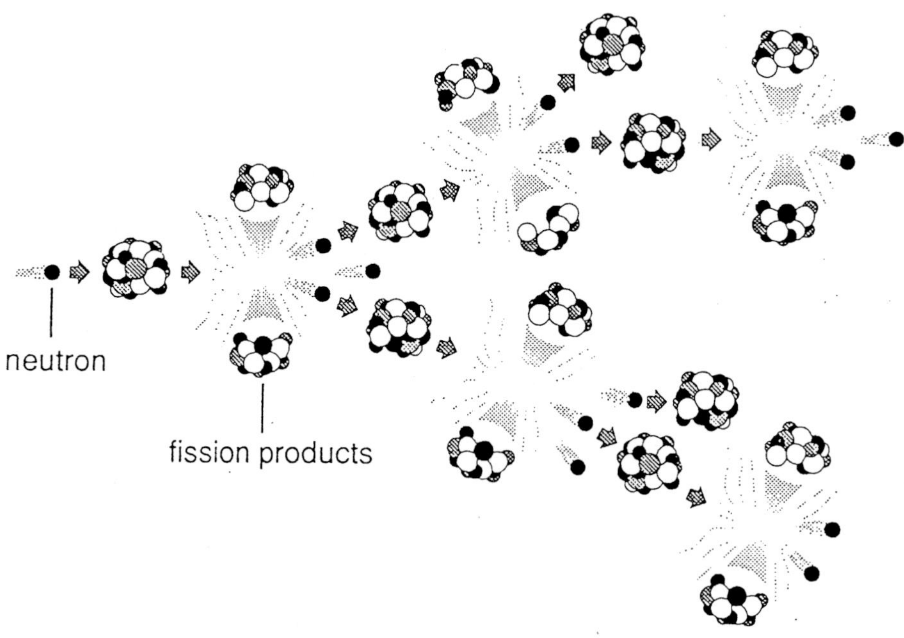

Fig. 111.1 A nuclear fission chain reaction.

of the patient's enforced stay in hospital, preferably less than 1 week;

- emit particulate radiation with a maximum tissue penetration equivalent to the dimensions of the lesions;
- possess specific activity in the medium to high range – although when used in conjunction with a monoclonal antibody vehicle may be required in a **carrier-free** state (this term implies that little or no non-radioactive forms of the element are present to contaminate the radioactive species);
- concomitantly emit gamma-rays in order to facilitate the visualization of the extent to which the radionuclide has concentrated in the target tissues.

From a population of more than 2300 possible radionuclides only a handful come close to satisfying the selection criteria for a diagnostic agent. Of these, reactor-produced technetium-99m (^{99m}Tc) is pre-eminent, being used in more than 80% of the investigative procedures performed on an estimated 100 000 patients worldwide each day. After ^{99m}Tc a series of cyclotron-produced radionuclides, such as thallium-201 (^{201}Tl), gallium-67 (^{67}Ga), indium-111 (^{111}In) and iodine-123 (^{123}I), find widespread application in visualization procedures.

A slightly wider range of radionuclides is being used or proposed for therapeutic purposes. Well-established examples are iodine-131 (^{131}I), phosphorus-32 (^{32}P) and yttrium-90 (^{90}Y). Several other radionuclides are under investigation for possible application in the future. Examples of these are samarium-153 (^{153}Sm), rhenium-186 and rhenium-188 (^{186}Re, ^{188}Re), dysprosium-165 (^{165}Dy) and holmium-166 (^{166}Ho).

● How do we obtain useful radionuclides?

▲ A number of radionuclides are found in terrestrial substances as very ancient remnants of the time when the earth was formed. In addition, some radionuclides are continually added to the earth's biosphere by the interaction of cosmic radiation with atmospheric elements (e.g. nitrogen). However, none of these substances satisfies the nuclear medicine selection criteria, and as a result naturally occurring radionuclides are not selected for use in clinical nuclear medicine.

The radionuclides that are used in diagnostic and therapeutic nuclear medicine are man-made, using a nuclear reactor or a cyclotron. The two routes to artificial radioactivity proceed in opposite directions, for which the following general observations may be made:

- In a reactor a target is bombarded with neutrons to produce a radioactive species whose nuclei contain extra neutrons.
- In a cyclotron a target is bombarded with charged particles (most commonly protons) to produce a radioactive species whose nuclei contain a deficiency of neutrons (i.e. an excess of protons).
- Most reactor-produced radionuclides emit beta-radiation as they spontaneously decay.
- Most cyclotron radionuclides emit positrons or capture an orbital electron as they spontaneously decay.
- Some reactor radionuclides and some cyclotron radionuclides essentially emit only gamma-rays as they decay. These service the needs of diagnostic nuclear medicine procedures.
- The therapeutic radionuclides are almost exclusively produced in a nuclear reactor.
- The radionuclides used in positron emission tomography are produced in a cyclotron.

REACTOR PRODUCTION

● How does a nuclear reactor work?

▲ Although certain elements at the heavy end of the periodic table exhibit the property of spontaneous nuclear fission, it is more usual for this phenomenon to be brought about by the neutron bombardment of predisposed (so-called '**fissile**') isotopes of **uranium** and **plutonium**. In the fission process the uranium atom is split into two fragments, a large amount of energy is released and 2–3 free neutrons are produced.

Neutrons have no electric charge and will readily interact with the nuclei of other substances they encounter and be absorbed. Of course, when the neutrons react with other uranium atoms further fission occurs to produce more neutrons. These secondary neutrons are capable of causing even more fission events and a chain reaction is produced, releasing a very large amount of energy in an extremely short period of time.

A nuclear reactor is a device in which a uranium chain reaction occurs at a slow and controlled rate. Control of the fission process ensures that a balance is maintained between the rate of production of free neutrons and the loss of neutrons to parasitic absorptions such that there is just a sufficient flux of neutrons to maintain the fission chain reaction.

While some reactors are operated to convert the released atomic energy into electricity, others are specifically designed to serve as **sources of neutrons** for a range of different applications. Most notable among this latter group is radioisotope production. When non-radioactive substances are exposed to a field of neutrons, a variety of nuclear reactions can be induced, leading to the production of radioactive substances.

In a nuclear reactor, facilities are provided for the insertion and subsequent removal of target substances (Fig. 111.2). The elemental composition of the target determines which radionuclide(s) is produced and the

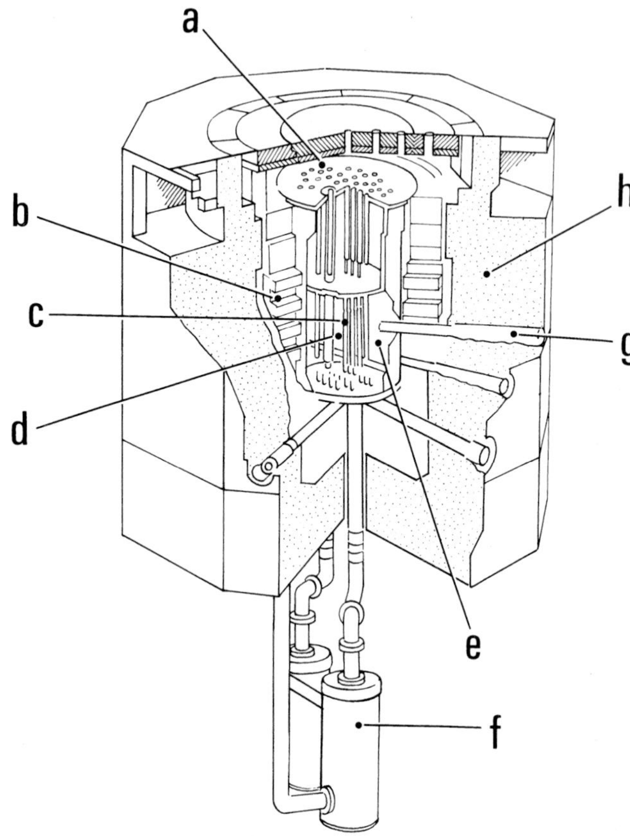

Fig. 111.2 A nuclear reactor for the production of radioisotopes. Identified features are: (a) vertical irradiation facility, (b) graphite neutron reflector, (c) assembly of uranium fuel elements, (d) intense flux of neutrons, (e) heavy water, neutron moderator and primary heat exchanger fluid, (f) bank of heat exchangers, (g) horizontal irradiation facility, (h) concrete biological shield.

period of exposure to neutrons governs the extent to which the target becomes radioactive.

The next step involves chemical processing of the target to extract the induced radioactivity.

● How are radionuclides produced in a reactor?

▲ In simple terms, when the nuclei of a target substance are bombarded by missile particles, a nuclear reaction occurs to produce a new radioactive substance. Symbolically the induced nuclear reaction may be written as in the following example:

$$^{23}\text{Na}\ (\text{n},\gamma)\ ^{24}\text{Na}$$

This is a typical nuclear reaction that occurs within a reactor where Na (sodium) is the target element (= product element), 23 is the target mass number and 24 is the product mass number and n is the bombarding particle (neutron) and γ is the immediate outgoing radiation (gamma-ray). Note that in the (n,γ) reaction only a very small proportion of the target nuclei are converted to the product radionuclide at the end of the bombardment. Because the product is chemically identical to the target, it cannot be separated from the bulk of the target. The (n,γ) reaction has the characteristic of producing a radioactive product of low specific activity, that is the radioactive product is diluted with a substantial proportion of its non-radioactive form.

However, the product radionuclide may spontaneously decay to form another by, say, the emission of a beta-particle. Symbolically, an example of this is:

$$^{130}\text{Te}\ (\text{n},\gamma)\ ^{131}\text{Te} \xrightarrow{\beta} {}^{131}\text{I}$$

In this sequence the end product is ^{131}I. Since tellurium (Te) and iodine (I) are different elements, their chemistries will be sufficiently distinct to permit the end product to be isolated. Now, providing no other forms of iodine are introduced into the system, ^{131}I should possess high specific activity (sometimes called 'no carrier added' or NCA).

Two other nuclear reactions performed with neutrons which are important in radionuclide production are the (n,p) reaction and nuclear fission.

A most important example of a (n,p) reaction occurs in the atmosphere, where nitrogen atoms are continuously bombarded with neutrons from outer space to produce carbon-14 (^{14}C; half-life 5730 years). The ^{14}C enters into the earth's carbon pool first as carbon dioxide and then it is photosynthesized into the plant world and finally enters the food chains of both animals and humans. As a consequence, every living creature or plant builds up an equilibrium level of ^{14}C radioactivity. This equilibrium is not altered until the organism dies and stops assimilating further ^{14}C. From that point on, the level of ^{14}C concentration in the remains acts as a built-in clock, revealing how long the organism has been dead; this is the principle behind **radiocarbon dating**.

$$^{14}\text{N}\ (\text{n,p})\ ^{14}\text{C}$$

The special features of the (n,p) reaction are that, following neutron bombardment of the nucleus, a proton is ejected. Therefore, while there is no overall change in mass, the product has an atomic number 1 less than the target substance. This change in atomic number implies that the product has different properties than the target and hence may be chemically separated at high specific activity.

A comparison of the (n,γ) and (n,p) nuclear reactions serves to exemplify how one radionuclide may be produced by different reactions

^{31}P (n,γ) ^{32}P	low specific activity
^{32}S (n,p) ^{32}P	high specific activity

The end use of the radionuclide would usually dictate which production route was chosen.

The use of nuclear fission to produce a range of radionuclides is also quite common. Fission products of uranium-235 include more than 360 radionuclides from about half the elements in the periodic table. The most probable fission products occur around the mass numbers 85 and 139. The fission fragments are radioactive with very short half-lives and undergo several radioactive decay transformations before a long-lived radionuclide or a stable nucleus is reached.

The most important fission product used in contemporary nuclear medicine is molybdenum-99 (^{99}Mo), which is the parent of technetium-99m (^{99m}Tc). In today's technology, the fission route to ^{99}Mo is preferred over the alternative neutron irradiation of the element molybdenum because it provides a product of much greater specific activity. However, this benefit is counterbalanced by the need to dispose of the other uranium fission products which remain as waste after the ^{99}Mo has been extracted. Newer technologies are being developed in the application of ^{99}Mo which are less sensitive to the degree of specific activity (see section on generators)

^{98}Mo (n,γ)^{99}Mo	low specific activity
^{235}U (n, fission) ^{99}Mo	high specific activity

The difference in specific activity has a major impact on the design of practical devices by which ^{99m}Tc is separated from ^{99}Mo.

CYCLOTRON PRODUCTION

● How does a cyclotron work?

▲ The cyclotron belongs to the class of machine called particle accelerators. These exist in two varieties, linear and cyclic. While simple in concept, the linear accelerator has a limited performance owing to constraints on the number of accelerating electrodes it can contain. The advantage of a cyclic accelerator is that particles can be made to travel many times around a central point, traversing the same accelerating electrodes to reach very high energies.

The charged particles are created by the ionization of a gas (hydrogen, deuterium or helium) and then are injected into the central region of an evacuated tank. In the tank the ions come under the influence of pairs of high-voltage electrodes, which oscillate in polarity at high radiofrequencies. The particles are accelerated each time they cross the electrode gap and begin to move with increasing speed. Perpendicular to the electrical field is a very strong magnetic field which constrains the accelerating particles into a circular path. An important characteristic of the cyclotron is that, as the particles speed up, the time they take to complete one circuit remains constant. This, of course, can only be achieved if the path taken by the particles increases in length with each circuit. Therefore in a cyclotron the beam of accelerating particles moves in an outwardly expanding spiral.

A common practice in modern cyclotrons is to accelerate negatively charged particles (e.g. the negative hydrogen ion, H^-, or negatively charged deuteron, D^-). This simplifies the extraction of the beam from the machine and thereby facilitates its efficient use in nuclear reactions. Passing the negatively charged beam through a graphite foil strips two electrons from each particle; they then become positively charged and immediately move into a new circular orbit with the opposite curvature. This change of motion is used to extract the beam through a port in the cyclotron tank and then by means of steering magnets the beam is directed towards a target (Fig. 111.3).

Bombardment of the target material by the beam of particles causes a nuclear reaction to take place, producing a radionuclide.

● How are radionuclides produced in a cyclotron?

▲ The production of radioactivity by means of a cyclotron is similar to its reactor counterpart in that it involves bombarding a target with missile particles to induce a nuclear reaction. However, it differs greatly in the ease with which it can be achieved. Whereas the neutron, carrying no charge, can react readily with the target, the positively charged particles employed in the cyclotron are repelled by the target nuclei. This coulombic repulsion can be overcome by increasing the energy of the bombarding particles; a typical proton-induced nuclear reaction has a threshold energy barrier of millions of electron volts (compared with a neutron reaction, where energies as low as 0.025 eV suffice). The cyclotron is the means by which the charged particle missiles are accelerated to the energies necessary to bring about the desired nuclear reaction.

A much greater number of different nuclear reactions are possible with a cyclotron than with a reactor, if the machine is capable of providing particles of high enough energy. Some cyclotrons are capable of being switched to accelerating more than one type of particle, thereby further expanding the possible productive repertoire.

A particularly important group of radionuclides are those which emit positrons, as these can be used in positron emission tomography (PET). For these radionuclides a cyclotron is essential, e.g.

^{14}N (p,α) ^{11}C	$t_{1/2}$ = 20 min
^{16}O (p,α) ^{13}N	$t_{1/2}$ = 10 min
^{16}O (p,pn) ^{15}O	$t_{1/2}$ = 2 min
^{18}O (p,n) ^{18}F	$t_{1/2}$ = 110 min

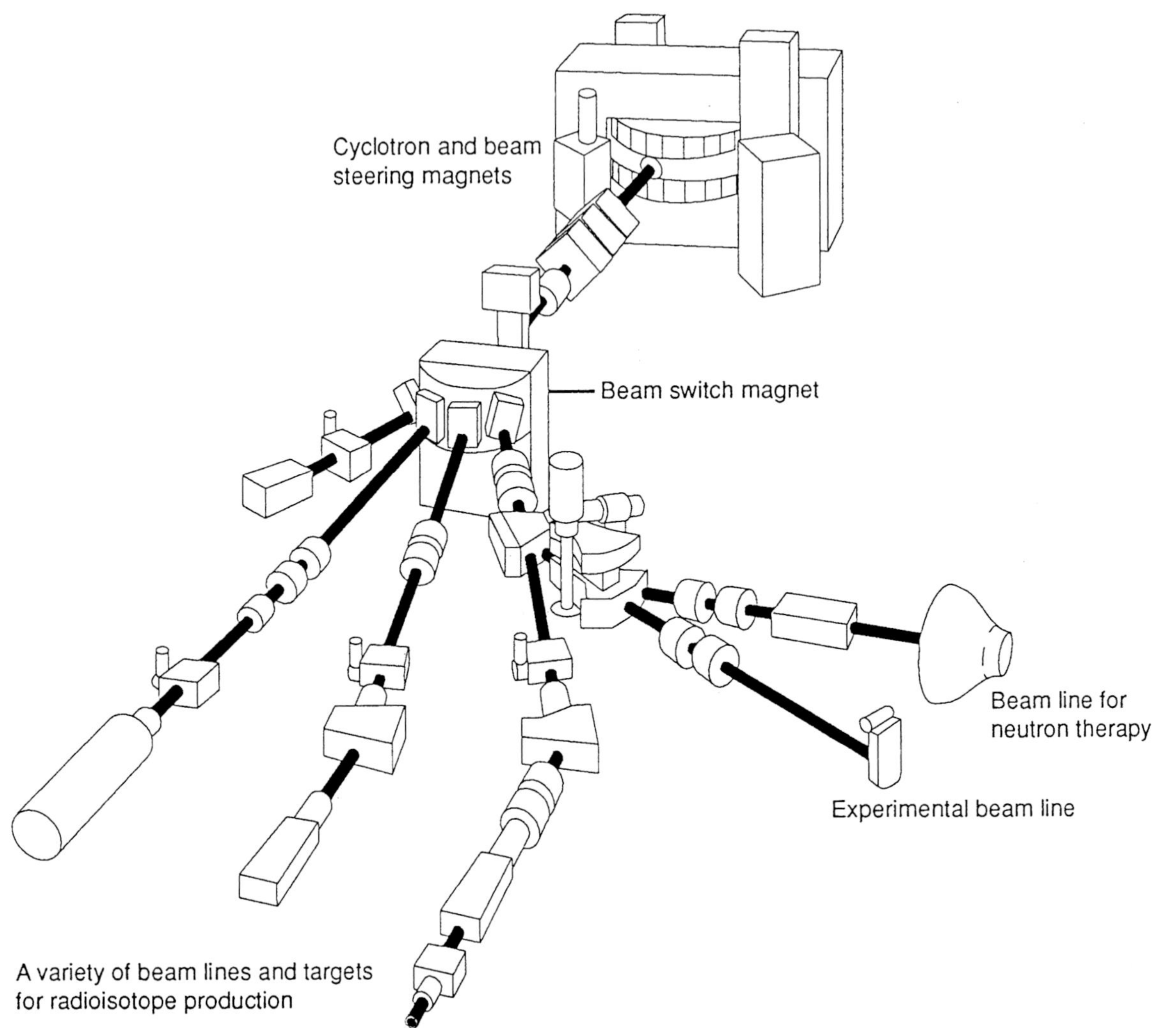

Fig. 111.3 An example of a multipurpose cyclotron dedicated to medical applications.

Some cyclotron radionuclides decay by capturing an electron orbiting the nucleus. When this occurs it is followed by the emission of radiation that is characteristic of the element produced by the decay. Thallium-201 (^{201}Tl) is a typical example of this type of radionuclide

$$^{203}\text{Tl (p,3n)} \rightarrow {}^{201}\text{Pb} \rightarrow {}^{201}\text{Tl} \rightarrow {}^{201}\text{Hg}$$
$$t_{1/2} = 9.4\ \text{h} \quad t_{1/2} = 74\ \text{h}$$

from which the principal emission is the Hg X-ray.

Other gamma-emitting radionuclides produced by cyclotrons and applied in biomedical investigations are ^{67}Ga, ^{111}In and ^{123}I.

LOGISTICS OF SUPPLY

● What is a generator?

▲ In general, the application of a short-lived radionuclide is restricted to a locale close to its source; the shorter the half-life the closer to the source are the practical distribution limits. Therefore in defining the infrastructure necessary to cover a national nuclear medicine service, the application of the first selection criterion on half-life implies the need to have several sites for the manufacture and processing of radionuclides. While this is still the case for the ultrashort-lived radionuclides used in PET, fortunately for the development of general nuclear medicine there is another way in which a limited number of short-lived radionuclides can be made more widely available.

Whenever a long-lived radionuclide (**parent**) decays to form a shorter lived radionuclide (**daughter**) and a suitable means exists for separating the two species, then the parent radioisotope can serve as a transportable source of the daughter radionuclide.

This general principle was first used for radon-222 ($t_{1/2}$= 3.8 days) from radium-226 ($t_{1/2}$ = 1600 years) and then early in nuclear medicine for iodine-132 ($t_{1/2}$= 2.3 h) from tellurium-132 ($t_{1/2}$ = 78 h).

The most important generator system is that used for provision of ^{99m}Tc from the fission product ^{99}Mo. This system allows hospitals to have daily access to ^{99m}Tc, with its short half-life of 6 h, through the once-weekly delivery of ^{99}Mo (half-life of 66 h). The ^{99}Mo is provided in a generator system which permits extraction of the ^{99m}Tc by simple column chromatography.

Within a ^{99m}Tc generator system, the radioactivities of both ^{99}Mo and ^{99m}Tc are continually changing. While the ^{99}Mo level is diminishing because of radioactive decay, the ^{99m}Tc is simultaneously influenced by both growth and decay effects. The level of ^{99m}Tc within the generator system follows a complex exponential function of time. Figure 111.4 indicates how the radioactivity of the ^{99m}Tc grows to a maximum value and then gradually decays. Before the maximum value, ^{99m}Tc is growing into the system faster than it is decaying – as a result there is a progressive build-up of the level of ^{99m}Tc. After the maximum value, the ^{99m}Tc growth rate equals its decay rate. However, from this point on, the growth rate of ^{99m}Tc gets progressively smaller as the parent ^{99}Mo decays away. The overall net effect is to establish an equilibrium (so called transient equilibrium) in which the ratio of ^{99}Mo activity : ^{99m}Tc activity remains at a constant value.

When ^{99m}Tc is removed from the ^{99}Mo–^{99m}Tc system, more ^{99m}Tc grows back because the rate of decay of ^{99m}Tc is now less than its rate of growth. The relative level of ^{99m}Tc must increase until the equilibrium condition is re-established. The growth, removal and regrowth of ^{99m}Tc in the generator is a cycle that can be repeated indefinitely. The life of the ^{99m}Tc generator is between 3 and 5 ^{99}Mo half-lives, after which time the level of ^{99m}Tc becomes too low for practical application. The method by which ^{99m}Tc may be removed (separated, milked) from the ^{99}Mo contained in the generator can be based on differences in the chemical or physical properties of molybdenum and technetium. The most common method is a chemical one, i.e. column chromatography, in which molybdate (^{99}Mo) is immobilized on an alumina column. The passage of a saline solution through the column will remove (elute) the ^{99m}Tc as a sodium pertechnetate solution. Other generators have been developed to utilize (n,γ) ^{99}Mo. It is not practical to use column chromatography to separate ^{99m}Tc from this grade of ^{99}Mo. The low specific activity would require the use of very large columns of absorbent material (usually alumina) to produce only very dilute ^{99m}Tc solutions. However, using the techniques of solvent extraction, sublimation or gel chromatography ^{99m}Tc can be successfully extracted from (n,γ) ^{99}Mo. The disadvantage of the methods for extracting ^{99m}Tc from low specific activity ^{99}Mo is that they involve large and complex equipment which requires operating skills and facilities not usually found within the clinical environment. On the other hand, such methods are suited for use in a **centralized radiopharmacy** from which the separated ^{99m}Tc may subsequently be transferred to a regional group of hospitals for immediate clinical application; this type of ^{99m}Tc is commonly referred to as '**instant ^{99m}Tc**'.

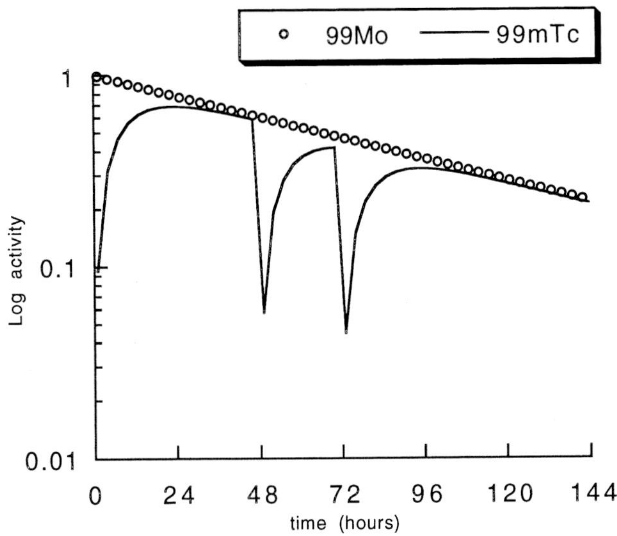

Fig. 111.4 The principle of the technetium generator. ^{99}Mo decays with a half-life of 66 h to ^{99m}Tc. The activity of ^{99m}Tc builds up until an equilibrium is reached, maximum activity being reached in 23 h. Each time the generator is milked the ^{99m}Tc activity re-establishes equilibrium with the parent activity.

● How are radiopharmaceuticals produced?

▲ When a radionuclide is used as a tracer in medicine, it is usual for it to be presented in a specific chemical form which controls its biological fate when administered (usually intravenously) to the patient. This presentation is referred to as a **radiopharmaceutical**. A particular radionuclide may be presented in a number of active forms, each designed to target specific tissues in the human body. It is implicit in the formulation of a radiopharmaceutical that it possess all the necessary attributes of purity, stability and freedom from undesirable by-products. Like other drug substances, a radiopharmaceutical must be proved safe and clinically effective through extended clinical trials prior to it being approved for general use.

A radiopharmaceutical is the end product of chemical processing performed on the target substance after it has been irradiated in a cyclotron or a nuclear reactor. Most commonly the preparation of a radiopharmaceutical involves:

- extracting the radionuclide from the bulk of the target substance;
- purification to remove unwanted chemical and radionuclidic impurities;
- chemical conversion of the pure radionuclide into a biologically specific form (a particular radionuclide may be presented in several active forms each targeting specific groups of tissues in the human body);
- addition of the necessary excipients to make the preparation suitable for administration to patients;
- testing the quality of the final product.

While radiopharmaceuticals must comply with all the normal pharmacopoeial requirements, their production must also contend with radiological safety demands and with half-life constraints. Problems are encountered with the radiopharmaceuticals used in positron emission tomography (PET). The extreme short half-lives (minutes) of PET radiopharmaceuticals require the adoption of special automated procedures for both production and quality control and demand that manufacture be placed close to the site of application.

FURTHER READING

The reader is referred to several general texts[1–3,4] for more detailed information on radioisotope production.

ACKNOWLEDGEMENT

The authors wish to acknowledge the assistance given by Gay Hawkins in the preparation of the text and the many helpful comments and suggestions she made for improving its clarity of expression.

REFERENCES

1. Friedlander G, Kennedy J W, Macias E S, Miller J M 1981 Nuclear and radiochemistry, 3rd edn. John Wiley, New York.
2. Helus F (ed.) 1983 Radionuclides production. CRC Press, Boca Raton
3. Parker R P, Smith P H S, Taylor D M 1984 Basic science of nuclear medicine, 2nd edn. Churchill Livingstone, Edinburgh
4. Theobald A E (ed.) 1985 Radiopharmacy and radiopharmaceuticals. Taylor & Francis, London

112. Basic science: radiochemistry

Richmond J. Baker

INTRODUCTION

● What types of radiopharmaceuticals are available for nuclear medicine studies?

▲ The term 'radiopharmaceutical' now has widespread acceptance in nuclear medicine, although these preparations are perhaps better described as 'radiodiagnostic agents'. The active ingredient, that is the actual radiolabelled chemical, is usually present in minute amounts, typically less than a nanogram and far below the amount necessary to initiate any physiological response in an individual. In most instances, there is a large molar excess of the non-radioactive component, be it protein, ligand or other carrier that may be necessary to stabilize the preparation, but again these substances are usually present at concentrations well below those which are active physiologically. The exception, perhaps, is the rare occasion on which a radiopharmaceutical is administered to a patient who has a hypersensitivity towards some component and may exhibit a typical allergic response.[1,2] In addition, a number of therapy radiopharmaceuticals have been designed to have cytotoxic properties by virtue of the particulate radiation emitted from their nuclei.

In designing radiopharmaceuticals, use is made of both physical and chemical properties to direct them to the target organ or tissue.[3] The various types of radiopharmaceuticals used for diagnostic purposes are summarized in Table 112.1.

Recent developments in the design and application of new radiopharmaceuticals are discussed in a comprehensive review by Verbruggen.[4]

RADIOPHARMACEUTICAL PRINCIPLES

● How do technetium-99m cold kits work?

▲ Technetium-99m cold kits are a versatile means of enabling the preparation of a wide variety of products in situations remote from laboratory facilities. The kit consists of a glass vial containing specified quantities of reagents, which are usually freeze dried in situ but may be in the form of a frozen solution. Figure 112.1 illustrates diagrammatically the essential components of a kit to which ^{99m}Tc pertechnetate has been added.

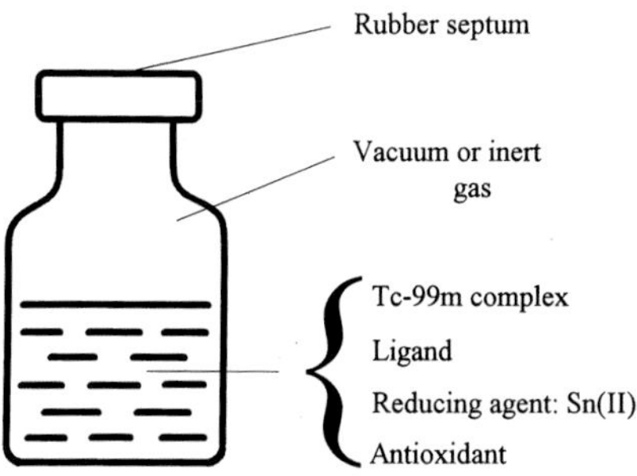

Fig. 112.1 Reagent vial or 'kit' for the preparation of ^{99m}Tc radiopharmaceuticals. The vial is inactive before the addition of ^{99m}Tc pertechnetate obtained from the technetium generator.

The biodistribution of the labelled product depends on the nature of the ligand present. The technique is also applicable to the labelling of insoluble particles. For labelling to occur, ^{99m}Tc must be reduced from oxidation state (VII) to lower oxidation states, usually (III) or (IV), which undergo complex formation with the ligand, e.g. DTPA, MDP, PYP, DISIDA, etc.

The reducing agent employed is usually tin(II) in the form of stannous chloride or stannous fluoride. Tin is a relatively non-toxic element in this form but may cause difficulties because of the ready formation of colloidal hydroxide or hydrated oxides, so that the formation of a soluble tin(II) complex is usually essential to avoid this problem.

Successful production and marketing of a cold kit product is greatly aided by the establishment of a long shelf-life, ideally in the order of 12 months or more. To prevent atmospheric oxidation of tin(II), the reagents are usually freeze dried and packed under vacuum or an inert gas such as nitrogen. The presence of an antioxidant (ascorbic acid or gentisic acid are most frequently used[5]) may improve long-term stability and also retard oxidation

Table 112.1 Classification of diagnostic radiopharmaceuticals

Type	Label	Example/use
Particulate		
Colloids	^{99m}Tc	Sulphur or phytate colloids accumulate in liver, spleen, bone marrow
Macroaggregates	^{99m}Tc	Albumin macroaggregates for lung imaging
Red cells	^{99m}Tc	Blood pool visualization
	^{51}Cr	Red cell survival, mass, etc.
Leucocytes	^{111}In, ^{99m}Tc	Accumulate at sites of infection
Platelets	^{111}In	Accumulate on thrombi
Heat-damaged red cells	^{99m}Tc	Spherocytes accumulate in spleen
Labelled proteins	^{99m}Tc, ^{111}In, ^{131}I	Albumin, immunoglobulins, monoclonal antibodies
Labelled peptides	^{111}In, ^{123}I	Somatostatin analogues
^{99m}Tc complexes	^{99m}Tc	
^{99m}Tc-essential		
Anionic		HIDA analogues for biliary; MAG_3 for renal studies
Neutral		HMPAO for cerebral studies, labelled leucocytes
Cationic		Isonitrile complexes for cardiac studies
^{99m}Tc-labelled		MDP for bone; PYP for blood pool, infarcts
Other ^{99m}Tc compounds		Pertechnetate for thyroid, Meckel's, etc.; Technegas for lung ventilation
Metal ions	^{201}Tl, ^{67}Ga, ^{51}Cr, ^{111}In	TlCl for cardiac, tumour; Ga-citrate for tumour; $CrCl_3$ and $InCl_3$ for protein labelling
Miscelaneous metal complexes	^{57}Co, ^{58}Co	Vitamin B_{12} absorption
	^{111}In	Oxinate complex for cell labelling
Non-metallic	^{131}I	Iodide for thyroid studies, labelled compounds e.g. metaiodobenzylguanidine
	^{123}I	Labelled compounds, e.g. iodoamphetamine
	^{125}I	Protein labelling, e.g. for RIA
	^{133}Xe	Gas for lung ventilation
Positron emitters	^{11}C	Many labelled compounds
	^{13}N	Ammonia for cardiac studies
	^{15}O	O_2, CO_2, H_2O for blood flow and metabolic studies
	^{18}F	Fluorodeoxyglucose for cerebral, cardiac and tumour metabolic studies
	^{68}Ga	Generator-produced positron emitter

of the labelled product. For example, ^{99m}Tc-MDP prepared without antioxidant may show uptake in thyroid and stomach in patients whose doses are withdrawn from a kit prepared several hours earlier. This problem is caused by the formation of free ^{99m}Tc pertechnetate and may be eliminated if an antioxidant is included in the formulation.[6]

● What factors determine the biodistribution of particulate radiopharmaceuticals?

▲ Particulate radiopharmaceuticals comprise radioactive colloids, macroaggregates and labelled blood cells. The smaller sized colloids, as exemplified by ^{99m}Tc antimony sulphide (which has a mean particle size of approximately 10 nm[7]) demonstrate migration in the lymphatic system and accumulation in the lymph nodes when injected subdermally. When injected intravenously, this colloid has a longer retention time in the blood and reduced uptake in liver and spleen compared with larger sized colloids. There is also higher uptake in the bone marrow.

As the particle size is increased, blood clearance is faster and liver uptake increases, but colloids at the smaller end of the range still have low splenic uptake. This behaviour is shown by ^{99m}Tc phytate when injected without added calcium, leading to in vivo formation of colloidal particles by reaction with plasma calcium ions. However, good splenic uptake is observed when particles are in the size range 100–1000 nm (0.1–1 μm), as occurs when ^{99m}Tc calcium phytate is preformed before injection.[8]

Once the particle size exceeds about 8 μm (the diameter of a red cell) they become trapped in the capillaries of the lungs. Since particles used for lung scanning are usually much larger than this (generally 20–40 μm), they become trapped in somewhat larger vessels, the precapillary arterioles.

The biodistribution of viable labelled blood cells is determined principally by their physiological properties. Thus, labelled red cells remain in the circulation. Labelling these cells with a longer lived radionuclide such as ^{51}Cr in the form of sodium chromate is a method which is widely used to determine their survival time in vivo.[9] For short-term studies, red cells are usually labelled with ^{99m}Tc after incubation with stannous ions, either in vivo or in vitro. These techniques are suitable for studies such as cardiac blood pool imaging, but there may be some elution of the label over longer periods. When heated to 50°C, labelled red cells form spherocytes, which are selectively removed from the circulation by the spleen. Prolonged heating may damage the cells so severely that they fragment, causing liver uptake.

Platelets labelled with ^{111}In via the oxinate complex remain in the circulation and can be used for the localization of thrombi. Leucocytes can also be labelled with ^{111}In or with a ^{99m}Tc colloid by making use of their propensity to phagocytose bacteria and other particles of the appropriate size. During the labelling procedure, leucocytes may become activated and may marginate in the lungs on reinjection, but should return to the circulation within an hour or so. Overly vigorous handling during labelling can cause the cells to aggregate, leading to the appearance of radioactive foci in the lungs which are retained for long periods.

● **What is the difference between radionuclidic, radiochemical, chemical and biological purity?**

▲ The monographs for radiopharmaceuticals found in national pharmacopoeias lay down specifications for purity from a number of different aspects. It is useful to discuss this with reference to ^{99m}Tc pertechnetate eluted from a generator.

Radiochemical purity

Unwanted or different chemical forms containing the radionuclide of interest are known as radiochemical impurities. Thus, ^{99m}Tc pertechnetate and $^{99m}TcO_2$ are both radiochemicals and the proportion of the latter can be determined by paper chromatography. The *British Pharmacopoeia* (BP) specifies that not less than 95% of the ^{99m}Tc radioactivity must be in the form of the pertechnetate ion.

Radionuclidic purity

This term refers to the presence of radionuclides other than the one of interest. The BP lays down limits for the gamma-emitting impurities ^{99}Mo, ^{131}I, ^{103}Ru and other gamma-emitters. Limits for the beta-emitters ^{89}Sr and ^{90}Sr and total alpha-emitters are also specified. Accurate determination of gamma-emitting radionuclidic impurities requires the use of gamma spectrometry on a suitably decayed sample. A less accurate method is to measure the fresh eluate in a lead pot using the '^{99}Mo assay' setting on a dose calibrator. This enables shielding of the 140 keV gamma emission of ^{99m}Tc but allows measurement of the more penetrating 740 and 780 keV emissions of ^{99}Mo. However, the method is not selective and will include all impurities with more energetic emissions.

Chemical purity

Non-radioactive chemical species in the product are referred to as chemical impurities. In ^{99m}Tc generator eluate the principal undesirable chemical contaminant is likely to be aluminium in the form of Al^{3+}, which, if it exceeds the specified limit of 10 μg/ml, may cause agglutination of red cells or the aggregation of colloidal preparations. The aluminium impurity arises from degradation of the alumina column retaining adsorbed ^{99}Mo and may be determined colorimetrically.

Biological purity

This is concerned with the presence of contaminating micro-organisms (sterility) or products of their growth (pyrogenicity). Products specified as sterile or pyrogen free must undergo testing in accordance with methods laid down in the national pharmacopoeia.[10] Current requirements are for the product to be incubated for 14 days with media proven to support the growth of both aerobic and anaerobic micro-organisms.

Pyrogens are water-soluble, heat-stable metabolic products of the growth of micro-organisms which produce the typical pyrogenic reaction (sweating, nausea, headache, elevated temperature, etc.) following intravenous injection. Pyrogen testing is frequently done in rabbits, in which the rectal temperature is measured before and after injection. Another method, the *Limulus* test, is now recognized as an alternative. This test makes use of the formation of a gel when *Limulus* (horseshoe crab) amoebocyte lysate (LAL) is mixed with pyrogens. The LAL test is much more sensitive than the rabbit test and can give an estimate of the quantity of pyrogen present. It is particularly valuable for the testing of products intended for intrathecal use.

TECHNETIUM RADIOCHEMISTRY

● **What is the significance of the oxidation state of technetium in ^{99m}Tc radiopharmaceuticals?**

▲ The oxidation state of an element in its various compounds is an important chemical property which determines the type of compound or ion formed. It is defined as the number of electrons lost or gained in the formation of a cation (positively charged) or anion (negatively charged). Transition metals, which include technetium, are characterized by their ability to exist in a number of oxidation states, each with a distinct electronic configuration. Technetium has been identified in its various compounds as having oxidation states with values from (–I) to (VII).[11,12] The latter is the most stable state, which occurs in the pertechnetate ion TcO_4^-. In this form,

^{99m}Tc is not particularly reactive and must be reduced (by the addition of electrons) to lower oxidation states which are able to combine with ligands to form complexes. Unfortunately, most of these complexes containing reduced technetium are also sensitive to oxidation by atmospheric oxygen and must be contained in an evacuated vial or stored under nitrogen to retard the formation of ^{99m}Tc pertechnetate as a radiochemical impurity. For this reason, the shelf-life of kits and the reconstituted shelf-life established by the manufacturer should always be observed.

As discussed above, the reducing agent most often employed in ^{99m}Tc radiopharmaceuticals is the tin(II) ion, which provides a source of electrons as it becomes oxidized to the tin(IV) (stannic) ion:

$$Sn(II) \rightarrow Sn(IV) + 2e^-$$

Other methods of reduction have been used when required in particular circumstances. These include electrolytic, the use of sodium borohydride and the use of organic reducing agents such as pyridoxal and formamidine sulphinic acid. Most of these methods do not have the advantage shown by Sn(II) in that reduction is not 'instant' but requires some form of laboratory manipulation, e.g. pH adjustment or heating.

Changing the oxidation state enables the preparation of many different compounds with potentially different biological properties. Very low oxidation states may be stabilized by special ligands, including isonitriles and phosphines, which have electronic orbitals arranged to accept excess electron density from the metal ion. Even with the same ligand, different oxidation states will produce compounds with different biological properties. As an example, the ^{99m}Tc complex formed with meso-2,3-dimercaptosuccinic acid (DMSA) at acid pH contains Tc in the (III) oxidation state [^{99m}Tc(III)-DMSA], which is localized principally in the renal cortex. When the preparation is carried out at pH 8, a different complex is formed, identified as containing ^{99m}Tc in the (V) state.[13] This complex is mainly excreted in the urine but also has the ability to concentrate in certain tumours, particularly thyroid medullary carcinoma.

• Why are ^{99m}Tc and ^{131}I not interchangeable as labels?

▲ Different types of molecule require different strategies for the introduction of non-isotopic labels. Although ^{99m}Tc can be used to 'label' many substances ranging from simple ions (e.g. pyrophosphate) to complex molecules such as proteins, binding requires the presence of donor atoms arranged to form a chelating function. In the case of small molecules, complex formation usually nullifies the biological properties of the ligand because the positively charged metal ion will have a perturbing effect on the electron cloud of the ligand and higher order complexes (2:1 or 3:1 ligand–metal ratio) are likely to be formed. These factors will be pronounced in small complexes but may not affect the properties of larger peptides or proteins to such a marked extent unless the metal ion occupies active sites or a high metal–protein ratio is used.

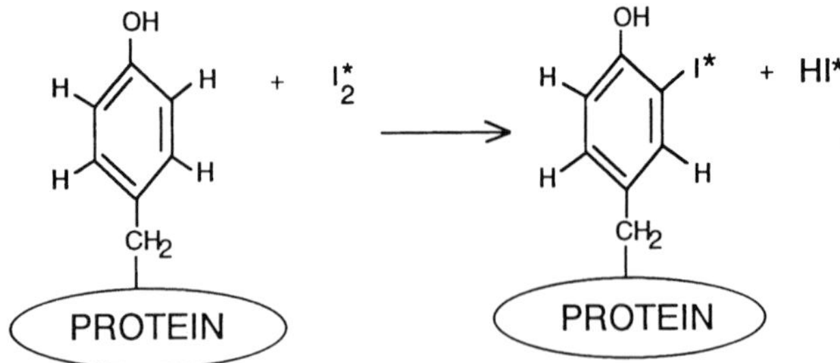

Fig. 112.2 Iodination of proteins by the direct method usually proceeds by substitution of radioiodine in the aromatic ring of tyrosine with the liberation of hydrogen iodide.

The introduction of iodine as ^{131}I or other iodine isotope requires a different binding mechanism. As a non-metal, iodine is not able to utilize chelate functions but is reactive towards substitution of atoms in the molecule, resulting in direct binding to carbon atoms. The C–I bond has greater stability when binding occurs in an aromatic ring system. In particular, the benzene ring in tyrosine residues is the main site of iodination in proteins, as shown in Figure 112.2.

Owing to the formation of HI, the maximum yield of labelled product obtained by the direct method is 50%. Better yields are possible if radioactive iodine monochloride is used or if radioiodine is generated in situ in the reaction vial by the use of chloramine-T, a weak oxidizing agent capable of oxidizing iodide to iodine.[14] More sophisticated methods make use of a prelabelled reactive intermediate such as the Bolton–Hunter reagent, which couples to the free amino groups of proteins by an acylation reaction mechanism.[15]

As with metallic radionuclides, the incorporation of too many iodide atoms in a protein may have a perturbing effect on its biological properties. Such effects may be minimized by the use of high specific activity radioiodine, enabling reduction of the iodine–protein ratio. For many proteins, care must be taken not to cause denaturation by the use of too vigorous reagents or conditions.

• How does the Technegas generator work? What is known about the nature of the product?

▲ Technegas is a new product for lung ventilation studies available from a commercial generator developed in Australia.[16] It is produced by heating ^{99m}Tc pertechnetate in a graphite crucible by means of an electric current, in a pure argon atmosphere. When the temperature reaches

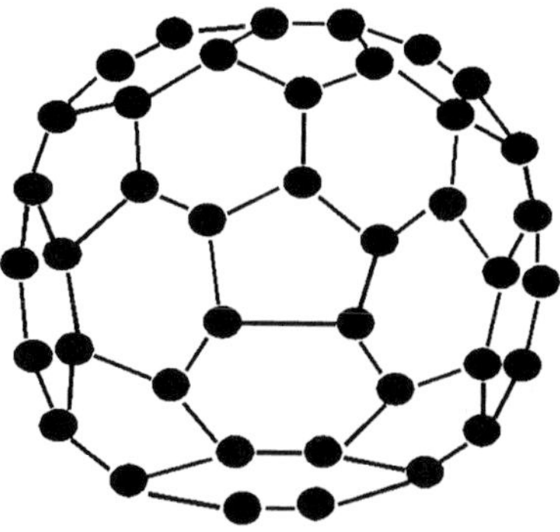

Fig. 112.3 Hemispherical view of the C_{60} fullerene molecule showing structural arrangement of the carbon atoms. The hollow sphere is capable of occluding metal atoms or ions.

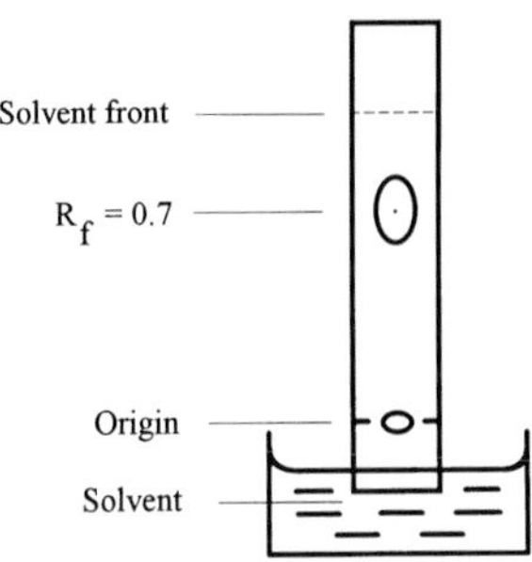

Fig. 112.4 Technique for ascending chromatography on paper or ITLC medium. A closed container is necessary to prevent evaporation, particularly if volatile solvents are used.

2400°C, ^{99m}Tc radioactivity is volatilized in association with carbon from the crucible in the form of a microaerosol. This 'gas' is not particularly stable as it undergoes coalescence and deposition on the sides of the containing vessel, so that it must be administered to the patient within 10 min of generation. When breathed, the radioactivity is deposited and retained in the alveoli, enabling multiple views of the lungs to be accumulated at leisure.

When the argon contains 3% oxygen, a different product is formed. Known as Pertechnegas, this product has been identified as ^{99m}Tc pertechnetate. It is also deposited in the lungs but undergoes diffusion into the blood, enabling lung washout curves to be recorded.

At this stage, the nature of Technegas is not known with certainty. However, the method of preparation has many similarities to that recently described for the preparation of C_{60} fullerene, a newly identified form of elemental carbon which has a spherical arrangement of atoms in a structure analogous to that of a soccer ball.[17] A large number of fullerenes have been identified, but C_{60} appears to be one of the most common and most stable. The spherical cage has been shown to be able to occlude metal ions, and this is one possible explanation for the formation of Technegas. The structure of this molecule is illustrated in Figure 112.3.

Recent work has identified the presence of fullerenes in the film deposited on a probe tip positioned over the graphite crucible under conditions used for the production of Technegas but not when 3% oxygen is present in the argon.[18] Alternative possibilities, such as a sandwich structure containing technetium atoms between layers of graphite lattice, have not yet been excluded.

RADIOCHEMICAL ANALYSIS

● What techniques can be used to determine the radiochemical purity of radiopharmaceuticals?

▲ *Chromatography*

The technique of most value for the determination of radiochemical purity is undoubtedly chromatography.[19] A small volume of the test solution is applied at the origin, near one end of a support medium, which is often filter paper. However, instant thin-layer chromatography medium impregnated with silica gel (ITLC-SG) has many advantages, including faster development times and, frequently, improved separations. The chromatogram is developed by allowing a solvent or mixture of solvents to migrate along the strip. After a convenient migration distance has been reached, the solvent front is marked and the strip dried ready for counting. It is generally convenient to cut the strip into segments so that a histogram of radioactivity distribution is obtained.

Partition of solutes is achieved by a process of selective adsorption on the support medium in conjunction with their solubility in the developing solvent. The position to which a solute migrates is constant for any particular system and is defined by the R_f (ratio of fronts) value.

$$R_f = \frac{\text{Distance migrated by solute}}{\text{Distance migrated by solvent}}$$

The R_f value ranges from 0 (no migration) to 1.0 (migration at the solvent front). Systems which produce intermediate R_f values are desirable but not always achievable.

The chromatogram should be run in a closed system so that the air is saturated with solvent vapour. It is usually run in the ascending mode (Figure 112.4) but can be arranged to run descendingly by using a wick to a solvent reservoir. To obtain a full chromatographic analysis, it may be necessary to run chromatograms in more than one system. For example, the analysis of ^{99m}Tc-MDP requires chromatograms to be run on ITLC-SG with acetone (system A) and ITLC-SG with saline (system B). The behaviour of ^{99m}Tc radioactivity in each system is shown in Figure 112.5.

In system A, ^{99m}Tc pertechnetate migrates at the solvent front (R_f = 1.0), while ^{99m}Tc-MDP and insoluble $^{99m}TcO_2$ remain at the origin (R_f = 0). System B enables the separation of $^{99m}TcO_2$ from the components which are soluble in saline, i.e. $^{99m}TcO_4^-$ and ^{99m}Tc-MDP, both of which migrate at the solvent front. The two systems there-

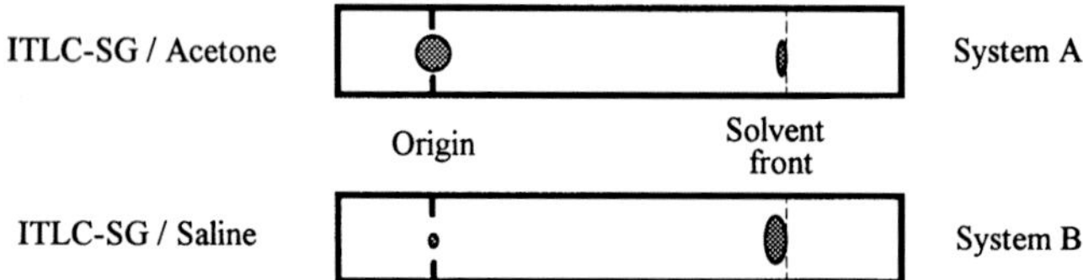

Fig. 112.5 Chromatographic analysis of ^{99m}Tc-MDP, showing migration of ^{99m}Tc radioactivity. In system A, ^{99m}Tc pertechnetate migrates at the solvent front, leaving ^{99m}Tc-MDP and $^{99m}TcO_2$ colloid at the origin, while in system B only the $^{99m}TcO_2$ remains at the origin.

fore enable determination of the radiochemical impurities $^{99m}TcO_4^-$ and $^{99m}TcO_2$ and, by difference from 100, the radiochemical purity of ^{99m}Tc-MDP.

The above procedure is readily adaptable to the use of short lengths of media (mini-strips) which can be developed rapidly in a small tube or glass jar.[20] Cutting the strips midway between the origin and solvent front will enable determination of radioactivity in each segment. This technique is sufficiently accurate for the routine analysis of ^{99m}Tc-MDP and other radiopharmaceuticals behaving in a similar fashion, but is not suitable for use when components have intermediate R_f values. Thus, the determination of radiochemical purity of ^{131}I-MIBG requires the use of a longer strip of filter paper developed in the solvent mixture *n*-butanol, acetic acid and water in the ratio 60:15:25, in which ^{131}I-MIBG has $R_f = 0.9–1.0$ and free ^{131}I iodide has $R_f = 0.3–0.5$.

Correct technique is particularly important in the chromatography of ^{99m}Tc radiopharmaceuticals, as the potential for atmospheric oxidation of the product on the strip is very high. If this occurs, an inaccurately high percentage of $^{99m}TcO_4^-$ content will be found and there may be severe streaking along the strip. It is therefore very important never to use a source of hot air, such as a hair dryer or oven, to dry the spot before development. Better results are usually obtained with the spot run wet, but if this is not satisfactory a locally directed current of nitrogen gas can be used for drying.

Although chromatography has wide application in radiopharmacy, there are situations where alternative techniques are required. Most commonly these include electrophoresis, gel filtration, high-performance liquid chromatography (HPLC) and solvent extraction. A brief description of each technique and its application is given here.

Electrophoresis

The principle utilized in electrophoresis is the property of charged molecules (ions) to migrate in an electric field. The rate of migration depends on both the charge and size of the molecule. The apparatus, shown diagrammatically in Figure 112.6, consists of a direct-current power supply, capable of providing a potential difference of 400 V or more, connected via an electrolyte buffer solution to either end of a strip of support medium, which may be cellulose acetate or filter paper.

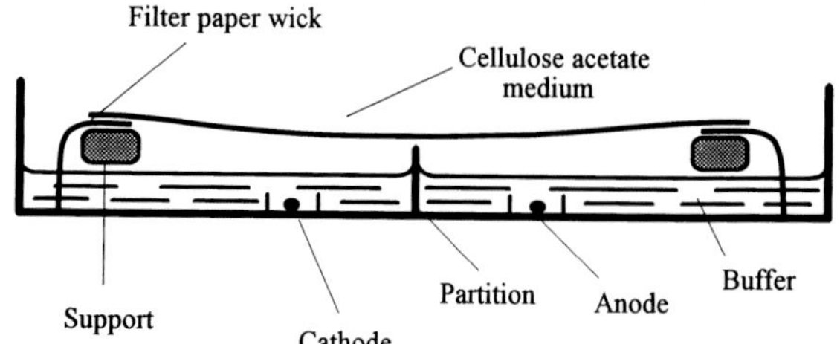

Fig. 112.6 Section through a basic electrophoresis chamber. Direct current is applied to the cathode (–ve electrode) and anode (+ve electrode) enabling migration of radioactive ions applied to the cellulose acetate medium.

One of the most common buffers is a sodium barbitone/barbituric acid mixture of pH 8.6, as used for the separation of proteins. This buffer is also suitable for the analysis of many radiopharmaceuticals, including those containing ^{99m}Tc. Being a small ion, ^{99m}Tc pertechnetate migrates rapidly and is readily separated from larger negatively charged complexes such as ^{99m}Tc-DTPA or insoluble $^{99m}TcO_2$, which remains at the origin.[21] After the run, the strip can be dried, cut and counted as with a chromatogram.

Electrophoresis is a particularly useful technique for separating mixtures of ^{99m}Tc pertechnetate and ^{99m}Tc complexes which are lipid soluble, e.g. ^{99m}Tc-DISIDA. Both will migrate at the solvent front in organic solvents such as acetone, but are easily resolved using electrophoresis. It is also a useful method for the analysis of radioiodinated compounds because the free iodide ion moves rapidly and may cleanly separate from the labelled product in a very short time, usually less than 10 min.

Gel filtration

This technique can be used for both quantitative separations and analytical purposes. When a mixture of solutes is passed down a column of suitable medium, such as the cross-linked dextran Sephadex, small molecules are able to penetrate pores in the polymeric structure and are selectively retarded as the mixture is eluted. Larger molecules are eluted from the column first and may be collected in specific fractions. By this means, mixtures of proteins can be separated and the purification of iodination reaction mixtures is readily accomplished. Sephadex is available in various grades from which the most appropriate for the separation can be selected. Figure 112.7 shows a typical elution profile which could be obtained from the purification of iodinated human serum albumin. Note that the high molecular weight product is eluted first followed by the small radioiodide ion present as an impurity.

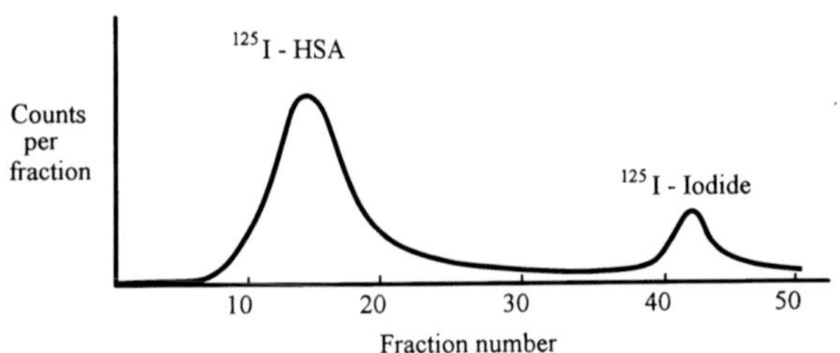

Fig. 112.7 Typical elution profile from the gel filtration purification of human serum albumin labelled with iodine-125. The high molecular weight protein is excluded from the gel and appears in the early fractions, while the much smaller iodide ion migrates more slowly down the column and appears in the eluate later.

Care should be exercised when Sephadex separation of ^{99m}Tc radiopharmaceuticals is envisaged. It has been shown that weaker complexes such as those formed by MDP or PYP may dissociate on the column, producing erroneous results. This effect may be minimized by using a solution of the ligand to elute the column or selecting an alternative non-complexing medium such as a polyacrylamide gel.

High-performance liquid chromatography

HPLC is a more recent development of column chromatography that utilizes densely packed columns of adsorbent through which the liquid phase is forced at high pressure. As the various components of the sample are eluted from the column, they pass through a detector which produces a response, usually presented in the form of a graph. The detector may be sensitive to radiation or may utilize some physical property of the analyte such as light absorption at a specific wavelength. The equipment is expensive, requiring specialized high-pressure pumps, injectors and columns, but can enable separations not achievable by any other means.

The stationary phase, contained in the column, most frequently consists of beads of silica to which is bonded an organic silane containing long-chain (C_{18}) carbon groups, although many other types are available. These include preparative as well as analytical columns.

As an example of its versatility, HPLC has been used to separate the bone agent ^{99m}Tc-MDP, prepared by borohydride reduction, into several different components.[22] As with column chromatography, any new application should be carefully evaluated to ensure that dissociation does not occur on the column and thereby introduce artifacts into the results. It has also been observed that stannous ions from tin(II)-reduced ^{99m}Tc preparations can be retained on the column and produce anomalous results for ^{99m}Tc pertechnetate content when subsequent analyses are performed.[23]

Solvent extraction

When two immiscible solvents are shaken together, any solute present will distribute between the two phases according to its solubility in each phase. An equilibrium is reached which is governed by the partition coefficient, *D*.

$$D = \frac{\text{Concentration in organic phase}}{\text{Concentration in aqueous phase}}$$

A molecule which is lipid soluble may have $D = 100$ or more so that it becomes highly concentrated in the organic phase. If the solvent is volatile, e.g. ether or chloroform, the solute can be readily recovered by distillation or evaporation.

This technique is widely used in all forms of chemistry. In radiopharmacy, two common applications will be mentioned. The first involves the separation of ^{99m}Tc pertechnetate from large-volume solutions of low specific activity ^{99}Mo dissolved in strongly alkaline solution, e.g. 5 M potassium hydroxide. When extracted with methyl ethyl ketone, ^{99m}Tc pertechnetate dissolves in the organic phase and can be recovered by evaporation to dryness.[24] This method has been used on a large scale to prepare ^{99m}Tc pertechnetate for radiopharmaceutical purposes.

The second application is for the rapid analysis of ^{99m}Tc-HMPAO by the extraction of this lipid-soluble complex from saline solution into ethyl acetate or ether.[25] The two phases can be mixed in a test tube using a vortex mixer then separated and counted in a dose calibrator. Only a small aliquot of the preparation is required and the result can be rapidly obtained before significant decomposition into the hydrophilic secondary complex occurs.

METAL COMPLEXES

● **What are metal complexes and why are they important to radiopharmacy?**

▲ It will be appreciated that most of the radionuclides used in nuclear medicine are radioisotopes of metal ions, principally ^{99m}Tc, ^{111}In, ^{67}Ga, ^{201}Tl, ^{51}Cr and ^{57}Co, which account for the majority of studies carried out in most departments. Although selected on the basis of favourable physical characteristics, the chemical properties of these radionuclides have played a vital role in the development of new and improved techniques. Many metal ions have useful biological properties in their own right, but the principal means of modifying their behaviour at our disposal is the formation of metal complexes with suitable molecules called ligands. Coordination chemistry is the branch of science devoted to this topic, which has wide-ranging applications from mineral processing to chemotherapy.

In order to form a complex in aqueous solution, ligand molecules must contain elements or ions capable of donating a pair of electrons to vacant metal orbitals, leading to the formation of a coordinate bond. The elements O, N, S and Cl are the most common donors. Important ligand groups containing these elements include H_2O, OH^-, $-COO^-$, $-NH_2$, CN^-, $-SH$, NCS^-, Cl^-, etc. Enough of these monodentate ligands bind to the metal ion to satisfy the typical coordination number of the ion. This is the number of ligand atoms bound, which is usually four or six for most transition metal ions. For example, when these ions are dissolved in water, they exist in the form of the hexaquo ions $[M(H_2O)_6]^{n+}$ and complex formation with other ligands involves displacement reactions in which water molecules are progressively replaced by stronger ligands. This has important consequences both for the thermodynamic stability constant governing the reaction

$$[M(H_2O)_6]^{n+} + L = [M(H_2O)_5L]^{n+} + H_2O$$

and also the kinetics of this process, which may be fast (labile complex) or slow (inert complex).

Since ligands can be either neutral or negatively charged, when they are bound to a metal ion the overall charge of the complex will be determined by the oxidation state or charge of the metal ion and the number of ligands bound. Thus, a complex may be cationic, e.g. $[Co^{III}(NH_3)_6]^{3+}$; neutral, e.g. $[Co^{III}(NH_3)_3Cl_3]$; or anionic, e.g. $[Co^{III}(NH_3)_2Cl_4]^-$. All of these can be isolated from solution under the appropriate conditions.

The coordination number (CN) also determines the stereochemistry, i.e. the spatial configuration of the groups surrounding the metal ion. The above examples have CN = 6, which leads to the formation of a regular octahedron in which the ligand atoms are placed at the six vertices of an octahedron. Other common stereochemistries are: for CN = 4, either square planar or tetrahedral; and for CN = 5, pyramidal. Such arrangements enable the existence of structural and optical isomeric forms, which can frequently be isolated when the central metal ion is inert and structural rearrangements are slow.

The presence of more than one donor atom in a molecule having the correct stereochemistry enables each of these atoms to bind to the metal ion, resulting in a ring structure known as a chelate ring. Such a ring will usually contain five or six members, including the metal, as these configurations produce less strain because the bonding angles are closest to the ideal. A chelate ring will also confer stability on the complex. It can be appreciated that for the complex to dissociate it will be necessary for both ends of the ligand molecule to break their bonds to the metal ion at the same time. As the number of chelate rings in a molecule is increased, the stability of the complex is also increased.

The importance of the above principles is well illustrated by reference to the structure of the ^{51}Cr complex of ethylenediaminetetraacetic acid (EDTA), which has been widely used for the estimation of glomerular filtration rate. The structure of this complex is shown in Figure 112.8.

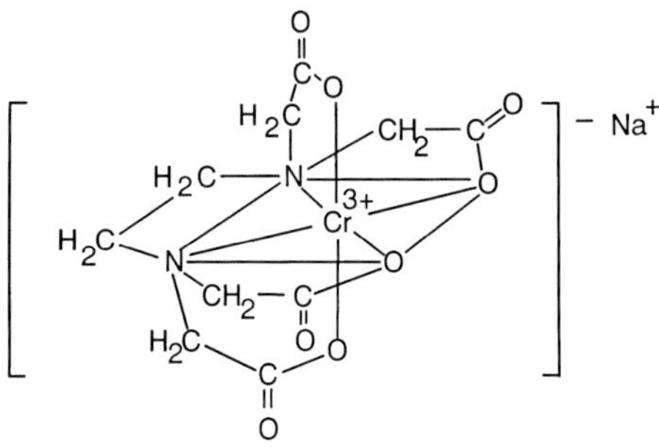

Fig. 112.8 Structure of the chromium–EDTA complex. The multidentate EDTA ligand occupies the vertices of a regular octahedron around the Cr(III) ion producing a very stable complex having overall negative charge.

EDTA contains two nitrogen atoms and four carboxyl groups. Each of the latter must be ionized before coordination to the metal is possible. The four negative charges on the ligand and the three positive charges on chromium(III) result in an overall charge of –1 for the complex. The coordinating atoms or ions each occupy the octahedral vertices around the Cr(III) ion and the ligand structure is such that a total of five five-membered chelate rings are formed, resulting in a high overall stability constant for this complex. In addition Cr(III) is a kinetically inert ion, meaning that once formed the complex will not easily undergo ligand substitution reactions. The negative charge confers solubility in aqueous media and assists excretion by the renal route. The complex is sufficiently stable to allow sterilization by autoclaving and following injection is excreted quantitatively in the urine. It does not undergo dissociation in vivo, which could occur with weaker complexes, leading to the deposition of toxic metal ions in tissues.

● What is a bifunctional chelating agent?

▲ A molecule which possesses both a chelating function and a means of changing the biodistribution is known as a bifunctional chelating agent. The biological properties are frequently varied by changing the lipophilicity of substituents attached to the molecule. Excellent examples of this effect are found in the biliary imaging agents based on the ^{99m}Tc chelates of substituted iminodiacetic acid (HIDA) ligands of the type shown in Figure 112.9. Following reduction with tin(II), ^{99m}Tc reacts with these ligands to form complexes with the structure illustrated in Figure 112.10.[26]

These are examples of so-called 'technetium-essential' complexes, in which the biological properties are dependent on the complex as a whole and may be considerably different from that of the components, as opposed to the 'technetium-tagged' radiopharmaceuticals, which include labelled colloids, particles and cells.

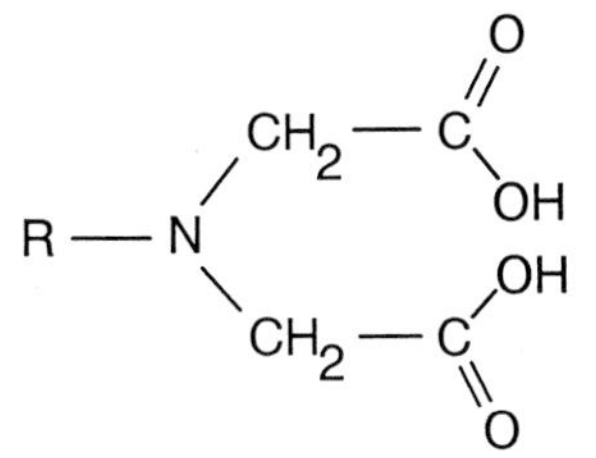

Fig. 112.9 General structure for tridentate iminodiacetic acid ligands capable of binding to metal ions via two ionized carboxyl oxygens and the imino nitrogen atom.

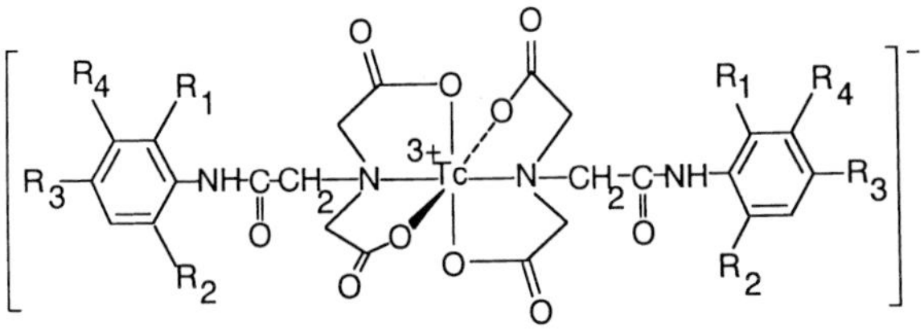

Fig. 112.10 Structure of the ^{99m}Tc-HIDA complexes. Two molecules of tridentate ligand are bound to the ^{99m}Tc(III) ion in an octrahedral configuration. The biological properties are largely governed by the lipophilicity of the R-groups attached to the benzene ring and the overall negative charge.

If the R-group in the iminodiacetic acid formula above is a methyl group, the ^{99m}Tc complex is almost entirely excreted in the urine. However, the introduction of a lipophilic benzene ring into the molecule produces a substantial biliary excreted component. The proportion of this component and the kinetics of excretion can be fine tuned by changing the nature of the groups R_1, R_2 and R_3 in Figure 112.10. In this manner, the three main biliary agents in clinical use have been developed. These are:

Diethyl-IDA $R_1 = R_2 = C_2H_5$-, $R_3 = R_4 =$ H-
DISIDA $R_1 = R_2 = (CH_3)_2CH$-, $R_3 = R_4 =$ H-
Mebrofenin $R_1 = R_2 = R_3 = CH_3$-, $R_4 =$ Br-

The ^{99m}Tc complexes of all three are easily prepared by tin(II) reduction via instant labelling kits in high yield. Although a small proportion of the dose appears in the urine with diethyl-IDA and DISIDA (disofenin), biliary excretion with mebrofenin is virtually quantitative. This compound also shows fast kinetics and is resistant to competition for hepatobiliary excretion from bilirubin.[27]

● What factors determine the biodistribution of metal chelates?

▲ When a metal complex is injected intravenously, a number of factors are involved in determining its eventual biological behaviour. Principal among these is competition for the metal ion by naturally occurring ligands. The various body fluids and tissues contain numerous substances capable of binding metal ions, including amino acids, peptides, proteins, nucleotides, etc. Very often, there are carrier proteins with highly specific metal binding properties, e.g. transferrin for iron(III), ceruloplasmin for copper(II), which bind the metal very strongly and are capable of undergoing ligand exchange with weaker complexes. Other factors to consider include the possibility of replacement of the central metal ion by endogenous metal ions which are capable of forming more stable complexes with the ligand. Varying conditions of pH or redox potential may also have a pronounced effect on the way the complex behaves in vivo.

It is important to note that the biodistribution of these complexes can also be dependent on the quantity injected.[28] Thus, high specific activity complexes may behave differently to low specific activity complexes, which contain larger quantities of non-radioactive metal. Even a very small proportion of the complex dissociating will enable saturation of the metal binding sites in tissues, leading to changes in the biodistribution.

As discussed above, the weaker complexes of radioactive metal ions usually have biodistributions similar to the free metal ion, i.e. that shown by its simple salts. Fortunately, this behaviour is not followed by ions which are characterized by their kinetic inertness. Such ions include Cr(III) and Tc(V),[12] particularly when the latter is present as the oxospecies $Tc = O^{3+}$ and $O = Tc = O^{+}$. Because they are slow to react, even though they may have low thermodynamic stability, complexes of very weak ligands such as gluconate, pyrophosphate, methylenediphosphonate, etc., have *unique* biological properties which enable the diversity of nuclear medicine studies available today.

Given that a complex must be stable, inert or preferably both to be distributed in the body without dissociation, a number of generalizations can be made concerning factors which affect its behaviour.

Molecular weight

Substances with low molecular weight, less than about 500, tend to be excreted by the kidneys. Between 500 and 1000, biliary excretion is favoured. High molecular weight substances tend to be retained in the circulation.

Charge

Neutral molecules are frequently lipid soluble and may penetrate cell membranes, as occurs with ^{111}In oxinate when used for cell labelling, or with ^{99m}Tc-HMPAO used for cerebral perfusion studies. Both of these complexes undergo dissociation or reaction inside the cell, leading to the formation of species which are unable to diffuse out of the cell.

Negatively charged molecules, e.g. those containing COO^- or SO_3^- groups are hydrophilic and tend to be excreted by the kidneys.

Positively charged complexes, particularly if they also contain lipophilic substituents, are localized in muscle, including the myocardium, as occurs with the ^{99m}Tc(I)-isonitrile complexes of the type $[Tc(CN\text{-}R)_6]^+$.

Presence of ring structures

Biliary excretion is promoted by the presence of aromatic or chelate rings in the molecule, especially if they occur in more than one plane. If the molecule also contains hydrophilic groups, particularly if they are well separated from the lipophilic groups, biliary excretion is again aided. All of these conditions are met in the ^{99m}Tc complexes of substituted iminodiacetic acid ligands.[26,29]

REFERENCES

1. Ramos-Gabatin A, Orzel J A, Maloney T R, Murnane J E, Borchert R D 1986 Severe systemic reaction to diphosphonate bone imaging agents: skin testing to predict allergic response and a safe alternative agent. J Nucl Med 27: 1432–1435
2. Keeling D H, Sampson C B 1984 Adverse reactions to radiopharmaceuticals. United Kingdom 1977–1983. Br J Radiol 57: 1091–1096
3. Saha G B 1979 Fundamentals of nuclear pharmacy. Springer, New York
4. Verbruggen A M 1990 Radiopharmaceuticals: state of the art. Eur J Nucl Med 17: 346–364
5. Tofe A J, Francis M D 1976 In vitro stabilisation of low-tin bone imaging agent (^{99m}Tc-Sn-HEDP) by ascorbic acid. J Nucl Med 17: 820–825
6. Beightol R W, Cochrane J 1983 Radiochemical analysis of commercial MDP bone kits. J Nucl Med Tech 11: 173–176
7. Warbick A, Ege G N, Henkelman R M, Maier G, Lyster D M 1977 An evaluation of radiocolloid particle sizing techniques. J Nucl Med 18: 827–834
8. Campbell J, Bellen J C, Baker R J, Cook D J 1981 Technetium-99m calcium phytate – optimisation of calcium content for liver and spleen scintigraphy (concise communication). J Nucl Med 22: 157–160
9. Gray S J, Stirling K 1980 The tagging of red cells and plasma proteins with radioactive chromium. J Clin Invest 29: 1604–1613
10. Karesh S M 1989 Sterility and pyrogen testing of radiopharmaceuticals. J Nucl Med Tech 17: 156–159
11. Jones A G, Davison A 1982 The chemistry of technetium I, II, III and IV. Int J Appl Radiat Isot 33: 867–874
12. Jones A G, Davison A 1982 The relevance of basic technetium chemistry to nuclear medicine. J Nucl Med 23: 1041–1043
13. Blower P J, Singh J, Clark S E M 1991 The chemical identity of pentavalent technetium-99m-dimercaptosuccinic acid. J Nucl Med 32: 845–849
14. Kowalsky R J, Perry J R 1987 Radiopharmaceuticals in nuclear medicine practice. Appleton & Lange, Norwalk, CT
15. Bolton A E, Hunter W M 1973 The labeling of proteins to high specific radioactivities by conjugation to an I-125 containing acylating agent. Biochem J 133: 529–539
16. Burch W M, Sullivan P J, McLaren C J 1986 Technegas – a new ventilation agent for lung scanning. Nucl Med Commun 7: 865–871
17. Kroto H W, Allaf A W, Balm S P 1991 C_{60}: Buckminsterfullerene. Chem Rev 91: 1213–1235
18. Mackey D W J, Willett G D, Fisher K J 1993 The observation of fullerenes in a technegas lung ventilation unit. J Nucl Med 34: 232P
19. Robbins P J 1984 Chromatography of technetium-99m radiopharmaceuticals – a practical guide. Society of Nuclear Medicine, New York
20. Zimmer A M, Pavel D G 1977 Rapid miniaturized chromatographic quality control procedures for Tc-99m radiopharmaceuticals. J Nucl Med 18: 1230–1233
21. Baker R J, Diamanti C I, Goodwin D A, Meares C F 1981 Technetium complexes of EDTA analogs: studies of the radiochemistry and biodistribution. Int J Nucl Med Biol 8: 159–169
22. Tanabe S, Zodda J P, Deutsch E, Heineman W R 1983 The effect of pH on the formation of Tc($NaBH_4$)MDP radiopharmaceutical analogues. Int J Appl Radiat Isot 34: 1577–1584
23. Hung J C, Corlija M, Volkert W A, Holmes R A 1988 Kinetic analysis of technetium-99m d,1,-HM-PAO decomposition in aqueous media. J Nucl Med 29: 1568–1576
24. Baker R J 1971 A system for the routine production of concentrated technetium-99m by solvent extraction of molybdenum-99. Int J Appl Radiat Isot 22: 483–485
25. Ballinger J R, Reid R H, Gulenchyn K Y 1988 Radiochemical purity of [^{99m}Tc]HM-PAO. J Nucl Med 29: 572–573
26. Chervu L R, Nunn A D, Loberg M D 1982 Radiopharmaceuticals for hepatobiliary imaging. Sem Nucl Med 12: 5–17
27. Nunn A D, Loberg M D, Conley R A 1983 A structure–distribution relationship approach leading to the development of Tc-99m mebrofenin: an improved cholescintigraphic agent. J Nucl Med 24: 423–430
28. Fornasiero D, Bellen J C, Baker R J, Chatterton B E 1987 Paramagnetic complexes of manganese(II), iron(III) and gadolinium(III) as contrast agents for magnetic resonance imaging. The influence of stability constants on the biodistribution of radioactive aminopolycarboxylate complexes. Invest Radiol 22: 322–327
29. Firnau G 1976 Why do Tc-99m-chelates work for cholescintigraphy? Eur J Nucl Med 1: 137–139

113. Basic science: radiopharmacy

Peter G. Yeates Richmond J. Baker

CELL LABELLING TECHNIQUES

● **What are the common problems encountered in the preparation of radiolabelled cells for diagnostic studies?**

▲ *^{99m}Tc erythrocytes (^{99m}Tc-RBC)*

There are three general procedures used clinically to label red blood cells. These are referred to as **in vitro** (totally outside the body), **in vivo** (totally inside the body) and '**in vivtro**' (performed both inside and outside the body, frequently called the 'modified in vivo method'[1]). The last two procedures are illustrated schematically in Figure 113.1. Each procedure utilizes the fact that stannous tin (stabilized in the form of a complex) binds strongly to the haemoglobin of red cells where, following incubation, it reduces ^{99m}Tc pertechnetate, which diffuses across the cell membrane. Ultimately the reduced ^{99m}Tc becomes bound to haemoglobin and is held firmly in the cell.

To ensure optimal and reproducible labelling efficiency, adherence to recommended levels of stannous ion and incubation times are critical. If too little stannous complex is used and there is insufficient present to reduce all the added ^{99m}Tc pertechnetate, there will be problems owing to free activity at scanning. Alternatively, if too much is used, excess stannous tin may be present extracellularly and will reduce added ^{99m}Tc pertechnetate at the radiolabelling step, making it unavailable to the red cells. The latter problem is more likely to occur with the in vitro procedure but is rarely encountered when the stannous complex is injected directly into the body because of the large number of red cells present. Excess stannous tin also undergoes renal excretion and adsorption to the skeletal system.[2] The recommended stannous levels for the different procedures are shown in Table 113.1.

Table 113.1 Recommended levels of stannous tin for ^{99m}Tc-red cell labelling procedures

	In vivo	In vitro	In vivtro
Recommended Sn^{2+} level	10–20 μg/kg body weight	50 μg/3ml whole blood	10–20 μg/kg body weight
Available products	Sn^{2+}-PYP Sn^{2+}-MDP	Sn^{2+} citrate	Sn^{2+}-PYP Sn^{2+}-MDP

A number of stannous preparations are available commercially for the specific purpose of red cell labelling. These include the complexes of medronate (MDP), pyrophosphate, citrate, etc. It is important to calculate the correct volume post reconstitution so that the desired quantity of stannous ions can be administered. Consider a vial containing, say, 5.1 mg of stannous fluoride and 4.7 mg of sodium medronate which is reconstituted with 6 ml of 0.9% sodium chloride BP. We are performing an in vivo study on a 70 kg patient using a recommended stannous level of 15 μg per kg body weight. To determine the required volume to be drawn up, firstly calculate the required amount of stannous ions, which is $0.015 \times 70 = 1.05$ mg. The formula weight of SnF_2 is $118.7 + (2 \times 18.9) = 156.5$, therefore the fraction of Sn^{2+} in SnF_2 is $118.7 / 156.5 = 0.758$. Hence, the amount of stannous ion in the vial is $5.1 \times 0.758 = 3.87$ mg. At reconstitution, 3.87 mg of Sn^{2+} is contained in 6.0 ml of solution. If the patient dose is 1.05 mg of Sn^{2+}, then the volume required is $(1.05 / 3.87) \times 6.0 = 1.6$ ml.

Irrespective of the method of labelling chosen, adherence to incubation times is critical as RBC uptake of both Sn^{2+} and ^{99m}Tc pertechnetate is largely dependent on diffusion gradients. Typical incubation times of 10–20 min are used for each step.[1]

Maintenance of good 'hot lab' housekeeping will ultimately ensure high-quality images. Stannous radiopharmaceutical kits should be kept away from direct sunlight to minimize degradation, while adherence to the manufacturer's storage and reconstitution directions will ensure that the correct amount of Sn^{2+} is present. In difficult patients (e.g. in vivtro label in a renal dialysis patient) consideration may be given to performing a premixing step prior to injection, i.e. before injecting the Sn^{2+} complex, draw 2–4 ml of patient blood into the syringe and then reinject slowly.

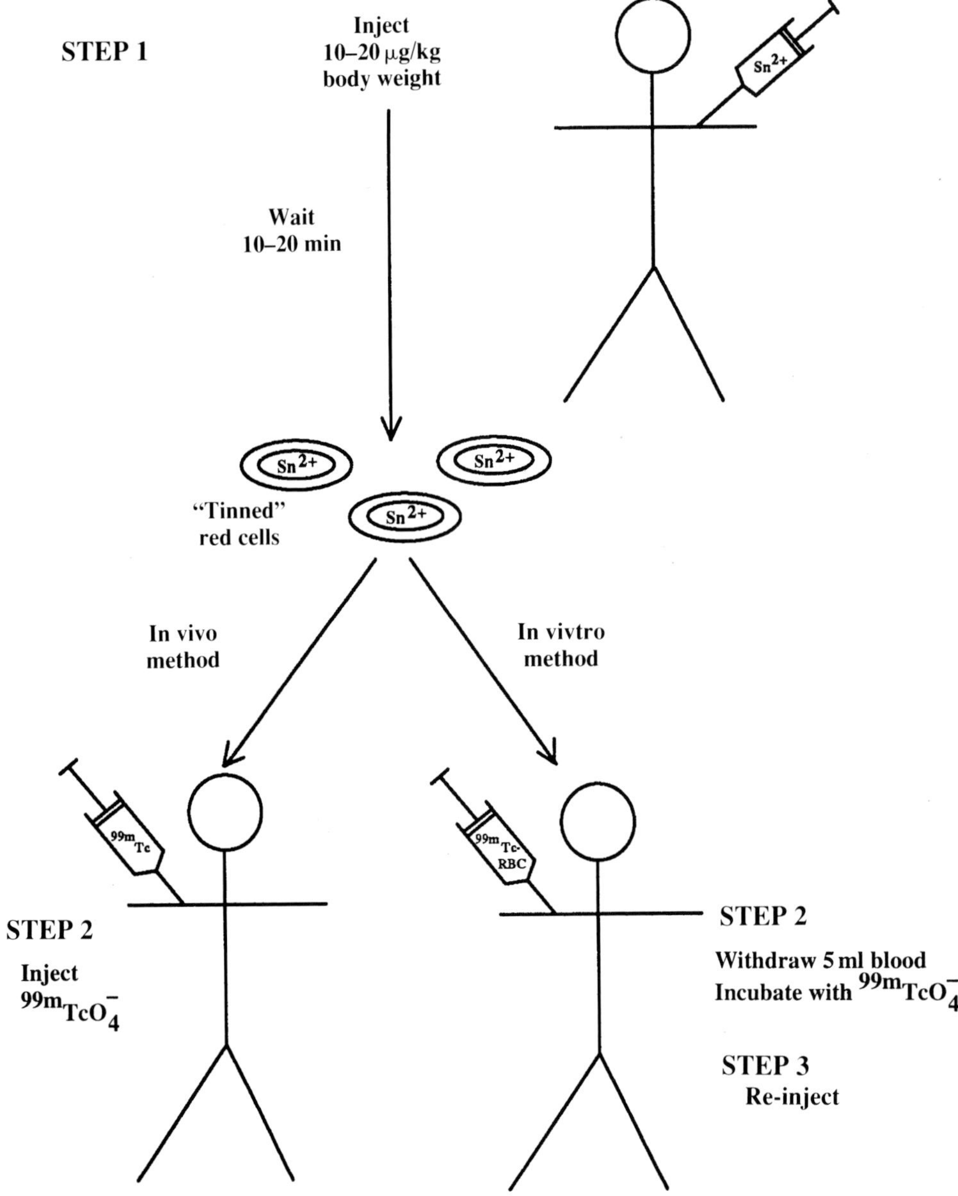

Fig. 113.1 Labelling of red blood cells by the in vivo and 'in vivtro' techniques.

^{111}In leucocytes

The radiopharmaceutical of choice, ^{111}In oxine, exhibits non-specific cell radiolabelling properties and undergoes trans-chelation in the presence of plasma to form non-diffusible ^{111}In transferrin. These special features of ^{111}In oxine require that the designated cell population be isolated prior to radiolabelling in the absence of plasma. The non-specific nature of ^{111}In oxine means that both the rate and extent of radiolabelling will be dependent on the cell concentration, i.e. the higher the cell concentration at the addition of ^{111}In oxine, the higher the labelling efficiency with time.

These special restrictions require a skilled operator to perform multiple isolation and manipulation steps while ensuring maintenance of cell viability and product sterility. In order to protect the operator from biological hazards, a biological containment cabinet (class II or III) or similar is suggested. Needle-stick injuries are eliminated by the use of flexible plastic mixing cannulas in all manipulation steps.

If a sedimentation agent is used to aid in cell purification procedures, the operator should ensure that after mixing it with blood residual air bubbles are removed, as they lead to unwanted cellular contamination. Obviously, the chosen labelling procedure must ensure that all remnants of the sedimentation agent are removed prior to patient reinjection. It is recommended that, if an i.v. line is used to reinject the labelled leucocytes, the line is flushed free of residual medication as instances of cellular aggregation have been observed.

The presence of plasma at the radiolabelling step is one of the most common reasons for poor labelling efficiency (Figure 113.2). One must weigh the advantages of multiple washing steps against potential loss of cell viability, particularly as the latter decreases with increasing time outside plasma and with the number of centrifugation steps used. Excessive centrifugation speed results in heavy cellular pelleting and a reduction in cell viability. Uneven distribution of radioactivity within the cellular suspension can occur if the cellular pellet is inadequately resuspended prior to the addition of ^{111}In oxine. Equally important is poor cellular resuspension before patient reinjection, leading to potential lung uptake due to microemboli. A mixing cannula fitted to a syringe is ideal for cellular resuspension (Figure 113.3).

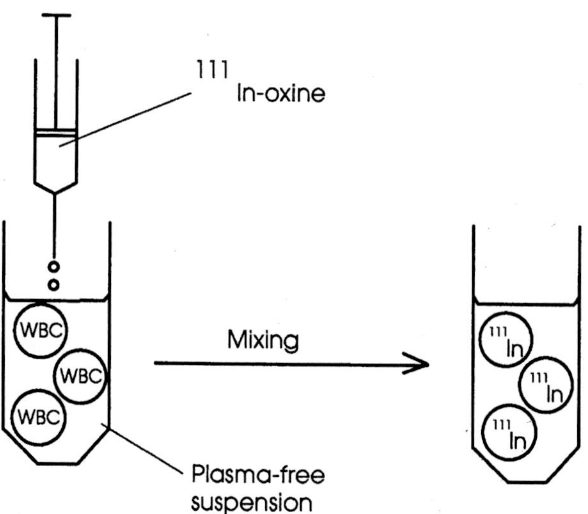

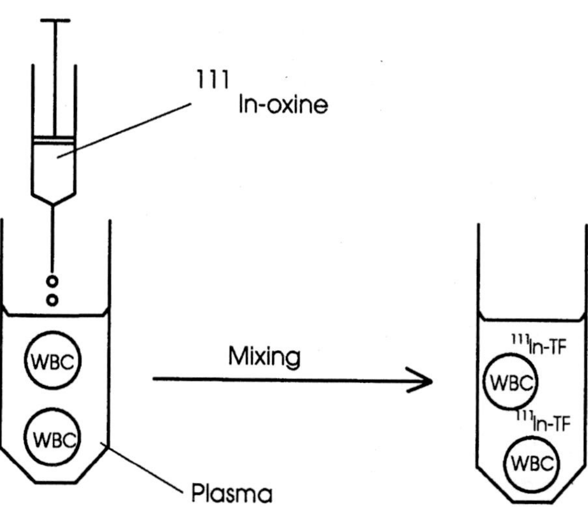

Fig. 113.2 Leucocyte labelling with ^{111}In oxine must be carried out in a plasma-free environment to achieve high labelling efficiency, but cell viability may be affected. Cells should be returned to plasma as soon as possible after the radiolabelling step.

- **What environment and precautions are necessary for the safe radiolabelling and reinjection of patients cells?**

▲ Clinical diagnosis with radiolabelled cells frequently involves in vitro manipulation of the patient's blood, as the non-specific nature of the labelling radiopharmaceutical requires isolation of the cell types from whole blood. In order to meet this requirement, operator methodology must be designed to maintain cell viability and sterility, while avoiding operator exposure to biological and radiation hazards. As a general rule, all blood and body fluids should be treated as potentially infectious.

Manipulation of blood should be performed in an approved containment cabinet (e.g. biological safety cabinet class II or similar) specifically designed and operated to minimize cross-contamination between the patient's blood sample, the operator and the immediate environment.[3–5] At minimum, the biological safety cabinet should be located in a low-traffic room, where the effect of exterior air movement will not impact on airflow pattern within the cabinet. Large objects should not be placed on the cabinet's workbench without due regard to their effect on the cabinet airflow pattern and hence containment function. Paramount to safe laboratory practice is proper utilization of the cabinet's airflow to ensure maintenance of product sterility and operator protection, particularly from generated aerosols which may contain blood-borne pathogens. Operators should remain gloved and gowned during all steps of the radio-

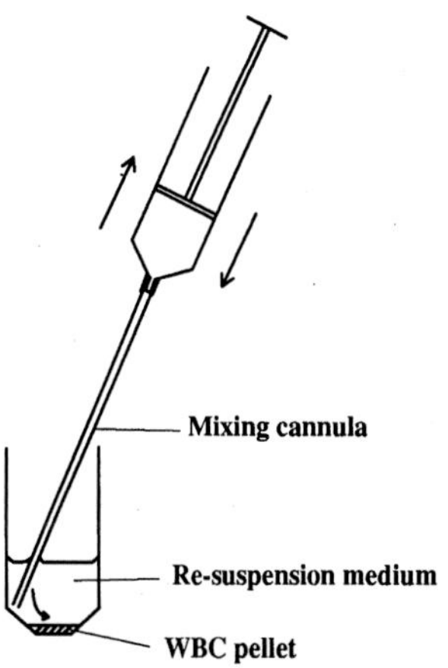

Fig. 113.3 In order to minimize operator biological exposure and eliminate needle-stick injuries, radiolabelling steps are performed in open containers (Falcon tubes), using plastic mixing cannulas attached to syringes to manipulate or resuspend cells. By repeatedly forcing medium over the WBC pellet, the cells are dispersed. Frothing must be avoided. A containment device equivalent to a biological safety cabinet class II or III is essential.

labelling procedure. Garments should be continuous fronted and of the low-linting type to reduce particulate contamination. Mask and eye protection are indicated for procedures that are likely to generate droplets of blood or body fluids which may enter the mouth, nostrils or eyes.[3,4] Routine use of needles during cell manipulation should be discouraged and replaced with plastic mixing cannulas (or similar) where possible. If needle use is essential, an approved recapping device should be used.[3,4]

Standard operating procedures (SOPs) must be in place to ensure that radiolabelled cells are returned to the correct patient otherwise the consequences may be catastrophic, especially if the cells are infected with HIV or hepatitis. SOPs should ensure that:

- Patients are identified with a unique nuclear medicine wrist badge, clearly marked with patient name, date and scan type.
- A single technician is responsible for the whole procedure including withdrawal of blood, radiolabelling and reinjection.
- Only one cell labelling procedure is carried out at any one time.
- During radiolabelling, the patient should remain in a designated area.
- At reinjection, the patient's identity is independently checked by two different people.

If sedimentation agents are used, the radiolabelling procedure should be validated for the absence of the agent in the final injectable cell suspension. Where cells are isolated using differential centrifugation, the cell suspension should be visually checked for signs of clumping prior to patient reinjection. Light microscopy is often useful in this regard.

Equally important are confirmation of cell viability post radiolabelling and radiolabelling efficiency, especially if new staff are being trained or new methodology is introduced. The activity of the dose must be calibrated prior to patient reinjection.

The reinjection of radiolabelled cells should be performed slowly, as this limits the volume of the injectate administered if an adverse drug reaction (ADR) is encountered. If pre-existing drug administration lines are used, they must be flushed with isotonic saline to remove residual traces of patient medication which may interact with the labelled cells, e.g. magnesium salts, 5% dextrose, etc. The quality of the patient injectate is totally dependent on the manipulative skills of the operator.

● What is the principle behind radiolabelling leucocytes with ^{111}In oxine? Are there any tricks to the radiolabelling methodology?

▲ ^{111}In oxine is a lipid-soluble complex that penetrates the cell membranes indiscriminately, requiring the desired cell type to be isolated from whole blood before labelling proceeds. Minor red blood cell (RBC) contamination is tolerable, as ^{111}In oxine has a reduced affinity for this cell, which is related to the RBC's lack of nucleus and lower intracellular protein concentration. Because of the low stability of the indium–oxine complex, high labelling efficiency can only be accomplished in the absence of plasma, as ^{111}In freely trans-chelates from oxine to the plasma metal-binding protein transferrin (Figure 113.2). The resulting complex, ^{111}In-TF, does not permeate cell membranes, reducing labelling efficiency. However long incubation times away from plasma should be avoided owing to problems of altered cellular viability.

Complicated leucocyte separation techniques should be avoided, as clinical studies have shown no real advantage of ^{111}In granulocytes versus ^{111}In mixed leucocytes. Where patients exhibit elevated erythrocyte sedimentation rates, simple gravity sedimentation of anticoagulated whole blood over 60 min is sufficient to harvest leucocytes for radiolabelling. To remove the variability in leucocyte separation with time, sedimentation agents (6% hydroxyethyl starch, 2% methycellulose, dextran) are added to increase erythrocyte sedimentation. Either method results in a plasma-based supernatant containing approximately 70% of the original leucocytes, but contaminated with 1–4 RBCs per WBC as well as the majority of platelets. Red cells may be lysed following the addition of hypotonic saline or ammonium chloride, however problems of altered leucocyte viability, evidenced by increased uptake by the reticular endothelial system, are often found. Whatever procedure is ultimately chosen, problems of ADR may be encountered if all traces of sedimentation agent are not removed at the time of reinjection. Acid citrate dextrose (ACD) is the preferred anticoagulant, as heparin appears to activate the WBC, while EDTA promotes trans-chelation, resulting in the formation ^{111}In EDTA.

Platelets, plasma and sedimentation agent contamination are largely removed from the cellular mixture by simple differential centrifugation, resulting in a pellet consisting of WBCs and RBCs. After discarding the supernatant, the WBC/RBC pellet is resuspended in 20 ml of 0.9% sodium chloride BP and centrifuged again, to ensure complete removal of contaminants. The WBC/RBC pellet is then resuspended ready for radiolabelling with ^{111}In oxine. Because cellular radiolabelling is dependent on diffusion, one would expect higher labelling efficiency when concentrated cellular suspensions are used. The final labelling volume can be altered according to the size of the WBC pellet initially isolated.

As is usually the situation, expertise in the radiolabelling of blood cells can only be achieved with considerable practice. In Table 113.2, a number of tips are presented which will be of assistance to operators performing this procedure.

Table 113.2 Useful tips for cell labelling procedures

Area	Tip
Sedimentation agents	After mixing the sedimentation agent with blood, remove all air bubbles from the meniscus. This minimizes RBC contamination as RBCs are trapped around the air bubble. During the incubation period, keep the blood sample vertical in a holder and left untouched. At the end of the incubation period, unscrew the lid with minimal movement
Plasma removal techniques	During removal of the plasma supernatant from the WBC/RBC pellet, use a syringe fitted with a plastic mixing cannula. All movements should be slow and controlled. Do not attempt to remove all the plasma after the first wash, as this disrupts the WBC/RBC pellet leading to leucocyte loss. The next wash overcomes this problem
Leucocyte concentration	Adjust the leucocyte concentration according to the number of leucocytes isolated, as dilute leucocyte solutions produce low labelling efficiency
Manipulation techniques	Overvigorous manipulation procedures reduce cellular viability. Excessive centrifugation speeds result in heavy pelleting of leucocytes. Use the movement of fluid up and down the syringe/cannula to resuspend the cell pellet. In terms of sensitivity RBCs > leucocytes >>> platelets in their ability to withstand overvigorous treatment

PRACTICAL CONSIDERATIONS

● What is the best way to ensure high radiochemical purity of ^{99m}Tc exametazime at reconstitution?

▲ ^{99m}Tc exametazime (^{99m}Tc-HMPAO) is a lipophilic complex used clinically for the evaluation of cerebral perfusion studies and the radiolabelling of mixed leucocytes.[6] Each vial contains lyophilized stannous exametazime complex in an atmosphere of nitrogen, which forms a basic solution of pH 9 following reconstitution with ^{99m}Tc pertechnetate. The maximum amount of tin present (stannous plus stannic) is only 4.4 μg. The unusually low stannous ion content is related to the difficulty of maintaining stannous ion solubility at pH 9 (which is necessary for optimal radiolabelling) and the destabilizing effect that excess unreacted Sn^{2+} has on the formed ^{99m}Tc exametazime complex.[7] Stannous ions promote the formation of an unwanted less lipophilic complex, commonly termed secondary ^{99m}Tc exametazime complex, together with free ^{99m}Tc pertechnetate. The reaction is quite rapid, resulting in a post-reconstitution expiry of only 30 min to ensure that the expiry specification of greater than 80% primary complex present is met.

As a consequence of this formulation, the product is susceptible to the level of carrier ^{99}Tc and trace levels of oxidants caused by radiolysis contained in the generator eluate at reconstitution. Both of these species consume stannous ions, resulting in a lower yield of the primary complex and increasing the amount of free ^{99m}Tc pertechnetate present. In order to reduce their combined detrimental effect, the manufacturer recommends that a freshly sourced eluate be used which satisfies the following conditions:

1. The generator must be eluted within the past 24 h.
2. The resulting eluate has a 2 h expiry. Where the eluate is sourced from a dry bed column, the expiry time of the eluate may be extended.
3. The activity added to the vial at reconstitution should not exceed 1.1 GBq.

In the clinical situation, experience has indicated that tight controls on the eluate are required to ensure a high, reproducible radiochemical purity of ^{99m}Tc exametazime. One should consider adopting an expiry time that includes both the time the eluate has been in contact with the generator column since the last elution and the age of the eluate post elution. Restricting this expiry time to a total of 6 h minimizes both the level of trace oxidants and carrier ^{99}Tc present in the eluate. A proposed generator elution schedule is shown in Table 113.3.

Under the above conditions, the radiochemical purity of ^{99m}Tc exametazime should routinely exceed 80% with a post-reconstitution expiry time of 30 min. Failure to follow these simple rules is likely to result in low and variable radiochemical yields.

In an effort to further limit the amount of trace oxidants contained in the reconstitution eluate, Bayne et al[8] and Millar[9] suggest the addition of sodium iodide. In this system, any oxidizing species present preferentially reacts with the added iodide, thus preserving the stannous ion for the reduction of ^{99m}Tc pertechnetate. A recent report by Weisner et al[10] indicates that a small quantity of cobalt chloride added to the vial immediately after reconstitution will stabilize the product for up to 5 h, but the mechanism of this effect is not known with certainty.

● What are the recommended storage conditions for multidose vials from which patient doses are withdrawn over a number of hours or days?

▲ Most commercial radiopharmaceuticals have recommended storage temperatures ranging from 2 to 25°C for

Table 113.3 Elution schedule for a ^{99m}Tc generator used for ^{99m}Tc exametazime reconstitution

Elution day	Elution time	Time since previous elution (h)	Expiry time of eluate	Reason
Monday	08.00 h	72*	Not useable	^{99}Tc/^{99m}Tc ratio is 12 at 08.00 h
	10.00 h	2	14.00 h	^{99}Tc/^{99m}Tc ratio is 0.3 at 10.00 h

* New generator, not eluted since Friday (72 h build-up time).

reconstituted ^{99m}Tc radiopharmaceuticals and opened or unopened vials of longer lived products such as indium-111 oxine, thallium-201 chloride, gallium-67 citrate, etc. In terms of practicality, room temperature storage in the hot laboratory, behind lead glass shields in lead pots, allows easy access and minimizes manipulation of the radiopharmaceutical during preparation of patient doses. This is particularly true when chemical stability of the preparation is unaffected at room temperature. However, room temperature storage can provide an ideal environment for microbial growth, which could produce dire consequences in the compromised patient. To minimize the risk of microbial bioburden, a lower storage temperature, usually 4°C, is preferred.

One should only advocate room temperature storage if each hot lab technician is fully conversant with the principles of aseptic technique. Simple rules based on the gloved operator using 70% alcohol to sanitize the surface of the septum before withdrawing a patient dose are mandatory. Equally important is maintenance of the septum integrity by minimizing the number of entries and using the smallest gauge needle possible, otherwise room air can be sucked into the vial as a consequence of the negative pressure created on removal of the dose. These points are critical as most hot labs are not located in controlled environments, i.e. clean rooms, thus the load of viable and non-viable particles in the air may be high. These issues are particularly important with products which do not contain a bacteriostat and have shelf-lives of several days, e.g. ^{67}Ga citrate. With ^{99m}Tc radiopharmaceuticals there is the additional concern that oxidation can occur in the presence of air. The incidence of microbial contamination can be gauged by routine retrospective stasis testing of used radiopharmaceutical vials, in which nutrient broth is added to the vial and incubated. The presence of microbial contamination is then a marker of operator competence.

In the absence of a controlled environment, the dispensing area should be located in the cleanest part of the hot lab, well away from sinks, open windows, doorways and paperwork. In recent years, a number of commercial firms have marketed containment devices (class II or III) which provide an adequately shielded sterile work area for patient dose dispensing.

● Should colloidal/particulate radiopharmaceuticals be inverted prior to patient dose withdrawal?

▲ The particulate or tagged radiopharmaceuticals used in nuclear medicine belong to the general classification of dispersed systems, which consist of particulate matter distributed throughout a dispersion medium. There are three classifications, namely molecular, colloidal and coarse dispersions. Although the size limits are somewhat arbitrary, the characteristics for the last two are tabulated in Table 113.4. For particles less than 1 μm there is no evidence to suggest that individual radioactive particles settle out of solution at 1 g, and thus vial inversion is not required prior to dispensing a patient radiopharmaceutical dose. This class includes ^{99m}Tc-Sb_2S_3 and the liver/spleen imaging agents, ^{99m}Tc-SnO and ^{99m}Tc sulphur colloid. In fact, these particles are kept in suspension as a result of Brownian motion. Stabilizing agents have been added by the manufacturer to prevent further growth and settling of the particles during storage.

In the case of ^{99m}Tc-MAA, individual particles are unable to remain suspended and settle out relatively quickly in the original storage vial or in the syringe prior to injection. In both cases, it is advisable that the vial or syringe be gently inverted to ensure uniform distribution of the particles.

Table 113.4 Physical properties of particulate radiopharmaceuticals

Class	Particle size range	System characteristics	Radiopharmaceutical and particle size range
Colloidal dispersion	0.5–50 nm	Diffuse very slowly, but unable to pass through semi-permeable membranes. Visible by electron microscopy	^{99m}Tc-Sb_2S_3 (3–20 nm)
Pseudo-colloidal dispersion	0.05–1 μm	Limited diffusion capability	^{99m}Tc-SnO colloid ^{99m}Tc sulphur colloid ^{99m}Tc calcium-phytate (0.1–1 μm)
Coarse dispersion	>1 μm	Unable to diffuse, settle with time Visible under light microscope	^{99m}Tc-MAA (10–40 μm)

PHARMACOLOGICAL INTERVENTIONS

● What are the dosages, method of administration and side-effects of the more common pharmaceuticals used diagnostically to modify the in vivo behaviour of radiopharmaceuticals?

▲ Pharmacological intervention in nuclear medicine is used to modify the normal behaviour of radiopharmaceuticals in a predictable manner.[11,12] Selected examples are listed in Table 113.5.

Myocardial interventions

Pharmacological coronary intervention (stress) using dipyridamole or adenosine provides an acceptable alternative in those patients who are unable to exercise adequately during radiodiagnosis of coronary artery

Table 113.5 Pharmacological intervention in scan procedures

Pharmaceutical	Dosage and administration route	Side-effects
Dipyridamole (Persantin)	i.v. infusion of 0.142 mg/kg/min over 4 min with patient supine. Non-responders have dose plus 25%	Chest pain, headache, dizziness and ECG ST-T changes (7.5%) Occasional reports of myocardial infarction and acute bronchospasm
Adenosine	i.v. infusion of 0.14 mg/kg min for 6 mins	Chest, throat and jaw pain. Headache, flushing and ischaemic electrocardiographic changes
Frusemide (Lasix)	0.3–0.5 mg/kg to a maximum of 40 mg Paediatric doses are calculated by weight	Rare, but typically related to extended therapy
Captopril (Captoten)	25 mg orally, 60 min before injection of ^{99m}Tc-DTPA	Transient hypotension, taste impairment and minor dermatological manifestations
CSK (Sincalide) (Kinevac)	i.v. infusion of 0.02 μg/kg over 3 min	GIT symptoms of abdominal discomfort or pain, or an urge to defecate, frequently accompany the injection of Sincalide. Nausea, dizziness and flushing occur occasionally
Morphine BP	0.04 mg/kg administered i.v.	Respiratory depression, anxiety, constipation, headache, depression of cough reflex, interference with thermal regulation and oliguria Evidence of histamine release such as urticaria, wheals and / or local tissue irritation may occur
Acetazolamide (Diamox)	500 –1000 mg i.v.	Slight discomfort to light-headedness, transient paresis in the distal limbs and around the mouth, and a short-acting diuretic effect

disease.[13-16] Studies are performed under medical supervision and may include monitoring of the patient's heart rate, blood pressure and electrocardiogram. Careful screening of patient medication and social habits are required before administration, as aminophylline, theophylline (and xanthine derivatives), caffeine, etc; are direct antagonists to the dilatory mechanism of dipyridamole and adenosine.[17] Typically, theophylline preparations are withheld for 48 h, while caffeine-containing foods, drinks and medications are withheld for 24 h.

Dipyridamole (Persantin). This is a potent coronary vasodilator (Vd) which produces a prolonged and one to twofold increase in coronary blood flow at 5–8 min post infusion. Maximal Vd effect may last for 10–30 min and is mediated by an increase in endogenous adenosine by blockage of adenosine receptors in myocardial artery walls. Low-level exercise (isometric handgrips, low-level treadmill) has been suggested to enhance the Vd activity of dipyridamole.

Most side-effects are dose related and can be reversed in 1–3 min with an i.v. bolus dose of aminophylline (50–75 mg). Because dipyridamole has the longer biological half-life, a second infusion of 250–500 mg of aminophylline in normal saline may be required. Dipyridamole solution is irritating and is diluted 1:2 with saline prior to infusion. It should never be mixed with other drugs.

Adenosine. This drug produces a direct dilation of coronary vessels within 2 min of administration, resulting in an approximate fourfold increase in coronary flow. The vasodilatory effect can be simply reversed by terminating the infusion, as adenosine has a biological half-life of 2–10 s. Adenosine provides no significant advantage over dipyridamole, as thallium-201 myocardial uptake reaches a plateau at higher blood flow rates.

Renal interventions

Frusemide (Lasix). This is a high-ceiling diuretic that inhibits sodium and chloride reabsorption in the proximal and distal tubules and loop of Henle, leading to increased urine production. Frusemide is contraindicated in patients who are dehydrated or hypotensive and may aggravate hypokalaemia and other electrolyte imbalances.

Diuretic radionuclide urography is used to distinguish an obstructed from non-obstructed dilated renal collecting system after visualization of the collecting structures. Prolonged activity is seen in the renal collecting system on the non-obstructed side, which can be removed by increased urine flow following injection of frusemide. If the urinary system is obstructed, diuretic stress is unable to remove the urine activity.

Captopril (Captoten). This is an angiotensin-converting enzyme (ACE) inhibitor which is used to evaluate renovascular hypertension and obstructive uropathy.[18-20] In patients with unilateral renal artery stenosis, glomerular filtration rate (GFR) measurements are performed before and after administration of captopril. With ACE inhibition, efferent arterioles are unable to constrict to maintain adequate perfusion (filtration) pressure, resulting in a decrease in GFR in those kidneys supplied by stenotic arteries.

Hepatobiliary interventions

Morphine sulphate. Morphine is most commonly used in the diagnosis of cystic duct patency, as it enhances the sphincter of Oddi tone, resulting in increased intraluminal common bile duct pressure. If the cystic duct is non-obstructed and/or the gall bladder is functionally obstructed by sludge, the hepatobiliary radiopharmaceutical is forced into the gall bladder.

Cholecystokinin (Kinevac, Sincalide). The endogenous hormone cholecystokinin or the active C-terminal octapeptide fragment (Sincalide) is used to contract the gall bladder. Cholecystokinin provides a more predictable response (timing of effect, type and magnitude of response) than the standard fatty meal, reaching a maximum effect 5–15 min post injection. It has an approximate biological half-life of 1–3 min and should be used with caution in patients with heart disease or suspected duodenal, gastric or pyloric ulcer.

Cerebral interventions

Acetazolamine (Diamox). This is a carbonic anhydrase inhibitor which, following injection, provides a vasodilatory stimulus through dilation of normal cerebral arteries, without changing cerebral flow. It is used in the assessment of regional cerebral blood flow (rCBF) reserve, e.g. area of stenosis versus normal vessel. In normal patients, rCBF may increase by 5–70%, most frequently between 20 and 35%. At 25 min post injection 75% maximal dilation is achieved.

ADVERSE REACTIONS

● **What is an adverse drug reaction (ADR) and what data should be recorded? Are ADRs more common with any particular radiopharmaceutical?**

▲ Adverse drug reactions, although rare, do occur with radiopharmaceuticals, having an estimated prevalence of 1–6 per 100 000 administrations.[21–23] Keeling[21] suggests that the true prevalence may be as high as 1 per 2000 injections, as only a small minority are actually reported. Minor physiological disturbances requiring minimal treatment predominate, although severe ADRs have occurred, e.g. overchelation of CSF calcium and magnesium with trisodium DTPA.[24] Fatalities have been associated with denatured serum albumin.[21]

The Society of Hospital Pharmacists of Australia (SHPA)[25] defines a suspected ADR as a 'response to a drug that is noxious and unintended and one which occurs in humans at doses used for prophylaxis, diagnosis or treatment of a disease'. Such responses may manifest themselves as alterations of anatomical, physiological or metabolic function as indicated by physical signs, symptoms and/or laboratory tests. The literature now refers to an ADR as an adverse drug experience (ADE), although in the following discussion ADR will be used. Direct application of the SHPA definition poses some interpretive difficulties as instances of altered biological distribution (e.g. excessive thyroid uptake on a bone scan) and faulty administration technique (e.g. tissued injections) are in the true sense an ADR. Cordova et al[23] redefine the radiopharmaceutical ADR as: 'any unexpected or unusual and undesirable clinical manifestation due to the vehicle carrying the radionuclide, not the radiation itself, excluding the effects of poor injection technique and overdosage'.

Most ADRs are classified as idiopathic hypersensitivity reactions (type B) and are principally related to the carrier ligand (vehicle) rather than to the labelling radionuclide. Skin problems typically include erythema and local or generalized rash (macular or urticarial) with itching, while vasomotor effects include fainting, sweating, malaise, nausea, vomiting and mild hypotension etc., with an expected onset several hours post administration, possibly lasting up to 48 h. Treatment with a non-sedative antihistamine is often helpful.[21,23]

With substantial improvements in radiopharmaceutical formulations and legislative adherence to Code of Good Manufacturing Practice, ADRs are now principally related to clinical use, rather than to any particular radiopharmaceutical. This is highlighted in the study by Keeling[21] for the period 1982–87, in which it was reported that 35% of ADRs were due to technetium diphosphonate compounds and 24% to ^{99m}Tc-DTPA. Bone scans in the UK accounted for 25% of all nuclear medicine procedures. ADRs have also been reported with technetium-labelled colloids, albumin particulates, gallium-67 citrate and thallium-201. In the case of labelled leucocytes and platelets, the possibility of residual contamination with sedimentation agents such as methylcellulose and poor operator technique should not be discounted. Unfortunately, limited information is available to enable segregation of minor from severe ADRs associated with the radiopharmaceutical administered.

There is a clear need to document these events correctly. The SHPA suggests three phases of ADR management.[25] The first involves assessment and correlation of the event, which requires documentation of patient particulars, drug details (both the drug in question and concomitant medication) and a description of the ADR. When describing an ADR, information relating to the type of reaction, onset and duration, complications and sequelae, treatment and outcome and relevant laboratory data all form vital pieces of the documentation. The next step is to document patient management, including treatment of symptoms and possible implications of readministration of the radiopharmaceutical. The last phase is to ensure that all suspected reactions are reported to medical staff, entered in patient notes and that the appropriate regulatory authority is notified.

REFERENCES

1. Kelly M J, Cowie A R, Antonio A, Barton H, Kalff V 1992 An assessment of factors which influence the effectiveness of the modified in vivo technetium-99m-erythrocyte labeling technique in clinical use. J Nucl Med 33: 2222–2225
2. Dewanjee M K, Wahner H W 1979 Pharmacodynamics of stannous chelates administered with ^{99m}Tc-labeled chelates. Radiology 132: 711–716
3. Yeates P 1991 Guidelines for in vitro/in vivo manipulation and radiolabelling of blood cells for patient re-injection. Australia and New Zealand Society of Nuclear Medicine Radiopharmacy Group, Sydney
4. Zabel P, Robichaud N, Hiltz A 1993 Personnel and product protection during manipulation of blood products. J Nucl Med Tech 21: 33–37
5. Zabel P, Robichaud N, Hiltz A 1982 Facilities and equipment for aseptic and safe handling of blood products. J Nucl Med Tech 10: 236–241
6. Spinnelli F, Milella M, Sara R 1990 The usefulness of the 1-hour technetium-99m-HMPAO leukocyte scan in the early diagnosis of acute abdominal sepsis. J Nucl Med 31: 1743
7. Hung J C, Corlija M, Volkert W A, Holmes R A 1988 Kinetic analysis of technetium-99m d,1-HMPAO decomposition in aqueous media. J Nucl Med 29: 1568–1576
8. Bayne V J, Forster A M, Tyrrell D A 1989 Use of sodium iodide to overcome the eluate age restriction for Ceretec reconstitution. Nucl Med Commun 10: 29–33
9. Millar A M 1992 A routine method for using sodium iodide to stabilise sodium pertechnetate[^{99m}Tc] dispensed for the preparation of ^{99m}Tc-exametazime. Nucl Med Commun 13: 306–311
10. Weisner P S, Bower G R, Dollimore L A, Forster A M, Higley B, Storey A E 1993 A method for stabilising technetium-99m exametazime prepared from a commercial kit. Eur J Nucl Med 20: 661–666
11. Cherico V V, Frater S I 1988 Pharmacologic interactions in interventional nuclear medicine. J Nucl Med Tech 16: 39–41
12. Freeman L M, Blaufox D M (eds) 1991 Interventions in nuclear medicine. Semin Nucl Med 21
13. Pounds B K, Moore W H, Ladwig E J, Blust J S, Viguet M G, Blust M J, Dhekne R D 1990 Dipyridamole thallium imaging. J Nucl Med Tech 18: 165–174
14. Rockett J F, Magill L H, Loveless V S, Murray G L 1990 Intravenous dipyridamole thallium-201 SPECT imaging methodology, applications and interpretations. Clin Nucl Med 15: 712–725
15. La Bonte C, Lette J, Cerino M, Gagnon A, Waters D 1991 Dipyridamole – thallium imaging: minimum dose requirements. Canada J Cardiol 7: 295–297
16. De Puey G E, Ronzanski A 1991 Pharmacological and other nonexercise alternatives to exercise testing to evaluate myocardial perfusion and left ventricular function with radionuclides. Semin Nucl Med 21: 92–101
17. Smits P, Aengevaeren W R, Corstens F H, Thien T 1989 Caffeine reduces dipyridamole-induced myocardial ischemia. J Nucl Med 30: 1723–1726
18. Heel R C, Brogden R N, Speight T M, Avery G S 1980 Captopril. A preliminary review of its pharmacological properties and therapeutic efficiency. Drugs 20: 409–452
19. Harris C, Smith G H 1981 Captopril (Capoten, E R Squibb and Sons). Drug Intelligence Clin Pharm 15: 932–939
20. Venkata C, Ram S 1982 Captopril. Arch Intern Med 142: 914–916
21. Keeling D H 1988 Adverse reactions to radiopharmaceuticals and their reporting. Aust NZ Nucl Med 3/19: 12
22. Keeling D H, Sampson C B 1984 Adverse reactions to radiopharmaceuticals. United Kingdom 1977–1983. Br J Radiol 57: 1091–1096
23. Cordova A M, Hladik W B, Rhodes B A 1984 Validation and characterisation of adverse reactions to radiopharmaceuticals. Noninvasive Medical Imaging 1: 17–24
24. Chatterton B E, Burrow D D 1979 Tetanic reaction to the intrathecal administration of ^{169}Yb-DTPA as a CSF transport marker associated with spontaneous hypoliquorrhoea. Aust NZ J Med 9: 630
25. Martin E D, May F, Coulthard K, Doecke C, Maloney T, Sansom L 1984 SPHA policy guidelines for the practice of clinical pharmacy. Aust J Hosp Pharm 14: 7–8

114. Radiation protection and dosimetry in clinical practice

John Cormack   Jocelyn E. C. Towson   Margaret A. Flower

INTRODUCTION AND TERMINOLOGY

The topic of radiation biology and protection in nuclear medicine ranges from the biological mechanisms of radiation damage and the mathematical computation of risk to the more mundane and practical details of monitoring, legislation and simple protection measures. This chapter addresses common queries relating to clinical practice, including internal dosimetry and the conceptual basis of radiation safety.

● Why are several different terms used for 'radiation dose'?

▲ Many quantities and units have been developed over the years by the International Commission on Radiological Protection (ICRP), the International Commission on Radiation Units and Measurements (ICRU) and similar bodies. Some of these are rather specialized, and are only likely to be used by persons with a specific interest in radiation protection. The following quantities are in 'everyday' use for distinct purposes in a medical imaging environment.

Activity (A)

The activity of a radioactive substance is measured in terms of the rate at which the nuclei of its radioactive atoms disintegrate. The unit of activity is the becquerel (Bq), which is the quantity of radioactive material in which one atom is transformed per second.

Radiation exposure

Radiation exposure is a measure of the intensity of the radiation field to which an individual or an object is exposed. For X-rays and gamma-rays, exposure is precisely defined[1] in terms of the amount of ionization produced in air by the radiation source. It is measured in units of coulombs per kilogram (C/kg) of air at NTP, and is directly related to the radiation fluence (X-ray or gamma-ray photons per unit area) and the radiation energy fluence (X-ray or gamma-ray energy incident on a unit area).

Air kerma

Air kerma is used as an alternative to radiation exposure. Kerma is an acronym for *k*inetic *e*nergy *r*eleased per unit *ma*ss. One unit of air kerma represents a transfer of 1 joule per kilogram from the radiation beam to the air. The air kerma rate at a fixed distance, *r*, from a 'point' radioactive source of known activity, *A*, is constant and given by

$$\text{Air kerma rate} = \frac{\Gamma_\delta A}{r^2} \tag{1}$$

This is the well-known **inverse square law**, which states that the air kerma or exposure rate is proportional to the activity of the source, and inversely proportional to the square of the distance from the (point) source. Values of the air kerma rate constant, Γ_δ (where the subscript indicates that only energy released by photons of energy greater than δ keV is considered), are given in Table 114.1 for radionuclides commonly used in nuclear medicine.[2]

Table 114.1 Air kerma rate and equivalent dose rate at 1 m from a 1 GBq point source of some of the radionuclides commonly used in nuclear medicine (Extracted from data compiled by Wasserman & Gruenewald[2])

Nuclide	Air kerma rate constant, Γ_{20} (m^2 μGy/GBq h)	Equivalent dose rate constant in soft tissue (m^2 μSv/GBq h)
^{11}C, ^{13}N, ^{15}O	140	154
^{18}F	135	149
^{57}Co	13.7	15.1
^{67}Ga	18.9	20.8
^{99m}Tc	14.2	15.6
^{111}In	76.5	84.2
^{123}I	36.1	39.7
^{125}I	33.3	36.6
^{131}I	51.0	56.1
^{201}Tl	10.6	11.7

Absorbed dose (D)

For all types of radiation, absorbed dose is a measure of the amount of energy from the radiation field which is deposited in unit mass of an absorbing material. The SI unit of absorbed dose is the joule per kilogram, and is called the gray (Gy). Most doses encountered in diagnostic imaging are of the order of milligrays (mGy) or micrograys (μGy). If the attenuation characteristics of the absorbing material are known, absorbed dose can be calculated from radiation exposure, and vice versa.

Equivalent dose (H)

Equivalent dose is a quantity which takes into account the relative biological damage produced in tissue by different types of radiation. Even when the energy deposition is equal at a macroscopic level (that is, the absorbed dose is the same), different types and energies of radiation will produce different amounts of biological damage. The actual damage produced per gray will depend on the **linear energy transfer** (LET) of the radiation, or density of ionization produced at a microscopic level by each radiation particle as it traverses through tissue.

The equivalent dose, *H*, is obtained by multiplying the absorbed dose, *D*, by a **radiation weighting factor** W_R, which takes account of the **relative biological effectiveness** (RBE) of each type of radiation. A radiation weighting factor of 1 is assigned to low-LET radiation, including X-rays and gamma-rays of all energies. Radiation weighting factors for other radiations are based on their observed RBE values (Table 114.2). The unit of equivalent dose is the joule per kilogram and is called the sievert (Sv).

For the ionizing radiations used in medical imaging, W_R is equal to 1 so that the equivalent dose in sieverts is numerically equal to the absorbed dose in grays. Most equivalent doses encountered in diagnostic imaging procedures will be in the millisievert (mSv) or microsievert (μSv) range. For radiation protection purposes, the equivalent dose rate in soft tissue in μSv/h for external exposure from a point source can be estimated from the data in Table 114.1, at a given distance and the inverse square law.

Table 114.2 Radiation weighting factors for different types and energies of radiation used in the calculation of equivalent dose[3]

Radiation type and energy range	Radiation weighting factor (W_R)
X-rays and gamma-rays, all energies	1
Electrons and muons, all energies	1
Neutrons	
< 10 ke V	5
10–100 keV	10
> 100 keV to 2 Mev	20
>2–20 MeV	10
>20 MeV	5
Protons, other than recoil protons, > 2 MeV	5
Alpha-particles, fission fragments, heavy nuclei	20

Effective dose (E)

The ICRP has developed this risk-related parameter to describe the overall effect of non-homogeneous dose distributions, taking into account the relative radiosensitivity of each organ and tissue.[3] The effective dose, *E*, is obtained by calculating a weighted average of the equivalent doses received by each organ or tissue in the body which has been irradiated:

$$E = \sum_T W_T H_T \quad (2)$$

where W_T is the **tissue weighting factor** for organ *T*, H_T is the equivalent dose received by organ or tissue *T* and

$$\sum_T W_T = 1 \quad (3)$$

Organs or tissues which are at higher risk from radiation will have higher weighting factors (Table 114.3). Effective dose is also expressed in sieverts.

Effective dose is similar, in terms of overall risk, to a uniform whole-body exposure in which each organ receives an equivalent dose equal to the effective dose. It is used extensively in radiation protection, and is also useful for categorizing diagnostic imaging procedures.[4–7] Because of the averaging procedures involved, however, some caution needs to be exercised in applying effective dose to individual patients or workers, where it may only be interpreted as an approximate indicator of risk.[8–10]

Factors for converting units between the SI and non-SI systems are given in Table 114.4.

Table 114.3 Tissue and organ weighting factors used in the calculation of effective dose[3]

Organ or tissue	Tissue weighting factor (W_T)
Gonads*	0.2
Red bone marrow	0.12
Colon	0.12
Lung	0.12
Stomach	0.12
Bladder	0.05
Breast	0.05
Liver	0.05
Oesophagus	0.05
Thyroid	0.05
Skin	0.01
Bone surface	0.01
Remainder	0.05
Total	1.0

*Includes severe hereditary disorders expressed over all generations.

Table 114.4 Conversions between various units used in radiation protection

Physical quantity	SI unit	Non-SI unit	Relationship
Activity	becquerel	curie (Ci)	1 Bq=2.7×10^{-11} Ci 1 Ci=3.7×10^{10} Bq
Exposure	coulomb/kg	roentgen (R)	1 R=2.58×10^{-4}C/kg 1 C/kg = 3.88×10^{3}R
Absorbed dose	gray (1 J/kg)	rad	1 Gy=100 rad 1 rad=10 mGy
Equivalent dose	sievert	rem	1 Sv=100 rem 1 rem=10 mSv

BIOLOGICAL EFFECTS OF EXPOSURE TO LOW-LEVEL IONIZING RADIATION

The detrimental effects of low-level radiation on human health have been extensively studied, and are summarized by Smith.[11] Epidemiological data from atom bomb populations (Japanese and Marshall Islanders), medical exposure (diagnosis and therapy) and occupational exposure are the subject of ongoing review.[3,12–15] For additional information there are several excellent texts at various levels.[16–19]

At medium to high dose levels, **deterministic** effects occur. These are characterized by a threshold dose below which the effect is not seen, a short latent period and a severity that depends on the dose. At low levels of radiation exposure, radiation damage is **stochastic**, or statistical in nature: it is possible to predict the proportion of a given population of exposed persons who will be affected, but impossible to predict precisely which particular individuals will succumb. There is no demonstrable threshold dose, and the damage presents as a small increment in normal or spontaneous incidence, expressed after a long latent period.

Somatic damage refers to effects in the tissues of the irradiated individual, while **genetic damage** refers to harm affecting future generations.

● Which deterministic effects are relevant to clinical nuclear medicine?

▲ Deterministic effects occur when there has been a loss of tissue function, usually as a result of cell death or loss of mitotic potential. The number of cells affected increases rapidly with dose, impaired tissue function becoming evident above a threshold dose which is tissue specific. Diagnostic nuclear medicine procedures are below dose thresholds for deterministic effects, whereas dose thresholds are exploited in radionuclide therapy, when ideally they are exceeded for the target tissue alone. Dose thresholds are influenced by dose rate, lower dose rates allowing time for cellular repopulation and repair mechanisms to act. Dose delivery is protracted in radionuclide therapy because of radiopharmaceutical biokinetics and radionuclide decay, and this helps to reduce the likelihood and severity of concomitant tissue damage. In radiotherapy, the same effect is achieved by fractionation of the exposure to minimize unwanted side-effects.

Threshold doses for most tissues range upwards from a few grays delivered as a single dose, and 0.5 Gy/year from protracted exposure (Table 114.5). The bone marrow, testis[20] and lens of the eye[21] are the most sensitive tissues for deterministic effects. Although the skin is not particularly radiosensitive, it is of interest in nuclear medicine because of the possibility of accidental high exposure from localized skin contamination. The threshold for transient ulceration from 'hot particle' exposure is estimated as about 1 Gy, at a depth of 100–150 mm and averaged over 1 cm^2.[22]

● What are the stochastic effects of radiation?

▲ Stochastic effects occur when the cell is modified by damage to its DNA but remains viable, the harm eventually being expressed through cell proliferation. Cancer, after a latency period of many years (2–10 years for leukaemia, 10–40 years for solid tumours), and severe hereditary disorders are the two stochastic effects of concern; any lifespan shortening at low doses is attributable to cancer. The risk of cancer, more so than severe hereditary disorders, is at the core of the radiation protection system for staff and patients.

The risk of radiogenic cancer is tissue dependent, tissues with high cell turnover being more susceptible, and also depends on age and sex. Its expression may be related to the spontaneous incidence of cancer in the population. In most instances, the risk will be expressed as a lifetime morbidity or mortality risk, not to be confused with the per annum risk often quoted for morbidity and mortality from other causes. The risk coefficient may be averaged over age and sex for the population in question, or it may be partitioned into different age and sex groups for more accurate estimation of the risk to an individual.

Genetic risk can be looked at in two ways; in terms of its effect on the descendants of the irradiated individual, or in

Table 114.5 Threshold doses for deterministic effects in the more radiosensitive tissues and organs[3]

Tissue and effect	Equivalent dose, brief exposure (Sv)	Equivalent dose rate, protracted exposure (Sv/year)
Testes		
Temporary sterility	0.15	0.4
Permanent sterility	>3.5	2.0
Ovaries		
Sterility	>2.5	>0.2
Lens of eye		
Detectable opacities	>0.5	>0.1
Visual impairment (cataract)	>2.0	>0.15
Bone marrow		
Haematopoiesis fall	>0.5	>0.4

terms of its effect on the community as a whole, when the average risk to the total gene pool is the relevant factor. In order for a radiation dose to have a genetic effect (i.e. be genetically significant), the dose must be to the gonads (germ cells) of a person or persons of reproductive capacity. For an exposed population, the genetically significant dose will depend on the average gonad dose of the population, the fraction of the population who are of child-bearing age and the average number of offspring produced. For an exposed individual, the genetically significant dose will be zero if the gonads receive no radiation dose or if the person exposed is unable to have children.

● What evidence is there that low-level radiation can cause cancer?

▲ It is not possible to determine directly the incidence rate of cancer and severe hereditary disorders at the very low doses at which these stochastic effects are presumed to occur. Carcinogenic and mutagenic changes produced by radiation are indistinguishable from those occurring spontaneously, and experimental data are not available in man. Current risk estimates for humans are mostly obtained from data on the Hiroshima and Nagasaki atomic bomb victims, although data from persons exposed during the Chernobyl disaster will undoubtedly accumulate over time. The data from the Japanese Life Span Study (LSS) are significant at the 95% level only for doses in excess of 200 mSv. Some 90 000 people are included in this study. In the review to 1986, of the 6000 cancers which had occurred, 260 solid tumours and 80 leukaemias were attributed to radiation. The ICRP has updated its risk estimates for radiation induced cancer, allowing for the fact that the Japanese data are incomplete, and extending the risk estimates for general application to other populations.[3]

For the purposes of radiation protection, the dose–response curve for radiation induced cancer is assumed to be linear at low doses, with no threshold. However, the shape of the curve may be better described by a linear–quadratic function, and consequently the risk coefficient or slope at very low doses would be less than the value obtained from observations at high doses. The ICRP has selected a **dose and dose rate effectiveness factor** (DDREF) of 2 which, when applied to the lifetime risk of 10%/Sv obtained from the Japanese data at high doses and dose rate, results in a nominal risk of 5%/Sv for low-dose, low dose rate exposure. For a working population (with no young individuals in the greatest risk brackets), the figure is 4%/Sv.[3] The risk to individual body organs and tissues is given in Table 114.6.[3] For some cancers (e.g. the thyroid) the risk of cancer induction is high, but the mortality rate is relatively low owing to a better survival rate.

A better estimate of the risk to an individual can be calculated from age and sex specific data. Figure 114.1 shows the attributable lifetime risk per sievert for males and females as a function of age at the time of exposure. The risk is highest for the younger age groups and decreases progressively until about the age of 35. There is a slight increase up to the age of 55 as the baseline cancer rates increase, then a progressive fall-off with age because there is less time for expression of the risk. Children aged 15 years and less have a risk that is nearly double the average; persons of age 75 or more have a risk which is less than half the average. Females are slightly more at risk than males, but the difference is only of the order of 6%. On these figures, an effective dose of 5 mSv, typical of nuclear medicine procedures, would result in an additional fatal cancer risk of 1 in 4000 on average, 1 in 2000 in those less than 15 years old and 1 in 8000 in those more than 70 years old.

Table 114.6 Lifetime risk of fatal cancer in general population from low-dose exposure[3]

	Probability of fatal cancer (10^{-4}/Sv), lethality fraction in parenthesis*				
Bladder	30	(0.50)	Oesophagus	30	(0.95)
Bone marrow	50	(0.99)	Ovary	10	(0.70)
Bone surface	5	(0.70)	Skin	2	(0.002)
Breast	20	(0.50)	Stomach	110	(0.90)
Colon	85	(0.55)	Thyroid†	8	(0.10)
Liver	15	(0.95)	Remainder	50	
Lung	85	(0.95)	**Total**	**500**	

*The lethality fraction, taken from US data of Mettler & Sinclair in ICRP60,[3] allows calculation of total radiogenic cancer incidence.
†The fatal cancer risk estimate is 0.075×10^{-2}/Gy at high doses, used here without DDREF because of the presumed linear response of the thyroid to external radiation.

● Is it possible to estimate the probability that a particular cancer was caused by a previous radiation exposure?

▲ For exposures of staff and patients involved in diag-

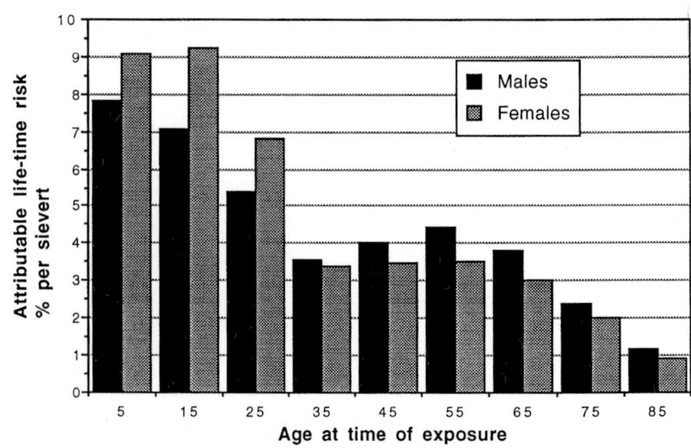

Fig. 114.1 Attributable lifetime risk of fatal cancer as a function of age and sex at time of exposure. Adapted from data in BEIR V,[14] normalizing to an age and sex-averaged risk of 5%/Sv.

nostic imaging, the a priori probability of cancer will be very small, and is calculated in order to allow these persons to comprehend the magnitude of their risk and make subjective risk–benefit decisions. In the event of an exposed person being diagnosed with a cancer, however, the perspective changes, and the question may arise as to whether this cancer is radiation induced or spontaneous. It is possible to estimate the a posteriori probability that radiation caused a particular cancer, by a method known as **probability of causation** (PC).[23,24] Calculated values of PC will be dependent on the type of cancer, the sex of the person and age at the time of diagnosis and the time elapsed since the radiation exposure. Tables have been compiled[25] which allow PC values for various cancers to be readily determined. Even if the a priori risks are quite small, the probability of causation (PC) can be quite large if the baseline (or spontaneous) cancer incidence rates are low.

It should be noted that although probabilistic estimates of causation such as these are useful, they will not necessarily be accepted as prima facie evidence in a court of law. The relevance of probability of causation analysis to intentional radiation exposure in medicine is vigorously contested.[26–28]

● What are the hereditary risks from radiation?

▲ Studies in plants and animals have shown that radiation can cause both point mutations and chromosome aberrations leading to hereditary disorders. However, no increase in genetic disorders has been observed in any studies of humans exposed to radiation, including the offspring of the Japanese survivors (who received an average gonadal dose of 0.5 Sv).[29]

Only the risk of **severe hereditary disorders** is considered for the purposes of radiation protection. The ICRP used animal data and the Japanese data as a lower bound when estimating the risk of mutations and chromosome aberrations from low-dose, low dose rate and low-LET radiation. A value of 1%/Sv was selected for the risk of severe hereditary disorders in all successive generations.[3] This risk is apportioned equally between mutations and chromosome aberrations, on the one hand, and multifactorial hereditary disorders – those caused by interactions of genetic and environmental factors, often expressed in middle age – on the other. For a working population the risk is 0.6%/Sv (because of the lower proportion of persons of reproductive capacity). Similarly, the risk for subgroups of reproductive age can be estimated from the proportion of the population in this category. For individuals of reproductive capacity, the actual hereditary risk will depend on the genetically significant dose to that individual. This dose may be two or more times the genetically significant dose to the population, resulting in a proportionally higher hereditary risk.

● What are 'nominal probability coefficients'?

▲ The concept of 'detriment' is used by the ICRP to cover both the probability of occurrence and the severity of stochastic radiation effects. Detriment has four components: the risk of fatal cancer, a weighted risk of non-fatal cancer, a weighted risk of severe hereditary disorders and a weighting for the years of life lost from fatal cancer and severe hereditary disorders. The resulting nominal probability coefficients are shown in Table 114.7. The tissue weighting factors used in the calculation of effective dose (see Table 114.3) are based on the distribution of detriment among the various tissues and organs of the body.

● What are the risks of radiation to the developing embryo/fetus?

▲ The increased radiosensitivity of the embryo and fetus is widely recognized, and gives cause for caution on the part of the nuclear medicine physician and anxiety on the part of the patient. A knowledge of the potential risks of irradiation during pregnancy and an estimation of the absorbed dose to the embryo/fetus in individual circumstances are essential for informed decision making and counselling of affected patients.

The effects of radiation during pregnancy are very dependent on the stage of gestation and the level of exposure[3,11,30] and are shown in Table 114.8. During the preimplantation (0–10 days post conception) and implantation (10–14 days) stages, radiation may cause death of the zygote or embryo. This appears to be an 'all or none' effect, and a surviving embryo will go on to develop normally. Major organogenesis in the embryo occurs during the gestation period from 15 to 50 days, when radiation can cause abnormalities such as malformation, cataracts and growth retardation. For the period from 8 to 15 weeks, and to a lesser extent from 16 to 25 weeks, radiation may cause severe mental retardation (SMR). All of these effects appear to be deterministic, requiring minimum threshold doses ranging upwards from about 100 mSv. There is debate on whether there is in fact a threshold for SMR,[31] and so for protection purposes it may be prudent to assume there is none.

Stochastic effects from low-level exposure of the embryo/fetus are important, just as they are for adults.

Table 114.7 Nominal probability coefficients for radiation detriment at low doses[3]

	Detriment (%/Sv)			
Exposed population	Fatal cancer	Non-fatal cancer	Severe hereditary effects	Total
Adult workers	4.0	0.8	0.8	5.6
Whole population	5.0	1.0	1.3	7.3

Table 114.8 Radiation risks to the embryo or fetus

Effect	Stage of gestation (weeks post conception)	Risk (%/Sv)	Threshold (mSv)
Lethality*	1–3 inclusive	Minimal	
Congenital malformations, growth retardation*	4–7 inclusive	50	>100
Severe mental retardation†	8–15 inclusive	40	–
Reduced IQ†	8–15 inclusive	30 pts/Sv	–
Severe mental retardation†	16–25 inclusive	10	>200
Cancer	4 until term		
Childhood (<15 yrs), all		6	–
fatal‡		3	–
Lifetime*		12	–
Hereditable disease‡	4 until term	2.4	

*ICRP 60.[3]
†Schull.[31]
‡Cox & MGibbon.[30]

There is evidence of an increased risk of cancer (including leukaemia) subsequent to prenatal exposure,[32,33] and excess cancers may continue to be observed beyond childhood.[34] The risk of radiogenic cancer in an exposed embryo or fetus, as in children, is greater than in an adult, and the increase may be relatively greater for exposure during the first trimester of pregnancy.[35,36] Another possible stochastic effect is intellectual impairment, with a downward shift in IQ estimated at 30 points/Sv.[3] The magnitude of this effect is consistent with the postulated threshold for SMR. For exposure in the range of 1–5 mSv, typical of diagnostic nuclear medicine studies, any such deficit would be very subtle indeed.

RADIATION PROTECTION GUIDELINES

● How are radiation protection guidelines determined?

▲ The International Commission on Radiological Protection (ICRP) is an international body of radiation experts which examines and reports on radiation protection issues. Over the years since its inception in 1928, the ICRP has developed a system of radiation protection which has gained widespread acceptance. Its various recommendations and guidelines form the basis of legislation in many countries.

The general philosophy of the ICRP's system of protection can be summarized under two broad categories:

1. **Practices,** i.e. current and proposed uses of radiation. These should be subject to three main criteria.
   - Justification: The net benefit to the exposed individual or society should at least offset the radiation detriment.
   - Optimization: The size of any exposure and the number of people exposed should be kept as low as reasonably achievable, economic and social factors being taken into account (the ALARA principle).
   - Limitation: The exposure of individuals, excluding that from medical practices, should be subject to dose limits. The risk (i.e. likelihood and detriment) of potential exposures should also be controlled.
2. **Interventions,** i.e. measures to reduce exposure from existing sources of radiation. These should be subject to similar criteria.
   - Justification: The potential benefit of the proposed intervention must warrant any possible harmful effects and economic costs.
   - Optimization: The proposed intervention should be optimized in terms of form, scale and duration.

The modification of dwellings to reduce indoor radon concentration and the pharmacological blocking of unwanted thyroid uptake of radioiodine are examples which lend themselves to intervention analysis.

● What limits are there on radiation exposure of radiation workers and others?

▲ The ICRP has recommended dose limits[3] (see Table 114.9) for exposure of radiation workers and members of the public.

Limits for **radiation workers** are intended to prevent the occurrence of deterministic effects – particularly to the skin and lens of the eye – and to limit the occurrence of stochastic effects, such as cancer and hereditary disorders, to levels at which the risk is regarded as acceptable. It is not intended that the occupational dose limits should be seen as an acceptable target, but rather as levels which are only just tolerable. A useful ICRP concept is the **dose constraint**; in this context the constraint serves as a guide as to what should be readily achievable in a well-managed operation. For nuclear medicine and radiology practice, on occupational dose constraint of 5 mSv/year would be reasonable.

The ICRP has also recommended the following supplementary dose limit for **pregnant workers,**[3] which is

Table 114.9 Recommended dose limits for exposure of radiation workers and members of the public[3]

	Dose limit (mSv/year)	
Application	Occupational	Public
Effective dose	20, averaged over 5 years and not > 50 mSv/year	1, averaged over 5 years
Equivalent dose		
Lens of eye	150	15
Hands, feet	500	
Skin (averaged over 1 cm^2)	500	50

intended to keep the dose to the fetus below 1 mSv, similar to the limit for a member of the public:

- The equivalent dose to the surface of the maternal abdomen should not exceed 2 mSv.
- The maternal intake of radionuclides should not exceed about 1/20 of the limit allowed for radiation workers.
- The mother's employment should not carry a significant probability of high accidental exposures and intakes.

Policy on the last of these points, if not defined by the regulatory agency, should be determined locally, preferably in consultation with a radiation safety officer.[37] For example, pregnant staff might not be required to care for a patient who has received a large dose of activity for radionuclide therapy, or perform lung ventilation studies, or be responsible for the large-scale preparation of radiopharmaceuticals.[38] Nonetheless, a pregnant staff member should not hesitate to provide assistance in the unlikely event of a radioactive patient requiring prompt medical attention for a life-threatening emergency. The risk to the fetus from a brief exposure in these circumstances is extremely small and is outweighed by the obvious potential benefit. The ICRP emphasizes that a properly implemented system of radiation protection, including source constraints, should usually be adequate for the protection of female staff who may not yet know they are pregnant – or for that matter for male staff concerned about germ cell exposure in the period before they conceive children – without need for specific restrictions on that person's employment.

The limit of 1 mSv/year for **members of the public** is even more stringent. It was chosen to ensure a low detriment (even for a continuous exposure of 5 mSv/year the mortality is very small) and having regard to natural background levels. The dose limit refers to practices which will increase exposure over the natural background level, not to exposures from sources such as radon in dwellings where protection can only be achieved by intervention. The public dose limit affects nuclear medicine practice in a number of ways, for example in determining how long a radionuclide therapy patient might need to be accommodated in an isolation ward, or how much distance and shielding is needed between radionuclide therapy beds and adjacent areas, or when suggesting how long after a radionuclide therapy dose a patient should wait before attempting to become pregnant in order to limit the conceptus dose to 1 mSv.[5] The ICRP has made a useful exclusion in its classification of members of the public by regarding the exposure of **friends or relatives assisting in the patient's treatment** as 'medical', and therefore not subject to the dose limits. The onus for controlling the exposure to such individuals clearly rests with the treating physician.

● How can radiation doses be placed in perspective for staff, research volunteers and patients?

▲ To those who are unfamiliar with radiation units, a radiation dose quoted in isolation is virtually meaningless. With no comprehension as to the size of the unit, and no frame of reference, it is difficult to judge whether the dose, and its associated hazard, is large, intermediate or small. The nuclear medicine practitioner should be able to communicate effectively with patients on the issue of radiation risk.[39] The following data and information from Clarke[40] and other sources may be useful in placing a radiation dose in perspective:

Doses in medical imaging

No limits or constraints are set for doses for diagnostic or therapeutic procedures, apart from general compliance with the ALARA principle and a requirement that risk–benefit factors be considered.

The effective dose from diagnostic nuclear medicine procedures is typically in the range 1–10 mSv,[41,42] with one survey reporting an average effective dose of 3.3 mSv. The dose from diagnostic radiology procedures is generally a little lower, with the exception of fluoroscopic procedures. Figure 114.2 illustrates the range of effective doses encountered in nuclear medicine and diagnostic X-ray procedures, along with some other miscellaneous landmark values.

Comparison with natural background sources of radiation

A large proportion of the average annual effective dose received by the population results from environmental radiation. Typically, environmental radiation amounts to around 2–3 mSv/year, or about 86% of the global per capita radiation dose. Environmental radiation will vary widely from location to location, depending on altitude and the abundance of natural radioactive ores in rocks and soil.[12,40,43] Each member of the world population is

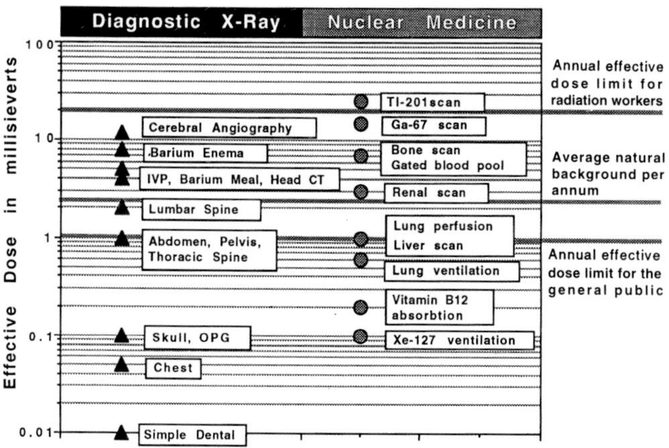

Fig. 114.2 Simplified comparison of effective dose ranges in diagnostic nuclear medicine and radiology procedures.

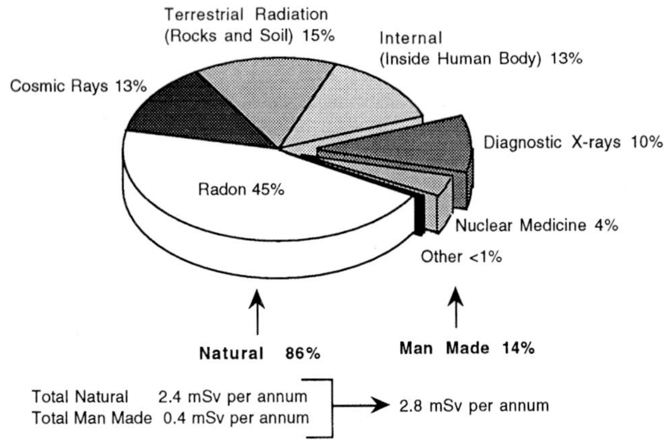

Fig. 114.3 Annual effective dose received by an average member of the world population.

exposed, on average, to 2.4 mSv of unavoidable ionizing radiation every year.

An additional 14% (0.4 mSv) of the average annual exposure is man-made, consisting of around 10% from diagnostic X-rays and 4% from nuclear medicine procedures, though again this is highly variable depending on local practice,[41,44] and a small amount from miscellaneous sources. Figure 114.3 shows a breakdown of the effective doses from various sources. The large component arising from radon gas in homes and workplaces has only come to light comparatively recently.[45]

Comparison with other risks

Perhaps the best method of placing a radiation dose in perspective is to convert the dose to an absolute risk which can be compared with some of the other risks normally encountered in life. The average lifetime risk from a known low-level radiation exposure can be approximated by multiplying the effective dose in mSv by the fatal cancer risk coefficient value of 5×10^{-5}. An alternative method of expressing the absolute risk is to use **loss of life expectancy** (LLE). This gives a little more information than a straight risk figure, in that it takes into account the temporal distribution of the risk. A risk which is expressed early in life, for example, will result in a much bigger LLE than the same risk expressed over the last decades of life. The average loss of life expectancy for a population exposed to a single dose of radiation ranges from about 1 year/Sv at high doses and dose rates, down to about 0.5 year/Sv at the lower doses normally encountered in diagnostic medical procedures. LLE has a drawback for risk comparisons, in that it is derived from the average of a large number of persons whose life expectancy is unaffected by the exposure and a much smaller number who lose a significant amount of time – typically around 15 years – as a result of a radiation-induced cancer.

Once the absolute risk or LLE from a given radiation exposure has been calculated, it can be compared with values from other sources,[46–49] many of which are far greater (Table 114.10).

Table 114.10 Comparison of various risks in terms of loss of life expectancy (LLE) (adapted from data of Cohen[47])

Risk	LLE (lost life expectancy, in days)
Cigarette smoking (male) – one or more packs per day	2441
Poor social connections	1644
Heart disease	1607
Cancer (all types)	1247
15% overweight	777
Alcohol abuse	365
Motor vehicle accident	205
Air travel (scheduled airline, 400 000 km over 40 years)	64
Passive smoking	50
Medical radiation (2 mSv/year over working life)	17
Asthma	11.3
Medical radiation (single exposure of 10 mSv)	2
Lightning strike	1.1
Earthquakes and volcanoes	0.13
Airbag in car	−50
Coronary pacemaker	−180

Comparison with other occupations

For a radiation worker in a nuclear medicine department, the annual effective dose received is generally of the order of 2 mSv. If this dose is received every year of a person's working life (assumed to be from age 18 to age 65), the average annual risk is 0.8 in 10 000 which is equivalent to a total lifetime risk of 3.7 in 1000 and an LLE of 17 days.[3] Unlike many other occupational hazards, the risk from continuous occupational radiation exposure peaks in the seventh, eighth and ninth decades of life. This risk compares favourably with many other occupations (see Table 114.11). It is interesting to note that the most hazardous occupation is *no* occupation (that is, unemployment).

Table 114.11 Comparison of various occupations in terms of loss of life expectancy (LLE) (adapted from data by Cohen[47])

Occupation	LLE (lost life expectancy, in days)
Unemployment	500
Agirculture	320
Construction	227
Mines, quarries	167
Transportation, utility	160
All	60
Government	60
Medical radiation worker (5 mSv/year over working life)	42
Manufacturing	40
Trade	27
Services	27
Medical radiation worker (2 mSv/year over working life)	17

Table 114.12 Natural prevalence/incidence of risks relevant to radiation protection

Risk	Natural prevalence/incidence (%)
Cancer mortality	
Lifetime*	<25
Childhood < 15 years†	0.077
Genetic disorders*	8
Autosomal dominant and X linked	1.0
Autosomal recessive	0.25
Chromosomal	0.38
Multifactorial	6.5
Pregnancy	
Spontaneous abortion	10–20
Congenital abnormalities*	6
Mental retardation‡	3

*ICRP 60.[3]
†Cox & McGibbon.[30]
‡Schull.[31]

Comparison with natural disease prevalence

Estimates of the local prevalence of cancer, hereditary disease and problems related to pregnancy (Table 114.12) can provide a background against which radiogenic incidence can be evaluated. The fact that the natural prevalence is generally much higher than the radiation risk of diagnostic procedures in clinical practice does not detract from the need to adhere to the ALARA philosophy.

INTERNAL DOSIMETRY

● How do you find out how much radiation dose is received from radionuclides in the body?

▲ Catalogues of absorbed doses to patients from radiopharmaceuticals have been published by the ICRP,[6] and these have been kept up to date as new radiopharmaceuticals are introduced.[7] These doses are listed for a range of ages and for different routes of administration. Absorbed doses are also quoted on package inserts by radiopharmaceutical companies.

The method of calculating absorbed dose delivered internally has been developed over many years by the **Medical Internal Radiation Dose** (MIRD) committee of the American Society of Nuclear Medicine.[50] The aim of this committee was to develop a dosimetry system (now called the MIRD schema) for diagnostic nuclear medicine. However, the methods have also been applied in radionuclide therapy and in internal contamination. A program called MIRDOSE for calculating absorbed doses is available from Oak Ridge National Laboratory. This is particularly useful when dealing with new radiopharmaceuticals or when special biokinetic models need to be considered (for example with haemodialysis patients).

● How is the internal radiation dose calculated using the MIRD schema?

▲ In the MIRD schema the body is considered as a combination of **source organs** (i.e. those with significant uptake of the radiopharmaceutical) and of **target organs** (i.e. those being irradiated by source organs), as shown in Figure 114.4. For each pair of source and target organs, the following equation is used to calculate the absorbed dose, $D_{t \leftarrow s}$ (in Gy), to a target organ from activity in a source organ:

$$D_{t \leftarrow s} = \tilde{A}_s S_{t \leftarrow s} \quad (4)$$

where $\tilde{A}_s$ is the cumulated activity in the source (in Bq/s) and $S_{t \leftarrow s}$ is the mean dose to the target per unit cumulated activity in the source (in Gy/Bq/s).

The **cumulated activity**, $\tilde{A}_s$, is the total number of radioactive disintegrations which occur in the source organ, and depends on: the activity administered; the uptake of, retention by, and excretion from the organ; and the physical decay of the radionuclide.

S-factors have been tabulated for a variety of radionuclides and for different source/target configurations in both standard man[51] and children.[52]

The total dose to a single organ arising from radiation emitted by several source organs is simply the sum of the absorbed doses from all the source organs. Figure 114.5 is a flow chart which summarizes how the MIRD schema is applied in practice.

● How is the cumulated activity, $\tilde{A}_s$, in equation 4 determined?

▲ $\tilde{A}_s$ is equal to the time integral of the activity in the source organ:

$$\tilde{A}_s = \int_0^{\infty} A_s(t)\mathrm{d}t \quad (5)$$

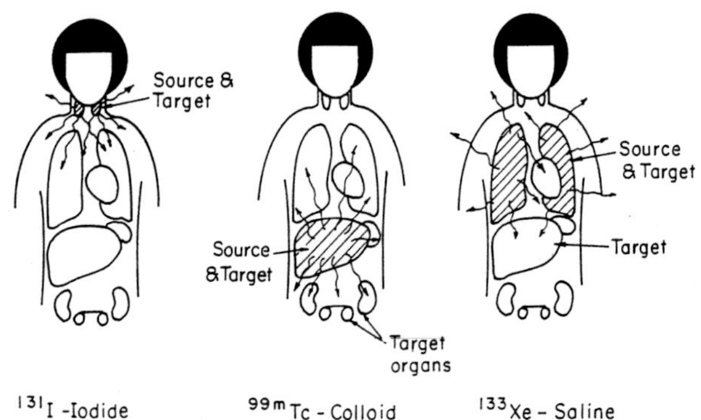

Fig. 114.4 Schematic illustrating the concept of source and target organs. In each of the examples only one source organ is shown, but in practice there may be multiple source organs. (A) Thyroid as source organ. (B) Liver as source organ. (C) Lungs as source organ. (Reproduced with permission from Loevinger et al.[50])

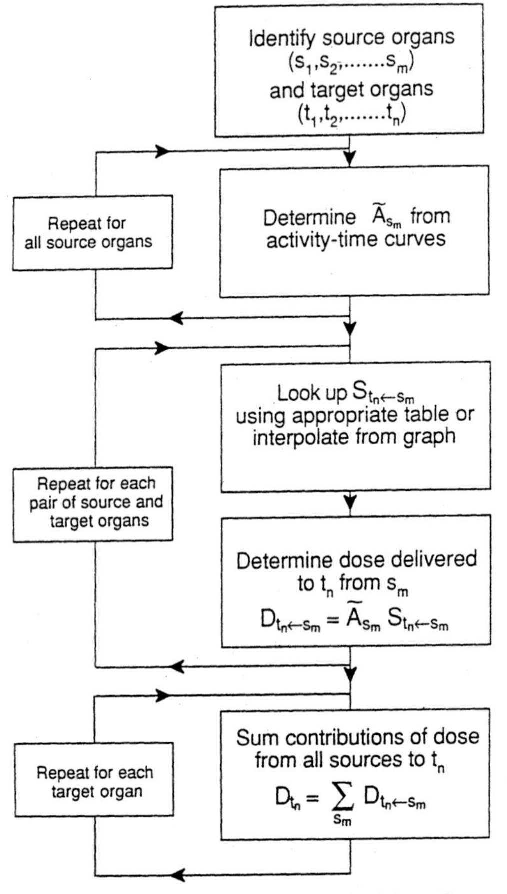

Fig. 114.5 Flow chart illustrating MIRD methodology. See text for definition of terminology.

which is the area under the activity–time curve, $A_s(t)$, for that organ. Some biological data are available[6,7] for the determination of cumulated activities. If the required biological data are unavailable or inapplicable, sequential measurements of the activity, $A_s(t)$, at various times t in each source organ of interest are required to determine $\tilde{A}_s$. Region of interest analysis on opposing planar views using a gamma-camera is a common method used to assess organ uptake (Ch. 108). Counts in the patient images are compared with counts in the images of a phantom which simulates the patient geometry and contains a known amount of the appropriate radionuclide. Corrections are needed for background activity in tissues surrounding the organ of interest and for variations in patient and source thickness. Single photon emission computerized tomography (SPECT) can also be used for the determination of $A_s(t)$ (Ch. 109).

When considering the whole body as the source organ, $\tilde{A}_S$ is determined from sequential measurements with a calibrated whole-body counter. When the radionuclide is not uniformly distributed in the body, the basic MIRD equations need to be modified[53] so that the dose to a target organ is not overestimated. Without the modifications, which require the whole body to be considered as the sum of the individual source organs plus the 'rest of body', the amount of radionuclide in a target organ would be included twice.

In addition to in vivo imaging and counting techniques, pharmacokinetic data can be obtained by sampling body fluids (e.g. blood and urine). These data are representative of 'rest of body' clearance and useful when considering the blood and urine as source organs.[54,55]

Before leaving this question, it is worth introducing the concept of the **residence time,** τ, which is defined as the average time that the administered activity spends in the source organ, and is given by

$$\tau = \frac{\tilde{A}_s}{A_a} \tag{6}$$

where A_a is the administered activity. Residence time is a useful concept as it is often convenient to express the dose to a target organ in terms of dose per unit administered activity ($D_{t \leftarrow s}/A_a$). From equations 4 and 6 it can be seen that

$$\frac{D_{t \leftarrow s}}{A_a} = \tau\, S_{t \leftarrow s} \tag{7}$$

● How are the *S*-values in equations 4 and 7 determined?

▲ The mean dose per unit cumulated activity, $S_{t \leftarrow s}$ (in Gy/Bq s), is defined by

$$S_{t \leftarrow s} = \frac{1}{m_t} \sum_i \Delta_i \Phi_i \tag{8}$$

where m_t is the mass of the target organ (in kg), Δ_i is the **equilibrium absorbed dose constant** for radiation of type i, or the mean energy per nuclear disintegration (in Gy kg/B s) and $ø_i$ is the **absorbed fraction**, defined as the fraction of the radiation of type i emitted from the source and absorbed by the target.

Values of Δ_i and the **specific absorbed fraction** ($\mathit{\Phi}_i = \Phi_i/m_t$), derived from Monte Carlo calculations, can be found from MIRD tables[56,57] for various radionuclides and pairs of source and target organs. For non-penetrating radiation such as beta-rays, the absorbed fraction is 1. For penetrating radiation including gamma-photons, the absorbed fraction may be quite small, particularly for small organs. For example, 95% of the absorbed dose to the thyroid from self-irradiation from ^{131}I activity in the thyroid is due to non-penetrating beta-radiation.

S-factors are strongly dependent on the mass of the target organ. Hence a small error in m_t may result in a large error in $S_{t \leftarrow s}$ and $D_{t \leftarrow s}$. In nuclear medicine procedures involving children, appropriate S-values can be obtained by interpolation from a plot of S-values against m_t using data tabulated for standard children[52] and standard man.[51]

X-ray computerized tomography (CT), magnetic resonance imaging and ultrasound, all with excellent spatial resolution, offer the means of obtaining very precise measurements of the anatomical volume of an organ. However, if the radiopharmaceutical is not uniformly distributed macroscopically within this volume, these alternative imaging modalities would overestimate the mass of tissue within which the radionuclide is concentrated. It is particularly difficult to determine accurately the mass of disseminated tissues, for example in radioimmunotherapy.

Nuclear medicine imaging is the only means of assessing in vivo the functioning volume (and hence mass) of tissue which is the parameter required for dosimetry calculations. The accuracy with which the functioning volume can be determined depends on its size relative to the spatial resolution of the imaging system and on the radionuclide involved. The best approach is to determine the radioactive concentration using a high-resolution SPECT or PET system if available (preferably with resolutions <10 mm and <5 mm respectively), rather than to assess m_t and $A_s(t)$ separately. In general, limitations in spatial resolution (in both planar and tomographic imaging) result in underestimates of tissue dose, unless a correction using the recovery coefficient[58] can be made (Ch. 109).

● What are the limitations of the MIRD method?

▲ Firstly, tabulated doses do not apply to all patients. In the MIRD schema it is assumed that the shape, size and position of the organs are as represented by the standard, 70 kg, hermaphrodite human phantom.[57] The patient's condition may result in enlarged organs which will alter their relative positions. Instead of using tabulated *S*-factors these factors should be reassessed using the appropriate values for the parameters m_t and ϕ_i in equation 8. Diseased organs can result in both increased or decreased uptake of activity and changes in the residence time compared with standard values so these factors should also be considered when assessing the dose to patients. The absorbed doses published by ICRP[6,7] do include tables relating to some abnormal physiology (e.g. abnormal renal function, diffuse liver disease, occlusion of cystic or common bile duct, different levels of thyroid uptake). The MIRD schema assumes that the activity is uniformly distributed in the source organ. Certain pathologies could result in non-uniform distribution of radioisotope in the source organs, which would alter the dose delivered to target organs.

Furthermore, the MIRD schema calculates each dose to the target organ as an average, without permitting the determination of a maximum or minimum dose to each target organ considered. The accuracy with which the absorbed dose can be estimated depends on the accuracy with which the parameters $\tilde{A}_s$ and $S_{t\leftarrow s}$ can be determined in practice. That is, the dose estimates are no more accurate than the biological and physical data used for the calculations. The MIRD schema has severe limitations when the isotope distribution in the source/target organ is non-uniform and particularly if the isotope is an Auger electron emitter. An alternative microdosimetric approach is required in this situation.

Table 114.13 Absorbed doses and effective dose from various radiopharmaceuticals

Radio pharmaceutical	Activity* (MBq)	Absorbed dose† (mGy)						Eff. dose‡ (mSv)
		Red marrow	Breast	Uterus	Thyroid	Ovaries	Testes	
^{51}Cr red cells	4	0.6	0.4	0.3	0.5	0.3	0.3	1.3
^{67}Ga citrate	150	28.5	9.3	11.9	8.4	12.3	8.6	16.5
^{99m}Tc colloid	80 (static)	0.9	0.2	0.2	0.06	0.2	0.05	0.7
	200 (SPECT)	2.2	0.5	0.4	0.2	0.4	0.1	1.8
^{99m}Tc-DMSA	80	0.5	0.1	0.4	0.09	0.3	0.1	0.7
^{99m}Tc-DTPA	300	0.8	0.3	2.4	0.2	1.3	0.8	1.6
^{99m}Tc-HIDA	150	1.1	0.09	2.0	0.02	3.0	0.2	2.3
^{99m}Tc-HMPAO	500 (SPECT)	1.7	1.0	3.3	13.0	3.3	1.2	4.6
^{99m}Tc-HSA	40	0.3	0.2	0.2	0.2	0.2	0.1	0.4
^{99m}Tc-MAA	100	0.4	0.6	0.2	0.2	0.2	0.1	1.1
^{99m}Tc pertechnetate§	500 (static)	2.3	1.3	3.3	1.1	2.4	1.6	6.0
	800 (SPECT)	3.6	2.0	5.3	1.7	3.8	2.6	9.6
^{99m}Tc phosphonate	600	5.8	0.5	3.7	0.6	2.1	1.4	3.5
^{111}In platelets	20	7.2	2.0	1.9	1.6	2.0	0.9	1.0
^{111}In white cells	40	27.6	3.6	4.8	2.4	4.8	1.8	1.9
^{123}I-MIBG §	400	3.7	2.5	4.4	1.7	3.2	2.2	5.6
^{131}I-MIBG §	20	1.3	1.4	1.6	1.0	1.3	1.2	2.8
^{201}Tl chloride	80	14.4	2.2	4.0	20.0	9.6	44.8	18.4

*Maximum usual activity per test, as recommended by ARSAC.[60]
†Data from ICRP.[6,7]
‡Data from Johansson et al.[59]
§With blocking agent.

● What are typical radiation doses for nuclear medicine diagnostic procedures?

▲ A few examples of absorbed doses which are delivered from radiopharmaceuticals in common use are listed in Table 114.13, together with the effective doses.[6,7,59]

RADIATION RISK CONSIDERATIONS FOR PATIENTS, BABIES AND CHILDREN

● What is the absorbed dose to an embryo or fetus following the administration of a radiopharmaceutical to a pregnant woman?

▲ There are several practical difficulties in estimating the radiation dose to an embryo or fetus. One is the lack of knowledge of radiopharmaceutical biokinetics in regard to placental transfer and fetal biodistribution.[61] Some data are available from animal studies, for example the uptake in the fetoplacental unit of ionic gallium and indium bound to transferrin.[62] In general, placental transfer of a substance in the maternal bloodstream may be expected when the molecular weight is less than 600 daltons.[63] Where the radiopharmaceutical is known not to cross the placenta, the fetal dose may be approximated by the dose to the uterus. Where there is placental transfer, the dose to maternal tissues and organs may be taken as representative of the dose to the corresponding fetal organs and tissues.[6]

The calculation of absorbed dose according to MIRD principles requires an estimate of the specific absorbed fraction (S) applicable to the relative geometries of source and target organs. A number of approaches have been used to derive S-factors for the embryo/fetus.[64,65] S-factors for fetal organs at ages of 3, 6 and 9 months, taking account of the displacement of maternal organs, are being determined by the MIRD Committee. Table 114.14 lists the dose to the conceptus (approximated by the dose to the uterus in the first three months of pregnancy) from various radiopharmaceuticals administered to the mother.

Table 114.14 Absorbed dose to conceptus from radiopharmaceuticals administered to mother (data from ICRP,[5] assuming no placental transfer and approximating by dose to uterus)

Radiopharmaceutical	Conceptus dose, 0–3 months (mGy per MBq administered to mother)
^{99m}Tc phosphate, phosphonate	6.1×10^{-3}
^{99m}Tc DTPA	7.9×10^{-3}
^{99m}Tc DMSA	4.6×10^{-3}
^{99m}Tc pertechnetate (unblocked thyroid)	8.1×10^{-3}
^{99m}Tc colloid	1.9×10^{-3}
^{99m}Tc microspheres	2.4×10^{-3}
^{99m}Tc aerosol (fast lung clearance)	5.9×10^{-3}
^{99m}Tc aerosol (slow lung clearance)	1.7×10^{-3}
^{99m}Tc red blood cells	4.7×10^{-3}
^{201}Tl chloride	5.0×10^{-2}
^{111}In white blood cells	1.2×10^{-1}
^{67}Ga citrate	7.9×10^{-2}
^{123}I iodide (35% thyroid uptake)	1.4×10^{-2}
^{131}I iodide (35% thyroid uptake)	5.0×10^{-2}
^{18}F fluorodeoxyglucose	2.0×10^{-2}

● Should nuclear medicine procedures be performed on pregnant patients?

▲ A nuclear medicine study of a pregnant patient may be contemplated on clinical grounds. The risk of the radiation exposure to the fetus should be viewed against the potential benefit of the study and the normal risks of pregnancy and childhood (Table 114.12).[66,67] A decision may be taken not to proceed with the study, but to rely on other clinical investigations which do not use ionizing radiation. Alternatively, the study may be performed if it appears that the additional risks of radiation exposure are outweighed by the potential benefits from the information the study can provide. In this case, steps should be taken to minimize the exposure of the embryo or fetus.[60] For example, it may be possible to defer the study until a later stage of gestation, when the risks are less. The amount of activity used should be reduced to the minimum required to obtain adequate study quality. Any dose to the fetus exceeding 0.5 mSv requires careful justification, and the study should not result in an absorbed dose of more than 1–2 mSv. When the radiopharmaceutical is excreted by the kidneys, the patient should be well hydrated and encouraged to void frequently. This will substantially reduce the exposure from nearby bladder contents.[68,69] Where possible, radiopharmaceutical forms such as pertechnetate or gallium citrate which concentrate in the placenta should be avoided, particularly if they subsequently undergo selective uptake in fetal organs.

Lung scanning for suspected pulmonary embolus provides a good illustration of a risk–benefit assessment.[70,71] It may be possible to limit the dose to the conceptus by performing a perfusion scan only without a ventilation scan, and by administering less than the usual amount of activity. For an activity of 80 MBq of ^{99m}Tc microspheres administered to the mother and taking the radiation dose to the conceptus as 2.4×10^{-3} mSv/MBq, the risk of fatal childhood cancer from the fetal dose of 0.2 mSv would be less than 1 in 100 000, compared with the normal prevalence of approximately 0.08% or 8 in 10 000, and the far more serious risk of pulmonary embolism.

● What precautions should be taken concerning radionuclide therapy and pregnancy?

▲ Radionuclide therapy is *not* indicated in pregnancy and

should be avoided. The radiation dose to the embryo/fetus may result in an increased risk of childhood cancer, and in certain applications may approach threshold levels for deterministic radiation effects such as depression of fetal thyroid function. Many physicians adopt the precaution of performing a pregnancy test immediately prior to the administration of therapy doses to women who could be pregnant. At the initial interview, the patient should be made aware of the need to avoid pregnancy until treatment is completed, preferably until the dose to the conceptus would be less than 1 mSv. For thyroid cancer patients, this might extend until there is no scan evidence of functioning thyroid tissue which might require an ablative dose of ^{131}I.[72] There have been a number of instances in which ^{131}I treatment of hyperthyroidism was performed in patients who happened to be pregnant at the time, one review[73] showing no increase in fetal loss, congenital abnormalities or childhood cancer. However, hypothyroidism following prenatal exposure to ^{131}I has been reported, and the need for prompt intervention to prevent cretinism has been noted.[74] The fetal thyroid concentrates iodide from about the 10th week of gestation, with the fetal thyroid dose estimated to peak during the fifth month of pregnancy at about 580 mGy per MBq of ^{131}I administered to the mother.[75] The maximum fetal whole-body dose from ^{131}I treatment of maternal hyperthyroidism has been estimated at 8×10^{-2} mGy/MBq, occurring during the first month of pregnancy.[76]

● What can be done about inadvertent exposure of an embryo or fetus?

▲ Where appropriate, female patients should be asked if they think they might be pregnant, before any radiopharmaceutical is administered. A sign should be displayed prominently in patient waiting areas, clearly stating (in several languages if necessary) the need for patients to inform staff of any pregnancy before commencing the study. Occasionally, unintended exposure of an embryo may occur if the pregnancy is not recognized at the time (an occult pregnancy rate of 4% in women of childbearing capacity has been reported[77]), or is not notified to staff by the patient. The patient should be counselled immediately about the level of risk. For diagnostic procedures, reassurance is appropriate. In some instances, hydration and frequent voiding, or use of a blocking agent to prevent uptake by thyroid-seeking radiopharmaceuticals, may be useful dose-minimizing measures. All instances of prenatal exposure should be fully documented in the patient's medical record.

Following any inadvertent exposure, the question of terminating the pregnancy may be raised by a concerned parent. Termination is virtually never warranted at the low dose levels of diagnostic procedures. After misadministration of a therapy dose to a pregnant patient an immediate assessment of all radiation risks to the fetus is required, although with the possible exception of large activities of ^{131}I it would be unusual for the radiation dose to reach the range at which deterministic fetal damage may occur. Discussion with the parents about possible intervention should include risk assessment based on realistic dose estimates, to be considered along with individual circumstances such as medical, social and personal factors.

● How 'safe' are nuclear medicine procedures in children?

▲ Because the risk of radiation-induced cancer is greater in the young, particular care is taken to see that radiation doses are kept as low as possible. *S*-factors for children are available for the calculation of absorbed dose.[52] Information on radiopharmaceutical behaviour specific to children is also required. Uptake may be greater, for example iodide in the infant thyroid, and ^{67}Ga citrate and ^{99m}Tc phosphonates in the long-bone epiphyses.[78,79] Metabolism and excretion are frequently more rapid than in the adult, although many paediatric procedures are requested to investigate obstructed flow, for example of urine[80] or cerebrospinal fluid, in which the radiation dose is increased.

Administered activity (and hence radiation dose) should be kept to a minimum consistent with adequate information density on images. For static imaging, reduction of activity in proportion to body weight is simplest and appropriate, although it will underestimate the activity required in some imaging procedures in very young children. For dynamic studies, or SPECT imaging, larger activities may need to be administered, the minimum amount being determined by the requisite information density per frame or slice of the study.

The absorbed dose should be estimated for the activity administered in every paediatric procedure. In most instances, the absorbed dose will be as high as that for the equivalent procedure in an adult, and, in some instances, much higher. Given the increased radiosensitivity of children, the associated radiation risk is therefore likely to be several times higher in a child than in an adult. In properly referred patients, the risk will be offset by the clinical utility of the study and the potential benefit to the patient (which in terms of quality-adjusted life years is likely to be greater for a child than an adult). For further information, readers are referred to the ARSAC Guide[60] and articles by Shore & Hendee[81] and Mountford.[82,83]

● What precautions are needed for patients caring for infants and small children?

▲ *Close contact care*

Parents caring for young children and infants may spend a considerable amount of time cuddling their children. As a

Table 114.15 Maximum measured dose rates at time of departure from nuclear medicine department (adapted from data of Harding et al,[84] Mountford et al[85])

Procedure (no. of patients)	Radionuclide	Time between dose administration and measurement (h)	Maximum dose rate μSv/h per MBq administered)		
			0.1 m	0.5 m	1.0 m
Static renal (3)	^{99m}Tc	3.1	0.1	0.02	0.01
Dynamic renal (5)	^{99m}Tc	0.5	0.3	0.08	0.01
Bone (37)	^{99m}Tc	3.2	0.2	0.06	0.01
Lung *V/Q*(5)	^{99m}Tc	0.3/2.2	0.2	0.04	0.01
Thyroid (2)	^{99m}Tc	0.5	0.3	0.06	0.01
Liver (3)	^{99m}Tc	0.7	0.3	0.07	0.01
Marrow (3)	^{99m}Tc	1.3	0.4	0.07	0.01
Brain (9)	^{99m}Tc	1.8	0.2	0.06	0.01
Thyroid (2)	^{123}I	0.5	0.6	0.1	0.03
Leucocyte (3)	^{111}In	28.0 (second scan)	1.5	0.2	0.05
Cardiac (1)	^{201}Tl	4.6	0.02	0.009	0.007
Gastric emptying (2)	^{113m}In	0.2	0.03	0.03	0.03
Gallium (2)	^{67}Ga	0.2	0.16	0.03	0.01
Therapy iodine (5)	^{131}I	<1	0.53	0.1	0.024

Table 114.16 Effective exposure times for close contact between an infant and its parent (adapted from data by Mountford[83]). For use with the data in Table 114.15 for estimation of the total close contact dose.

Radiopharmaceutical	Effective exposure time (h)
^{99m}Tc (all compounds)	2
^{123}I iodide (euthyroid)	2
^{123}I iodide (hyperthyroid)	3
^{131}I iodide (euthyroid)	16
^{131}I iodide (hyperthroid)	18
^{123}I-MIBG	2
^{131}I-MIBG	7
^{111}In leucocytes	21
^{201}Tl chloride	18
^{75}Se selenomethionine	340
^{67}Ga citrate	19
^{113m}In (all compounds)	1
^{90}Y colloid	20
^{32}P phosphate	80
^{89}Sr chloride	370

consequence, these children will be exposed to close contact (0.1 m) dose rates, which can either be measured or estimated from data such as those given in Table 114.15.[84–86] The total close contact dose can be estimated by multiplying the administered activity by the dose rate at 0.1 m (Table 114.15) and the effective exposure time, based on a reasonable pattern of contact, given in Table 114.16.[83] If this exceeds 1 mSv (or any other desired dose limit) some restriction of close contact with the infant for a period of time may be advised.

For radiopharmaceuticals administered in typically used diagnostic amounts, close contact doses to children will rarely exceed 1 mSv, and special restrictions will not be required. One notable exception is that of ^{111}In leucocytes,[87] for which administration of activities in excess of 30 MBq can lead to an estimated close contact dose greater than 1 mSv. ^{131}I iodide, often used in amounts up to 400 MBq for the detection of thyroid metastases, may also lead to close contact doses exceeding 1 mSv if the administered activity exceeds 100 MBq.

Breast feeding

If ingestion of radioactivity in breast milk is a possibility, an estimate of the potential radiation dose to the child must be made and breast feeding may need to be suspended until levels of radioactivity in the breast milk have fallen to acceptable levels. If the suspension time is very long, breast feeding may have to stop. The risk of radiation to the child must be weighed against the benefits of breast feeding and the possible trauma to both mother and child, including interference with the establishment of the milk supply in the post-partum patient. Data on the secretion of radiopharmaceuticals in breast milk can be found in a number of reviews.[5,88–92]

Mountford & Coakley[92] provide a flexible set of criteria based on a realistic model which assumes breast feeding of a newborn infant at 4-hourly intervals, with the first feed taking place 3 h after administration of the radiopharmaceutical to the mother. Among the parameters derived are the effective half-life in milk ($_mt_{1/2}$), the effective dose to the infant (E) per unit activity administered to the mother and the period (T_s) for which breast feeding must be suspended if the total effective dose to the infant is to be kept below 1 mSv. Table 114.17 lists the values of these parameters for various radiopharmaceuticals. For ^{201}Tl, calculations are based on data given in a paper by Murphy et al.[93]

It is most important that breast-feeding patients be identified before the administration of a radiopharmaceutical.[94] If it is decided to proceed with the investigation, the child should be breast fed between 30 and 60 min beforehand. Practical and technical aspects of nuclear medicine procedures on breast-feeding patients are discussed admirably in a short article by Hogg.[95]

Table 114.17 Effective dose to infant per unit activity administered to mother, breast-feeding suspension periods and other parameters associated with the administration of radiopharmaceuticals to breast-feeding patients[92]

Radiopharmaceutical	Effective half-life in milk (h)*	Effective dose to infant per MBq to mother (mSv)	Administered activity (MBq)	Suspension period (h)†	Category
$^{99m}TcO_4^-$	5.3	0.092	800	36	3
^{99m}Tc-MAA	7.9	0.015	80	6	2
^{99m}Tc erythrocytes	7.7	0.003	800	13	3
^{99m}Tc-DTPA	4.4	4.2×10^{-5}	800	None	1
^{99m}Tc-DMSA	5.9	8.4×10^{-5}	80	None	1
^{99m}Tc glucoheptonate	4.0	1.5×10^{-4}	800	None	1
^{99m}Tc-MDP	5.1	1.0×10^{-4}	600	None	1
^{99m}Tc-HDP	5.1	5.9×10^{-5}	600	None	1
^{99m}Tc-HMDP	4.1	5.3×10^{-5}	600	None	1
^{123}I iodide	5.8	0.06	20	5	3
^{123}I-IOH	4.9	0.09	20	8	3
^{123}I-IOH	4.8	4.2	2	18	3
^{125}I fibrinogen	80	26	4	540	4
^{125}I-HSA	72	35	0.2	206	4
^{131}I iodide	142	113	40	1727	4
^{131}I-IOH	5.8	12	2	30	3
^{75}Se methionine	79	5.9	10	467	4
^{67}Ga citrate	68	0.5	150	427	4
^{111}In leucocytes	134	0.026	40	None	1
^{51}Cr-EDTA	11	3.6×10^{-4}	3	None	1
^{201}Tl	362	0.0132	111	203	4

*Maximum value of longest half-life component.
†Suspension required if effective dose to infant is to be limited to 1 mSv.
Category 1 Suspension not essential except possibly for short period for reassurance of mother.
Category 2 Suspension for period indicated.
Category 3 Suspension for period indicated, with measurement of samples to ensure radioactive concentration in milk is sufficiently low to resume feeding.
Category 4 Cessation of feeding as the period of suspension would be very long. If mother insists on maintaining her milk supply, treat as category 3.

● Can any harm result from an extravasated injection of a radiopharmaceutical?

▲ Occasionally difficulty will be experienced with an intravenous injection, resulting in the local deposition of some or all of the radiopharmaceutical. In some cases, the absorbed dose to the skin may exceed the threshold for deterministic radiation damage. The dose will be high for radiopharmaceuticals with slow tissue clearance, such as colloidal, water-insoluble or intracellularly localized material, and those with a long physical half-life and emitting non-penetrating radiation such as beta-particles and internal conversion or Auger electrons.

^{201}Tl chloride decays by electron capture with the subsequent emission of Auger electrons (as do ^{67}Ga and ^{111}In), and it also undergoes rapid cellular uptake. Anecdotal evidence suggests that a subcutaneous deposition of 100 MBq of this radiopharmaceutical can cause harm; ulceration at the injection site has been reported two years after the accidental subcutaneous injection of 74 MBq, with an absorbed dose estimate of 200 Gy.[96] Pruritis and erythema have been observed 20 days after the subcutaneous injection of 34 MBq of ^{131}I iodocholesterol, with the dose estimate ranging from 490 to 245 Gy for an assumed skin target thickness of 5–10 mm.[97] The dose to a 5 g mass of tissue from infiltrated injections of ^{67}Ga, ^{201}Tl and ^{99m}Tc, estimated from clearance studies in animals, was said to be less than the skin erythema dose for ^{32}P of 10 Gy.[98] Dose estimates for a number of radionuclides are given by Hoop[99] from a model of Shapiro et al,[100] which assumes all the radiopharmaceutical has been locally deposited in a volume equal to the volume of the injection, with no biological clearance.

If a large amount of an injection has been deposited subcutaneously, an estimation of the maximum skin dose can be obtained as described by Hoop.[99] If this is significant, further measurements can be made to obtain an indication of the amount of activity at the site, and the clearance rate. The incident should be noted in the patient's medical record, and the patient should be asked to return for investigation if any unexpected skin reaction occurs at the site of injection over the following 2 years.[96]

● What side-effects are associated with radionuclide therapy?

▲ In general, side-effects and long-term complications are minimal. A brief summary is given here, but see

Chapters 72–76 and the review by Hoefnagel[101] for more detailed discussions of potential side-effects.

Long-term follow-up studies on ^{131}I therapy for thyroid carcinoma have shown that chronic side-effects include haematological effects, pneumonitis and lung fibrosis, fertility disorders, induction of leukaemia and other secondary cancers. However, the haematological effects are moderate provided the whole-body dose is kept below 1 Gy per treatment, and the other long-term effects occur rarely. Acute side-effects include nausea and vomiting, sialadenitis, temporary painful swelling of metastases, thyroid storm and bone marrow suppression.

Induction of acute leukaemia is a possible long-term effect (in about 6% of patients) following the treatment of polycythaemia vera with ^{32}P orthophosphate. However, the UK Polycythaemia Vera Study Group found that this occurred more frequently with chlorambucil chemotherapy than after ^{32}P therapy. Vascular complications (bleeding and thromboembolism) can occur following treatment with ^{32}P.

Long-term follow-up is not yet available for the newer therapy radiopharmaceuticals. However, several limiting factors have been noted for radioimmunotherapy: acute toxicity (including fever, nausea, bronchospasm) can occur; human anti-mouse antibody (HAMA) response prevents subsequent follow-up treatment; and bone marrow toxicity has been reported.

● **What guidelines should be followed for the irradiation of volunteers in research studies?**

▲ The ICRP regards the irradiation of volunteers in research studies as a medical exposure, and not subject to defined dose limits as for the exposure of radiation workers and the public. However, the risks and potential benefit of any proposed exposure for research purposes should be subject to independent review, for example by a local ethics committee.[7] Approval is usually conditional on:

- a written protocol for the study;
- radiation dose constraints appropriate to adults, children, infants and fetuses (effective dose for diagnostic studies, equivalent dose for higher exposure levels);
- referral to an external agency of proposals above the dose constraints;
- information to the volunteer as part of the process of seeking informed, willing consent to participate in the study;
- age restrictions unless this is inconsistent with the purpose of the study;
- exclusion of children and pregnant women, unless there is clearly a benefit to the individual;
- minimal number of subjects.

Table 114.18 Radiation risk assessment for adult volunteers in research protocols.[7] Note the corresponding detriment (fatal and non-fatal cancers and hereditary disorders) per unit dose is 2–3 times greater in children than in adults, and 5–10 times smaller in those over 50 years of age than in young adults

Level of risk	Category	Effective dose (mSv)	Required benefit for approval
Trivial ($<10^{-4}$)	I	<0.1	Minor, e.g. increase knowledge
Minor ($\sim 10^{-4}$)	IIa	0.1–1	Intermediate, e.g. increase knowledge leading to health benefit
Intermediate ($\sim 10^{-3}$)	IIb	1–10	
Moderate ($>10^{-3}$)	III	>10	Substantial benefit to volunteer

Guidance on the conduct of radiation research proposals is provided by the ICRP,[7] including a broad categorization of the radiation dose to the subject as initially proposed by the World Health Organization, which can be useful for evaluating the risks and benefits of a proposal (see Table 114.18).

RADIATION RISK FACTORS FOR STAFF AND OTHER PERSONS

● **What sort of hazard is a nuclear medicine patient to others?**

▲ The patient is a potential source of external exposure to others in the vicinity. As a rough approximation, the dose rate may be estimated by assuming that the radioactivity in the patient is a 'point source', which is a good approximation at a distance of 2 m or more. Calculations such as these will tend to overestimate the exposure because of attenuation of radiation in the patient and distribution of the activity throughout the body organs and tissues. Point source and patient exposures for some commonly used radionuclides are given in Table 114.19[102] (see also Table 114.15).

Table 114.19 Dose rates from point sources and patients (adapted from Williams[102])

Radionuclide	Half-life	Equivalent dose rate at 1 m (μSv/h per MBq)	
		Point source	Patient (mean)
^{18}F	110 min	0.149*	–
^{51}Cr	27.7 days	0.005	0.0025
^{67}Ga	78.1 h	0.028	0.011
^{99m}Tc	6.02 h	0.020	0.0075
^{111}In	2.8 days	0.086	0.03
^{123}I	13 h	0.041	0.015
^{131}I	8.06 days	0.058	0.023
^{133}Xe	5.3 days	0.014	0.0055
^{201}Tl	73.1 h	0.014	0.0038

*Datum from Wasserman & Gruenewald.[2]

Nuclear medicine staff

By far the greater part of the radiation dose to staff comes from external exposure rather than contamination. Much of this is due to patient handling, and will depend on the workload. A weighted average figure of 1.5 μSv per procedure has been estimated for typical British work patterns and workloads (see Table 114.20).[37] A nuclear medicine technologist performing eight varying procedures per day would receive, on average, a dose of 12 μSv per day, corresponding to 2.9 mSv per year, an estimate that agrees with the reported values of a typical monitoring program.[103] Some PET examinations can result in quite high exposures to staff; values of between 17 μSv and 50 μSv per procedure have been reported by McCormack & Miklos.[104]

Internal exposure may result from personal contamination, which is most likely to occur during the preparation and administration of radiopharmaceuticals. Small body burdens of ^{99m}Tc have been found in nuclear medicine staff, mostly acquired during lung ventilation procedures, but the effective dose from this source was only 0.01–0.1 mSv/year.[105] These results are reassuring, but it is important to remember that contamination compromises study quality as well as radiation safety. Skin or eye contamination by beta-emitting radionuclides or solutions of very high radioactive concentration, such as a ^{99m}Tc generator eluate, could result in high localized doses[106] (Table 114.21). Decontamination methods in general are described by Mountford,[107] and for skin by Merrick et al.[108]

The handling of radioiodines requires particular attention to ventilation, contamination control and monitoring. Protection measures are beyond the scope of this section; reference should be made to guides such as that by Prime.[109] Following a significant contamination incident, thyroid uptake of radioiodine can be blocked by the prompt administration of 100–300 mg of stable iodine, subject to clinical considerations such as age and possible allergy, goitre or hyperthyroidism. Administration of stable iodine beyond 12 h after the incident will have little effect, and may in fact prolong the retention of radioiodine already accumulated in the thyroid.[74,110–112]

Table 114.20 Radiation doses to nuclear medicine technologists from various procedures, based on typical UK work pattern and workload[37]

Procedure	Administered activity (MBq)	Average dose to technologist (μSv)	Average dose to technologist (μSv/GBq)	Procedures/ year (× 1000)
Bone	500	1.0	2	143.5
Brain	500	5.3	11	17.9
Lung	100	1.3	6.5	51.9
Liver	70	0.3	4.3	7.2
Gated RBC cardiac	800	3.5	4.4	15.6
Renal: DTPA	100	0.8	8	19.2
Renal: MAG3	200	0.8	4	9.0
GI bleed	200	3.0	15	–

Average = 1.5 μSv per procedure.

Table 114.21 Skin contamination: beta dose rates at various depths in water beneath a contamination of 1 Bq distributed uniformly over a 1 cm^2 circular area on an air/water boundary (Data from Cross et al[106])

Radionuclide	Dose rate (nGy/h, 1 Bq/cm^2) at skin depth of		
	0.07 mm	0.4 mm	3 mm
^{11}C	1632	752	0.7
^{18}F	1574	458	–
^{32}P	1726	990	90
^{67}Ga	293	–	–
^{89}Sr	1667	887	55
^{90}Y	1756	1049	200
^{99m}Tc	207	–	–
^{111}In	295	12	–
^{123}I	305	–	–
^{131}I	1319	303	–
^{201}Tl	208	–	–

Nursing staff

The dose to nursing staff from patients returning to the ward after a nuclear medicine procedure depends on the radiopharmaceutical administered, its activity and the degree of care required by the patient. In caring for a bone scan patient, for example, to whom 550 MBq ^{99m}Tc-MDP has been administered, nursing staff will receive a maximum of 114 μSv if the patient is totally helpless, but only 2–4 μSv if the patient is largely self-caring. At most, for nurses spending long periods of time near helpless patients (but excluding ICU patients), the maximum dose has been estimated at around 150 μSv per shift.[85] Fortunately, many nuclear medicine patients need little nursing care and doses are at the lower end of the above range, usually less than 20 μSv per patient.[113]

Because of nursing rosters and the relatively small number of nuclear medicine patients in wards, most members of the nursing staff will encounter only a small number of nuclear medicine patients in any one year, and the average annual radiation dose to nursing staff in the ward should be quite small. Nevertheless, administrative procedures should be set in place to make nursing staff aware of patients to whom radioactive materials have been administered and procedures (such as staff rotation for intensive nursing care of therapy patients) which can be used to minimize exposure.[84]

Others

The radiation doses to patient escorts, relatives and others in a nuclear medicine waiting room have been estimated by Harding et al.[114] In the worst situation, of a person sitting next to a bone scan patient for 3 h, the radiation dose was 33 μSv or approximately 3% of the recommended dose limit for members of the public. The radiation dose to a typical departmental porter transporting nuclear medicine patients is estimated to be about 0.1 mSv per month.[113] Ultrasonographers carrying out examinations on nuclear medicine patients may receive doses up to 25 μSv in some instances,[115] but this exposure can often be avoided by carrying out the ultrasound examination before the nuclear medicine procedure, or deferring it until another day. External exposure of clinical biochemistry staff from radioactive blood and urine samples from nuclear medicine patients is negligible, of the order of 0.02 mSv per month for all urine samples and 0.002 mSv per month from all blood samples from nuclear medicine patients.[113]

● Is their any risk to the patient's family and colleagues?

▲ When a patient leaves hospital, family members or colleagues may ask 'What radiation dose will I receive from this person?' The 'worst case' dose that any other person might receive is the close contact dose to a frequently cuddled child of the patient discussed above, which will not exceed 1 mSv for most procedures involving diagnostic quantities of radionuclides (with the exception of ^{111}In leucocytes in activities exceeding about 30 MBq and ^{131}I iodide in activities exceeding 100 MBq). The highest such dose has been estimated at around 240 μSv,[85] and it is highly unlikely that other persons will receive a radiation dose anywhere near the 1 mSv limit recommended for members of the public. Special advice, such as 'avoiding unnecessary contact with children', which may unduly alarm an already anxious patient, will generally be unnecessary and may, in fact, be counter to the spirit of ALARA.

● What are the hazards of radioactive contamination from nuclear medicine patients?

▲ Contamination of other persons from radioactivity in the body fluids of diagnostic nuclear medicine patients returning home or to the ward is not a significant hazard. Careful personal hygiene is all that is required from all concerned. Contamination of equipment by diagnostic nuclear medicine patients who subsequently receive dialysis has been found to be negligible.[116] Blood samples taken for laboratory analysis also represent a minimal contamination hazard. Where radioimmunoassay is to be carried out, the amount of activity in the blood can interfere with sample counting; deferral of such tests for a day or so after the nuclear medicine procedure may be necessary.

● What special precautions are required for therapy patients?

▲ The radiation exposure near therapy patients can be estimated in the same way as that for diagnostic patients[86,117] The dose rate at 0.5 m from a patient to whom 5 GBq of ^{131}I iodide has been administered, for example, will be about 500 μSv per hour immediately after the radioactive material has been given. At this dose rate, the 1 mSv limit for members of the public will be exceeded in 2 h; at 0.1 m, this time will be even shorter, of the order of 20 min. Some degree of isolation, for example by hospitalization, is usually recommended for therapy patients with more than a defined amount of certain radionuclides in their body.

During the 'isolation phase', strict protocols regarding nursing care are followed and visiting rights are generally restricted to short stays, with children and pregnant women excluded. Following this period, restrictions on certain activities will still apply[60,118] (see Table 114.22). The time for which various restrictions will apply varies widely and will depend on the clinical status of the patient (for example, hyperthyroid or hypothyroid). The residual activity in the patient can be estimated from time to time by comparing the exposure rate at a fixed distance (usually 2 or more metres from the patient) with the exposure rate

Table 114.22 Suggested radioactivity levels above which restrictions apply to patients having radionuclide therapy[60,118]

Restriction	Activity (MBq) above which restrictions apply for			
	^{131}I iodide	^{198}Au colloid	^{90}Y colloid	^{32}P phosphate
Radiosensitive work Non-essential contact with young children	30	30	100	300
Return to work where there is close contact with others	150	150	500	1500
Return to work where there is negligible contact with others Travel by public transport	400	400	1500	4500
Discharge from isolation care Travel by private transport	800	800	3000	9000

measured a short time after administration of the radionuclide, before any excretion has taken place.

On discharge from hospital, the patient should be advised about precautions to follow for a further period.[60,119–121] These will apply until the activity in the patient has decayed to levels which are unlikely to present any significant risk to other persons (often chosen as the levels at which continuing exposure will not lead to a dose exceeding 1 mSv).

Varying amounts of a radionuclide which has been administered to a nuclear medicine patient will be excreted in sweat, saliva, urine, faeces and even expired air. Vomitus may also be contaminated. Radioactive urine is the main contributor to contamination for many radiopharmaceuticals, particularly ^{131}I iodide. Private toilet facilities should be provided for an iodine therapy patient in isolation care. Buchan & Brindle,[122] in a study of patients who returned home after administration of between 150 and 750 MBq of ^{131}I, found negligible amounts of ^{131}I in the thyroid of 39 relatives living at home with the patients. The results of this study have been confirmed by others,[123,124] suggesting that radioactive contamination from patients is unlikely to present an appreciable hazard to other persons if normal hygiene procedures are followed. Although surface contamination can be found on and around patients following administration of high-dose radioactive iodine therapy,[125] there is little evidence to suggest that this is transferred to medical staff, nursing staff or any other persons in amounts likely to present an appreciable hazard.[126]

● What precautions are required in medical emergencies?

▲ Medical emergencies such as cardiac arrest or emergency surgery of a nuclear medicine patient may require response from staff who are not familiar with the nature and level of hazard or the precautions required. Little time may be available for prior consultation with nuclear medicine staff, particularly for incidents occurring outside normal working hours. In the case of patients who have had diagnostic nuclear medicine procedures the risk is negligible.

For patients who have been given therapeutic quantities of radionuclides, the risk to staff providing emergency care such as cardiopulmonary resuscitation is very small and more than offset by the potential benefit to the patient. The main message should be that the radiation risk is never high enough to prevent staff – even those who are pregnant – from responding promptly to a clinical emergency in the usual way. Even when working at 0.5 m from a patient with 5 GBq of ^{131}I for half an hour, the accumulated dose to a staff member would be of the order of 0.25 mSv, well within the ICRP's recommended annual limit of 1 mSv for members of the public. Ward staff familiar with the patient should be able to help prevent personal contamination and unnecessary exposure, without compromising patient care.

Table 114.23 Limits on cadaver activity levels[119]

Radionuclide	Autopsy or embalming (MBq)	Burial (MBq)	Cremation (MBq)
^{32}P	100	2000	30
^{89}Sr	50	2000	20
^{90}Y	200	2000	70
^{131}I	10	400	400
^{198}Au colloid	400	400	100

Preliminary planning for possible emergencies is particularly important when caring for therapy patients. Problems may be avoided by measures such as the use of identity wrist bands or similar to ensure ready identification of the patient's radioactive status, and the availability of resuscitation facemasks and Lugol's iodine or other thyroid-blocking agents when caring for ^{131}I patients.

● What special precautions are required following the death of a radioactive patient?

▲ There have been a number of instances of patients dying after radionuclide therapy, although 'in principle, radionuclide therapy is not given to moribund patients'.[119] The risk of death in patients being treated for thyroid disease is small; it may be greater for other radionuclide therapies, such as in patients having palliation for bony metastases, or those in clinical trials who may be selected on the basis of end-stage disease. Consultation with health physics and pathology staff is required. Guidance on levels of activity above which special consideration should be given to the handling of corpses is given by Godden[118] (see Table 114.23). Below these levels, the general precautions followed in autopsy and embalming procedures will provide adequate protection. Detailed procedures for autopsy, embalming, cremation and burial are given by the NCRP.[119]

REFERENCES

1. International Commission on Radiological Units 1980 Radiation quantities and units. ICRU Report Number 33. ICRU Publications, Washington, DC
2. Wasserman I, Gruenewald W 1988 Air kerma rate constants for radionuclides. Eur J Nucl Med 14: 569–571
3. International Commission on Radiological Protection 1991 1990 Recommendations of the International Commission on Radiological Protection. ICRP Publication 60. Ann ICRP 21(1–3)
4. Johansson L 1985 Patient irradiation in diagnostic nuclear

medicine: assessment of absorbed dose and effective dose equivalent. University of Gothenburg: Gothenburg
5. International Commission on Radiological Protection 1987 Protection of the patient in nuclear medicine. ICRP Publication 52. Ann ICRP 17(4)
6. International Commission on Radiological Protection 1987 Radiation dose to patients from radiopharmaceuticals. ICRP Publication 53. Ann ICRP 18(1–4)
7. International Commission on Radiological Protection 1991 Radiological protection in biomedical research. ICRP Publication 62. Ann ICRP 22(3)
8. Poston J W 1993 Application of the effective dose equivalent to nuclear medicine patients. J Nucl Med 34: 714–716
9. Beninson D, Sowby D 1985 Age and sex dependent weighting factors for medical irradiation. Radiat Protect Dosim 11: 57–60
10. Mettler F, Davis M, Moseley R, Kelsey C 1986 The effect of utilising age and sex dependent factors for calculating detriment from medical irradiation. Radiat Protect Dosim 15: 269–271
11. Smith H 1992 The detrimental health effects of ionizing radiation. Nucl Med Commun 13: 4–10
12. United Nations Scientific Committee on the Effects of Atomic Radiation (UNSCEAR) 1988 Sources, effects and risks of ionizing radiation. United Nations Publications, New York
13. National Council on Radiation Protection and Measurements 1993 Risk estimates for radiation protection. NCRP Report No. 115. NCRP, Bethesda, MD
14. National Academy of Sciences 1990 Health effects of exposure to low levels of ionizing radiation. BEIR V Report. National Academy Press, Washington, DC
15. International Commission on Radiological Protection 1991 Risks associated with ionising radiations. Ann ICRP 22(1)
16. United Nations 1986 Radiation doses, effects, risks. London: United Nations Publications, London
17. Mettler F A, Moseley R D 1985 Medical effects of ionizing radiation. Grune & Stratton, London
18. Brill B (ed.) 1985 Low-level radiation effects: a fact book. Society of Nuclear Medicine, New York
19. Webster E W 1986 A primer on low-level ionizing radiation and its biological effects. AAPM Report No. 18. American Institute of Physics, New York, p 103
20. Ash P 1980 The influence of radiation on fertility in man. Br J Radiol 53: 271–278
21. Otake M, Schull W 1990 Radiation-related posterior lenticular opacities in Hiroshima and Nagasaki atomic bomb survivors based on the DS86 dosimetry system. Radiat Res 121: 3–13
22. Hopewell J 1991 Biological effects of irradiation on skin and recommended dose limits. Radiat Protect Dosim 39(1/3): 11–24
23. National Council on Radiation Protection and Measurements 1993 The probability that a particular malignancy may have been caused by a specified irradiation. NCRP Statement No. 7. Health Phys 64: 545–548
24. Breitenstein B D 1988 The probability that a specific cancer and a specified radiation exposure are causally related. Health Phys 2: 397–398
25. National Institutes of Health 1985 Report of the National Institutes of Health Ad Hoc Working Group to Develop Radioepidemiological Tables. US Government Printing Office, Washington, DC
26. Gray J E 1993 Clinical viewpoint in NCRP probability of causation. Statement. Health Phys 64: 550–551
27. Saenger E L 1993 Reflections on NCRP Statement No. 7. Health Phys 64: 549
28. Jose D E 1993 Probability of causation. Health Phys 64: 549–550
29. Sankaranarayanan K 1991 Genetic effects of ionising radiation in man. Ann ICRP 22: 75–94
30. Cox R, McGibbon B 1992 Medical exposures: advice on exposure to ionising radiation of pregnant women. National Radiological Protection Board, Chilton
31. Schull W J 1991 Ionizing radiation and the developing human brain. Ann ICRP 22: 95
32. Mole R H 1987 Irradiation of the embryo and fetus. Br J Radiol 60: 17–31
33. Mole R H 1990 Fetal dosimetry by UNSCEAR and risk coefficients for childhood cancer following diagnostic radiology in pregnancy. J Radiol Prot 10: 199–203
34. Yoshimoto Y, Kato H, Schull W 1988 Risk of cancer among children exposed in utero to a-bomb radiations, 1950–1984. Lancet 2: 665–669
35. Gilman E, Kneale G, Knox E, Stewart A 1988 Pregnancy, X-rays and childhood cancers: effects of exposure age and radiation dose. J Radiol Prot 8: 3–8
36. Knox E G, Stewart A M, Kneale G W, Gilman E A 1987 Prenatal irradiation and childhood cancer. J Soc Radiol Prot 7: 177–189
37. Clarke E A, W.H.T, Notghi A, Harding L K 1992 Radiation doses from nuclear medicine patients to an imaging technologist: relation to ICRP recommendations for pregnant workers. Nucl Med Commun 13: 795–798
38. Harding L, Mountford P 1993 Editorial. Pregnant employees in a nuclear medicine department. Nucl Med Commun 14: 345–346
39. Coakley A 1990 Risks, their explanation, and written consent for nuclear medicine procedures. Nucl Med Commun 11: 819–822
40. Clarke R H 1991 The causes and consequences of human exposure to ionising radiation. Radiat Protect Dosim 36: 73–77
41. Bennett B G 1991 Exposures from medical radiation world-wide. Radiat Protect Dosim 36: 237–242
42. Elliot A T, Shields R A 1993 UK nuclear medicine survey, 1989/90. Nucl Med Commun 14: 360–364
43. National Council on Radiation Protection and Measurements 1987 Ionizing radiation exposures of the population of the United States. NCRP Report No. 93. National Council on Radiation Protection and Measurements, Washington, DC
44. Colmanet S F, Samuels D L 1993 Diagnostic radiopharmaceutical dose estimate to the Australian population. Health Phys 64: 375–380
45. Hendee W R, Doege T C 1988 Origin and health risks of indoor radon. Semin Nucl Med 18: 3–9
46. Cohen B L, Lee I S 1979 A catalog of risks. Health Phys 36: 707–722
47. Cohen B L 1991 Catalog of risks extended and updated. Health Phys 61: 317–335
48. Pochin E E 1987 Radiation risks in perspective. Br J Radiol 60: 42–50
49. Hamilton L D 1980 Comparative risks from different energy systems: evolution of the methods of studies. International Atomic Energy Agency Bulletin 22(5/6): 35–71
50. Loevinger R, Budinger T F, Watson E E (eds) 1989 MIRD primer for absorbed dose calculations. Society of Nuclear Medicine, New York
51. Snyder W S, Ford M R, Warner G G, Watson S B 1975 'S', Absorbed dose per unit cumulated activity for selected radionuclides and organs. MIRD Pamphlet No. 11. Society of Nuclear Medicine, New York
52. National Council on Radiation Protection and Measurements 1983 Protection in nuclear medicine and ultrasound diagnostic procedures in children. NCRP Report No. 73. NCRP, Washington, DC
53. Cloutier R J, Watson E E, Rohrer R H, Smith E M 1973 Calculating the radiation dose to an organ. J Nucl Med 14: 53–55
54. Akabani G, Poston J W 1991 Absorbed dose calculations to blood and blood vessels for internally deposited radionuclides. J Nucl Med 32: 830–834
55. Thomas S R, Stabin M G, Chen C T, Samaratunga R C 1992 A dynamic urinary bladder model for dose calculations. MIRD Pamphlet No. 14. J Nucl Med 33: 783–801
56. Dillman L T, Von der Lage F C 1975 Radionuclide decay schemes and nuclear parameters for use in radiation dose estimation. MIRD Pamphlet No. 10. Society of Nuclear Medicine, New York
57. Snyder W S, Ford M R, Warner G G 1978 Estimates of specific absorbed fractions for photon sources uniformly distributed in organs of a heterogeneous phantom. MIRD Pamphlet No. 5, revised. Society of Nuclear Medicine, New York
58. Hoffman E J, Huang S, Phelps M E 1979 Quantitation on positron emission tomography. 1. Effect of object size. J Comput Assist Tomogr 3: 299–308
59. Johansson L, Mattsson S, Nosslin B, Leide-Svegborn S 1992

Effective dose from radiopharmaceuticals. Eur J Nucl Med 19: 933–938
60. Administration of Radioactive Substances Advisory Committee (ARSAC) 1993 Notes for guidance on the administration of radioactive substances to persons for purposes of diagnosis, treatment or research. Department of Health and Social Security, London
61. Roedler H D 1987 Assessment of fetal activity concentration and fetal dose for selected radionuclides based on animal and human data. In: Gerber G B, Metivier H, Smith H (eds) Age related factors in radionuclide metabolism and dosimetry. Martinus Nijhoff, Dordrecht, pp 327–337
62. Lathrop K A, Tsui B M, Harper P V 1992 Distribution of ionic indium and gallium in pregnant and non-pregnant animals. In: Watson E E, Schlafke-Stelson A T (eds) 5th International Radiopharmaceutical Dosimetry Symposium. Oak Ridge Associated Universities, Oak Ridge, pp 167–178
63. Mirkin B L 1973 Maternal and fetal distribution of drugs in pregnancy. Clin Pharmacol Ther 14: 643
64. Elsasser U, Henrichs K, Kaul A, Reddy A R, Roedler H D 1985 Specific absorbed fractions and S-factors for calculating absorbed dose to embryo and fetus. 4th International Radiopharmaceutical Dosimetry Symposium. Oak Ridge Associated Universities, Oak Ridge, pp 155–166
65. Smith E M, Warner G G 1976 Estimates of radiation dose to the embryo from nuclear medicine procedures. J Nucl Med 17: 836–839
66. Mountford P 1989 Foetal risks following antenatal radionuclide administration. Nucl Med Commun 10: 79–81
67. Mountford P, Harding L 1993 Nuclear medicine and the pregnant patient (editorial). Nucl Med Commun 14: 625–627
68. Cloutier R J, Smith S A, Watson E E, Snyder W S, Warner G G 1973 Dose to the fetus from radionuclides in the bladder. Health Phys 25: 147–161
69. Husak V, Wiedermann M 1980 Radiation absorbed dose estimates to the embryo from some nuclear medicine procedures. Eur J Nucl Med 5: 205–207
70. Marcus C S, Mason G R, Kuperus J H, Mena I 1985 Pulmonary imaging in pregnancy – maternal risk and fetal dosimetry. Clin Nucl Med 10: 1–4
71. Ponto J A 1985 Fetal dosimetry from pulmonary imaging in pregnancy – revised estimates. Clin Nucl Med 10: 108–109
72. Casara D, Rubello D, Saladini G et al 1993 Pregnancy after high therapeutic doses of iodine-131 in differentiated thyroid cancer: potential risks and recommendations. Eur J Nucl Med 20: 192–194
73. Sakar S, Beierwaltes W, Gill S, Cowley B 1976 Subsequent fertility and birth histories of children and adolescents treated with ^{131}I for thyroid cancer. J Nucl Med 17: 460–464
74. National Council on Radiation Protection and Measurements 1977 Protection of the thyroid gland in the event of releases of radioiodine. NCRP Report No. 55. NCRP, Bethesda, MD
75. Watson E E 1992 Radiation absorbed dose to the human fetal thyroid. In: Watson E E, Schlafke-Stelson A T (eds) 5th International Radiopharmaceutical Dosimetry Symposium. Oak Ridge Associated Universities, Oak Ridge, pp 179–187
76. Stabin M G, Watson E E, Marcus C S, Salk R D 1991 Radiation dosimetry for the adult female and fetus from iodine-131 administration in hyperthyroidism. J Nucl Med 32: 808–813
77. Block I 1977 Routine pregnancy testing: better safe than sorry. Hospitals 51: 94
78. Thomas S 1978 Dose to the metaphyseal growth complexes in children undergoing ^{99m}Tc-EDHP bone scans. Radiology 126: 193–195
79. Thomas S, Gelfand M, Burns S, Purdom R, Kereiakes J, Maxon H 1983 Radiation absorbed dose estimates for the liver, spleen, and metaphyseal growth complexes in children undergoing gallium-67 citrate scanning. Radiology 146: 817–820
80. Marcus C, Kuperus J 1985 Pediatric renal iodine-123 orthoiodohippurate dosimetry. J Nucl Med 26: 1211–1214
81. Shore R, Hendee W 1986 Radiopharmaceutical dosage selection for pediatric nuclear medicine. J Nucl Med 27: 287–298
82. Mountford P 1990 Paediatric radiopharmaceutical dosimetry (editorial). Nucl Med Commun 11: 339–342
83. Mountford P J 1991 Parental and paediatric radiation protection. In: Goldstone K E, Jackson P C, Myers M J, Simpson A E (eds) Radiation protection in nuclear medicine and pathology. The Institute of Physical Sciences in Medicine, York, pp 52–74
84. Harding L K, Mostafa A B, Roden L, Williams N 1985 Dose rates from patients having nuclear medicine investigations. Nucl Med Commun 6: 191–194
85. Mountford P J, O'Doherty M J, Forge N I, Jeffries A, Coakley A J 1991 Radiation dose rates from adult patients undergoing nuclear medicine investigations. Nucl Med Commun 12: 767–777
86. O'Doherty M J, Kettle A G, Eustance C N P, Mountford P J, Coakley A J 1993 Radiation dose rates from adult patients receiving I-131 therapy for thyrotoxicosis. Nucl Med Commun 14: 160–168
87. Mountford P J, Coakley A J 1989 Body surface dosimetry following re-injection of In-111 leucocytes. Nucl Med Commun 10: 497–501
88. Hospital Physicists' Association 1984 Radiation protection procedures in the use of Tc-99m. Topic Group Report No. 39. Hospital Physicists' Association, London
89. Ahlgren L, Ivarsonn S, Johansson L, Mattsson S, Nosslin B 1985 Excretion of radionuclides in human breast milk after the administration of radiopharmaceuticals. J Nucl Med 26: 1085–1089
90. Romney B M, Nickoloff E L, Esser P D, Alderson P O 1986 Radionuclide administration to nursing mothers: mathematically derived guidelines. Radiology 160: 549–554
91. Mountford P J, Coakley A J 1986 Guidelines for breast feeding following maternal radiopharmaceutical administration. Nucl Med Commun 7: 399–401
92. Mountford P J, Coakley A J 1989 A review of the secretion of radioactivity in human breast milk: data, quantitative analysis and recommendations. Nucl Med Commun 10: 15–27
93. Murphy P H, Beasley C W, Moore W H, Stabin M G 1989 Thallium-201 in human milk: observations and radiological consequences. Health Phys 56: 539–541
94. Anonymous 1991 Baby radiation error leads to fine. Radiography Today, September: p 1
95. Hogg P 1991 Taken in with the mother's milk. Radiography Today, September, pp 42–43
96. Piers D, Beekhuis H 1987 Local radiation dose from extravasal Tl-201. J Nucl Med 28: 684
97. Breen S, Driedger A 1991 Radiation injury from interstitial injection of iodine-131-iodocholesterol. J Nucl Med 32: 892
98. Castronovo F, McKusick K, Strauss H 1988 The infiltrated radiopharmaceutical injection: dosimetric considerations. Eur J Nucl Med 14: 93–97
99. Hoop B 1991 The infiltrated radiopharmaceutical injection: risk considerations. J Nucl Med 32: 890–891
100. Shapiro B, Pillay M, Cos P 1987 Dosimetric consequences of interstitial extravasations following IV administration of a radiopharmaceutical. Eur J Nucl Med 12: 522–523
101. Hoefnagel C R 1991 Radionuclide therapy revisited. Eur J Nucl Med 18: 408–431
102. Williams E D 1991 Imaging and other diagnostic and research *in vivo* procedures. In: Goldstone K E, Jackson P C, Myers M J, Simpson A E (eds) Radiation protection in nuclear medicine and pathology. The Institute of Physical Sciences in Medicine, York, pp 35–51
103. Morris N D 1992 Personal radiation monitoring and assessment of doses received by radiation workers (1991). Australian Radiation Laboratory, Melbourne
104. McCormack V A, Miklos J A 1993 Radiation dose to positron emission tomography technologists during quantitative versus qualitative studies. J Nucl Med 34: 769–772
105. Smith T 1984 Internal exposure of patients and staff in diagnostic nuclear medicine procedures. J Soc Radiol Prot 4(2): 45–57
106. Cross W G, Freedman N O, Wong P Y 1992 Beta ray dose distributions from skin contamination. Radiat Protect Dosim 40: 149–162
107. Mountford P 1991 Techniques for radioactive decontamination in nuclear medicine. Semin Nucl Med 21: 82–89

108. Merrick M, Simpson J, Liddell S 1982 Skin decontamination – a comparison of four methods. Br J Radiol 55: 317–318
109. Prime D 1985 Health physics aspects of the use of radioiodines. In: Hughes D (ed) Occupational Health Monographs. Science Reviews, H and H Scientific Consultants, Leeds, p 55
110. Wolff J 1980 Physiological aspects of iodide excess in relation to radiation protection. J Mol Med 4: 151–165
111. Crocker D 1984 Nuclear reactor accidents – the use of KI as a blocking agent against radioiodine uptake in the thyroid – a review. Health Phys 46: 1265–1279
112. Bhattacharyya M, Breitenstein B, Metivier H, Muggenburg B, Stradling G, Volf V 1992 Methods of treatment. In: Gerber G, Thomas R (eds) Guidebook for the treatment of accidental internal radionuclide contamination of workers. Ashford: Nuclear Technology, Ashford, pp 27–36
113. Harding L K, Mostafa A B, Thomson W H 1990 Staff radiation doses associated with nuclear medicine procedures – a review of some recent measurements. Nucl Med Commun 11: 271–277
114. Harding L K, Harding N J, Warren H, Mills A, Thomson W H 1990 The radiation dose to accompanying nurses, relatives and other patients in a nuclear medicine waiting room. Nucl Med Commun 11: 17–22
115. Hvard A C 1989 The unseen hazards of ultrasound. Br J Radiol 62: 295–296
116. Serrano A, Olson A, Man C, Galonsky R, Stein R 1991 Contamination and radiation exposure from Tl-201 in patients undergoing dialysis after a nuclear medicine study. Health Phys 60: 365–366
117. Castronovo F P, Robert A B, Veilleux N M 1982 Dosimetric considerations while attending hospitalized I-131 therapy patients. J Nucl Med Technol 10: 157–160
118. Godden T J 1991 Therapeutic uses of unsealed radionuclides. In: Goldstone K E, Jackson P C, Myers M J, Simpson A E (eds) Radiation protection in nuclear medicine and pathology. Institute of Physical Sciences in Medicine, York, pp 13–34
119. National Council on Radiation Protection and Measurements 1970 Precautions in the management of patients who have received therapeutic amounts of radionuclides. NCRP Report No. 37. NCRP, Washington, DC
120. Culver C M, Dworkin H J 1991 Radiation safety considerations for post-iodine hyperthyroid therapy. J Nucl Med 32: 169–173
121. Culver C M, Dworkin H J 1992 Radiation safety considerations for post-iodine-131 thyroid cancer therapy. J Nucl Med 33: 1402–1405
122. Buchan R C T, Brindle J M 1970 Radioiodine therapy to outpatients – the contamination hazard. Br J Radiol 43: 479–482
123. Jacobsen A P, Plato P M, Toeroek D 1978 Contamination of the home environment by patients treated with iodine-131. Am J Public Health 68: 225–230
124. Allen H C J, Zelenski J P 1992 430 non-hospitalised thyroid cancer patients treated with single doses of 40–400 mCi (abstract). J Nucl Med 33: 784
125. Ibis E, Wilson C R, Collier B D, Akansel G, Isitman A T, Yoss R G 1992 I-131 contamination from thyroid cancer patients. J Nucl Med 33: 2110–2115
126. Beierwaltes W, Widman J 1992 How harmful to others are iodine-131 treated patients? J Nucl Med 33: 2116–2117

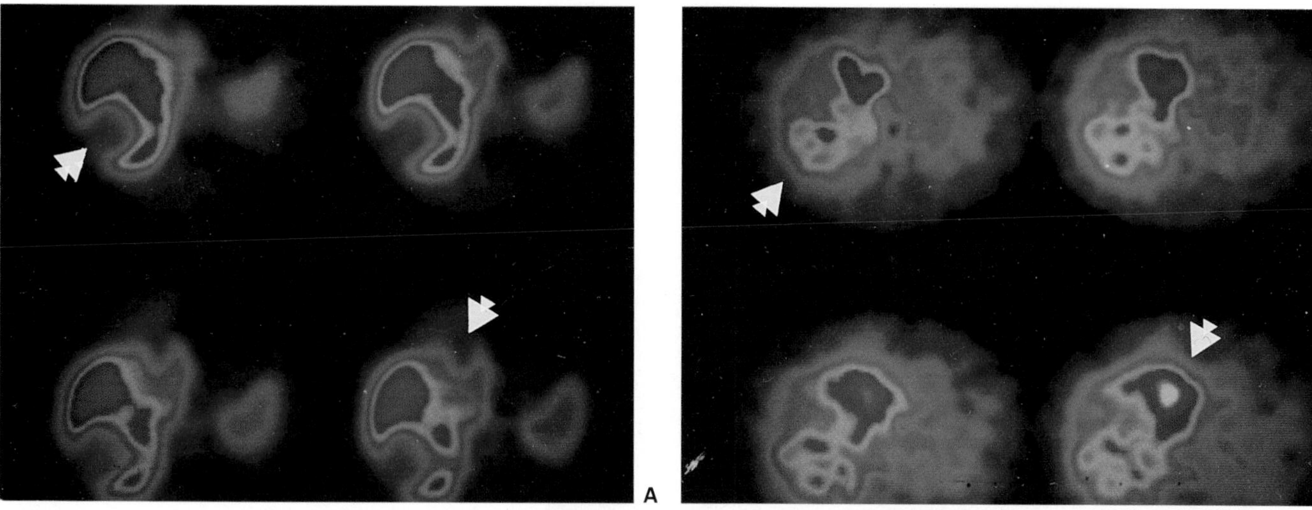

Fig. 65.7 Liver metastases from gastric carcinoid (relapsed after gastrectomy) in a 51-year-old man. The cold defects of uptake demonstrated on ^{99m}Tc colloid liver SPECT (transaxial sections) in both lobes (A) and on ^{123}I-MIBG SPECT appear to take up the tracer intensively, though inhomogeneously (B). (See text, p. 753)

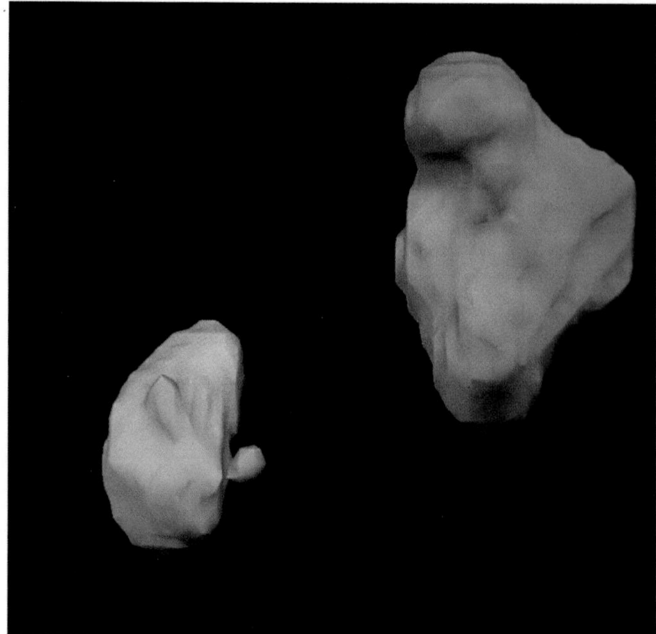

Fig. 66.3 (B) Three-dimensional reconstruction from a three-head camera (Picker Prism 3000) of the abdomen of the same patient. The spleen and left kidney are depicted in green, the insulinoma and right kidney in pink. (See text, p. 758)

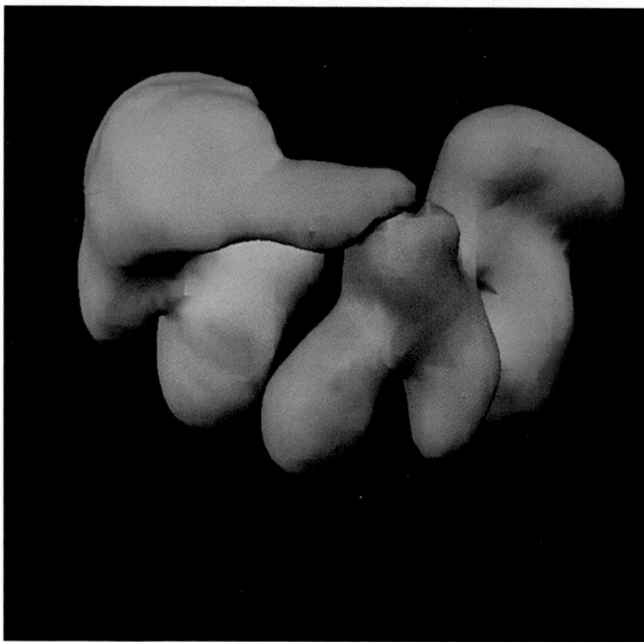

Fig. 66.6 (B) Three-dimensional reconstruction from a three-head camera (Picker Prism 3000) of the abdomen of the same patient. The liver, right kidney, spleen and left kidney are in orange, yellow, green and green-blue respectively. The tumour mass in purple to blue is also clearly visualized. (See text, p. 761)

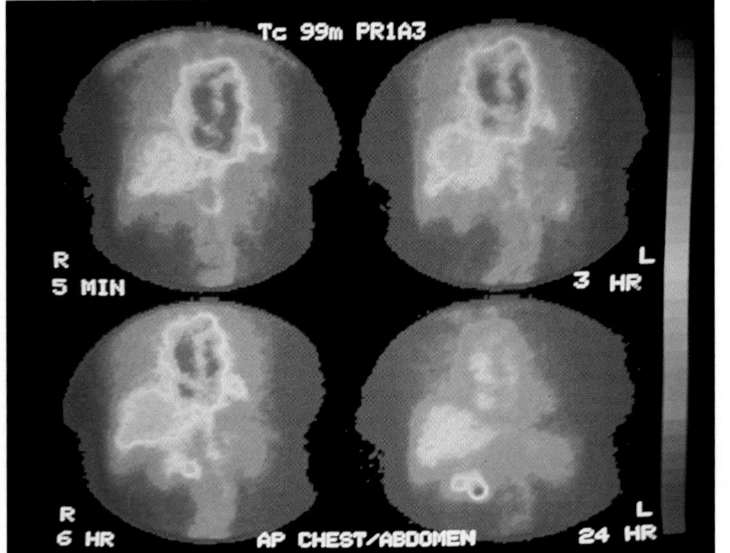

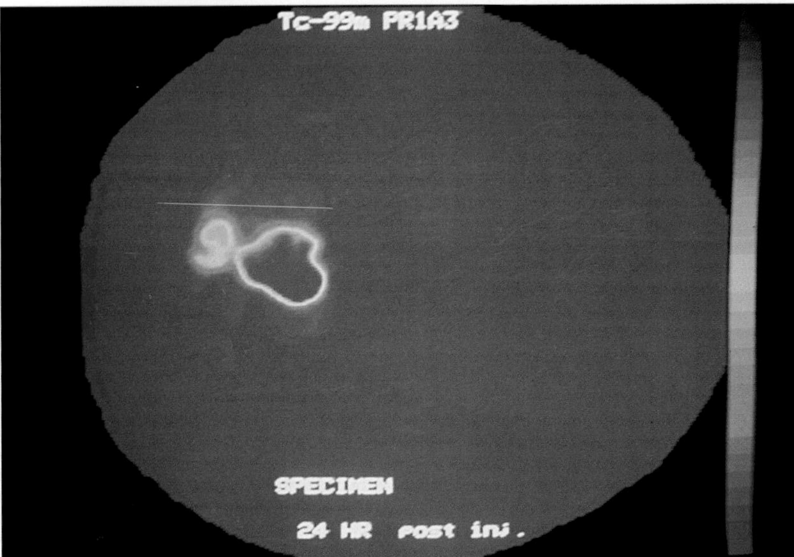

Fig. 68.2 Colon cancer: (A) RIS with ^{99m}Tc PRIA3 (ICRF) was undertaken in a man with carcinoma of the transverse colon starting the day before surgery. Anterior views of the upper abdomen are shown at 5 min top left, 3 h top right, 6 h bottom left and 24 h bottom right. The blood pool, initially red, decreases with time to yellow; the liver, yellow, stays much the same with time; an area of abnormal uptake inferior to the liver first appears at 6 h, yellow, and increases in uptake at 24 h, red, so that it is more active than the adjacent liver. This is specific uptake increasing with time in the colon carcinoma.
(B) Image of the surgical specimen on the same day as the 24 h image. The tumour, red and yellow, has high uptake compared to the mucosa, blue, tumour to mucosa ratio 63:1. 0.014% of the injected dose was in the tumour. Note no lymph nodes are seen in the specimen, none was involved with tumour, Duke's B. (See text, p. 785)

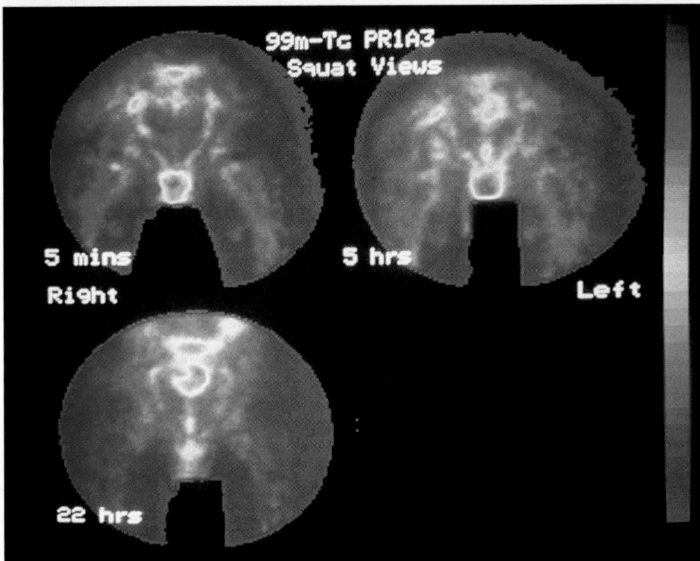

Fig. 68.3 Rectal cancer: RIS with ^{99m}Tc PRIA3. Squat views at 5 min top left, 5 h top right and 22 h bottom left. Uptake is seen in the scrotum at 5 min anteriorly but the pre-sacral area shows no uptake. At 5 h in addition to the scrotal and bladder activity, pre-sacral uptake is seen. At 22 h scrotal and bladder activity is reduced and pre-sacral uptake is further increased. A rectosigmoid adenocarcinoma, moderately differentiated, Dukes B, was resected. (Reproduced with permission from Eur J Nucl Med.) (See text, p. 785)

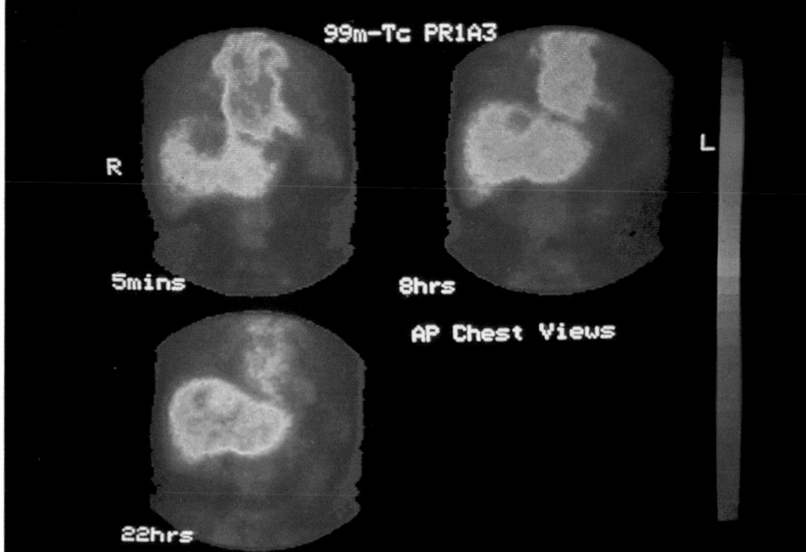

Fig. 68.4 Liver metastases: a 63-year-old man had rectal adenocarcinoma with a solitary hepatic metastasis 1 year previously. Anterior resection, chemotherapy and laser treatment of the liver metastasis was undertaken. X-ray CT of the liver metastasis showed complete necrosis and normal liver and abdomen èlsewhere. It was thought that the laser treatment was a success. RIS with ^{99m}Tc-PRIA3 (ICRF) was performed. Anterior views of the upper abdomen top left 5 min, top right 8 h, bottom left 22 h. A large defect in the superior part of the right lobe and a small defect superiorly at the tip of the left lobe are seen on the 10 min image. Both show increasing uptake around the defects with time, indicating viable metastases. The defect of the right lobe appears to diminish in size with time and that in the left lobe becomes similar to the normal liver. (Reproduced with permission from Eur J Nucl Med). (See text, p. 785)

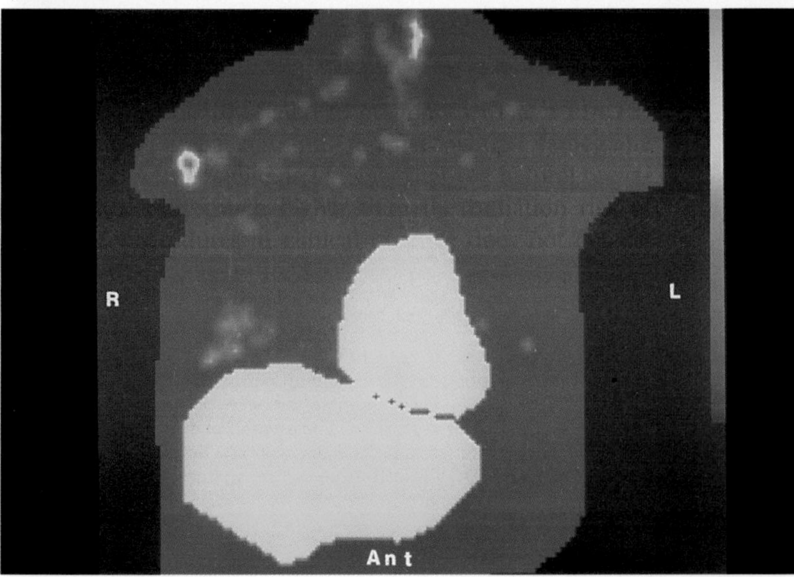

Fig. 68.5 Breast cancer: a woman with carcinoma evident clinically and on mammography in the right breast had RIS with ^{99m}Tc-SM3 (ICRF) before surgery to determine node involvement. Kinetic analysis with probability mapping was undertaken on the 10 min and 24 h anterior view images. The heart and liver are masked in yellow, the left breast and axilla are normal in dark blue ($P>0.05$ for change). The right breast shows significant uptake over an area ($P<0.05$ light blue) and the right axilla shows highly significant uptake ($P<0.001$ red). Changes in the neck and throat area are to be discounted because of movement. Involvement of right axillary nodes was confirmed at surgery. (See text, p. 787)

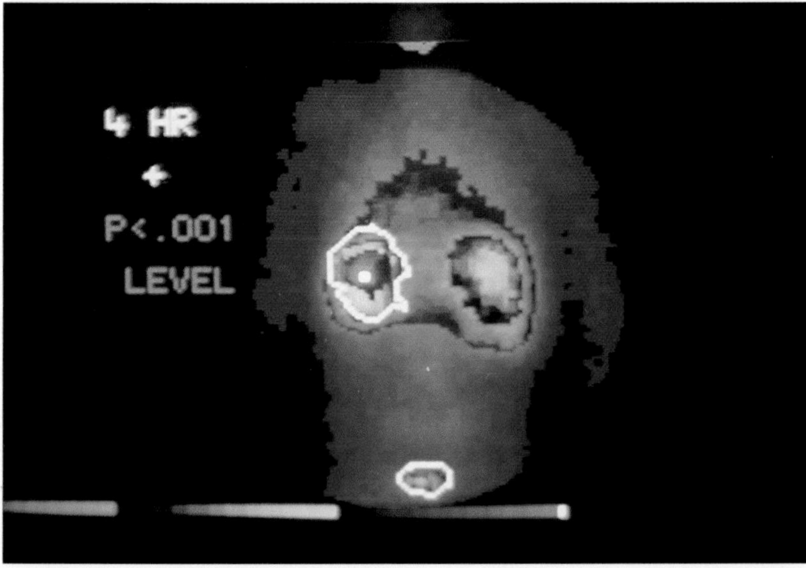

Fig. 68.10 Neuroblastoma: RIS with ^{99m}Tc-UJ13A (ICRF). Posterior view of a 4-year-old child at 4 h. Visual display shows the tumour superior to the spleen in red, the spleen, liver and bladder in yellow and green, and tissue background activity in blue. Kinetic analysis with probability mapping of the 10 min and 4 h images is displayed as a white contour at sites of significant change between the two images: the tumour site and urinary excretion of activity into the bladder. (See text, p. 794)

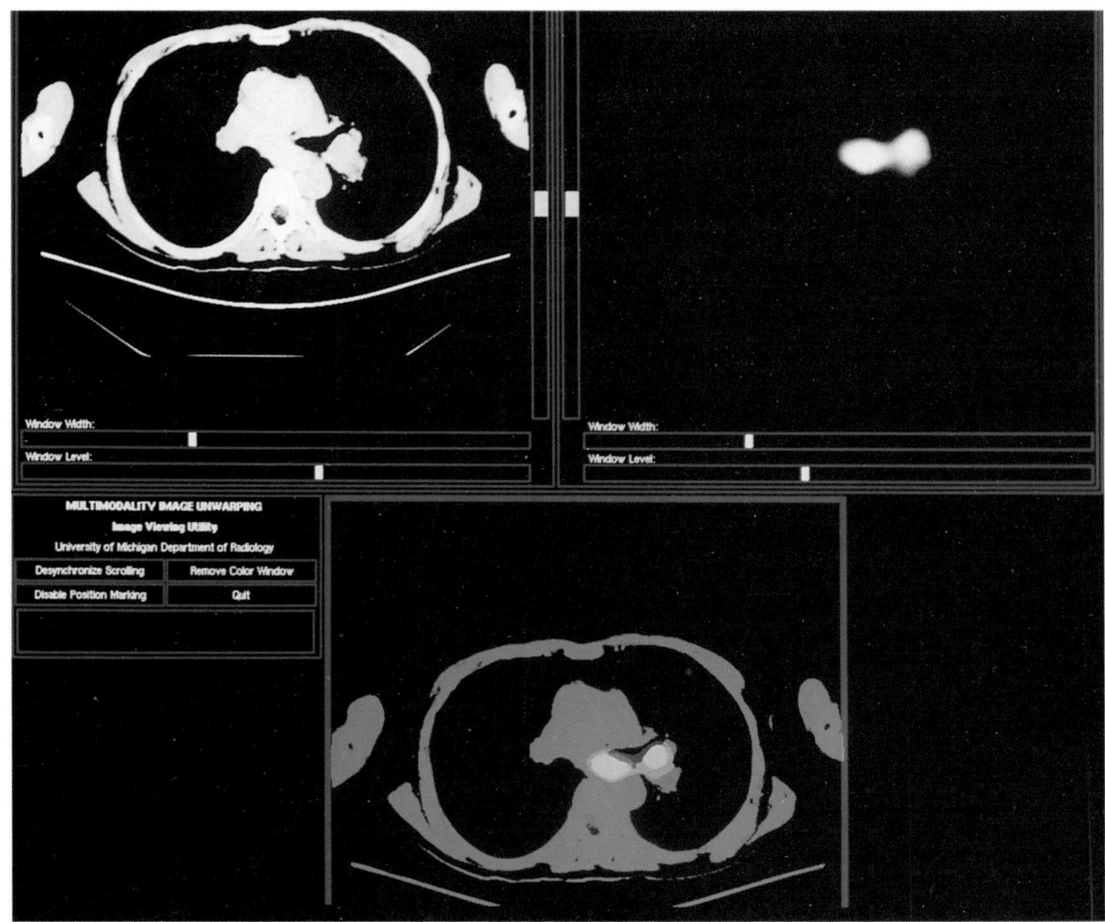

Fig. 69.3 Intense FDG uptake is seen into enlarged lymph nodes in a patient with non-small cell lung carcinoma. These lymph nodes were proven to be involved with cancer at surgery. The method of display here is that of an 'anatometabolic' image (see text). Top left: CT. Top right: FDG PET. Bottom centre: anatometabolic image. (See text, p. 808)

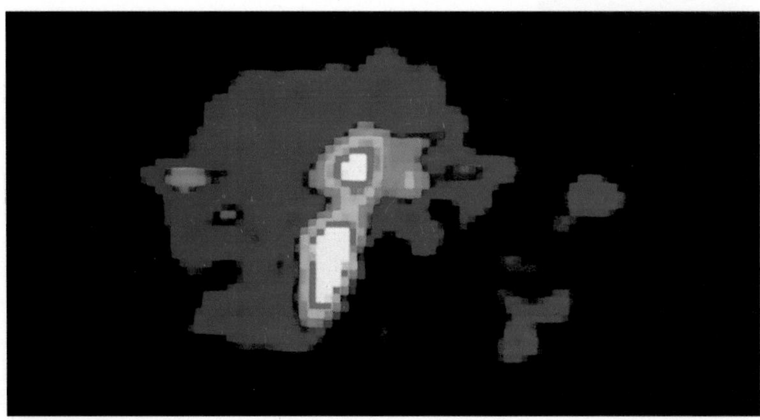

Fig. 69.7 Transverse FDG PET image demonstrates intense uptake immediately posterior to the liver and just above the right kidney. Intense uptake was seen, despite the fact that this represents a low grade lymphoma. (See text, p. 813)

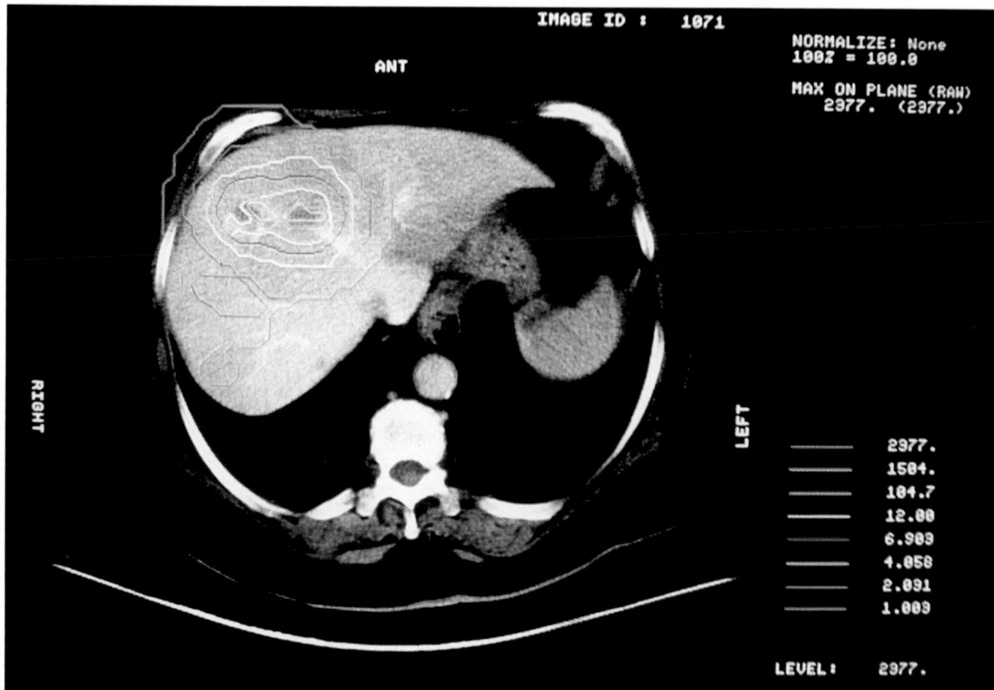

Fig. 71.4 Isodose contours superimposed on a CT image through the liver. The dose values (in cGy) assigned to each isodose contour arise from a cumulated activity concentration of 740 GBq s/ml in the two tumours seen in the anterior portion of the liver and in a third tumour seen in a different slice. (Reproduced with permission from Sgouros et al.[11]) (See text, p. 831)

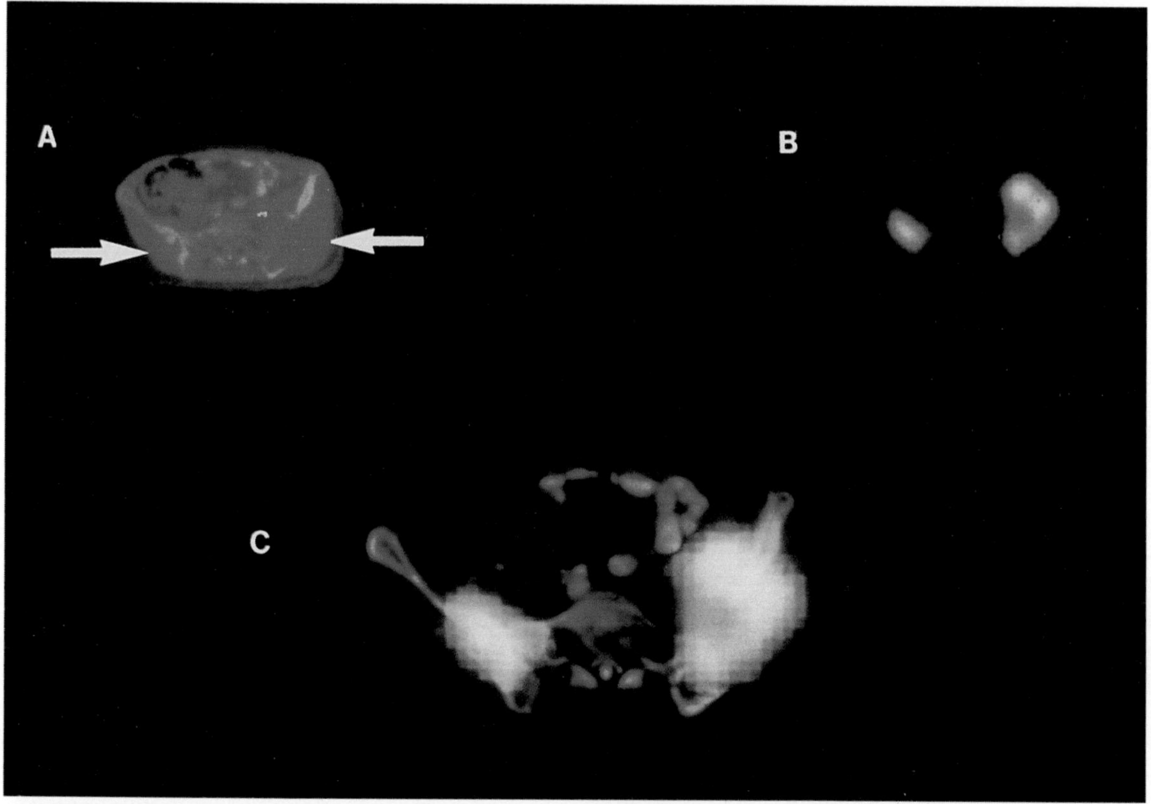

Fig. 74.10 The use of combined imaging, using computerized tomography (CT) to provide a map of attenuation coefficients for [^{123}I]MIBG single photon emission tomography (SPECT). **A** CT scan of pelvis showing tumour infiltration of the right acetabulum and left ilium (arrowed). **B** Corresponding SPECT [^{123}I]MIBG image. **C** CT/SPECT overlay confirming functioning phaeochromocytoma at tumour sites shown on CT. (See text, p. 858)

A

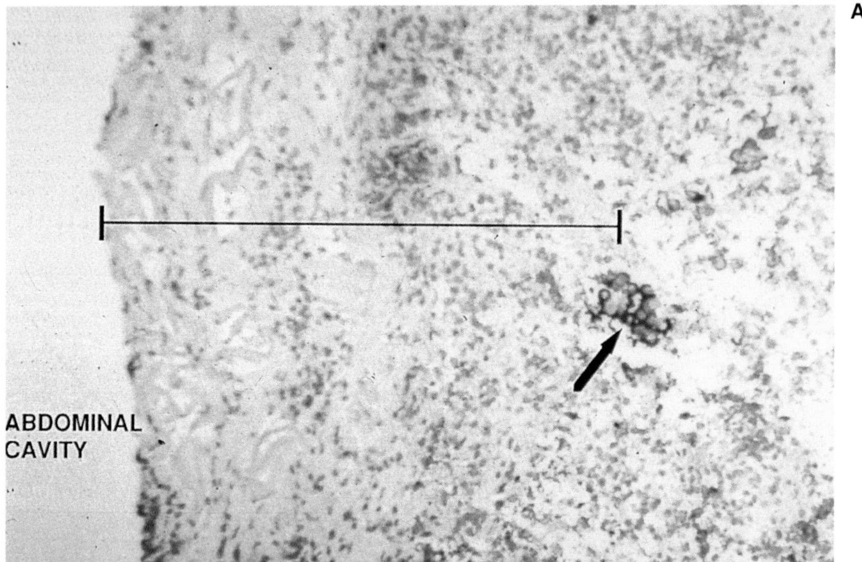

B

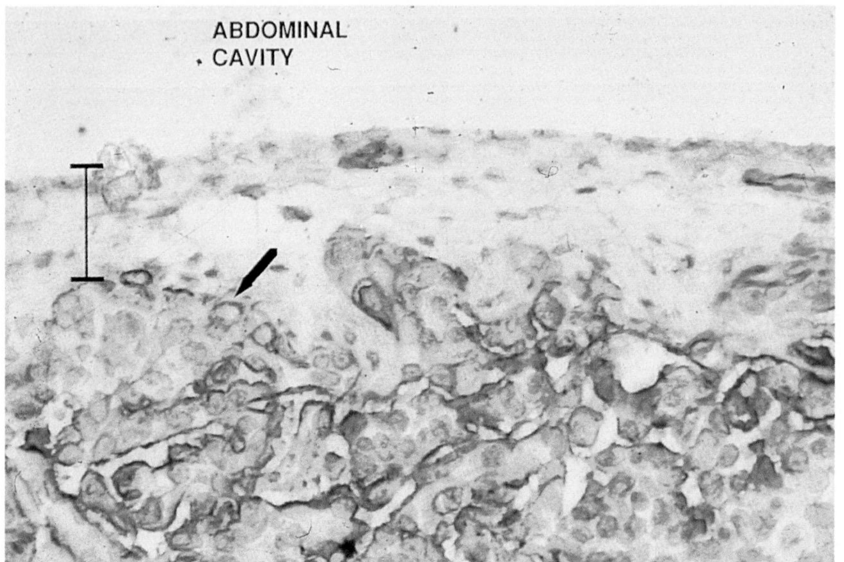

C

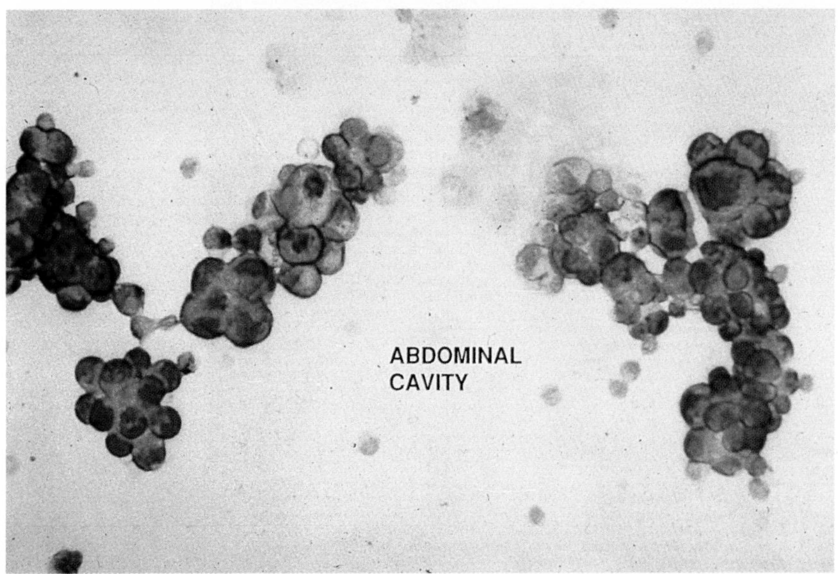

Fig. 75.1 Immunohistochemical pattern of CA 125 antigenic expression in large (>1 cm diameter) serous ovarian carcinomas (A), macroscopic (<0.5 cm diameter) tumours (B) and in microscopic (<0.5 mm diameter) clusters of malignant cells (C). For macroscopic tumours the accessibility of antibody fragments to tumour cells (brown colour) is limited by the thickness of connective tissue located between the abdominal cavity (in which the radioantibody is infused) and the tumour cells expressing the antigen (as indicated by solid line). (Reproduced with permission from Chatel et al.[7]) (See text, p. 866)

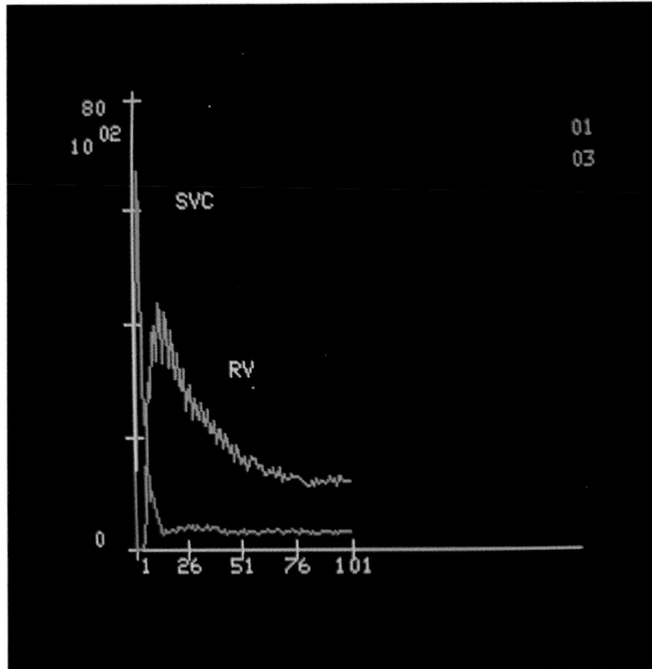

Fig. 90.3 First pass radionuclide angiocardiography. Activity time curves from a subject with tricuspid regurgitation. Top = Right ventricle. Bottom = Superior vena cava. After a satisfactory bolus injection, the effect of the tricuspid regurgitation is to spread out the bolus. (See text, p. 1072)

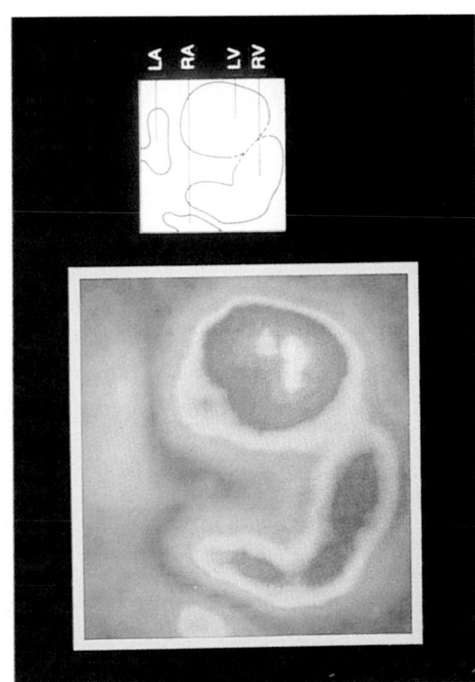

Fig. 90.5 Equilibrium radionuclide angiocardiography. Amplitude image; normal subject. Each pixel is colour coded according to the Fourier amplitude of its time activity curve. Ventricular regions with good contraction manifest high values of amplitude and are shown in red. In this example, there are high values of amplitude across both left and right ventricles. (Reproduced with permission from *Nuclear Cardiology*.) (See text, p. 1076)

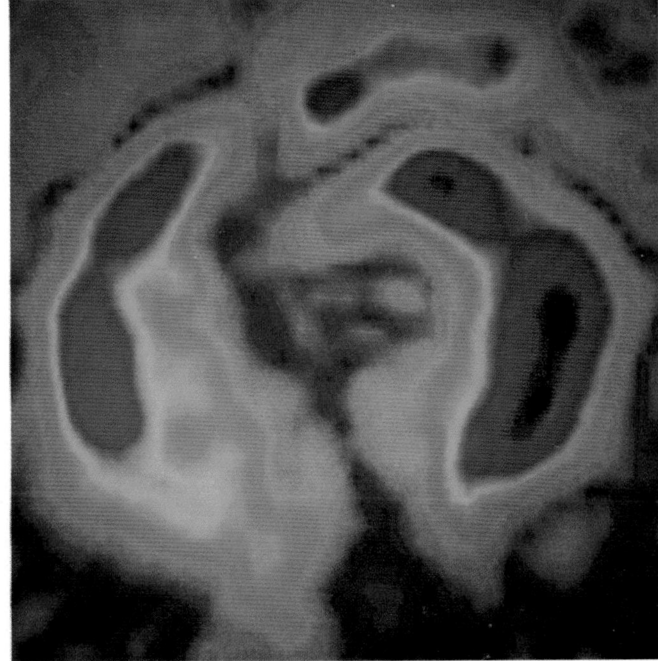

Fig. 90.6 Equilibrium radionuclide angiocardiography. Amplitude image; septal infarction. High values of amplitude are apparent in the lateral region of the left ventricle and throughout the right ventricle. The interventricular septal and apical regions of the left ventricle have very low values of amplitude, suggesting akinesis. (See text, p. 1076)

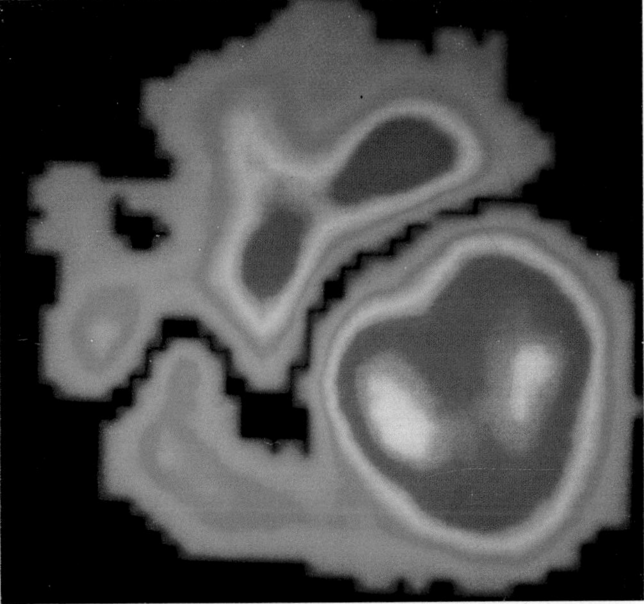

Fig. 90.7 Equilibrium radionuclide angiocardiography. Amplitude image; mitral regurgitation. The left ventricle is enlarged. Much higher values of amplitude are apparent in the left ventricle than in the right, reflecting the much higher left ventricular stroke volume. (See text, p. 1076)

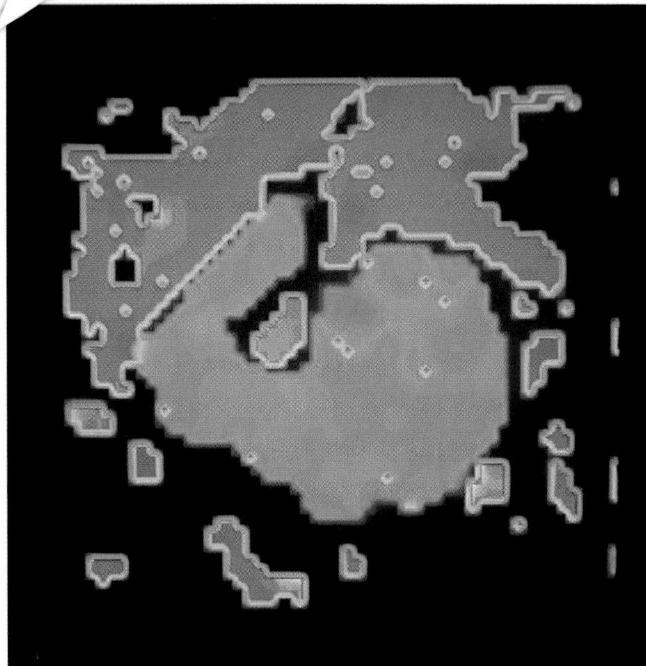

Fig. 90.8 Equilibrium radionuclide angiocardiography. Phase image; normal subject. Each pixel is colour coded according to the Fourier phase of its time activity curve. Regions, such as normal ventricles, which empty relatively early in the cardiac cycle have low phase values and are coloured blue or green; regions, such as atria and great vessels, which empty relatively late during the cardiac cycle are coloured red. (See text, p. 1076)

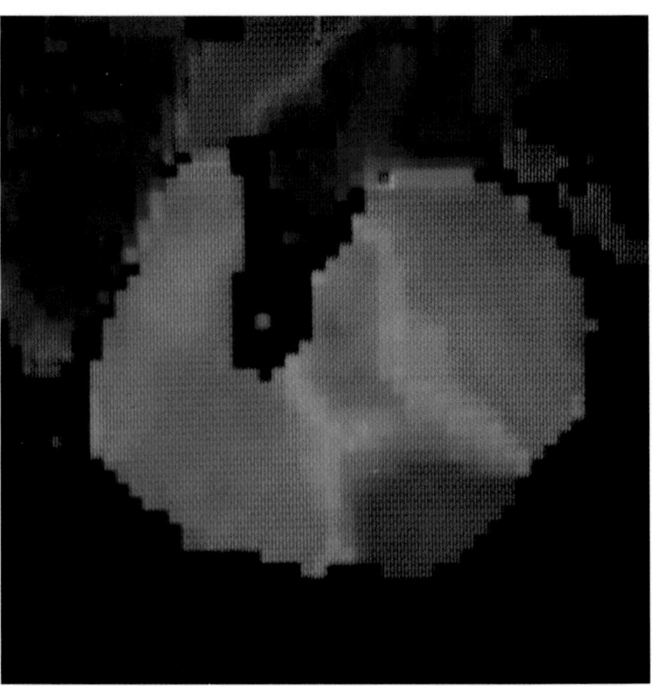

Fig. 90.9 Equilibrium radionuclide angiocardiography. Phase image; septal infarction and apical aneurysm. Intermediate (yellow) and high (red) phase values are seen within the left ventricle. The high values at the left ventricular apex reflect paradoxical emptying typical of an aneurysm. In such cases, it it possible to calculate an ejection fraction from that portion of the ventricle which contracts normally as well as the left ventricle as a whole. In this case the left ventricular ejection fraction was 19% and that of the contractile segment 36%. After removal of the aneurysm, left ventricular ejection fraction was 33%. (See text, p. 1076)

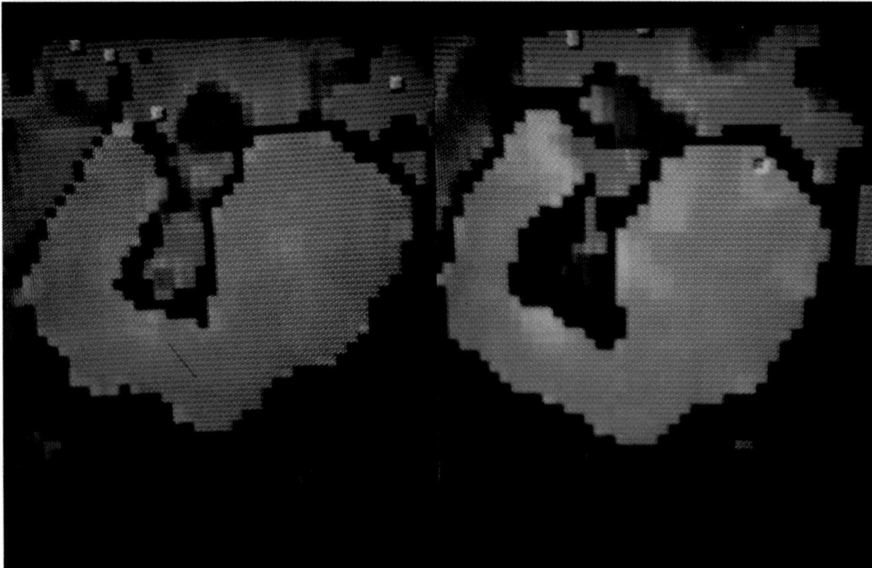

Fig. 90.10 Equilibrium radionuclide angiocardiography. Phase image; pre-excitation. Phase images are shown from the same subject with Wolff-Parkinson-White syndrome during normally conducted sinus rhythm (left) and pre-excitation (right). When the by-pass is conducting, two areas of very early activation of the left ventricle (light blue) can be seen high on the lateral wall. (See text p. 1076)

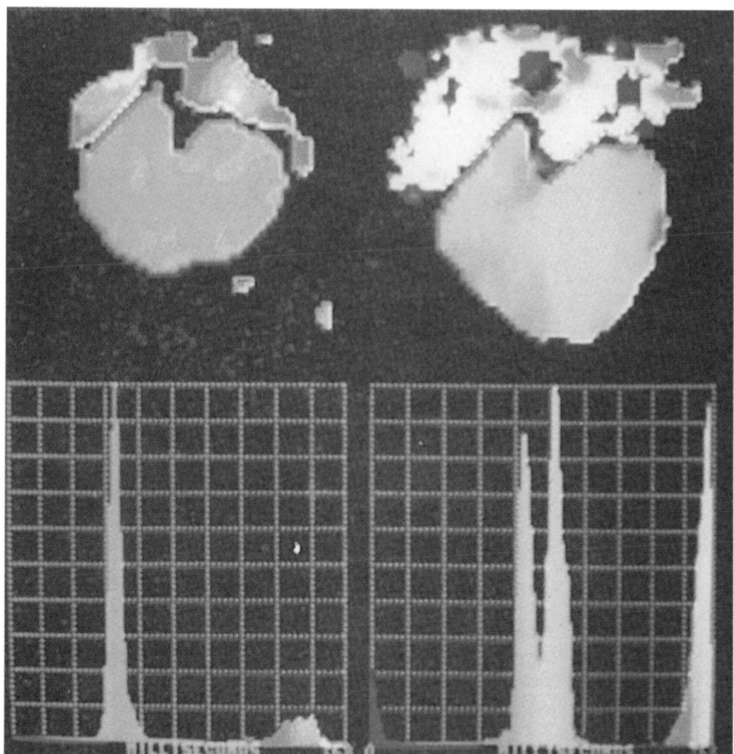

Fig. 90.11 Equilibrium radionuclide angiocardiography. Phase image; quantitative analysis. Phase images (top) are shown from a normal subject (left) and from one with left bundle branch block (right). Below each phase image is a histogram of phase values from that image. In the normal subject there is a narrow peak at low values of phase, reflecting uniform, early emptying of both ventricles. A minor peak of high values reflects atrial emptying. In left bundle branch block, intermediate values of phase are apparent throughout the left ventricle, reflecting delayed emptying. On the histogram, there are two peaks within the low phase values, the lowest corresponding to right and the higher to left ventricular phase values. Once again, high phase values corresponding to atrial emptying are easily distinguished. Such histograms can be used to analyse the distribution of phase values within a particular ventricle also. (Reproduced with permission from *Nuclear Cardiology*.) (See text, p. 1076)

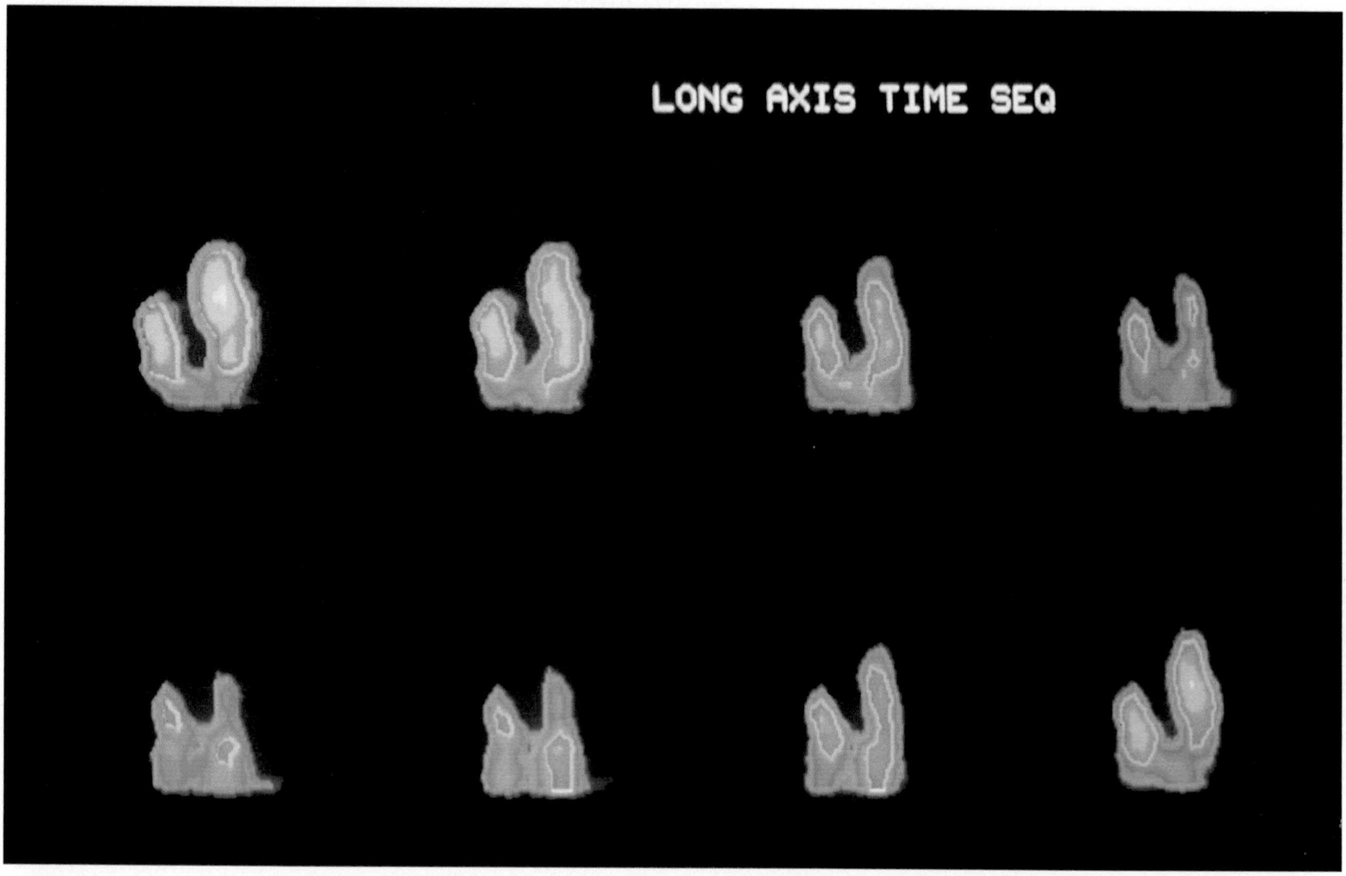

Fig. 90.12 Gated blood pool tomography. Reconstructed tomogram in the horizontal long axis view; normal subject. In each of the 8 views shown, the projection is the same. The series of images starts as end-diastole and represents a single cardiac cycle. The left ventricle lies on the left and it is separated from the right by a space which corresponds to the interventricular septum. Emptying of both ventricles is normal. (See text, p. 1079)

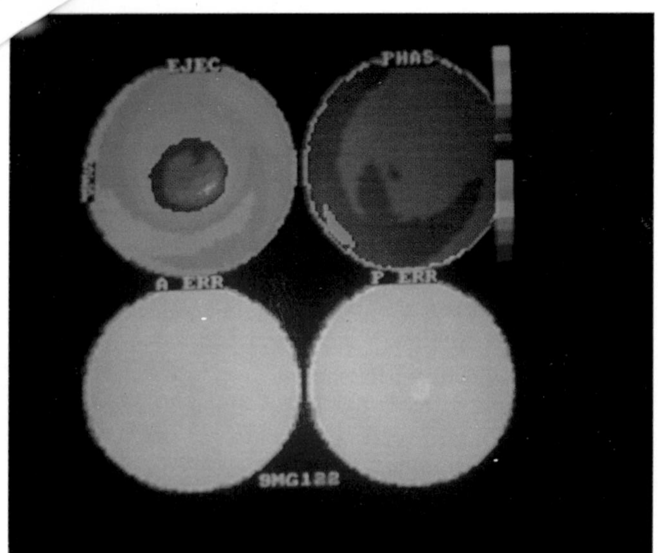

Fig. 90.13 Gated blood pool tomography. 'Bull's eye' display of wall motion; normal subject. In the 'bull's eye' display, the left ventricle is represented as if its apex were at the centre of the display and as if its base were around the periphery. The upper portion of each display represents the anterior wall, the left portion the interventricular septum, the right portion the lateral wall and the lower portion the inferior wall. Here, Fourier amplitude and phase have been used to describe wall motion. The top left image shows the distribution of amplitude values, maximal at the apex (red), and the top right phase values. Below, these amplitude and phase values have been compared to the normal range; the uniform blue colour confirms that all values of amplitude and phase are normal. (See text, p. 1079)

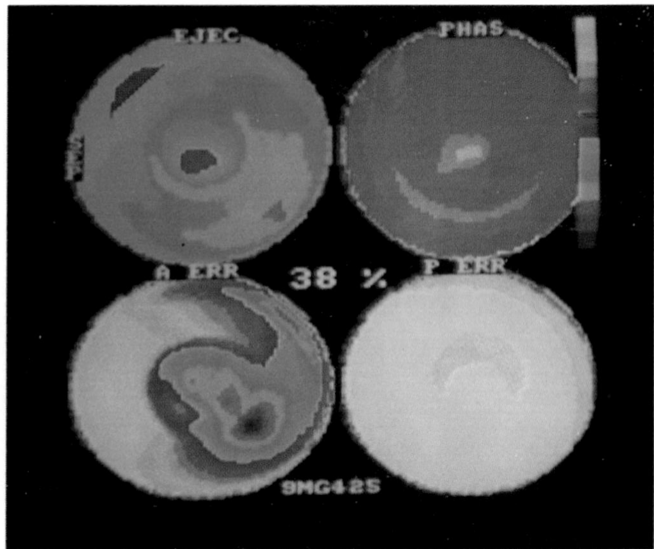

Fig. 90.14 Gated blood pool tomography. 'Bull's eye' display of wall motion; inferolateral infarction. The format is the same as that of Fig. 90.13. There is some heterogeneity of amplitude values in particular. Comparison with the normal range shows abnormal amplitude, corresponding to akinesis, in the inferolateral region of the left ventricle. In this case, phase values are relatively normal. (See text, p. 1079)

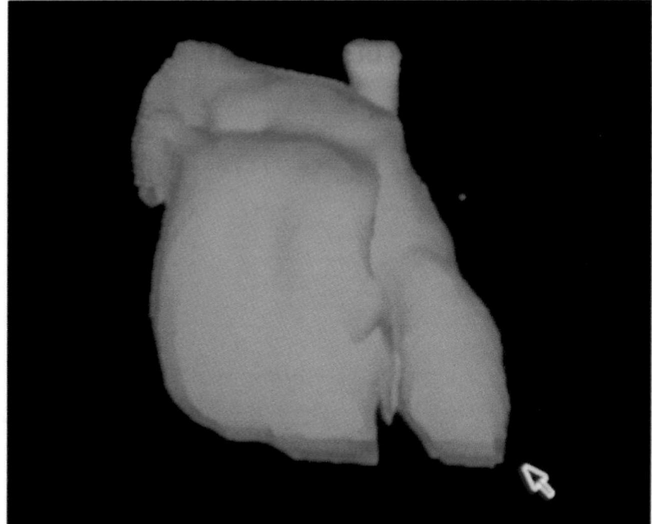

Fig. 90.15 Gated blood pool tomography. Three dimensional reconstruction; normal subject. The 'bull's eye' display is a useful way of showing three dimensional information in a ready format, but it does lead to a certain degree of distortion. The tomographic data can also be reconstructed into the type of solid body display shown here. Motion can be superimposed and the display can be rotated, permitting observation of the beating heart in any orientation. Here, the heart is viewed in the right anterior oblique projection. The right ventricle is seen on the left and the left ventricle (arrowed) on the right of the image. (See text, p. 1079)

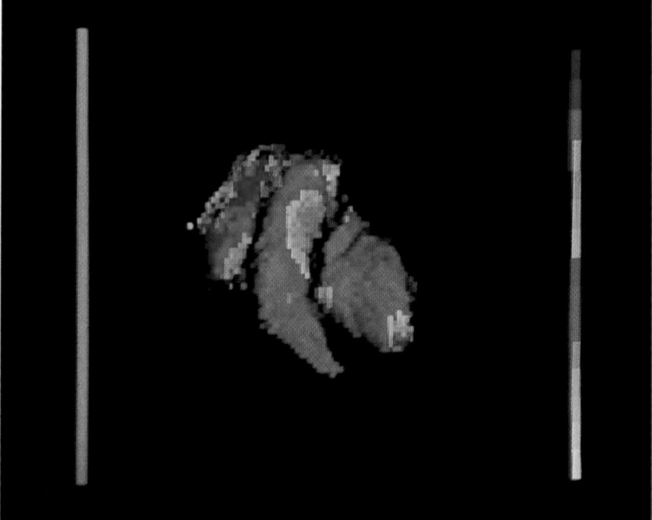

Fig. 90.16 Gated blood pool tomography. Three dimensional reconstruction; phase display — left ventricular infarction. The left anterior oblique projection has been chosen and phase values have been superimposed. In this colour scale, low phase values are seen red or green and high phase values blue. High phase values are apparent within the right atrium and at the apex of the left ventricle, the latter representing infarction and possibly a small aneurysm. (See text, p. 1079)

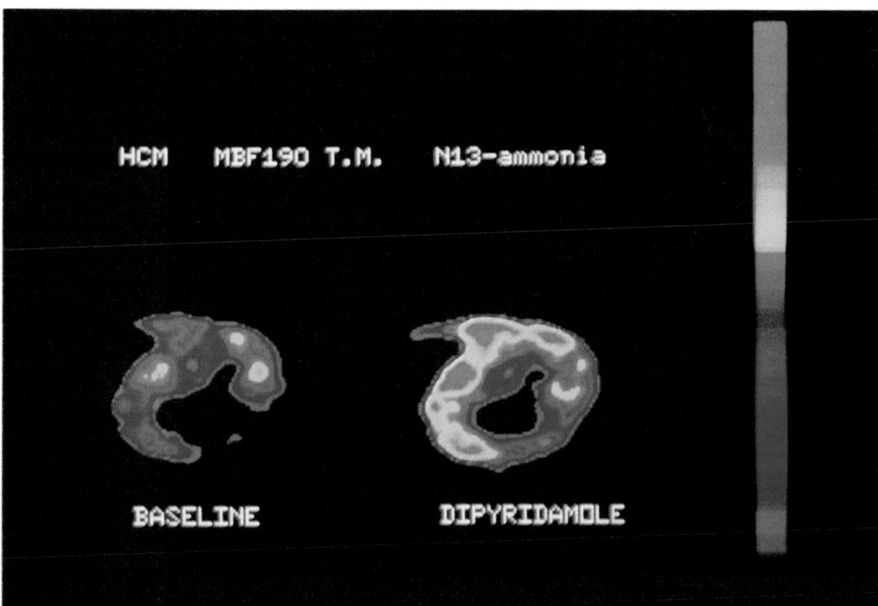

Fig. 92.7 Transaxial images of the heart obtained with $^{13}NH_3$ in a patient with hypertrophic cardiomyopathy at baseline and following i.v. dipyridamole (0.56 mg/kg). The extraordinary thickness (39 mm) of the interventricular septum (9 to 1 o'clock position) allowed the assessment of transmural flow distribution. The subendocardial/subepicardial flow ratio which was 1.01 at baseline, decreased to 0.69 following dipyridamole suggesting subendocardial underperfusion. (See text, p. 1104)

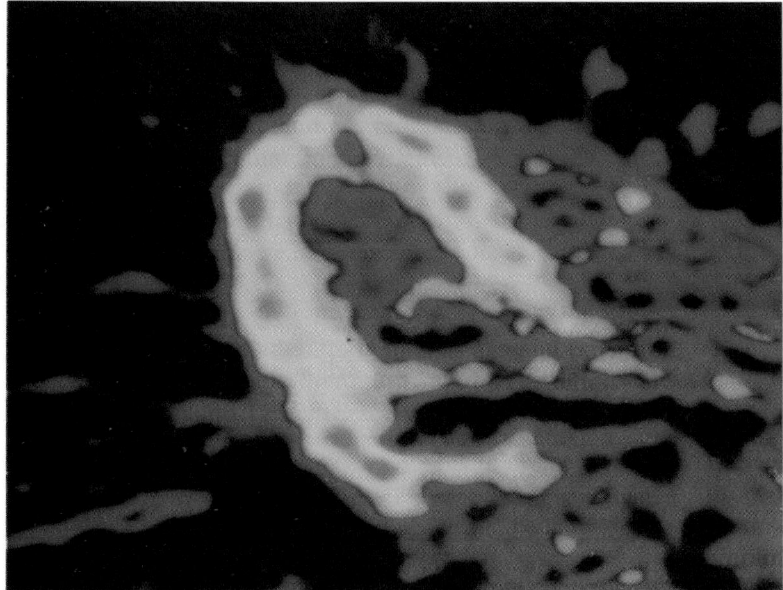

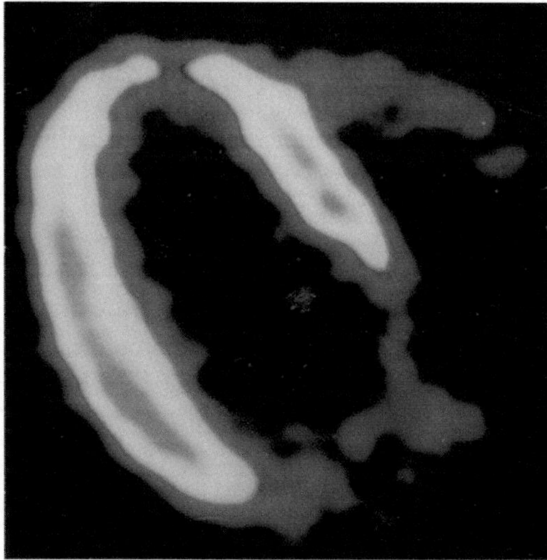

Fig. 92.10 An example pf transaxial image of the heart in a patient with coronary artery disease obtained with 18F-fluorodeoxyglucose and PET during euglycaemic-hyperinsulinaemic clamp. (Reprinted with permission from Knuuti et al 1992 J Nucl Med 33: 1255–1262) (See text, p. 1106)

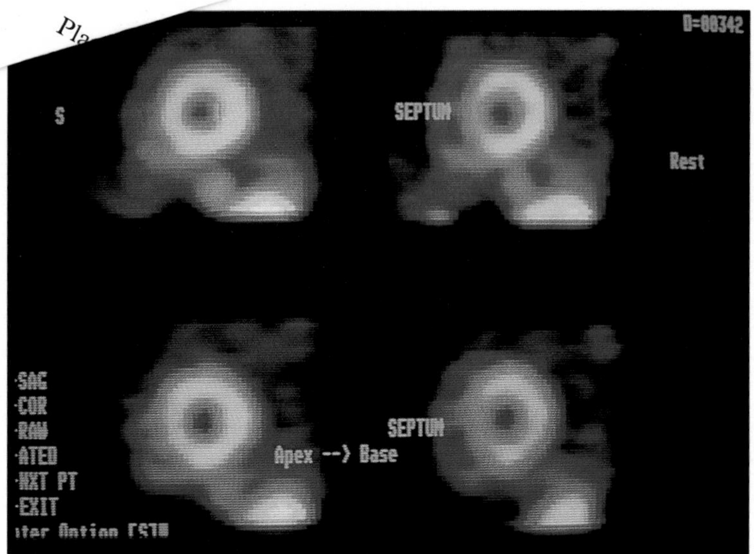

Fig. 94.2 SPECT [^{99m}Tc] sestamibi images from a subject with a very low probability of coronary artery disease. This short-axis tomogram demonstrates the normal variation of the membranous portion of the upper septum in the most basal short-axis slice. (See text, p. 1132)

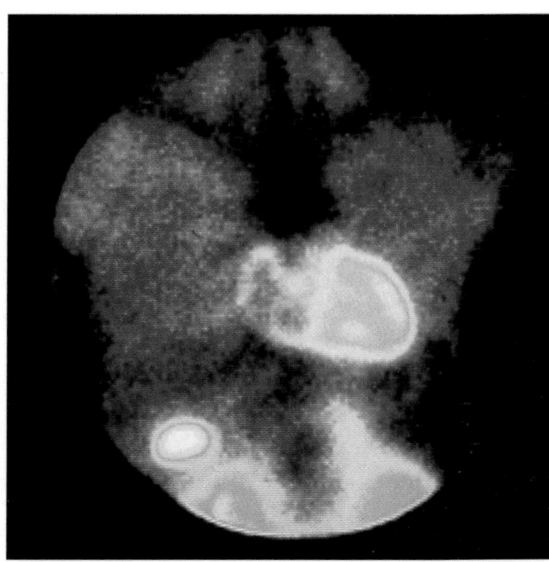

Fig. 94.3 Normal variation apical thinning in a large field-of-view anterior planar SPECT [^{99m}Tc] sestamibi image from a subject with a low probability of coronary artery disease. Apical thinning may at times be quite prominent. (See text, p. 1132)

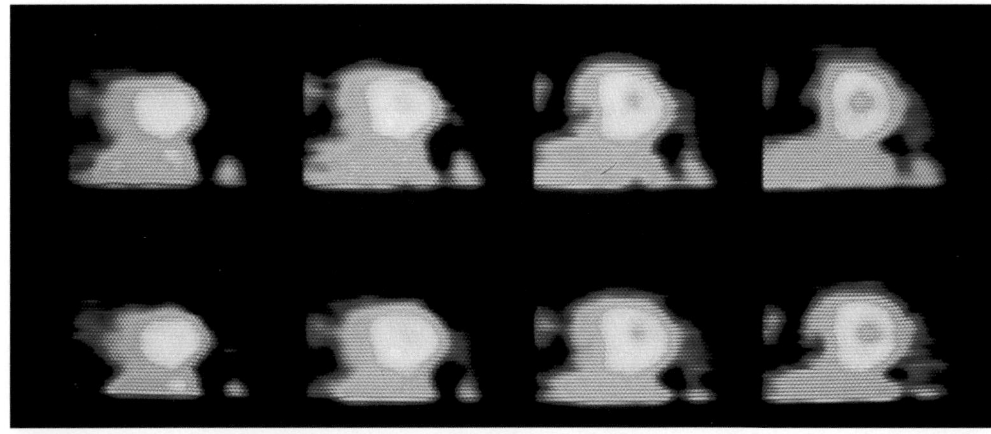

Fig. 94.4B An apparent anterolateral wall mild irreversible defect caused by breast attenuation. With SPECT imaging, breast attenuation is more difficult to recognize in the final processed images, and a review of the cine-projection data is important. (See text, p. 1132)

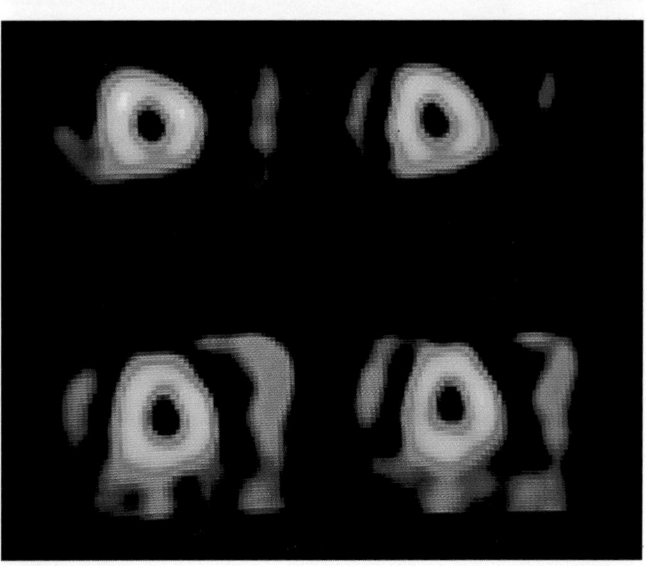

Fig. 94.5 Short-axis SPECT ^{201}Tl images from a young, highly trained normal subject demonstrating an apparent reversible inferior defect, due to inferior attenuation in the stress images (top row) and possible 'upward creep'. See text (p. 1134) for details.

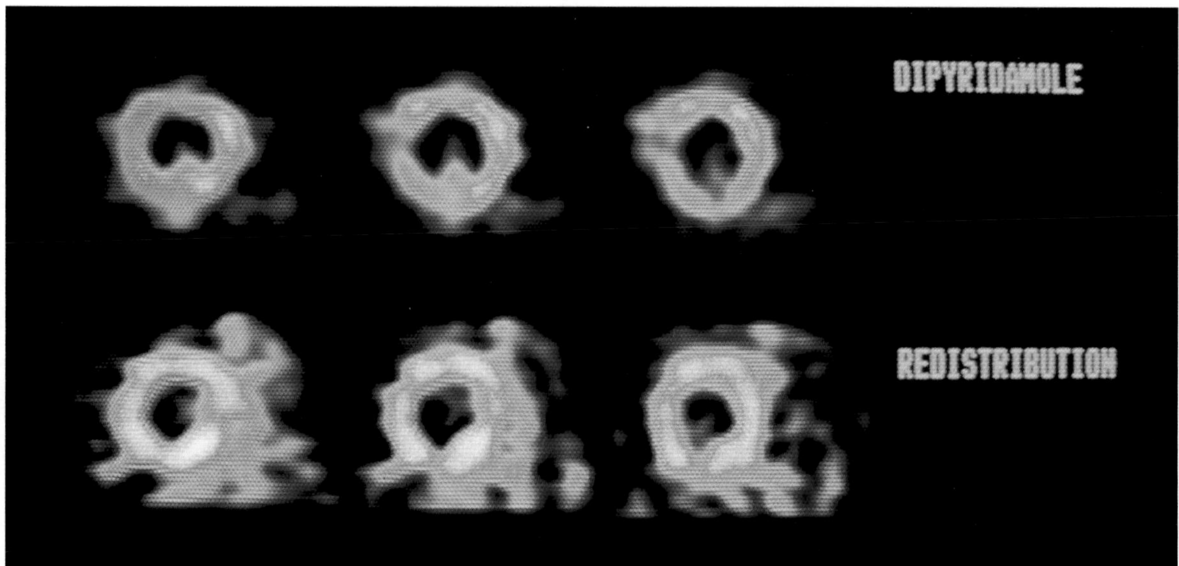

Fig. 94.8B Short-axis ^{201}Tl SPECT images following dipyridamole (top) and redistribution (bottom) in a patient with idiopathic dilated cardiomyopathy and normal epicardial arteries. Multiple reversible defects are apparent. (See text, p. 1136)

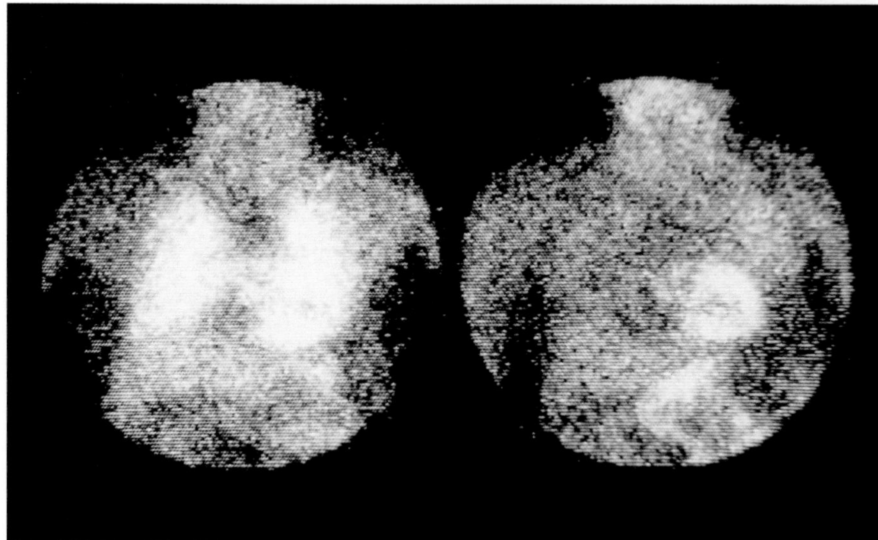

Fig. 94.9 Large field of view anterior planar images immediately following treadmill exercise (left) and 4 h later for comparison (right) demonstrating marked pulmonary uptake of ^{201}Tl in a patient ultimately found to have three-vessel coronary artery disease. (See text, p. 1139)

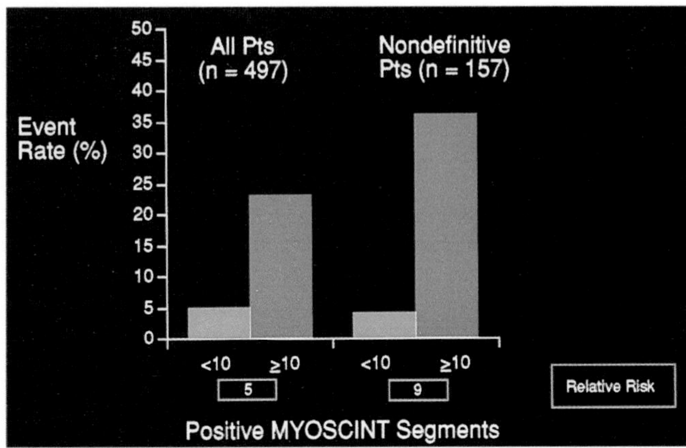

Fig. 99.7 Risk of cardiac death or non-fatal myocardial infarction, predicted by the extent of [^{111}In]antimyosin uptake in all patients and a subgroup of patients with non-definitive evidence of myocardial infarction. (See text, p. 1213)

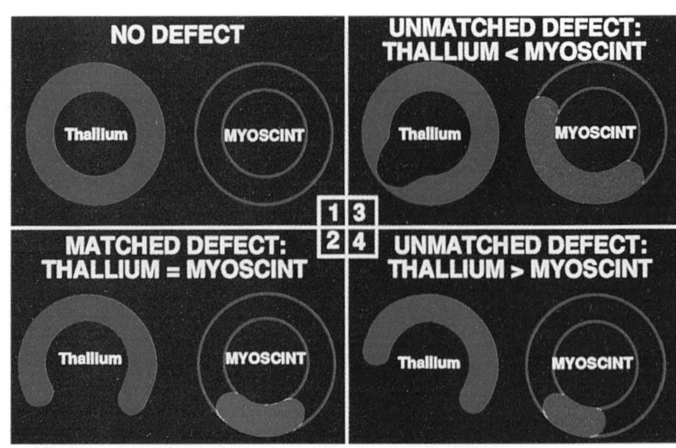

Fig. 99.8 Diagrammatic representation of dual isotope (^{201}Tl and [^{111}In]antimyosin) image patterns. (See text, p. 1214)

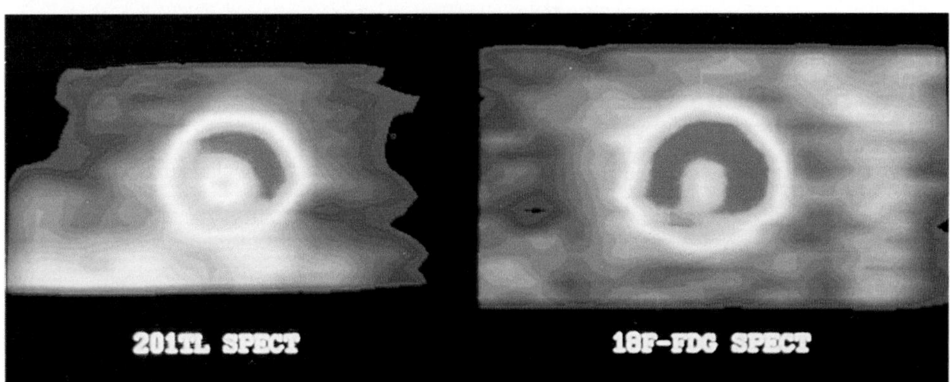

Fig. 102.10 ^{201}Tl and FDG uptake in a SPECT study of a patient with a previous inderoseptal infarction. Especially in the septal area, FDG uptake is preserved. (See text, p. 1246)

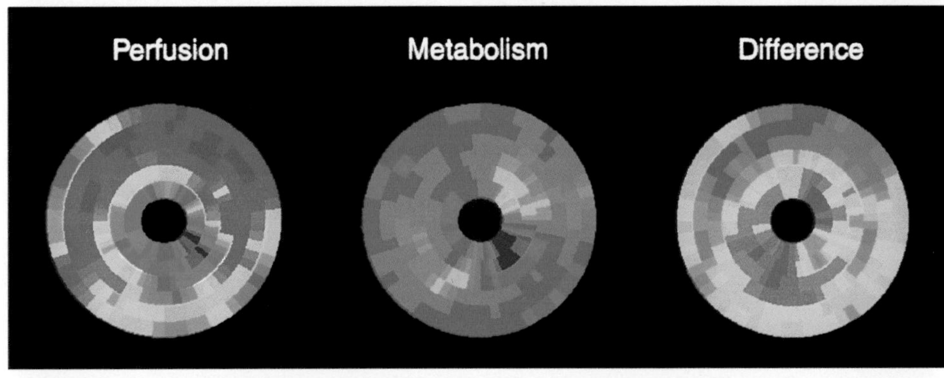

Fig. 103.6 Polar map displays of perfusion metabolism in a patient with reduced blood flow in the inferior wall (blue). Note the homogeneous [^{18}F]DG uptake as seen on the polar map of metabolism. The difference polar map (left) reveals a blood flow–glucose metabolism mismatch (red). (See text, pp 1258–59)

Fig. 103.7 Polar map displays of perfusion and metabolism in a patient with LAD disease. Note the extensive perfusion abnormality affecting the anterior wall. The metabolism polar map indicates a concordant zone of decreased [^{18}F]DG uptake (dark blue). Accordingly, the difference polar map fails to reveal a blood flow–metabolism mismatch. The polar maps at the bottom depict a blood flow–metabolism match. As noted on the polar map of myocardial perfusion, blood flow is decreased in the inferior wall. This is associated with a concordant reduction in [^{18}F]DG uptake. Accordingly, the difference polar may as shown on the right does not reveal any regional increases in the difference in the uptake of [^{18}F]DG and [^{13}N]ammonia. (See text, pp 1258–59)

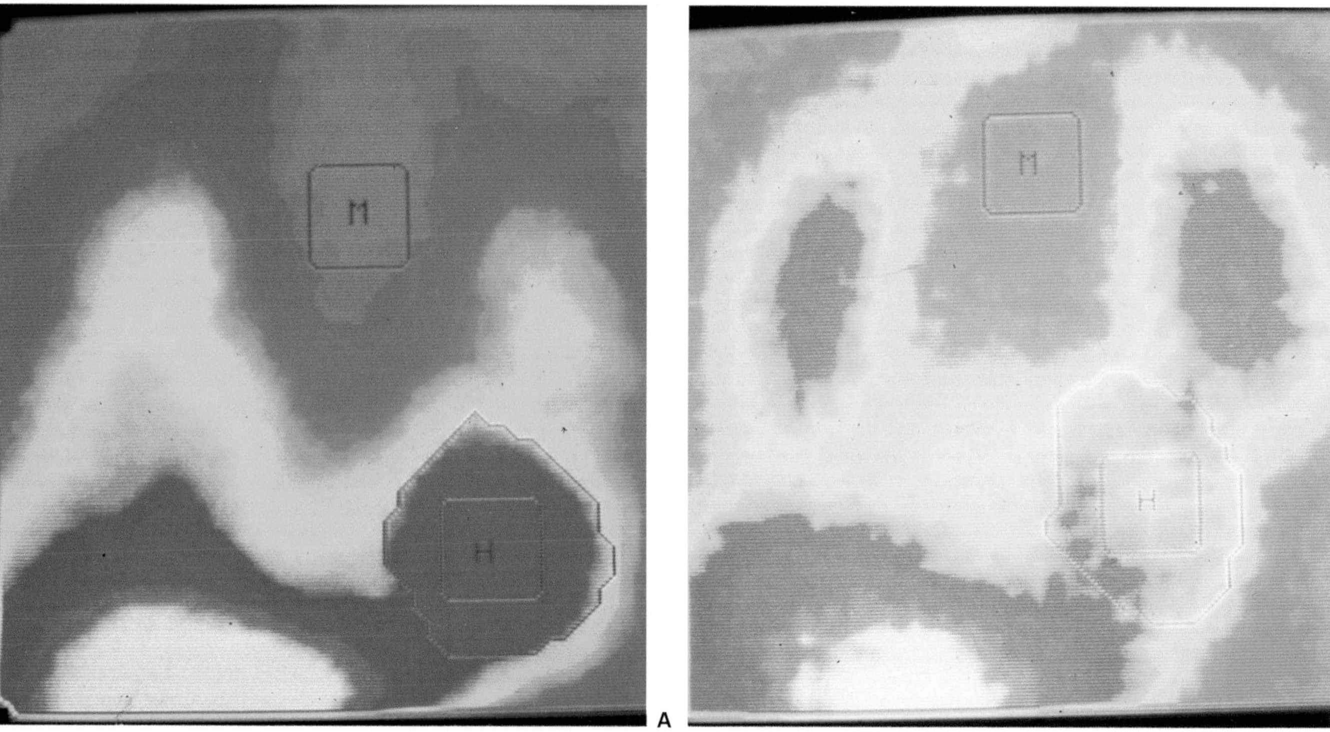

Fig. 104.1 Scintigraphic images obtained 4 h after injection of 3–4 mCi of [^{123}I]MIBG (anterior view of the chest). Cardiac MIBG uptake is quantified as the ratio of heart (H) activity to mediastinal activity (M). **A** Control subject. **B** Patient with moderate congestive heart failure: a decrease in myocardial MIBG uptake is clearly seen. (See text, p. 1265)

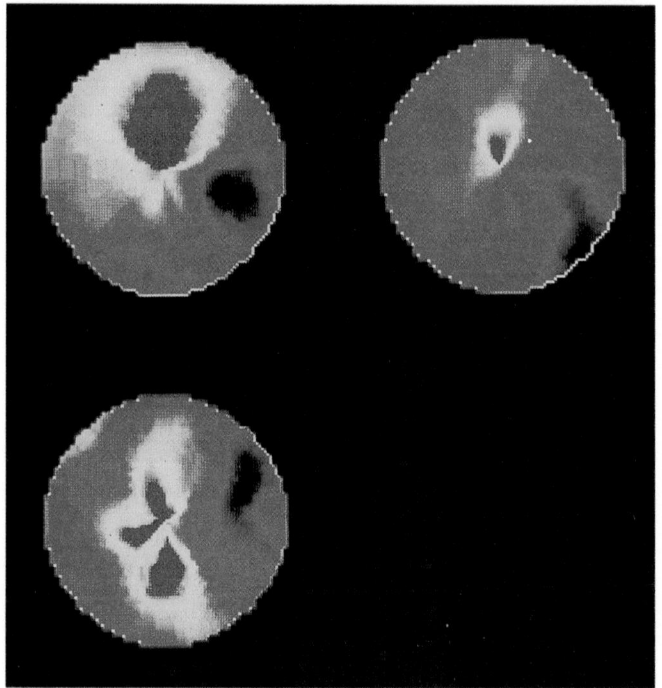

Fig. 104.2 ^{201}Tl and [^{123}I]MIBG 'bull's eye' images of a patient with a left anterior descending coronary artery stenosis. Post-exercise ^{201}Tl image (upper left) shows a large anterior defect which 'fills-in' on 3 h delayed images (upper right). On the [^{123}I]MIBG image, acquired 5 h after exercise, the defect is much larger than on the delayed perfusion bull's eye. (See text, p. 1266)

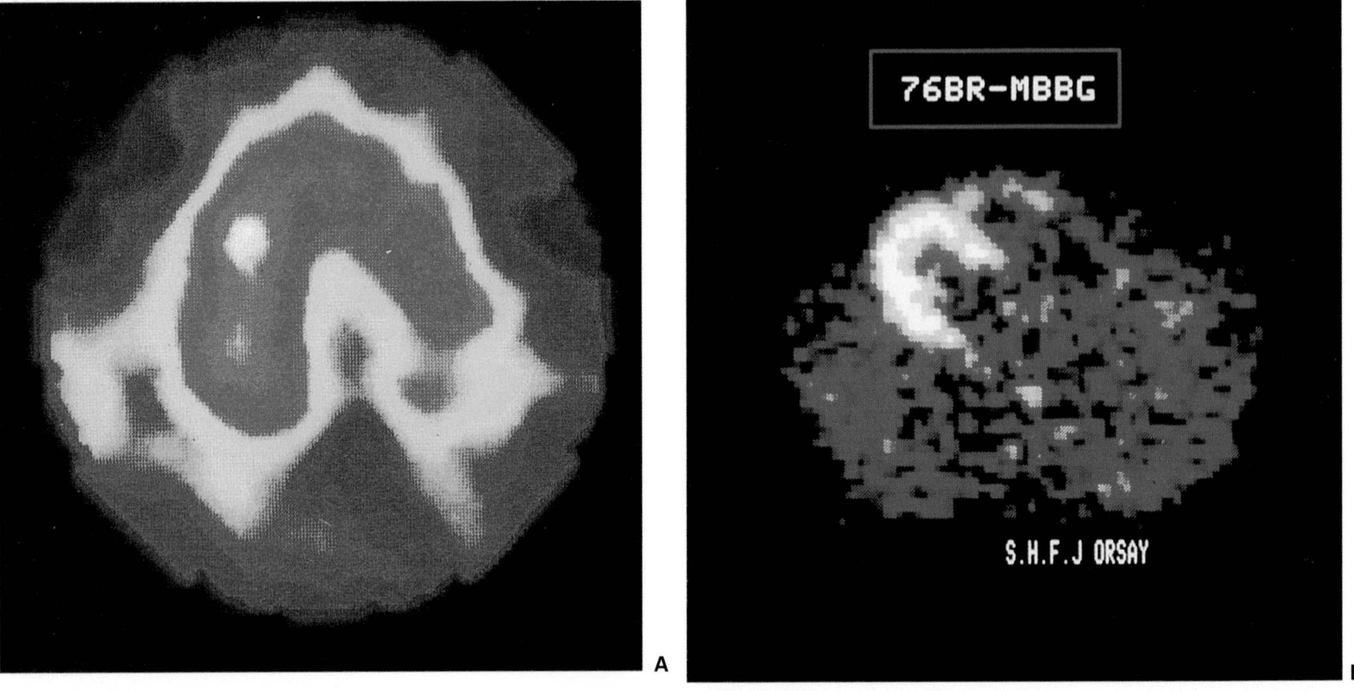

Fig. 104.3 SPET image obtained after injection of 3–4 mCi of [^{123}I]MIBG (**A**) in a patient with a primary hypertrophic cardiomyopathy (mainly septal hypertrophy). Single static PET image obtained after injection of 1 mCi of [^{76}Br]MBBG (**B**) in a control subject. Acquisition duration was 60 min. (See text, p. 1266)

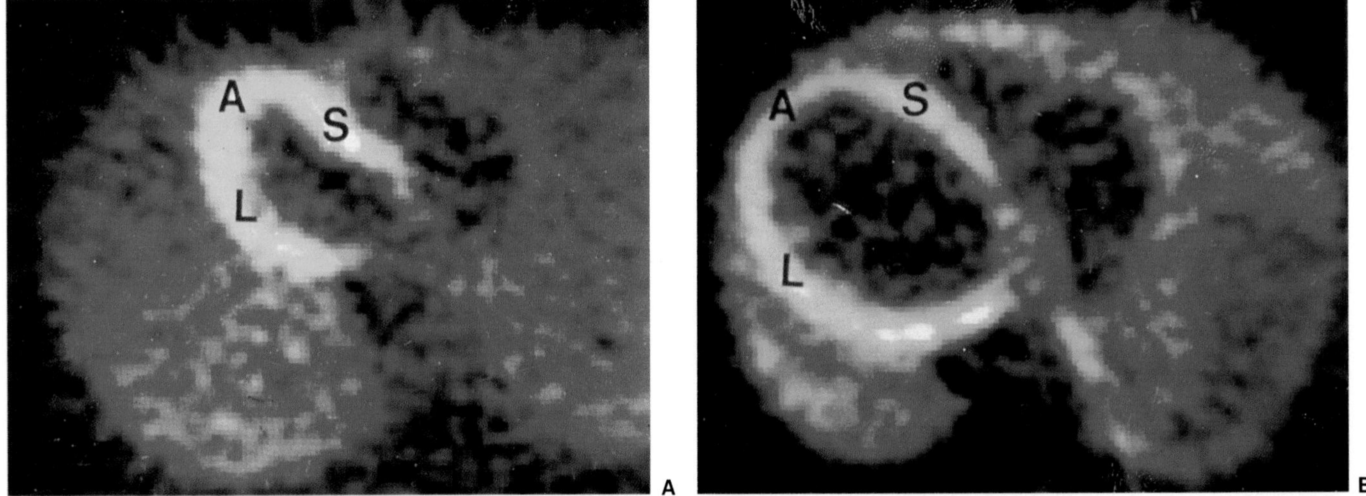

Fig. 104.5 PET slices showing the myocardial distribution of [^{11}C]CGP 12177 in a control subject (**A**) and in a patient with congestive heart failure (**B**). The images are scaled to their own maximum, therefore they do not show the two-fold decrease in beta-adrenergic receptor density calculated from the dynamic series. (See text, p. 1268)

Index